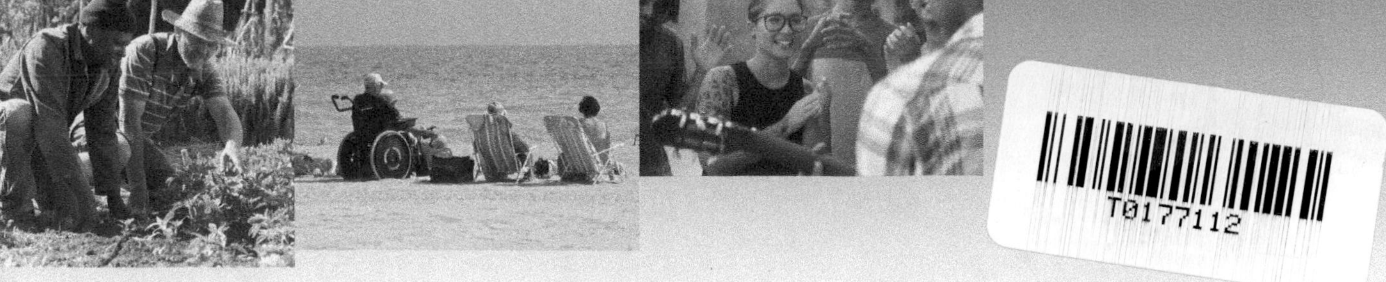

Occupational Therapy
in Community and Population Health Practice

THIRD EDITION

Marjorie E. Scaffa, PhD, OTR/L, FAOTA
Professor Emeritus and Founding Chair
Department of Occupational Therapy
Pat Capps Covey College of Allied Health Professions
University of South Alabama
Mobile, Alabama

S. Maggie Reitz, PhD, OTR/L, FAOTA
Vice Provost
Office of the Provost
Towson University
Professor
Department of Occupational Therapy and
Occupational Science
Towson University
Towson, Maryland

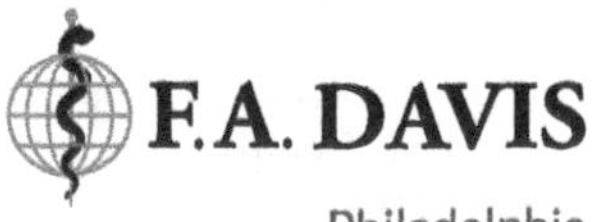

Philadelphia

F. A. Davis Company
1915 Arch Street
Philadelphia, PA 19103
www.fadavis.com

Printed in the United States of America

Last digit indicates print number: 10 9 8 7 6 5 4

Senior Acquisitions Editor: Christa A. Fratantoro
Manager of Content Development: George W. Lang
Developmental Editor: Jill Rembetski
Content Project Manager: Megan Suermann
Art and Design Manager: Carolyn O'Brien

Library of Congress Cataloging-in-Publication Data

Names: Scaffa, Marjorie E., author. | Reitz, S. Maggie, author.
Title: Occupational therapy in community and population health practice / Marjorie E. Scaffa, S. Maggie Reitz.
Other titles: Occupational therapy in community-based practice settings
Description: Third edition. | Philadelphia : F.A. Davis, 2020. | Preceded by Occupational therapy in community-based practice settings / Marjorie E. Scaffa, S. Maggie Reitz. 2nd ed. c2014. | Includes bibliographical references and index. | Summary: "This book combines the areas of occupational therapists and health educators. It is clearly and straightforwardly an occupational therapy text with an appreciation of the importance of populations and community as a context for health. The third edition aims to be a useful with a more developed discussion of the issues related to present-day community and population health practice in occupational therapy"—Provided by publisher.
Identifiers: LCCN 2019046782 (print) | LCCN 2019046783 (ebook) | ISBN 9780803675629 (library binding) | ISBN 9780803675636 (ebook)
Subjects: MESH: Occupational Therapy—methods | Community Health Services | Population Health
Classification: LCC RM735 (print) | LCC RM735 (ebook) | NLM WB 555 | DDC 615.8/515—dc23
LC record available at https://lccn.loc.gov/2019046782
LC ebook record available at https://lccn.loc.gov/2019046783

Occupational Therapy
in Community and Population Health Practice

THIRD EDITION

For all those special people
who see what others ignore,
embrace what others fear,
and create new paths that others can follow.

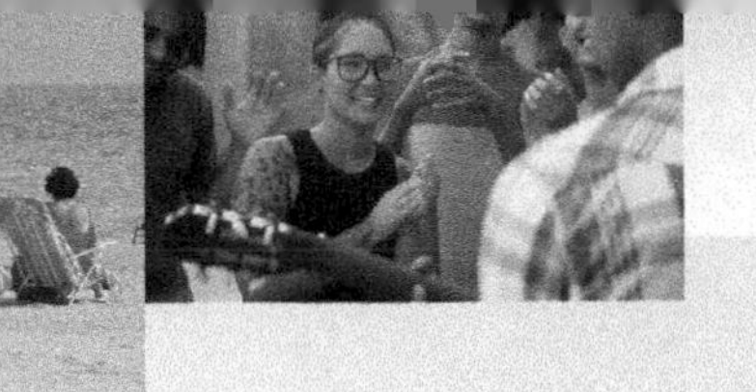

Dedication

This text is dedicated to the memory of Dr. Gary Kielhofner (1949–2010), scholar, teacher, mentor, and friend. His extraordinary contributions to occupational therapy education, research, and practice are unparalleled.

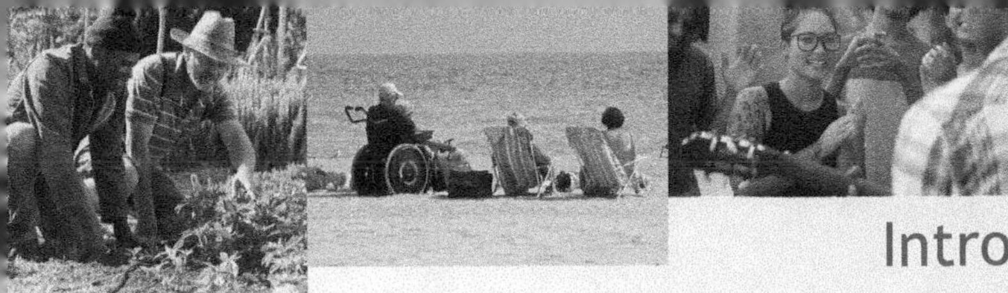

Introduction to the Foreword

This is the foreword that appeared in the first edition of this text, published in 2001. It is particularly meaningful to me because it was written by Dr. Gary Kielhofner, my occupational therapy professor and mentor. Dr. Kielhofner died in September 2010 after a short battle with cancer, but his legacy lives on in the many students he taught and the professionals he mentored. For this reason, in this third edition we have chosen to retain this foreword and the dedication from the second edition in honor of Dr. Kielhofner.

—Marjorie E. Scaffa, PhD, OTR, FAOTA

Foreword

Twenty-five years ago, I collaborated on my first publication with one of my mentors, Florence Cromwell. The paper described preparation of occupational therapy students to work in community settings (Cromwell and Kielhofner, 1976). I had the good fortune of working with a mentor who appreciated that much of the future of occupational therapy would be in community practice. A quarter century ago, this was still a new idea.

In the intervening period, a number of changes in health care, health demographics, and funding of health services have made community-based practice not only common but the most promising direction for the future of practice in occupational therapy.

It gives me great satisfaction to see that one of my former students has gone on to edit the first comprehensive volume in community practice. It is even more gratifying to note the scope and quality of chapters that make up this ambitious volume. Community practice means much more than physical placement in a community setting. Importantly, it represents a different paradigm of care than seen in traditional hospital and rehabilitation settings. The therapist working in the community most likely works in an organization whose philosophy, reimbursement, and expectations for practice are much different from traditional medically defined settings. Moreover, the voices and viewpoints of those served will often carry much more weight than in a traditional setting. Therapists who wish to be effective in community practice must be prepared to take on new roles, to take unusual risks, and to envision service in creative ways. Thus, although community practice is not as anomalous as it was 25 years ago, it still represents new territory for most of occupational therapy.

Marjorie Scaffa and her colleagues have assembled a remarkable set of resources for the occupational therapist in community practice. The scope and depth of the chapters make this at once an authoritative work on community practice and an invaluable collection of resources.

—Gary Kielhofner, DrPH, OTR

Cromwell, F. S., and Kielhofner, G. (1976). An educational strategy for occupational therapy community service. American Journal of Occupational Therapy, 30, *629–633.*

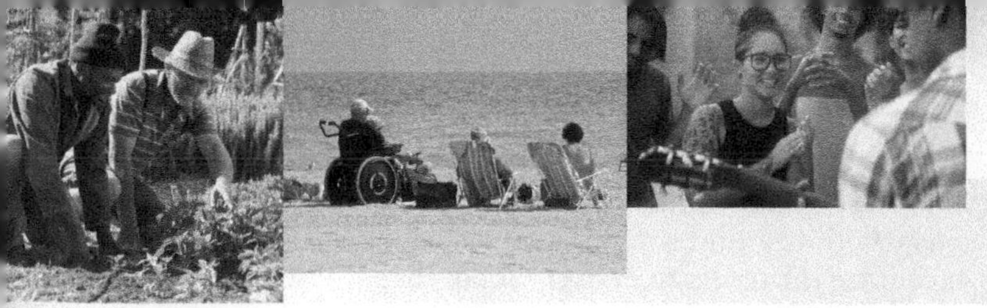

Preface

This book is the culmination of one aspect of the professional journey of Marjorie Scaffa that started when she was an undergraduate major in psychology with a minor in health education and continued on during an entry-level master's program to become an occupational therapist. During her years as an occupational therapy student at Virginia Commonwealth University, she was introduced to the model of human occupation by Dr. Kielhofner and became increasingly excited about its potential for practice in nonmedical settings. When given the opportunity to choose a topic for a paper, Marjorie wrote about occupational therapy's role in community health, and the seeds of what would later become this book were sown.

As a practicing occupational therapist, she gained experience in a variety of settings but was most energized and excited by home health practice. Providing services in the home enabled her to become part of a client's daily life context in which the person participated in self-care, work, and leisure. Marjorie was impressed by how much more meaningful occupations were to individuals and their families in real-life environments.

Through our practice and further education, we both came to believe firmly that if occupation could restore function and enhance the quality of life for individuals with disabilities and their families, it could also be used to prevent injuries and promote health in communities and among populations. Thus began our quests for doctorates in health education and community health. We quickly realized that much of what we had learned in occupational therapy would be useful in community-based prevention and health promotion but that we needed to become acculturated to the mind-set and conceptual frameworks of health educators and public health specialists, which were quite different from those of occupational therapy practitioners. We were exposed to planning, implementing, and evaluating preventive interventions directed at groups and populations rather than rehabilitative interventions directed at individuals.

Over time we were able to assimilate both of our professional identities as occupational therapists and health educators, which enabled us to envision the second edition and now the third edition of this book. It is clearly and straightforwardly an occupational therapy text with an appreciation of the importance of populations and community as a context for health.

We hope that you find this third edition of the book to be a useful and more developed discussion of the issues related to present-day community and population health practice in occupational therapy.

The first section of this edition has been reimagined and now includes a chapter on population health by Hocking and Wilcock. Four new chapters emerged from topics previously identified as trends in the future directions chapter in the second edition; two of these new chapters discuss transition services for children, one addresses telehealth, and one covers marginalized populations and issues of occupational justice. Additional new chapters on health professional well-being; needs of the homeless; transition of military Veterans into civilian life; disaster preparedness, response, and recovery; and violence prevention and mitigation exemplify how the profession's contributions to community and population health and well-being have significantly expanded since the first edition of this book.

Chapters carried over from the second edition have been substantially revised to include updated content and graphics. All chapters, both new and recurring, now include the feature "Engage Your Brain," designed to encourage the reader to actively apply chapter content. Returning features include learning outcomes, key terms, learning activities, and a summary, which in this edition directly links to the learning outcomes. Chapters in sections III through VIII include case studies, as in the second edition, but now also include a "Program Showcase" that details the development and assessment of a relevant practice example. The third edition ends once again with a chapter focusing on future trends in community and population health practice.

The book remains designed as a textbook for entry-level occupational therapy students, but it also proves useful to practitioners wishing to facilitate a transition from medical model practice to community and population health practice. We are grateful for the opportunity to participate in and contribute to the profession's expanding role in prevention, health promotion, and community and population health.

—Marjorie E. Scaffa and
S. Maggie Reitz

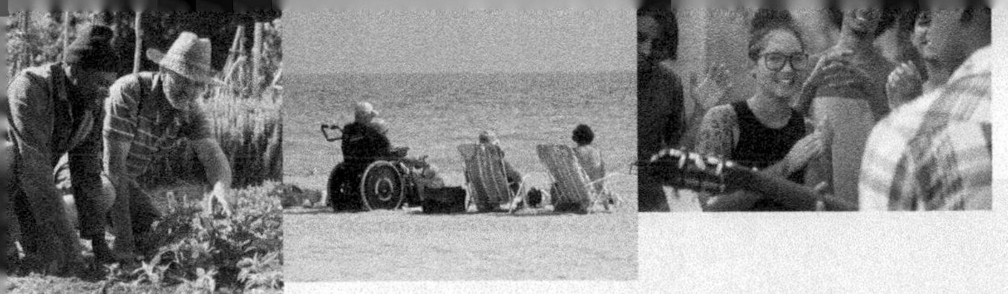

Contributors

Abigail Baxter, PhD
Professor of Education
Department of Leadership and Teacher Education
University of South Alabama
Mobile, Alabama

Peter Bowman, OTD, MHS, OTR/L, OT (C), Dip COT
Professor Emeritus
Division of Occupational Therapy
Medical University of South Carolina
Charleston, South Carolina

Susan Cahill, PhD, OTR/L, FAOTA
Associate Professor and Program Director
Occupational Therapy Program
Lewis University
Romeoville, Illinois

S. Blaise Chromiak, MD
Family Practice Physician
Mobile County Health Department
Mobile, Alabama

Leah K. Cox, PhD
Vice President of Inclusion and Institutional Equity
Towson University
Towson, Maryland

Lisa Crabtree, PhD, OTR/L, FAOTA
Associate Professor
Department of Occupational Therapy and Occupational Science
Towson University
Towson, Maryland

Patricia A. Crist, PhD, OTR, FAOTA
Academic Consultant and Professional Development Coach
Owner, Life Enhancement and Accessible Places
Glendale, Arizona

Janet V. DeLany, DEd, OTR/L, FAOTA
Professor Emeritus
Department of Occupational Therapy and Occupational Science
Towson University
Towson, Maryland

Barbara Demchick, ScD, OTR/L, FAOTA
Clinical Associate Professor
Department of Occupational Therapy and Occupational Science
Towson University
Towson, Maryland

Anne E. Dickerson, PhD, OTR/L, SCDCM, FAOTA, FGSA
Professor
Department of Occupational Therapy
East Carolina University
Greenville, North Carolina

Camille Dieterle, OTD, OTR/L
Associate Professor
Mrs. T. H. Chan Division of Occupational Science and Occupational Therapy
University of Southern California
Los Angeles, California

Joy D. Doll, OTD, OTR/L
Associate Professor and Executive Director
Center for Interprofessional Practice, Education, and Research
Department of Occupational Therapy
Creighton University
Omaha, Nebraska

Anna Domina, OTD, OTR/L
Vice Chair and Assistant Professor
Department of Occupational Therapy
Creighton University
Omaha, Nebraska

David Ensminger, PhD
Associate Professor
Teaching and Learning and Research Methods
School of Education
Loyola University Chicago
Chicago, Illinois

Kathleen Flecky, OTD, OTR/L
Associate Professor
Department of Occupational Therapy
Creighton University
Omaha, Nebraska

Rita P. Fleming-Castaldy, OTL, PhD, FAOTA
Professor Emeritus
Department of Occupational Therapy
The University of Scranton
Scranton, Pennsylvania

Jeremy Fletcher, PT, DPT, OCS
Major, U.S. Army Reserve
Assistant Professor
Department of Physical Therapy
Pat Capps Covey College of Allied Health Professions
University of South Alabama
Mobile, Alabama

Trish H. Foley, MOT, OTL, CAPS
Director of Community Services
Independence Now Inc.
Silver Spring, Maryland

Sarah Anne Hewitt, BA
Graduate Student
Department of Occupational Therapy and Occupational Science
Towson University
Towson, Maryland

Clare Hocking, PhD, MHSc(OT), AdvDipOT, DipOT
Professor
Auckland University of Technology
Auckland, New Zealand

Wendy M. Holmes, PhD, OTR/L
Adjunct Professor
School of Occupational Therapy
Brenau University
Gainesville, Georgia

Amanda C. Jozkowski, PhD, OTR/L
Assistant Professor
Department of Occupational Therapy and Occupational Science
Towson University
Towson, Maryland

Stephen B. Kern, PhD, OTR/L, FAOTA
Professor and Director
Master of Science Program in Occupational Therapy, Center City Campus
Department of Occupational Therapy
Thomas Jefferson University
Philadelphia, Pennsylvania

Kevin Kilkuskie, BA, MAT
Master of Science in Occupational Therapy Student
Department of Occupational Therapy
Thomas Jefferson University
Philadelphia, Pennsylvania

John F. Kilpatrick, MSW
Lieutenant Colonel, U.S. Army Reserve
Executive Director
Veterans Recovery Resources
Mobile, Alabama

M. Beth Merryman, PhD, OTR/L, FAOTA
Professor and Chair
Department of Occupational Therapy and Occupational Science
Towson University
Towson, Maryland

Michelle Messer, OTD, OTR/L, BCPR
Assistant Professor and Capstone Coordinator
Department of Occupational Therapy
St. Catherine University
St. Paul, Minnesota

Lynne Murphy, EdD, OTR/L
Assistant Professor
Department of Occupational Therapy
East Carolina University
Greenville, North Carolina

Anton Nguyen, BA
Master of Science in Occupational Therapy Student
Department of Occupational Therapy
Thomas Jefferson University
Philadelphia, Pennsylvania

Ranelle Nissen, PhD, OTR/L
Associate Professor
Department of Occupational Therapy
University of South Dakota
Vermillion, South Dakota

Thaddeus Parker, MS, OTR/L
Occupational Therapist
Huntsville, Alabama

Gabriella Santos, BS
Master of Science in Occupational Therapy Student
Department of Occupational Therapy
Thomas Jefferson University
Philadelphia, Pennsylvania

Janie B. Scott, MA, OT/L, FAOTA
Occupational Therapy and Aging in Place Consultant
Columbia, Maryland

Francine M. Seruya, PhD, OTR/L
Program Director and Professor
Graduate Occupational Therapy Program
Mercy College
Dobbs Ferry, New York

Kendra Heatwole Shank, PhD, OTR/L
Assistant Professor
Department of Occupational Therapy and Occupational Science
Towson University
Towson, Maryland

Jillian Silveira, OTR/L
LGBT Veteran Care Coordinator
VA Maryland Health Care System
Baltimore, Maryland

Betsey C. Smith, PhD, OTR/L
Senior Associate Dean
School of Health Sciences
Quinnipiac University
Hamden, Connecticut

Theresa M. Smith, PhD, OTR/L, CLVT
Associate Professor
School of Occupational Therapy
Texas Woman's University
Houston, Texas

Toni Thompson, DrOT, OTR/L, C/NDT
Adjunct Professor and Senior Instructor
TherapyED
Nova Southeastern University
Fort Lauderdale, Florida

Sally Wasmuth, PhD, OTR
Assistant Professor
Department of Occupational Therapy
Indiana University–Purdue University Indianapolis
Indianapolis, Indiana

Ann Allart Wilcock, PhD, BAppScOT, GradDipPH, FCOT
Honorary Professor
Deakin University
Geelong, Australia

Donna A. Wooster, PhD, OTR/L, BCP
Associate Professor and Chair
Department of Occupational Therapy
University of South Alabama
Mobile, Alabama

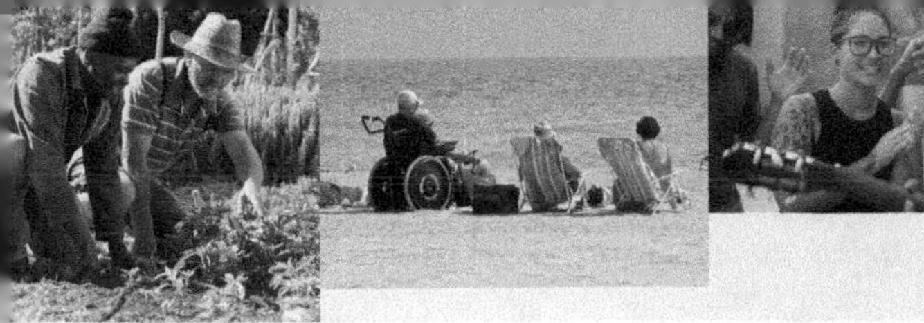

Reviewers

Christine Berg, PhD, OTR/L, FAOTA
Associate Professor
Program in Occupational Therapy
School of Medicine
Washington University in St. Louis
St. Louis, Missouri

Rebecca Birkenmeier, OTD, OTR/L
Assistant Professor of Occupational Therapy
Occupational Therapy
Maryville University
St. Louis, Missouri

Nicole Boyington, OTD, MOT, OTR/L, CLT
Academic Fieldwork Coordinator and Assistant Professor
Occupational Therapy Department
Mount Mary University
Milwaukee, Wisconsin

Elizabeth Cara, PhD, OTR/L, MFCC
Emeritus Professor
Occupational Therapy
San José State University
San Jose, California

Lisa Crabtree, PhD, OTR/L, FAOTA
Associate Professor
Department of Occupational Therapy and Occupational Science
Towson University
Towson, Maryland

Mariana D'Amico, EdD, OTR/L, FAOTA
Associate Professor
Occupational Therapy
Nova Southeastern University
Tampa, Florida

Janet V. DeLany, DEd, OTR/L, FAOTA
Professor Emeritus
Department of Occupational Therapy and Occupational Science
Towson University
Towson, Maryland

Jewell Dickson, OTD, MHP, OTR/L, ATP
Assistant Professor
Department of Occupational Therapy
Alabama State University
Montgomery, Alabama

Carolyn R. Dorfman, PhD, OTR/L
Assistant Professor
The College of St. Scholastica
Duluth, Minnesota

Julie Dorsey, OTD, OTR/L, CEAS
Associate Professor
Department of Occupational Therapy
Ithaca College
Ithaca, New York

Christopher Eidson, MS, OTR/L
Assistant Professor
Department of Occupational Therapy
The University of Alabama at Birmingham
Birmingham, Alabama

Cynthia Evetts, PhD, OTR
Director and Associate Professor
School of Occupational Therapy
Texas Woman's University
Denton, Texas

Sarah E. Fabrizi, PhD, OTR/L
Instructor
Department of Rehabilitation Sciences
Florida Gulf Coast University
Fort Myers, Florida

Kathleen Flecky, OTD, OTR/L
Associate Professor
Department of Occupational Therapy
Creighton University
Omaha, Nebraska

Rita P. Fleming-Castaldy, OTL, PhD, FAOTA
Professor Emeritus
Department of Occupational Therapy
The University of Scranton
Scranton, Pennsylvania

Karen P. Funk, OTD, OTR
Clinical Associate Professor and Program Chair
University of Texas at El Paso
El Paso, Texas

Mary Gavacs, MEd, OTR/L
Director
Occupational Therapy Assistant Program
Instructor
Occupational Therapy
Mercyhurst University
Erie, Pennsylvania

Lynn Gitlow, PhD, OTR/L, ATP
Associate Professor
Department of Occupational Therapy
Ithaca College
Ithaca, New York

Laura Green, MOT, OTR/L
Assistant Professor and Program Director
Occupational Therapy Assistant Program
Kirkwood Community College
Hiawatha, Iowa

Barbara Haase, MHS, OTR/L, FAOTA
Director
Occupational Therapy Assistant Program
EHOVE Career Center
Lorain County Community College
Milan, Ohio

David Haynes, DHS, MBA, OTR
Program Director
Master of Science in Occupational Therapy Program
Jefferson College of Health Sciences
Roanoke, Virginia

Susanne Higgins, OTD, OTR/L, CHT
Assistant Professor
Occupational Therapy
Midwestern University
Glendale, Arizona

Angela Hissong, DEd, OTR/L, CMCP, CMMT, CIR
Senior Instructor
Occupational Therapy
Health and Human Development
Pennsylvania State University
University Park, Pennsylvania

Mary-Ellen Johnson, OTD, MAHSM, OTR/L
Clinical Assistant Professor
Graduate Program in Occupational Therapy
Sacred Heart University
Fairfield, Connecticut

Michele Karnes, EdD, OT
Assistant Professor
Occupational Therapy
D'Youville College
Buffalo, New York

Pamalyn J. Kearney, EdD, OTR/L
Department Chair and Associate Professor
Department of Occupational Therapy
Augusta University
Augusta, Georgia

Melissa Khosla, MS, OTD, OTR/L
Clinical Coordinator and Assistant Professor
Department of Occupational Therapy
Indiana Wesleyan University
Marion, Indiana

Annmarie Kinsella, OTD, MS, OTR/L
Assistant Professor
Occupational Therapy
Utica College
Utica, New York

Nancy Krolikowski, MS, OTR/L, CHT
OTA Program Director and Assistant Professor
South University
Virginia Beach, Virginia

Julie Kugel, OTD, MOT, OTR/L
Associate Professor and OTD Program Director
Occupational Therapy
Loma Linda University
Loma Linda, California

Leanne Leclair, BHSc(OT), MSc, PhD
Associate Professor
Occupational Therapy
University of Manitoba
Manitoba, Canada

Susan Leech, EdD, OT
Assistant Professor
University of Texas at El Paso
El Paso, Texas

Amy Mahle, MHA, COTA/L, ROH
Program Chair
Occupational Therapy Assistant Program
Rowan-Cabarrus Community College
Salisbury, North Carolina

Catherine McNeil, MS, OTR/L
Assistant Professor
Worcester State University
Worcester, Massachusetts

Rochelle J. Mendonca, PhD, OTR/L
Assistant Professor
Rehabilitation and Regenerative Medicine
Columbia University
New York, New York

Christine Merchant, PhD, OTR/L
Associate Professor
Occupational Therapy
Midwestern University
Glendale, Arizona

Whitney Lucas Molitor, OTD, OTR/L, BCG
Assistant Professor
Department of Occupational Therapy
University of South Dakota
Vermillion, South Dakota

Jaime Muñoz, PhD, OTR/L, FAOTA
Department Chair and Associate Professor
Department of Occupational Therapy
Duquesne University
Pittsburgh, Pennsylvania

Peggy Neufeld, PhD, OTR/L, FAOTA
Adjunct Faculty
Program in Occupational Therapy
Washington University in St. Louis
St. Louis, Missouri

Meryl Marger Picard, PhD, MSW, OTR
Assistant Professor
Department of Occupational Therapy
Seton Hall University
South Orange, New Jersey

Patricia J. Precin, PhD, OTR/L, FAOTA
Assistant Professor
Occupational Therapy
Department of Rehabilitation and Regenerative Medicine
Vagelos College of Physicians and Surgeons
Columbia University
New York, New York

Christine Privott, PhD, OTR/L
Professor
Occupational Science and Occupational Therapy
Eastern Kentucky University
Richmond, Kentucky

Monika Robinson, DrOT, OTR/L
Assistant Professor
Occupational Therapy Department
Midwestern University
Downers Grove, Illinois

Eva L. Rodriguez, PhD, OTR
Associate Professor
Department of Occupational Therapy
York College/City University of New York
Jamaica, New York

Penny Rogers, DHA, MAT, OTR/L
Associate Professor and Capstone Coordinator
Department of Occupational Therapy
University of Mississippi Medical Center
Jackson, Mississippi

Sandra L. Rogers, PhD, OTR/L
Program Chair and Associate Professor
Occupational Therapy Program
Rutgers University
Newark, New Jersey

Veronica Rowe, PhD, OTR/L, CBIST, FNAP
Assistant Professor
Occupational Therapy
University of Central Arkansas
Conway, Arkansas

Jacquelyn M. Sample, DrOT, MEd, OTR/L
Clinical Instructor
Occupational Therapy Assistant Program
Missouri Health Professions Consortium
University of Missouri
Columbia, Missouri

Jennifer J. Saylor, MEd, OT/L
Program Director and Fieldwork Coordinator
New Hampshire Community Technical College
Claremont, New Hampshire

Stacy Smallfield, DrOT, MSOT, OTR/L, BCG, FAOTA
Associate Professor
Occupational Therapy and Medicine
Program in Occupational Therapy
Washington University School of Medicine
St. Louis, Missouri

Yvonne Swinth, PhD, OTR/L, FAOTA
Professor and Program Director
School of Occupational Therapy
University of Puget Sound
Tacoma, Washington

Joan Temple, MEd, OTR
Academic Fieldwork Coordinator and Clinical Assistant
Health Professions
University of Wisconsin–La Crosse
La Crosse, Wisconsin

Christine Urish, PhD, OTR/L, BCMH, FAOTA
Professor
Occupational Therapy
St. Ambrose University
Davenport, Iowa

Shelley L. Wallock, DrPH, OTR/L
Assistant Professor
Occupational Therapy
Thomas Jefferson University
Philadelphia, Pennsylvania

Suzanne M. White, MA, OTR/L, FAOTA
Clinical Associate Professor
Occupational Therapy Program
SUNY Downstate Medical Center
Brooklyn, New York

Kirsten Wilbur, EdD, OTR/L
Clinical Assistant Professor
School of Occupational Therapy
University of Puget Sound
Tacoma, Washington

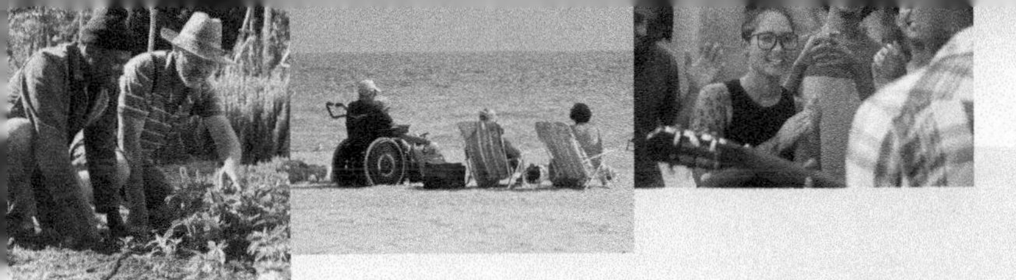

Acknowledgments

The third edition of this text would not have been possible without the encouragement and assistance of many people who share our enthusiasm for community and population health practice. We would first like to acknowledge our universities, the University of South Alabama and Towson University, for their support. Several students were valuable contributors to the production of this book, including Charlotte Brown, Chenise Calhoun, Kristen Gittings, Bridget Graef, Katie Lowe, Meheret Messelwork, Taryn Painter, and Jennifer Perea-Lopez from Towson University.

We are also indebted to the fine staff at the F. A. Davis Company, especially Christa Fratantoro, senior acquisitions editor, for her encouragement and unwavering faith in our work and Jill Rembetski, freelance developmental editor, for her exceptional guidance and assistance throughout the project.

And last, but certainly not least, we would like to acknowledge the support of family and friends. We are fortunate to have understanding, caring, and thoughtful people in our lives, as we could not have completed this textbook without their assistance. However, our spouses, Blaise Chromiak and Fred Reitz, deserve the South Alabama Jaguar and Towson Tiger share of our gratitude and love for their patience as this project continued evolving into a third edition that finally came to fruition.

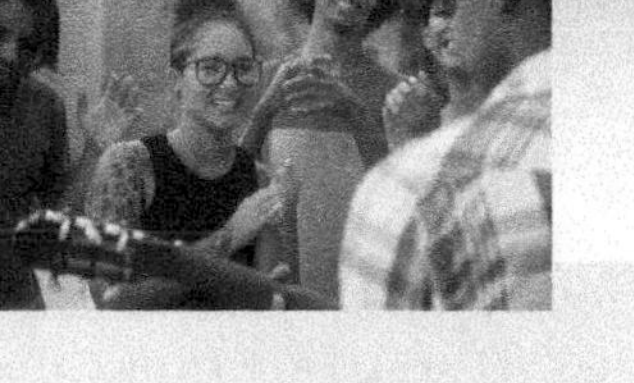

Contents

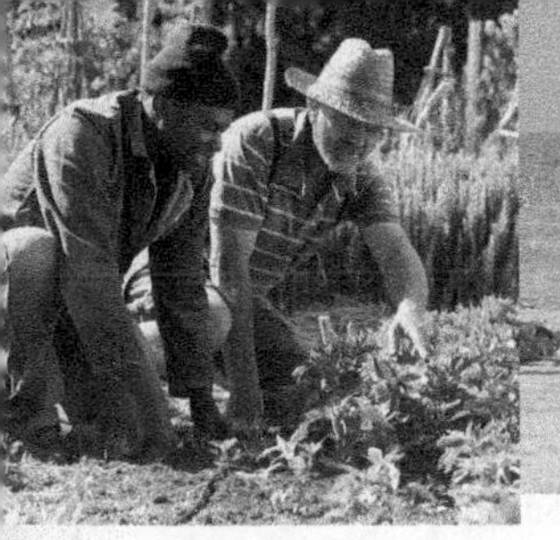
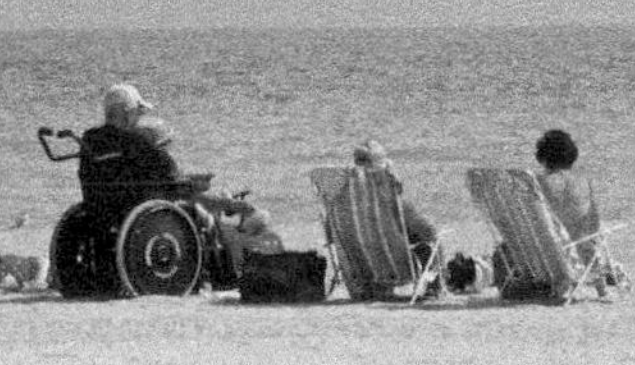
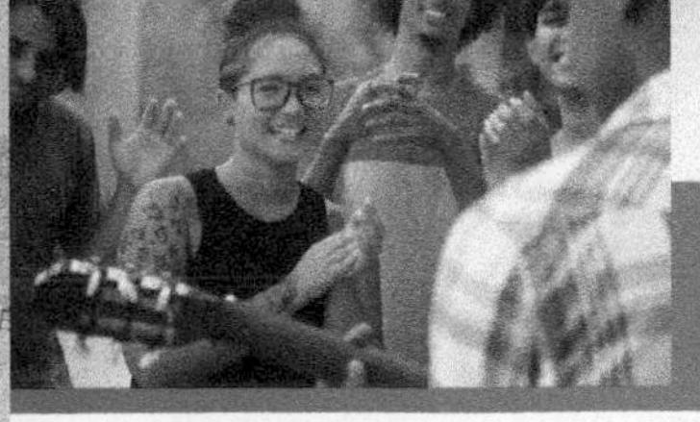

SECTION I

Basic Principles and Relevant Issues

Chapter 1

Historical and Philosophical Perspectives of Community and Population Health Practice

Marjorie E. Scaffa, PhD, OTR/L, FAOTA, and S. Maggie Reitz, PhD, OTR/L, FAOTA

We know what we are, but we know not what we may be.
—Shakespeare

Learning Outcomes

This chapter is designed to enable the reader to:

1-1 Describe the history of community and population health practice in occupational therapy.
1-2 Describe the variety of roles for occupational therapy practitioners in community and population health practice.
1-3 Describe the characteristics of effective community and population health practitioners.
1-4 Describe the history of paradigm shifts in occupational therapy.
1-5 Identify key characteristics of a community and population health practice paradigm for occupational therapy.

Key Terms

Client-centered approach
Community
Community-based practice
Community-centered initiative/intervention
Community health promotion
Community-level intervention
Dynamic systems approach
Ecological approach
Health
Paradigm
Paradigm shift
Population
Population health
Strengths-based

Introduction

In 2017, the profession of occupational therapy and the American Occupational Therapy Association (AOTA) turned 100 years of age. In order to set a course for the future and to celebrate the profession's history, the AOTA developed a *Centennial Vision* document that stated: "We envision that occupational therapy is a powerful, widely recognized, science-driven, and evidence-based profession with a globally connected and diverse workforce meeting society's occupational needs" (Baum, 2006, p. 610). This statement has been updated in the document *Vision 2025* and now reads, "Occupational therapy maximizes health, well-being, and quality of life for all people, populations, and communities through effective solutions that facilitate participation in everyday living" (AOTA, 2017, p. 1).

A community and population health practice (CPHP) paradigm is entirely consistent with these visions. For example, expanding community-based occupational therapy services and population health interventions makes occupational therapy more visible, thereby enhancing understanding and recognition of the profession. An improved awareness of occupational therapy may also increase consumer demand for services. If occupational therapy practitioners are working in more varied settings and providing needed services, then more opportunities to influence policies and take on leadership roles may result. Practicing in the community and with various populations increases involvement with other professionals and assists in building alliances that also may expand the profession's power base. In addition, CPHP enables the development of a variety of new roles for occupational therapy practitioners. Finally, because community practice occurs in environments where people work, play, go to school, and participate in activities of daily living, the profession is more likely to be aware of and meet society's occupational needs.

Occupational therapy as a profession has the opportunity to respond to and help resolve social and health problems of the 21st century, including poverty, homelessness, addiction, depression, joblessness, chronic disease and disability, unintentional injury, violence and abuse, and social discrimination and stigma. Meeting the occupational needs of society will require not only the provision of occupational therapy services to individuals and families in community-based settings but also the provision of occupational therapy services to organizations, communities, and populations.

An overview of CPHP for occupational therapy is provided in this chapter. Also included are a review of the historical perspectives of CPHP, an identification of the various roles associated with these practices, and a description of the necessary characteristics for effective practice. The major paradigm shifts in occupational therapy, highlighting the impact of systems theory, are presented. Concluding the chapter is a discussion of the CPHP paradigm as a client-centered approach to practice.

Historical Perspectives of Community and Population Health Practice[1]

Community-based practice and population health are not new concepts in occupational therapy (Table 1-1). During the profession's inception, the community was a primary site of service provision, and military personnel and individuals with mental illness were the populations of focus of occupational therapy.

Early Community and Prevention Practice

Two founders of the profession, George Barton and Eleanor Clarke Slagle, developed community-based programs in the early 1900s. Barton, who was disabled by tuberculosis (TB) and a foot amputation, established Consolation House in New York in 1914. The program used occupations to enable convalescents to return to productive living (Punwar, 1994; Sabonis-Chafee, 1989). Barton's establishment of Consolation House in 1914 is the earliest example of community-based occupational therapy practice within the United States (Scaffa, 2001; Scaffa and Brownson, 2005).

The doors of Consolation House opened on March 7, 1914, after extensive alterations. In an article

1. Portions of this section first appeared in Reitz, S. M. (2010). Historical and philosophical perspectives in occupational therapy's role in health and promotion. In M. E. Scaffa, S. M. Reitz, and M. A. Pizzi (Eds.), *Occupational therapy in the promotion of health and wellness* (pp. 1–21). Philadelphia, PA: F. A. Davis.

Table 1-1 Historical Time Line of Community and Population Health Practice in Occupational Therapy

Date	Event
1914	George Barton establishes Consolation House in New York.
1915	Eleanor Clarke Slagle establishes the work program at Hull House in Chicago.
1937	Humphreys advocates community treatment for persons with developmental disabilities.
1938	Banyai advocates following tuberculosis patients into the community after discharge from sanitariums.
1940	The AOTA reports on roundtable discussions held at the national conference on the role of occupational therapy in community health.
1968	Bockhoven suggests that occupational therapy take responsibility for community occupational development.
1969–1973	In the United States, West, Reilly, and Mosey describe the need for occupational therapy services in the community.
1972	Llorens describes a community-based program in San Francisco for pregnant teenagers.
1972	Finn argues that the profession move beyond the role of therapist to "health agent."
1973	Hasselkus and Kiernat describe an independent living program for the elderly.
1974	The AOTA Task Force on Target Populations expands the role of the profession to include health promotion and disability prevention.
1977	Laukaran describes the major obstacles to community-based practice.
1982	Kirchman, Reichenback, and Giambalvo describe a prevention program for the well elderly.
1997	Well Elderly Study published in the *Journal of the American Medical Association.*
2006	Accreditation Council for Occupational Therapy Education (ACOTE) standards revised, with increased emphasis on health promotion and population-based services.
2006	The AOTA adopts the *2017 Centennial Vision.*
2016	The AOTA adopts *Vision 2025.* Populations are identified as a potential recipient of services.

commemorating the AOTA's 50th anniversary, Barton's wife, Isabel, described the alterations and the dedication of the Consolation House (Barton, 1968). The alterations included a 6-foot tub, which Barton installed against the advice of the plumber. After many months at a sanatorium, Barton desired the opportunity to "stretch out" while bathing. The parlor of the house was turned into an office that housed books related to occupational therapy, as well as a glass case exhibiting patients' craftwork. The décor of Consolation House was heavily influenced by the Arts and Crafts Movement of the early 1900s (Krieger, 2001).

The first floor of an old red barn on the property was converted into a workshop, and the second floor became a studio. Barton acquired a vacant lot adjacent to the house and subdivided it into three sections: a vegetable garden, a grass lawn, and an area containing flowering shrubbery and a hammock. The house provided tools for engaging in a variety of occupations, and "experimental projects were carried out in the quest for new occupations to be offered to incapacitated individuals" (Barton, 1968, p. 342). An example of one of the many "experiments" conducted in the garden area was growing calabash, with the expectation that patients could turn them into pipes. The philosophy of George Barton and Consolation House can best be expressed through his words:

raise the cry that it is time for humanity to cease regarding the hospital as a door closing upon a life which is past, and to regard it henceforth as a door opening upon a life which is to come . . . filled with the joy of hope for a better job, or a job done better. (Barton, 1914, cited by Quiroga, 1995, p.134)

Eleanor Clarke Slagle was hired in 1915 to develop a program to provide persons with mental and/or physical disabilities an opportunity to work and become self-sufficient. The project was funded by philanthropic contributions and was located at Hull House, a settlement house in Chicago. In its first year of operation, the program served 77 persons who developed manual skills and received wages for their work. The goods produced in the workshop included baskets, needlework, rugs, simple cabinets, and toys (Reed and Sanderson, 1999).

In the United States, occupational therapy's early work in prevention focused on the deterrence of infectious disease such as TB. Diaz (1932) described her efforts to organize a preventorium in Puerto Rico for children of parents with TB with the goal of decreasing the children's risk of contracting the disease. The board of directors of an association for the prevention of TB among children contacted Diaz to organize a new facility to house and care for 50 children between the ages of 2 and 10. Diaz performed a variety of administrative functions, including developing a daily regimen of habit training and occupations that included "marching, sunbaths, singing, folk dancing, rest in bed, storytelling, calisthenics, outdoor games, daily prayers, personal habits . . . academic classes, and some craft work" (Diaz, 1932, p. 200). Within a 1-year period, the progress of the children was reported as "remarkable. They entered the institution in very bad condition: undernourished, unhealthy, and with little or no discipline. They were returned quite different" (Diaz, 1932, p. 201).

Banyai (1938) wrote about the care individuals with TB were receiving while residing in sanitariums.

Engage Your Brain 1-1

What role could occupational therapy play in an interdisciplinary type of community-based or population health TB preventive action? Where in the United States and abroad would this type of intervention be most needed?

While acknowledging the importance of occupational therapy intervention in the institution, she emphasized the need to follow the patient into the community. The ultimate goal was to restore the individual to a satisfactory level of social and economic functioning. Banyai (1938) believed that this required the occupational therapist to work with the person in the community after discharge from the institution.

In 1947, the director of the Philadelphia Committee for the Prevention of Blindness discussed the need for interdisciplinary collaboration to prevent blindness through combating its three primary causes: venereal disease, now referred to as *sexually transmitted infection;* glaucoma; and accidents (Carpenter, 1947). Carpenter believed occupational therapists, due to their interactions with families, had a key role in the early screening of visual problems in children and their parents (Reitz, 1992). Specifically, occupational therapists were encouraged to look for and intervene when symptoms of congenital syphilis or ineffective home remedies for injured eyes were present or if they heard reports of family members or neighbors seeing colored rings around lights at night. Occupational therapists were also encouraged to take advantage of being in the community as an opportunity to minimize adverse health conditions and prevent future illness in other family or community members, thereby joining the public health team.

The professional literature of the 1960s suggests that the field was on the verge of expanding its services outside of traditional medical settings (Laukaran, 1977). West (1969) asserted that "the traditional role of the occupational therapist, that of the reintegration of social function, is not a hospital service but rather a function that can be best filled in the community" (p. 231). Reilly (1971) advocated that the future growth of the profession was predicated on the transition of occupational therapy services from the hospital to the community. The focus of occupational therapy, in her view, should be to develop experiences and programs in the individual's community environment that enhance adaptive competencies. This broader perspective requires the professional to provide therapeutic programming in the individual's milieu, including the home, school, workplace, and community.

In spite of these early admonitions to focus on broader health needs and services outside of institutional settings, the move to community-based practice was short-lived and very limited in scope. In the 1970s and 1980s, examples of outreach into the community included an independent living project for the elderly (Hasselkus and Kiernat, 1973), a project for pregnant teenage girls (Llorens, 1972), and prevention services for the well elderly (Kirchman, Reichenback, and Giambalvo, 1982). According to Laukaran (1977), three major obstacles to community-based practice existed at that time. These barriers were practical constraints, historical factors within the discipline, and gaps in knowledge and theory related to community-based practice. The practical constraints were related to the limited number of opportunities for community-based practice at that time and the public perception of occupational therapy as a medical discipline. Historically, occupational therapy practitioners' professional identities had been associated with work in medical institutions. In addition, professional education programs emphasized preparation for practice in medical rather than community-based settings. Laukaran (1977) noted that some theoretical frameworks of that era (e.g., occupational behavior, biopsychosocial, and developmental models) were compatible with community-based practice. However, these early models were inadequate in providing guidelines and rationales for services in community settings.

Some of these same obstacles exist today, albeit in different forms. Opportunities for utilizing occupational therapy expertise in community or population health practice are limitless but typically not designated as occupational therapy positions. For the profession to move into these arenas, practitioners must seek out positions that, although not labeled "occupational therapy," could benefit from the unique contributions of the discipline. The perception of occupational therapy as strictly a medical discipline continues to exist both outside and within the profession. The identity of "medical professional" is an alluring one, as in the past it denoted an aura of legitimacy. Many occupational therapy practitioners today are reluctant to "let go" of this restrictive image in favor of a more broadly defined role. In addition, professional preparation programs are slow to shift focus. However, many educators concur that the future of the profession will largely be determined by its ability to expand the scope of practice into community-based settings (Holmes and Scaffa, 2009a). Many more theoretical frameworks exist today than existed in the 1960s. These models, based on the work of previous theorists, are readily applicable to CPHP. Some of these theories and models are described in Chapter 3.

Interestingly, one of the boldest predictions and the strongest support for the validity of occupational therapy services in the community came from a physician in 1968. Bockhoven (1968) suggested a new role for occupational therapists, described as "taking responsibility for community occupational development, alongside the businessman, city planner and the economist . . . to support growth of respect for human individuality in occupation" (p. 25). The AOTA (1974) Task Force on Target Populations redefined occupational therapy as "the science of using occupation as a health determinant" (p. 158). This definition advanced the notion that occupational therapy was not limited to the seriously or chronically ill but could also remediate mild to moderate impairments and contribute to health promotion and disability prevention.

Finn (1972), in the 1971 Eleanor Clarke Slagle Lecture, stated: "In order for a profession to maintain its relevancy it must be responsive to the trends of the times. . . . Occupational therapists are being asked to move beyond the role of therapist to that of health agent. This expansion in role identity will require a reinterpretation of current knowledge, the addition of new knowledge and skills, and the revision of the educational process" (p. 59).

These words are still true today. The expanded role of health agent requires practitioners to move into the community and provide a continuum of services; these include prevention, health promotion, and population health, in addition to the intervention services typically provided by the profession. Health agent is more than "therapist." Other roles, such as consultant, advocate, community organizer, program developer, and case manager, are also included.

Military and the Use of Occupation in Population Health

Military leaders have long recognized the benefits of using occupation to improve their armies. These occupations have primarily included physical activities for conditioning and the prevention of injury (Kavasch and Baar, 1999; Levin, 1937) and for entertainment, such as that provided by the United Service Organizations (USO, 2019) since 1941 to prevent boredom and maintain morale.

However, occupation does not appear to have been used for the rehabilitation of soldiers until World Wars I and II. The rehabilitation efforts described below were aimed at the individual needs of soldiers but were also part of a broader societal intervention through governmental policies and programs, which can be considered forms of population-based health promotion.

"During World War I, it was found in Germany, France, and England that much could be done to recondition the wounded by means of occupation" (Dunton, 1954, p. 5). Early in World War I, before the United States entered the conflict, leaders in countries already involved were concerned about the prospect of large numbers of wounded and their need for rehabilitation (Willard and Cox, 1979). The previous system of pensioning injured veterans for life was not going to be economically feasible. Thus, there was great interest in ensuring the self-sufficiency of these soldiers (Christensen, 1991).

At the onset of World War I, British physicians began to see a cluster of symptoms that became known as shell shock. At first, these symptoms were blamed on exposure to the deafening sounds of shells and grenades exploding. Later, it was understood that the symptoms were caused by the horrific living conditions endured during trench warfare, which included spending weeks at a time in rat-infested, corpse-laden, and flooded trenches.

In 1918, Dunton became president of the National Society for the Promotion of Occupational Therapy at the group's second annual meeting. At that meeting, he shared the Europeans' success in using occupation to treat shell shock and stressed the need for the United States to prepare well-trained occupational workers for the eventual war effort (Peloquin, 1991). Within months, the United States entered World War I, and recruitment and education for reconstruction aides began (Dunton, 1954; Peloquin, 1991; Willard and Cox, 1979). Recovering soldiers in World Wars I and II received instructions in basket weaving, woodwork, and other occupations to facilitate their recovery from physical injuries and from psychosocial dysfunction caused by the horrors of war (McDaniel, 1968). Figure 1-1 shows an example of an occupational therapy workshop in a U.S. Army hospital in France during World War I. As often happens, knowledge gained in war can later be used to favorably affect the health and well-being of nonmilitary populations.

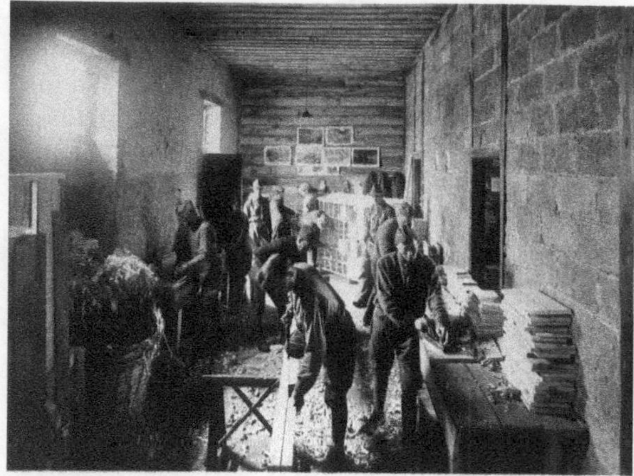

Figure 1-1 Base Hospital No. 9., Chateauroux, France, woodwork. *(Courtesy of the National Library of Medicine Collection. Appears as Figure 24 in "Occupational Therapists Before World War II [1917–40]," by M. L. McDaniel, in H. S. Lee and M. L. McDaniel [Eds.],* Army Medical Specialist Corps *[pp. 69–97], Washington, DC: Office of the Surgeon General, Department of the Army.)*

Definitions of Terms

To conceptualize and operationalize CPHP in occupational therapy, definitions of various terms have been adopted for the purposes of this textbook. These terms include health, community, community-based practice, community health promotion, community-level intervention, community-centered initiatives/interventions, population, and population health.

Health

Health is defined as the ability to "realize aspirations, to satisfy needs, and to change or cope with the environment. Therefore, health is seen as a resource for everyday life . . . a positive concept emphasizing social and personal resources, as well as physical capacities. . . . The fundamental conditions and resources for health are peace, shelter, education, food, income, a stable ecosystem, sustainable resources, social justice and equity" (World Health Organization [WHO], 1986, p. 1).

Community

Community means different things to different people. No single definition appears to capture the richness and diversity of the term, but considering the following definitions provides a broad and comprehensive perspective. Community refers to "noninstitutional aggregations of people linked together for common goals or other purposes" (Green and Raeburn, 1990, p. 41). It is the "space where people think for themselves, dream their dreams, and come together to create and celebrate their common humanity" (O'Connell, 1988, p. 31). The WHO (1998) defines a community as "a specific group of people, often living in the same geographical area, who share a common culture, values and norms, are arranged in a social structure according to relationships, which the community has developed over a period of time" (p. 5).

The community or neighborhood setting is a vital part of growing up, raising families, and meeting the many challenges and stresses of modern life (Warren and Warren, 1979). According to Nisbit (1972), people do not come together in community relationships merely to be together; they come together to do something that cannot easily be done in isolation.

Community-Based Practice

Community-based practice is more comprehensive than simply providing rehabilitation services in a community setting. Community-based practice includes a broad range of health-related services: prevention and health promotion, acute and chronic medical care, habilitation and rehabilitation, and direct and indirect service provision, all of which are provided in community settings. Community in this framework "means more than a geographic location for practice, but includes an orientation to collective health, social priorities, and different modes of service provision" (Kniepmann, 1997, p. 540). Community models are responsive to individual and family health needs in homes, workplaces, and community agencies. In this way, interventions are contextually embedded. The goal in community-based practice is for the client and the practitioner to become integral parts of the community. Some hospitals and rehabilitation centers provide field trips in the community for patients or clients and health fairs for community members, but these activities are not considered community-based services. They are more appropriately referred to as community outreach (Robnett, 1997).

Community Health Promotion

Community health promotion can be defined as "any combination of educational and social supports for people taking greater control of, and improving their own or the health of a geographically defined area" (Green and Ottoson, 1999, p. 729). Educational programs may be directed at individuals, families, groups, or communities through schools, work sites, organizations, and/or mass media. Social approaches focus on organizational, legal, political, and economic changes that support health and well-being. "Organized community effort is the key to community health. There are some things the individual can do entirely alone, but many health benefits can be obtained only through united community effort" (Green and Anderson, 1982, p. 4).

Community-Level Intervention

Community-level interventions "attempt to modify the socio-cultural, political, economic and environmental context of the community to achieve health goals" (Scaffa and Brownson, 2005, p. 485). These are population-based approaches to health and do not focus on individual health behavior change. Community-level interventions are directed at having an impact on systems that affect health in communities. Often initiated by health-care and government agencies, they typically involve community organization strategies. Decisions are often based on the source of funding, and planning is done by a "lead" agency. The professional serves as an expert in a leadership capacity.

Community-Centered Initiatives/Interventions

Community-centered initiatives/interventions are often generated by leaders and members of the community and typically utilize existing community resources. Community coalitions form to identify common concerns and needs and to design approaches to solve community problems. Community-centered interventions follow the principles of client-centered practice in which the client is the entire community. In this way, community-centered initiatives promote community participation, the exchange of information, and community autonomy. The role of the professional is as a consultant, facilitator, and mentor in the community. Occupational therapists can participate in community-centered initiatives by "identifying occupational risk factors, engaging in problem-solving and proposing and implementing solutions" that meet the community's unique occupational needs (Scaffa and Brownson, 2005, p. 485).

Population

According to the AOTA, a population is a "collective of groups of individuals living in a similar locale—e.g., city, state, or country—or sharing the same or like characteristics or concerns" (2014, p. S3). The authors of this chapter have conceptualized a broader definition—**population** is viewed as an aggregate of people who may or may not know each other but share at least one common characteristic such as age, race, ethnicity, gender, health habit or condition, geographic location, cultural identity, socioeconomic status, or education level.

Population Health

David Kindig and Greg Stoddart sought to define and provide a rationale for their definition of what was a "relatively new term" in 2003—**population health.** They defined it as "the health outcome of a group of individuals, including the distribution of such outcomes within the group" (Kindig and Stoddart, 2003, p. 380). This view has evolved. According to the Centers for Disease Control and Prevention (CDC, 2019), population health is an approach wherein the distribution of health outcomes within a population and local priorities determine areas to address through interdisciplinary collaboration, including nontraditional partners such as universities and industry. A further broadening of this definition is needed to address the occupational needs of populations and for populations that are broad and not isolated to one geographical area. The authors thus define population health as a collaborative, interdisciplinary approach that includes advocacy; program development, implementation, and evaluation; and policy revision and development to maximize health equity and occupational justice in a population based on the social and health determinants and priorities of that population.

Trends and Roles in Community-Based Practice

The AOTA (2015a) Salary and Workforce Survey indicated that 1.9% of occupational therapy practitioners work in a community setting such as an "adult day care program, area agency on aging, community residential care facility, environmental modification program/services, group home, independent-living center, low vision program, prevention/wellness program, retirement/assisted living, senior center, and supervised housing" (p. 16). More occupational therapists were reported to work in the community (2%) versus occupational therapy assistants (1.7%). In addition to the community, 1.6% of occupational therapy practitioners work in settings characterized as "other," including "driving program, industrial rehabilitation/work programs, sheltered workshop, supported employment," among others, all of which are community-based (p. 16). A total of 4.3% of occupational therapy practitioners work in early intervention programs, and another 6.3% work in home health. Thus, the data reveal that approximately 14% of occupational therapy practitioners work in community settings. This figure does not include occupational therapy practitioners who work in community-based mental health programs.

The overall median annual compensation for occupational therapists working in community settings was $70,000, which was the same for the "typical" occupational therapists working full-time.

This demonstrates that the common perception that occupational therapists in community settings earn far less than their counterparts in more traditional settings is a myth. Gender differences in pay (i.e., men being paid more than women) were greatest in home health and nonexistent in community employment (AOTA, 2015a).

Role Descriptions

Occupational therapy practitioners have a significant role to play in supporting individuals in their homes and workplaces, facilitating their independence, and promoting their integration into the community (Stalker, Jones, and Ritchie, 1996). More than 50 years ago, West (1967) described her vision of the changing responsibility of occupational therapists to the community. This vision acknowledged the newly emerging focus on prevention and health promotion in medicine and the impact this new focus would have on practice settings, roles, and responsibilities. West (1967) predicted that as a result of the change in focus, practice would move into new settings—"namely, the communities in which our potential patients live, work and play" (p. 312). She described four emerging roles that at the time were adding new dimensions to the traditional role of the clinically based occupational therapist: evaluator, consultant, supervisor, and researcher.

Other roles that community-based practitioners may fulfill include program planners and evaluators, staff trainers, community health advisors, policymakers, and primary care providers. Practitioners in the community may function as community health advocates, consultants, case managers, entrepreneurs, supervisors, and program managers. It is important for community-based practitioners in these roles to develop networks of support and collaboration with other occupational therapy practitioners, health and social service professionals, and community leaders.

Community Health Advocate

As a community health advocate, practitioners identify the social, physical, emotional, medical, educational, and occupational needs of community members for optimal functioning and advocate for services to meet those needs. In addition, practitioners act as advocates and lobbyists by providing input and shaping legislation and government policies, thereby affecting local and national physical and mental health issues and changing environmental conditions to promote health.

Consultant

Occupational therapy practitioners in the role of consultant provide information and expert advice regarding program development and evaluation, supervisory models, organizational issues, and/or clinical concerns. Consultation is "an interactive process of helping others solve existing or potential problems by identifying and analyzing issues, developing strategies to address problems and preventing future problems from occurring" (Epstein and Jaffe, 2003, p. 260). Consultation services are most often utilized when new programs are being developed or undergoing significant change and may be short-term or long-term, depending on the needs of the program. Within the community, occupational therapy practitioners can act as consultants to a variety of groups, such as the Scouts or Boys and Girls Clubs, adult education programs, adult day care, transitional living programs, independent living centers, community development and housing agencies, health departments, military bases and organizations, and work site safety and health programs.

Case Manager

As a case manager, a practitioner coordinates the provision of services; advises the consumer, family, or caregiver; evaluates financial resources; and advocates for needed services. Case management requires a professional who has ample clinical experience, understands reimbursement mechanisms, and has good organizational skills. Frequently, the qualifications and duties of case managers are dictated by state regulations. Occupational therapy practitioners are most often designated as case managers in mental health and children and youth practice areas.

Although the primary role of case managers is to ensure access to community services and resources, they may also assist in the development of independent living skills (e.g., money management, social interaction, and cognitive skills such as decision-making and problem-solving). Occupational therapists are qualified by their education and training to serve as case managers and/or to supervise others in case management positions.

Private Practice Owner/Entrepreneur

An occupational therapy entrepreneur is "an individual who organizes a business venture, manages its operation, and assumes the risks associated with the business" (Vaughn and Sladyk, 2011, p. 167). The entrepreneur may own a private practice, provide services on a contractual basis, and/or function as a consultant. In order for entrepreneurs to be successful, they must be able to assess and respond to the unique needs of their communities. Changing demographics, including the significant growth of the aging population, will provide a variety of opportunities for occupational therapy entrepreneurs. In order to be successful, entrepreneurs must have a wide range of skills, including financial management, marketing, leadership, and organizational and team-building skills (Vaughn and Sladyk, 2011). A broad overview of entrepreneurship is provided in Chapter 8.

Supervisor

Supervisors typically manage and are responsible for all the activities of their team members. A supervisor sets up work schedules, delegates tasks, recruits and trains employees, and conducts performance appraisals. In occupational therapy practice, supervision "is a process aimed at ensuring the safe and effective delivery of occupational therapy services and fostering professional competence and development" (AOTA, 2015b, p. S16). The role of an occupational therapy supervisor varies from facility to facility but generally includes training and evaluating staff and fieldwork students, developing and reviewing intervention plans and other documentation, solving problems as needed, and contributing to budget and program development. Supervisors typically do not have final budgetary or personnel authority but assume responsibility for the day-to-day operations of the program.

Program Managers

Program managers are responsible for the overall design, development, function, and evaluation of a program; budgeting; and staff hiring and supervision. Many occupational therapists have served as program managers in community settings (Fazio, 2008). Program managers conduct needs assessments, SWOT (strengths, weaknesses, opportunities, threats) analyses, strategic planning, and program development functions. Occupational therapists not in positions officially designated as program managers may be asked to expand existing programs or develop new programs to meet client needs. Program managers in community-based settings tend to "use a more interactive approach that promotes open communication, feedback and collaboration than managers in more traditional, institutionally-driven medical settings" (Scaffa, Doll, Estes, and Holmes, 2011, p. 320).

Engage Your Brain 1-2

Which principle from the AOTA (2015c) *Occupational Therapy Code of Ethics (2015)* would be most applicable to community and population health programming?

Characteristics of Effective Community-Based Occupational Therapy Practitioners

According to Learnard, "occupational therapy in community health is both an art and a science" (Robnett, 1997, p. 30). In addition to the typical occupational therapy focus on enhancing function through task analysis and the modification of important life tasks and the environment, occupational therapists in community-based practice need a variety of other skills and attributes. According to Robnett (1997), Learnard believes effective community-based therapists exemplify the following characteristics:

- A sense of positive hopefulness
- An understanding of individuals in their specific personal circumstances
- The creativity to envision a variety of possibilities
- The ability to set aside one's cultural, personal, and professional biases and respect individual choices rather than passing judgment

Holmes and Scaffa (2009b) studied 23 occupational therapists working in emerging practice areas and attempted to identify the competencies needed to work in new or underdeveloped practice settings. The competencies were identified through the use of the Delphi technique of forecasting, whereby respondents have multiple opportunities to identify, rate, and rank the characteristics they deem essential for emerging practice. The competencies and characteristics were classified into five categories used in the AOTA (1999) *Standards for Continuing Competence* that were most current at the time. The most recent revision of this official document (AOTA, 2015d) has essentially the same categories, which include:

1. Knowledge required for multiple roles
2. Critical reasoning necessary for decision-making in those roles
3. Interpersonal abilities to establish effective relationships with others
4. Performance skills and proficiencies necessary for practice
5. Ethical reasoning required for responsible decision-making

A sixth category—traits, qualities, and characteristics—was added based on the Delphi panel responses. The competencies and characteristics identified by the Delphi panel are listed in Box 1-1 (Holmes and Scaffa, 2009b).

In addition, the following attributes and skills are recommended for those contemplating practice in community settings:

- Comfort with indirect service provision
- Grant-writing skills
- Networking skills
- Organizational skills
- Professional autonomy
- Program-planning and evaluation skills
- Public relations skills

Paradigm Shifts in Occupational Therapy

A **paradigm** is a conceptual framework that allows the explanation and investigation of phenomena. Kuhn (1970) defined a paradigm as "universally recognized scientific achievements that for a time provide model problems and solutions to a community of practitioners" (p. viii). Paradigms have two essential characteristics. They are (a) sufficiently unprecedented scientific achievements that draw many constituents from competing areas of inquiry and (b) adequately open-ended enough to allow for the exploration of solutions to a variety of problems. A paradigm is a world view that characterizes a particular group or discipline that has common interests. It is a "consensus-determined matrix of the most fundamental beliefs or assumptions of a field" (Kielhofner, 1983, p. 6). A profession or discipline-specific paradigm determines:

- How professionals view their phenomenon of interest
- What puzzles, problems, or questions practitioners will seek out in their work
- What solutions will emerge
- What goals will be set for the direction of the profession

A paradigm is the "cultural core of the discipline" and "provides professional identity" (Kielhofner, 1997, p. 17).

Kuhn (1970) asserted that change within a discipline or profession does not occur gradually. Rather, it occurs very dramatically. When a discipline abandons one view of the world for another, it has undergone a revolution, a drastic conceptual restructuring, called a **paradigm shift.** Often, there is much resistance to paradigm shifts and to those initiating them. Paradigm shifts dramatically change the existing rules, create new trends, and trigger innovations. Paradigm shifts occur in four stages: preparadigm, paradigm, crisis, and return to paradigm.

Kielhofner conducted a historical examination of paradigm shifts in occupational therapy (see Fig. 1-2). According to Kielhofner (1983), the preparadigm stage in occupational therapy traces its roots to the moral treatment movement with its humanistic focus. Moral treatment proponents advocated that the treatment of persons with mental illness should emphasize a daily routine of occupations in a family-like atmosphere (Neidstadt and Crepeau, 1998). Participation in occupations was believed to normalize disorganized habits and behaviors (Kielhofner, 1997). During the 18th and 19th centuries, the moral treatment philosophy was

Box 1-1 Competencies and Characteristics Needed for Emerging Practice Areas

Listed in order of importance ratings

Knowledge Competencies*

Occupation-based practice for evaluation and intervention
Philosophy of occupational therapy
Occupational therapy models and frames of reference applied to intervention
Principles of client-centered practice
Occupational therapy practice framework: domain and process
Core values of occupational therapy
Program development
Potential occupational therapy role and contribution in the practice area
Community systems
Public health principles and practice models

Performance Skills Competencies

Envision occupational therapy roles and service possibilities
Implement client-centered practices
Assess, evaluate, and provide intervention for occupational issues
Work collaboratively with others
Identify and access available resources
Search, analyze, and synthesize evidence-based research for emerging practice
Seek opportunities to demonstrate and use skills to meet clients' needs
Select, administer, and interpret evaluation results for a variety of practice areas
Conduct comprehensive task and activity analyses
Provide consultation to groups and individuals

Critical Reasoning Competencies*

Reason holistically
Translate theory into practice
Solve problems
Use clinical reasoning for client services
Think outside the box
Use good judgment—know when to seek assistance
Think abstractly
Complete a SWOT analysis

Ethical Reasoning Competencies*

Self-assessment of strengths and needs for ongoing professional development
Principles of social justice
Principles of occupational justice

Interpersonal Abilities Competencies*

Listen actively
Communicate occupational therapy concepts to a variety of audiences
Establish relationships with stakeholders and community leaders
Network effectively with other professionals
Demonstrate cultural competence
Establish and maintain relationships with professionals
Seek mentors within and outside of the occupational therapy profession
Understand and use language and terms of other professions
Negotiate effectively
Ask for feedback, advice, and assistance from colleagues and friends

Traits, Qualities, and Characteristics

Self-starter, self-directed
Adaptable to new situations
Able to step outside of the medical model
Self-confident
Persevering, determined, and persistent
Flexible
Tolerant of ambiguity
An independent worker
Creative
Able to challenge the status quo

Category headings* from "Standards for Continuing Competence," by the American Occupational Therapy Association, 1999, *American Journal of Occupational Therapy, 53,* 559–560.
Data from "An Exploratory Study of Competencies for Emerging Practice in Occupational Therapy," by W. H. Holmes and M. E. Scaffa, 2009, *Journal of Allied Health, 38*(2), 81–90.

competing with a pathology-oriented approach in the treatment of the mentally ill.

During the first four decades of the 20th century, a remarkable degree of consensus emerged among practitioners and in the literature regarding "occupation" as the central phenomenon of interest. Although the paradigm of occupation originated in the mental health arena, it was easily applicable to physical disabilities. Occupation referred to the balance of work, play, self-care, and rest. Occupational

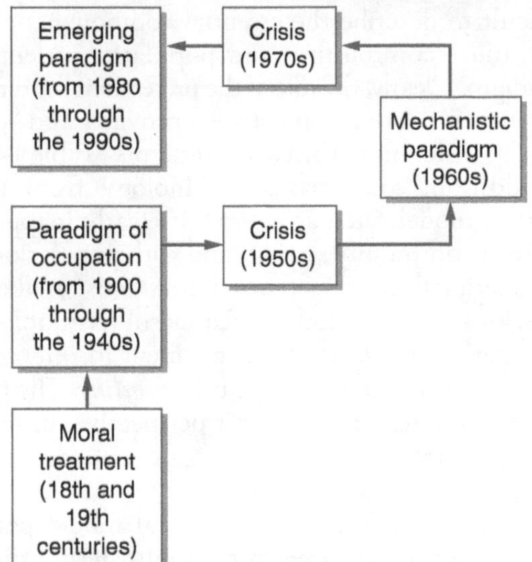

Figure 1-2 Paradigm shifts in occupational therapy. *(From* Conceptual Foundations of Occupational Therapy *[2nd ed., p. 48], by G. Kielhofner, 1997, Philadelphia, PA: F. A. Davis. Used with permission.)*

therapists of the time viewed the individual holistically, comprising both mind and body, participating in daily tasks in interactions with different environments. Occupations were graded according to the individual's capabilities. Persons progressed from simple activities that stimulated the senses to more demanding occupations requiring concentration and skill (Kielhofner, 1997).

The first paradigm crisis is evident in the professional literature of the late 1940s and early 1950s, when increasing pressure from medicine to be more scientific led to the questioning of the paradigm of occupation. The literature began to favor kinesiological, neurophysiological, and psychoanalytic approaches to occupational therapy practice. The Great Depression of the 1930s caused much job insecurity, compelling occupational therapy to develop a closer relationship with medicine. The American Medical Association began accrediting occupational therapy educational programs. Occupational therapy practice began to align itself more closely with the medical model and adopted the medical paradigm of reductionism with few modifications (Kielhofner, 1983).

The reductionist, or mechanistic, paradigm of the 1960s asserted that by focusing on the inner mechanisms of disease and disability (i.e., neurophysiology, anatomy, kinesiology, and psychoanalysis), occupational therapy could actually alter function and thereby gain professional respect as a scientific discipline. The early paradigm of occupation had a holistic appreciation of the occupational nature of human life. The new paradigm provided a more in-depth view and shifted professional thinking from the gestalt to a reductionist focus on parts. The medical model, or reductionist paradigm, was not simply added to the paradigm of occupation; the former replaced the latter, and as a result, the focus of occupational therapy practice changed dramatically in the 1960s and 1970s. Practitioners dropped "occupations" from therapy in favor of exercise, talk groups, specialized treatment techniques, and modalities (Kielhofner, 1983).

The reductionist, or mechanistic, paradigm was not, and is not, altogether negative. New assistive devices and technology, new techniques (e.g., sensory integration and neurodevelopmental treatment), and greater respect from the medical community emerged from this approach. The major loss was the profession's commitment to the occupational nature of human beings and the importance of occupation as a therapeutic medium. Without this common theme of early practice, the specialty areas within the field began to drift apart, leading to a second paradigm crisis.

This second paradigm crisis, which occurred in the 1970s, was precipitated by the recognition that reductionism was an inadequate framework for understanding the complexities of human occupational behavior. Awareness grew that the problems of the chronically disabled could not be solved by technology alone. In addition, occupational therapists expressed dissatisfaction over a loss of professional identity, a fragmented ideology, and a lack of professional unity (Kielhofner, 1983, 1997).

According to Kielhofner (2004), a new paradigm has emerged that recommits itself to the core construct of occupation and attempts to regain the profession's identity and holistic orientation. This paradigm is characterized by a synthesis of useful concepts from the mechanistic paradigm with contemporary knowledge of occupation from many disciplines. In addition, the new paradigm utilizes a systems perspective. An underlying assumption of "systems theory is that no system (e.g., cell, person, or organization) can be fully explained by examining the component parts of which it is made" (Kielhofner, 2004, p. 66). A systems viewpoint emphasizes that occupational performance results from the dynamic interaction between the person, the environmental context, and the occupations in which the person engages. In addition, it allows for a more complex perspective on factors that have an impact on occupational performance and therefore offers a broader range of potential solutions to occupational performance problems. The purpose of occupational therapy in this perspective is to provide "opportunities and environmental resources that support the emergence of new patterns of performance and participation in everyday life" (Kielhofner, 2004, p. 66).

Engage Your Brain 1-3

How might occupational therapy theories and models be affected by paradigm shifts?

Community and Population Health Practice Paradigm

CPHP is more than just a decentralization of services through outreach into the community and across communities, states, and nations. It includes a focus on community and population health in addition to individual health. Functioning effectively in the community and with populations requires a range of new roles for the practitioner and a unique set of knowledge, skills, and attitudes (Wiemer and West, 1970). A key difference between the model of community health espoused by Wiemer and West (1970) and the model currently being proposed is that Wiemer and West suggested community health was merely an extension of the medical model into community-based settings. The current belief is that community health requires a paradigm different from that of the medical model—that is, a reductionist perspective, a shift to a new way of thinking. This new paradigm is, however, consistent with the early foundations of occupational therapy and represents a return to the early principles of the profession.

Though it is easy to critique the limitations of medical models of health-care delivery, it is far more difficult to describe the essential components of a new, more community- and population-oriented paradigm. Clearly, the role of the professional and the therapeutic relationship between provider and "patient" is different in the two paradigms (Table 1-2). In addition, some basic terminology from the medical model, such as *patient,* is clearly inappropriate in community settings and with populations. Occupational therapy practitioners must make a conscious effort to modify their use of terminology from patient to *client,* from treatment to *intervention,* and from reimbursement to *funding.* The use of medical language can limit perspective, unnecessarily narrow professional focus, and decrease the ability to perceive options.

In the transition from a medical model paradigm, professionals need to relinquish responsibility, power, and control to the recipient of services: client, community member, or population. Clients are the experts regarding their situation, needs, and desires. Therefore, the client makes the decisions regarding the services utilized. For community or population health practice to be successful, planning must be coordinated with and through a variety of agencies, organizations, and individuals in the community or population. The impact of culture must also be recognized, appreciated, and incorporated into service delivery. Ultimately, the professional reports to the client, who is both the recipient and evaluator of the services provided.

Table 1-2 Contrasting Paradigms

Medical Model	Community Model
Professional is responsible	Community member is responsible
Professional has power	Community member has power
Professional makes decisions	Community member makes decisions
Professional is the "expert"	Community member is the "expert"
Professional answers to the agency	Professional answers to the consumer
Planning is fragmented	Planning is coordinated
Culture is denied	Culture is appreciated

Health professionals function as facilitators whose role is to build and reinforce capacity and develop leadership in others. This requires humility, the ability to share successes with others, and patience. Successful practice in the community and with populations requires more time than in the typical clinical setting, as consensus must be developed and resources identified and obtained to support individuals and groups in maintaining a satisfying lifestyle in the community of their choice.

Evaluation of individuals in the community should include aspects of the domain of occupational therapy: "Occupations, client factors, performance skills, performance patterns, and context and environment" (AOTA, 2014, p. S4). Client factors are often the primary focus in the medical model. In CPHP, the areas of occupation including activities of daily living, instrumental activities of daily living, rest/sleep, work, education, play/leisure, social participation, and contexts/environment take on much more significance. If the focus of intervention is not the individual but rather a collection of individuals—for example, a family, a community, or some subpopulation of a community, such as members of a senior center—then the evaluation process must be much broader in scope. Evaluation in community settings, often referred to as needs assessment, requires attention to the population to be served and the context in which the services will be delivered (Box 1-2). Intervention planning utilizes the information generated from the comprehensive needs assessment, and potential programs of services are identified with input from the intended service recipients and community organizations. Community institutions, such as schools, churches, mosques, temples, social organizations, health-care providers, and political entities, are all part of the context of service and therefore are integral components of evaluation and intervention. The process of program development is described in detail in Chapters 5 and 6 and program evaluation in Chapter 7.

Box 1-2 Assessment of Population and Context

- **I.** Assessment of the population:
  - **A.** General demographics (age, gender, diagnoses, etc.)
  - **B.** Current and anticipated living and working environments and role expectations
  - **C.** Current performance in areas of activities of daily living, instrumental activities of daily living, work, education, sleep/rest, play/leisure, and social participation
  - **D.** General performance component assets and deficits
  - **E.** Significance of these factors with respect to community members' goals and needs
- **II.** Assessment of the context:
  - **A.** General characteristics of the agency/program (mission, goals, etc.)
  - **B.** Characteristics of the physical environment
  - **C.** Characteristics of the social environment/milieu (norms, emotional and cultural climate, etc.)
  - **D.** Availability of resources (space, materials, staff, etc.)
  - **E.** Significance of these factors with respect to community members' goals and needs

Characteristics of a Community and Population Health Practice Paradigm

A well-developed CPHP paradigm can enhance the likelihood of achieving *Vision 2025*. The following are some preliminary suggestions on the nature of a CPHP paradigm. The emerging paradigm has the following characteristics:

- Client-centered
- Occupation-based
- Supported with evidence
- Based on dynamic systems theory
- Ecologically sound
- Strengths-based

Client-Centered

A CPHP paradigm requires a **client-centered approach** that "promotes participation, exchange of information, client decision-making, and respect for choice" and "focuses on the issues which are most important to the person and his or her family" (Law, 1998, preface). The collaborative process is designed to enable the client to identify occupational performance problems, engage in problem-solving, and propose solutions that meet his or her unique individual needs and circumstances. The occupational therapist is a facilitator, educator, and mentor in the process (Law, 1998). A client-centered model has three key elements:

- It considers the values, goals, roles, activities, and tasks of the person, group, or community.
- It involves the client as an active participant in the entire process of needs assessment, intervention planning, implementation, and evaluation.
- It establishes a partnership between the client and practitioner that enables the client to assume responsibility for the process and the outcome of services (Baum, Bass-Haugen, and Christiansen, 2005).

A client in the CPHP paradigm may be an individual, a family, a group, an organization, a community, or a population (AOTA, 2014). Regardless of the type of client identified, the principles of client-centered practice are still relevant.

Occupation-Based

A CPHP paradigm in occupational therapy should be occupation-based. The focus on occupation is what makes the profession's contribution to health and well-being unique and valuable. Occupation-based refers to using the client's engagement in occupation as a means of both evaluation and intervention. Occupational performance is evaluated through observation. Intervention utilizes occupational engagement as the therapeutic agent. In this way, occupational performance and participation are contextualized in their transactions with real-world environments. In addition to the objective aspects of occupational performance in context, the client's subjective experience (i.e., feelings of pleasure, productivity, and restoration) is also important (Fisher, 2014).

Supported With Evidence

Demonstrating the effectiveness and efficiency of occupational therapy services through research enhances the profession's credibility. Scientific evidence provides data for decision-making regarding the importance and changeability of risk factors and the appropriateness of specific interventions. Evidence-based decision-making is the "process of coming to a conclusion or making a judgment that combines clinical expertise, patient concerns, and evidence gathered from scientific literature to arrive at best practice recommendations" (Abreu and Chang, 2011, p. 331). According to Holm (2000), evidence-based practitioners:

- Examine what they do by asking questions
- Take the time to find the best evidence to guide their practice
- Appraise the evidence carefully
- Use the evidence to "do the right things right"
- Evaluate the impact of their evidence-based practices

Based on Dynamic Systems Theory

Communities function as systems; therefore, a dynamic systems perspective is extremely useful in conceptualizing community practice. According to Capra (1982, p. 43), systems theory "looks at the world in terms of the inter-relatedness and interdependence of all phenomenon, and in this framework an integrated whole whose properties cannot be reduced to those of its parts is called a system." Dynamic systems are characterized by complete interconnectedness. This means that all variables are interrelated and that a change in one variable affects all other variables that are part of the system. In addition, dynamic systems are nested; every system is part of another larger system, with the same dynamic principles operating at each level. Subsystems settle into preferred, although not predictable, patterns called attractor states. Attractor states are temporary, with various strengths. The development of dynamic systems is in part dependent on initial states. Minor differences in the beginning can become huge effects with dramatic consequences in the long term. Dynamic systems are constantly developing and changing through interactions with their environment and through internal reorganization (De Bot, Lowie, and Verspoor, 2007). Relationships among variables in dynamic systems are governed by heterarchy. Heterarchy refers to "the relation of elements to one another when they are unranked, or when they possess the potential for being ranked in a number of different ways, depending on systemic requirements" (Crumley, 2005, p. 39). Throughout history,

> *people have organized themselves into families, institutions, communities, and societies to exercise*

more control over the environment and over the behavior of each other. Rules of behavior become community norms that are transmitted from one generation to another as culture. Culture defines acceptable social organization (family interaction patterns, roles and responsibilities of institutions and leaders, and the functions of government) as well as individual behavior. The influence of all these cultural, economic, organizational, and institutional forces on the environment, on individual behavior, and on health may be referred to as the social history of health. (Green and Anderson, 1982, p. 22)

A **dynamic systems approach** recognizes the complexity of the social history of health and provides a framework for assessment and intervention at various levels of systems, including individual, interpersonal, organizational, community, and public policy levels. The focus of intervention in community practice might be the individual recipient of service. However, just as frequently, if not more frequently, the focus of intervention is the family or the community as a whole. Individuals are embedded in a number of systems that must be addressed even when the focus of intervention is at the individual level. For example, an individual's level of self-fulfillment and independence in the community may well be more a function of environmental, institutional, and social barriers than the individual's disability itself. Therefore, intervention may focus on several levels of systems simultaneously. According to dynamic systems theory, if one component of a system changes, "a chain reaction of adaptations and adjustments is created in other parts of the system" (Scaffa and Brownson, 2005, p. 482). Interventions to improve health and well-being are most effective when multiple components of a dynamic system are targeted. This creates a synergistic effect that resonates throughout all aspects of a community or population.

Ecologically Sound

An **ecological approach** considers the client embedded in and interacting with a variety of environments and contexts. This perspective requires the occupational therapy practitioner to consider both the client's capabilities and constraints and the environmental enablers and barriers. Client capabilities may include psychological, physiological, cognitive, neurobehavioral, and spiritual assets. Environmental enablers may include cultural and social, policy, socioeconomic, and built and natural environmental resources (Baum et al., 2005). Client constraints may include poor health status, occupational risk factors, and occupational performance limitations. Environmental barriers may include poverty, lack of natural and built environmental resources, economic recession, high unemployment rates, inadequate public transportation, and lack of access to social and occupational participation. Recognizing the interdependence between the client and the social and physical environment is critical to effective community practice.

Strengths-Based

Finally, a CPHP paradigm for occupational therapy is **strengths-based,** meaning that the focus is on what clients can do—their assets, talents, resources, and capabilities—and not simply the clients' deficits or functional limitations. A strength is the ability to consistently perform in a high-quality manner in a particular activity. A talent is a naturally occurring pattern of thought, feeling, or behavior that can be used productively. A strengths-based approach to intervention assesses the client's inherent strengths and talents and then incorporates these into the intervention process to facilitate occupational engagement and empowerment. A strengths-based model avoids the use of stigmatizing labels; reduces the sense of victimization; and fosters hope, growth, and self-efficacy. The development of strengths can be conceptualized as a three-step process:

1. Identifying strengths and talents
2. Incorporating these strengths and talents into the client's view of self
3. Changing behavior

Behavior change may include acquiring knowledge to enhance strengths and talents, sharing one's talents with others, and creating and implementing strategies to maximize one's strengths and utilize them more consistently. A focus on the development of strengths increases life satisfaction and productivity (Hodges and Clifton, 2004).

The basic underlying tenets of the emerging CPHP paradigm can be summarized as follows:

- Occupational therapy is best provided "in vivo" where people play, work, go to school, participate in social interactions, and engage in activities of daily living (Scaffa, 2001).
- Participation in occupations that structure everyday life promotes health and well-being and enhances quality of life (AOTA, 2014).
- Occupational risk factors—for example, occupational deprivation, occupational alienation, and occupational imbalance—predispose individuals, families, groups, communities, and populations to illness, disability, and dysfunction (AOTA, 2013; Wilcock, 2006).
- The physical, social, cultural, personal, temporal, and virtual environments influence occupational choice, priorities, and organization, as well as quality and satisfaction with occupational performance (AOTA, 2014).
- Habits, routines, roles, and rituals are performance patterns that have an impact on occupational participation (AOTA, 2014).
- Engagement in occupation contributes to occupational identity and self-efficacy (AOTA, 2014).
- People have the right to fully participate in their communities and engage in occupations of their choice that provide purpose and meaning in their lives (AOTA, 2014).
- Health and health behaviors are influenced by a variety of factors: personal, social, economic, and ecological (USDHHS, 2019).
- Social isolation, low educational attainment, poverty, violence, pollution, crime, and discrimination are all threats to individual and community health and well-being (USDHHS, 2019).
- The reduction of occupational risk factors and the enhancement of occupational resilience factors can improve the health and well-being of individuals, families, and communities (Scaffa and Brownson, 2005).

The occupational therapy profession must reinterpret and expand its knowledge base to support community and population health initiatives as well as think creatively and develop new models of practice appropriate for community-based settings. As occupational therapy services in the community increase and as practitioners become more comfortable with indirect service provision and designing interventions for populations, the paradigm of CPHP will evolve.

Looking Ahead

Over 35 years ago, Dasler (1984) stated that occupational therapists, regardless of their area of practice, should focus their attention on creating and filling more positions in community-based settings. She believed that practitioners should adapt their roles and skills to fit with the community environment outside of the medical setting. Dasler (1984) referred to this as the "deinstitutionalization of the occupational therapist" (p. 31). Fidler (2000) echoed this sentiment when she stated, "As a profession, our single focus on and identity as a therapy, as a remedial rehabilitation service, has, I believe, significantly hampered our development. This narrow identity has, over many years, hindered our discovery and validation of the rich and broad dimensions of occupation" (p. 99).

For the future, Fidler (2000) envisioned an "occupationalist" who, in addition to rehabilitation services, provides health promotion services and programs of prevention, lifestyle counseling, and learning enhancement and participates in organizational, institutional, and community planning and design. If occupational therapy practitioners continue to resist the move into community-based settings, where their services are most needed, in favor of hospital and clinic environments, then the future of the profession will surely be unnecessarily limited.

In 1972, Finn suggested a number of issues that need to be addressed as the profession moves from an emphasis on medical and clinical services to community and population health services. An updated interpretation of these issues follows. Occupational therapy practitioners need to:

- Gain knowledge about community organizations and institutions and how they operate
- Acquire a thorough understanding of the unique services they can offer in community

settings and be able to communicate these services clearly
- Develop strategies to translate knowledge into actual programs that are responsive to community needs
- Prepare to take risks when faced with challenges in unfamiliar environments
- Learn to relate to and communicate effectively with nonmedical personnel and avoid the use of professional jargon
- Offer services to a community rather than waiting for services to be solicited
- Develop the role of health agent while maintaining professional identity and appreciate the opportunities for personal and professional growth in the experience

Occupational therapy philosophy and services are very compatible with community and population health service provision. However, the paradigm of direct service provision to individuals in clinical settings is inadequate for these emerging areas of practice in the community. The old paradigms are insufficient for identifying relevant issues and solving the problems associated with community and population practice. Learning from other disciplines, which have had a community or population focus for all or most of their existence (e.g., sociology, social psychology, public health, and community health education), can be a powerful tool in facilitating occupational therapy's expansion into the community.

Now is the time for occupational therapy practitioners to move ahead with confidence. If the profession fails to assume the dynamic, new roles emerging in the community, other professions will surely replace it. All occupational therapy practitioners, educators, and students are critical links in this monumental paradigm shift in the profession. With vision and creativity, the profession's potential contribution to communities, populations, and society is limitless.

Summary

- While few occupational therapy practitioners are currently engaged in either community-based or population health service delivery, at the profession's inception, this area was the core of practice.
- Community-based practitioners may fulfill a variety of roles, including consultant, program planner, manager, evaluator, staff supervisor and trainer, community health advocate, case manager, entrepreneur, and primary care provider.
- In addition to the basic competencies required of all occupational therapy practitioners, supplementary attributes and skills are recommended for those contemplating CPHP. These include but are not limited to comfort with indirect service provision, grant-writing skills, networking skills, professional confidence and autonomy, public relations skills, and program-planning and evaluation skills.
- There have been a number of paradigm shifts in the profession of occupational therapy, from the original paradigm focused on occupation to the reductionist paradigm of medicine, to the current paradigm that synthesizes the two. As more practitioners move into CPHP, a new paradigm is needed.
- It is suggested that this new CPHP paradigm be client-centered, occupation-based, supported with evidence, founded on dynamic systems theory, ecologically sound, and strengths-based.

Learning Activities

1. Review issues of *Occupational Therapy and Rehabilitation* or *American Journal of Occupational Therapy* from the 1930s to the 1950s for articles about community-based, occupation-based, or population health programs. Read at least three articles and determine whether there is still a need for that type of service delivery.
2. Interview an occupational therapist in community practice regarding the skills, abilities, and characteristics a person needs to be successful in providing community-based services. Assess your own readiness to practice in community settings. What do you need to learn to be able to make this transition?
3. In pairs or small groups, write a brief article for *OT Practice* describing the benefits for clients and practitioners of providing community-based

services and the barriers to developing occupation-based community programs.

4. Pay particular attention to your local news for a week and identify at least two community or population health problems that could be addressed by occupational therapy practitioners. Describe the populations and communities affected and the environmental and contextual characteristics that contribute to the health problems. Who would you contact in order to investigate volunteer or paid employment opportunities to help solve one or both of the health problems?

REFERENCES

Abreu, B. C., and Chang, P-F. J. (2011). Evidence-based practice. In K. Jacobs and G. McCormack (Eds.), *The occupational therapy manager* (5th ed., pp. 331–347). Bethesda, MD: AOTA Press.

American Occupational Therapy Association. (1974). Task force on target populations: Report of the task force on target populations, report I. *American Journal of Occupational Therapy, 28,* 158–163.

American Occupational Therapy Association. (1999). Standards for continuing competence. *American Journal of Occupational Therapy, 53,* 559–560.

American Occupational Therapy Association. (2013). Occupational therapy in the promotion of health and well-being. *American Journal of Occupational Therapy, 67*(6 Suppl.), S47–S59. doi:10.5014/ajot.2013.67S47

American Occupational Therapy Association. (2014). Occupational therapy practice framework: Domain and process (3rd ed.). *American Journal of Occupational Therapy, 68*(Suppl. 1), S1–S48. doi:10.5014/ajot.2014.682006

American Occupational Therapy Association. (2015a). *2015 AOTA salary and workforce survey.* Bethesda, MD: AOTA Press.

American Occupational Therapy Association. (2015b). Guidelines for supervision, roles, and responsibilities during the delivery of occupational therapy services. *American Journal of Occupational Therapy, 63*(6), 797–803.

American Occupational Therapy Association. (2015c). Occupational therapy code of ethics (2015). *American Journal of Occupational Therapy, 69*(6 Suppl. 3), 6913410030. http://dx.doi.org/10.5014/ajot.2015.696S03

American Occupational Therapy Association. (2015d). Standards for continuing competence. *American Journal of Occupational Therapy, 69*(6 Suppl. 3), 1–3.

American Occupational Therapy Association. (2017). Vision 2025. *American Journal of Occupational Therapy, 71,* 7103420010. doi:10.5014/ajot.2017.713002

Banyai, A. L. (1938). Modern trends in the treatment of tuberculosis. *Occupational Therapy in Rehabilitation, 17,* 245–254.

Barker, J. A. (1992). *Future edge.* New York, NY: William Morrow.

Barton, I. (1968). Consolation house, fifty years ago. *American Journal of Occupational Therapy, 2*(4), 340–345.

Baum, C., Bass-Haugen, J., and Christiansen, C. (2005). Person-environment-occupation-performance: A model for planning interventions for individuals and organizations. In C. H. Christiansen, C. M. Baum, and J. Bass-Haugen, *Occupational therapy: Performance, participation and well-being* (pp. 373–385). Thorofare, NJ: SLACK.

Baum, M. C. (2006). Presidential address, 2006 centennial challenges, millennium opportunities. *American Journal of Occupational Therapy, 60*(6), 609–616.

Bockhoven, J. S. (1968). Challenge of the new clinical approaches. *American Journal of Occupational Therapy, 22,* 23–25.

Capra, F. (1982). *The turning point.* New York, NY: Bantam.

Carpenter, E. M. (1947). Considerations for prevention of blindness and conservation of vision. *American Journal of Occupational Therapy, 1*(6), 348–351.

Centers for Disease Control and Prevention. (2019). *Population Health Training in Place Program (PH-IPP).* Retrieved from www.cdc.gov/pophealthtraining/whatis.html

Christensen, E. (1991). *A proud heritage: The American Occupational Therapy Association at seventy-five.* Rockville, MD: American Occupational Therapy Association.

Crumley, C. L. (2005). Remember how to organize: Heterarchy across disciplines. In C. S. Beekman and W. W. Baden (Eds.), *Nonlinear models for archaeology and anthropology* (pp. 35–50). Burlington, VT: Ashgate.

Dasler, P. J. (1984). Deinstitutionalizing the occupational therapist. *Occupational Therapy in Health Care, 1*(1), 31–40.

De Bot, K., Lowie, W. and Verspoor, M. (2007). A dynamic systems theory approach to second language acquisition. *Bilingualism: Language and Cognition, 10*(1), 7–21.

Diaz, M. P. (1932). Organizing a preventorium for children. *Occupational Therapy and Rehabilitation, 11*(3), 199–201.

Dunton, W. R. (1954). History and development of occupational therapy. In H. S. Willard and C. S. Spackman (Eds.), *Principles of occupational therapy* (2nd ed., pp. 1–10). Philadelphia, PA: Lippincott.

Epstein, C. F., and Jaffe, E. G. (2003). Consultation: Collaborative interventions for change. In G. McCormack, E. G. Jaffe, and M. Goodman-Levy (Eds.), *The occupational therapy manager* (4th ed., pp. 259–286). Bethesda, MD: AOTA Press.

Fazio, L. (2008). *Developing occupation-entered programs for the community.* Upper Saddle River, NJ: Pearson-Prentice-Hill.

Fidler, G. S. (2000). Beyond the therapy model: Building our future. *American Journal of Occupational Therapy, 54*(1), 99–101.

Finn, G. L. (1972). The occupational therapist in prevention programs. *American Journal of Occupational Therapy, 26,* 59–66.

Fisher, A. G. (2014). Occupation-centred, occupation-based, occupation-focused: Same, same or different? *Scandinavian Journal of Occupational Therapy, 21,* 96–107.

Green, L. W., and Anderson, C. L. (1982). *Community health* (4th ed.). St. Louis, MO: Mosby.

Green, L. W., and Ottoson, J. M. (1999). *Community and population health* (8th ed.). Boston, MA: McGraw-Hill.

Green, L. W., and Raeburn, J. (1990). Contemporary developments in health promotion, definitions and challenges. In N. Bracht (Ed.), *Health promotion at the community level* (pp. 29–44). Newbury Park, CA: Sage.

Hodges, T. D., and Clifton, D. O. (2004). Strengths-based development in practice. In P. A. Linley and S. Joseph (Eds.), *Positive psychology in practice.* Hoboken, NJ: John Wiley and Sons.

Holm, M. B. (2000). Our mandate for the new millennium: Evidence-based practice. *American Journal of Occupational Therapy, 54*(6), 575–585.

Holmes, W. M., and Scaffa, M. E. (2009a). The nature of emerging practice in occupational therapy: A pilot study. *Occupational Therapy in Health Care, 23*(3), 189–206.

Holmes, W. M., and Scaffa, M. E. (2009b). An exploratory study of competencies for emerging practice in occupational therapy. *Journal of Allied Health, 38*(2), 81–90.

Kavasch, E. B., and Baar, K. (1999). *American Indian healing arts.* New York, NY: Bantam Books.

Kielhofner, G. (1983). *Health through occupation: Theory and practice in occupational therapy.* Philadelphia, PA: F. A. Davis.

Kielhofner, G. (1997). *Conceptual foundations of occupational therapy* (2nd ed.). Philadelphia, PA: F. A. Davis.

Kielhofner, G. (2004). *Conceptual foundations of occupational therapy* (3rd ed.). Philadelphia, PA: F. A. Davis.

Kindig, D., and Stoddart, G. (2003). What is population health? *American Journal of Public Health, 93*(3), 380–383.

Kneipmann, K. (1997). Prevention of disability and maintenance of health. In C. Christiansen and C. Baum (Eds.), *Occupational therapy: Enabling function and wellbeing* (pp. 531–555). Thorofare, NJ: SLACK.

Krieger, D. (2001, Winter). Something old, something new. *USC Trojan Family Magazine.* Retrieved from www.usc.edu/dept/pubrel/trojan_family/winter01/therapy/something.html

Kuhn, T. S. (1970). *The structure of scientific revolutions* (2nd ed.). Chicago, IL: University of Chicago Press.

Laukaran, V. H. (1977). Toward a model of occupational therapy for community health. *American Journal of Occupational Therapy, 31*(2), 71–74.

Law, M. (Ed.). (1998). *Client-centered occupational therapy.* Thorofare, NJ: SLACK.

Levin, H. L. (1937). Occupational and recreational therapy among the ancients. *Occupational Therapy and Rehabilitation, 17*(5), 311–316.

McDaniel, M. L. (1968). Occupational therapists before World War II (1917–40). In H. S. Lee and M. L. McDaniel (Eds.), *Army Medical Specialist Corps* (pp. 69–97). Washington, DC: Office of the Surgeon General, Department of the Army. Retrieved from http://history.amedd.army.mil/booksdocs/histories/ArmyMedicalSpecialistCorps/chapter4.htm

Neidstadt, M. E., and Crepeau, E. B. (1998). *Willard and Spackman's occupational therapy* (9th ed.). Philadelphia, PA: Lippincott.

Nisbit, R. (1972). *Quest for community.* New York, NY: Oxford.

O'Connell, M. (1988). *The gift of hospitality: Opening the doors of community life to people with disabilities.* Evanston, IL: Center for Urban Affairs and Policy Research, Northwestern University.

Peloquin, S. M. (1991). Looking back—occupational therapy: Individual and collective understandings of the founders, part 2. *American Journal of Occupational Therapy, 45,* 733–44.

Punwar, A. J. (1994). *Occupational therapy: Principles and practice* (2nd ed.). Baltimore, MD: Williams and Wilkins.

Quiroga, V. A. M. (1995). *Occupational therapy: The first 30 years—1900 to 1930.* Bethesda, MD: American Occupational Therapy Association.

Reed, K. L., and Sanderson, S. N. (1999). *Concepts of occupational therapy* (4th ed.). Philadelphia, PA: Lippincott.

Reilly, M. (1971). The modernization of occupational therapy. *American Journal of Occupational Therapy, 25,* 243–246.

Reitz, S. M. (1992). A historical review of occupational therapy's role in preventive health and wellness. *American Journal of Occupational Therapy, 46,* 50–55.

Reitz, S. M. (2010). Historical and philosophical perspectives in occupational therapy's role in health and promotion. In M. E. Scaffa, S. M. Reitz, and M. A. Pizzi (Eds.), *Occupational therapy in community-based practice settings* (pp. 1–21). Philadelphia, PA: F. A. Davis.

Robnett, R. (1997). Paradigms of community practice. *OT Practice, 2*(5), 30–35.

Sabonis-Chafee, B. (1989). *Occupational therapy: Introductory concepts.* St. Louis, MO: Mosby.

Scaffa, M. E. (2001). *Occupational therapy in community-based practice settings.* Philadelphia, PA: F. A. Davis.

Scaffa, M. E., and Brownson, C. (2005). Occupational therapy interventions: Community health approaches. In C. Christiansen and C. Baum (Eds.), *Occupational therapy: Performance, participation and well-being.* Thorofare, NJ: SLACK.

Scaffa, M. E., Doll, J., Estes, R., and Holmes, W. (2011). Managing programs in emerging practice areas. In K. Jacobs and G. McCormack (Eds.), *The occupational therapy manager* (5th ed., pp. 311–327). Bethesda, MD: AOTA Press.

Stalker, K., Jones, C., and Ritchie, P. (1996). All change? The role and tasks of community occupational therapists in Scotland. *British Journal of Occupational Therapy, 59*(3), 104–108.

United Service Organizations (2019). *About us: The organization.* Retrieved from www.uso.org/about

U.S. Department of Health and Human Services. (2019). *Social determinants of health.* Retrieved from www.healthypeople.gov/2020/topics-objectives/topic/social-determinants-of-health

Vaughn, L., and Sladyk, K. (2011). Entrepreneurship. In K. Jacobs and G. McCormack (Eds.), *The occupational therapy manager* (5th ed., pp. 167–178). Bethesda, MD: AOTA Press.

Warren, R., and Warren, D. (1979). *The neighborhood organizer's handbook.* Notre Dame, IN: University of Notre Dame.

West, W. A. (1967). The occupational therapist's changing responsibility to the community. *American Journal of Occupational Therapy, 21,* 312–316.

West, W. A. (1969). The growing importance of prevention. *American Journal of Occupational Therapy, 23,* 226–231.

Wiemer, R. B., and West, W. A. (1970). Occupational therapy in community health care. *American Journal of Occupational Therapy, 24,* 323–328.

Wilcock, A. A. (2006). *An occupational perspective of health.* Thorofare, NJ: SLACK.

Willard, H., and Cox, B. (1979). A profile of occupational therapy and occupational therapy practice [An interview of H. Willard by B. Cox]. In *Occupational therapy: 2001* (pp. 69–70). Rockville, MD: American Occupational Therapy Association.

World Health Organization. (1986). *Ottawa charter for health promotion.* Retrieved from http://euro.who.int/__data/assets/pdf_file/0004/129532/Ottawa_Charter.pdf

World Health Organization. Division of Health Promotion, Education, and Communication. (1998). *Health promotion glossary.* Geneva, Switzerland: World Health Organization. Retrieved from http://apps.who.int/iris/handle/10665/64546

Chapter 2

Community and Population Health Concepts

Marjorie E. Scaffa, PhD, OTR/L, FAOTA

The greatness of a community is most accurately measured by the compassionate actions of its members.

—Coretta Scott King

Learning Outcomes

This chapter is designed to enable the reader to:

2-1 Discuss the rationale for occupational therapy participation in community and population health practice.

2-2 Identify the social determinants of health in a community.

2-3 Describe the contributions occupational therapy can make to achieve the goals of *Healthy People 2020.*

2-4 Describe the basic constructs associated with community and population health, prevention, and health promotion.

2-5 Discuss occupational therapy's role within the context of health promotion, community health practice, and population health practice.

2-6 Describe the community-centered practice framework and its application to community and population health.

Key Terms

Client
Community health
Community health interventions
Determinants of health
Epidemiology
Health disparities
Health promotion
Incidence
Occupational justice
Population health
Prevalence
Prevention
Preventive occupation
Primary prevention
Public health
Resiliency factors
Risk factors
Secondary prevention
Social determinants of health
Tertiary prevention

Introduction

The profession's participation in community and population health efforts is affirmed in *Vision 2025* and in the *Occupational Therapy Framework: Domain and Process* (American Occupational Therapy Association [AOTA], 2014). *Vision 2025* states, "Occupational therapy maximizes health, well-being, and quality of life for all people, populations, and communities through effective solutions that facilitate participation in everyday living" (AOTA, 2018, p. 18). This new vision for the profession emphasizes the value of occupational therapy services for communities and populations. In addition, the *Framework* provides a broad definition of an occupational therapy **client** as a

> person or persons (including those involved in the care of a client), group (collective of individuals, e.g., families, workers, students, or *community* members), or *population* (collective of groups or individuals living in a similar locale—e.g., city, state, or country—or sharing the same or like concerns). (AOTA, 2014, p. S41; italics added)

In the *Framework,* health promotion and disability prevention are described as approaches to intervention. Health promotion, from an occupational therapy perspective, is an intervention approach that can be used for anyone, with or without a disability, and is "designed to provide enriched contextual and activity experiences that will enhance performance for all people in the natural contexts of life" (AOTA, 2014, p. S33). Disability prevention in the *Framework* is an intervention approach used with persons and populations at risk for occupational dysfunction and is "designed to prevent the occurrence or evolution of barriers to performance in context. Interventions may be directed at client, context, or activity variables" (AOTA, 2014, p. S33).

Additionally, health management and maintenance are identified within the domain of occupational therapy as instrumental activities of daily living. Health and wellness, participation, prevention, quality of life, and occupational justice are just a few of the outcomes that can result from the application of occupational therapy to community and population health needs (AOTA, 2014). **Occupational justice** refers to "access to and participation in the full range of meaningful and enriching occupations afforded to others, including opportunities for social inclusion and the resources to participate in occupations to satisfy personal, health, and societal needs" (AOTA, 2014, p. S43).

Engage Your Brain 2-1

Which principles from the AOTA (2015) *Occupational Therapy Code of Ethics (2015)* make occupational justice an ethical imperative for occupational therapy practitioners?

Although having a sound knowledge base in occupational therapy is likely, the reader may be less familiar with the areas of community and population health. This chapter presents the underlying constructs and principles of community and population health as a foundation for providing occupational therapy in this practice area. It begins with a discussion of key community and population health constructs such as health promotion, prevention, risk factors, and epidemiology. Following this are descriptions of roles that may be assumed by occupational therapy practitioners and strategies that may be implemented to improve the health of communities and populations. A perspective on global and national health provides background and a context for occupational therapy in community and population health practice.

A Global Perspective: World Health Organization

The World Health Organization (WHO) established the Commission on Social Determinants of Health (CSDH) in 2005 to develop strategies on reducing health inequities. Health inequities exist both within and between countries, with a 40-year life expectancy difference between the richest and poorest countries. The CSDH concluded that health inequities are not inevitable; they are due mainly to policy failures and inequities in daily living conditions, access to power, and participation in society. These differences are often due to inequities in the social determinants of health. **Social determinants of health** are the conditions into which a person is born (e.g., social, economic, and physical) that have an impact on health, functioning, and quality of life (U.S. Department of Health and Human Services [USDHHS], 2019a).

The CSDH proposed three overarching recommendations: (1) improve daily living conditions; (2) address the inequitable distribution of power, money, and other resources; and (3) measure the problem and evaluate outcomes of intervention (WHO, 2009). Nine key themes with implementation strategies were identified, including:

- Early child development
- Globalization

- Health systems
- Employment conditions
- Social exclusion
- Women and gender equity
- Urbanization
- Priority public health conditions
- Measurement and evidence

At the 2011 World Conference on Social Determinants of Health in Brazil, sponsored by the WHO, heads of governments and government representatives reaffirmed the belief that

> *health inequities within and between countries are politically, socially and economically unacceptable, as well as unfair and largely avoidable, and that the promotion of health equity is essential to sustainable development and to a better quality of life and well-being for all, which in turn can contribute to peace and security. (WHO, 2011, para. 4)*

The participants pledged to collectively take global action on the social determinants of health in order to create vibrant, inclusive, and healthy communities.

The WHO has released a five-year strategic plan—the *13th General Programme of Work 2019–2023.* The plan focuses on 10 identified threats to global health. These include, in no particular order:

- Air pollution and climate change
- Noncommunicable chronic diseases, such as diabetes, cancer, and heart disease
- Global influenza pandemics
- Fragile and vulnerable settings such those dealing with drought, famine, conflict, and population displacement
- Antimicrobial resistance
- Ebola and other high-threat pathogens
- Weak primary health-care systems
- Decreased public acceptance of vaccines
- Dengue fever
- HIV (WHO, 2019)

A National Perspective: Healthy People

In 1979, the Surgeon General's office, in the U.S. Department of Health, Education, and Welfare (now the USDHHS), published a document titled *Healthy People.* This document was designed to identify national health goals and discuss health promotion and disease prevention in the United States. The concept underlying *Healthy People* came from Canada's *LaLonde Report,* a document published in 1974 describing the health status of Canadians (LaLonde, 1974). The *Healthy People* document (U.S. Department of Health, Education, and Welfare, 1979) emphasized the importance of lifestyle changes in reducing morbidity and mortality rates. Five major health goals for the nation were identified and categorized according to life span—that is, one major goal was identified for each age group (i.e., infants, children, adolescents and young adults, adults, and older adults). Goals, several subgoals, and other problems experienced by each age group also were presented. Approximately every 10 years, *Healthy People,* the plan for the nation's health, is updated and revised based on accumulated health data. See Table 2-1 for a brief history and timeline of the *Healthy People* document.

Healthy People 2020 (*HP 2020*) has four goals:

- "Attain high-quality, longer lives free of preventable disease, disability, and premature death.
- Achieve health equity, eliminate disparities, and improve health of all groups.
- Create social and physical environments that promote good health for all.
- Promote quality of life, healthy development, and healthy behaviors across all life stages." (USDHHS, n.d.a., p. 1)

A major focus of *HP 2020* is to eliminate health disparities and achieve health equity. **Health disparities** are

> *a particular type of health difference that is closely linked with social, economic, and/or environmental disadvantage. Health disparities adversely affect groups of people who have systematically experienced greater obstacles to health based on their racial or ethnic group; religion; socioeconomic status; gender; age; mental health; cognitive, sensory, or physical disability; sexual orientation or gender identity; geographic location; or other characteristics historically linked to discrimination or exclusion. (USDHHS, 2011b, para. 6)*

Persons with disabilities are at particular risk for experiencing health disparities. The secondary

Table 2-1 *Healthy People* Timeline

Title	Date Released	Goal(s)	Description
Healthy People	1979	Reduce morbidity and mortality	Five major health goals categorized by age group
Healthy People 2000	1990	• Increase the span of healthy life • Reduce health disparities • Achieve access to preventive health services for all (USDHHS, 1990)	22 priority areas identified, increased emphasis on social and environmental factors, data collection system created to monitor progress
Healthy People 2010	2000	• Increase quality and years of healthy life • Eliminate health disparities (USDHHS, 2000)	467 objectives in 28 topic areas, increased emphasis on healthy communities, recognition that individual health is dependent to some degree on the physical and social environments that exist in the community, provided a framework for interdisciplinary collaboration in health promotion
Healthy People 2020	2010	• "Attain high-quality, longer lives free of preventable disease, disability, injury, and premature death. • Achieve health equity, eliminate disparities, and improve the health of all groups. • Create social and physical environments that promote good health for all. • Promote quality of life, healthy development, and healthy behaviors across all life stages" (USDHHS, 2011a, para. 5).	More than 1,200 objectives in 42 topic areas Added concept of determinants of health
Healthy People 2030	Currently under development	• "Attain healthy, thriving lives and well-being, free of preventable disease, disability, injury and premature death. • Eliminate health disparities, achieve health equity, and attain health literacy to improve the health and well-being of all. • Create social, physical, and economic environments that promote attaining full potential for health and well-being for all. • Promote healthy development, healthy behaviors and well-being across all life stages. • Engage leadership, key constituents, and the public across multiple sectors to take action and design policies that improve the health and well-being of all" (USDHHS, 2019b, para. 15).	

Box 2-1 Social Determinants of Health

Economic Stability
- Employment
- Food insecurity
- Housing instability
- Poverty

Education
- Language and literacy
- Early childhood education and development
- High school graduation
- Enrollment in higher education

Social and Community Context
- Civic participation
- Social cohesion
- Discrimination
- Incarceration

Health and Health Care
- Access to health care
- Access to primary care
- Health literacy

Neighborhood and Built Environment
- Access to healthy goods
- Crime and violence
- Environmental conditions
- Quality of housing

Social determinants of health in *Healthy People 2020,* by the U.S. Department of Health and Human Services, 2019.

conditions (e.g., obesity, anxiety, depression, unemployment, and social isolation) that contribute to health disparities are frequently preventable (Drum, Krahn, Culley, and Hammond, 2005). Achieving health equity will require a coordinated and concerted effort to address the complex social, economic, educational, and environmental factors that produce health disparities, as well as to increase access to health care.

In *HP 2020,* the range of factors that influence health status, or the **determinants of health,** fall into five broad categories: policy-making, social factors, health services, individual behavior, and biology and genetics. Individual and population health are influenced by the interrelationships among these factors. Interventions that target multiple determinants of health are likely to be more effective than programs that address single factors. Social factors, or social determinants of health, are organized into five key areas: economic stability, education, social and community context, health and health care, and neighborhood and built environment (USDHHS, 2019a). Each of these five areas have multiple components that are targets for intervention (see Box 2-1).

Engage Your Brain 2-2

Which of the social determinants of health might occupational therapy address, and what types of interventions might be developed?

The long-range goals, topic areas, and measures of progress included in *HP 2020* provide an action-oriented foundation for occupational therapy practitioners to consider in all phases of evaluation and intervention. There are 42 topic areas identified in the *HP 2020* document (see Box 2-2). These topical areas are sets of health objectives that have been grouped to bring attention and focus to the needs of certain populations or needs specific to each condition. Health objectives are assigned to particular federal agencies to develop, track, monitor, maintain, and periodically report to the public the status of each. A significant number of the health objectives for the nation outlined in *HP 2020* specifically address the needs of the population of persons with disabilities. Box 2-3 contains examples of these objectives, many of which are directly relevant for occupational therapy intervention.

Ultimately, the goal of *HP 2020* is to provide data and tools to enable practitioners and communities across the nation to easily integrate services and intervention efforts. In order to meet population health goals, a framework for implementation is included in *HP 2020: MAP-IT* (mobilize, assess, plan, implement, and track; USDHHS, 2010b). The *MAP-IT* guide, available online, includes information on conducting a community needs assessment, a brief overview of *Healthy People 2020,* and tools for assessing and tracking progress.

Healthy People 2030 (*HP 2030*) is currently under development. The mission of *HP 2030* is "to promote, strengthen, and evaluate the Nation's efforts to improve the health and well-being of all

Box 2-2 *Healthy People 2020* Focus Areas

Access to health services
Adolescent health
Arthritis, osteoporosis, and chronic back conditions
Blood disorders and blood safety
Cancer
Chronic kidney disease
Dementias, including Alzheimer's disease
Diabetes
Disability and disability health
Early and middle childhood
Educational and community-based programs
Environmental health
Family planning
Food safety
Genomics
Global health
Health-care-associated infections
Health communication and health information technology
Health-related quality of life and well-being
Hearing and other sensory or communication disorders
Heart disease and stroke
HIV
Immunization and infectious diseases
Injury and violence prevention
Lesbian, gay, bisexual, and transgender health
Maternal, infant, and child health
Medical product safety
Mental health and mental disorders
Nutrition and weight status
Occupational safety and health
Older adults
Oral health
Physical activity
Preparedness
Public health infrastructure
Respiratory diseases
Sexually transmitted diseases
Sleep health
Social determinants of health
Substance abuse
Tobacco use
Vision

Data from *Healthy People 2020,* by the U.S. Department of Health and Human Services, Office of Disease Prevention and Health Promotion, ODPHP Publication No. B0132, 2010.

people" (USDHHS, 2019b, para. 13). The overarching goals include the following:

- "Attain healthy, thriving lives and well-being, free of preventable disease, disability, injury and premature death.
- Eliminate health disparities, achieve health equity, and attain health literacy to improve the health and well-being of all.
- Create social, physical, and economic environments that promote attaining full potential for health and well-being for all.
- Promote healthy development, healthy behaviors and well-being across all life stages.
- Engage leadership, key constituents, and the public across multiple sectors to take action and design policies that improve the health and well-being of all." (USDHHS, 2019b, para. 15)

Clearly, *HP 2030* is a population health approach addressing the health of the nation.

Population Health

Confusion exists among the terms **population health, public health,** and **community health** as there is a lack of consensus on definitions in the literature. However, Kindig (n.d.) conceptualizes **public health** as "the critical functions of state and local health departments such as preventing epidemics [e.g., infectious disease outbreaks], containing environmental hazards [e.g., drinking water contamination], and encouraging healthy behaviors [e.g., smoking cessation]" (para. 1). Other public health functions may include workplace injury prevention and safety standards, provision of vaccinations, and policy advocacy, such as for seatbelt laws and nutritious school lunches. In other words, public health could be construed as a set of approaches used to improve the health of a population.

The U.S. Surgeon General oversees the national Public Health Service and an elite group of nearly 7,000 public health officers in the Commissioned Corps working throughout the federal government (USDHHS, n.d.b.). Public health departments are

Box 2-3 Selected Objectives Addressing the Needs of People With Disabilities

The overall goal in this focus area is to promote the health and well-being of people with disabilities. Objectives designed to address this goal include:

- DH-1: Include in the core of *Healthy People 2020* population data systems a standardized set of questions that identify "people with disabilities."
- DH-2: Increase the number of tribes, states, and the District of Columbia that have public health surveillance and health promotion programs for people with disabilities and caregivers.
- DH-3: Increase the proportion of U.S. master of public health (MPH) programs that offer graduate-level courses in disability and health.
- DH-4: Reduce the proportion of people with disabilities who report delays in receiving primary and periodic preventive care due to specific barriers.
- DH-7: Reduce the proportion of older adults with disabilities who use inappropriate medications.
- DH-8: Reduce the proportion of people with disabilities who report physical or program barriers to local health and wellness programs.
- DH-9: Reduce the proportion of people with disabilities who encounter barriers to participating in home, school, work, or community activities.
- DH-10: Reduce the proportion of people with disabilities who report barriers to obtaining the assistive devices, service animals, technology services, and accessible technologies they need.
- DH-11: Increase the proportion of newly constructed and retrofitted U.S. homes and residential buildings that have visitable features.
- DH-13: Increase the proportion of people with disabilities who participate in social, spiritual, recreational, community, and civic activities to the degree they wish.
- DH-14: Increase the proportion of children and youth with disabilities who spend at least 80% of their time in regular education programs.
- DH-16: Increase employment among people with disabilities.
- DH-17: Increase the proportion of adults with disabilities who report sufficient social and emotional support.
- DH-18: Reduce the proportion of people with disabilities who report serious psychological distress.
- DH-19: Reduce the proportion of people with disabilities who experience nonfatal, unintentional injuries that require medical care.
- DH-20: Increase the proportion of children with disabilities, birth through age 2 years, who receive early intervention services in home or community-based settings.

Data from *Healthy People 2020,* by the U.S. Department of Health and Human Services, Office of Disease Prevention and Health Promotion, ODPHP Publication No. B0132, 2010.

governmental agencies responsible for implementing these approaches in their states and local districts. Although public health is concerned with optimizing the health status of populations, its functions are subsumed under the larger construct of population health. Population health addresses broader determinants of health such as education, poverty, and health care, which are typically outside the scope of public health authority and responsibility (Kindig, n.d.).

For the purposes of this text, the editors define **population health** from an occupational therapy perspective, as a collaborative, interdisciplinary approach that includes advocacy; program development, implementation, and evaluation; and policy revision and development to maximize health equity and occupational justice in a population based on the social and health determinants and priorities of that population.

Epidemiology

The fundamental scientific basis of population and public health is **epidemiology,** the study of the distribution, frequencies, and determinants of disease, injury, and disability in human populations (MacMahon and Trichopoulos, 1996). Epidemiologists use health statistics, including measures of incidence and prevalence, to estimate disease, injury, and disability in a variety of population groups; analyze health trends; plan and evaluate population and public health initiatives; and make informed health policy decisions. **Incidence** refers to the number of new cases of disease, injury, or disability within a specified time frame, typically a year. **Prevalence** refers to the total number of cases of disease, injury, or disability in a community, city, state, or nation existing at one point in time (Pickett and Hanlon, 1990).

According to Pickett and Hanlon (1990), preventive interventions attempt to reduce the incidence rate of a disease or an injury, and early detection procedures and rapid treatments attempt to reduce the duration of illness. Either strategy would result in a decreased prevalence rate. Combining the two strategies of prevention and early detection is the most effective approach to reducing overall prevalence.

Population health practitioners are also very interested in risk factors, both modifiable and nonmodifiable, that compromise health. **Risk factors** are those precursors that increase an individual's or population's vulnerability to developing a disease or disability or sustaining an injury (Scaffa, 1998). Often when people hear or use the term *risk factor,* they are thinking of a physical condition that contributes to a disease. For example, diabetes, smoking, high cholesterol, hypertension, and obesity are risk factors that can contribute to cardiovascular disease. However, risk factors are not just physical, behavioral, or genetic. They can also be social, economic, political, and environmental. Some risk factors are considered *causal* because the health problem cannot occur in the absence of the risk factor. Other risk factors are considered *contributory* because they interact with other risk factors, leading to the development, exacerbation, or maintenance of disease, injury, or disability (Scaffa, 1998).

In addition to considering risk factors, population health practitioners attempt to increase resiliency or the protective factors that contribute to improved health and well-being. **Resiliency factors** are those precursors that appear to increase an individual's or population's resistance to developing a disease or disability or sustaining an injury (Scaffa, 1998). Resiliency factors may include the individual's genetic composition, personality, and health behavior patterns and social factors such as peer and family relationships and environmental and institutional supports for health. Population health interventions attempt to modify all types of risk factors and strengthen resiliency or protective factors to enhance the overall health and well-being of populations.

Community Health

Typically, when people use the terms *community* and *health,* they assume others define the words in the same manner. In reality, definitions can vary widely. To avoid misunderstandings, these two words are defined here for this discussion. Community refers to "noninstitutional aggregations of people linked together for common goals or other purposes" (Green and Raeburn, 1990, p. 41). Inherent is the idea that a community does not have to be composed of individuals within a particular geographical region. Communities may be "religious, professional, cultural, political, recreational, and a myriad of others based on groups of people with common bonds" (Rhynders and Scaffa, 2010, p. 209). Communities are dynamic entities that evolve with the changing characteristics of their members. **Community health** refers to the physical, emotional, social, and spiritual well-being of a group of people who are linked together in some way, possibly through geographical proximity or shared interests.

A community-based approach can be optimal when providing prevention and health-care services to individuals. Social support, the ability to reach many consumers, targeted interventions that meet specific community needs, active community involvement, community-driven priorities, and the potential for a systems approach in which problems can be addressed at multiple levels are included. A systems-oriented approach allows all involved to see the big picture and better understand relationships, connections, and dependencies. Because consequences and interactions are integral components, employing a systems view is helpful when trying to prioritize community needs and determine solutions to problems.

Community health interventions can be defined as "any combination of educational, social, and environmental supports for behavior conducive to health" (Green and Anderson, 1982, p. 3). Also, according to Green and Anderson (1982, pp. 3–4):

> *Educational interventions may be directed at high-risk individuals, families, or groups or at whole communities through mass media, schools, worksites, and organizations. Social interventions may include economic, political, legal, and organizational changes designed to support actions conducive to*

health. Environmental supports include the structure and distribution of physical, chemical, and biological resources, and facilities and substances required for people to protect their health. The health behavior of a community includes the actions of the people whose health is in question and the actions of community decision makers, professionals, peers, teachers, employers, parents and others who may influence health behaviors, resources or services in the community.

Engage Your Brain 2-3

What occupation-based theories are most appropriate for community health interventions and why?

Community health interventions can be described on a continuum from community-based to community-level to community-centered (Scaffa and Brownson, 2005). Community-based interventions are health services provided in community settings targeted at individuals and families in order to improve health and facilitate health behavior change. Community-level interventions seek to modify the norms and behaviors of a population and improve health through sociocultural, political, economic, and environmental changes. Community-centered interventions are population-based approaches that are initiated and driven by the community itself, using existing resources and seeking external support as needed. The goal of community health is that each member of the community experiences a level of well-being and vitality, enabling everyone to choose, participate in, and enjoy the activities of the community (Scaffa and Brownson, 2005). Health promotion and prevention strategies are used to enhance community and population health.

Health Promotion and Prevention

Health promotion is defined as any planned combination of educational, political, regulatory, environmental, and organizational supports for actions and conditions of living conducive to the health of individuals, families, communities, and populations (Green and Kreuter, 1991). More simply, it is "the process of enabling people to increase control over, and to improve, their health" (WHO, 1986, p. 1). Health promotion is concerned with creating the conditions necessary for health, including "peace, shelter, education, food, income, a stable ecosystem, sustainable resources, social justice, and equity" (Trentham and Cockburn, 2005, p. 441). Health promotion encompasses strategies affecting all societal levels, including individuals, groups, organizations, communities, and government policy-makers.

According to Wilcock (2006):

Following an occupation-focused health promotion approach to well-being embraces a belief that the potential range of what people can do, be, and strive to become is the primary concern and that health is a by-product. A varied and full occupational lifestyle will coincidentally maintain and improve health and well-being if it enables people to be creative and adventurous physically mentally and socially. (p. 315)

Health promotion, management, and maintenance require the implementation of strategies to prevent disease, disability, and injury in individuals and populations.

Prevention refers to "anticipatory action taken to reduce the possibility of an event or condition from occurring or developing, or to minimize the damage that may result from the event or condition if it does occur" (Pickett and Hanlon, 1990, p. 81). When applying the term to population health, prevention refers to reducing the likelihood of the occurrence of disease/disability or inhibiting its progression to achieve optimal health and enhance quality of life.

Levels of Prevention

Specifically, the three levels of prevention are primary, secondary, and tertiary. Each level focuses on preventing health problems at a particular point along the continuum of the illness/injury process.

Primary prevention focuses on healthy individuals who potentially could be at risk for a particular health problem. The goal is to prevent the health problem or injury from occurring by taking steps to maintain one's current healthy status and reduce susceptibility and exposure to health hazards. For example, an already healthy person could continue to eat nutritious foods in the proper quantities and exercise regularly. Doing so could potentially avert obesity, diabetes, or cardiovascular disease. Another primary prevention strategy is to always wear a seat belt while in a motor vehicle, possibly avoiding or reducing injury if a crash occurs.

Secondary prevention focuses on early detection and intervention in the case of disease, injury, or health hazards that have already occurred. The goal is to slow the progression and prevent complications, reinjury, recurrence, and/or disability. Arresting or reversing communicability is also a focus because early treatment of an infectious disease will limit exposure to others, and containment may prevent an outbreak. An example of secondary prevention is an individual with hypertension exercising and maintaining an optimal weight to achieve normal blood pressure readings and thus reduce the risk of myocardial infarction (MI) and cerebrovascular accident (CVA).

Tertiary prevention, the third level, refers to measures used in the advanced stages of disease to limit disability and other complications. Tertiary prevention is implemented when a person is already ill or impaired, and the initial damage has already occurred. The goal is to restore as much functionality as possible, rehabilitate the individual, and attempt to prevent further damage. This level of prevention is the most familiar to occupational therapy practitioners. For example, occupational therapy practitioners routinely teach joint protection techniques to individuals with rheumatoid arthritis to prevent deformity and to enhance their ability to complete desired occupations with less pain. Energy conservation techniques are taught to individuals with cardiac conditions to prevent overexertion during the performance of occupations.

Improving Community and Population Health Through Occupation

Wilcock (1998) defines health from an occupational perspective as

> *the absence of illness, but not necessarily disability; a balance of physical, mental and social wellbeing attained through socially valued and individually meaningful occupation; enhancement of capacities and opportunity to strive for individual potential; community cohesion and opportunity; and social integration, support and justice, all within and as part of a sustainable ecology. (p. 110)*

Seligman (2011) proposes that well-being is a state of flourishing that consists of five elements: positive emotion, engagement, positive relationships, meaning, and accomplishment. This perspective suggests that occupation is a fundamental process for achieving health and well-being by facilitating engagement, meaning, and accomplishment. According to Wilcock (2005), the "occupations that will have the most obvious effects on wellbeing are those that are socially sanctioned and valued and that enable people freedom to effectively use physical and mental capacities in combination with social activity" (p. 153).

One approach to improving the health of individuals, communities, and populations is to decrease occupational risk factors and increase occupational resiliency factors. Occupational risk factors may "result from or lead to the development of other risk factors, which in turn result in larger health and social problems" (AOTA, 2013, p. S50). Occupational risk factors to health can result from less than optimal use, choice, opportunity, or balance in occupation. Risk factors for occupational dysfunction and poor health include occupational imbalance, occupational deprivation, and occupational alienation (Wilcock, 1998), as well as occupational delay, occupational interruption, and occupational disparities (Bass-Haugen, Henderson, Larson, and Matuska, 2005). These risk factors are described in Box 2-4. Occupational resiliency factors that could be developed or enhanced include occupational adaptation, occupational coherence, occupational competence, occupational continuity, occupational identity, occupational orchestration, and occupational self-efficacy. These resiliency factors are described in Box 2-5.

Occupational therapy practice is based on the premise that participation in meaningful occupations can improve occupational performance and overall health and well-being. Therefore, **preventive occupation** can be characterized as the application of occupational science in the prevention of

Box 2-4 Occupational Risk Factors

- **Occupational alienation:** "Sense of isolation, powerlessness, frustration, loss of control, and estrangement from society or self as a result of engagement in occupation that does not satisfy inner needs" (Wilcock, 2006, p. 343). Tasks that are perceived as stressful, meaningless, or boring may result in an experience of occupational alienation.
- **Occupational delay:** Occupational development that does not follow the typical schedule for the acquisition of occupational skills and is associated with occupational performance deficits (Bass-Haugen, Henderson, Larson, and Matuska, 2005).
- **Occupational deprivation:** "Deprivation of occupational choice and diversity because of circumstances beyond the control of individuals or communities" (Wilcock, 2005, p. 343). Conditions that lead to occupational deprivation may include poor health, disability, lack of transportation, isolation, and homelessness.
- **Occupational disparities:** Inequalities or differences in occupational patterns among populations that are often the result of occupational injustice (Bass-Haugen et al., 2005).
- **Occupational imbalance:** "A lack of balance or disproportion of occupation resulting in decreased well-being" (Wilcock, 2006, p. 343). Occupational patterns that fail to meet an individual's physical and/or psychosocial needs, resulting in stress and a negative impact on health.
- **Occupational interruption:** A temporary interference with occupational performance or participation as a result of a change in personal, social, or environmental factors (Bass-Haugen et al., 2005).

Box 2-5 Occupational Resiliency Factors

- **Occupational adaptation:** The ability to adjust and respond to challenges and changes in circumstances that require modifications in occupational performance or participation (Schultz, 2014).
- **Occupational coherence:** Engagement in occupations that are integrated, consistent, and congruent with one's current and aspirational occupational roles.
- **Occupational continuity:** Engagement in valued and meaningful occupations that provide a continuous sense of occupational identity throughout one's life.
- **Occupational competence:** "The degree to which one is able to sustain a pattern of occupational participation that reflects one's occupational identity" (Schell, Gillen, and Scaffa, 2014, p. 1237).
- **Occupational identity:** A "composite sense of who one is and wishes to become as an occupational being generated from one's history of occupational participation" (Schell et al., 2014, p. 1238).
- **Occupational orchestration:** "The capacity of individuals to enact their occupations on a daily basis to meet their own needs and the expectations of the many environments in which they are required to function" (Schell et al., 2014, p. 1238).
- **Occupational self-efficacy:** The belief in one's capacity to perform occupations to meet one's own needs and the demands of the environment.

disease and disability and the promotion of health and well-being of individuals and communities through meaningful engagement in occupations. An excellent example of the power of preventive occupation was demonstrated in a comprehensive research project, commonly referred to as the Well Elderly Study, conducted at the University of Southern California (Clark et al., 1997). This randomized, controlled trial, involving 361 men and women aged 60 years or older living independently in the community, was designed to evaluate the effectiveness of a preventive occupational therapy program. The main outcome measures of interest were "physical and social function, self-rated health, life satisfaction and depressive symptoms" (Clark et al., 1997, p. 1321). Older adults receiving occupational therapy services demonstrated improved vitality, physical and social functioning, life satisfaction, and general mental health. A 6-month follow-up assessment indicated that 90% of the therapeutic gains had been maintained (Clark et al., 2001). A replication of this study with a more diverse population found that occupational therapy was a cost-effective approach to enhance the health and well-being of older adults (Clark et al., 2012).

Role of Occupational Therapy in Community and Population Health

The AOTA (2013) supports and promotes the involvement of occupational therapy professionals in the design and implementation of health promotion and prevention services. Health promotion services may address the needs of individuals, families, groups, organizations, communities, and populations. The goals of occupational therapy in health promotion and prevention are to:

- Prevent or reduce the incidence of illness or disease, accidents, injuries, and disabilities in the population
- Reduce health disparities among racial and ethnic minorities and other underserved populations
- Enhance mental health, resiliency, and quality of life
- Prevent secondary conditions and improve the overall health and well-being of people with chronic conditions or disabilities and their caregivers
- Promote healthy living practices, social participation, occupational justice, and healthy communities, with respect for cross-cultural issues and concerns (AOTA, 2013, S48)

Occupational therapy practitioners may assume any combination of three major roles in community and population health, health promotion, and disease/disability prevention. The first role is to promote healthy lifestyles for all clients, their families, communities, and populations. Lifestyle risk factors, such as tobacco use, unhealthy diet, physical inactivity, and substance abuse, are important to address in all encounters with clients. However, these lifestyle concerns are often overlooked for persons with disabilities. Standard health promotion programs and services may be inappropriate for persons with disabilities. Occupational therapy practitioners are capable of adapting these programs to meet the special needs of individuals living with disabling conditions and their caregivers.

The second role is to infuse occupation into existing health promotion efforts developed by experts in areas such as health education, nutrition, and exercise. For example, when working with a person with a lower-extremity amputation due to diabetes, the occupational therapy practitioner may focus on the occupation of meal preparation using foods and preparation methods recommended in the nutritionist's health promotion program. This enables the achievement of the goal of functional independence in the kitchen while reinforcing the importance of proper nutrition for the prevention of further disability.

The third role is to develop and implement occupation-based community and population health promotion interventions, targeting a variety of constituencies, including individuals (both with and without disabilities), groups, organizations, communities, populations, and governmental policies. A variety of examples of occupation-focused health promotion interventions are listed in Box 2-6.

Philosophically, occupational therapy and community and population health are quite compatible and even complementary. Occupational therapy practitioners can learn much from collaboration with public health, health promotion, and health education professionals in terms of primary and secondary prevention strategies and community and population health initiatives. In addition, population health programs and public health initiatives can benefit from the unique occupational science perspective that occupational therapy practitioners can provide.

Changes in demographics, including the rapid growth in the number of elderly who are at risk for injuries, illnesses, and disabilities, provide an opportunity for occupational therapy practitioners to expand their role in health promotion and disease/disability prevention. As in all areas of practice, community and population health promotion interventions should be based on the best available evidence. Funding for community and population health programs "can come from governmental agencies, foundations, nonprofit organizations, insurance companies, and large corporations" (AOTA, 2013, p. S52), as well as fees-for-service. Most community and population health programs rely on multiple sources of funding.

Although occupational therapy practitioners have the basic competencies to design and implement occupation-based health promotion interventions,

Box 2-6 Examples of Occupation-Based Community and Population Health Interventions

Organizational-level interventions
- Consultation with industrial managers regarding the benefits of ergonomic workspace design and worksite injury prevention strategies
- Disability awareness training for service industry personnel, such as those who work for airlines, hotels, restaurants, etc.

Community-level interventions
- Modification of community recreational facilities to increase accessibility for persons with disabilities
- Staff and volunteer training for special-needs shelters during disasters

Population-level interventions
- Implementation of a depression-screening program for new mothers for the purpose of developing prevention and early intervention programs
- Development and implementation of chronic disease self-management programs addressing obesity, diabetes, and other chronic health conditions to reduce health disparities within local public health clinics

Governmental policy interventions
- Promotion of barrier-free, universal design environments to enable full community participation for persons of all ages and abilities
- Lobbying for public funds to support community-based mental health programs for veterans

continuing education to acquire specialized knowledge and skills is required for this practice area (Scaffa, Van Slyke, and Brownson, 2008). Providing community-centered occupational therapy services is a challenge, and occupation-based models to guide the development and implementation of interventions are lacking. Hyett, Kenny, and Dickson-Swift (2018) have proposed a conceptual framework to address this void.

A Community-Centered Practice Framework

According to Hyett et al. (2018), community-centered occupational therapy practice facilitates the achievement of the community's occupational goals and enables community participation. Community engagement is both a process and an outcome of occupation-based, community-centered practice.

The community-centered practice framework (CCPF) was developed based on principles derived from qualitative multicase research. The CCPF consists of four components, or phases: community identity, community occupations, community resources and barriers, and participation enablement. Identifying the characteristics and dimensions of community identity, community occupations, and resources and barriers to community participation enables occupational therapy practitioners to develop and implement appropriate strategies and interventions to empower communities to achieve their occupational goals and facilitate community participation.

The first component, community identity, is defined by the individuals, groups, organizations, and social networks that are members of the community. Community membership is fluid and changes over time. Members have particular social roles that support the community's shared purpose and goals. Other factors associated with community identity include geographic location, climate, the natural and built environment, population characteristics, and sociocultural elements (Hyett et al., 2018).

The second component of the CCPF, community occupations, are those occupations that are important and meaningful to the community as a whole. Community occupations provide a sense of meaning and purpose, community identity, and belonging. Community members participate in co-occupations or collective occupations to move in the direction of their shared goals, with everyone drawing on "diverse skill sets, knowledge, experiences, and expertise" (Hyett et al., 2018, p. 8). Co-occupation is an occupational science construct that refers to two or more people engaging in an occupation in a shared social, temporal, and spatial environment with cooperative intentionality. Collective occupations are "community occupations with socio-political intentions" (Hyett et al., 2018, p. 8).

Community resources and barriers, the third component of the CCPF, emphasizes the importance of identifying factors that facilitate and inhibit community participation. Resources and barriers exist in the community member, the community occupation, and the community environment and context. Resources and social capital are forms of power that flow among community members, groups, organizations, and institutions. Resources must be mobilized and power shared in order for community goals to be achieved.

The fourth and final component of the CCPF is participation enablement. Occupational therapy can enable community-level occupational participation through a variety of strategies. These may include:

- "Building and sustaining partnerships,
- Recruiting, educating and supporting volunteers,
- Increasing the community's public profile and attracting members/funders,
- Negotiating and advocating with power holders, and coaching community members to complete applications for grants and/or council permits" (Hyett et al., 2018, p. 11).

This occupation-focused CCPF can assist occupational therapy practitioners and students with understanding, conceptualizing, and implementing community and population health interventions.

Summary

- There is clear evidence and support for occupational therapy participation in community and population health initiatives in the AOTA *Vision 2025,* the *Framework,* and other AOTA official documents.
- As outlined in *HP 2020,* the social determinants of health include economic stability, education, social and community context, health and health care, and the neighborhood and built environment. Many of these are amenable to occupational therapy intervention.
- There are 42 topic areas and more than 1,200 objectives in *HP 2020,* including specific objectives related to people with disabilities. There are nearly an infinite number of opportunities for occupational therapy involvement.
- It is important for occupational therapy practitioners to be cognizant of the terminology, constructs, and principles of community and population health. These include but are not limited to epidemiological concepts, levels of prevention, and determinants of health.
- Occupational therapy practitioners have three main roles in community and population health: promoting healthy lifestyles for all clients, infusing an occupational science perspective into existing health promotion initiatives, and developing and implementing occupation-based community and population health interventions.
- The CCPF developed by Hyett et al. (2018) is an occupation-based approach to needs assessment and program development that has broad-based application in community and population health practice.

Learning Activities

1. Select a population in a specific geographic area and search for information on the health needs of this population. Identify potential occupational risk factors for this population and occupational therapy interventions to address these risk factors.
2. Apply the four components or phases of the CCPF to the same (or a different) population as in Learning Activity 1. Describe the community's identity, occupations, and factors that facilitate and inhibit occupational participation. What enabling strategies might you use to enhance community occupational participation?
3. Visit your local public health department and identify the programs and services it provides. Consider how an occupational therapy practitioner might be integrated into one or more of these programs and services.

REFERENCES

American Occupational Therapy Association. (2013). Occupational therapy in the promotion of health and well-being. *American Journal of Occupational Therapy, 67*(6), S47–S59.

American Occupational Therapy Association. (2014). Occupational therapy practice framework: Domain and process (3rd ed.). *American Journal of Occupational Therapy, 68,* S1–S48. doi:10.5014/ajot.2014.682006

American Occupational Therapy Association. (2015). Occupational therapy code of ethics (2015). *American Journal of Occupational*

Therapy, 69(Suppl. 3), 6913410030. http://dx.doi.org/10.5014/ajot.2015.696S03

American Occupational Therapy Association. (2018). Vision 2025. *OT Practice, 23*(1), 18–19.

Bass-Haugen, J., Henderson, M. L., Larson, B. A., and Matuska, K. (2005). Occupational issues of concern in populations. In C. H. Christiansen, C. M. Baum, and J. Bass-Haugen (Eds.), *Occupational therapy: Performance, participation and well-being* (3rd ed.). Thorofare, NJ: SLACK.

Clark, F., Azen, S. P., Carlson, M., Mandel, D., LaBree, L., Hay, J., et al. (2001). Embedding health-promoting changes into the daily lives of independent-living older adults: Long-term follow-up of occupational therapy intervention. *Journal of Gerontology: Psychological Sciences, 56,* 60–63.

Clark, F., Azen, S. P., Zemke, R., Jackson, J., Carlson, M., Mandel, D., Hay, J., Josephson, K., Cherry, B., Hessel, C., Palmer, J., and Lipson, L. (1997). Occupational therapy for independent living older adults: A randomized controlled trial. *Journal of the American Medical Association, 278,* 1321–1326.

Clark, F., Jackson, J., Carlson, M., Chou, C., Cherry, B. J., Jordan-Marsh, M., . . . Azen, S. P. (2012). Effectiveness of a lifestyle intervention in promoting the well-being of independently living older people: Results of the Well Elderly 2 randomized controlled trial. *Journal of Epidemiology and Community Health, 66,* 782–790. doi.org/10.1136/jech.2009.099754

Drum, C. E., Krahn, G., Culley, C., and Hammond, L. (2005). Recognizing and responding to the health disparities of people with disabilities. *Californian Journal of Health Promotion, 3,* 29–42.

Green, L. W., and Anderson, C. L. (1982). *Community health.* St. Louis, MO: Mosby.

Green, L. W., and Kreuter, M. W. (1991). *Health promotion planning: An educational and environmental approach* (2nd ed.). Mountainview, CA: Mayfield.

Green, L. W., and Raeburn, J. (1990). Contemporary developments in health promotion, definitions and challenges. In N. Bracht (Ed.), *Health promotion at the community level* (pp. 29–44). Newbury Park, CA: Sage.

Hyett, N., Kenny, A., and Dickson-Swift, V. (2018). Re-imagining occupational therapy clients as communities: Presenting the community-centred practice framework. *Scandinavian Journal of Occupational Therapy.* doi:10.1080/11038128.2017.1423374

Kindig, D. A. (n.d.). What is the difference between population health and public health? *Improving Population Health: Policy, Practice, Research.* Retrieved from www.improvingpopulationhealth.org/blog/what-is-the-difference-between-population-health-and-public-health.html

LaLonde, M. (1974). *A new perspective on the health of Canadians: A working document.* Ottawa, Canada: Ministry of National Health and Welfare.

Los Angeles Times. (2000). *King's widow urges acts of compassion.* Retrieved from http://articles.latimes.com/2000/jan/17/news/mn-54832

MacMahon, B., and Trichopoulos, D. (1996). *Epidemiology principles and methods.* Boston, MA: Little, Brown.

Pickett, G., and Hanlon, J. J. (1990). *Public health: Administration and practice.* St. Louis, MO: Times Mirror/Mosby.

Rhynders, P. A., and Scaffa, M. E. (2010). Enhancing community health through community partnerships. In M. Scaffa, S. M. Reitz, and M. Pizzi (Eds.), *Occupational therapy in the promotion of health and wellness* (pp. 208–224). Philadelphia, PA: F. A. Davis.

Scaffa, M. E. (1998). Adolescents and alcohol use. In A. Henderson, S. Champlin, and W. Evashwick (Eds.), *Promoting teen health: Linking schools, health organizations and community* (pp. 78–99). Thousand Oaks, CA: Sage.

Scaffa, M. E., and Brownson, C. (2005). Occupational therapy interventions: Community health approaches. In C. H. Christiansen, C. M. Baum, and J. Bass-Haugen (Eds.), *Occupational therapy: Performance, participation and well-being* (3rd ed., pp. 477–488). Thorofare, NJ: SLACK.

Scaffa, M. E., Van Slyke, N., and Brownson, C. A. (2008). Occupational therapy in the promotion of health and the prevention of disease and disability. *American Journal of Occupational Therapy, 62*(6), 694–703.

Schell, B. A., Gillen, G., and Scaffa, M. E. (2014). *Willard and Spackman's Occupational Therapy* (12th ed.). Philadelphia, PA: Wolters Kluwer.

Schultz, S. W. (2014). Theory of Occupational Adaptation. In B. A. Schell, G. Gillen, and M. E. Scaffa (Eds.), *Willard and Spackman's Occupational Therapy* (12th ed., pp. 527–540). Philadelphia, PA: Wolters Kluwer.

Seligman, M. (2011). *Flourish: A visionary new understanding of happiness and well-being.* New York, NY: Free Press.

Trentham, B., and Cockburn, L. (2005). Participatory action research: Creating new knowledge and opportunities for occupational engagement. In F. Kronenberg, S. Simo Algado, and N. Pollard (Eds.), *Occupational therapy without borders: Learning from the spirit of survivors* (pp. 440–453). Philadelphia, PA: Churchill Livingstone.

U.S. Department of Health and Human Services. (n.d.a). *The vision, mission and goals of Healthy People 2020.* Retrieved from www.healthypeople.gov/sites/default/files/HP2020Framework.pdf

U.S. Department of Health and Human Services. (n.d.b.). *About the Office of the Surgeon General.* Retrieved from www.surgeongeneral.gov/about/index.html

U.S. Department of Health and Human Services. (1990). *Healthy People 2000: National health promotion and disease prevention objectives* (Publication No. 017-001-00474-0). Washington, DC: U.S. Government Printing Office.

U.S. Department of Health and Human Services. (2000). *Healthy People 2010* (2nd ed.). Washington, DC: U.S. Government Printing Office.

U.S. Department of Health and Human Services. (2010a). *Healthy People 2020* (ODPHP Publication No. B0132). Retrieved from http://healthypeople.gov

U.S. Department of Health and Human Services. (2010b). *Implementing Healthy People 2020.* Retrieved from http://healthypeople.gov/2020/implementing/default.aspx

U.S. Department of Health and Human Services. (2011a). *About Healthy People.* Retrieved from http://healthypeople.gov/2020/about/default.aspx

U.S. Department of Health and Human Services. (2011b). *Disparities.* Retrieved from http://healthypeople.gov/2020/about/DisparitiesAbout.aspx

U.S. Department of Health and Human Services. (2019a). Social determinants of health. *Healthy People 2020.* Retrieved from www.healthypeople.gov/2020/topics-objectives/topic/social-determinants-of-health

U.S. Department of Health and Human Services. (2019b). *Healthy People 2030 Framework.* Retrieved from www.healthypeople.gov/2020/about-healthy-people/development-healthy-people-2030/framework

U.S. Department of Health, Education, and Welfare. (1979). *Healthy people: Surgeon general's report on health promotion/disease prevention* (Publication No. 79-55071). Washington, DC: U.S. Government Printing Office.

Wilcock, A. A. (1998). *An occupational perspective of health.* Thorofare, NJ: SLACK.

Wilcock, A. A. (2005). Relationship of occupations to health and well-being. In C. H. Christiansen, C. M. Baum, and J. Bass-Haugen (Eds.), *Occupational therapy: Performance, participation and well-being* (3rd ed., pp. 134–164). Thorofare, NJ: SLACK.

Wilcock, A. A. (2006). *An occupational perspective of health* (2nd ed.). Thorofare, NJ: SLACK.

World Health Organization. (1986). *The Ottawa charter for health promotion.* Retrieved from http://who.int/healthpromotion/conferences/previous/ottawa/en/

World Health Organization. (2009). *Commission on Social Determinants of Health: Report by the secretariat.* Retrieved from https://apps.who.int/iris/handle/10665/2189

World Health Organization. (2011). *Rio political declaration on social determinants of health.* Retrieved from http://who.int/sdhconference/declaration/Rio_political_declaration.pdf

World Health Organization. (2019). *Ten threats to global health in 2019.* Retrieved from www.who.int/emergencies/ten-threats-to-global-health-in-2019

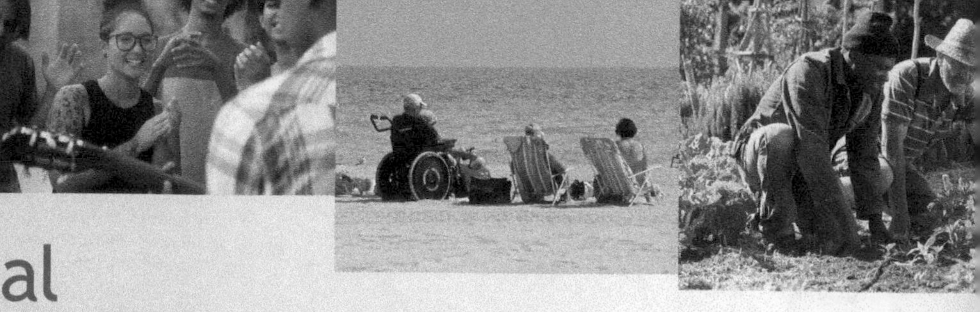

Chapter 3

Theoretical Frameworks for Community-Based Practice

M. Beth Merryman, PhD, OTR/L, FAOTA, Kendra Heatwole Shank, PhD, OTR/L, and S. Maggie Reitz, PhD, OTR/L, FAOTA

Public health service should be as fully organized and as universally incorporated into our governmental system as is public education. The returns are thousand fold in economic benefits, and infinitely more in reduction of suffering and promotion of human happiness.

—Herbert Hoover

Learning Outcomes

This chapter is designed to enable the reader to:

3-1 Appreciate the need for occupational therapy practitioners to be knowledgeable and competent in the use of theory in community-based and population-based health practice.

3-2 Compare and contrast the constructs and principles of a variety of theoretical frameworks in order to select one or more to support program development and evaluation in community-based and population-based health practice.

3-3 Apply the principles of occupation-based frameworks to address the occupational needs of communities and diverse populations through evidence-based program development and implementation.

3-4 Utilize theoretical frameworks to assess community-based and population-based programs.

3-5 Describe the general characteristics and principles of theories from related disciplines that may be used in community-based and population-based practice.

3-6 Apply the principles of a combination of occupation-based frameworks and other theoretical frameworks to address the occupational needs of communities and diverse populations through evidence-based program development and implementation.

Key Terms

Adaptive cycle
Creativity
Enabling factors
Functional coordination
Growth
Habituation
Human agency
Individualism
Maladaptive cycle
Occupational ecology
Occupational injustice
Outcome expectations
Performance capacity
Pragmatism
Predisposing factors
Problematic situation
Reciprocal determinism
Reinforcing factors

Relapse
Self-efficacy
Trajectory of change
Transaction
Volition

Introduction

The American Occupational Therapy Association (AOTA, 2017c) launched *Vision 2025* to highlight the development of leaders that use evidence-based practice to collaborate and provide culturally responsive interventions at the individual, community, and population level. The utilization of theory is the first step in a profession's quest to be both science-driven and evidence based. A well-developed theoretical foundation for community-based and population health–based practice is essential for a variety of reasons. Theories and models provide the foundation and context for basic and applied research, program design, implementation, and evaluation. This chapter presents a review of a few select theoretical frameworks from occupational therapy and occupational science, public health, and health education that can be applied to community-based and population-based practice. Theoretical frameworks such as these and others can be used to assist communities in their efforts to improve residents' occupational performance, health and wellness, quality of life, participation, role competence, well-being, and occupational justice. These outcomes are consistent with those of occupational therapy, as detailed in the AOTA (2014) *Occupational Therapy Practice Framework: Domain and Process.*

In the current climate of rapid change and the need to justify and substantiate the value of occupational therapy, knowledge of theory is essential. Established and evolving theoretical frameworks are well suited to support occupational therapy's role in health-care institutions and in the community. However, before selecting a theoretical framework, it is important to consider the variety of theories and models that are available. It is important to consider other frameworks that potentially can be blended with occupation-based frameworks in order to provide the best theoretical support of community-based and population health practice.

A theory "is a systematic way of understanding events or situations" that describes the relationships between the constructs, concepts, and principles on which it is built (National Cancer Institute [NCI], 2005, p. 4). Humans use theory to link an event or behavior to antecedent factors whether or not those factors are directly observable (Miller and Schwartz, 2004). A well-constructed theory satisfies four basic criteria:

- Fit
- Understanding
- Generality
- Control

For a theory to have a good *fit,* it must reflect the everyday reality of the phenomenon it is designed to represent. *Understanding* refers to the need for the theory to be rational, logical, and make sense both to the researcher/theorist and to the community involved in the initiative. *Generality* means that a well-developed theory is comprehensive and includes sufficient variation to provide applicability to a diversity of contexts. Lastly, it should allow for a degree of *control* over the phenomenon in question (Strauss and Corbin, 1990).

Many theoretical frameworks are available to occupational therapy practitioners as they engage in community-based and population health occupational therapy practice. These include the frameworks and perspectives from the discipline of occupational science as well as conceptual practice models from occupational therapy. Theories and models from health education, health psychology, and public health can also be helpful guides for community-based practice. While the occupation-based theoretical frameworks provide the lens through which the occupational therapy practitioner defines the issue/need/problem, non-occupation-based theories and models assist with understanding barriers and supports to engagement and participation.

Selected Occupation-Based Frameworks

A description of occupation-based frameworks from occupational therapy and occupational science literature that apply to community-based practice follows. This selection is not exhaustive of all relevant approaches but rather is a sampling to illustrate how occupation-based frameworks offer a foundation for identifying and defining the problem or issue. Readers are encouraged to conduct an independent analysis to determine the most appropriate model to address the health needs of each unique community or population.

The three models discussed in this chapter were selected due to their applicability for use in community-based practice at both the individual and population levels. The model of human occupation (MOHO; Kielhofner and Burke, 1980) was one of the first clearly articulated occupation-based models. Using a systems approach to identify occupation-based problems and provide focus for intervention, this model was among the first to explicitly embrace the potential for prevention as well as both individual- or community-level intervention within the occupational therapy scope of practice. The transactional perspective of occupation (TPO) developed by Dickie, Cutchin, and Humphrey (2006) represents the evolution of the contribution of occupational science to the understanding of occupation as both a means and an end in daily life. The argument that occupation is embedded in the multidimensional environment has broad implications for community practice, including how problems are identified and interventions aimed. Wilcock's contribution (i.e., doing, being, belonging, becoming) to community practice evolved from her own scholarly inquiries into the relationship between occupation and health. Her embrace of the World Health Organization (WHO) principles of health frame the concepts of "doing, being, belonging, and becoming" that are central to the four occupation-based health frameworks presented in this text (Wilcock, 1999, 2006). These community health–oriented occupational perspectives have evolved to include the occupational ecosustainable community development approach, occupational justice approach, occupation-focused prevention of illness and disability approach, and the occupation-focused health promotion approach (Wilcock and Hocking, 2015). Each approach embraces participatory action methods involving affected community members to define needs and generate the best solution (Wilcock and Hocking, 2015). The use of participatory methods also aligns with the use of insights from the non-occupation-based frameworks identified in this chapter that serve to increase awareness and engage community members in the change process.

Model of Human Occupation

The MOHO was developed by Kielhofner and Burke (1980) to provide a link between practice and Reilly's theory of occupational behavior (Scott, Miller, and Walker, 2004) and was later influenced by dynamic systems theory. Kielhofner spearheaded the continued evolution of the MOHO over a 40-year period. The MOHO explains how the human system selects and performs occupations and how this is influenced through ongoing interaction with the environment, as well as the "dynamic and reciprocal" interaction between the environment and the three other elements of the model—volition, habituation, and performance capacity (Taylor, 2017b, viii). This model can be applied to a client who is an individual, family, community, or population. In each situation, the client receives input from the environment as well as the other three elements. Each of these three elements—volition, habituation, and performance capacity—plays an important role in occupation-based decision-making.

Performance Capacity

Performance capacity involves the interplay of the client's physical, physiological, and cognitive capacities, which are observable and objectively measured with the equally important client's subjective experiences and perspectives (Tham, Erikson, Fallaphour, Taylor, and Kielhofner, 2017). The primary function of this subsystem is to produce "the actions required to accomplish occupation" (Kielhofner, 1997, p. 194), which allows the individual, family, community, or population to meet the demands of both the environment and the remaining two elements.

Habituation

Habituation is the "internalized readiness to exhibit consistent patterns of behavior guided . . . by habits and roles and fitted to the characteristics of the routine temporal physical and social environments" (Kielhofner, 2017, p. 52). The maintenance of these patterns occurs through the development and refinement of habits and internalized roles (e.g., worker, student, parent, and spouse). Habits and internalized roles provide humans with a sense of order and predictability. In addition, they allow humans to be energy and time efficient. An example of a healthy habituation subsystem is an individual or community that routinely engages in physical activity.

Volition

Volition, the third element, describes what motivates the individual, community, or population to engage in behaviors. This element is composed of three "structural components: personal causation, values, and interests" (Kielhofner and Burke, 1980, p. 576). Kielhofner and Burke (1985) defined personal causation as "a collection of beliefs and expectations which a person holds about his or her effectiveness in the environment" (p. 15). These beliefs include "belief in skill, belief in efficacy of skill, expectancy of success/failure, and internal/external control" (Kielhofner and Burke, 1985, p. 16). In addition, Kielhofner and Burke (1985) view values as "images of what is good, right and/or important" (p. 17), whereas interests concern the self-knowledge of occupations that provide pleasure to the individual. This self-knowledge includes the ability to recognize patterns of enjoyed occupations and an understanding of which occupations evoke more potency of interest than others. Through the years, the description of the components of the environment was modified to reflect both the continued development of the model and the influence of other theorists. In the current language of the MOHO (Taylor, 2017b), the environment consists of physical, social, and occupational aspects. Humans and their occupation-based decision-making are also influenced by local, national, and international cultural norms, political situations, and financial resources. The environment both "affords" and "presses" the individual (Kielhofner, 1997), meaning that it simultaneously facilitates and constrains the human system. Two related constructs that explain how the human system changes within, and in response to, the environment over time are also important to consider when applying this model in the community. These constructs are the trajectory of change and adaptive and maladaptive cycles. The **trajectory of change** is the self-transformation of the system over time. An **adaptive cycle** supports the individual in satisfying internal demands as well as the demands of the environment (Kielhofner and Burke, 1980). Kielhofner described a **maladaptive cycle** as failing "to meet one or both" of the internal or environmental demands just mentioned (1980, p. 737). It is possible, however, to reverse a maladaptive cycle and encourage the development of an adaptive cycle. Successful change is dependent on the incorporation of new actions and their associated positive subjective feelings over time into revised routinized habits and patterns of healthy occupation-based decision-making (Taylor, 2017b).

The MOHO has been applied to interventions with individuals with a variety of health conditions and situations ranging from AIDS, borderline personality disorder, blindness, posttraumatic stress disorder (PTSD), and stroke, among others (de las heras de Pablo, Abelenda, and Parkinson, 2017). In addition, the model has been successfully used in prevention efforts and in community-based health promotion programming (de las heras de Pablo et al., 2017). Occupational therapy practitioners can access a list of validated MOHO assessments, programs and interventions, and evidence-based literature on the MOHO through the MOHO Clearinghouse (Taylor, 2017a). Figure 3-1 illustrates a simplified adaptation of the MOHO for use as a community empowerment model (Reitz, 1990), in which the recipient of services is the community rather than an individual or family. Case Study 3-1 presents an application of this model in a community setting using the adapted MOHO depicted in Figure 3-1.

Transactional Perspective of Occupation

The TPO (Cutchin and Dickie, 2013; Dickie et al., 2006) grew from the discipline of occupational science and inquiry about the fundamental nature of

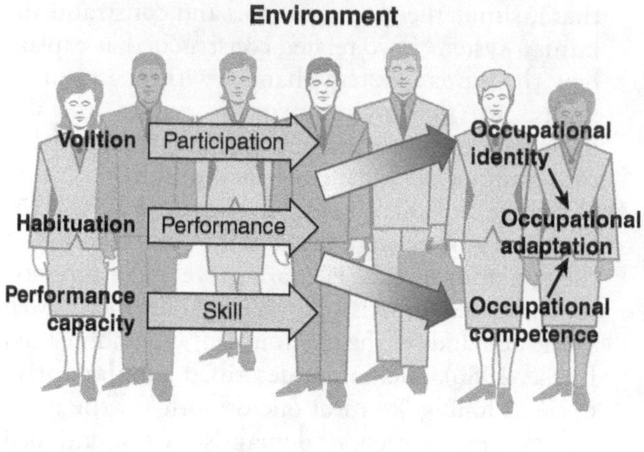

Figure 3-1 The model of human occupation as a framework for use in community-based practice. *(Adapted from* Model of Human Occupation: Theory and Application *[3rd ed., p. 121], by G. Kielhofner, 2002, Baltimore, MD: Lippincott Williams and Wilkins.)*

occupation. Grounded in the **pragmatism** of John Dewey (1977), whose writings also influenced founders of occupational therapy such as Adolf Meyer (Cutchin, 2004), this perspective represents a general shift away from a systems view, in which there are many different elements, and toward a focus on holism and the interconnections of people, places, mind, body, and contexts. The TPO posits that occupations are part of the **transaction** of persons and environments—part of the connective relationships that join people and their environments. From this vantage, occupation is defined as "a type of relational action through which habit, context, and creativity are coordinated toward a provisional yet particular meaningful outcome that is always in process" (Cutchin, Aldrich, Bailliard, and Coppola, 2008, p. 164). In other words, occupation is a relationship of many factors, shaped by values, and not just an isolated and individual "performance." Aspects of this definition will be explained further below.

One of the primary implications of this perspective is that it challenges the long-held **individualism** in therapy—a view of individuals as containers of meaning and motivation who exist inside various contexts and act and react with these contexts through their own agency—that was prevalent in many theories and frameworks within occupational therapy in the late 20th century. Dickie et al. (2006) argued that while an understanding of individual experiences and meaning is important, many other dimensions of occupation need to be considered in order to have a holistic understanding of how human action contributes to health and well-being.

Since the introduction of the TPO, researchers in occupational science have begun to more deeply examine the sociocultural, historical, temporal, and environmental aspects of occupation. This theoretical framework has grounded the development of knowledge about occupation itself and has repeatedly revealed and emphasized the highly social and contextualized nature of occupation. Because these widely recognized social and contextual factors extend beyond the individual, the TPO is particularly well suited to inform group, community, and population-level efforts to maximize well-being through occupation.

The four key concepts from the TPO that lay a foundation for application to community practice are problematic situations, functional coordination, creativity, and growth. After explaining these four concepts, this chapter will outline several ways in which the TPO supports and enhances community-based practice.

Problematic Situations

Fritz and Cutchin (2017) defined a **problematic situation** as a context "that, because of change, demands attention, reflection, and action" (p. 452). Problematic situations are familiar to occupational therapy practitioners since they may result from an injury or illness, a change in the demands of the environment, a habit or routine that is no longer working or satisfying, or a shift in the meaning attributed to an occupation. Problematic situations happen when participation in occupation—no matter the reason—is disrupted. Occupational participation can become problematic due to policy changes, a new living situation, a worsening chronic condition, a change in relationship among family or friends, or even a change in the geography or built environment of the community (e.g., a new bus stop or stoplight). Because the relationship among several dimensions can affect occupations in complex ways, occupational therapy practitioners need to take a broad view in considering what elements contribute to a problematic situation.

Functional Coordination

Functional coordination is the ongoing process of resolving problematic situations. When a problematic situation is encountered, it necessitates coordination through action in the world (Garrison, 2001). This coordination is an active process of *doing* occupation and is similar to a therapeutic process in which clients learn, practice, relearn, transfer and apply skills, and modify the environment and aspects of performance to support participation. However, coordination happens *through* occupations, not just *toward* occupation. Adopting a TPO, functional coordination can be seen as the recognition that a problem unfolds in a specific context (i.e., the problematic situation), and therefore solutions must be infused by the meaning, values, and experiences of that whole situation.

As compared to the idea of adaptation, which is typically used to describe a discrete change in person, environment, or task aimed at achieving a new equilibrium, the concept of functional coordination is a change that occurs *among* elements and is never complete. The process of doing, learning, modifying, adjusting, negotiating, and integrating is ongoing since change is constant. As Dickie et al. (2006) explained, occupations can be seen as the transactions that join all these elements, through which people coordinate and recoordinate themselves and their worlds. For example, several clients attending a community cooking program are disengaged and occasionally disruptive. Using TPO, the occupational therapy practitioner might support the clients' participation by considering the type of food being prepared, the characteristics of other group members, the previous roles and routines related to cooking, and the social and geographical food norms. This reflection and a review of the shared goals of the group could help the disengaged clients recoordinate with the shared cooking occupation. Since problematic situations are multifaceted and arise through a specific time and place (Cutchin, 2004), solutions must also be multifaceted and relevant to the whole situation.

Creativity

Due to the complex holism of problematic situations and the ongoing and situated processes of functional coordination, Dewey (Fesmire, 2003) and others (Cutchin et al., 2008) have emphasized the necessity of **creativity.** In the context of occupation-centered practice, creativity also looks like imagination: imagining what is possible when outcomes are uncertain (Cutchin, 2001) and using creative means, including trial and error, to find the ways that an occupational breakdown can be transformed. This concept of creativity is not only consistent with the long-standing professional identity of occupational therapy practitioners but is also connected to the pragmatist philosophers' thoughts about solutions. Creativity is necessary because the "right" solution is not always foreseeable. Instead, solutions—the ways in which problems are functionally recoordinated—should be evaluated based on how effective they are in solving the issue. From a transactional perspective, any aspect of the person-place relationship can be a source of creativity and intervention.

Growth

Finally, the concept of ***growth*** is important in the TPO. Growth refers to the "forward lean" of action (Cutchin, 2001), or the idea that occupational transactions are future-oriented (Heatwole Shank and Cutchin, 2016). This concept has two facets. First, this future orientation, described by Dewey as "ends in view" (Aldrich, 2008), relates back to the view that occupations are shaped by values and perceived meaning, including imagined possibilities for the future participation of individuals and groups. For example, the ability of children with physical disabilities to have a playground that enables a full range of outdoor free play activities might be seen as an "end in view" toward which the community needs to grow. Second, growth also implies a process that does not end. Like any growing organism, while we may observe specific milestones or achievements, the trajectory of growth does not happen in increments and plateaus but rather with continuity and fluctuations over time. The concept of growth as applied to a community setting suggests that therapists shift away from the language of goals-to-be-achieved and toward the focus on growth that is ongoing, progressive, and sustainable within the holistic situation. In the example of the playground, a redesigned accessible playground might raise awareness and spur efforts to improve the accessibility of other local businesses or may become a meeting site for ongoing work by disability advocacy groups in that community.

This theoretical framework supports and enhances community-based practice in several ways. First, the TPO embraces complexity and holism by foregrounding the influence and relationships among history, sociocultural context, various stakeholders, the physical setting, goals and visions for the future, and community norms and values. The real-world complexity of community practice benefits from a framework in which these dimensions are integrated not just as part of the problematic situation but also, potentially, as part of the solution (e.g., Jones, Hocking, and McPherson, 2017). Second, habits and situated patterns of participation can be leveraged for health promotion in ways that target groups and communities, not just individuals. Since there is less focus on individual "agency" and more of a recognition that actions and values are shaped by context (Fritz and Cutchin, 2017), the potential for interventions to transcend the individual maximize the reach and potency of occupational therapy practice. And third, the explicit focus on occupation and the promotion of participation by individuals, groups, and communities grounds a practice that can address issues of justice and equity (Bailliard and Aldrich, 2016). The TPO emphasizes the centrality of occupation in the ways that humans and their worlds relate. Community-based and population health occupational therapy can therefore leverage occupation to identify problems, develop and implement creative solutions, and partner with individuals and agencies to maximize growth toward the envisioned and desired participation of clients. This occupation-based framework can be complemented by other frameworks and intervention models.

Wilcock Doing, Being, Belonging, Becoming

Occupation-based frameworks for community practice have evolved over the past decade. Wilcock is an occupational therapist and scientist internationally recognized for her contributions to understanding the relationship between occupation and health, specifically through "doing, being, belonging and becoming" (Wilcock, 2006; Wilcock and Hocking, 2015). These complex constructs are action focused and enacted by humans not only to survive but to thrive in an environment of sustainability and justice for all. Definitions of these constructs appear in Box 3-1.

The action focus involves a process of identifying and clarifying the issue; collaborating to explore with those affected using contextual research; engaging in participatory action, including reflection and modification; and participating in ongoing negotiated change (Wilcock and Hocking, 2015, p. 410). In this manner, Wilcock's approach reflects an orientation consistent with the participatory action research on empowering marginalized populations, specifically those affected by policy change, in the definition of the problem and design of the best solution (Hammel, Jones, Gossett, and Morgan, 2006; Knightbridge, King, and Rolfe, 2006).

Box 3-1 Wilcock's Framework for Health (Wilcock, 1999, 2007; Wilcock and Hocking, 2015)

Doing:	Synonym for occupation; humans have innate need; grounded in biological needs; shape cultural experiences and community structures
Being:	One's awareness and capacity; how people feel about what they do; bidirectional influence of consciousness and occupational choices
Belonging:	Importance of relationships to physical/mental/social health; shared sense of community, identity, and interconnectedness
Becoming:	Notion of ongoing nature of growth/change/transformation; future orientation of self-potential; grounded in doing, being, and belonging; facilitates well-being

Wilcock and Hocking (2015) articulated four occupation-focused approaches to addressing population health. These approaches include the occupational ecosustainable community development approach, the occupational justice approach, the occupation-focused prevention of illness and disability approach, and the occupation-focused health promotion approach. Each of the four approaches follows WHO directives relative to population health and are action focused.

Occupational Ecosustainable Community Development Approach

The occupational ecosustainable community development approach purports that healthy relationships are necessary for sustainability and broadly identifies relationships between humans and environments. The term **occupational ecology** describes the need to restore balance with the natural environment, and Wilcock expresses concern about the loss of routine connection with the natural environment through many contemporary work and daily routines. This framework espouses three main ideas:

- Occupation includes all that people do, and the skills of the community are needed to address issues of inequity.
- There is a need to sustain healthy relationships between all organisms.
- Community involvement is necessary to support equitable and sustainable well-being for all (Wilcock, 2006; Wilcock and Hocking, 2015).

An example of community practice using this model would be one that uses culturally congruent methods in the long term to address the social factors of a population, such as a food desert in which healthy, less-processed food is unavailable to a community, and involves the community in both problem identification and resolution.

Occupational Justice Approach

The occupational justice approach first affirms that people are occupational in nature and that engagement and participation in individual and collective environments is critical to well-being. In addition, this approach states that people have a right to occupational engagement and participation in their environments of choice. This approach states that an **occupational injustice** exists when an individual or group is prevented from exercising these rights due to social, political, and/or economic policies and practices. Mere inconvenience or missed opportunity does not meet the standard for an injustice. Rather, ongoing deprivation that limits potential or puts one at risk in terms of personal safety is an example. A community-based occupational therapy application of this approach could be exploring the employment conditions of undocumented workers or those on disability who work without the protections that a formal job title "on the books" affords. This type of work arrangement creates vulnerability and opportunities for exploitation such as excessive hours, unsafe working conditions, unfair pay, or sexual harassment. Interventions often include advocacy strategies that aim to influence policies or practices for a marginalized group, again collaborating with those affected by the injustice in an emancipatory and empowering manner. The Adverse Childhood Experiences (ACEs) Study linking cumulative childhood exposure to trauma such as domestic violence, active substance abuse, or homelessness to the risk of mental health challenges, such as attempted suicide (Dube et al., 2001), has changed the approach to school-based mental health programs in the United States. Whiteford and Townsend's (2011) participatory occupational justice framework (POJF) provides a six-step process for employing this approach, including analyzing resources through a needs assessment; articulating a justice-based framework; analyzing occupational injustices; articulating a program design including expected outcomes; developing a participatory means to evaluate them; and finalizing the planning, implementation, and evaluation of the program. The POJF is discussed in more detail in Chapter 22.

Occupation-Focused Prevention of Illness and Disability Approach

The occupation-focused prevention of illness and disability approach considers occupation as a contributing factor to illness and recovery. Wilcock (2006) critiques the current medical model and health-care delivery system as deficient in describing and diagnosing ill health, as well as in prescribing healthful means to improve quality of life. She suggests a broader approach to diagnosis, including epidemiological attention to occupational and social risk factors. An example might be a community in which the predominant employer leaves the country for cheaper means of production, resulting in sustained poverty and job loss and leading to a reduction in the social capital and resources needed to maintain individual and community health. This approach is relevant not only for individual-level intervention but also for communities and populations since it reflects the broad interests of epidemiology and the risk factors that are present in the broader social environment.

Occupation-Focused Health Promotion Approach

The occupation-focused health promotion approach is an occupation-based orientation to health promotion. This approach is congruent with those of health education and preventive medicine and emphasizes achieving well-being. Individual-level interventions may focus on maximizing well-being and quality of life by aiding the individual in identifying meaning and purpose in adhering to a healthy eating and physical activity plan. A group- or community-level intervention may include workplace consultation to address positive mental health and fitness as a means of employee retention. The focus is on a multidimensional definition of health and well-being to encompass not only physical but also social and emotional factors and the broad role of the environment to support or prevent the adoption of health behaviors. This approach may be relevant to address the relationship between poverty and other social factors of health, as well as successful child development and healthy aging.

Engage Your Brain 3-1

How are these occupation-based theories similar and different?

Selected Non-Occupation-Based Frameworks

The occupational therapy profession can draw on the expertise of individuals conducting research on community empowerment initiatives in the fields of public health and health education. Political activism and the generation of research evidence supporting the efficacy of occupational therapy interventions in community-based and population-based practice will increase the likelihood that occupational therapy contributions will be valued in the public health arena.

Community-based and population health practice often involves a team approach wherein the membership of the team does not conform to the familiar hospital- or school-based interdisciplinary team. Often, health educators, community organizers, and politicians are potential community-based team members who may work together on a community initiative. Many of these professionals share a common language that is represented in the models from other disciplines presented in this chapter. It is hoped that exposure to these models will facilitate interdisciplinary work in the community by occupational therapy practitioners

When working in community practice, an occupational therapy practitioner's focus is to assist an individual or group to define an occupational need, generate the best-fitting solution, implement it, and assess its effectiveness. While the occupation-based frameworks provide the lens for occupational therapy involvement, non-occupation-based theories and models assist in other ways. This includes describing action, such as how behavior changes or how individuals are motivated to change. Since the 1950s, the fields of health education, public health, and health psychology have been developing and employing models to explain why people do or do not engage in health behaviors. Many theories are referenced in the health education and public health literature, but one of the most frequently cited is social cognitive theory (SCT; Bandura, 1977).

The following section will briefly describe this theory, as well as four additional models, including:

- Health belief model (HBM; Rosenstock, Strecher, and Becker, 1994)
- Transtheoretical model of health behavior change (TMHBC; Prochaska and DiClemente, 1983, 1992)
- PRECEDE-PROCEED framework (Green and Kreuter, 1991, 2005)
- Diffusion of innovations model (Rogers, 2003)

The HBM is a model of the precursors of health behavior, while the TMHBC change explains the stages people experience as they seek to change their health behavior (McKenzie, Neiger, and Thackeray, 2009). The PRECEDE-PROCEED framework is a program-planning and evaluation tool, while diffusion of innovations is a health communications approach, the diffusion of innovation model (Rogers, 2003).

Social Cognitive Theory

Bandura (2004) described the core determinants of health behaviors, the mechanisms through which these core determinants work, and the application of SCT to prevention and health promotion practices. The core determinants of health behaviors include knowledge of the health risks and benefits of various behaviors, perceived self-efficacy, outcome expectations, self-determined health goals and strategies, and perceived facilitators and impediments to health behavior change. In addition, the SCT relies on the postulate of **reciprocal determinism,** which is present when there is a continuous, interdependent interaction among the person, the person's behavior, and the environment. The relative contribution of each of these factors in the determination of an outcome differs according to the setting and the behavior in question (Bandura, 1977).

Knowledge of the health effects of various behaviors is a necessary, but not sufficient, precondition for change. Other factors are also involved. Individuals' perception that they will be able to successfully perform a specific behavior, or perceived self-efficacy, plays a central role in motivation for change (Bandura, 2004). **Self-efficacy** is the belief in one's own competence and power to execute an action that will achieve a desired outcome. These efficacy beliefs have a profound impact on goal setting and aspirations. According to Bandura (2004, p. 145), "the stronger the perceived self-efficacy, the higher the goals people set for themselves and the firmer their commitment to them."

Self-efficacy is derived from personal performance attainments, vicarious experiences, verbal persuasion, and emotional arousal. The successful accomplishment of a behavior enhances one's expectation for future endeavors. The more similar the current task to tasks performed successfully in the past, the greater the efficacy expectations will be. Observations of others who are perceived as similar to oneself engaging in activities and achieving the desired outcome can also increase one's expectations for accomplishment. According to SCT, verbal encouragement, receipt of permission to attempt a specific behavior, and a perceived physiological and emotional state that is conducive to the successful execution of a task will also enhance an individual's confidence and self-efficacy relative to that behavior.

Health behavior change is also mediated by expectancies. According to Bandura (1977), **outcome expectations** are the individual's belief that a given behavior will lead to specific outcomes. The following are the three types of outcome expectations:

- Physical outcomes: the pleasurable and/or aversive effects of the health behavior
- Social outcomes: the social approval and/or disapproval the behavior evokes
- Self-evaluative outcomes: the degree of satisfaction and/or self-worth the person derives from his or her health behavior and/or health status (Bandura, 2004)

Finally, personal values and goals, as well as perceived facilitators and barriers, affect health behavior. **Human agency,** or the ability to intentionally create and influence one's future, enables goal setting, behavior change, and environmental adaptation (Bandura, 2006). Barriers, obstacles, and impediments to health behavior and health behavior change may be personal, social, economic, and environmental. Persons with high levels of self-efficacy are more likely to perceive obstacles as surmountable, while persons with low levels of self-efficacy quickly become discouraged in the face of adversity (Bandura, 2004).

Behavior change, in the SCT paradigm, can be achieved in the following ways: directly, by the reinforcement of particular behaviors; indirectly, through social modeling or observing someone else being reinforced for the behavior; and through self-regulation, with the individual monitoring and providing a self-reward (Wilroy and Turner, 2016; Parcel and Baranowski, 1981).

When adopting this theory for an individual rather than a population-based approach, Bandura (2004) recommends a stepwise strategy, tailoring the strategy to the particular level of self-efficacy and outcome expectations of the individual. For example, persons with high levels of self-efficacy and positive outcome expectations will require minimal guidance to achieve health behavior change. However, persons who have doubts about their self-efficacy and the outcomes of their behaviors will need more guidance, support, and modeling. Persons with low levels of self-efficacy and negative outcome expectations will require considerable structure and personal guidance, as well as the incorporation of the routine occupational therapy principle of "the just right challenge" in order to build confidence through experiences of behavioral success.

In general, the SCT provides a unique perspective for community-based and population-based practice. The constructs of self-efficacy, outcome expectations, behavioral capability, modeling, reciprocal determinism, and self-control appear to be particularly relevant for the development of occupational therapy interventions.

Health Belief Model

The HBM describes the relationships between a person's beliefs about health and her or his health-specific behaviors. The beliefs that mediate health behavior are, according to the model, perceived susceptibility, severity, benefits, and barriers. Box 3-2 defines these terms and cues to action. In addition to the beliefs just mentioned, cues to action are viewed as necessary triggers of behavior. These cues may be internal, such as perceptions of pain, or external, such as feedback from a health-care provider (Rosenstock, 1974) or the media.

According to the model, in order for a person to take action to avoid illness or trauma, several beliefs must be present. For example, individuals must believe they are personally susceptible to the disease, illness, or trauma and that the health problem is severe enough to have a negative impact on their life. They must also believe that taking specific actions would have beneficial effects and that there are more benefits to action than barriers. In addition, if they are in an environment that supports positive action, they will be more likely to engage in the health behavior (Rosenstock, 1974).

The HBM has been used with a variety of populations and a diversity of health topics, including mammogram screening (Wang et al., 2008), diabetes self-management adherence (Bereolos, 2007), health habits of college students (Deshpande, Basil, and Basil, 2009), and osteoporosis prevention (Johnson, McLeod, Kennedy, and McLeod, 2008).

A recent study using the HBM of inpatients to be discharged to the community identified the main predictors of patient safety practices as perceived threat and self-efficacy (Bishop, Baker, Boyle, and MacKinnon, 2015). Another study explored participation by people with lower extremity injuries in a prevention program (Hartley, Hoch, and Cramer, 2018). Among the findings were the need to plan effectively, such as designing the assessment tool, identifying behavioral determinants, and piloting the materials, implying that there is a challenge to conduct research in routine clinical practice. A community-based study of physical activity engagement by people with mental illness using the HBM identified that perceived barriers to access had the greatest impact on likelihood to engage in physical activity, as the barriers decreased self-efficacy, the greatest predictor of engagement (Mo, Chong, Mak, Wong, and Lau, 2016).

Perceived threat, which encompasses perceived susceptibility, has been suggested as an important first cognitive step in the health-action link described by this model. Figure 3-2 presents an adapted schematic representation of the updated HBM as applied to the goal of increasing physical activity.

Box 3-2 Health Belief Model Constructs and Definitions

- ***Perceived susceptibility*** is a person's subjective impression of the risk of a disease, illness, trauma, or negative health experience/health condition.
- ***Perceived severity*** refers to the convictions a person holds regarding the degree of seriousness of a given health problem.
- ***Perceived benefits*** are the beliefs a person has regarding the availability and effectiveness of a variety of possible actions in reducing the threat of an illness, trauma, or negative health experience/health condition.
- ***Perceived barriers*** are the costs or negative aspects associated with engaging in a specific health or preventive behavior.
- ***Cues to action*** are defined as instigating events that stimulate the initiation of a behavior.

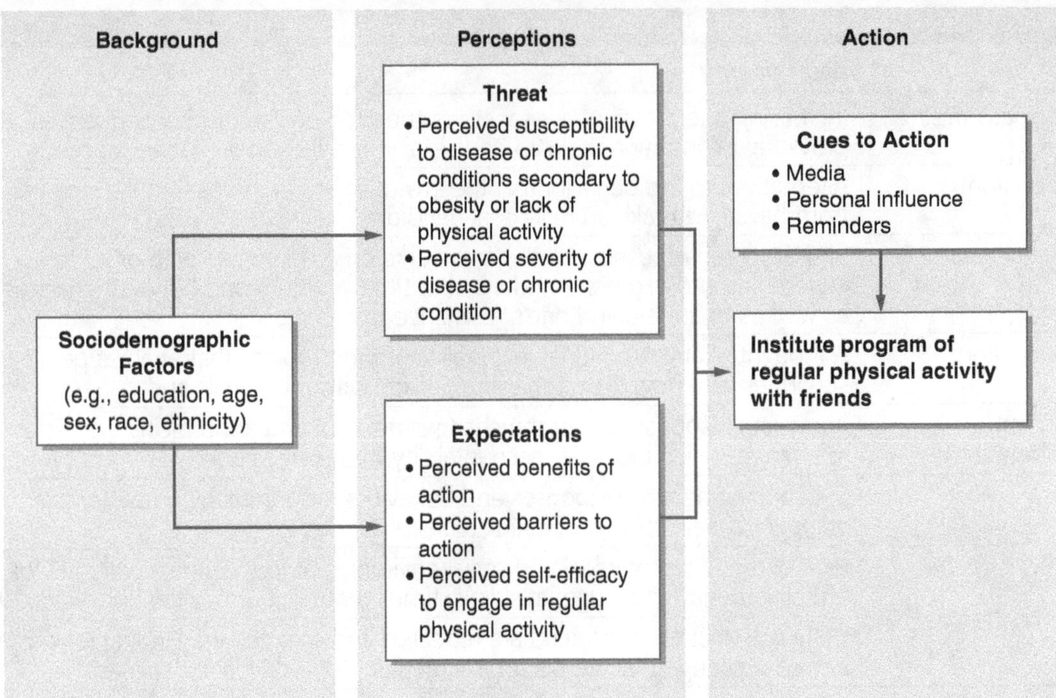

Figure 3-2 Adapted from the revised health belief model as a framework to investigate compliance with required physical activity. *(From "The Health Belief Model and HIV Risk Behavior Change," by I. M. Rosenstock, V. J. Strecher, and M. H. Becker, in R. J. DiClemente and J. L. Peterson [Eds.],* Preventing AIDS: Theories and Methods for Behavioral Interventions *[p. 11], 1994, New York, NY: Plenum, p. 11.)*

Transtheoretical Model of Health Behavior Change

The TMHBC, also referred to as the stages of change model, is a complex model consisting of stages (precontemplation, contemplation, preparation, action, maintenance, and relapse/recycling) and processes of change (Prochaska, Norcross, and DiClemente, 1994). The stages are depicted in Figure 3-3, and the processes are described in Table 3-1.

The precontemplation stage refers to the individual's inability to identify that he or she has a problem and, as a result, has no intention of changing his or her behavior. In the contemplation stage, the individual can identify and acknowledge a problem behavior and is motivated to remedy it. The preparation stage is characterized by planning for change, acquiring needed resources to facilitate the behavior change, and making declarations about intentions to change to family and friends. The action

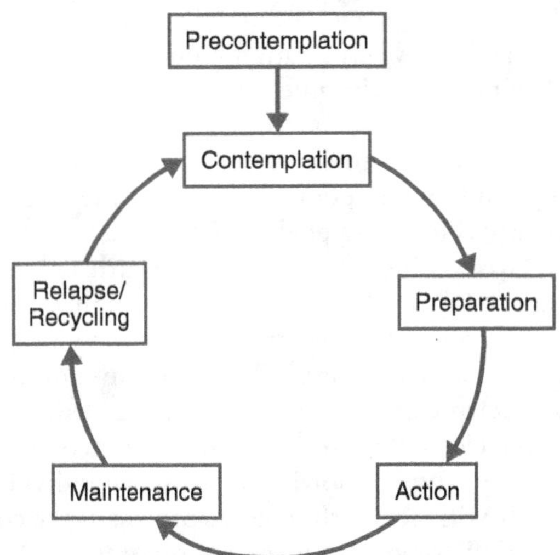

Figure 3-3 Stages of change from the transtheoretical model. *(Data from* Changing for Good: A Revolutionary Six-Stage Program for Overcoming Bad Habits and Moving Your Life Positively Forward, *by J. O. Prochaska, J. C. Norcross, and C. C. DiClemente, 1994, New York, NY: Avon Books.)*

Table 3-1 Processes Associated With the Transtheoretical Model

Process	Description
Consciousness-raising	Increasing one's level of awareness of the problem and its consequences, providing information that can be useful in the behavior change process.
Social liberation	Alternatives to the behavior that the environment provides that free the person from having to make an individual decision.
Emotional arousal	Similar to consciousness-raising but works on a deeper level in order to experience and express emotions about the problem and behavior changes, as well as to understand one's resistance to change.
Self-reevaluation	A thoughtful and emotional reappraisal of the problem that enables people to see when and how their behavior conflicts with their goals and values.
Commitment (or self-liberation)	Accepting responsibility for the changes needed and announcing one's decision to change, which increases accountability for taking action.
Countering	Substituting healthy responses and behaviors for unhealthy ones—for example, going for a walk instead of eating a piece of cake.
Environment control	Restructuring the physical and social environment to maximize potential for effective behavior change; avoiding stimuli that elicit unhealthy behaviors.
Rewards	Behaviors that are reinforced are repeated and maintained. Finding rewards for behavior change that are personally meaningful is critical for success.
Helping relationships	Soliciting, accepting, and receiving support and other types of assistance from significant others in one's life, including friends, family, colleagues, clergy, and health-care professionals.

Data from *Changing for Good: A Revolutionary Six-Stage Program for Overcoming Bad Habits and Moving Your Life Positively Forward,* by J. O. Prochaska, J. C. Norcross, and C. C. DiClemente, 1994, New York, NY: Avon Books.

stage involves overtly changing one's behavior and modifying the environment to facilitate and maintain the change. The maintenance stage requires a long-term commitment to sustain the behavior change and to incorporate it into one's lifestyle permanently (Prochaska et al., 1994).

Relapse is included, as many health behavior changes, such as those relating to substance abuse and addiction, follow a pattern of initiation, relapse, and reinitiation of change. It is important not to interpret relapse as a failure but to acknowledge it as a natural element in the long-term process of health behavior change. Following a relapse, an individual typically will reenter the change process at the contemplation, preparation, or action stages. Those practitioners working in addictions embrace the model's circular nature as a strength, whereby an individual can enter the cycle at any point, and repeated attempts to change behavior, or "recycle," are possible.

The broad change processes listed in Table 3-1 should not be confused with techniques. There are potentially hundreds of techniques associated with the processes of change. Research indicates that many methods for implementing change processes can be effective; individuals who believe they have the autonomy and power to change their lives are the most likely to initiate and maintain a change, and tailoring the techniques employed to the individual's preferences and needs enhances the probability of successful long-term behavior change (Prochaska et al., 1994).

For example, a study using this model to explore behavior change for people with eating disorders found that self-referral positively correlated with motivation for treatment. The model contributed to understanding the importance of motivation and emotions to behavior change in this population (Hasler, Delsignore, Milos, Buddeberg, and Schnyder, 2014). Another study used the model to encourage home safety modifications with community-dwelling adults and found that the action-oriented stages were associated with more modifications (McNulty, Johnson, Poole, and Winkle, 2003). Hammond, Young, and Kidao (2004) conducted a study on the effectiveness of a pragmatic occupational therapy program that was developed over a period of years for clients with rheumatoid arthritis. From this experience, the researchers came to realize that the program may have been more effective had it been theory-based and matched to the client's readiness for change, an important construct of the transtheoretical model.

PRECEDE-PROCEED Planning Model

The PRECEDE model was developed as a planning model for health education based on principles, both theoretical and applied, from epidemiology, education, administration, and the social/behavioral sciences. In the PRECEDE-PROCEED framework, PRECEDE stands for predisposing, reinforcing, and enabling causes in educational diagnosis and evaluation. PROCEED represents the policy, regulatory, and organizational constructs in educational and environmental development (Green and Kreuter, 1991). Figure 3-4 illustrates the complete PRECEDE-PROCEED framework.

The PRECEDE portion of the framework is readily applicable across a variety of settings, providing structure and organization to health education program planning and evaluation. Application of this approach occurs in several phases and involves the diagnoses of variables in four domains: social, epidemiological, educational and ecological, and administrative and policy (Green and Kreuter, 2005). The approach is unique in that it begins with the desired final outcome and works backward, taking into account factors that must precede a certain result.

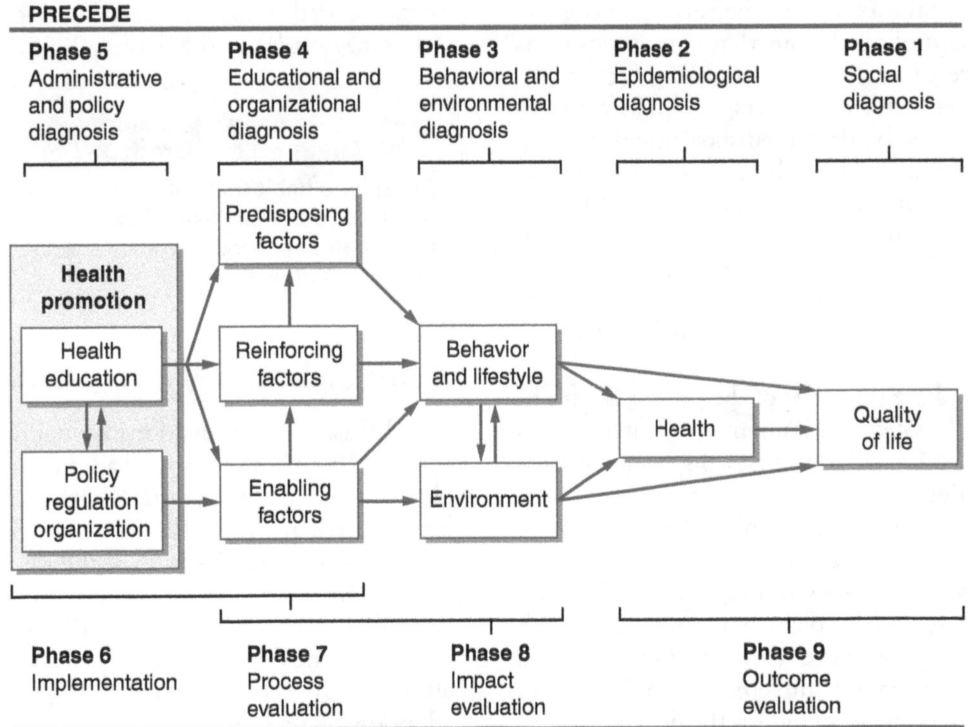

Figure 3-4 The PRECEDE-PROCEED model. *(From* Health Promotion Planning: An Educational and Ecological Approach *[4th ed., p. 17], by Lawrence W. Green and Marshall W. Kreuter, 2005, New York, NY: McGraw-Hill. Reprinted with permission.)*

Phase 1, social assessment, is an analysis of the social problems that exist in a community, which is a necessary step in assessing the quality of life of the target population. The purpose of this phase is to ascertain the relationship between a given health problem and the social problems and priorities of the population. Phase 2, epidemiological, and phase 3, behavioral and environmental assessment, are evaluations of the health problems associated with the community's quality of life. These phases include a review of vital indicators such as morbidity, mortality, fertility, and disability rates along with behavioral and environmental indicators (Green and Kreuter, 2005). Environmental assessment is an evaluation of the health problems associated with the community's quality of life.

In phase 4, educational and organizational assessment, resources, and barriers are differentiated by three categories of influence: predisposing, enabling, and reinforcing factors. **Predisposing factors** provide the motivation or rationale for the behavior(s)—for example, knowledge, attitudes, values, and beliefs. **Reinforcing factors** supply the reward, incentive, or punishment of a behavior that contributes to its maintenance or extinction. **Enabling factors** include personal skills and assets as well as community resources and barriers. Predisposing and enabling factors are antecedent to the health behavior and allow the behavior to occur. Each group of factors is analyzed in terms of importance and changeability, and priorities are established for the intervention. Based on the nature of the targets for intervention, educational methodologies are selected (Green and Kreuter, 2005).

The final phase (phase 5) of the process is administrative and policy assessment and intervention alignment, which includes reviewing budgetary implications; identifying and allocating other types of resources, including time; defining the nature of any cooperative agreements; and assessing the availability of and gaps in policies and regulations. Gaps in, and barriers to, the implementation of the health promotion program need to be addressed at this stage, prior to program implementation. These and subsequent steps are essential for the development of an ethical, evidence-based program. Neglect of this important step can doom an otherwise viable intervention to failure. After this phase is completed, the PROCEED portion of the model is activated.

The PROCEED phase follows the four phases of the PRECEDE portion and includes the implementation of the program (i.e., phase 6) as well as three phases of evaluation. The goal of the PROCEED portion is to monitor the program processes in order to make adjustments as needed to ensure quality as program implementation continues. The three types of evaluation include process (phase 7), impact (phase 8), and outcome (phase 9) evaluations (Green and Kreuter, 2005).

The PRECEDE-PROCEED planning framework has been used to develop a wide variety of community and population health programs (Green and Kreuter, 2005). While this planning framework has not been widely used in occupational therapy, it has been used by an interdisciplinary team with members from a variety of health professions and disciplines, among them occupational therapy, to conduct a systematic literature review. The team used the PRECEDE portion of the PRECEDE-PROCEED framework to systematically investigate the literature and report risk and protective factors related to driving safety among older adults (Classen, Awadzi, and Mkanta, 2008).

Engage Your Brain 3-2

Consider a habit that you would like to quit or one that you would like to start. Which model or combination of models might assist you in planning your actions?

Diffusion of Innovations Model

The diffusion of innovations model developed by Rogers (2003) is a very useful adjunct to specific occupation or health theories (Reitz, Scaffa, Campbell, and Rhynders, 2010). Whereas specific health or occupation theories inform the development of an effective structure and content for the program, the diffusion of innovations model provides a guide on how to most efficiently communicate the availability of the intervention (i.e., diffusion) and the adoption of new behaviors (i.e., innovation). The factors that influence the speed of behavior adoption appear in Table 3-2, together with questions to address in order to maximize success in communicating the message.

Table 3-2 Key Attributes Affecting the Speed and Extent of an Innovations Diffusion

Attribute	Key Question
Relative advantage	Is the innovation better than what it will replace?
Compatibility	Does the innovation fit with the intended audience?
Complexity	Is the innovation easy to use?
Trialability	Can the innovation be tried before making a decision to adopt?
Observability	Are the results of the innovation observable and easily measurable?

From *Theory at a Glance* (2nd ed., p. 28), by National Cancer Institute, 2005, Bethesda, MD: National Institutes of Health.

The AOTA promotes a population-based health promotion initiative developed by Jacobs (Yamkovenko, 2010) to promote the healthy wearing of backpacks worn to school. In this backpack awareness program, the answer to each of these questions would be yes. The innovation (e.g., limiting weight and using both padded shoulder straps), once tried, is more comfortable and will affect the daily lives of the intended participants; the innovation is easy to use and easy to try; and it is easy to see other influential people adopting the innovation (Rhynders, 2010). Whereas specific health or occupation theories inform the development of an effective structure and content for the program, the diffusion of innovations model provides a guide on how to most efficiently communicate the availability of the intervention and the adoption of new behaviors.

According to Rogers, people vary in their readiness to adopt new behaviors (NCI, 2005; Rogers, 2003). Rogers found that people, following a normal distribution, will fall into one of five categories of adopters: innovators, early adopters, early majority adopters, late majority adopters, or laggards. Most people fall into the early majority adopters or late majority adopters categories. Fewer individuals are classified as early adopters or laggards. The rarest categories are those on either end of the distribution, the innovators (i.e., those first to adopt) and the laggards (i.e., the last to adopt). Early adopters are often seen as trendsetters; once a trend becomes popular, people who often lag in trying new things may eventually adopt the innovation (NCI, 2005; Rogers, 2003).

Engage Your Brain 3-3

When a new health trend is circulating on media platforms or when a new piece of technology is released, would you consider yourself an early adopter, early majority adopter, late majority adopter, or a laggard? What influences the timing of your adoption?

Whereas there is tremendous potential to use this theory to disseminate occupational therapy health promotion strategies (Reitz et al., 2010), there is little evidence in the literature. However, the theory has been used to develop recommendations for increasing the compatibility of reported research evidence for use by occupational therapists (Sudsawad, 2005) and to explore adherence to intervention guidelines for low back pain by physical therapists (Harting, Rutten, Rutten, and Kremers, 2009). This theory is often used to explore the adoption of technological innovations in health care, such as electronic scheduling by patients (Zhang, Yu, Yan, and Spil, 2015). In each case, the importance of data collection to understand the characteristics of users of the innovation is critical to understand and design effective adoption behaviors. In the case of the adoption of health-related technology, for example, researchers found that the low value placed on technology as a means to communicate, a familiar alternative to make an appointment, and the low technological skill level of potential adopters were all barriers to adoption.

Summary

- For occupational therapy to reach its potential in the community, its practitioners must possess the knowledge and expertise to join together with a varied group of stakeholders, gatekeepers, community members, and other health professionals to creatively and cost-effectively facilitate the achievement of the health goals of diverse communities.

- A variety of theoretical frameworks are available for occupational therapy practitioners to use in community and population-based programs. Careful review and comparison of the principles of the theoretical framework can facilitate a selection that tailors the fit to the unique characteristics of the community or population.
- Occupation-based frameworks have much to offer decision-makers and occupational therapy practitioners in relation to the occupational needs of people involved in programs and affected by policies, given the link between occupational engagement and health and well-being.
- As in all areas of occupational therapy practice, outcomes research is needed to evaluate the efficacy of interventions. This is particularly true in community-based practice.
- Non-occupation-based theories inform important aspects of program impact for communities and populations, such as how to engage and sustain involvement in behavior change.
- A combination of occupation-based frameworks and those of other disciplines can optimize efforts for communities and populations to make sustainable health behavior change.

CASE STUDIES

CASE STUDY 3-1 Population Approach to Violence Prevention

Benita, an occupational therapy practitioner employed by a school system, has been asked by the Parent Teacher Student Association (PTSA) to assist a task force with the development of a violence (i.e., perpetrators from outside the school community) and bullying (i.e., perpetrators from within the school community) prevention program in the county's only high school. In this example, the community's volition has already been enacted through making the decision to address its concern with the development of a task force. Thus, the community is already exhibiting "community causation" by identifying the problem and believing it has the power to take steps to accomplish the goal of improving school and student safety.

The actual steps the community or PTSA decides to take are greatly influenced by the community's cultural norms (e.g., values and interests), as well as the habits and roles of its members. Working collaboratively with opinion leaders from the PTSA and school professionals, Benita assists the community with identifying key values and interests that influence decision-making relative to changes in the structure of the school and community habits. The community collectively determines if (a) bullying or the potential of an active shooter is more of a priority and (b) the relative priorities of potentially conflicting values. For example, the community will need to weigh the value it places on personal freedom against the value it places on student safety and comfort when deciding whether to require students to wear identification or to install security cameras.

An online survey followed by focus groups can be a useful approach to aid the community's decision-making. In addressing the habituation level of this model, Benita, in collaboration with the PTSA Task Force, will identify potentially dangerous habits (e.g., propping open exterior doors on balmy days; no barrier to prevent visitors from bypassing the front office to sign in) and roles (e.g., the identification of disengaged students with no apparent role in the school community). In addition, the task force community's skills and skill constituents would be determined and listed. This analysis would then be used to facilitate the community's current skills (e.g., competent and effective student leaders) to maximize habit and role performance as well as identify necessary skills requiring development in order to achieve the goals of the program. As a next step, Benita orients the task force to the PRECEDE-PROCEED model, which will help in the identification of the community's capacity and other information and resources that can be used to support program development and evaluation.

CASE STUDY 3-1 Population Approach to Violence Prevention

Discussion Questions

1. What AOTA and USDHHS resources could Benita use to share with the task force to inform its decision-making and efforts?
2. Which AOTA (2015) core values and ethical principles could assist Benita in her work with this population?
3. What violence prevention resources and programming are available at your university or college? How might these resources and programming be enhanced with an occupation-based theoretical approach?

CASE STUDY 3-2 Individual Approach for Violence Prevention

This individual level of intervention is derived from the population approach described above. Benita will establish outreach services for students who are identified as at risk and/or disengaged from the online surveys, focus groups, or personal referrals from students themselves, school personnel, or parents. Benita will use Wilcock's occupation, environment, and community development approach to engage key participants in designing an intervention that contributes to a healthy school environment in which all feel valued and included (Wilcock and Hocking, 2015). As part of her needs assessment, she will observe school routines, such as arrival and dismissal, as well as recess and cafeteria time. In addition, Benita will meet with a range of constituent groups and individuals in a variety of ways to ensure that multiple points of view are included in a potential solution.

The individual-level approach involves adopting the Comfortable Cafeteria program (Bazyk, Demerjian, Horvath, and Doxsey, 2018) so that all students can benefit during the school day. The targeted students identified as disengaged will receive intervention that addresses their engagement and feelings of belonging in the school community. They will work in occupational therapy groups intended to build their interpersonal and problem-solving skills to design the area and plan activities, emphasizing a tiered approach in alignment with a public health framework (Bazyk, 2011). The eventual program will have multiple aspects, and the objective is to establish a sustainable school cafeteria culture that is inclusive to all members of the community.

Discussion Questions

1. What AOTA, state, and national resources could Benita use to share with the task force to inform its decision-making and efforts?
2. What potential ethical dilemmas could arise while implementing the Comfortable Cafeteria program?
3. Which other theories described in this chapter could be used to support or evaluate the Comfortable Cafeteria program? How did you arrive at your selection?

Learning Activities

1. Review recent issues of *OT Practice* for articles about community-based, occupation-based, or population health programs. Read at least three articles and determine whether the programs were theory-based. If a theory was not mentioned, reflect on the description of the program and identify possible theories and constructs from those theories that could be used to support the implementation or evaluation of the program.

2. Concerned about a recent fatal bike crash, an occupational therapy student joins with a health education student to design a program to increase bicycle helmet usage on their college campus. Identify and describe how the students could use constructs from one or more theories in the program development and evaluation plan.
3. After graduation you have contracted to work with a health educator to develop a falls prevention program on a cruise ship that caters to older adults. Identify and describe how you would use constructs from one or more theories in your program. Draw a sketch of the theory and the corresponding constructs.
4. Many examples of effective community-based interventions are identified in AOTA's critically appraised topics (CATs). Consider how characteristics of these interventions are consistent with the occupation-based theories introduced in this chapter. Using the terminology of these three theories, can you describe in your own words how the problems were identified and interventions were designed to support participation in the following examples?
   - Multifactorial approaches for fall prevention for community-dwelling older adults (AOTA, 2017a): www.aota.org/Practice/Productive-Aging/Evidence-based/CAT-PA-Falls-Multifactorial.aspx
   - Support group interventions that include a virtual element for Alzheimer's caregivers (AOTA, 2017b): www.aota.org/Practice/Productive-Aging/Evidence-based/CAT-Group-ALZ.aspx
   - The policy implications, community partnerships, and program development of community mobility interventions (AOTA, 2013): www.aota.org/~/media/Corporate/Files/Secure/Practice/CCL/Low-Vision/Community%20Mobility.pdf

REFERENCES

Aldrich, R. M. (2008). From complexity theory to transactionalism: Moving occupational science forward in theorizing the complexities of behavior. *Journal of Occupational Science, 15*(3), 147–156.

American Occupational Therapy Association. (2013). *Driving and community mobility for older adults.* Retrieved from www.aota.org/~/media/Corporate/Files/Secure/Practice/CCL/Low-Vision/Community%20Mobility

American Occupational Therapy Association. (2014). Occupational therapy practice framework: Domain and process (3rd ed.). *American Journal of Occupational Therapy, 68*(Suppl. 1), S1–S48. doi:10.5014/ajot.2014.682006 *68*(Suppl. 1), S1–S48. doi:10.5014/ajot.2014.682006

American Occupational Therapy Association. (2015). Occupational therapy code of ethics (2015). *American Journal of Occupational Therapy, 69*(Suppl. 3), 6913410030. http://dx.doi.org/10.5014/ajot.2015.696S03

American Occupational Therapy Association. (2017a). *Critically appraised topic: Evidence for the effect of multifactorial fall-prevention interventions on community-dwelling older adults.* Retrieved from www.aota.org/Practice/Productive-Aging/Evidence-based/CAT-PA-Falls-Multifactorial.aspx

American Occupational Therapy Association. (2017b). *Evidence for the effect of group interventions for caregivers of people with dementia.* Retrieved from www.aota.org/~/media/Corporate/Files/Secure/Practice/CCL/Alz/AlzCATs2016/Alz_Group_Interventions_mini_CAT.pdf

American Occupational Therapy Association. (2017c). Vision 2025. *American Journal of Occupational Therapy, 71,* 7103420010. doi:10.5014/ajot.2017.713002

Bailliard, A., and Aldrich, R. M. (2016). Occupational justice in everyday occupational therapy practice. In D. Sakellariou and N. Polland (Eds.), *Occupational therapies without borders: Integrating justice with practice* (2nd ed., 83–94). Oxford, UK: Elsevier.

Bandura, A. (1977). *Social learning theory.* Upper Saddle River, NJ: Prentice Hall.

Bandura, A. (2004). Health promotion by social cognitive means. *Health Education and Behavior, 31*(2), 143–164.

Bandura, A. (2006). Toward a psychology of human agency. *Perspectives on Psychological Science, 1*(2), 164–180.

Bazyk, S. (2011). Occupational therapy process: A public health approach to promoting mental health in children and youth. In S. Bazyk (Ed.), *Mental health promotion, prevention, and intervention with children and youth: A guiding framework for occupational therapy* (pp. 21–43). Bethesda, MD: American Occupational Therapy Association.

Bazyk, S., Demerjian, L., Horvath, F. and Doxsey, L. (2018). The Comfortable Cafeteria Program for promoting student participation and enjoyment: An outcome study. *American Journal of Occupational Therapy, 72*(3): 7203205060p1. doi:10.5014/ajot.2018.025379

Bereolos, N. M. (2007). *The role of acculturation in the health belief model for Mexican-Americans with type II diabetes* [Abstract]. Denton, TX. Retrieved from UNT Digital Library http://digital.library.unt.edu/ark:/67531/metadc4001/http://digital.library.unt.edu/ark:/67531/metadc4001/

Bishop, A. C., Baker, G. R., Boyle, T. A., and MacKinnon, N. J. (2015). Using the health belief model to explain patient involvement in patient safety. *Health Expectations, 18*(6), 3019–3033. doi:10.1111/hex.12286

Brainy quote. (2018). *Herbert Hoover quotes.* Retrieved from https://www.brainyquote.com/quotes/herbert_hoover_756126

Classen, S., Awadzi, K. D., and Mkanta, W. W. (2008). Person-vehicle-environment interactions predicting crash-related injury among older drivers. *American Journal of Occupational Therapy, 62,* 580–587.

Cutchin, M. P. (2001). Deweyan integration: Moving beyond place attachment in elderly migration theory. *International Journal of Aging and Human Development, 52,* 29–44. http://dx.doi.org/10.2190/af2d-a0t4-q14c-1rtw

Cutchin, M. P. (2004). Using Deweyan philosophy to rename and reframe adaptation-to-environment. *American Journal of Occupational Therapy, 58,* 303–312.

Cutchin, M. P., Aldrich, R. M., Bailliard, A. L., and Coppola, S. (2008). Action theories for occupational science: The contributions of Dewey and Bourdieu. *Journal of Occupational Science, 15*(3), 157–165. doi:10.1080/14427591.2008.9686625(3)

Cutchin, M. P., and Dickie, V. A. (2013). *Transactional perspectives on occupation.* Dordrecht, NL: Springer.

de las heras de Pablo, C-G., Abelenda, J., and Parkinson, S. (2017). MOHO-based program development. In R. R. Taylor (Ed.), *Kielhofner's model of human occupation* (5th ed., pp. 397–417). Philadelphia, PA: Wolters Kluwer.

Deshpande, S., Basil, M. D., and Basil, D. Z. (2009). Factors influencing healthy eating habits among college students: An application of the health belief model. *Health Marketing Quarterly, 26*(2), 145–164.

Dewey, R. E. (1977). *The philosophy of John Dewey: A critical exposition of his method, metaphysics, and theory of knowledge.* The Hague, NL: Martinus Nijhoff.

Dickie, V., Cutchin, M. P., and Humphrey, R. (2006). Occupation as transactional experience: A critique of individualism in occupational science. *Journal of Occupational Science, 13*(1), 83–93. doi:10.1080/14427591.2006.9686573

Dube, S. R., Anda, R. F., Felitti, V. J., Chapman, D. P., Williamson, D. F., and Giles, W. H. (2001). Childhood abuse, household dysfunction, and the risk of attempted suicide throughout the lifespan. *Journal of the American Medical Association, 286*(24), 3089–3096.

Fesmire, S. (2003). *John Dewey and moral imagination: Pragmatism in ethics.* Bloomington: Indiana University Press.

Fritz, H., and Cutchin, M. P. (2017). The transactional perspective on occupation: A way to transcend the individual in health promotion interventions and research. *Journal of Occupational Science, 24*(4), 446–457. doi:10.1080/14427591.2017.1366354

Garrison, J. (2001). An introduction to Dewey's theory of functional "trans-action": An alternative paradigm for activity theory. *Mind, Culture, and Activity, 8*(4), 275–296. http://dx.doi.org/10.1207/S15327884MCA0804_02

Green, L. W., and Kreuter, M. W. (1991). *Health promotion planning: An educational and environmental approach* (2nd ed.). Mountainview, CA: Mayfield.

Green, L. W., and Kreuter, M. W. (2005). *Health promotion planning: An educational and ecological approach* (4th ed.). New York, NY: McGraw-Hill.

Hammel, J., Jones, R., Gossett, A., and Morgan, A. (2006). Examining barriers and supports to community living and participation after a stroke from a participatory action research approach. *Topics in Stroke Rehabilitation, 13*(3), 43–58.

Hammond, A., Young, A., and Kidao, R. (2004). A randomized controlled trial of occupational therapy for people with early rheumatoid arthritis. *Annals of the Rheumatic Diseases, 63,* 23–30.

Harting, J., Rutten, G. M., Rutten, S. T., and Kremers, S. P. (2009). A qualitative application of the diffusion of innovations theory to examine determinants of guideline adherence among physical therapists. *Physical Therapy, 89*(3), 221–232.

Hartley, E. M., Hoch, M. C., and Cramer, R. J. (2018). Health belief model and theory of planned behavior: A theoretical approach for enhancing lower extremity injury prevention program participation. *International Journal of Athletic Therapy and Training, 23*(1), 16–20. doi:10.1123/ijatt.2017-0016

Hasler, G., Delsignore, A., Milos, G., Buddeberg, C., and Schnyder, U. (2014). Application of Prochaska's transtheoretical model of change to patients with eating disorders. *Journal of Psychosomatic Research, 57*(1), 67–72. doi:10.1016/S0022-3999(03)00562-2

Heatwole Shank, K., and Cutchin, M. P. (2016). Processes of developing "community livability" in older age. *Journal of Aging Studies, 39,* 66–72. doi:10.1016/j.jaging.2016.11.001.

Johnson, C. S., McLeod, W., Kennedy, L., and McLeod, K. (2008). Osteoporosis health beliefs among younger and older men and women. *Health Education and Behavior, 35*(5), 721–733.

Jones, M., Hocking, C., and McPherson, K. (2017). Communities with participation-enabling skills: A study of children with traumatic brain injury and their shared occupations. *Journal of Occupational Science, 24*(1), 88–104. doi:10.1080/14427591.2016.1224444

Kielhofner, G. (1980). A model of human occupation, part 3: Benign and vicious cycles. *American Journal of Occupational Therapy, 34*(11), 731–737.

Kielhofner, G. (1997). *Conceptual foundations of occupational therapy* (2nd ed.). Philadelphia, PA: F. A. Davis.

Kielhofner, G. (2002). *A model of human occupation: Theory and application* (3rd ed.). Baltimore, MD: Lippincott Williams and Wilkins.

Kielhofner, G. (2017). Habitation: Patterns of daily occupation. In R. R. Taylor (Ed.), *Kielhofner's model of human occupation* (5th ed., pp. 51–67). Philadelphia, PA: Wolters Kluwer.

Kielhofner, G., and Burke, J. (1980). A model of human occupation, part 1: Conceptual framework and content. *American Journal of Occupational Therapy, 34,* 572–581.

Kielhofner, G., and Burke, J. (1985). Components and determinants of human occupation. In G. Kielhofner (Ed.), *A model of human occupation: Theory and application* (pp. 12–36). Baltimore, MA: Williams and Wilkins.

Knightbridge, S. M., King, R., and Rolfe, T. J. (2006). Using participatory action research in a community-based initiative addressing complex mental health needs. *Australian and New Zealand Journal of Psychiatry, 40*(4), 325–332. https://doi.org/10.1080/j.1440-1614.2006.01798.x

McKenzie, J. F., Neiger, B. L., and Thackeray, R. (2009). *Planning, implementing, and evaluating health promotion programs: A primer* (5th ed.). San Francisco, CA: Pearson Benjamin Cummings.

McNulty, M. C., Johnson, J., Poole, J. L., and Winkle, M. (2003). Using the transtheoretical model of change to implement home safety modifications with community-dwelling older adults: An exploratory study. *Physical and Occupational Therapy in Geriatrics, 21*(4), 53–66.

Miller, R. J., and Schwartz, K. (2004). What is theory, and why does it matter? In K. F. Walker and F. M. Ludwig (Eds.), *Perspectives on theory for the practice of occupational therapy* (3rd ed., pp. 1–26). Austin, TX: PRO-ED.

Mo, P. K. H., Chong, E. S. K., Mak, W. W. S., Wong, S. Y .S., and Lau, J. T. F. (2016). Physical activity in people with mental illness in Hong Kong: Application of the health belief model. *Journal of Sport and Exercise Psychology, 38*(2), 203–208.

National Cancer Institute. (2005). *Theory at a glance* (2nd ed.). Bethesda, MD: National Institutes of Health. Retrieved from www.cancer.gov/publications/health-communication/pink-book.pdf

Parcel, G. S., and Baranowski, T. (1981). Social learning theory and health education. *Health Education, 12,* 14–18.

Prochaska, J. O., and DiClemente, C. C. (1983). Stages and processes of self-change of smoking: Toward an integrative model of change. *Journal of Counseling and Clinical Psychology, 51*(3), 390–395.

Prochaska, J. O., and DiClemente, C. C. (1992). Stages of change in the modification of behavior problems. In M. Hersen, R. M. Eisler, and P. M. Miller (Eds.), *Progress in behavior modification* (pp. 184–214). Sycamore, IL: Sycamore.

Prochaska, J. O., Norcross, J. C., and DiClemente, C. C. (1994). *Changing for good: A revolutionary six-stage program for overcoming bad habits and moving your life positively forward.* New York, NY: Avon Books.

Reitz, S. M. (1990, Fall). *Community development model: An application of the model of human occupation.* Unpublished paper for Health 688Community Health Issues for Minority Populations, University of Maryland, College Park.

Reitz, S. M., Scaffa, M. E., Campbell, R. M., and Rhynders, P. A. (2010). Health behavior frameworks for health promotion practice. In M. E. Scaffa, S. M. Reitz, and M. A. Pizzi (Eds.), *Occupational therapy in the promotion of health and wellness* (pp. 46–69). Philadelphia, PA: F. A. Davis.

Rhynders, P. A. (2010). Health behavior frameworks for health promotion practice. In M. E. Scaffa, S. M. Reitz, and M. A. Pizzi (Eds.), *Occupational therapy in the promotion of health and wellness* (pp. 46–69). Philadelphia, PA: F. A. Davis.

Rogers, E. M. (2003). *Diffusion of innovations* (5th ed.). New York, NY: Free Press.

Rosenstock, I. (1974). Historical origins of the health belief model. In M. Becker (Ed.), *The health belief model and personal behavior.* Thorofare, NJ: SLACK.

Rosenstock, I. M., Strecher, V. J., and Becker, M. H. (1994). The health belief model and HIV risk behavior change. In R. J. DiClemente and J. L. Peterson (Eds.), *Preventing AIDS: Theories and methods for behavioral interventions* (pp. 5–24). New York, NY: Plenum.

Scott, P., Miller, R. J., and Walker, K. F. (2004). Gary Kielhofner. In K. F. Walker and F. M. Ludwig (Eds.), *Perspectives on theory for the practice of occupational therapy* (3rd ed., pp. 267–325). Austin, TX: PRO-ED.

Strauss, A., and Corbin, J. (1990). *Basics of qualitative research: Grounded theory procedures and techniques.* London, England: Sage.

Sudsawad, P. (2005). Concepts in clinical scholarship—a conceptual framework to increase usability of outcome research for evidence-based practice. *American Journal of Occupational Therapy, 59,* 351–355.

Taylor, R. R. (2017a). Introduction to the UIC MOHO Clearing House and MOHOWeb website. In R. R. Taylor (Ed.), *Kielhofner's model of human occupation* (pp. 486–489, 5th ed.). Philadelphia, PA: Wolters Kluwer.

Taylor, R. R. (2017b). Preface and editorial introduction to the 5th edition. In R. R. Taylor (Ed.), *Kielhofner's model of human occupation* (5th ed., pp. vii–ix). Philadelphia, PA: Wolters Kluwer.

Tham, K., Erikson, A., Fallaphour, M., Taylor, R. R., and Kielhofner, G. (2017). Performance capacity and the lived body. In R. R. Taylor (Ed.), *Kielhofner's model of human occupation* (5th ed., pp. 74–90). Philadelphia, PA: Wolters Kluwer.

Wang, J. H., Liang, W., Schwartz, M. D., Lee, M. M., Kreling, B., and Mandelblatt, J. S. (2008). Development and evaluation of a culturally tailored educational video: Changing breast cancer-related behaviors in Chinese women. *Health Education and Behavior, 35*(6), 806–820.

Whiteford, G., and Townsend, E. (2011). Participatory occupational justice framework (POJF): Enabling occupational participation and inclusion. In F. Kronenburg, N. Pollard, and D. Sakellariou (Eds.), *Occupational therapies without borders: Volume 2—toward an ecology of occupation-based practices* (pp. 65–84). New York, NY: Elsevier.

Wilcock, A. A. (1999). Reflections on doing, being and becoming. *Australian Occupational Therapy Journal, 46*(1), 1–11.

Wilcock, A. A. (2006). *An occupational perspective of health* (2nd ed.). Thorofare, NJ: SLACK.

Wilcock, A. A. (2007). Occupation and health: Are they one and the same? *Journal of Occupational Science, 14*(1), 3–8.

Wilcock, A. A., and Hocking, C. (2015). An occupational perspective of health. Thorofare, NJ: SLACK.

Wilroy, J., and Turner, L. (2016). Utilizing social cognitive theory to enhance physical activity among people with spinal cord injuries. *American Journal of Health Studies, 31*(3), 123–131.

Yamkovenko, S. (2010). Backpack awareness day for people of all ages. American Occupational Therapy Association. Retrieved from http://aota.org/News/Consumer/Backpack-Day.aspx

Zhang, X., Yu, P., Yan, Y., and Spil, I. T. (2015). Using diffusion of innovation theory to understand the factors impacting patient acceptance and use of consumer e-health innovations: A case study in a primary care clinic. *BMC Health Services Research, 15*(71), 1–15. https://doi.org/10.1186/s12913-015-0726-2

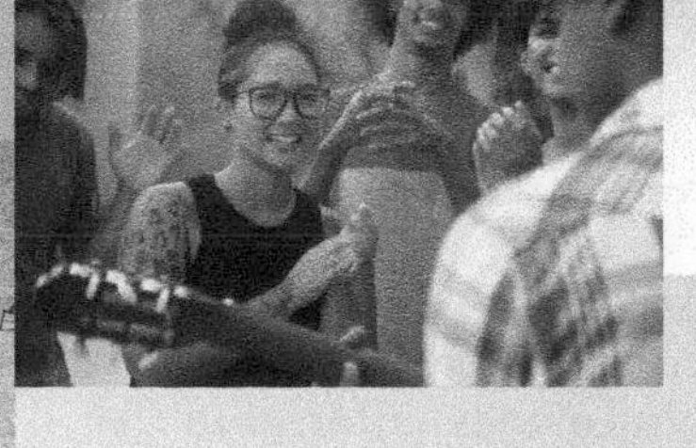

Chapter 4

Population Health: An Occupational Perspective

Clare Hocking, PhD, MHSc(OT), AdvDipOT, DipOT, and
Ann A. Wilcock, PhD, BAppScOT, GradDipPH, FCOT

Professional and social groups, and health personnel have a major responsibility to mediate between differing interests in society for the pursuit of health. Health promotion strategies and programmes should be adapted to local needs and possibilities of individual countries and regions to take into account differing social, cultural and economic systems.

—World Health Organization, 1986

Learning Outcomes

This chapter is designed to enable the reader to:

4-1 Understand health and ill-health from a population-based occupational perspective as distinct from an individualistic medical perspective.

4-2 Understand the sociopolitical factors that lead to unfair distribution, shortage, or lack of opportunity for populations to experience meaningful and satisfying lifestyles.

4-3 Appreciate diverse occupational issues and resultant health consequences for population groups across the globe.

4-4 Promote the general recognition of occupational justice as a specific aspect of social justice, particularly in relation to population health (Wilcock and Hocking, 2015).

4-5 Promote occupations to develop a sense of doing, being, belonging, and becoming at a community level.

4-6 Apply the participatory occupational justice framework to collaborate with disadvantaged populations and groups to develop capabilities and opportunities to do, be, belong, and become.

Key Terms

Balanced lifestyle
Becoming
Being
Belonging
Doing
Health inequities
Lifestyle
Occupational balance
Occupational justice
Participatory occupational justice framework

Introduction

The World Health Organization (WHO) explained in the Ottawa Charter (1986) that, as well as individuals, groups of people "must be able to identify and to realize aspirations" if they are "to reach a state of complete physical, mental and social well-being" (p. 1). The intent behind shifting the focus from securing the health of individuals to the well-being of groups, communities, and populations is more than simply a matter of scale. Where an individual focus is well suited to curative interventions, population health demands efforts to actively promote the well-being of the whole population, alongside working to eliminate threats to the health of groups with identified risk factors (Wilcock and Hocking, 2015). In taking a preventive approach, the architects of the Ottawa Charter recognized that health resources internationally would not stretch to providing high-quality medical services to populations globally and, perhaps more important, that people working to realize individual and communal aspirations actively maintain their own health if circumstances allow.

Aligned with the idea that human well-being and aspirations work in tandem, the Ottawa Charter asserts that "health is created and lived by people within the settings of their everyday life; where they learn, work, play, and love" (WHO, 1986, p. 2). The charter thus explicitly acknowledges the health consequences of the things people do on an ongoing basis—across the spectrum of educational, productive, and playful occupations, including those that express love of other people, animals, and the natural world. Recognition that where people do things, the settings of everyday occupation, also plays a part in generating good or ill-health is amplified by the WHO's (2013) Healthy Settings approach to population health. Once again, the WHO is lifting the gaze from narrowly focusing on patients receiving health care to considering everyone who occupies a hospital or any other setting, be it a city, village, community, island, market, school, workplace, home, aged care facility, prison, or natural setting.

This chapter explores population health from an occupational perspective, attending to the things people routinely do and the settings in which they do them. The discussion is underpinned by the concept of social determinants of health—the socially modifiable factors that cause some sectors of society to enjoy long and healthful lives, while others do not. Health inequities are considered from the perspective of occupational balance, as the outcome of doing, being, belonging, and becoming, and as an occupational justice issue. To begin, the concept of population health is outlined.

An Overview of Population Health

Population health is, potentially, an all-encompassing field of virtually everything that medical care aimed solely at treating illness is not. While no universally agreed upon definition exists, there is general consensus that it covers a broad canvas including clinical care, social services, and environmental interventions based on the current understanding of the determinants of health that emerged in the latter half of the 20th century. One widely adopted view, based on a review of definitions proposed by health policy organizations and scholarly articles, describes population health as the "health outcomes of a group of individuals, including the distribution of such outcomes within the group" (Kindig and Stoddart, 2003, p. 380). How that plays out depends on the health outcome of concern and how broadly or narrowly the group in question is defined. The population referred to may be all the citizens of a country or geographic region, members of a specific community, or people with a shared characteristic (e.g., age, gender, ethnicity, income level) or may be identified according to a diagnosis or because its members receive care from a specific health-care provider.

Irrespective of how the group is defined, the most pressing question is why some sectors of the population are healthier and live longer than others (Young, 1998). Indeed, the main challenge for population health is the significant differences in health that currently exist between socioeconomic groups. Population health experts acknowledge that **health inequities,** such as higher morbidity and mortality rates, are caused by inequalities in education, job choice, and income, as well as differential access to transportation, housing, healthy physical environments, and public safety (National Academies of Sciences, Engineering, and Medicine, 2017). These issues could be lessened by the "active engagement of many policy sectors, not only of the public health and health care systems but also of many other policy sectors, including education, social security, working life, city planning" (Mackenbach, Meerding, and Kunst, 2011, p. 412).

The consequences of inaction are substantial. In 2004, deaths attributable to health inequalities in the European Union (EU) were estimated at 707,000 per year, and the prevalent cases of illness "that can be attributed to health inequalities is estimated to be more than 33 million" (Mackenbach et al., 2011, p. 415). Given the current refugee crisis overwhelming the EU, this situation has likely worsened. It is now understood that improving population health requires a commitment to health equity, as well as a holistic focus on both the social and biological determinants of health (Diez Roux, 2016). Framing health in terms of equity causes a shift of attention, from broad-based interventions that aim to improve the health status of the population at large to targeting those groups and communities most affected by disparities in social, economic, and physical environments—that is, the extrinsic and potentially modifiable factors that cause ill-health.

Those factors include all forms of discrimination, overcrowding, homelessness and displacement, high levels of alcohol and drug abuse, domestic and neighborhood violence, armed conflict, child labor, human trafficking and modern-day slavery, lack of access to clean water and healthy food, inadequate sanitation, poor-quality housing, famine, exposure to disease-carrying organisms, natural and man-made disasters, pollution, and other forms of environmental degradation (Wilcock and Hocking, 2015). Exposure to such health threats is commonly associated with absolute poverty (i.e., living on less than US $1.90 per person per day; World Bank, 2015) or relative poverty, which is more typical in countries with wide income disparities (Perry, 2014), as well as with being female or having a disability. In many cases, the root causes are intertwined with historical injustices, including the oppression of women and minority groups, colonization, and repressive political regimes with apartheid policies, in addition to systemic corruption, the rise of neoliberal politics, the imposition of economic sanctions, and forced and voluntary migration.

> **Engage Your Brain 4-1**
>
> Which principles in the American Occupational Therapy Association's (2015) *Occupational Therapy Code of Ethics (2015)* address health inequities? What is the role of the occupational therapy practitioner in addressing health inequities and occupational injustice?

The scope of population health initiatives thus encompasses proactive approaches to provide the very basics of healthy living—clean air and water, sanitation, nutritious food, safety, and shelter. Equally important to these biological necessities, health and well-being depend on the social, economic, and environmental conditions in which people live. Addressing the question of what constitutes "sufficient" conditions for well-being and thus when societies should intervene to improve the conditions in which people live and work, Amartya Sen (1999) defined a minimally decent life as "avoiding escapable morbidity and premature mortality, etc., to [attaining] more complex achievements such as being happy, having self-respect, taking part in the life of the community, and so on" (p. 39). While a minimally decent life falls short of the lofty goal envisioned in the Ottawa Charter (1986) of individuals, groups, and populations enjoying "complete physical, mental and social wellbeing" (p. 1), it directs population health policy-makers and practitioners to focus on groups and communities in the most vulnerable circumstances.

In the spirit of occupational therapy practitioners becoming active in improving population health, the American Occupational Therapy Foundation (2003) drew attention to the United Nations (UN) Millennium Development Goals to:

1. Eradicate extreme poverty and hunger
2. Achieve universal primary education
3. Promote gender equality and empower women
4. Reduce child mortality
5. Improve maternal health
6. Combat HIV/AIDS, malaria, and other diseases
7. Ensure environmental sustainability
8. Develop a global partnership for development

The foundation's interest in population health has not yet manifest in wide-ranging, well-recognized programs or multidisciplinary actions that address the occupational nature of health and illness. More attention to, and advocacy for, population health is a necessity. Toward that end, this chapter bridges the gap between the Millennium Development Goals and the occupational perspective of health and well-being more familiar to occupational therapy practitioners.

Engage Your Brain 4-2

What competencies are needed to address the United Nations Millennium Development Goals through an occupational perspective?

Occupational Perspective of Population Health

In promoting an occupational perspective of population health, the perspective needs to be that if all "economic and social activity has the capacity to influence health outcomes" (Woodley, 2001, p. 7), then population health is involved with every occupation that bears on people's well-being. Support for an occupational, as distinct from a singularly social, economic, environmental, or biological, perspective on population health comes from evidence of the health advantages of traditional occupational lifestyles. For instance, nomadic populations, such as First Nation Australians, derived health advantages from periodically shifting camps as they sought out seasonal food supplies. Relocation avoided the health problems associated with permanent settlements, such as depletion of essential food sources, sedentary lifestyles, and the buildup of disease organisms due to unhygienic waste disposal systems, while also providing adventure and enhancing mutual support and bonding among members of the group (King-Boyes, 1977). Similarly, the virtual absence of heart disease, cancer, diabetes, obesity, and dementia among present-day hunter-gatherer tribes has been attributed to the match between humans' biological characteristics and their lifestyle and diet (McMichael, 2001).

Further evidence that shared occupational patterns have an impact on population health is provided by archaeological research. For example, population health sharply declined when humans transitioned from nomadic foraging to settled agricultural lifestyles approximately 12,000 years ago. Skeletal evidence points to considerably higher levels of dental decay and arthritis, along with a decrease of several inches in stature, than in the immediately preceding generations, which is consistent with less diverse diets and periodic crop failures (Diamond, 2002; McMichael, 2001). As agricultural and animal husbandry techniques advanced and food sources became more secure, people were able to live together in much higher numbers than previously. Inevitably, the rise of villages, towns, and cities led to hyperinfestations of disease organisms, with consequent outbreaks of leprosy, malaria, diphtheria, smallpox, scarlet fever, tuberculosis, syphilis, typhus, and bubonic plague (Munford, 1963).

Industrialization, which enabled the mass production of cheap consumer goods and thus destroyed the livelihood of large numbers of people engaged in cottage industries, is a further example of a large-scale shift in people's everyday occupations with an immediate impact on population health. No longer able to support themselves by handcrafting objects using traditional tools and techniques, many thousands of people were forced to move to cities to seek employment. The combination of separation from friends and relations; overcrowded, unsanitary living conditions and the consumption of rotten food, forced on them by starvation-level wages; long hours of heavy labor; and workplace accidents (Eversley, 1965; Wilcock and Hocking, 2015) amounted to rates of disease and injury that can only be termed a population health disaster.

Further evidence supporting the utility of an occupational perspective of population health is provided by occupational medicine, which is concerned with health in the workplace. While there are recorded examples of occupations directly conferring health benefits to a subpopulation of workers, such as the immunity to smallpox observed among milkmaids who had been exposed to cowpox (Glynn and Glynn, 2004), there are many more examples of causative links between specific trades and disfiguring or lethal health conditions. "Black lung" among coal miners and "mad hatter" disease, the result of mercury and lead poisoning from the process used to turn fur into felt, are widely recognized examples. Further historical examples are found in Oakley's (2018) book, *Women, Peace and Welfare,* which catalogs the appalling working conditions of certain classes of American and British women employed in industrial settings in the late 19th and early 20th centuries. Among others, Oakley reports accounts of the following:

- Women in fish-curing sheds standing in filthy salty water, their hands and shins covered in exposed sores
- Match girls inhaling phosphorous in the process of making and packing matches and developing "phossy jaw," a lethal form of bone cancer that turned the sides of their faces green and black and caused foul-smelling pus to ooze out as their jawbones gradually decayed
- Laundresses being scalded by boiling water, burned by irons, and caught in mangling (wringing) and starching machines
- Women working in the pottery industry, often dismissed by medics as "hysterical," who suffered lead poisoning from inhaling and absorbing lead dust through the pores of their skin

Despite such evidence, a general lack of awareness of the relationship of occupation and population health was still apparent late into the 20th century, perhaps because of the overmedicalized understanding of health prevalent in Western, and possibly other, societies. For instance, a small-scale study of 100 Australians aged over 60 years found that the majority did not associate occupations over their lifetimes with their health status (Wilcock, 1990). The more recent emphasis at international and governmental levels on the necessity of physical exercise to avoid obesity and a range of noncommunicable diseases may be changing that perception. However, the focus on physical exercise demonstrates the general lack of understanding of the complex relationship of well-being and the things people do over their life spans, including occupations that are not physically taxing. Accordingly, drawing on the ideas presented here, an occupational perspective of population health can bring valuable new insights to explain why the health and well-being of some groups of people are under threat, while other communities of people lead long and satisfying lives.

Population Health as Doing, Being, Belonging, and Becoming

In the discussion thus far, population health has been considered largely in terms of what people do—and by extension, what they do not do, whether because they lack the requisite knowledge, skill, self-perception, or resources or because their participation is subtly discouraged or more actively barred. The discussion now expands to also consider "what the doing does," or the sense of being, belonging, and becoming that people derive from the things they do (Wilcock, 2007). Each of these concepts is discussed in turn in relation to well-being; the first will be doing. **Doing** refers to everything of meaning that people do in their daily lives (Wilcock and Hocking, 2015).

When members of a group of people have a similar pattern of occupations, their daily round of activities is commonly referred to as a **lifestyle.** Determining whether the lifestyles available to, condoned by, or forced onto a group of people support health and well-being is not as simple as adding up all the things they do. The variety, intensity, duration, timing, purpose, and subjective experience of occupations are also important. The concept of balance is useful in bringing such considerations together. An **occupational balance** has traditionally been conceptualized in terms of engaging in relatively equal amounts of work, self-care, rest, and leisure occupations. From this perspective, it seems reasonable to suggest that people's well-being can be ascertained by finding out how much of each type of occupation they typically do, including whether they have sufficient periods of rest and sleep to meet biological needs.

Although individuals have preferences for their optimal balance of occupations, it is possible to apply the concept of balance to groups of people with similar patterns of occupation, relative to groups with different occupational patterns. For example, knowledge of working mothers doing a "second shift" comprising housework, childcare, grocery shopping, and family activity scheduling, in addition to their paid work role, is so commonplace that a Google search generated over 1 million hits. Compared to working fathers, the two "shifts" these women work each day can scarcely be described as a balanced lifestyle, even for the most organized women. Occupational scientists have documented other lifestyles that appear equally imbalanced:

- Shift workers who compromise their sleeping schedules in order to fulfill family and social obligations (Walker, 1996)

- Homeless people who have daily routines but report doing things just to fill their time (Thomas, Gray, and McGinty, 2017)
- People with mental illness who spend comparatively more time sleeping or engaged in relatively unfulfilling self-care occupations than others (Eklund, Erlandsson, and Leufstadius, 2010)
- Professional musicians who continue to devote hours to practicing and performing music, even after they develop painful musculoskeletal conditions that indicate the need for rest (Guptill, 2012)

As these examples illustrate, an imbalance of occupations measured in terms of doing "too much" or "too little" of particular kinds of activities provides some insight into the well-being of specific groups. Disruptions to sleep patterns also come to light as a factor in at least two of the imbalanced patterns of work, self-care, rest, and leisure described.

Thinking about occupational balance in terms of work, rest, and so on is, however, problematic. From a research and practical standpoint, that way of categorizing doing is slippery because people categorize their occupations differently; what is work for some groups might be leisure for others (Christiansen, 1994). In addition, categorizing occupation in accordance with Western understandings of the nature of doing creates a culturally uncertain basis for applying the concept of balance to non-Western populations. For example, the separation of work and leisure, the Protestant valuing of work over leisure, or the Marxist concept of work as onerous may not be applicable in Eastern contexts.

Matuska and Christiansen's (2008) model of lifestyle balance offers an alternate conceptualization of balance that potentially renders it more universally relevant. The model proposes that a **balanced lifestyle,** defined as one that is satisfying, meaningful, and sustainable, is achieved when people's occupations:

- Meet basic needs for sustained biological health and physical safety
- Enact "rewarding and self-affirming relationships"
- Make them "feel interested, engaged, challenged and competent"
- "Create meaning and a positive personal identity"
- "Organize time and energy" to achieve important goals and values (Wagman, Håkansson, Matuska, Björklund, and Falkmer, 2012, pp. 109–110)

Elements of doing, being, belonging, and becoming are readily discernible in this prescription. Enacting relationships through doing connects occupation to experiences of **belonging,** defined as being accepted by others and feeling secure in relationships and connected to place. At a population level, this might be experienced and expressed as the level of group cohesion, the network of relationships holding a community together, and the collective occupations that create bonds and a sense of common identity and shared history. In indigenous populations, such ideas might manifest as a deep sense of connection to land and the responsibility of caring for its well-being. Occupations that create meaning and align with values link us to the spiritual dimension of life, fostering contemplation and an existential sense of "being." **Being** refers to people's essential nature—that is, what drives them to do things (Wilcock and Hocking, 2015). At a group or population level, this might be evident in shared creation myths, value systems, or tolerance for different ways of "being" in the world.

Becoming, in an occupational sense, relates to people's development over their lifetimes. When people's repertoire of occupations includes those that generate feelings of competence in the present moment while challenging them to do and be more and to organize future occupations to achieve goals, there is a sense of becoming more; of fulfilling people's occupational potential (Asaba and Wicks, 2010) to become what they have the capacity to be (Wilcock and Hocking, 2015). At a population level, becoming relates to equitable opportunities for all groups within society to learn, work, play, and love (WHO, 1986). The kinds of occupations available, and thus the kinds of people the population can become, are largely determined by the economic basis of a society and how well its educational system equips people to participate in culturally valued occupations. The distribution of those opportunities across different sectors of society is determined by regulations and social mores specifying who can do what and thus the opportunities that are opened up or closed down for specific populations or groups. See Table 4-1 for a detailed analysis of the alignment between doing, being, belonging, and becoming and a balanced lifestyle.

To summarize to this point, the concept of lifestyle balance can be as equally applied to groups of people living a similar lifestyle as it can to individuals. Lifestyle balance can be operationalized as doing, being, belonging, and becoming. That suggests that the occupational well-being of a group or population can be appraised by considering its opportunities to do, be, belong, and become and whether it can convert those opportunities into a satisfying, meaningful, and sustainable lifestyle that supports health and well-being in the long term (Sen, 1999). To further this idea, the occupational science literature will be reviewed for research evidence that doing, being, belonging, and becoming support population health, while barriers to any or all of these aspects of doing can threaten the health of affected groups.

Understanding and Promoting Population Health

In truth, doing, being, belonging, and becoming are inseparable. However, in the discussion that follows, these elements of occupation are artificially teased apart to demonstrate the value of an occupational perspective to understanding population health issues and envisaging effective interventions. The approach described considers the health and well-being of groups and communities in vulnerable circumstances in terms of their opportunities to do, be, belong, and become.

Doing

Multiple factors have the potential to disrupt or deprive groups of people of occupations they value. Members of a subgroup of North Americans with osteoarthritis of the knee, for example, described their symptoms as limiting engagement in occupation to the point where their identity was threatened. As their occupational losses mounted and strategies that had helped them participate became ineffective, they reached a "tipping point" at which they decided to seek knee joint replacement surgery (Man, Davis, Webster, and Polatajko, 2017). In a very different context, Palestinian olive growers living under military occupation were actively prevented from planting, tending, and harvesting olives by the Israeli Defense Forces and settlers. Rather than give up or retreat, they practiced acts of resistance, including recruiting international volunteers to assist with the work and act as witnesses to incidents of aggression (Simaan, 2017). As these very different examples illustrate, taking heed of patterns of eroding, lost, or blocked occupations may assist with understanding threats to population health, identifying pivotal points at which members of the population are prepared to take action, and determining why people persist with their actions, even against great odds of failure.

An occupational perspective also opens up new possibilities for effective preventive interventions. Such was the case in the Well Elderly Study, a large-scale intervention to promote occupational well-being among low-income older residents of downtown Los Angeles. Designed by occupational science faculty at the University of Southern California, exploratory research underpinning the program identified personal and community factors that explained the participants' progressive withdrawal from stimulating occupations while suggesting the knowledge, experiences, and motivation that would propel them toward active participation in meaningful occupations and improved health status (Jackson, Carlson, Mandel, Zemke, and Clark, 1998).

Being

Digital technologies are now a pervasive aspect of many people's daily lives, but what of those born decades before computers, smartphones, and Internet banking were even imagined? A small-scale study in Sweden found that older adults who used electronic devices to manage everyday tasks and communicate with friends and family had encompassed digital participation as part of their identity (Fischl, Asaba, and Nilsson, 2017). Through the technologies, they experienced meaning in daily life. Moreover, they were not passive users; rather, they actively managed their online identities. The mastery of digital technologies had become an integrated part

Table 4-1 Doing, Being, Belonging, and Becoming in Relation to Lifestyle Balance and Population Health

Wilcock's Dimensions of Occupation	Definition (Wilcock and Hocking, 2015)	Matuska and Christiansen's Model of Lifestyle Balance (2008)	Application at a Population Level
Doing	Everything of meaning that people do in their daily lives Enabled by humans' biological heritage (upright stance, binocular vision, opposable thumbs, capacity for language, etc.) The means of meeting survival needs Exists on a continuum with rest/sleep An important determinant of health and illness	Sustain biological health and physical safety (e.g., gather food, construct shelter and clothing) Organize time and energy (including time for restoration and sleep)	Collective occupations and traditions Typical lifestyles
Being	People's essential nature, what drives them to do things Relates to roles (being a parent, student, breadwinner) and to reflection/contemplation/stillness Includes the need for meaning, satisfaction, purpose	Feel interested, engaged, challenged, and competent Experience meaning Achieve values	Creation myths Shared value systems Tolerance for diverse ways of "being"
Belonging	Being recognized as a member of a group, community, or having ties to a place Provides feelings of connection, attachment, being cared for and wanted, sharing interests and commitments, reciprocity, intimacy Context of expressing empathy, willingness to follow directions or take the lead, a sense of humor Shaped by social conventions, behavioral norms, rituals, celebrations Always provisional or in process; connections are forged, developed, and terminated	Enact rewarding and self-affirming relationships	Create group cohesion and a sense of community through collective occupations (e.g., traditions) Sense of having a shared occupational history In indigenous populations, a spiritual connection to land with a sense of responsibility for caring for its well-being
Becoming	What people have the capacity to become, occupational potential Relates to talents, aptitudes, and experience Achieved through doing; thus stunted by occupational barriers Might be incremental or transformational An ever-incomplete process	Create a positive personal identity Achieve important goals	Equitable occupational possibilities, as determined by legal, economic, educational, employment, and other systems

of their being. Not all older adults, however, access digital technologies. Contrary to their expectations, Kottorp and colleagues (2016) found that poverty, rather than cognitive impairment, was the primary barrier to the ownership and use of digital technologies among older adults in Sweden. As everyday processes, from shopping to banking to contacting health services to maintaining relationships, become increasingly digital, being excluded from this increasingly vital means of "being" in the 21st century signals a population health threat for low-income as well as cognitively impaired older adults. Recognition of that threat is a first step toward addressing the needs of these specific populations to "be" citizens of the 21st century.

Belonging

The natural state for human beings is to belong to family groups and, beyond that, to the greater society. Groups and communities excluded from mainstream society, therefore, are extremely vulnerable to poor health outcomes. Instances of groups that do not "belong" to the society in which they live have been documented in the occupational science literature. Two examples are the South American women employed as domestic workers in Spain (Rivas-Quarneti, Movilla-Fernández, and Magalhães, 2018) and the Romanians begging on the streets in Sweden (Johansson, Fristedt, Boström, Björklund, and Wagman, 2018). Both groups face very limited opportunities to secure dignified work and thus lack opportunities to use their full capabilities. Their only available means of earning a living is physically arduous and carries the risk of abusive behaviors from citizens of the country. While their situation is eased by contact with compatriots and family at home, daily life is highly stressful and demeaning, with little recourse to legal protections.

In comparison, Norwegian children with disabilities have legislation protecting their right to inclusion in organized sports. In that context, participation can be an experience of acceptance of differences in capacity and of being encouraged and appreciated (Asbjørnslett and Bekken, 2016). While inclusion does not change the fact of disability, feelings of belonging actively support well-being.

Becoming

All people have the potential to develop over their lifetimes. Circumstances, however, thwart that potential for many millions of people. The plight of asylum seekers held in camps while their applications for citizenship are considered is a well-documented example. For many of those in Australian detention centers, having nothing to do is deeply distressing; life is on hold, and the motivation and ability to prepare for the future ebbs away (Crawford, Turpin, Nayar, Steel, and Durand, 2016). Occupational deprivation is also true in the U.S. prison system and can be a hindrance to successful community integration upon release (Smith et al., 2018). While youths raised in marginalized communities in postapartheid South Africa do have choices about what to do and become, their circumstances and occupational experiences channel them into intergenerational educational underachievement, poorly paid jobs, and drug abuse (Galvaan, 2015). In contrast, Canadian youths with and without disabilities who secure a role as a volunteer are more fortunate. They report that the experience enhances their occupational potential, as they both develop skills relevant to future employment and achieve greater clarity about their intended career pathway (Lindsay, Chan, Cancelliere, and Mistry, 2018). The outcomes for these populations are thus markedly different.

Context

As this discussion illustrates, approaching population health issues from an occupational perspective means being concerned with the capability of disadvantaged groups to do, be, and become and their opportunities to belong. In addition, reflection on the evidence provided here underscores the importance of the occupational setting in determining the health of the whole population or groups within it. For instance, the earliest evidence of human habitation is tied to the extended territory needed to support a nomadic lifestyle and the fertile plains that enabled the emergence of agricultural lifestyles. More recently, the squalor of rapidly growing industrial cities and the often dark and dangerous conditions endured by sweat laborers had a documented impact on population health. In the present day, the setting where population health is created might be a city street where someone is begging for a living, households employing immigrant workers, a marginalized neighborhood, or a government-run institution.

Settings shape people's occupational endeavors and aspirations, as well as determine who is present. For example, settings might include parents and children in playgrounds, factory workers and factory floor supervisors, or a cross section of society at a church service. Diverse groups within a setting can be distinguished by their demographic profile, whether by age, gender, educational achievements, social circumstances, cultural background, level of authority, or economic resources. It is a short step from observing differences between groups to acknowledging the inequities that ensure some fare better than others, in terms of having equitable opportunities to do, be, belong, and become; a balanced repertoire of occupations; and the possibility of securing positive health and well-being.

Engage Your Brain 4-3

What are the similarities and differences between the doing, being, belonging, becoming model described in this chapter and other occupational therapy theories and models?

Occupational Justice and Population Health

As defined by the World Federation of Occupational Therapists (2006), **occupational justice** asserts that people "have the right to participate in a range of occupations that enable them to flourish, fulfil their potential and experience satisfaction in a way consistent with their culture and beliefs" (p. 1). When viewed as efforts to enhance the health of all citizens, it is not immediately evident that population health is an issue of social or occupational justice. The government-sponsored dissemination of information about the benefits of exercise is one example. The message applies to young and old, rich and poor. Yet opportunities to act on that advice are not equally distributed. It is an occupational injustice and a social justice issue in that some sectors of society are severely disadvantaged by factors that are within the powers of a society to put right.

For example, children living in low-income households have multiple reasons for not being as physically active as more affluent children. There are obvious problems with funding sports equipment, club memberships, and transport to sports practices and events. There are also neighborhood factors (e.g., a reduced number of and poor-quality recreational facilities) and competing priorities (e.g., supporting the family by babysitting younger siblings, providing caregiving services, and working to contribute to the family income) (Stalsberg and Pedersen, 2010). In addition, children in low-income families are more likely to be obese and thus discouraged from joining in with physically demanding occupations because of the embarrassment experienced when changing into sports clothing (Murtagh, Dixey, and Rudolf, 2006) and the risk of being teased or bullied for their weight when they do join in (Edmunds, 2000).

Even where a contravention of human rights would be difficult to argue, it is believed that some form of occupational disadvantage or injustice is most likely present in population health issues. Accordingly, where disparities in doing, being, belonging, and becoming that pose a population health risk are identified, Townsend and Whiteford's (2005) **participatory occupational justice framework** (POJF) is advocated as the basis for developing occupationally focused interventions (see Fig. 4-1 and Chapter 3).

The POJF is designed to provide a reflective and collaborative process to address occupational injustices. While not prescriptive, it is a means "to raise consciousness of occupational injustice, engage collaboratively with partners, mediate on an agreed plan, strategize how to find resources, support implementation and continuous evaluation, and inspire advocacy for sustainability or closure" (Whiteford, Jones, Rahal, and Suleman, 2018, p. 498). With its emphasis on working in partnership with identified populations and other agencies, focus on participation (understood in this context to mean social inclusion), and philosophy of empowering marginalized populations, the POJF is well aligned with the WHO's (2013) key principles for creating healthy settings, community participation, partnership,

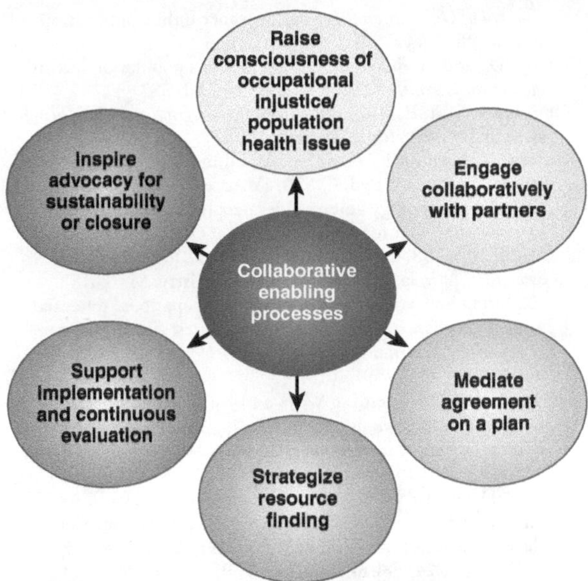

Figure 4-1 The participatory occupational justice framework. *(Adapted from "The Participatory Occupational Justice Framework as a Tool for Change: Three Contrasting Case Narratives," by G. Whiteford, K. Jones, C. Rahal, and A. Suleman, 2018,* Journal of Occupational Science, *25[4], 498. Reprinted with permission.)*

empowerment, and equity. It is readily applicable to the development of population health initiatives.

Summary

- Understanding people as occupational beings brings a valuable new insight to population health and is consistent with and operationalizes the tenets of the Ottawa Charter in its assertion that health is created where people learn, work, play, and love.
- Viewing population health from a perspective of doing, being, belonging, and becoming sheds light on the nature and extent of systemic challenges to population health, such as health inequities and occupational injustice.
- An occupational perspective provides clarity about the population health implications of what groups of people have opportunities to do (participation or exclusion), the existential outcomes of doing (meaning, values), whether their doing enhances belonging (positive relationships, connection), and how people develop and change over time as a result of the things they do (identity, self-respect, competence).
- In addition, an occupational perspective directly informs action: what groups of people, population health advocates, and societies as a whole might do differently to create better health and change the situations in which they live.
- Informed by the notion of balanced lifestyles and armed with the participatory occupational justice framework, occupational therapy practitioners have the tools necessary to work collaboratively to develop programs that will enhance the well-being of populations in vulnerable circumstances.

Learning Activities

1. Think about the lifestyles of diverse people in your community. Select one group to focus on. It might be working mothers of young children, shift workers, older adults who report being lonely, or a marginalized group (see Chapter 22) exposed to daily stressors. Gather information from research and social media about their lifestyle and compare that to Matuska and Christiansen's (2008) model of lifestyle balance. Describe, in occupational terms, aspects of their lifestyle that support health and well-being and aspects that might put their well-being at risk.
2. Using the information you have about the group you selected in Learning Activity 1, describe their current life in terms of doing, being, belonging, and becoming. If you do not have adequate knowledge about some aspects, build an argument about how that information might inform your understanding of that population's well-being and suggest ways you might access further data.
3. Locate an article that describes an occupational injustice and list the negative impacts on health and welfare for the population described. Guided by the participatory occupational justice framework, map out actions you might take toward enhancing the health of that population.

REFERENCES

American Occupational Therapy Association. (2015). Occupational therapy code of ethics (2015). *American Journal of Occupational Therapy, 69*(Suppl. 3), 6913410030. http://dx.doi.org/10.5014/ajot.2015.696S03

American Occupational Therapy Foundation. (2003). *Wilma L. West Library resource notes: Global poverty.* Retrieved from www.aotf.org/Portals/0/documents/Resources-WLWLibrary/Resource%20Notes/AOTF%20WLW%20Library%20Resource%20Notes%20-%20global%20poverty.pdf

Asaba, E., and Wicks, A. (2010). Occupational terminology: Occupational potential. *Journal of Occupational Science, 17*(2), 120–124. doi:10.1080/14427591.2010.9686683

Asbjørnslett, M., and Bekken, W. (2016). Openness to difference: Inclusion in sports occupations for children with (dis)abilities. *Journal of Occupational Science, 23*(4), 434–445. doi:10.1080/14427591.2016.1199389

Christiansen, C. (1994). Classification and study in occupation: A review and discussion of taxonomies. *Journal of Occupational Science: Australia, 1*(3), 3–20. doi:10.1080/14427591.1994.9686382

Crawford, E., Turpin, M., Nayar, S., Steel, E., and Durand, J-L. (2016). The structural-personal interaction: Occupational deprivation and asylum seekers in Australia. *Journal of Occupational Science, 23*(3), 321–338. doi:10.1080/14427591.2016.1153510

Diamond, J. (2002). Evolution, consequences and future of plant and animal domestication. *Nature, 418,* 700–707.

Diez Roux, A. V. (2016). On the distinction—or lack of distinction—between population health and public health. *American Journal of Public Health, 106,* 619–620.

Edmunds, L. (2000). *Primary prevention in children at risk of obesity as adults* (Unpublished doctoral thesis). University of Exeter, United Kingdom.

Eklund, M., Erlandsson, L-K., and Leufstadius, C. (2010). Time use in relation to valued and satisfying occupations among people with persistent mental illness: Exploring occupational balance. *Journal of Occupational Science, 17*(4), 231–238. doi:10.1080/14427591.2010.9686700

Eversley, D. E. C. (1965). Epidemiology as social history. In C. A. Creighton (Ed.), *History of epidemics in Britain* (2nd ed., pp. 1–35). London, England: Cassell.

Fischl, C., Asaba, C., and Nilsson, I. (2017). Exploring potential in participation mediated by digital technology among older adults. *Journal of Occupational Science, 24*(3), 314–326. doi:10.1080/14427591.2017.1340905

Galvaan, R. (2015). The contextually situated nature of occupational choice: Marginalised young adolescents' experiences in South Africa. *Journal of Occupational Science, 22*(1), 39–53. doi:10.1080/14427591.2014.912124

Glynn, I., and Glynn, J. (2004). *The life and death of smallpox.* Cambridge, United Kingdom: Cambridge University Press.

Guptill, C. (2012). Injured professional musicians and the complex relationship between occupation and health. *Journal of Occupational Science, 19*(3), 258–270. doi:10.1080/14427591.2012.670901

Jackson, J., Carlson, M., Mandel, D., Zemke, R., and Clark, F. (1998). Occupation in lifestyle redesign: The well elderly study occupational therapy program. *American Journal of Occupational Therapy, 52*(5), 326–336. doi:10.5014/ajot.1998.52.5.326

Johansson, A., Fristedt, S., Boström, M., Björklund, A., and Wagman, P. (2018). Occupational challenges and adaptations of vulnerable EU citizens from Romania begging in Sweden. *Journal of Occupational Science.* Advance online publication. doi:10.1080/14427591.2018.1557071

Kindig, D., and Stoddart, G. (2003). What is population health? *American Journal of Public Health, 93,* 380–383.

King-Boyes, M. J. E. (1977). *Patterns of aboriginal culture: Then and now.* Sydney, Australia: McGraw-Hill.

Kottorp, A., Nygård, L., Hedman, A., Öhman, A., Malinowsky, C., Rosenberg, L., . . . Ryd, C. (2016). Access to and use of everyday technology among older people: An occupational justice issue—but for whom? *Journal of Occupational Science, 23*(3), 382–388. doi:10.1080/14427591.2016.1151457

Lindsay, S., Chan, E., Cancelliere, S., and Mistry, M. (2018). Exploring how volunteer work shapes occupational potential among youths with and without disabilities: A qualitative comparison. *Journal of Occupational Science, 25*(3), 322–336. doi:10.1080/14427591.2018.1490339

Mackenbach, J. P., Meerding W. J., and Kunst, A. E. (2011). Economic implications of health inequalities in the European Union. *Journal of Epidemiology and Community Health, 65*(5), 412–419. doi:10.1136/jech.2010.112680

Man, A., Davis, A., Webster, F., and Polatajko, H. (2017). Awaiting knee joint replacement surgery: An occupational perspective on the experience of osteoarthritis. *Journal of Occupational Science, 24*(2), 216–224. doi:10.1080/14427591.2017.1315832

Matuska, K. M., and Christiansen, C. H. (2008). A proposed model of lifestyle balance. *Journal of Occupational Science, 15*(1), 9–19. doi:10.1080/14427591.2008.9686602

McMichael, T. (2001). *Human frontiers, environments and disease: Past patterns, uncertain futures.* Cambridge, United Kingdom: Cambridge University Press.

Munford, L. (1963). *The condition of man.* London, England: Heinemann.

Murtagh, J., Dixey, R., and Rudolf, M. (2006). A qualitative investigation into the levers and barriers to weight loss in children: Opinions of obese children. *Archives of Disease in Childhood, 91*(11), 920–923. doi:10.1136/adc.2005.085712

National Academies of Sciences, Engineering, and Medicine. (2017). *Communities in action: Pathways to health equity.* Washington, DC: National Academies Press. doi:10.17226/24624

Oakley, A. (2018). *Women, peace and welfare: A suppressed history of social reform, 1880–1920.* Bristol, United Kingdom: Policy Press.

Perry, B. (2014). *Household incomes in New Zealand: Trends in indicators of inequality and hardship 1982 to 2013.* New Zealand Ministry of Social Development. Retrieved from www.msd.govt.nz/about-msd-and-our-work/publications-resources/monitoring/household-incomes/index.html

Rivas-Quarneti, N., Movilla-Fernández, M-J., and Magalhães, L. (2018). Immigrant women's occupational struggles during the socioeconomic crisis in Spain: Broadening occupational justice conceptualization. *Journal of Occupational Science, 25*(1), 6–18. doi:10.1080/14427591.2017.1366355

Sen, A. (1999). *Development as freedom.* Oxford, United Kingdom: Oxford University Press.

Simaan, J. (2017). Olive growing in Palestine: A decolonial ethnographic study of collective daily-forms-of-resistance. *Journal of Occupational Science, 24*(4), 510–523. doi:10.1080/14427591.2017.1378119

Smith, J., Gonzalez, J, Jordan, A., Herd, H., Hutter, C., and Karimabadi, M. (2018). Occupational barriers during incarceration and quality of life. *American Journal of Occupational Therapy, 72,* 7211505100p/1. doi:10.5014/ajot.2018.7251-PO3015

Stalsberg, R., and Pedersen, A. (2010). Effects of socioeconomic status on the physical activity in adolescents: A systematic review of the evidence. *Scandinavian Journal of Medicine and Science in Sports, 20*(3), 368–383. doi:10.1111/j.1600-0838.2009.01047.x

Thomas, Y., Gray, M. A., and McGinty, S. (2017). The occupational wellbeing of people experiencing homelessness. *Journal of Occupational Science, 24*(2), 181–192. doi:10.1080/14427591.2017.1301828

Townsend, E., and Whiteford, G. (2005). A participatory occupational justice framework: Population-based processes of practice. In F. Kronenberg, S. Simo Algado, and N. Pollard (Eds.), *Occupational therapy without borders: Learning from the spirit of survivors* (pp. 110–126). Edinburgh, United Kingdom: Elsevier Churchill Livingstone.

Wagman, P., Håkansson, C., Matuska, K. M., Björklund, A., and Falkmer, T. (2012). Validating the model of lifestyle balance on a working Swedish population. *Journal of Occupational Science, 19*(2), 106–114. doi:10.1080/14427591.2011.575760

Walker, C. (1996). Shift work: In search of the workers' perspective. *Journal of Occupational Science, 3*(3), 99–103. doi:10.1080/14427591.1996.9686413

Whiteford, G., Jones, K., Rahal, C., and Suleman, A. (2018). The participatory occupational justice framework as a tool for change: Three contrasting case narratives. *Journal of Occupational Science, 25*(4), 497–508. doi:10.1080/14427591.2018.1504607

Wilcock, A. A. (1990). *Retrospective study of elderly people's perceptions of the relationship between their lives, occupations and health.* [Unpublished research data]. Adelaide: University of South Australia.

Wilcock, A. A. (2007). Occupation and health: Are they one and the same? *Journal of Occupational Science, 14*(1), 3–8. doi:10.1080/14427591.2007.9686577

Wilcock, A. A., and Hocking, C. (2015). *An occupational perspective of health* (3rd ed.). Thorofare, NJ: Slack.

Woodley, P. (2001). *Occasional papers: Health financing series* (Vol. 7). National Population Health Planning Branch, Commonwealth Department of Health and Aged Health Financing and Population Health. Australian Government Department of Health: Canberra, Australia.

World Bank. (2015). *Ending extreme poverty and sharing prosperity: Progress and policies.* Retrieved from www.worldbank.org/en/research/brief/policy-research-note-03-ending-extreme-poverty-and-sharing-prosperity-progress-and-policies

World Federation of Occupational Therapists. (2006). *Position statement: Human rights.* Available from www.wfot.org/AboutUs/PositionStatements.aspx

World Health Organization. (2013). *Healthy settings.* Retrieved from www.who.int/healthy_settings/en/

World Health Organization and Health and Welfare Canada, Canadian Public Health Association. (1986). *Ottawa Charter for health promotion.* Ottawa, Canada: World Health Organization. Retrieved from www.who.int/healthpromotion/conferences/previous/ottawa/en/

Young, T. K. (1998). *Population health: Concepts and methods.* New York, NY: Oxford University Press.

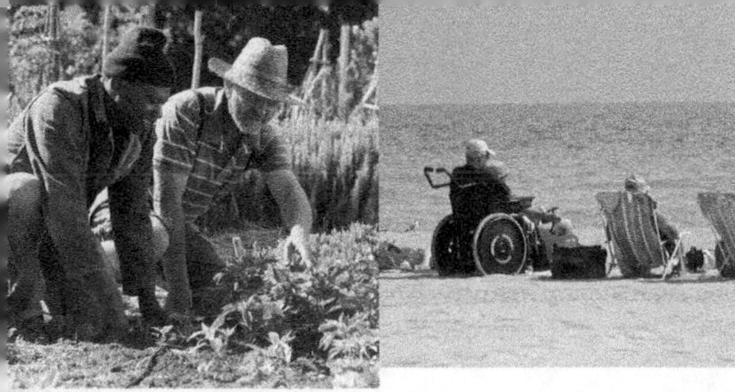

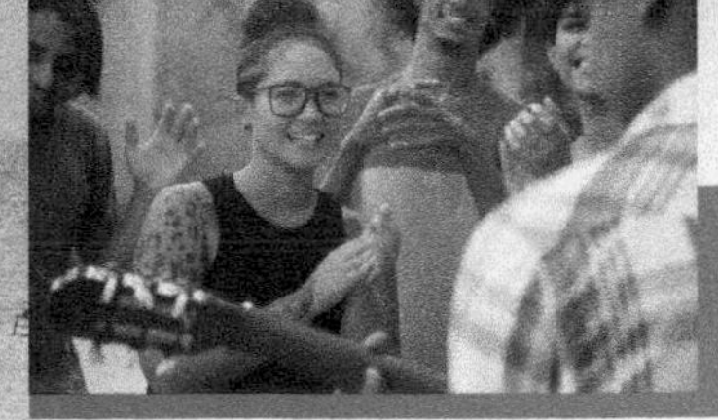

SECTION II

Community-Based and Population Health Program Development

Chapter 5

Program Planning and Needs Assessment

Kathleen Flecky, OTD, OTR/L, Joy Doll, OTD, OTR/L,
Marjorie E. Scaffa, PhD, OTR/L, FAOTA

To build collaborative models of consumer-driven, community-based practice, we need to focus on a communication process that helps us understand other persons' unique culture and priorities for life occupations as well as meaning associated with past experiences, current situations, and hopes for the future.

—Ann Grady (2017), 1994 Eleanor Clarke Slagle Lecture

Learning Outcomes

This chapter is designed to enable the reader to:

5-1 Describe the occupational therapy practitioner's role in community and population health program development and needs assessment.
5-2 Identify the seven principles common to all planning models.
5-3 Explain how the needs assessment process is similar to the occupational therapy evaluation process.
5-4 Explain the three steps of a needs assessment.
5-5 Describe the importance of primary and secondary data collection to the needs assessment process.

5-6 Explain why community-based programs need to be grounded in theory and based on the best available evidence.

5-7 Discuss the relationship of evidence and program planning.

Key Terms

Evidence
Evidence-based planning for health
Interprofessional teamwork
Interventions
Key informants
Needs assessment
Political activities of daily living
Preplanning
Program
Program development
Quadruple Aim
Stakeholders
Secondary data
Sustainability
Systematic reviews
Target population
Theory
Triple Aim

Introduction

Occupational therapy practitioners play a key role in community-based programming to meet individual, group, and population occupational and health needs. The American Occupational Therapy Association (AOTA) illustrates the importance of occupational therapy practitioners to promote health and wellness, enhance participation, and advocate for quality of life and occupational justice for populations through its *Occupational Therapy Practice Framework: Domain and Process* (AOTA, 2014). As skilled professionals in the analysis of occupational performance, habits, routines, and roles within the context of meaningful environments, occupational therapy practitioners are well placed to contribute in all areas of community health programming (Bass and Baker, 2017). Population health was initially described by Kindig and Stoddart (2003) as "the health outcomes of a group of individuals, including the distribution of such outcomes within the group" (p. 381). Occupational therapy practitioners can play a key role in population health, as it is framed around a holistic focus on the social determinants of health and the health priorities of individuals, families, and groups within health systems (Minnesota Department of Health, Center for Public Health Nursing, n.d.). The National Academy of Medicine made recommendations for all health professions to become familiar with population health concepts no matter their practice arena (Shortell, 2013).

With growing concerns about health-care costs and access to care, health promotion and disease/injury prevention activities will likely play a major role in the future of health services in the United States (Institute of Medicine [IOM], 2015a). The goal of the **Triple Aim** is to enhance the care experience, improve the health of populations, and reduce health-care costs (Institute for Healthcare Improvement, 2018). Innovative and creative strategies to meet the Triple Aim provide opportunities to explore new ways of delivering health care. Bodenheimer and Sinsky (2014) introduced the concept of the **Quadruple Aim,** building on the Triple Aim by adding the dimension of health-care provider well-being as a means of improving health-care delivery. This addition recognizes not only the wellness of the population but also the well-being of practitioners themselves, as engaged community members and workers in their communities.

Along with an interest in population health, a resurgence in team-based interprofessional work has taken hold as an influential strategy to ensure the health system, whether clinical or community-based, can address population health issues (IOM, 2015b). With a unique perspective on the role of occupation in health, occupational therapy practitioners are important interprofessional team members in community-based health education and population health interventions. **Interprofessional teamwork** is defined as "the levels of cooperation, coordination and collaboration characterizing the relationships between professions in delivering patient-centered care" (American Association of Colleges of Nursing et al., 2011, p. 2). With health-care delivery and accountability systems in a state of constant change, interprofessional collaboration is becoming the new norm in accountable care and a best practice for addressing population health (IOM, 2015b; Nester, 2016).

This chapter is part of the overall aim of section II (Chapters 5–8) to describe important concepts and processes in the development, implementation, and evaluation of community and population health programs and interventions. Specifically, this chapter provides the reader with an opportunity to develop knowledge and skills in program planning and needs assessment to contribute to community and population health, whether the client is an individual, a group, a community, or a target population. As noted by Braveman (2016), "Practitioners must understand and perform in ways that showcase how their perspective and approaches add distinct value to achieving population health as well as individual goals" (p. 3).

What is a community-based program? A **program** is a "planned, coordinated group of activities, procedures, etc., often for a specific purpose or outcome; it addresses a specific need, problem or situation, shows what activities have taken place and reports what measurable changes have occurred" (Rutgers Cooperative Extension, 2007, p. 5). Sometimes referred to as **interventions,** programs are systematic efforts to achieve preplanned objectives such as changes in knowledge, attitudes, skills, and behaviors to maintain or improve function and/or health. These interventions can occur across many settings, some of which are community-based, such as schools, work sites, and community agencies.

For example, one of the authors worked with the local safety council to address an increased incidence in the number of older adult fall visits to local emergency departments reportedly caused by tripping over pets. The occupational therapist worked with the safety council and local animal shelters to develop an educational fall prevention program. In community-based occupational therapy, the concept of occupation-based practice is still applied, but the concept is broadened and the intervention is delivered to a population as identified in the example provided.

Other differences include the underlying philosophy and location of community-based programs. There are subtle distinctions in community programs—for example, a *community-based* program describes where the program occurs: in the community (Issel and Wells, 2018). A *community-focused* program is developed to have an impact on the community as a whole, and a *community-driven* program is designed with community members very involved in the inception, implementation, and evaluation of a program, and thus, they drive the process (Issel and Wells, 2018). The fall prevention educational intervention with the safety council was developed as a community-focused program in response to a local concern by the safety council and emergency room professionals. The case provided at the end of this chapter follows a community-driven approach.

Program development, including planning and developing implementation and evaluation strategies, emerged in the 1980s as a key component of health education and health promotion (Timmreck, 2003). Program development is a process involving continuous cycles of needs assessment, planning the intervention, implementation, and evaluation with feedback at each step to revise or improve previous steps, as depicted in Figure 5-1 (Dignan and Carr, 1992).

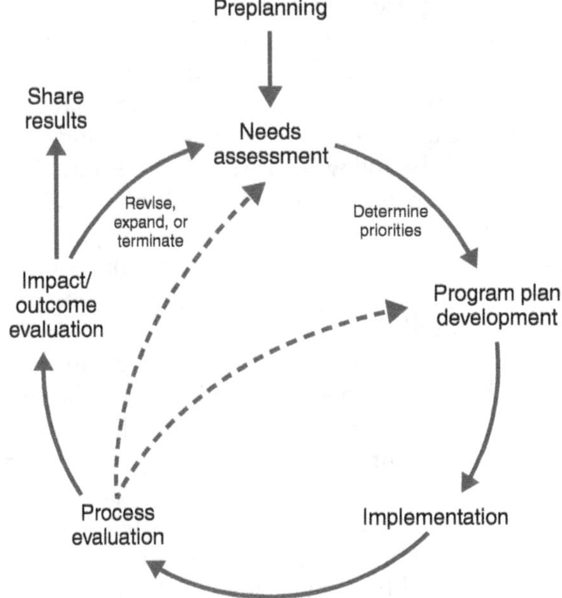

Figure 5-1 The cycle of program development.

The first half of this chapter begins with a discussion of the steps involved in developing community health and health promotion programs, beginning with the assessment of the needs and assets of the targeted population and the associated community. The chapter concludes with a review of theoretical foundations and models on which programs can be based.

Program Planning Principles and Best Practices

Program planning is an organized, systematic process of:

- Communicating with the targeted group, other team partners, and stakeholders
- Identifying community problems and issues
- Establishing priorities, objectives, and resources
- Designing, implementing, and evaluating program activities (Issel and Wells, 2018)

Although no perfect program-planning model exists, Breckon, Harvey, and Lancaster (1994) point to seven principles common to all planning models.

Preplanning

Preplanning is an important step that if overlooked can undermine the success of an otherwise effective intervention strategy. The preplanning phase considers who should be involved, when the planning should occur, what resources are needed, and what process will be followed. Internal and external resources are assessed, including attitudes, policies, available expertise, time, space, money, priorities, and fit with the organization's mission. Brainstorming is a great strategy to begin the preplanning process (Caldwell, Whitehead, Fleming, and Moes, 2008). Brainstorming can be formal or informal and is best when done with a group with the freedom to think and generate ideas. In addition, preplanning is essential to achieve the sustainability of a program. To make a program sustainable is to make it last. Sustainable programs are those that build a community's capacity to survive and thrive after the initial funding is gone (Edberg, 2015).

In the fall prevention and pets program, the safety council contacted the occupational therapist who had collaborated on other community-based fall prevention initiatives. The council asked her to join a task force. At the first task force meeting, the issue of older adult falls and pets was introduced as a concern, and the members initially discussed strategies through a simple brainstorming exercise. It was decided that the issue needed more investigation, and the first step would be to perform a community needs assessment.

Plan With People

Experience has demonstrated the vital importance of involving community members and stakeholders in the planning process. **Stakeholders** are "persons who may or may not benefit directly by being involved in the potential program, but who may have a stake in the program's outcome and often the ability to influence that outcome" (Scaffa and Reitz, 2013, p. 204). Knowing who the stakeholders are in a community and who should be at the table for initial planning is important. The best way to determine stakeholders is to ask community members. Stakeholders and community advocates are often known and recognized by many. When planning with people, two community health promotion principles are encompassed: relevance and participation. Similar to the concept of client-centeredness in occupational therapy, the principle of relevance, or "starting where the people are," is applied when program planners begin by considering the perceived needs of community residents rather than those of the planners or their organizations. This is supported by the ethical principle of autonomy in the AOTA *Occupational Therapy Code of Ethics (2015)*, as clients have the right to voice their needs, make choices, and be involved with decisions and actions that relate to their health and well-being (AOTA, 2015). In addition, building participation early on ensures that program development aligns with community needs and promotes the buy-in that will be critical for successful program implementation (Suarez-Balcazar, 2005) and sustainability.

Participation is essential for developing effective programs and is considered health enhancing. People meet and sustain their goals more effectively when they are active team members involved in the planning process (McKenzie, Neiger, and Thackeray, 2017; Minkler, 2014). Participation can range from responding to requests for feedback on program plans to taking an active role in designing, implementing, and evaluating program activities. Occupational therapy practitioners are particularly adept at engaging individuals in participation, a skill required for occupation-based practice delivery. Suarez-Balcazar (2005) identified clear roles for occupational therapy practitioners in engaging community members as change agents in developing relevant community programming, as advocates for the vulnerable, and as capacity builders. Due to the natural skill sets of occupational therapy practitioners, the ability to plan with people is a strong asset to community program development.

Planning with people also encompasses the concept of collaboration. Program planning generally begins with a group of people who have a vested interest in the issues. Hyett and colleagues (2016) acknowledged occupational therapy practitioners' ability to understand the influence of context on enablement and disablement, along with how values of social justice and human rights directly influence abilities to plan with community members. In addition, the skills of occupational therapy practitioners to coproduce occupations with clients provide a foundation for the collaboration necessary for community work. Working with people and agencies who have shared interests and goals offers many advantages: resources and workload can be shared, duplication of effort can be minimized, and more creative problem-solving can occur. The end result is a program that provides better service to the community for the long term.

For the fall prevention and pets program, the occupational therapist sought out individuals who were affected by falls due to pets, interviewing older adults with pets, caregivers, experts in pet safety at the local animal shelter, and emergency room professionals who had reported the concern. Talking with stakeholders ensured that the occupational therapist understood the issue from multiple perspectives and could involve a variety of experts in the intervention as needed.

Plan With Data

Sound planning decisions are based on a thorough knowledge of health goals and associated factors, the service area or site, the target population, social and environmental support systems, and existing or former programs addressing the same issue, as well success rates. When planning a program, epidemiological data and statistics to consider include prevalence, incidence, and the broader impact of the health issue on the community and its members. Prevalence is "the proportion of a population who have a specific characteristic in a given time period" (National Institute of Mental Health, 2017, para. 1). Incidence is the rate of a disease or disorder that is contextually based (Harvard T. H. Chan School of Public Health, 2018). Much of the quantitative information can be gathered from existing sources such as health departments, libraries, the National Center for Health Statistics, chambers of commerce, and health systems. Planners may also identify the need for additional data—perhaps more qualitative data that would help to identify attitudes, beliefs, or barriers. A review of available and gathered data provides a rich context in which planning and prioritizing can occur logically. Beyond statistical data, qualitative data can provide insights into the experience and can be collected through means like focus groups and town hall meetings.

In addition to interviewing stakeholders about the proposed fall prevention program, the occupational therapist also performed a literature review and explored local health statistics on the causes of falls in the older adult population. Although little literature existed on the issue of pets and falls, it was identified in statistics as a reported cause for falls among older adults (Stevens, Teh, and Haileysus, 2010).

Gaining a qualitative perspective can also begin to build trust with community members. Establishing a thorough understanding of the community's perceived needs will help establish an effective program. Building a relationship of mutual respect and reciprocity is an essential part of the planning process and is time well spent. Building a team with the targeted population and interprofessional members that has a shared vision, goal, and plan requires communication and collaboration on team member roles, areas of expertise, and skills (Issel and Wells, 2018). An occupational therapy practitioner can assume a variety of roles as a team member in planning a program (e.g., leader or administrator, developer, consultant, clinician, educator, or researcher; Doll, 2010). These roles are dynamic and can change within the life cycle of a program, depending on need.

The interviews conducted for the fall prevention program provided a qualitative perspective on the issue. In general, older adults reported understanding that pets caused falls but were fearful about admitting their pet could cause a fall due to a personal bond with the animal. Caregivers reported wanting companionship for the older adult, but many regretted the type of pet chosen, not realizing it could be a fall risk. The animal shelter workers reported having anxiety about matching a pet with an older adult but were hesitant to say anything because they believed it was not their place. All of this qualitative information directly influenced the design of the education that the team implemented.

Plan for Performance

The plan for performance principle speaks to long-range planning. Given that most serious health challenges will not completely disappear nor will community health goals be achieved with one program, approaching the planning process with the idea of permanence, or sustainability, makes sense. This includes considering how the program might be staffed and financed after the initial intervention or how it will be sustained, such as becoming incorporated as an integral part of an agency's services. Many factors influence **sustainability,** from financial resources to recruitment of participants to engagement of program staff. It is important to move the concept of program sustainability beyond simply financial and consider the multiple factors that affect a program's longevity (Barnett et al., 2004). A strong program planner considers sustainability and its application from the very beginning of planning.

In the fall prevention program, the local safety council was committed to delivering the educational information. The occupational therapist donated her time as an act of service to the safety council. In this example, sustainability is less of a concern but is still important to consider in any community program.

> **Engage Your Brain 5-1**
>
> Why is planning for sustainability an ethical imperative? Which principles of the AOTA *Occupational Therapy Code of Ethics (2015)* apply to sustainability?

Plan for Priorities

The most effective programs are those that address the greatest need and are designed or known to have the greatest effect within the given resources. Prioritization should flow naturally from planning with people and planning with data. Time for this activity needs to be built in to ensure continued community participation. Many strategies exist for prioritization, including activities like a strengths, opportunities, weaknesses, and threats (SWOT) analysis. A SWOT analysis is discussed more in-depth in Chapter 8. Another option involves the use of a logic model, a visual representation that describes the input, process, outputs, outcomes, and impacts as part of prioritization and planning (Kettner, Moroney, and Martin, 2017). Critically, all programs require a comprehensive needs assessment, and input from all stakeholders helps to ensure accurate prioritization of identified needs. The community needs assessment process will be addressed in further detail later in this chapter.

After the information was collected for the fall prevention program, the team, including members of the safety council, the occupational therapist, and members from the animal shelter, met several times as a task force to plan the priorities for the program. A SWOT was performed to ensure a holistic plan was developed to prevent older adult falls due to pets.

Plan for Evaluation

Evaluation is a continuous process of asking questions such as "Are we doing the right thing?" and "Are we doing things right?" and "What do we need to measure to know what and how we're doing?" These questions are usually answered through the systematic collection and analysis of program outcome data. Evaluation methods, depending on the goals and objectives of the program, should be built into the program design and spelled out in the program plan. In program planning, several key questions should be considered in evaluation planning. While the first consideration is grounded in the intended program outcomes, it should also focus on the process used to achieve the outcomes. Program evaluation is extensively discussed in Chapter 7. Once the needed information is determined, record-keeping systems and evaluation instruments need to be selected and put in place to ensure that data are properly collected. The planning process should address who will be responsible for both data collection and analysis. It should also establish time frames for all steps, including sharing results with the community. In the fall prevention program, evaluation was built into the website where the educational materials were housed. The safety council tracked the incidence of older adult falls due to pets to determine if any impact was being achieved in the community.

Plan for Measurable Outcomes

The last of the seven planning principles is to match clearly articulated and measurable program objectives with data against which to judge program accomplishments. The format for the objective and the evaluation should match. For example, if the objective of a program is to reduce the risk of falling, then the outcome would be stated in terms of risk reduction, not reduced mortality or reduced hospitalization.

Community Needs Assessment

In order to establish any program, a thorough and complete community needs assessment is critical. A community needs assessment moves beyond preplanning to explore existing data about the community, with identification of community issues and a review of resources. Identifying an issue to address can come from data, professional judgment, observation, existing literature, concerned individuals, or agencies. As health-care providers, occupational therapy practitioners can easily identify gaps, but it is critical in gap analysis that those identified match with community priorities to ensure programmatic success.

A community needs assessment answers the key questions of who, what, and why. For example, *who* are the key players (e.g., service receivers, community leaders, service providers, experts in the field, policy-makers, agency representatives) with a vested interest in the issue, *what* do they hope will come from the needs assessment, and *why*—what prompted their concern, and how important is it (Soriano, 2013)? Answers to these questions will help define the key questions for the needs assessment. Planning often occurs through a group of stakeholders forming a planning committee or task force, as mentioned in the fall prevention example. However broad or narrow the group, the perspectives of all stakeholders—particularly those of potential clients—must be considered and integrated into the planning process. Keep in mind who the occupational therapist collaborated with to gain multiple perspectives in the fall prevention example.

When gathering community members around the table, it is critical to allow adequate time for discussion and brainstorming. Finding a time that community members can meet and gather ensures a diversity of voices at the table. Identifying individuals who might be missing in the initial planning and seeking their perspective is important. These small details may not seem significant but can be critical in building a program truly focused on community need. In addition, naming the group as either a planning team or a task force may help clarify the intention to the members.

Every program-planning initiative is influenced by factors that can support or inhibit the process. Considering these internal and external factors early in the process is important to avoid unnecessary pitfalls. First, it is necessary to analyze a need for consistency or “fit” with the organization’s mission. Assuming it fits, how important is the need relative to other issues? Is there a commitment of time and resources to see the project through? What is the potential for effecting a positive change? What do the other stakeholders want or expect? Are there other programs addressing this issue of concern?

Analysis of these questions is best accomplished by occupational therapy practitioners and other members of the interprofessional team in collaboration with community members. Different perspectives are appreciated and recognized as valuable to the planning discussion. Team members must demonstrate openness and a willingness to listen to a diversity of ideas. Similar to building rapport in client interactions, the occupational therapy practitioner should translate these skills by building the respect and reciprocity needed in the context of program planning.

Teamwork also acknowledges that others may have expertise the occupational therapist does not.

For example, in the fall prevention program the occupational therapist did not have knowledge regarding the types of pets and breeds that are less likely to cause falls. Partnering with experts in pet care provided insight, ensuring that the education developed was meaningful and supported by all stakeholders.

The assessment of resources goes beyond the question of whether or not funding exists. Depending on the nature of the program being planned, other considerations should include location, space, materials, appropriately trained personnel, transportation for clients, and access to experts for certain phases of the process. Finally, preplanning should include an assessment of the existing regulations and policies that might have an impact on the issue or the approach(es) being considered.

Needs Assessment Process

A *need* is considered the gap or difference between the present state of affairs (what is) and some desired future state (what could or should be; Altschuld, 2015; Soriano, 2013). **Needs assessment** can be defined in many ways; for example, it is a "systematic identification of a population's needs or the assessment of individuals to determine the proper level of services needed" (National Library of Medicine, 2018, p. 1). Further, Soriano (2013) defined it as "a well-thought-out and impartial systematic effort to collect objective data or information that brings to light or enhances understanding of the need for services or programs" (p. 5). The needs assessment process is depicted in Figure 5-2. In essence, it is an analysis of a health problem or need based on information gathered about those with the need (target population) and the environment around them (environment, context). It is important to keep in mind that a needs assessment is a systematic process for collecting information about a targeted population and involves an understanding of the population needs and desires in the context of community issues.

Occupational therapy practitioners use both a target population and a systems approach in community assessment. In a needs assessment, the "client" is the **target population,** or a group of persons who share characteristics that identify them as the focus of health programming or have an unmet health need (AOTA, 2017a). In addition to the target population, the community is an essential stakeholder in the needs assessment process, as goals based on population needs are only realistic and meaningful if the community context is considered. Kretzmann and McKnight (1993) recognized that needs assessment is often focused on the deficiencies, gaps, or lack of abilities of the target population and local community, instead of on the abilities, capacities, and skills (i.e., assets) of these stakeholders. Individuals, local institutions, neighborhood groups, and nonprofit agencies have the potential to develop relationships around unmet needs and to share resources.

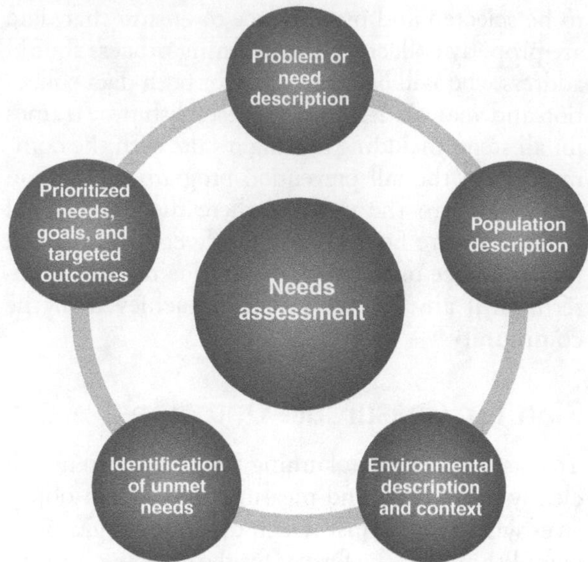

Figure 5-2 Needs assessment process.

Building on the work of Kretzmann and McKnight, Beaulieu (n.d.) described asset mapping as a process of identifying local community individuals, businesses, agencies, and government who offer assets for community planning in the form of skills, gifts, and resources for programming. In alignment with Kretzmann and McKnight (1993), occupational therapy practitioners are easily able to identify enablers and strengths among the community stakeholders, as this skill is common in patient interaction across practice areas. Again, translating skills from other practice settings is an asset in community programming.

In the fall prevention program, an asset-based approach was used by not simply labeling pet ownership as a fall risk. The program planners recognized the value of the companionship provided to older adults through relationships with pets. The program was designed around the benefits of pet companionship combined with mediating the potential fall risk of pets.

The needs assessment process can be viewed within three general steps that are essential regardless of the population, community, and need or the complexity of programming (Gilmore and Campbell, 2005; Hodges and Videto, 2011; Soriano, 2013). Figure 5-3 denotes the first step: describing the population, which involves gathering data to create an accurate picture of the target population and the need. In this step, it is important to elicit the voices of members of the target population through

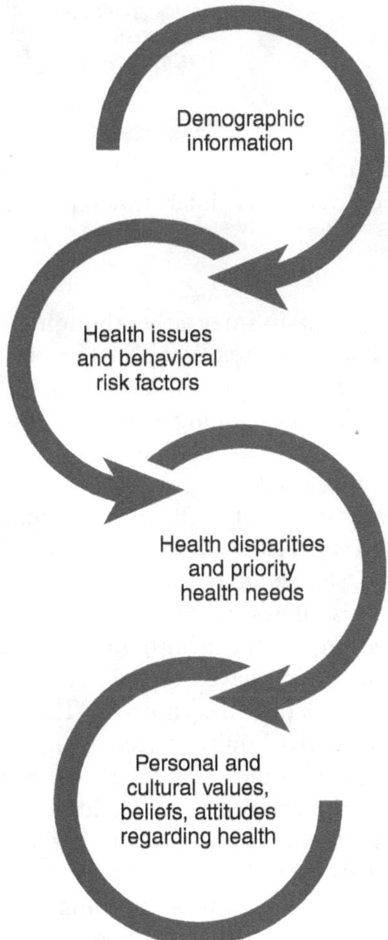

Figure 5-3 Needs assessment step 1: population description.

interviews, focus groups, or surveys to appreciate the complexities of their health needs through the collection of relevant demographic data and the identification of key health issues, behavioral health risk factors, health disparities and values, and beliefs and attitudes about health (Issel and Wells, 2018). As noted by Alley, Asomugha, Conway, and Sanghavi (2016), "In our current health system, patient health-related social needs frequently remain undetected and unaddressed" (p. 8).

This step in the needs assessment process illuminates the perspectives of members of the target population for programming in order to represent their heath needs authentically. Further, data from other key informants, such as community members, offer important viewpoints to confirm health needs, as in all the steps in the needs assessment process. **Key informants** are persons, typically formal or informal leaders, who have expert knowledge about a phenomenon of interest. In the fall prevention program, key informants included older adults, caregivers, safety council task force members, and staff from local pet shelters. The type of key informants involved will vary based on program and community needs.

Figure 5-4 illustrates the second step of the needs assessment process: describing the environment, which includes gathering data about the physical and social environment related to the target population. Using concepts based on Kretzmann and McKnight (1993) and Beaulieu (n.d.), this step involves the collection of information about the assets or strengths of the physical and social environments of the target population and the community, as well as the barriers or challenges of the physical and social environments. Collecting information from multiple key informants, as noted in step one, can provide multiple perspectives to bring an accurate picture of the physical and social environments. According to the AOTA (2014), context is a broader term that includes the physical and social environments, as well as other aspects of the environment that have an impact on occupational engagement, such as temporal and virtual contexts.

In addition, other aspects of environmental data that influence occupational performance, health programming, access to health care, health disparities, and health behaviors are socioeconomic and sociopolitical factors (Lysack and Adamo, 2014;

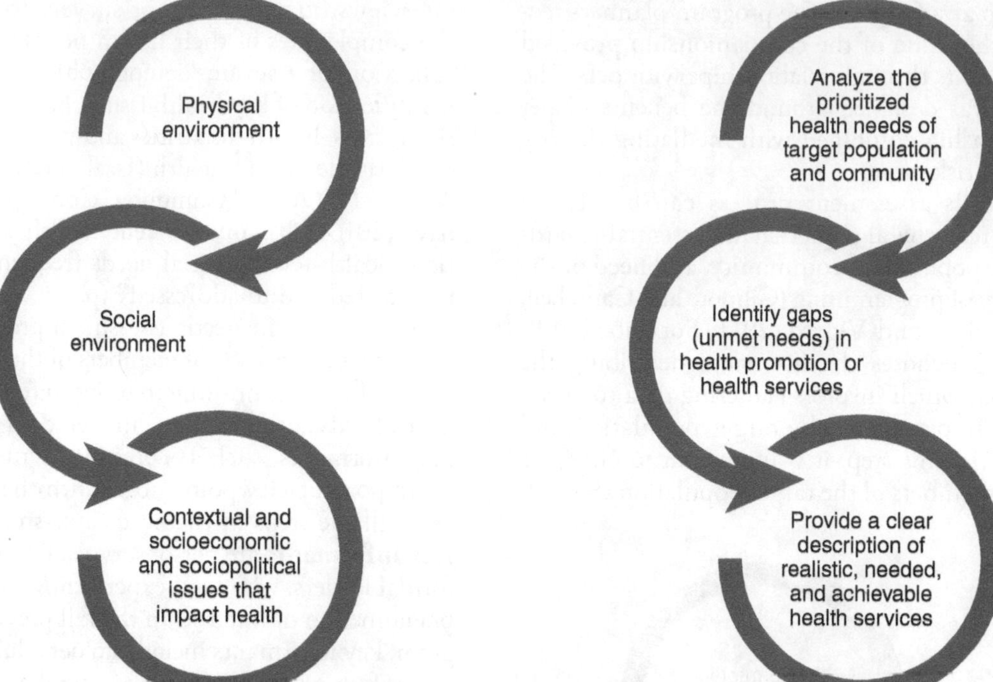

Figure 5-4 Needs assessment step 2: environmental description.

Figure 5-5 Needs assessment step 3: analysis of needs and priorities for intervention programming.

Nash, Fabius, Skoufalos, Clarke, and Horowitz, 2016). The social and political landscape influences the target population as **political activities of daily living** (pADL), or key issues and activities that persons in communities face to gain opportunities to fully participate in daily life (Kronenberg, Pollard, and Sakellariou, 2011). Population groups engage in acts of advocacy based on political values and systems in place in communities, and an awareness of pADLs can enhance authentic need assessment.

Engage Your Brain 5-2

What are the competencies needed to conduct a comprehensive needs assessment of a population?

Figure 5-5 highlights the third step of the needs assessment process—analysis of needs and priorities for intervention programming. This step represents a synthesis and an integrative thought and action process of analyzing collected data from steps one and two, prioritizing health needs, identifying unmet needs, and developing a clear and realistic picture of the potential, doable health services and programming needed (Centers for Disease Control and Prevention [CDC], 2013). An important part of this step is to reflect on the conflicting data gathered from stakeholders and gather more data if needed. This allows for the development of an accurate picture of the health needs of the target population when viewed as part of a larger community with its own health needs. Thus, the list of prioritized needs, unmet needs, and achievable health services would reflect both the target population and the community. In addition, a systematic literature review of local and national data on health needs, health disparities, and evidence of best practice in health programming adds an integrative approach to this third step and prepares for the program development and implementation steps (Minkler, 2014).

Developing an Occupational Profile

Occupational therapy practitioners focus on engagement in occupation and optimal occupational performance and health outcomes for target populations in the community. Developing an occupational profile is an important outcome of an occupational therapy evaluation (AOTA, 2014). For example, in conducting a needs assessment of young children in a preschool setting (the target population), a priority need identified from multiple data collection sources was a lack of healthy eating patterns for optimal child development. Data collected also indicated a need for the enhancement of primary caregiver and family social participation in the preschool. Statistical evidence for the community at large and community stakeholder data collection validated the need for health literacy regarding nutrition, healthy eating patterns, and more opportunities for social participation for young children and families. Figure 5-6 shows the similarities between the occupational therapy evaluation profile process and the needs assessment process.

If an occupational therapist was collaborating with an individual child and family to develop a

For Individual Client

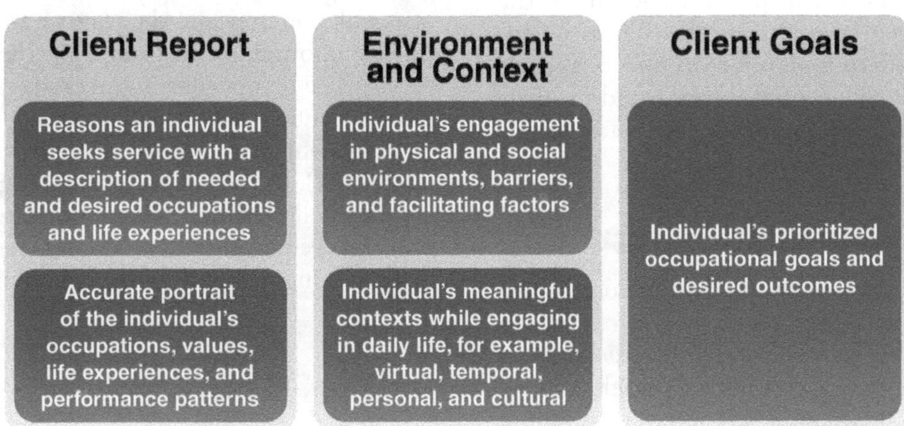

For Target Populations in a Community

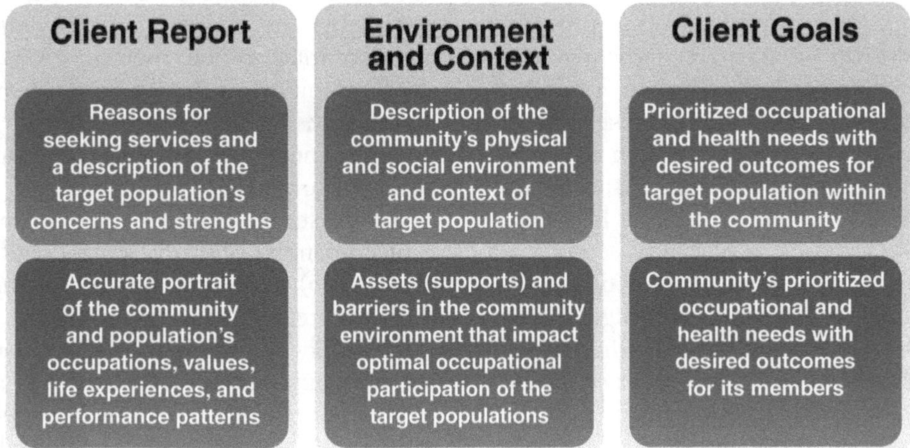

Figure 5-6 Occupational evaluation profile. (*Adapted from the AOTA* Occupational Profile Template [*2017b*].)

narrative for an occupational profile, data would be collected using the steps in the first part of Figure 5-6. Occupational performance strengths (assets) and concerns (barriers) would be identified and goals for enhancing healthy eating patterns and social participation in meaningful contexts may be identified.

In the second part of Figure 5-6, instead of an individual child as a client, the target of the data collection is the children who attend the preschool. Data related to the children as a group or population are collected and analyzed along with systems data about the community in which the children live. Data collection would include demographic information, health risk factors, socioeconomic information, and health disparities relevant to the children and their families. All of this data is analyzed and prioritized to develop occupational goals for the targeted group of children based on their health and occupational needs, in the context of the community's needs and resources.

Needs Assessment Data Collection

Key to the needs assessment process, as noted in the three steps previously described, is information collection. Information is the basis for decisions about the best use of resources to resolve high-priority needs for the target population in the community and is critical to program development. It is typically impossible to gather all the data desired to develop a program, as access to the target population, key stakeholders, funding, and time to complete a needs assessment are barriers. However, program planners should focus on accurate, authentic, relevant, and comprehensive data collection. Typically, in a needs assessment, information is gathered from key informants and stakeholders within the community, but environmental scanning and trends are also important to provide the larger landscape of health needs.

Before collecting new data, a review of the scientific and intervention literature for background on the issue of concern and for the identification of strategies that have been used in similar situations is necessary. Methods for gathering data vary. Some common data sources and data collection methods, such as secondary data, surveys, and group processes, are outlined in Table 5-1.

Use of Secondary Data

The use of secondary data is one of the simplest and most cost-effective methods to add to a community needs assessment. **Secondary data,** also called archival data, are existing data collected by agencies for other purposes (McKenzie et al., 2017; Prince, Dake, and Ward, 2017). Examples include birth and death records; census data; prevalence data on diseases, disability, illness, injury, and risk; demographic data; social indicators; and special surveys and reports. Secondary data are generally easy to obtain and particularly useful in the exploratory phase of the needs assessment process to determine what is already known about an issue. These data give a sense of the current status of the community or population and give the planner an idea of what further information to gather. By themselves, secondary data do not constitute a needs assessment. To provide context and client perspective, they are best used in conjunction with qualitative data (Prince et al., 2017). In the fall prevention program, secondary data collected through electronic health records from local emergency departments were key factors in identifying the need for the community program.

Role of Theories

In planning a program or service, planners make assumptions about the causes of the problem and the best ways to effect change. If those assumptions are not made in terms of an explicit theory or theories and there is no conceptual framework behind the choice of intervention, then there is no way to link the intervention to the intended outcome (Posavac and Carey, 1997). As a result, program design would be much less effective, and evaluation would be less informative.

Simply stated, a **theory** is an explanation of why a phenomenon occurs the way it does (Freudenberg et al., 1995). Good theories complement practical skills and technologies by taking the program beyond simply conducting activities to actually solving problems. Theories can provide answers to a program developer's questions about *why* people engage or do not engage in specific health behaviors and *how* to engage people in changing and maintaining behaviors. Programs devised to address

Table 5-1 Overview and Comparison of Commonly Used Data Collection Methods for Needs Assessment

Data Source/Method	Description	Resulting Information	Advantages	Disadvantages
Secondary (archival) data—i.e., records and logs, prior studies, demographic data, social indicators, risk-factor data, epidemiologic studies, census data, and rates under treatment	Existing data usually found in city, county, state, and national organizations and government bureaus	Quantitative data that help determine the status of a target population with regard to a need; may furnish information on causal or contributing factors	Relatively low in cost; generally available; minimal investment of time or staff; unbiased; complements other sources of data	No client input; possibly not representative for given target audience; technical assistance for statistical interpretation possibly needed
Survey methods, i.e., written questionnaire, face-to-face interview, telephone interview, and key informant interview	Techniques for gathering information directly from individuals using structured forms or protocols	Mainly qualitative—values, perceptions, opinions, judgments of importance, and observations	Client input achieved; quantitative data complemented	Generally more time- and labor-intensive than using secondary data sources
1. Written questionnaire			Easy to administer; relatively low in cost; time efficient; quantifiable; broad reach into community/target population	Possible low return rates; may not be representative; not useful for people who are illiterate or not fluent in English; prone to design problems; technical assistance for questionnaire construction and data processing/analysis possibly necessary
2. Face-to-face interview			High response rate; greater flexibility for answers and interviewer probing; opportunity to observe nonverbal responses; ability to include people who are illiterate or who have vision problems; rapport building	Smaller sample size; costly in terms of time and travel; trained interviewers required; possible difficulty with scheduling; time consuming; opportunity for bias; possibility to raise client expectations; data more difficult to interpret and summarize; technical assistance for questionnaire construction and data processing/analysis possibly necessary

(*Continued*)

Table 5-1 Overview and Comparison of Commonly Used Data Collection Methods for Needs Assessment—cont'd

Data Source/Method	Description	Resulting Information	Advantages	Disadvantages
3. Telephone interview			Easy to administer; no travel time and cost; perceived anonymity; fairly good response rate	Sampling challenges; may not be representative; not as suitable for long questionnaires; inability to observe nonverbal reactions; possible rise in client expectations; trained interviewers necessary to avoid bias; computer capability and technical assistance for questionnaire construction and data processing/analysis possibly needed
4. Key informant	Surveys (written and/or interview) of a select group of key community leaders, informal lay leaders, and professional persons who are aware of, and in touch with, the target population and the given issue		Limited number of participants necessary	Possible difficulty in identifying informal leaders; biased results possible; participants may have vested interests
Group processes—i.e., community forums, focus groups, and nominal group processes	Techniques that involve small or large groups of stakeholders (e.g., service receivers, service providers, experts in the field, policymakers, and agency representatives) in varying degrees of interaction	Mainly qualitative—opinions and expert judgments; group perceptions and perspectives regarding values, importance of need; information on causes/barriers; decisions on priorities; feedback or consensus on goals or courses of action	Opportunity for fluid, natural discussion around an issue; complementary to other data	

Table 5-1 Overview and Comparison of Commonly Used Data Collection Methods for Needs Assessment—cont'd

Data Source/Method	Description	Resulting Information	Advantages	Disadvantages
1. Community forum	An open public meeting with all interested parties invited; a large group discussion	Ideas and input from a broad segment of the population	Broad range of views and concerns provided; natural discussion format; facilitation of dialogue among people with different viewpoints	Possibly not reflective of opinions of general population; participation possibly low; domination by a few possible; difficult to analyze; logistics
2. Focus groups	Groups of 8 to 12 clients/ potential clients responding to a structured set of questions	Individual and group perspectives on a focused area or theme	Possible in-depth probing of themes	Skilled facilitators needed; technical assistance in data analysis possibly required; logistical challenges getting group together; groups variable, thus more than one needed for reliable results
3. Nominal group process	The most structured of the group methods; a combination of written responses, voting, and discussion used in small groups of 10 or less	Ranking by the group members of what they perceive to be the most important issues and/or solutions	Highly effective for getting at a large number of issues in a short amount of time; equitable participation	Expensive in terms of time and results; skilled leadership required; limited ability to generalize

expected behaviors according to a theory help to determine *what* factors to focus on in the evaluation (Posavac and Carey, 1997; van Ryn and Heaney, 1992).

No single theory exists on which to base health education and health promotion programs. Populations, environments, cultures, and health issues vary broadly, so different theories or different combinations of theories may be useful in addressing a particular issue. Some theories focus on individual behavior; others focus on groups, organizations, or communities as the unit of change. The dominant theories currently used in health education have roots in social psychology and focus on health behavior at the individual level. These include the health belief model and the transtheoretical model. Bridging the individual, group, and community levels is social learning theory, also called social cognitive theory. Theories that address organizations and communities include organizational change theory (Butterfoss, Kegler, and Francisco, 2008), community organization and empowerment (Wilson et al., 2008), and diffusion of innovations (Balas and Chapman, 2018). These theories provide a foundation for community program design and implementation. See Chapter 3 for a discussion of these and other theories that are useful for community and population health program planning.

Learning how to analyze a theory's fit with the identified issue or problem can be challenging. According to Glanz and Rimer (2005, p. 6), "a

Box 5-1 A Good Fit: Characteristics of a Useful Theory

A useful theory makes assumptions about a behavior, health problem, target population, or environment that is:

- Logical
- Consistent with everyday observations
- Similar to those used in previous successful programs
- Supported by past research in the same or related ideas

From *Theory at a Glance: A Guide for Health Promotion Practice* (2nd ed., p. 7), by K. Glanz and B. K. Rimer, 2005, Washington, DC: National Cancer Institute, U.S. Department of Health and Human Services, National Institutes of Health.

working knowledge of specific theories, and familiarity with how they have been applied in the past improves skill in this area." When selecting the best model, it is important to consider the characteristics outlined in Box 5-1 rather than prematurely selecting a theory that may be temporarily in vogue or a personal favorite. For more detail on the theories just described and others and for a better understanding of their applications, the reader is referred to Glanz and Rimer (2005) and Glanz, Rimer, and Viswanath (2015).

Engage Your Brain 5-3

Your local community has received funding for a wellness initiative for persons who are homeless. One of the goals of the initiative is to promote participation in a community garden located near a church where many persons who are homeless come to share a free lunchtime and dinner meal. How might you use an occupational therapy theoretical framework as a foundation for empowering community members and building community capacity to fund and oversee the garden? How could the garden be used not only to nourish persons who are homeless but also to increase the awareness of the local community of the needs of persons who are homeless and to empower persons who are homeless to participate in taking care of the garden?

Planning With Evidence

Community-based programs should be developed, implemented, and evaluated by applying principles of scientific reasoning and using appropriate theoretical frameworks and program-planning models (Brownson, Baker, Deshpande, and Gillespie, 2017; Glanz and Rimer, 2005). Program planning begins with the best evidence available. **Evidence** can be defined as data that inform decision-making. Evidence is rarely constant; it is always emergent. The best available evidence of yesterday may be totally irrelevant today. Evidence may be quantitative, or numeric, and qualitative in the form of narrative. **Evidence-based planning for health** is the "application of the best available information derived from clinical, epidemiological, administrative, demographic and other relevant sources and consultations to clearly describe current and desired outcomes for an identified population or organization" (Ardal, Butler, Edwards, and Lawrie, 2006, p. 1). Epidemiological and demographic data are information about a population usually derived from a census or survey. Administrative data are information about services provided and the activities of the health-care system. Consultation with experts can also be a source of evidence. Expert opinion should be sought when formulating questions, identifying sources of information and evidence, and interpreting the findings (Ardal et al., 2006).

No single type of evidence exists that is the most useful for planning health interventions. The type of information needed varies depending on the stage of the planning process. Decisions about program goals, objectives, and strategies ought to be grounded in established best practice, and interventions should be evidence-based. Effectiveness means that the intervention chosen has better results than the alternatives, including no intervention.

The World Health Organization (2012) has developed five criteria for evaluating the quality of evidence. These include:

- Proven validity of measurement instruments
- Quantified reliability of measurement instruments
- Comparability of measures over time and within populations

Box 5-2 Sources of Systematic Literature Reviews and Other Evidence

- Campbell Collaboration Library (www.campbellcollaboration.org/library)
- Centers for Disease Control and Prevention: Program Performance and Evaluation Office (www.cdc.gov/eval/tools/strategies/index.html)
- Centers for Medicare and Medicaid Services Healthy Aging Initiative—Evidence Reports (https://nfsi.org/wp-content/uploads/2013/10/medicare.pdf)
- Clinical Evidence (www.clinicalevidence.bmj.com)
- Cochrane Collaboration (www.cochrane.org)
- Community Tool Box (https://ctb.ku.edu/en)
- Community Commons (https://www.communitycommons.org)
- ERIC Digests (www.eric.ed.gov)
- Evidence-Based Mental Health (https://bestpractice.bmj.com/info/evidence-information)
- *Healthy People 2020* Evidence-Based Resources (www.healthypeople.gov/2020/topics-objectives/topic/educational-and-community-based-programs/ebrs)
- Joanna Briggs Institute Clinical Online Network of Evidence for Care and Therapeutics/JBI COnNECT (www.jbiconnect.org)
- National Guidelines Clearinghouse (www.ahrq.gov/gam/index.html)
- National Rehabilitation Information Center (www.naric.com)
- OT Seeker (www.otseeker.com)
- Substance Abuse and Mental Health Services Administration (www.samhsa.gov)
- The Community Guide (https://www.thecommunityguide.org/resources)

- Explicit data trail that clearly identifies how data were obtained and analyzed
- Consultation with relevant experts and authorities to understand and accurately interpret the data

According to Ardal et al. (2006), "an evidence base that has proven validity, quantified reliability, comparability, consultation with experts and an explicit data audit trail should lead to a plan that is valid, coherent and applicable" (p. 14). A plan is valid when the information and evidence gathered address relevant planning questions. A coherent plan explains the differences in the data and the conclusions in a way that can be understood. A plan is applicable if it identifies how change can be measured, provides information that informs decision-makers, captures relevant situational realities, and addresses sustainability.

Framing questions clearly is key to locating and using the right evidence. Finding and evaluating evidence can be time-intensive and requires some research expertise. **Systematic reviews** are often the most useful as they identify, assess, and synthesize research evidence from a number of individual research studies. A variety of sources of systematic reviews of research exist, some of which are listed in Box 5-2. Utilizing a range of information types and sources will create a comprehensive picture of the phenomenon of interest that results in a solid evidence base from which to make decisions and plan for the future.

To further establish the role of occupational therapy practitioners in community health, health promotion, and injury/disease prevention, more studies are needed to identify the occupational factors that affect health and well-being and to document the effectiveness of occupation-based community and population health promotion interventions.

By being skilled in the steps of program development, from preplanning to publication, occupational therapy practitioners can strengthen their position in the provision of health education and health promotion programs and increase their marketability in the evolving health-care arena.

Summary

- Program-planning best practices include preplanning, planning with people and data, planning for performance and priorities, planning for evaluation and measurable outcomes, and sustainability.
- The needs assessment process for a community or population parallels the occupational therapy evaluation profile process of an individual client.

- Community-based programs need to be grounded in theory and based on the best available evidence.
- Involving community stakeholders and members of the target population in the planning process is essential, as the AOTA *Occupational Therapy Code of Ethics (2015)* principle of autonomy promotes client centeredness in the community as a community-centered approach.

CASE STUDIES

CASE STUDY PART 1 Suicide Prevention in a Native American Community

Suicide prevention for youth in Native American communities is an important public health concern. Suicide is identified by the CDC as the second leading cause of death among Native Americans ages 10–34 and is 1.5 times higher than the national average (CDC, 2015). An occupational therapy practitioner playing both a professional and community role was invited to be part of a community coalition exploring ways to address suicide prevention on a reservation. The community was not only aware of national statistics but had also experienced a recent increase in suicide attempts and completions among middle and high school-aged youth. Through brainstorming, the community decided to pursue grant funding to develop programming for suicide prevention. One issue identified by youth was high levels of daily stress caused by family situations and the implications of poverty, along with the impact of historical trauma.

In a casual conversation, the occupational therapy practitioner mentioned that it might be helpful to teach the children stress management strategies in a fun and meaningful way. Through conversation, this evolved into identifying the opportunity to place stress management stations in two Native American schools, develop a curriculum, and train teachers and children how to monitor and use the stress management rooms and equipment. The coalition members asked the occupational therapy practitioner to help develop the tools as part of a federal grant application. The grant was written and funded, with the occupational therapy practitioner contributing the description of the proposed curriculum.

Community members, including the occupational therapist, set up stress reduction rooms in two Native American schools and developed a training manual. They implemented training and developed a tool for evaluation. The evaluation plan was multipronged, including posttraining surveys, focus groups with trainees, and a pre-post tool for youth to identify their levels of stress before and after the stress reduction experience. A small group of youths participated in the development of the youth tool, which was designed to be visual and culturally sensitive.

The remaining three chapters in this section will refer to this case as an example of how to successfully develop, fund, and implement a program to have an impact on a community need through an occupational therapy lens.

Discussion Questions and Application

1. What principles of program preplanning do you observe in this case?
2. Describe how theory influenced program development in this case.

The principles of program preplanning occurred because the occupational therapy practitioner was a valued and integrated member of the community. In this case, the occupational therapy practitioner was invited to the table as a valued stakeholder. Her perspective provided a foundation to design and implement a program to meet a community-identified need. In this case, the occupational therapy practitioner needed to become better informed about suicide prevention and the cultural implications. She wanted to develop a program that did not evoke further dependency on others and taught skills to manage stress not only to empower the community but to be sensitive to

CASE STUDY PART 1 Suicide Prevention in a Native American Community

the impact of historical trauma on the community. The intent was based on research on suicide prevention related to stress as an indicator for suicidal ideation and completion, with an occupation-based approach to teach positive stress management techniques to ensure improved stress modulation strategies (CDC, 2015). In addition, trauma-informed care was considered, and the occupational therapist and community members sought additional training in this approach to ensure a strong connection to trauma-informed concepts of care in the program design and implementation.

The program was designed to train community members to prevent dependency on the occupational therapist and to enhance community program ownership. In addition, the train-the-trainer approach provides a foundation for program sustainability by ensuring multiple community stakeholders can help implement the program. A manual was developed with descriptions of the stress management equipment, along with guidelines for proper use and equipment maintenance. In collaboration with the teachers, guidelines for use of the stress reduction rooms were developed. In addition, training was provided quarterly to teachers and the youth accessing the room. Evaluation was infused throughout the process. The evaluation strategies included conducting surveys to determine the effectiveness of the training, holding focus groups with teachers to gain their perspective on the effectiveness of the stress management rooms, and developing a tool, with input from the participants, to assess stress before and after the use of the stress management rooms. The program was developed in this way because the occupational therapy practitioner wanted to truly respect and integrate the community's cultural health beliefs.

Learning Activities

1. You have been contracted to provide occupational therapy services to children in a rural day-care setting. Many of the single, teenaged mothers have sought your advice on parenting. The day-care manager has secured funding to develop a parenting class and has hired you to develop and implement the program. What steps would you take to assess need? Who would you involve? What questions would you want answered?
2. How would you use occupational therapy constructs and theories to shape an intervention strategy for the teen mothers?
3. What types of needs assessment information would you collect from the population? Which data collection strategies would you use and why?

REFERENCES

Alley, D., Asomugha, C. N., Conway, P. H., and Sanghavi, D. M. (2016). Accountable health communities—addressing social needs through Medicare and Medicaid. *New England Journal of Medicine, 374*(1), 811.

Altschuld, J. W. (2015). *Bridging the gap between asset/capacity building and needs assessment: Concepts and practical applications.* Thousand Oaks, CA: Sage.

American Association of Colleges of Nursing, American Association of Colleges of Osteopathic Medicine, American Association of Colleges of Pharmacy, American Dental Education Association, Association of American Medical Colleges, and Association of Schools of Public Health. (2011). *Core competencies for interprofessional collaborative practice.* Retrieved from www.aacom.org/docs/default-source/insideome/ccrpt05-10-11.pdf?sfvrsn=77937f97_2

American Occupational Therapy Association. (2014). *Occupational therapy practice framework: Domain and process* (3rd ed.). Bethesda, MD: AOTA Press.

American Occupational Therapy Association. (2015). Occupational therapy code of ethics (2015). *American Occupational Therapy Association, 69*(Suppl. 3), 6913410030p1–6913410030p8. https:doi.org/10.5114/ajot.2015.696S03

American Occupational Therapy Association. (2017a). Vision 2025. *American Journal of Occupational Therapy, 71,* 7103420010.

American Occupational Therapy Association. (2017b). *Occupational profile template.* Retrieved from www.aota.org/~/media/Corporate/Files/Practice/Manage/Documentation/AOTA-Occupational-Profile-Template.pdf

Ardal, S., Butler, J., Edwards, R., and Lawrie, L. (2006). Evidence-based planning: Module 3. In *The health planner's toolkit.* Ontario, Canada: Health System Intelligence Project.

Balas, E. A., and Chapman, W. W. (2018). Road map for diffusion of innovation in health care. *Health Affairs, 37*(2), 198–204.

Barnett, L. M., Van Beurden, E., Eakin, E. G., Beard, J., Dietrich, U., and Newman, B. (2004). Program sustainability of a community-based intervention to prevent falls among older Australians. *Health Promotion International, 19*(3), 281–288.

Bass, J. D., and Baker, N. A. (2017). Occupational therapy and public health: Advancing research to improve population health and health equity. *OTJR: Occupation, Participation and Health, 37*(4), 175–177. https://doi.org/10.1177/1539449217773165

Beaulieu, L. J. (n.d.) *Mapping the assets of your community: A key component for building local capacity.* Retrieved from http://srdc.msstate.edu/publications/227/227_asset-mapping.pdf

Bodenheimer, T., and Sinsky, C. (2014). From triple to quadruple aim: Care of the patient requires care of the provider. *Annals of Family Medicine, 12*(6), 573–576.

Braveman, B. (2016). Health policy perspectives—population health and occupational therapy. *American Journal of Occupational Therapy, 70,* 7001090010. https://doi.org/10.5014/ajot.2016.701002

Breckon, D. J., Harvey, J. R., and Lancaster, R. B. (1994). *Community health education: Settings, roles, and skills for the 21st century.* Gaithersburg, MD: Aspen.

Brownson, R. C., Baker, E. A., Deshpande, A. D., and Gillespie, K. N. (2017). *Evidence-based public health* (3rd ed.). New York, NY: Oxford University Press.

Butterfoss, F. D., Kegler, M. C., and Francisco, W. T. (2008). Mobilizing organizations for health promotion: Theories of organizational change. In K. Glanz, B. K. Rimer, and K. Viswanath. *Health behavior and health education: Theory, research and practice* (4th ed.). San Francisco, CA: Jossey-Bass.

Caldwell, E., Whitehead, M., Fleming, J., and Moes, L. (2008). Evidence-based practice in everyday clinical practice: Strategies for change in a tertiary occupational therapy department. *Australian Occupational Therapy Journal, 55*(2), 79–84.

Centers for Disease Control and Prevention. (2013). *Community needs assessment: Participant workbook.* Retrieved from www.cdc.gov/globalhealth/healthprotection/fetp/training_modules/15/community-needs_pw_final_9252013.pdf

Centers for Disease Control and Prevention. (2015). *Suicide: Facts at a glance.* Retrieved from www.cdc.gov/violenceprevention/pdf/suicide-datasheet-a.pdf

Dignan, M. B., and Carr, P. A. (1992). *Program planning for health education and health promotion* (2nd ed.). Philadelphia, PA: Lea and Febiger.

Doll, J. D. (2010). *Program development and grant writing in occupational therapy: Making the connection.* Sudbury, MA: Jones and Bartlett.

Edberg, M. (2015). Community and populations as the focus of health promotion programs. In *Essentials of health behaviour: Social and behavioural theory in public health* (2nd ed., pp. 109–118). Burlington, MA: Jones and Bartlett.

Freudenberg, N., Eng, E., Flay, B., Parcel, G., Rogers, T., and Wallerstein, N. (1995). Strengthening individual and community capacity to prevent disease and promote health: In search of relevant theories and principles. *Health Education Quarterly, 22*(3), 290–306.

Gilmore, G. D., and Campbell, M. D. (2005). Group participation process: Nominal group. In *Needs and capacity assessment strategies for health education and health promotion* (pp. 88–97). Sudbury, MA: Jones and Bartlett.

Glanz, K., and Rimer, B. K. (2005). *Theory at a glance: A guide for health promotion practice* (2nd ed.). Washington, DC: National Cancer Institute, U.S. Department of Health and Human Services, National Institutes of Health.

Glanz, K., Rimer, B., and Viswanath, K. (Eds.). (2015). *Health behavior and health education: Theory, research, and practice* (4th ed.). San Francisco, CA: Jossey-Bass.

Grady, A. (2017). Building inclusive community: A challenge for occupational therapy. 1994 Eleanor Clarke Slagle Lecture. In R. Padilla and Y. Griffiths (Eds.), *A professional legacy: The Eleanor Clarke Slagle lectures in occupational therapy, 1955–2016* (Centennial ed., pp. 385–398). Bethesda, MD: AOTA Press.

Harvard T. H. Chan School of Public Health. (2018). *Prevalence and incidence defined.* Retrieved from www.hsph.harvard.edu/obesity-prevention-source/prevalence-incidence/

Hodges, B. C., and Videto, D. M. (2011). *Assessment and planning in health programs* (2nd ed.). Sudbury, MA: Jones and Bartlett.

Hyett, N., McKinstry, C. E., Kenny, A., and Dickson-Swift, V. (2016). Community-centred practice: Occupational therapists improving the health and wellbeing of populations. *Australian Occupational Therapy Journal, 63*(1), 5–8.

Institute for Healthcare Improvement. (2018). *IHI triple aim initiative.* Retrieved from www.ihi.org/Engage/Initiatives/TripleAim/Pages/default.aspx

Institute of Medicine. (2015a). *Building health workforce capacity through community-based health professional education: Workshop summary.* Washington, DC: National Academies Press.

Institute of Medicine. (2015b). *Measuring the impact of interprofessional education on collaborative practice and patient outcomes.* Washington, DC: National Academies Press.

Issel, L. M., and Wells, R. (2018). *Health program planning and evaluation: A practical systematic approach for community health* (4th ed.). Burlington, MA: Jones and Bartlett.

Kettner, P. M., Moroney, R. M., and Martin, L. L. (2017). *Designing and managing programs: An effectiveness-based approach* (5th ed.). SAGE Sourcebooks for the Human Services. Thousand Oaks, CA: Sage.

Kindig, D., and Stoddart, G. (2003). What is population health? *American Journal of Public Health, 93*(3), 380–383.

Kretzmann, J. P., and McKnight J. L. (1993). *Building communities from the inside out: A path toward finding and mobilizing a community's assets.* Skokie, IL: ACTA.

Kronenberg, F., Pollard, N., and Sakellariou, D. (Eds.). (2011). *Occupational therapies without borders: Towards an ecology of occupation-based practices* (Vol. 2). Amsterdam, Netherlands: Elsevier Health Sciences.

Lysack, C. L., and Adamo, D. E. (2014). Social, economic, and political factors that influence occupational performance. In B. A. B. Schell, G. Gillen, and M. E. Scaffa (Eds.), *Willard and Spackman's occupational therapy* (12th ed., pp. 188–201). Philadelphia, PA: Wolters Kluwer/Lippincott Williams and Wilkins.

McKenzie, J. F., Neiger, B. L., and Thackeray, R. (2017). *Planning, implementing, and evaluating health promotion programs: A primer* (7th ed.). Upper Saddle River, NJ: Pearson.

Minkler, M. (2014). *Community organizing and community building for health and welfare* (3rd ed.). New Brunswick, NJ: Rutgers University Press.

Minnesota Department of Health, Center for Public Health Nursing. (n.d.). *Definitions of Population Health.* Retrieved from www.health.state.mn.us/divs/opi/cd/phn/docs/0303phn_popbasedpractice.pdf

Nash, D. B., Fabius, R. J., Skoufalos, A., Clarke, J. L., and Horowitz, M. R. (2016). *Population health: Creating a culture of wellness* (2nd ed.). Burlington, MA: Jones and Bartlett.

National Institute of Mental Health. (2017). *What is prevalence?* Retrieved from www.nimh.nih.gov/health/statistics/what-is-prevalence.shtml

National Library of Medicine. (2018). *Needs Assessment MeSH Descriptor Data 2018.* Retrieved from https://meshb.nlm.nih.gov/record/ui?name=Needs%20Assessment

Nester, J. (2016). The importance of interprofessional practice and education in the era of accountable care. *North Carolina Medical Journal, 77*(2), 128–132. doi.org/10.18043/ncm.77.2.128

Posavac, E., and Carey, R. (1997). *Program evaluation: Methods and case studies* (5th ed.). Upper Saddle River, NJ: Prentice Hall.

Prince, J. H., Dake, J. A., and Ward, B. (2017). Assessing the needs of program participants. In C. I. Fertman and D. D. Allenworth (Eds.), *Health promotion programs: From theory to practice* (2nd ed., pp. 85–110). San Francisco, CA: Jossey Bass.

Rutgers Cooperative Extension. (2007). *Ten easy steps to program impact evaluation.* Retrieved from http://nacaa.com/ampic/2007/presentations/ten_easy_steps_to_program_impact_evaluation.pdf

Scaffa, M. E., and Reitz, S. M. (2013). *Occupational therapy in community-based practice settings* (2nd ed). Philadelphia, PA: F. A. Davis.

Shortell, S. M. (2013). A bold proposal for advancing population health. *NAM Perspectives.* Discussion Paper, National Academy of Medicine, Washington, DC. doi:10.31478/201308a

Simons-Morton, B. G., Greene, W. H., and Gottlieb, N. H. (1995). *Introduction to health education and health promotion.* Prospect Heights, IL: Waveland.

Soriano, F. L. (2013). *Conducting needs assessments: A multidisciplinary approach* (2nd ed). Thousand Oaks, CA: Sage.

Stevens, J. A., Teh, S. L., and Haileyesus, T. (2010). Dogs and cats as environmental fall hazards. *Journal of Safety Research, 41*(1), 69–73.

Suarez-Balcazar, Y. (2005). Empowerment and participatory evaluation of a community health intervention: Implications for occupational therapy. *OTJR: Occupation, Participation and Health, 25*(4), 133–142.

Timmreck, T. C. (2003). *Planning, program development, and evaluation* (2nd ed.). Boston, MA: Jones and Bartlett.

van Ryn, M., and Heaney, C. A. (1992). What's the use of theory? *Health Education Quarterly, 19*(3), 315–330.

Wilson, N., Minkler, M., Dasho, S., Wallerstein, N., and Martin, A. C. (2008). Getting to social action: The youth empowerment strategies (YES!) project. *Health Promotion Practice, 9*(4), 395–403.

Witkin, B. R., and Altschuld, J. W. (1995). *Planning and conducting needs assessments: A practical guide.* Thousand Oaks, CA: Sage.

World Health Organization. (2012). *WHO Handbook for Guideline Development.* WHO Press, World Health Organization, Geneva. Retrieved from http://apps.who.int/iris/bitstream/ 10665/75146/1/ 9789241548441_eng.pdf

Chapter 6

Program Design and Implementation

Joy D. Doll, OTD, OTR/L, and Anna Domina, OTD, OTR/L

Never doubt that a small group of thoughtful committed people can change the world. Indeed, it is the only thing that ever has.

—Margaret Meade

Learning Outcomes

This chapter is designed to enable the reader to:

6-1 Identify and discuss the similarities and differences between intervention planning for individuals and the development of community and population health initiatives.

6-2 Describe the best practices to use in the development of a mission statement.

6-3 Discuss the components of an implementation plan.

6-4 Describe the characteristics of an effective team and the stages of team development.

6-5 Discuss the importance of partnerships to a program's success.

6-6 Discuss the role of advisory boards, boards of directors, and community coalitions in relation to program management.

6-7 Identify and discuss issues related to program sustainability.

Key Terms

Advisory board
Board of directors
Community coalition
Goal
Implementation plan
Interprofessional collaborative practice
Mission statement
Objective
Partnerships
Psychological safety
SMART
Sustainability
Team
Vision statement

Introduction

Occupational therapy practitioners develop individualized intervention plans for their clients every day. Using clinical reasoning, the practitioner is able to determine which occupations will enable clients to reach their goals. In community practice settings, the occupational therapy practitioner utilizes these same skills and applies them in the context of a community to address the greater health needs of a population. Designing and implementing a program requires a similar thought process using reasoning skills to develop goals and objectives to implement a program. Many of the skills from practice with individuals can transfer to community practice. As indicated in Chapter 5, program development requires an occupational therapy practitioner to use a systems approach instead of an individual patient model (Fazio, 2017).

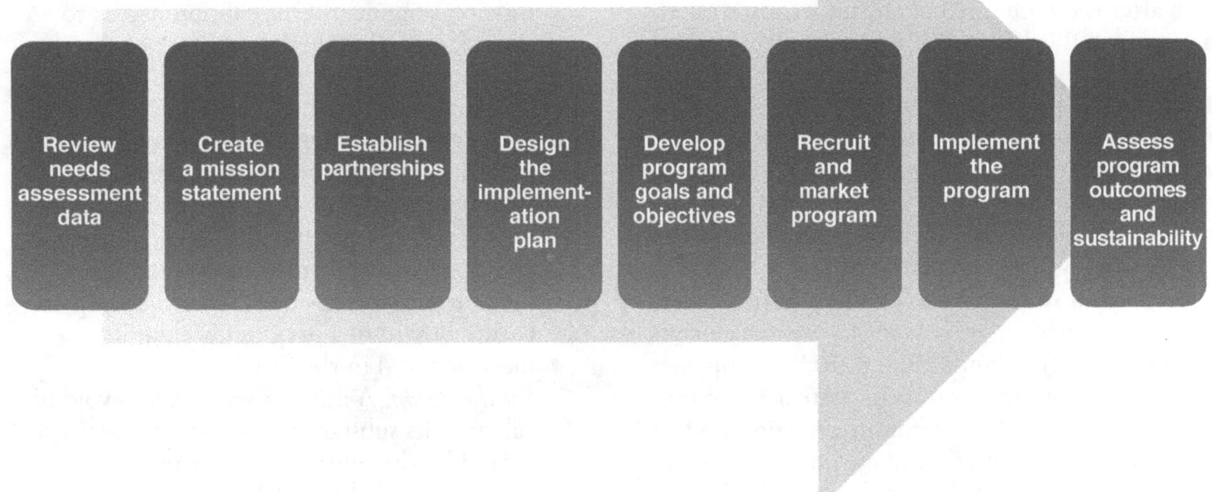

Figure 6-1 Program development and implementation process.

Chapter 5 provided a general overview of program development and the needs assessment process. This chapter will expand on this information by providing details regarding developing a mission statement and an implementation plan with goals and objectives. The chapter also reviews strategies for recruiting participants, developing teams, and establishing partnerships. In addition, recommendations for budgeting, program management, and program sustainability are presented. The strategies described in this chapter utilize a systems approach based on the occupational therapy practice framework (American Occupational Therapy Association [AOTA], 2014) and clinical reasoning models. Figure 6-1 summarizes the stages of community and population health program design and implementation.

Vision and Mission Statements

When beginning the process of developing and implementing a new program, the occupational therapy practitioner should have a clear understanding of the community or population and the type of program that should be developed. If the occupational therapy practitioner is developing a program within an existing organization, one of the first steps in program planning should be to review the organization's vision and mission statements. The practitioner should review needs assessment data to ensure that the program has a clear focus. Often program planners will compose a vision statement prior to the development of a mission statement. A **vision statement** outlines the "ideal state or ultimate level of achievement to which an organization aspires" (Strickland, 2011, p. 103). A vision statement is always something the program or organization is trying to attain. As described, it should be visionary. A vision statement should also be brief but capture the essence of the dreams of the organization or program. Most community organizations and corporations have vision and mission statements that can be easily accessed on their websites. Often, programs begin development with the overall vision and mission to provide direction and focus. Reviewing existing vision statements from other community organizations can help with brainstorming and forming the ideal vision statement. A vision statement is what the program or organization strives to be, and the profession of occupational therapy uses visioning on a national level to advance the profession. The AOTA used visioning with its well-known *Centennial Vision,* which transformed into *Vision 2025* after the centennial of the profession was celebrated in 2017. *Vision 2025* specifically mentions the value of the profession in community and population health practice by stating the following: "As an inclusive profession, occupational therapy maximizes health, well-being, and quality of life for all people, populations, and communities through effective solutions that facilitate participation in everyday living" (AOTA, 2017, p. 1).

A **mission statement** is "an organization's core, underlying purpose, or basis for its existence, focus and actions" (Strickland, 2011, p. 103). Companies and organizations utilize mission statements to provide employees with a common direction and to make consumers aware of the purpose of the company (Management Sciences for Health [MSH], 2010). A mission statement goes beyond simply educating workers and consumers; it acts as the driving force or motivation behind decisions, actions, and program development. Mission statements also imply future direction, indicating what the program hopes to accomplish over time (Ohio Literacy Resource Center, 2018).

The challenge to developing a mission statement is to describe a program and its values, purpose, and future direction in a few short sentences. The occupational therapy practitioner and team members should begin by finding current mission statements of organizations they believe are effective. Mission statements can easily be found on websites or in company materials. If the client is a nonprofit organization, the program developer may want to explore existing mission statements of other nonprofits as a starting point. The United Way can be a useful resource for identifying local nonprofit organizations.

The INSPIRE Model

The INSPIRE model by Li, Frohna, and Bostwick (2017) provides a useful framework for developing mission statements. It consists of seven components:

1. *Identify core values.* The purpose of a mission statement is to focus on the values and the premise of the program. The purpose is not to provide accolades to past successes or identify the reasons why the program was started. Identifying core professional values helps guide what is most relevant to the mission statement. One caution here is to avoid jargon that might confuse people who are unfamiliar with occupational therapy terminology.
2. *Name the population.* When an organization is working in the community, the mission statement should be collective and inclusive of those the program will serve. Including community members in developing the mission statement is one essential strategy to ensure buy-in to a program both at its inception and in the future.
3. *Set the vision.* A mission statement devoid of values lacks substance. The mission statement should be thoughtful and meaningful. It should elicit feelings of passion and offer an opportunity to articulate that passion for the program to others and to those being served.
4. *Plan how to achieve the mission.* Mission statements should be a brief snapshot that captures the essence of the program or organization. Ideal mission statements are captured in a few easily recalled sentences that are written clearly and concisely. The occupational therapy practitioner should consider the literacy level of the audience when drafting the mission statement. Careful editing is important, as grammatical and syntax errors in the mission statement can detract from the program and its purpose. Once the purpose is clear, it is essential to develop a plan and a time line for how the organization or program will achieve the mission over time.
5. *Identify activities that align with the mission.* The plan should focus on activities or events that align with the mission clearly and which can be implemented. A well-crafted mission statement will focus the organization and assist in making decisions that will support the achievement of goals in the implementation plan phase.
6. *Review, revise, and refine.* Continue to revise the mission statement until all parties are

satisfied and passionate about it (Doll, 2008). When designing a program, it is important to be thoughtful about a mission statement, as it is often one of the first aspects program participants may view. Furthermore, since the mission statement is included in reports and grant proposals, it needs to be representative of the program. Taking the time to ensure the mission statement clearly reflects the program can aid the program's sustainability.

7. *Enlist others.* One of the best strategies to developing a good mission statement is to seek advice and feedback. This advice should come from peers and community members. Seeking feedback ensures that others understand the intent of the program, which is the ultimate goal of the mission statement. The occupational therapy practitioner can ask others the following questions to help them evaluate the mission statement:
   - Does the mission statement reveal the values of the program?
   - What future direction does this mission statement indicate for this program?
   - Does the mission statement inspire? Why or why not?

Answers to these questions can provide feedback on the clarity and relevance of a mission statement. Mission statements are not created in isolation. The intent is to provide focus and direction for the community program. Team members and community stakeholders are invaluable in this process and will help drive the formation of the mission. After the mission statement has been established, the next step in program design is to develop an implementation plan that includes the program goals, objectives, and activities.

Implementation Plan

Traditionally, when designing and implementing a program, the occupational therapy practitioner considers what will make the program work and also be sustainable. This thought process aids in the development of a structured and relevant implementation plan. An **implementation plan** includes the goals, objectives, activities, and desired outcomes of the program. This could be formulated in a table similar to the example in Table 6-1. The plan should also identify:

- Who will be served by the program (target population)
- How the individuals being served will be recruited

Program qualifications that describe how and why an individual qualifies for the program and how an individual enters the program once qualification has been determined should also be included.

The development of an implementation plan is important to identify specifically how program goals and objectives will be realized. The plan provides a holistic approach for identifying the program's purpose, design, and implementation in one succinct document. According to Brownson (2001), an implementation plan "spells out the details of each procedure and activity necessary for successful execution of the program and specifies who is responsible for each" (p. 115). In the implementation plan, the details of who, what, when, where, and how need to be finalized for the program (Brownson, 2001; Chambless, 2003). The implementation plan usually contains a time line and persons responsible for addressing these goals to reach the program outcomes. An implementation plan allows the practitioner to map out the entire program in an effective and pragmatic manner. After completion, the implementation plan can be distributed to employees or even used for writing future grant proposals. Effective implementation plans help to ensure program success and sustainability. Table 6-1 outlines a sample program implementation plan.

Program implementation also requires thoughtful planning in order to maintain focus and ensure that activities are completed in a timely manner (Timmreck, 2003). Many organizations now use strategic planning for program implementation. This is a common method, and facilitators with expertise in strategic planning can be hired to assist with the process. Strategic planning is described in more detail in Chapter 8. A method for designing a strategic plan can include a logic model, which is described in detail in Chapter 7.

Ideally, implementation planning should be completed in a group environment to promote

Table 6-1 Sample Implementation Plan

Objectives	Intervention Activities	Measurement Activities to Determine Outcomes	Short-Term Outcomes	Long-Term Outcomes
Describe scopes of practice by the end of March	• Article on what constitutes scopes of practice • Internet research on licensing parameters for nurse/pharmacist/physician • Simulated patient scenario in which providers must refer to another professional • Interdisciplinary care plan	(a) Written exam (b) Care plan	(a) Knowledge of scope of practice/pharmacist/physician/nurse with 95% accuracy (b) Utilization of team resource on care plan per "scopes rubric"	Increased confidence in referral to another professional
Develop a marketable educational module focusing on interprofessional ad hoc team function by the end of May	• Develop a marketing plan	(a) Count the number of courses using the material (b) Count the number of learners using the material	Modules incorporated into the curricula of medicine, nursing, pharmacy	Modules used in all schools at the university
Develop and validate measurement tools related to individual professional performance	• Develop the instrument • Pilot the instrument with sufficient numbers to generate power to do measurement study	Conduct reliability study on instrument (e.g., item analysis, factor loading)	Obtain a reliability factor of X	Publish the instrument

Data from *Interdisciplinary Team Skills Development for Health Professional Students*, by C. G. Goulet, K. Begley, K. Gould, and J. D. Doll, 2008, Association for Prevention Teaching and Research. Awarded October 2008.

communication among team members, especially if a program is in development. Implementation planning provides an opportunity to clarify who will do what and when it will be done. Creating a document that outlines program activities ensures that all team members stay on track, communication flows smoothly, and the program goals and objectives are completed in an efficient manner. Implementation planning also allows the program team to plan and anticipate challenges in a proactive manner, which can have an impact on program success and sustainability (Timmreck, 2003).

Program Goals and Objectives

In program development, a **goal** is defined as "a statement of a quantifiable desired future state or condition" (Timmreck, 2003, p. 32). Goals are written to be long term and future-oriented, indicating a desired outcome (Doll, 2010). While goals capture intended outcomes of the program, **objectives** are more specific, identifying how goals will be met. Objectives are measurable, short term, and usually contain a time line for completion (Doll, 2010). Goals and objectives are different but complementary. Goals and objectives should indicate the program's priorities and intended outcomes, the communities' priorities, and the evaluation plan. A program can have multiple outcomes but should have a defined focus with prioritized outcomes. Too many goals and objectives can make a program appear incoherent and disconnected, posing challenges to successful completion. Drafting goals and objectives that are difficult to achieve makes a program appear disjointed and infeasible, which affects program sustainability and the ability to garner support for the program, especially financially.

Occupational therapy practitioners are familiar with goal and objective writing related to intervention planning; however, writing goals and objectives for a program requires a different perspective. Writing goals and objectives for a community program requires occupational therapy practitioners to think broadly and envision an overall outcome. In medical model patient care, the focus of goals is to enhance the well-being of an individual. In program planning for community practice, the focus is population-based, identifying how an intervention affects a group of individuals (Edberg, 2019). In community settings, occupational therapy practitioners need an expanded thought process that incorporates a population-based approach. Although this aspect of goal writing can be challenging, the process of goal writing is similar to that in other practice areas, just applied more broadly.

The mnemonic **SMART** can aid in writing appropriate program objectives (Doran, 1981). SMART stands for:

S = specific
M = measurable
A = attainable
R = relevant
T = timely

Program objectives should be *specific* to the program, identifying a *measurable* outcome. It is important that objectives are *attainable* and feasible, considering time lines, resources, and staffing. Goals and objectives should be developed with the targeted population to be served with a focus on the community needs identified in the assessment. Written goals and objectives should align with community needs and wants to ensure they are *relevant,* improving the likelihood of success. This concept follows the occupational therapy principle of client-centered practice applied to a program model (Scaffa and Brownson, 2014; Law, 1998; Sumsion, 2006). Goals and objectives that focus on community needs facilitate community buy-in and programmatic success, making them *timely*. See an example of a SMART program objective in Box 6-1.

The SMART approach is useful not only when drafting objectives but also when evaluating the match between objectives and program activities (Weis and Gantt, 2004). After drafting the goals and objectives, the team should design specific activities that address the goals and objectives. The program activities are exactly what will be done day to day in the program. Similar to the therapeutic occupations used to reach client goals, program activities are meant to achieve the desired program outcomes.

Box 6-1 Example of a SMART Objective

Program Objective: develop five group intervention plans for young children with hearing impairment in a community setting by the end of March.

This example objective follows the SMART mnemonic:

- **S**pecific: the goal provides a specific action, "develop five group intervention plans," that will be taken by the occupational therapy practitioner or team.
- **M**easurable: the goal can be measured by the achievement of the five group intervention plans being completed by the set time frame.
- **A**ttainable: this is a task that can be completed in a short period of time by the occupational therapy practitioner or team and would need to be completed prior to implementing the community group programming.
- **R**elevant: this goal supports the progression of future program planning and is therefore relevant to the implementation of the community-based program.
- **T**imely: the timeline associated with the goal is appropriate and timely based on the larger implementation plan for the program.

Another essential component of program planning beyond the goals and objectives is to identify programmatic roles. In the planning stage, the details of who will complete the program roles and responsibilities may not need to be identified, but consideration should be given to the potential roles and responsibilities required to make the program a success. Drafting job descriptions for both employees and volunteers provides program structure and improves the probability of successful implementation. Time lines should also be discussed and developed.

Including all of these aspects in the implementation plan provides a stable and sustainable program design. Such a plan guides implementation and ensures that the program remains aligned with its mission and purpose. The implementation plan should be tied clearly to the strategic and evaluation plan and used to aid in garnering funds, such as grants. The plan should be an active document that is reviewed regularly to ensure goals and objectives remain meaningful and relevant (Sand, 2005). A balanced plan should be dynamic and flexible enough to change but sufficiently stable to serve as a road map for program implementation.

Participant Recruitment

A key aspect of successful implementation is the recruitment of program participants. The recruitment and retention of program participants must be considered in the planning process and are crucial in program design. Inattention to this step can negatively affect the use and success of the program and ultimately result in a failure to meet the community's needs. Establishing referrals to the program requires the development of protocols and roles for each person involved in the program (Braveman, 2016). Policies and procedures are developed that outline how community members will access and benefit from the services. Eligibility requirements or stipulations for admission to the program need to be identified. The program team strategizes how to recruit participants and market to potential clients. For example, a nonprofit organization offers a health equipment recycling program that provides used health equipment to individuals in need. When promoting the program, identifying who is eligible to receive the equipment may need to be based on income, access to health insurance, or a vetting process to ensure those most in need benefit.

Developing a marketing plan will help to identify methods for recruitment. The marketing plan may be referred to as a community awareness campaign depending on the program and target audience. Whatever the title, the marketing of services needs to be considered in the program design. When marketing, the occupational therapy practitioner or program team should consider all necessary venues and utilize community resources such as partners, advisory boards, coalitions, community members, and participants.

In the marketing plan development process, the occupational therapy practitioner should take into account the services being provided, who will benefit from these services, and who needs to know about the services (Braveman, 2016). For example, the main targets for marketing the health equipment recycling program are social workers, occupational therapy practitioners, and physical therapy practitioners in various health-care, school, and community settings. These individuals may refer clients who cannot receive health equipment through insurance or cannot afford to pay for it themselves (Doll, 2010). In the health equipment recycling example, eligibility criteria for receiving the equipment would need to be explicit and included in marketing materials.

In other instances, programs may choose to target both health-care professionals and the general public through newspaper articles or television segments, such as with a community-based fall prevention and home safety program (Painter and Elliot, 2004). Many organizations now use social media and other relevant platforms to support marketing efforts. Inadequate participation and loss of funding can be an unfortunate consequence of poor marketing or community awareness. More strategies for marketing and outreach are described in Chapter 8.

Location and Space

Location and space for program implementation also need to be addressed in program development (Braveman, 2016). For some, these will not be of concern because the program is part of a larger organization that will donate or loan space for program implementation. This is the case for a program implemented in a hospital practice setting where meeting rooms may be available for a community outreach program. For example, a health system may offer conference or training rooms to community organizations as part of its mission to be a good partner. Program managers may need to make a formal request for such space and should follow the policies of the institution with which they partner.

For other programs that are not part of a larger organization, space and location are critical factors. If a paid space is necessary, this information must be included when budgeting and determining program costs. The program manager may need to work with a realtor to find an appropriate space and location for the program. Collaborating with other community institutions may also allow for shared costs of space. For example, faith communities (e.g., churches, temples, mosques) may be willing to donate space for health programming that benefits their constituents and the greater community (Swinney, Anson-Wonkka, Maki, and Corneau, 2001).

The health equipment recycling example began in a church basement and then grew into its own nonprofit community organization as demand for the program increased. This not only was cost-effective but demonstrated the good stewardship of resources and collaboration with community entities that community members value. The program outgrew a small storage closet in a faith community facility and was therefore moved to a more formal location. When this move occurred, space rental became a priority for the transforming program.

Local nonprofit agencies may also be willing to share space or provide space at a reduced cost in exchange for lower fees for participants or just as goodwill to the community. Universities and local libraries are other good options for exploring space utilization or partnering to offer a program. In addition, coworking spaces are now more common. In this case, space may be rented or used at a facility that exists to offer such space. Some examples include co-ops that offer affordable rates to community organizations with missions related to those of the co-op. Organizations that donate space can identify it as an in-kind donation, which may be of benefit to that organization. When lobbying an organization for space at a free or reduced cost, the occupational therapy practitioner should be able to articulate the benefits to the organization clearly. Developing a memorandum of understanding or a formal contract is recommended to establish an agreement about space, cost, and use.

When considering space for implementing a program, the program manager has to consider the needs of program participants. This includes liability issues, accessibility for participants, and the regulations and use of the space depending on program needs. Related to liability, the program budget should include insurance to cover the facility. For program success, consider accessibility to the location and space (Gitlow and Flecky, 2005). For example, if program participants are unable to drive, then considering a location close to public transportation is important. Other considerations include the availability of ramps, elevators, accessible entrances, parking, and lighting. Locations such as faith communities may not be as accessible as other public facilities, so it is important to consider these factors when choosing a location for the program. One of the challenges of the health equipment recycling program was its original location in a church basement storage closet. No elevator access was available, and staff had to constantly move equipment in and out of the cramped space. When the program moved, a priority of the program director was accessibility to the stored equipment and a showroom to promote dignity when participants came in to choose items. As programs grow and change, space needs and priorities also evolve.

Last, maintaining the space is important to consider in program planning. For example, if the space needs regular professional cleaning, then this must be considered in the budget during program planning. Each location and space will come with regulations, and it is essential to consider these in planning and budgeting. Furthermore, the amount of space and the time the space will be used need to be considered. In initial stages or with program growth, a change of space and location may be needed. Careful consideration of any change in location should be taken once a program has been established, as it can affect participants and overall program implementation.

Where to implement a program will depend on the needs of the program. Once a program has been implemented, challenges with space and location may arise. One method for strategizing is to build an assessment of the space and location into the program evaluation plan to continually assess the benefits and challenges of the place and location for the program. As described in the health equipment recycling program example, a showroom concept became important as a way to promote choice and dignity for clients, similar to a shopping experience in the community.

Supplies and Equipment

Each program will have a need for unique supplies and equipment. During program planning, brainstorming a list of supplies and equipment is critical to ensure the program has what is required for successful implementation (Braveman, 2016; Scaffa and Brownson, 2014; Fazio, 2017). Most programs have similar basic needs, such as computers and office supplies. However, programs will require specific supplies and equipment based on program demands. For example, the health equipment recycling program would require donations of equipment to ensure the ability to recycle to those in need. Donated equipment must be cleaned and sometimes repaired, which requires cleaning supplies and tools. In addition, supplies include consumables (e.g., office supplies), durable equipment (e.g., copy machine), and software (e.g., for tracking equipment or volunteer time). For the health equipment recycling program, a web-based inventory was purchased to help maintain records of donations and client requests if equipment was not available at the time requested.

Garnering supplies and equipment may be similar to garnering funds. Supplies may be donated, or equipment may already be purchased by an organization that will allow its use by a program. Strategies for garnering donations are discussed in Chapter 8. Otherwise, in the program development phase, the needed supplies and equipment will have to be identified and included in the budget.

Staffing and Personnel

The greatest resource of any program is the staff who make the program a success (Timmreck, 2003). When developing a program, it is important to consider what staffing and personnel are needed for successful program implementation. The team should recognize that what is ideal for a program may not be feasible, and staff may be responsible for multiple roles. For example, an occupational therapy practitioner may play many roles in a community setting. For a small program, the occupational therapy practitioner may be the program manager and the program evaluator. In a larger program, staff may be hired for specific roles in program management and evaluation. It is important to analyze what staff members are needed for the program to be successful. If the program has a large budget, then a bookkeeper will be critical to help maintain accurate records. Administrative and support staff may also be of benefit to help with appointments or with basic administrative tasks. If traditional occupational therapy services are offered and billing is necessary, then a staff member trained in billing and coding may be required. With program growth, more staff may be needed in the future. Basic human resources training will be a critical development area for the occupational therapy practitioner hiring and retaining staff.

Engage Your Brain 6-1

Identify a program you would like to develop. Brainstorm the staff you need for your program idea. If you cannot think of an idea, consider the health equipment recycling program. How many staff members do you need? What would you pay them? What qualifications do they need to implement the program?

Along with identifying and hiring staff, establishing an infrastructure for staff evaluation is critical to ensure that personnel are successful in their ability to engage in their roles and that the program runs smoothly. Staff members should be clear on expectations and their roles in any paid or volunteer positions. Management strategies should be implemented to support employee development. Each employee should have a professional development plan that aligns with the job description for the position and receive frequent feedback on performance and expectations for the role. A successful manager will facilitate an environment for employee growth and development. In any program, the manager should consider strategies to hire and retain the best employees for the roles needed to ensure programmatic success. A managerial role is challenging, and engaging a mentor to provide strong support can ensure the program team has the support it needs to be successful.

One way to clearly define staff roles is to develop job descriptions. Job descriptions have multiple purposes; they can be used for hiring, employee orientation, employee supervision and performance review, and salary considerations. A job description traditionally includes the job title, supervisor, summary of the job duties, and qualifications needed for the job. When developing job descriptions, the occupational therapy practitioner and the program team should start with the mission statement, which helps identify what values and goals are desired in employees. Next, they should analyze a potential job to identify the qualifications needed of a potential hire (MSH, 2010). Many samples of job descriptions exist online and can serve as templates for developing appropriate job descriptions for a program. Management of human resources is an essential piece of programming and when done well can result in a motivated and cohesive workforce (MSH, 2010).

If paid staffing is not an option, volunteers may be another choice in helping to implement a program. The use of volunteers in program implementation is a popular model to leverage resources and build social capital for a program's success (Finlayson, Baker, Rodman, and Herzberg, 2002). In academic-community partnerships, service learning has been demonstrated as one approach that uses student volunteers to help with program implementation (Gitlow and Flecky, 2010). Programs can tap into volunteer organizations, like Senior Corps or AmeriCorps, to garner volunteers to aid in program implementation or utilize community resources, such as the Council on Aging, for additional staff (Painter and Elliot, 2004; Simon, 2002; Simon and Wang, 2002). The recruitment and retention of volunteers can be challenging. Volunteers may benefit from a volunteer job description that outlines the desired time commitments and skill levels. Due to work and lifestyle, it is important to consider what types of volunteers may be available when needed for program implementation. Recently, many corporations now provide the benefit of allowing staff to engage in volunteer hours in their communities during the workweek. Connecting with participating companies can be an effective strategy for short, one-time events where volunteers are needed. In addition, connecting with local branches of organizations, such as United Way, that recruit volunteers can be helpful. Building in support and recognition for volunteers is important. Designing a program on volunteer efforts necessitates flexibility on the part of the program manager in order to be successful.

Compliance With Practice Regulations

As an occupational therapy practitioner, it is important to consider practice regulations when developing a program implementation plan. If using occupational therapy skills to design and implement the program, it is critical that the practitioner follow practice guidelines, including the differentiation of roles between the occupational therapist and occupational therapy assistant. Programs must fall within the occupational therapy scope of practice (AOTA, 2010) and always follow the *Occupational Therapy Code of Ethics (2015)* (AOTA, 2015). If occupational therapy practitioners have questions about whether the program falls within occupational therapy regulations, they should contact the state licensure board to ensure the program is in compliance. In the case that the program is engaged in billing and coding for services, reimbursement regulations should be followed at all times.

Engage Your Brain 6-2

From your understanding of the AOTA (2015) *Occupational Therapy Code of Ethics (2015),* what considerations should you take into account when designing a program with a vulnerable population? Consider the health equipment recycling program. Hint: What was the intent of a showroom concept?

Team Development

Due to its complicated nature, community practice cannot be done in isolation. Community programs require a team approach, making it necessary to create a strong team (Fazio, 2017). Developing a team to implement the program is an important aspect of program design and facilitates successful implementation. Being strategic with team development ensures that the program's implementation is not hindered by miscommunication or mistrust among team members. Occupational therapy practitioners can use their expertise in group processes to aid in team development and sustainability. In this situation, the occupational therapy practitioner may lead the team or become a member of a developing or existing team.

Due to the recent interest in interprofessional collaborative practice, teamwork has become increasingly valued as a core skill of health-care professionals (Interprofessional Education Collaborative, 2016). **Interprofessional collaborative practice** is defined as "when multiple health workers from different professional backgrounds work together with patients, families, carers and communities to deliver the highest quality of care" (World Health Organization, 2010, p. 7). An understanding of concepts from interprofessionalism in regard to team-based skills can be an asset in building a team for program development. A **team** consists of "two or more individuals with a high degree of interdependence geared toward the achievement of a goal or the completion of a task" (Weiss, Tilin, and Morgan, 2018; White and West, 2008, p. 3). A team differs from a group in the fact that teams are assembled with diverse perspectives to solve a problem, whereas groups are typically like-minded individuals with similar interests collaborating on a project (Drinka and Clark, 2016; Weiss et al., 2018). Teams make decisions, solve problems, develop a focus, and accomplish outcomes. In community practice, the team will include not only the occupational therapy practitioner and other experts but also community partners and community members. Using a team approach provides different perspectives on program design and implementation, enhances program success and sustainability, and expands expertise and resources (Doll, 2010).

Engage Your Brain 6-3

What competencies are required to work effectively as an interprofessional team member?

What competencies are required to work effectively as an interprofessional team member? Teams require time to develop. Multiple approaches to team development exist, including the process of forming, storming, norming, and performing (Blue et al., 2008). Another approach is forming, norming, confronting, performing, and leaving (Drinka and Clark, 2016). In the forming stage in both models, team members begin by getting to know one another and establishing goals for the team. Team members begin to explore what tasks they will undertake as part of the team. Trust has not yet developed, and some members will be uncertain how to proceed in the team.

Typically, if conflict exists at this stage, it is not discussed or addressed. Team strategies to promote the forming stage include participating in team-building activities, identifying ground rules for how team members want to interact, and beginning to bring up team issues in a safe environment. This last approach will later be discussed as a team development strategy.

In the norming stage, team members begin to voice their opinions about the team and its proposed tasks. The team wrestles with identity and goals as members may begin to disagree. Leaders may try to emerge, which can either help or hinder the team. Ground rules must be discussed and modified to promote ongoing team development. The structure of the team functions becomes clearer. Dysfunction can occur at this stage as team members negotiate goals and team member roles. However, this negotiation process is normal for a successful and effective team.

During the confronting stage, team members come to an agreement about the expectations for the team and its members, keeping in mind the mission and programming plan. Health-care professionals tend to be empathetic individuals and find discomfort in conflict engagement (Eichbaum, 2018). But without engaging in conflict, teams risk stagnation and becoming dysfunctional. Strategies to effectively engage conflict include establishing psychological safety. **Psychological safety** is defined as "a shared belief held by members of a team that the team is safe for interpersonal risk-taking" (Edmondson, 1999, p. 350). Psychological safety occurs when team members feel it is "safe" to bring up concerns without fear of negative repercussions. Leaders promote psychological safety through role modeling and being accepting of mistakes, along with a willingness to listen to concerns and following up with actions to address the concerns if relevant. Other strategies for helping a team evolve through conflict include diffusing hierarchies in the team when possible and embracing conflict as an opportunity to learn. In any team, the leader sets the tone and can help the team grow. The myth that all conflict should be resolved and all team members will be happy with the results of a conflict need to be overcome in any productive team (Eichbaum, 2018).

When the team evolves into performing, trust begins to develop, and team roles become clearly defined. In the performing stage, the team is able to complete goals successfully and effectively. The team is able to work together, without conflict, toward the team's goals (Blue et al., 2008). Team members are engaged, appreciating the differences in team member perspectives, and every member feels some sense of responsibility to the team outcome (Drinka and Clark, 2016). In the performing stage, it is important to celebrate team accomplishments and reinforce team behaviors that benefit the team.

In teams, stability is rare, and teams must have a plan when members leave and other members join. In some cases, a team can terminate due to the task being complete. Team members leave for a variety of reasons and factors. The loss of a valued team member should be acknowledged and celebrated. Orienting a new team member to the organization should be considered a team function (Drinka and Clark, 2016).

The key activities of a team include communication, decision-making, delegation, and problem-solving (White and West, 2008). These activities should be collectively accomplished in the collaborative model of a team in order to successfully design and implement a community program. Yet working in a team is challenging. According to Lencioni (2002), author of the *Five Dysfunctions of a Team,* a team becomes dysfunctional when there is an absence of trust, a fear of conflict, a lack of commitment, and inattention to results. These factors can destroy a team, which ultimately destroys a program or the ability to address a community need. The team should be aware of these challenges and develop plans to remedy them as they arise.

A program team will look different for each program, but having a collaborative and cooperative team can lead to success and ensure that the program operates to meet the community need. When building a team, the occupational therapy practitioner needs to identify who must be involved and when these individuals must be involved (Brooks, 2006). In some cases, bringing people in too late can be detrimental to the team and ultimately to program implementation. Ideally, team leaders avoid the common trap of inviting only like-minded individuals, as change and new ideas help a team grow.

Next, the team members should collectively define their purpose and goals for the program (Blue et al., 2008). During this process, team members will communicate and begin to build trust with one another. Team members should take time to identify what each brings to the group. Understanding roles and responsibilities is critical for team development. Team training and team building are important activities for any team to develop. These activities help in building trust early and in delegating responsibilities later.

In a team, power is shared, which is sometimes called distributive leadership (Brewer, Flavell, Trede, and Smith, 2016). When working in a community program, this is an especially important aspect to emphasize. In cases in which community members may be working with educated health-care professionals, community members may feel inadequate, leading to a lack of active participation. The team leader can identify the strengths and contributions of each member in initial team-building activities and publicly recognize members for what each brings to the effort (Israel, Eng, Schulz, and Parker, 2005). In addition, the team leader should explore leadership models to determine the best "fit" for the team (Brewer et al., 2016). As mentioned, teams should celebrate together. The focus of a team should be not only to address needs but also to celebrate when a challenge has successfully been tackled, individually or collectively. Taking the time to celebrate is crucial to ensuring ongoing commitment and making team members feel rewarded for their participation.

Teams need ongoing development and care, especially when team members change (Holtzclaw, Kenner, and Walden, 2009). Team dynamics can be challenging, but overcoming these challenges is possible with effective leadership. The processes of the team need to be clearly defined, including communication, decision-making processes, and problem-solving. One suggestion is to develop a dynamic team commitment or ground rules and allow team members to identify each of the processes required for the team to be successful. In this commitment, all members of the team agree on how the team and its members should function, ensuring buy-in and dispelling common team challenges. As a team changes and develops, the team must revisit its purpose and mission frequently to ensure success and effective outcomes (Blue et al., 2008).

Establishing Partnerships

In community practice, it is rare that a program occurs without connections to similar or complementary programs. In addition to building a team of individuals to implement the program, building community partnerships is equally important. **Partnerships** are entities "formed between two or more sectors to achieve a common goal that could not otherwise be accomplished separately" (Meade and Calvo, 2001, p. 1578). A common example of a partnership is an academic-community partnership, or community-campus partnership, which is a partnership between a university and a community organization (Drahota et al., 2016). Partnerships also help with marketing and recruiting participants that may be connected with other programs. Community organizations typically partner to help work toward community change, and, typically, the most successful partnerships include those that have a clear, collaborative focus, an action plan, and champions or leaders committed to having an impact on the community (University of Kansas, 2017).

Collaboration is the foundation of partnerships, and successful collaboration is fundamental to a partnership's success (Ansari, Phillips, and Hammick, 2001; Fazio, 2017). Occupational therapy practitioners already understand the concept of partnership as discussed in literature related to client-centered practice (Law, 1998). In these discussions, the practitioner is in partnership with the client to ensure the client's therapeutic goals are addressed (Law, 1998; Sumsion, 2006). Community partnerships maximize resources by utilizing the strengths of a mobilized group of people. In many cases, one program alone is unable to fully address a need, but in collaboration, such programs can address community needs more effectively and efficiently. Furthermore, partnerships created to address health-related issues can "aim to create a seamless system of relevant healthcare services for the community" (Meade and Calvo, 2001, p. 1578).

Partnerships form between groups or organizations. Occupational therapy practitioners can be involved in multiple ways in community partnerships, such as through academic-community partnerships, community coalition memberships, advisory board memberships, nonprofit board memberships, or simply as members of the community. Community partnerships, in themselves, may be complicated to develop and maintain (Becker, Israel, and Allen, 2005). As with the development of any team, a significant investment is required to develop trust and relationships and face the challenges necessary to collaborate effectively (Becker et al., 2005). Research has shown that developing and maintaining partnerships takes time, commitment, and open communication in order to develop the mutual trust required for true exchange in a partnership (Burhansstipanov, Dignan, Bad Wound, Tenney, and Vigil, 2000; Kagawa-Singer, 1997; Poole and Van Hook, 1997). Ideally, the collaborating occupational therapy practitioner will commit the time and problem-solving abilities needed to be an effective community partner. In addition, it is important to understand the change process and culture, as these factors directly influence community change (University of Kansas, 2017).

Partnerships can be very formal or very informal, depending on the partners involved, the community need, and the program. If partnerships are formal, the partners may develop a strategic plan identifying goals and objectives for the partners based on the program's mission (Becker et al., 2005). Formal agendas and meeting minutes should be maintained to track partners' efforts. In some cases, this documentation may be part of a program's evaluation plan and may provide valuable information for a grant report. Granting agencies that require partnerships will want documentation of the success of the partners in reaching their goals.

Developing community partnerships requires commitment. Occupational therapy practitioners can play critical roles in community practice using their expertise in occupation (Fazio, 2017).

However, there are many aspects of developing and maintaining a community partnership. Partnerships thoughtfully developed and managed can be a great asset to an underserved community.

Program Management

Programs are important to the communities they serve. In order to sustain programs and ensure they meet community needs, community members should be actively involved in the program. When designing and implementing a program, the practitioner should consider how community members will be involved in monitoring the program. Advisory boards are a model for including the community in program implementation and management.

An **advisory board** is a collection of community members who provide feedback to a program (MacQueen et al., 2001). These individuals may be community stakeholders and/or community members. The advisory board is a resource for the program team and connects the team with community members. Prior to convening an advisory board, the team should first establish the role of the advisory board, its goals, and a description of its members' roles. Advisory boards usually consist of experts who know the community and the organization, so these individuals can make recommendations and guide the organization or program. An advisory board displays quality assurance to the community by demonstrating that the organization is listening to the voice of the community. When inviting individuals to participate in an advisory board, the leader of the advisory board needs to ensure that participants are individuals who will provide constructive and critical feedback and have the time to devote to advisory board activities. Different from formal boards, advisory boards often do not include bylaws identifying who leads. The board members may decide the process of leadership as they engage and evolve together. Advisory boards typically do not meet often and do not require a significant amount of time, which is a benefit when recruiting members. Advisory boards are not the same as a board of directors used in a nonprofit model and do not necessarily require the same level of formality (Weis and Gantt, 2004). In some cases, a program may have a board of directors and an advisory board, depending on program needs.

A **board of directors** is a group of individuals who guide the organization in its mission, finances, and programming. Nonprofit agencies follow a model of including a board of directors to aid in planning and ensuring financial viability for the organization. Each board of directors has traditional officer roles, including president, vice president, treasurer, and secretary. Members of a board of directors are volunteers who have expertise and can aid the organization. The members of a board are fiscally responsible for the agency they support both in monetary donations and in expert guidance. Depending on the role of the manager in relation to the board, the manager should know how to work with the board and communicate with board members as necessary. An executive director of a nonprofit organization will work directly with the board, keeping it informed about the organization's functioning and development. Board members may also be expected to support the organization financially through donations.

A **community coalition** is "a group that involves multiple sectors of the community and comes together to address community needs and solve community problems" (Wolff, 2001, p. 166). Community coalitions are typically composed of active and engaged community members, often known as stakeholders or champions. Champions are individuals who are attracted to innovative practices and typically help advocate to others to implement change (May et al., 2007). Coalitions recognize community assets and come together to address community issues (Wolff, 2001). A community coalition is one strategy to engage the collective community in program development, implementation, management, and evaluation. Charters and organizational structures for coalitions vary but typically include a group of community members committed to civic engagement (Wolff, 2001).

Program Sustainability

A program's sustainability is crucial and should be part of the program design and implementation. Community programs are not meant to be static and are ever evolving. **Sustainability** is more than simply having the funding to continue a program and includes other factors that influence the program's ongoing success (Doll, 2010). Program sustainability in communities means going beyond program implementation to connect with the community and build capacity to engrain the program into the community (Edberg, 2019). Sustainable community programs are "endurable, livable, adaptable, and supportable" (Akerlund, 2000, p. 354).

Programs terminate for many reasons, including inadequate planning or a lack of prioritization for program sustainability, a lack of support for the program, a lack of funding, or poor economic times. In some underserved and diverse communities, mistrust of outside individuals, corporations, or government involvement and mistrust of health care in general are part of the community's dynamics. Developing a program that suddenly ends when grant funding ends sends a message to the community that the program was not really created for their benefit (Jensen and Royeen, 2001). These actions can lead to further mistrust and difficulty in forging future partnerships.

When addressing significant health issues in communities, sustainability can appear nearly impossible due to barriers and a lack of resources. Yet sustainability is possible if programs are well designed and complement the community's needs and capacities (Akerlund, 2000). Successful approaches to sustainability include ongoing evaluation, ongoing service development, program modification to meet community needs and desires, effective program marketing, and the use of capacity-building approaches (Gaines, Wold, Bean, Brannon, and Leary, 2004). Strategies for sustainability through program evaluation are discussed in Chapter 7.

Community programs also need to be flexible to be successful. Community programs should respond not only to community needs but also to social, economic, and environmental conditions that have an impact on both the community and the program (Brennan, Baker, and Metzler, 2008). Community programs are developed to address community needs, and sustainability is more likely when services are modified as community needs and desires change.

When addressing program sustainability, the following factors should be considered: effectiveness of the program, relationship with the community, anticipated duration of the program, funding, and staff expertise. Program effectiveness should be considered when developing a program plan through determining outcome measures that are a part of the evaluation plan (Painter and Elliot, 2004). Evaluation results will reveal if the program is really worth continuing, responds to community needs, or requires changes to be effective. In some instances, a program may be designed to meet a short-term community need in which sustainability may not be a strong consideration.

The length of the program is an important factor to consider. With most health-related community issues, a short-term solution will not be viable (Edberg, 2019; Timmreck, 2003). If the plan is to sustain the program for the long term, then goals and objectives need to be put into place that promote and suggest sustainability. If sustainability has not been considered in initial program development, the program team may need to revisit basic program development and redevelop components of the program for the long term.

The expertise of program staff is a very important factor in sustainability, especially because sustainability infers that programs change according to the community. Having staff who are flexible and able to offer expertise in multiple areas related to community issues is important in maintaining a successful program. Involving stakeholders from the community or hiring community members to implement the program enhances this aspect (Edberg, 2019). If funding staff salaries is difficult, then the program may choose to move toward a volunteer model instead. This strategy will depend on the program, the access to volunteers, and the community needs (Akerlund, 2000).

Obviously, funding plays a role in the ability of a program to sustain itself. Multiple strategies can be considered when exploring the financial sustainability of a program. If a program is initially grant funded, it must remain sustainable either by garnering outside funds or implementing a fee for services. If seeking funds from external sources, the program team will need a plan to either search for future grant funds or engage in fund-raising efforts. The team should conduct a cost-benefit analysis to demonstrate to potential and existing funders and donors the impact of the program and its relevance (Akerlund, 2000). The strategies for fund-raising are many and will differ based on the program's structure and needs.

Table 6-2 Program Design Checklist

The following checklist summarizes an overview of the action steps to consider in community-based program design.

Reflection Question	Action Step	Progress Note	Outcome Measure
What is the community need?	Establish a mission and vision for the program		
How can the identified community need be addressed?	Draft program goals		
What can be done to meet the goals of the program?	Draft program objectives complementary to goals		
Who will this program benefit?	Identify participant eligibility criteria		
How will community members know about the program?	Identify a marketing and recruitment strategy		
Where will the program be implemented?	Ascertain the most appropriate location for the program		
What is needed to help the program be successful?	List equipment needs for the program		
Who is needed for the program to be successful?	Name role of individuals who will help support the program		
How will the program be funded?	Consider the budget implications of the program		
How will personnel and volunteers be trained for the program?	Develop training materials		
How will the program be sustained?	Create a sustainability plan		
What else is needed?			

In addition to monetary contributions, fundraising may also seek services or supplies needed by the program. These "in-kind" services are provided free of cost to the program and can aid in balancing a program budget (Akerlund, 2000). Fundraising is often most successful when program staff have developed relationships with potential donors; sometimes this process is referred to as "friendraising" (Gottlieb, 2006). Chapter 8 explores funding for community programs in greater detail.

Developing a Sustainability Plan

One of the best ways to ensure the long-term maintenance of the program is to develop a sustainability plan (Doll, 2010). This is similar to the implementation plan but is future-oriented. It should encompass an overall strategy for program maintenance to keep the program going into the future (U.S. Department of Justice [USDJ], 2005). A sustainability plan is meant to be an action plan outlining specifically what needs to be done and who needs to do it in order to maintain the program. The plan should include goals, objectives, and action steps, including who will do what and a date for accomplishment (USDJ, 2005). All the aspects of this plan should be focused and geared toward sustainability rather than program implementation.

Sustainability planning should include identifying the challenges to sustainability. One question to pose is: What could cause the program or organization to not be able to sustain itself? Addressing this question is difficult but essential to the core of any sustainability plan. Identifying the challenges and barriers to sustainability allows the program team to develop approaches to effectively address them (Akerlund, 2000; Conrad, 2008). Planning for sustainability is an essential process for a program's survival. One approach is to develop a committee or task group focused specifically on sustainability (Akerlund, 2000). In some cases, these individuals may be volunteers or members of the program team. Sustainability planning should involve a group of community stakeholders and those who have a vision for the future. This group should include individuals who have used the services and directly benefited from them. Including input from community members ensures that the plan that is developed meets the needs and desires of the community and aids in establishing sustainability. Also, the plan needs to be practical and feasible to ensure success. This means that it does not include raising community fees by an exorbitant amount or proposing strategies that will ultimately lead to challenges rather than successes. The sustainability committee needs to continually search for and garner resources that will support the program. A program design checklist (Table 6-2) summarizes the action steps to consider in community and population health program design.

Summary

- Designing a community-based or population health program or initiative utilizes skills similar to those an occupational therapist uses in developing an individualized client intervention plan and can result in a means to address the greater health needs of a population or community.
- Program design requires the development of the program's vision, mission, and implementation plan.
- Team building, sustainability planning, and budgeting are important components of program design to ensure successful implementation.
- Program design requires the occupational therapy practitioner to envision how the program will work, who will be involved, who will benefit from services, and how the program will be funded.
- Through this process, the occupational therapy practitioner can take a programmatic idea and design a program with an interdisciplinary team that meets community needs to have an impact on occupation and quality of life.
- The occupational therapy practitioner needs to create a program design that once implemented is viable and sustainable.

CASE STUDIES

CASE STUDY PART 2 Suicide Prevention in a Native American Community

The training manual for the stress management room curriculum identified the following as the goal of the project:

> *The purpose of this project is to develop a comprehensive program that facilitates hope, self-concept, and engagement in meaningful activities based on cultural desires through a culturally appropriate stress management program in order to prevent suicide or suicidal behaviors or thoughts (Gutman, 2005). This program will focus on using occupational therapy evidence-based theoretical approaches including sensory integration and neuro-occupation, a heuristic model for framing occupational engagement and forming the occupational being through the integration of neuroscience, nonlinear dynamics and chaos theory. (Padilla and Peyton, 1997; Haltiwanger, Lazzarini, and Nazeran, 2007)*

CASE STUDY PART 2 Suicide Prevention in a Native American Community

Discussion Questions and Application

1. From this excerpt write one program goal with two to three program objectives you envision as being possible to achieve. Follow the best practices for goal and objective writing outlined in the chapter.
2. What occupational therapy theories or concepts could be used to support this program?
3. Identify in this case example how space and place played a role in program implementation.
   By using the existing school spaces, the occupational therapy practitioner collaborated with school administrators to identify the location of the stress management rooms; how equipment would be used, cleaned, and maintained; and when the rooms would be available for use. A check-out system for classroom use was also implemented. By using existing space and infrastructure, the occupational therapy practitioner simply had to collaborate with others on how best to use the space and equipment.
4. From reviewing the case, how do you think sustainability was considered in program design?
   Sustainability was important to this grant-funded project. The design of a curriculum and train-the-trainer model with the schools' teachers facilitates sustainability, as the program was not reliant on the occupational therapy practitioner. In addition, the equipment purchased was sufficiently durable to last beyond the grant period. The occupational therapist ensured that the stress-reduction equipment would be owned by the tribal community, so it would be available to them beyond the grant period. Policies and procedures for use of the stress-reduction rooms, developed with representatives from the school and community, also helped ensure consistency and sustainability. In addition, training multiple stakeholders ensured the program could be implemented by many and sustained beyond the grant period.

Learning Activities

1. Draft a mission statement for a potential program. Gather some vision and mission statements from corporations or local organization via the Internet. Compare and contrast your drafted vision and mission statements with those of other organizations.
2. Develop two to three program goals related to your potential program using the SMART mnemonic. Do your goals relate to your mission? Will an outside party understand the focus of your program by reviewing your mission statement and goals? Are your program goals measurable?
3. Contact local programs similar to your program idea and set up an interview with an employee. Find out more about the program, including staffing, budgeting, and supplies and equipment. Compare the results of this interview to your initial program ideas.
4. Create a sample implementation plan for your idea of a community-based program similar to what was presented in the chapter. Make sure to outline the objectives, activities, necessary staff, and short- and long-term outcomes for your implementation plan.
5. You are working with a team to develop a program for children in an after-school program for high-risk youth. You are applying your skills as an occupational therapist to this process in order to maximize the therapeutic aspects for the children and their families. How might you utilize the occupational therapy practice framework (AOTA, 2014) to support your program development plan for this population?

REFERENCES

Akerlund, K. M. (2000). Prevention program sustainability: The state's perspective. *Journal of Community Psychology, 28*(3), 353–362.

American Occupational Therapy Association. (2010). Scope of practice. *American Journal of Occupational Therapy, 64*(6), 389–396.

American Occupational Therapy Association. (2014). Occupational therapy practice framework: Domain and process (3rd ed.).

American Journal of Occupational Therapy, 68(Suppl. 1), S1–S48. http://dx.doi.org/10.5014/ajot.2014.682006

American Occupational Therapy Association. (2015). Occupational therapy code of ethics (2015). *American Journal of Occupational Therapy, 69*(Suppl. 3), 6913410030. http://dx.doi.org/10.5014/ajot.2015.696S03

American Occupational Therapy Association. (2017). Vision 2025. *American Journal of Occupational Therapy, 71,* 7103420010. https://doi.org/10.5014/ajot.2017.713002

Ansari, W. E., Phillips, C. J., and Hammick, M. (2001). Collaborating and partnerships: Developing the evidence base. *Health and Social Care in the Community, 9*(4), 215–227.

Becker, A. B., Israel, B. A., and Allen, A. J. (2005). Strategies and techniques for effective group process in CBPR partnerships. In B. A. Israel, E. Eng, A. J. Schulz, and E. A. Parker (Eds.). *Methods in community-based participatory research for health* (pp. 52–72). San Francisco, CA: Jossey-Bass.

Blue, A. V., Hamm, T. L., Harrison, D. S., Howell, D. W., Lancaster, C. J., Smith, T. G., West, V. T., and White, A. (2008). *Team skills handbook.* Charleston, SC: Medical University of South Carolina.

Braveman, B. (2016). *Leading and managing occupational therapy services: An evidence-based approach.* Philadelphia, PA: F. A. Davis.

Brennan, L. K., Baker, E. A., and Metzler M. (2008). *Promoting health equity: A resource to help communities address social determinants of health.* Atlanta, GA: U.S. Department of Health and Human Services, Centers for Disease Control and Prevention.

Brewer, M. L., Flavell, H. L., Trede, F., and Smith, M. (2016). A scoping review to understand "leadership" in interprofessional education and practice. *Journal of Interprofessional Care, 30*(4), 408415.

Brooks, D. M. (2006). *Grant writing made easy.* Paper presented at the E-Tech Conference, Columbus, OH.

Brownson, C. A. (2001). Program development for community health: Planning, implementation, and evaluation strategies. In M. Scaffa (Ed.), *Occupational therapy in community-based practice settings* (pp. 95–118). Philadelphia, PA: F. A. Davis.

Burhansstipanov, L., Dignan, M. B., Bad Wound, D., Tenney, M., and Vigil, G. (2000). Native American recruitment into breast cancer screening: The NAWWA project. *Cancer Education, 15,* 28–52.

Chambless, D. L. (2003). Hints for writing a NIMH grant. *Behavior Therapist, 26,* 258–261.

Conrad, P. (2008). To boldly go: A partnership enterprise to produce applied health and nursing services researchers in Canada. *Health Care Policy, 3,* 13–30.

Doll, J. D. (2008). Professional development: Growing as an occupational therapist. *Advance for Occupational Therapy Practitioners, 24*(5), 41–42.

Doll, J. D. (2010). *Program development and grant writing in occupational therapy: Making the connection.* Boston, MA: Jones and Bartlett.

Doran, G. T. (1981). There's a S.M.A.R.T. way to write management's goals and objectives. *Management Review, 70*(11), 35–36.

Drahota, A. M. Y., Meza, R. D., Brikho, B., Naaf, M., Estabillo, J. A., Gomez, E. D., . . . Aarons, G. A. (2016). Community-academic partnerships: A systematic review of the state of the literature and recommendations for future research. *Milbank Quarterly, 94*(1), 163–214.

Drinka, T. J., and Clark, P. G. (2016). *Healthcare teamwork: Interprofessional practice and education.* Santa Monica, CA: Prager.

Edberg, M. (2019). *Essentials of health behavior: Social and behavioral theory in public health* (3rd ed.). Boston, MA: Jones and Bartlett.

Edmondson, A. (1999). Psychological safety and learning behavior in work teams. *Administrative Science Quarterly, 44,* 350–383.

Eichbaum, Q. (2018). Collaboration and teamwork in the health professions: Rethinking the role of conflict. *Academic Medicine, 93*(4), 574–580.

Fazio, L. (2017). *Developing occupation-centered programs for the community* (3rd ed.). Upper Saddle River, NJ: Prentice Hall.

Finlayson, M., Baker, M., Rodman, L., and Herzberg, G. (2002). The process and outcomes of a multimethod needs assessment at a homeless shelter. *American Journal of Occupational Therapy, 56*(3), 313–321. doi:10.5014/ajot.56.3.313

Gaines, S. K., Wold, J. L., Bean, M. R., Brannon, C. G., and Leary, J. M. (2004). Partnership to build sustainable public health nurse child care health support. *Family and Community Health, 27*(4), 346–354.

Gitlow, L., and Flecky, K. (2005). Integrating disability studies concepts into occupational therapy education using service learning. *American Journal of Occupational Therapy, 59*(5), 546–553. doi:10.5014/ajot.59.5.546

Gitlow, L., and Flecky, K. (2010). *Service-learning in occupational therapy education.* Boston, MA: Jones and Bartlett.

Gottlieb, H. (2006). *Friendraising: Community engagement strategies for boards who hate fundraising but love making friends.* Tucson, AZ: Renaissance Press.

Goulet, C.G., Begley, K, Gould, K, and Doll, J.D. (2008). *Interdisciplinary Team Skills Development for Health Professional Students.* Grant proposal funded by the Association for Prevention Teaching and Research, October, 2008.

Gutman, S. A. (2005). Understanding suicide: What therapists should know. *Occupational Therapy in Mental Health, 21*(2), 55–77.

Haltiwanger, E., Lazzarini, I., and Nazeran, H. (2007). Application of nonlinear dynamics theory to neuro-occupation: A case study of alcoholism. *British Journal of Occupational Therapy, 70*(8), 349–357.

Holtzclaw, B. J., Kenner, C., and Walden, M. (2009). *Grant writing handbook for nurses* (2nd ed.). Boston, MA: Jones and Bartlett.

Interprofessional Education Collaborative. (2016). *Core competencies for interprofessional collaborative practice: 2016 update.* Washington, DC: Interprofessional Education Collaborative.

Israel, B. A., Eng, E., Schulz, A. J., and Parker, E. A. (2005). Introduction to method in community-based participatory research for health. In B. A. Israel, E. Eng, A. J. Schulz, and E. A. Parker (Eds.), *Methods in community-based participatory research for health.* San Francisco, CA: Jossey-Bass.

Jensen, G. M., and Royeen, C. B. (2001). Analysis of academic-community partnerships using the integration matrix. *Journal of Allied Health, 30,* 168–175.

Kagawa-Singer, M. (1997). Addressing issues for early detection and screening in ethnic populations. *Oncology Nursing Forum, 24*(10), 1705–1711.

Keys, D. (1982). *Earth at omega: Passage to planetization.* Wellesley, MA: Branden Books.

Law, M. C. (1998). *Client-centered occupational therapy.* Thorofare, NJ: SLACK.

Lencioni, P. (2002). *The five dysfunctions of a team: A leadership fable.* San Francisco, CA: Jossey-Bass.

Li, S. T. T., Frohna, J. G., and Bostwick, S. B. (2017). Using your personal mission statement to INSPIRE and achieve success. *Academic Pediatrics, 17*(2), 107–109.

MacQueen, K. M., McLellan, E., Metzger, D. S., Kegeles, S., Strauss, R. P., Scotti, R., Blanchard, L., and Trotter, R. T. (2001). What is community? An evidence-based definition for participatory public health. *American Journal of Public Health, 91*(12), 1929–1938.

Management Sciences for Health. (2010). *Health systems in action: An ehandbook for leaders and managers.* Cambridge, MA: Management Sciences for Health. Retrieved from www.msh.org/ resource-center/health-systems-in-action.cfm

May, C., Finch, T., Mair, F., Ballini, L., Dowrick, C., Eccles, M., . . . Rogers, A. (2007). Understanding the implementation of complex interventions in health care: The normalization process model. *BMC Health Services Research, 7*(1), 148.

Meade, C. D., and Calvo, A. (2001). Developing community-academic partnerships to enhance breast health among rural and Hispanic migrant and seasonal farmworker women. *Oncology Nursing Forum, 28*(10), 1577–1584.

Ohio Literacy Resource Center. (2018). *Leadership Development Institute: Personal mission statement.* Retrieved from http://literacy.kent.edu/Oasis/Leadership/mission.htm

Padilla, R., and Peyton, C. G. (1997). Neuro-occupation: Historical review and examples. In C. B. Royeen (Ed.), *Neuroscience occupation: Links to practice* (pp. 1–31). Bethesda, MD: American Occupational Therapy Association.

Painter, J., and Elliot, S. (2004). Developing and implementing a senior community based fall prevention and home safety program. *Occupational Therapy in Health Care, 18*(3), 21–32.

Poole, D., and Van Hook, M. (1997). Retooling for community health partnerships in primary care and prevention. *Health and Social Work, 22*(1), 2–4.

Sand, M. (2005). *How to manage an effective nonprofit organization: From writing and managing grants to fundraising, board development, and strategic planning.* Franklin Lakes, NJ: Career Press.

Scaffa, M. E. and Brownson, C. A. (2014). Program planning and needs assessment. In M. E. Scaffa and S. M. Reitz (Eds.), *Occupational therapy in community-based practice settings* (2nd ed., pp. 61–79). Philadelphia, PA: F.A. Davis.

Simon, C. A. (2002). Testing for bias in the impact of AmeriCorps service on volunteer participants: Evidence of success in achieving a neutrality program objective. *Public Administration Review, 62*(6), 670–678.

Simon, C. A., and Wang, C. (2002). The impact of AmeriCorps service on volunteer participants. *Administration and Society, 34*(5), 522–540.

Strickland, R. (2011). Strategic planning. In K. Jacobs and G. McCormack (Eds.), *The occupational therapy manager* (5th ed.). Bethesda, MD: AOTA Press.

Sumsion, T. (2006). *Client-centered practice in occupational therapy: A guide to implementation* (2nd ed.). Edinburgh, United Kingdom: Churchill Livingstone Elsevier.

Swinney, J., Anson-Wonkka, C., Maki, E., and Corneau, J. (2001). Community assessment: A church community and the parish nurse. *Public Health Nursing, 18*(1), 40–44. doi:10.1111/j.1525-1446.2001.00040.x

Timmreck, T. C. (2003). *Planning, program development and evaluation* (2nd ed.). Boston, MA: Jones and Bartlett.

University of Kansas Center for Community Health and Development. (2017). *Community toolbox.* Retrieved from https://ctb.ku.edu/en/table-of-contents

U.S. Department of Justice. (2005). *Developing a sustainability plan for weed and seed sites.* Retrieved from www.ilj.org/publications/docs/Developing_a_Sustainability_Plan_for_Weed_and_Seed_Sites.pdf

Weis, R. M., and Gantt, V. W. (2004). *Knowledge and skill development in non-profit organizations.* Peosta, IA: Eddie Bowers.

Weiss, D., Tilin, F. J., and Morgan, M. J. (2018). *The interprofessional health care team.* Boston, MA: Jones and Bartlett.

White, A., and West, V. (2008). *An introduction to teamwork.* Retrieved from http://academicdepartments.musc.edu/c3/presentations/teamskills_training.ppt

Wolff, T. (2001). Community coalition building—contemporary practice and research: Introduction. *American Journal of Community Psychology, 29*(2), 165–172.

World Health Organization. (2010). *Framework for action on interprofessional education and collaborative practice.* Geneva, Switzerland: World Health Organization.

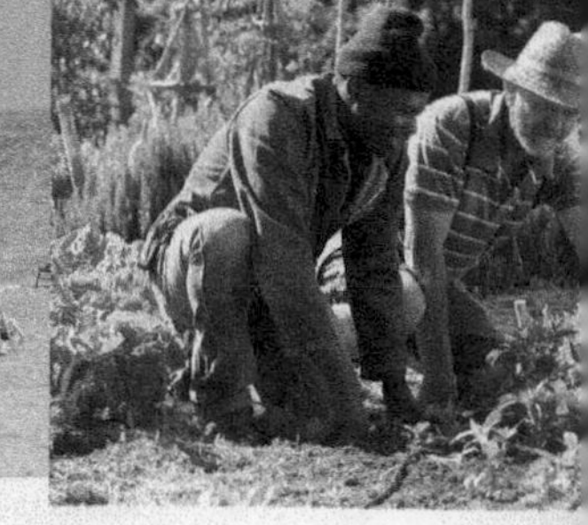

Chapter 7

Program Evaluation

David Ensminger, PhD, Marjorie E. Scaffa, PhD, OTR/L, FAOTA, Joy D. Doll, OTD, OTR/L, Michelle Messer, OTD, OTR/L, BCPR, and S. Maggie Reitz, PhD, OTR/L, FAOTA

What gets measured gets done. Measure the wrong things, and the wrong things get done.
—Michael Patton (2007, p. 110)

Learning Outcomes

This chapter is designed to enable the reader to:

7-1 Define the purposes of internal and external program evaluation.
7-2 Discuss the different types of program evaluations and when it is appropriate to use each type.
7-3 Compare and contrast four different approaches to program evaluation.
7-4 Explain the process of completing a program evaluation.
7-5 Discuss the value of evaluation results.
7-6 Discuss the importance of disseminating the results of program evaluation.
7-7 Identify ethical considerations when completing program evaluation.

Key Terms

Appreciative inquiry approach
Decision-oriented approach
External evaluation
Formative evaluation
Impact evaluation
Indicators
Internal evaluation
Logic model
Objectives approach
Outcome evaluation
Participatory approach
Process evaluation
Program evaluation
Return on investment
Stakeholders

Introduction

Program evaluation is used to make a judgment of the merit, worth, or value of a program. All programs, including community and population health programs, should include program evaluation as a key component to ensuring program success and sharing outcomes with community members. Program evaluation optimizes the collection of relevant data from various stakeholder groups and then facilitates the use of this information for decision-making and action (Yarbrough et al., 2011). Fink (2015) defines **program evaluation** as "an unbiased exploration of a program's merits, including its effectiveness, quality, and value. An effective program provides substantial benefits to individuals, communities, and societies and these benefits are greater than their human and financial costs" (p. 4). Program evaluation is critical to any program to demonstrate its outcomes and adjust the program to meet needs during implementation. Program evaluation differs from an occupational therapy evaluation, but the process is similar in that the intent is to demonstrate progress and outcomes. The application of program evaluation to community programs requires a program development and population health perspective, with thinking that differs from a typical patient evaluation.

Program evaluation is not a perfectly designed process, and it is not "one size fits all." When determining the evaluation plan, the occupational therapy practitioner must have a broad understanding of the program and what needs to be evaluated. Different types of evaluations may be appropriate at different times in program development and implementation. A well-thought-out evaluation plan is the best strategy to ensure a well-executed program evaluation (Doll, 2010). In addition, considerations related to who will conduct program evaluation—the "evaluator"—are important. If qualified personnel are available, an internal evaluation may be appropriate. Due to the expertise of occupational therapy practitioners in understanding how to design occupation-based interventions and measure outcomes, these same competencies can be applied to community and population health program evaluation.

Internal evaluation occurs when a member of the program team conducts the program evaluation. The role of program evaluation may exist as the primary role of the program team member or as a component. In a community program focused on recycling health equipment, for example, the occupational therapy practitioner could conduct an internal evaluation by surveying customers on how valued the service is and track the number of health equipment items donated and distributed to those in need.

For more rigorous program evaluation, external evaluation should be used. **External evaluation** occurs when an individual outside the program team, typically with program evaluation expertise, conducts the program evaluation. An example of external evaluation would be when a community health organization hires a nonprofit consulting firm to complete a review of its programming. This may be advantageous because the consulting firm will be unbiased in its evaluation and may be able to collect more informative data as an outside agency. Another example would be to engage a professional evaluator at a university, whose time can typically be purchased through a contract, to conduct the program evaluation.

Determining whether internal or external evaluation is appropriate for a program will depend on what needs to be evaluated and the rigor of program evaluation required. It will also depend on the breadth and depth of information desired by the program stakeholders. Each approach has strengths and challenges. Internal evaluation is typically more cost-effective but can be affected by bias, as the evaluator is closely tied to the program. If the internal evaluator is an occupational therapy practitioner, the understanding of the impact of occupation-based interventions may be advantageous. External evaluation ensures rigor and bias reduction. This option may come with a higher cost, and the evaluator may potentially lack familiarity with the program, which may create a barrier to assessing the program accurately and efficiently. The evaluator also may not have a strong understanding of the role of occupational therapy in community settings, which can be an opportunity or a challenge, depending on the situation. Program evaluation is critical to demonstrate success, to identify potential places for adjustments, and to promote program sustainability. It is also an important responsibility in community-based programs to report to the community the impact, value, and challenges of the program. Evaluation will ensure the program is meeting its aims and help identify areas of growth and change. The evaluation approach should be considered in detail and be a valued component of any program implementation.

Because program evaluators seek to provide useful information to various program partners, the evaluator, unlike other types of researchers, has many factors to balance when planning and executing a program assessment. This is most evident in determining the questions for the evaluation. Evaluators rely on stakeholders to help develop the essential questions that will be answered in the evaluation. **Stakeholders** are "individuals, groups or organizations that can affect or are affected by an evaluation process and/or its findings" (Bryson, Patton, and Bowman, 2011, p. 1). The degree of stakeholder involvement in the evaluation process is often dependent on the approach and can range from helping generate questions to full involvement in the collection, analysis, and reporting of results. Keep in mind that stakeholders may or may not have an understanding of the role of occupational therapy in the community, so education may need to be provided. Evaluators also differ from other researchers in that they consider the context to be a critical component of the research. As a result, there are limitations to generalizing the results from a program evaluation to other programs or contexts. In addition, evaluators make value statements related to the merit or worth of the program based on the data (Yarbrough et al., 2011).

The determination of a program's merit or worth is grounded in the perspective that programs should have some level of accountability to stakeholders and the community at large. Although public perception of the need for evaluations generally focuses on accountability in terms of program effects and efficiency, evaluations can also be conducted to support the development and improvement of a program or to further or deepen stakeholders' understanding of a program (Fink, 2015). The unique role of occupational therapy should also be strongly considered. With a focus on occupation-based interventions, it is a natural fit to involve community members and stakeholders in the program evaluation process. In addition, evaluation data should be publicly shared through public forums and end-of-year reports. If grant funding is involved, program evaluation will need to meet grant requirements as well. Although the notion of accountability suggests a decisive type of judgment, as will be explained in this chapter, the reporting of merit, worth, and value has different meanings depending on the purpose and focus of the evaluation, as well as the approach used to conduct the evaluation (Fink, 2015).

Engage Your Brain 7-1

You are part of a team developing a new program, and thus far the team has only established program objectives. At this stage, you suggest the team start planning for program evaluation. What reasons do you give for thinking about program evaluation so early in the development process?

Types of Program Evaluation

When designing or planning evaluations, evaluators work with key stakeholders and team members to determine the main purpose of an evaluation. An evaluation process provides valuable information that can assist stakeholders in making decisions and taking action regarding a program. It is often the nature of the decision made or action taken that helps form the purpose of an evaluation (Johnson and Christensen, 2017). In addition, program evaluation provides a foundation for accountability and sustainability. A program should meet the mission, and program evaluation provides a process for ensuring a program is meeting its mission (Hoefer, 2000). With stakeholders, several decisions should be made when designing the evaluation plan; these include the purpose of the plan, the users of the results, and the uses of evaluation outcomes (Salabarria-Peña, Apt, and Walsh, 2007). Since multiple types of program evaluation exist, the team should thoroughly vet each one to ensure an appropriate match to a program. Although approaches to evaluation may differ across the literature, the most commonly recognized types of evaluation include formative evaluation, process evaluation, outcome evaluation, and impact evaluation.

Formative evaluation is conducted to inform decisions or actions to be taken for either program implementation or program improvement. Typically, formative evaluation occurs at intervals throughout the program and acts as an advisory process. Thus, formative evaluation provides credible and relevant information concerning a program's theoretical framework, design, activities, and operation. These data assist stakeholders in making changes that will lead to improvements in the program's activities, practices, processes, or operations (Johnson and Christensen, 2017). Formative evaluation is often used after a pilot version of a program is executed in order to identify any modifications that may be necessary before full implementation of the program. For example, once the health equipment recycling program is implemented, formative evaluation strategies, such as interviews or feedback surveys, could be used to ensure that the recipients of the donations are satisfied with the process. In addition, formative evaluation will often enhance feasibility and program success (Centers for Disease

Control and Prevention [CDC], n.d.). Formative evaluation is typically used during program design or to adjust an existing program. Formative evaluation helps ensure successful program implementation and provides a platform for modification as needed to ensure success (Salabarria-Peña et al., 2007).

Process evaluation, also referred to as implementation evaluation, ensures that program activities have been implemented as intended by the program. It begins when program implementation begins and typically occurs periodically throughout the duration of the program (Salabarria-Peña et al., 2007). Process evaluation helps determine if the program is being delivered according to its design; it is truly focused on what went well in program implementation and what needs improvement so that program modification is possible. It is best evaluated through a "4W's" approach (i.e., who, what, when, and where; Salabarria-Peña et al., 2007). For example, imagine a program focused on fall prevention in the community. The program consists of screening, intervention, and follow-up. Process evaluation would occur during implementation of the program to ensure all three elements of the program are occurring as outlined when the program was developed.

Questions that drive implementation or process evaluations include:

- How well does the program reach its intended target populations?
- What are the barriers that prevent the program from operating as intended?
- What factors facilitate the implementation of the program?
- How well do the organizational processes support the program?
- To what extent is the program reaching intended outcomes?

Using the example of the health equipment recycling program, each of these questions can be addressed as follows:

- How well does the program reach its intended target populations? The program provides dual benefits by preventing health equipment from going to landfills and contributing to unnecessary waste and by providing health equipment to those in need who may not be able to access or afford it. To determine the program reach, process evaluation would identify how many pieces of equipment were donated and how many were distributed.
- What are the barriers that prevent the program from operating as intended? During the process evaluation of the health equipment loan program, a barrier that was identified was the lack of universal design and accessibility in the program's original location, a faith community basement closet. To accommodate, the program made a plan to move to a new, more accessible location. This issue was recognized when recipients were surveyed on their satisfaction with the program.
- What factors facilitate the implementation of the program? In the health equipment program example, referrals from community members and health-care professionals created a demand for health equipment that outpaced donations, and the program had to develop a wait list process.
- How well do the organizational processes support the program? The program, due to ongoing process evaluation, became more formal as time passed, adding processes like a tracking system for donations and equipment recipients.
- To what extent is the program reaching intended outcomes? The health equipment program goal was to fill a gap in services, and tracking the number of donations received and the equipment distributed was considered a measure of success.

An important part of process evaluation is relying on the evaluator to provide information that allows stakeholders to identify areas where program operation does not fit with the program design, to identify areas where program activities can be improved, and to identify and establish means for ongoing data collection related to program activities and outcomes (Barker, Pistrang, and Elliott, 2016).

Outcome evaluation, also known as effectiveness evaluation, explores the impact of a program on its participants or target population (Salabarria-Peña et al., 2007). For example, a program implementing diabetes prevention would typically evaluate hemoglobin A1C as a metric to determine if the program affected participants' health status. Outcome evaluation measures are focused on the program participants and vary based on the intended effect of the program on its participants. Outcome evaluation can explore knowledge, skills, behaviors, attitudes, perceptions, and awareness (Salabarria-Peña et al., 2007). Survey tools are often used in a pretest-posttest approach to collect outcome data. Typically, outcome evaluation identifies a baseline for the target population and the change to this baseline, if any, after program implementation. Outcome evaluation determines whether or not the expected effect is occurring (Salabarria-Peña et al., 2007).

Outcomes can be affected by a number of variables aside from the program intervention. For example, changes in economic or social conditions can influence health outcomes. Other programs with similar objectives may target the same population at the same time, which could influence the outcome. In addition, the normal development and maturation of participants, particularly children, could contribute to the outcome. Likewise, some program participants may have already been predisposed to the outcomes being measured and would have realized those positive outcomes without being exposed to the program interventions (Barker et al., 2016). Therefore, it is important to identify other possible factors that may have contributed to the results of the program's outcome evaluation.

Impact evaluation explores the overall impact of the program. It explores whether the program met its goals (Salabarria-Peña et al., 2007). It typically occurs toward or at the end of program implementation (Salabarria-Peña et al., 2007). Impact evaluation considers the broad outcomes of the program on the community. The questions that drive impact evaluations include:

- What effect does the program have on the health or social need(s) experienced by the population?
- To what extent can program outcomes be directly linked to program activities?

A well-conducted impact evaluation provides the foundation for sound policy-making. It describes whether the program had an impact, as well as how much of an impact and on whom. For example, impact evaluation on a new free health clinic would determine if and how the program goals were achieved and use this information to advocate for additional funding to continue to meet those program goals in the future.

In this impact evaluation process, the program may consider exploring the economic impact of the program, sometimes called economic evaluation (Salabarria-Peña et al., 2007). Considering factors like cost savings, return on investment, and reduction of wasted health-care services can truly demonstrate the power and purpose of a community program. **Return on investment** (ROI) explores the efficiency of an investment versus cost savings and identifies whether a service could be delivered at a lower cost (Millar and Hall, 2013). When considering these factors, ROI should be broadened beyond financial implications to review the positive impacts of workflows that save time and the improved processes that lead to higher satisfaction and improved productivity.

One way to include financial factors in an evaluation plan is to include a cost-benefit analysis. Here, the evaluator compares the benefits of the program, determined in a benefits analysis, to the actual costs of the program. When conducting a cost analysis, evaluators must examine all the costs associated with running the program, not simply the costs associated with direct services to the client (e.g., material resources, operation expenses, salaries and benefits of employees, loss of workdays for clients in the program). Questions that drive evaluations of fiscal efficiency include:

- What are the monetary values of the program outcomes?
- How do the benefits of the program compare to the cost of running the program?
- Which program is more cost-effective to run?

For example, in the health equipment recycling program, in order to sustain the program it was decided that equipment would be loaned and then returned. Participants were charged a nominal fee to rent or buy the equipment as needed to financially support the program. See Table 7-1 for comparisons of evaluation types and when to use them.

Any strong evaluation plan will consider the program and its intended impact on participants and

Table 7-1 Comparison of Evaluation Types

Evaluation Types	When to Use	What It Shows	Why It Is Useful
Formative evaluation Needs assessment	• During the development of a new program • When an existing program is being modified or is being used in a new setting or with a new population	• Whether the proposed program elements are likely to be needed, understood, and accepted by the population you want to reach • The extent to which an evaluation is possible, based on the goals and objectives	• It allows for modifications to be made to the plan before full implementation begins • Maximizes the likelihood the program will succeed
Process evaluation Program monitoring	• As soon as program implementation begins • During operation of an existing programi	• How well the program is working • The extent to which the program is being implemented as designed • Whether the program is accessible and acceptable to its target population	• Provides an early warning for any problems that may occur • Allows programs to monitor how well the program plans and activities are working
Outcome evaluation Objectives-based evaluation	• After the program has made contact with at least one person or group in the target population	• The degree to which the program is having an effect on the target population	• Tells whether the program is being effective in meeting its objectives
Economic evaluation Cost-benefit analysis Return on investment	• At the beginning of a program • During the operation of an existing program	• What resources are being used in the program and their costs (direct and indirect) compared to outcomes	• Provides program managers and funders a way to assess cost relative to effects
Impact evaluation	• During the operation of an existing program at appropriate intervals • At the end of a program	• The degree to which the program meets its ultimate goal	• Provides evidence for use in policy and funding decisions

From *Types of Evaluation,* by the Centers for Disease Control and Prevention, n.d.

the local community. In addition, the evaluation plan will be holistic, taking into consideration multiple evaluation aspects to ensure a comprehensive understanding of program impact. Multiple types of evaluation can take place at various points during the development and execution of a single program. Stakeholders can guide this process by helping to identify what outcomes are most meaningful to community members. When designing an evaluation plan, it is best to determine who needs, and would benefit from, the evaluation data.

Approaches to Program Evaluation

The field of program evaluation has been influenced by diverse epistemologies, beliefs, methodological views, values, and perspectives (Fink, 2015). These influences have shaped the approaches used by evaluators today. These varying approaches provide foundational perspectives on how evaluations can be conducted for different purposes. The authors of this chapter do not favor one approach but instead encourage evaluators to employ a contingency perspective when determining the methods and activities to be carried out in an evaluation.

Mistakenly viewed as the main goal of all evaluations, the **objectives approach** emphasizes the determination of the achievement of stated goals and objectives in the program design. The main activities in this approach are determining the goals and objectives of the program, including the development of specific operational definitions (i.e., specific behavioral or observational definitions) of the objectives. Whereas stakeholders may be involved in determining the objectives and providing operational definitions, typically in this approach the objectives are determined based on the mission and goals of the program, and in some cases specific objectives may already exist as part of the program documentation (Fitzpatrick, Sanders, and Worthen, 2011).

Once the objectives are determined, a method for measuring the objectives is agreed upon. The evaluator then collects the data from these measurements and compares the data collected to the specific goals and objectives. If a specific criterion of success has been established for an objective, then the data collected are compared to the predetermined criterion and directly tied to the program goals or objectives. For example, objective data on the efficacy of a bike safety program would likely include the number of participants who wear helmets with the correct fit. The criterion for success for this objective may be "75% of participants wear helmets that fit correctly." Discrepancies between the observed data and the stated objectives are interpreted to provide either formative or outcome information to stakeholders. For the objectivist approach, program value is directly related to the achievement of stated objectives, and quantitative methods are frequently used to specifically measure program outcomes (Fitzpatrick et al., 2011).

Strengths associated with the objectives approach include:

- It is easy to understand and carry out.
- Objectives are clear, leading to a simple way to define a program's success.
- Information concerning the achievement of program objectives is relevant to most stakeholder groups.

Weaknesses associated with this approach include:

- Program merit or worth is limited to the program objectives.
- No value is set for the objectives themselves.
- Outcomes or program values not related to objectives are often overlooked.
- Information concerning program planning and implementation is ignored.
- In many cases stakeholder involvement may be minimal (Fitzpatrick et al., 2011).

Although this approach is simple and provides valuable information about a program, it often provides limited information that stakeholders can use to improve programs. Even if objectives are a component of an evaluation plan, few evaluators rely solely on this approach when conducting an evaluation (Fitzpatrick et al., 2011).

Similar to the objectives approach, the **decision-oriented approach** examines program objectives; however, it also looks beyond programmatic outcomes and views the informational needs of program leaders and managers as a critical aspect of evaluation. This approach emphasizes providing useful information to managers or program directors in order to improve their decision-making. Evaluations must provide information about how the program operates, not simply whether objectives are being reached. In order to assist managers, the decision-oriented approach evaluates the context, planning, structure, resources, implementation, and organizational factors that have an impact on a program (Fitzpatrick et al., 2011). In this case, the bike safety program could use a decision-oriented approach by identifying additional information on participants who do not wear helmets that fit correctly. This approach may ask staff and volunteers to explain why they cannot successfully fit all participants, which provides the program with specific targets to improve upon. Understanding the reasons a population does not participate in the way the program intended can help to modify the program to ensure it is meeting community needs. This approach is consistent with the values of occupational therapy.

The strengths of the decision-oriented approach include:

- Collecting useful information to make informed decisions for the purpose of program changes

- Focusing of evaluation activities on specific program aspects (e.g., planning, structure, implementation)
- Emphasizing timely ongoing feedback through the life cycle of the program

Weaknesses of the decision-oriented approach include:

- Emphasis on a single stakeholder group's needs (i.e., managers) makes this approach undemocratic.
- There is a possibility that important information may not be gathered if the manager does not see its importance.
- The manager may fail to make decisions even when presented with relevant information.
- It can be costly to carry out an evaluation on all aspects of a program.
- Important decisions may be made in advance, which may ignore the organic nature of programs (Fitzpatrick et al., 2011).

The **participatory approach** emphasizes the formative purpose of evaluation. Similar to the decision-oriented approach in that both types emphasize the need to provide information for program improvement, the participatory approach, however, considers the information needs of all stakeholder groups rather than emphasizing the information needs of a specific stakeholder group. The involvement of all stakeholders is viewed as essential to the evaluation process in order to gain multiple perspectives on the program. Of all the approaches, the participatory approach places the most value on democratic principles, viewing the knowledge of those who carry out program activities (i.e., front-end users), clients, and program supervisors as critical when gathering information about a program and determining the merit or worth of the program (Fitzpatrick et al., 2011). Applying this approach to the bike safety example, a participatory approach would seek input and feedback from participants on what to evaluate and how to evaluate and the criteria for success. This approach encourages all participant viewpoints and aligns directly with the values of client-centered practice.

The strengths of this approach include:

- Involving a variety of stakeholder groups
- Recognizing that programs serve people and are run by people
- Bringing to light multiple accounts of the program
- Placing importance on democratic processes and the need for stakeholder dialogue
- Considering the complexity of programs
- Recognizing that one of the contextual elements of evaluations is that different stakeholder groups will have different evaluation questions and need different information

Weaknesses associated with this approach include:

- The subjective nature of these evaluations
- Stakeholders may not be familiar with evaluation approaches and choose metrics difficult to measure
- Emphasis on qualitative methods may cause concerns of evaluator bias
- Extensive cost and time associated with qualitative data collection and analysis (Fitzpatrick et al., 2011)

Engage Your Brain 7-2

Imagine the program developers of a new program are using a participatory approach to program evaluation. From whom should they seek input? What would be the benefit of gathering qualitative data from stakeholders?

An **appreciative inquiry (AI) approach** to evaluation focuses on organizational and program assets, as opposed to the identification of problems and deficits. The evaluation process attempts to discover what is working particularly well and then envisions what the future might be like if these positive attributes were to manifest themselves more frequently. AI is grounded in social constructivism, which reflects a belief that there is no single, objective reality but that many realities exist based on individuals' perceptions and shared understandings.

Cooperrider, Whitney, and Stavros (2008) described five principles for the practice of AI. These include the following:

- *Constructivist principle:* acceptance that multiple realities exist

- *Simultaneity principle:* inquiry and change are simultaneous, and therefore inquiry is intervention
- *Poetic principle:* an organization or program is continuously authoring its own story and can take the plotline in any direction at any time
- *Anticipatory principle:* the image an organization or program has about its future guides its current actions
- *Positive principle:* by focusing on positive experiences, participants become more motivated, inspired, and engaged

The most common method for conducting AI is referred to as the 4D model (discovery, dream, design, and destiny). The discovery phase of the process involves participants sharing stories about their peak experiences and *appreciating what is* currently good about the program or organization. Out of these stories, key themes are identified. In the dream phase, participants imagine themselves and their organization functioning at its best and envision *what might be,* developing a broad and holistic vision of a desirable future. In the design phase, the dream or vision is operationalized into *what should be* and coconstructed through the development of goals, strategies, processes, collaborations, and systems. The destiny phase involves implementing the strategies, monitoring progress, sustaining the change, and engaging in new AI dialogues. The 4D process is ongoing, iterative, cyclical, and highly participatory in nature (Coghlan, Preskill, and Catsambas, 2003). Applying this approach in the bike safety program would be to ask those with properly fitting helmets to engage in discussion that follows the 4D model or a similar model. In addition, this model also aligns nicely with the strengths-based approach of occupational therapy practice.

AI has the potential to contribute to evaluation practice in many ways. Coghlan et al. (2003) provide a list of situations in which AI might be most useful. These include:

- "Where there is a fear of or skepticism about evaluation"
- "When change needs to be accelerated"
- "When dialogue is critical to moving the organization forward"
- "When relationships among individuals and groups have deteriorated and there is a sense of hopelessness"
- "Where there is a desire to build a community of practice" (p. 19)

All evaluation approaches are concerned with the values and merit, or worth, of programs. However, they can differ in what elements of evaluation are emphasized (e.g., which stakeholders have more input, what information or data provide greater evidence, or what methods for collecting information are most important) and how program value is determined. These approaches emphasize different aspects of the evaluation process or the program; it is important to note that each approach has its own unique set of strengths and weaknesses. Evaluators should have an understanding of each approach, so they can effectively modify or combine approaches in order to meet the needs of stakeholders (Fitzpatrick et al., 2011). It is important to ensure that the occupational therapy contribution to the program is evaluated to determine its contribution to the overall success of the program. Occupational therapy theories can guide decisions regarding what and how to measure during various aspects of program evaluation (see Chapter 3).

Process for Completing Program Evaluation

Before beginning program evaluation, it is important to determine the focus of the evaluation. The evaluation process can be conceptualized in a variety of ways. One approach is organized around five focus areas (Rossi, Lipsey, and Henry, 2019), which include:

- Needs assessment (described previously in Chapter 6)
- Program theory
- Program implementation
- Program impact
- Program efficiency

Even though these five focus areas are distinct, it is helpful to understand the relationships among them. Social programs are developed to address specific needs or problems within a community, population, or society. Once the need or problem is defined, programs must develop theories that explain the cause-and-effect links between the need or problems and their potential resolutions. Program theory evaluations help stakeholders develop a clear and agreed-upon model of how the program is intended to operate in order to address an identified social need or problem. To achieve their intended outcomes, programs need to be implemented as they are described within a program theory. Implementation evaluations focus on evaluating the fidelity of program implementation in terms of design and logic models. Programs that are implemented correctly should produce outcomes that address the social need or problem. Impact evaluation can assess the cause-and-effect relationship between the need or societal program and the executed program results, and efficiency evaluation can determine if the value of the program to the community and the stakeholders was worth the investment or effort (Rossi et al., 2019). All five of these focus areas are important to address, and each lends itself to either summative or formative purposes.

In addition, the CDC (1999) offer a six-phase process to consider when creating and implementing a comprehensive evaluation plan:

- Engage stakeholders
- Describe the program
- Focus the evaluation design
- Gather credible evidence
- Justify conclusions
- Ensure use and share lessons learned

The first phase in the evaluation process, engaging stakeholders, is similar to building rapport in a traditional occupational therapy patient encounter. Evaluation done without input from community members will most likely not provide value or be recognized as valuable by the community or population. In program evaluation, engaging stakeholders means focusing on several key stakeholder groups, including individuals involved in the program design and implementation; individuals directly affected by the program, such as program participants; and those individuals who will use the program evaluation results. Diversity of thought is important, and a comprehensive approach will ensure that the evaluation plan considers multiple perspectives. Also, engaging stakeholders who have both a positive and negative perspective is important to ensure the evaluation is constructive, leading to program evolvement that continues to meet population health needs. For example, in the bike safety program, the stakeholders would likely include community members involved with bike safety, the school district, public health experts, the local safety council, city council members, and children and adults receiving helmets, to name a few.

In the CDC (1999) approach, the next phase focuses on describing the program. Stakeholders need to have a clear definition of the intent and value of the program in order to ensure the evaluation design or plan corresponds to program objectives. In the bike safety example, stakeholders should understand the program's mission and vision, along with the goals of the program and who in the community the program is intended to affect. With this knowledge, stakeholders can ensure the evaluation plan is meaningful both to the program and to the community. The program description should include the population health need being addressed, the intended program outcomes related to the population health need or issue, what activities will occur and what resources are needed to address the population health need, the stage of program development, and any contextual aspects influencing the program (e.g., economics and politics). In the bike safety exemplar, the focus could be on the prevention of head injuries and improved bike safety, with a broader intent to encourage engagement in healthy lifestyle activities like bike riding and a focus on sustainable approaches to transportation to support environmental protection. As indicated in the previous example, a program can address multiple population health issues, and the program evaluation should address these numerous aspects to demonstrate the impact of a program like bike safety on multiple population health concerns.

One common format used to visually represent the program description is a logic model. A **logic model** is a graphic representation, often a flowchart, used to describe a program, including relationships between activities, chronological sequencing, and intended outcomes. Logic models, because they often display program-planning, implementation, and evaluation processes simultaneously, can help a novice evaluator develop a comprehensive evaluation plan (Doll, 2010). Different logic model templates

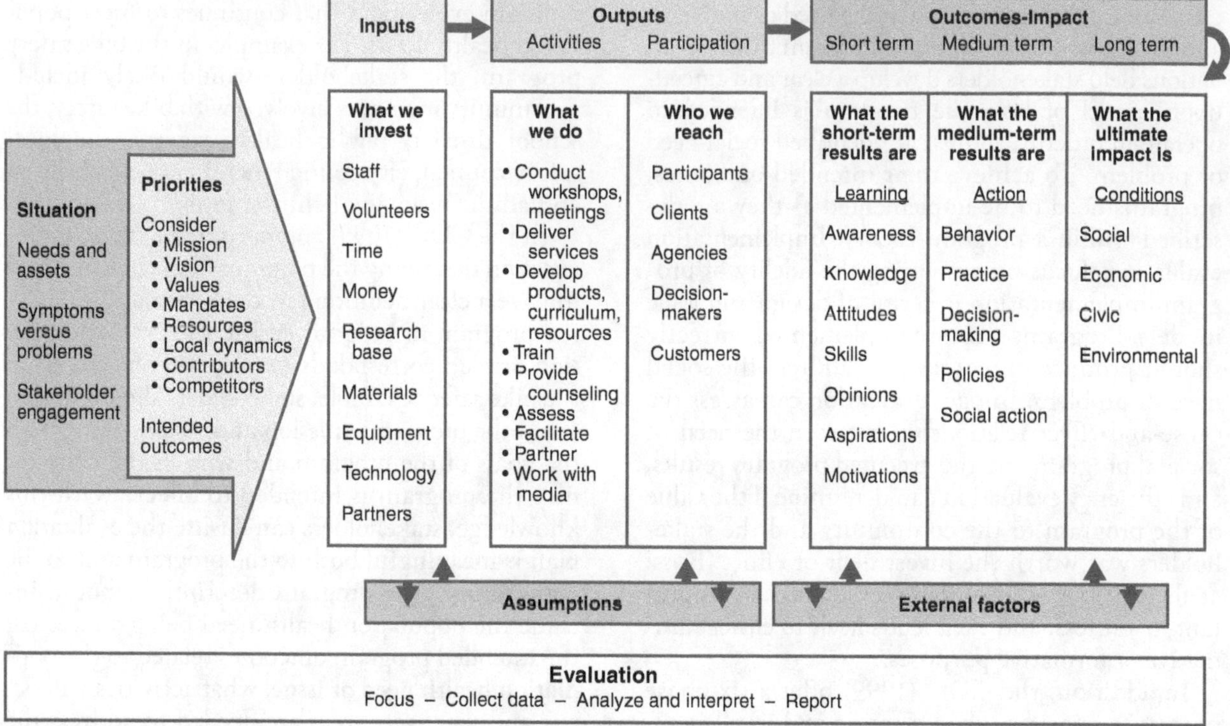

Figure 7-1 Example of a logic model. *(Courtesy of University of Wisconsin–Madison, Cooperative Extension.)*

exist and can be customized to programs to ensure all unique elements of a program are represented. See Figure 7-1 for an example of a logic model.

The next phase in the evaluation process focuses on the evaluation design or plan. The intent is to ensure the evaluation design is broad and meaningful to the program and its stakeholders. In this phase, the team identifies the aspects of the logic model and how these components will be evaluated. The evaluation plan includes the purpose of the evaluation; who will use the evaluation results and how the results will be used; the questions asked in the evaluation, along with the methods for obtaining data; and the resources needed to implement the evaluation plan. Purpose focuses on the overall intent of the evaluation plan. It is typically broad and lays the foundation for the plan. In the bike safety program, all of these elements could be mapped out as modeled in Table 7-2.

The next phase in the evaluation process is gathering credible evidence by ensuring the evaluation plan includes the collection of meaningful program information. In this step, the intent is to ensure that the evaluation outcomes are credible and of value to the stakeholders and the program itself. When addressing this aspect of the evaluation plan, consideration should be given to the following questions:

- How will indicators provide valuable data?
- Which sources will be used to gather the data?
- What efforts will be made to ensure the data collected are of appropriate quality and occur at an appropriate time line?
- What are the logistics of the data collection process?

Although this process may sound complex, it simply means taking the time to ensure that the evaluation process is well designed so multiple stakeholders can understand the approach and benefit from the process. In the bike safety example, if a survey is

Table 7-2 Evaluation Plan for Bike Safety Program

Evaluation Design	Bike Safety Program
Purpose	The intent of the bike safety program is to address the main population health issue of the prevention of head injuries related to bike riding for either recreation or transportation.
Users	The following individuals have been identified as critical users of the evaluation results to make programmatic decisions: • Program team • Board of directors • Community advisory board
Uses	The stakeholder groups identified as "users" will use the program evaluation results to make decisions to ensure the program achieves its goals related to bike safety.
Questions and data collection methods	The specific questions and methods would vary based on what the users decide, but an example would be a survey to participants.
Resources needed	The resources needed to implement such a survey would include software to develop the survey and send out to participants and data analysis software to analyze survey results

being used to collect information, the evaluation team should consider when the survey should be sent, to whom, and how the data will be analyzed to ensure fidelity to the process.

The next phase in the evaluation process is justifying the conclusions. Essentially, a clear rationale and explanation for the evaluation plan should be understood by multiple stakeholders. The intent here is to ensure that stakeholders can articulate the evaluation results correctly and meaningfully. Learning to articulate and explain the program, its intent, and its outcomes to multiple individuals is important for many reasons, including building program visibility, fundraising, and community support for the program. The intent of any evaluation plan is to use the results ultimately to support the program to continue to address its intended population health need. This includes considering how the evaluation plan results will be analyzed and synthesized and how recommendations are formed to continue to shape the program. For example, in the bike safety program, results from the survey indicate that children are adopting helmet use, but adults are less likely to adopt helmet use. The program team can use this information to reformat approaches to ensure adult community members increase bike helmet use.

Lastly, it is important to not just complete evaluation for the sake of evaluation. Intentional effort should be made to ensure that evaluation results and recommendations are shared and used in future program planning or program modification. In this step, deliberate consideration should be given to the following aspects: the evaluation design was implemented as intended, the results and recommendations are prepared and disseminated appropriately, and feedback and follow-up occur after results are shared. In addition, the evaluation results may need to be prepared in a variety of formats considering the reading level and health literacy of the recipients. The bike safety program may choose to produce an end-of-year report that summarizes the program outcomes and is placed on the program's website. This report would provide information on the program's mission, along with the evaluation outcomes and recommendations for the future of the program. An end-of-year report is a common approach used to share programmatic outcomes with the community, ensuring public access and transparency about the program's impact on the community and areas for improvement. The report can also be used to support fund-raising activities.

Program evaluation does not have to be complex, but it should be comprehensive. A program focused on addressing a significant population health need should follow one of the approaches described in this chapter. The stages and processes of each evaluation approach are not linear or step-based. Many aspects overlap and can be developed concurrently to ensure they complement one another and, taken together, are comprehensive. For occupational therapy practitioners, who are naturally holistic and occupation-based, this should be a familiar concept.

Planning for Program Evaluation

Planning an evaluation is best done prior to program implementation. The creation of an evaluation plan involves identifying stakeholders, developing evaluation questions, determining data needs, and choosing evaluation methods and instruments. Stakeholders should have a high level of interest in the outcome of the evaluation and substantial power to affect change. Not all stakeholders will participate equally. Some may only desire information, some may want to be consulted, others will be involved, and a few will collaborate as decision-makers (Bryson et al., 2011). The most difficult task in evaluation is often the development of clear, useful, and researchable evaluation questions. The information needs of program developers and managers change with varying organizational and environmental conditions. To develop appropriate program evaluation questions, aspects of the program being evaluated and the approach should first be identified. The team must also determine the method of data collection and the type of data that need to be collected to answer the evaluation questions (Bryson et al., 2011). If the method of program evaluation is determined during program planning, then pieces of program evaluation can be incorporated easily into program implementation. Being prepared for program evaluation from the outset can facilitate efficient, comprehensive, and timely evaluation (Doll, 2010).

Engage Your Brain 7-3

Think of an extracurricular activity in which you are or have engaged. What was the primary outcome, and how was it measured?

Collecting Evaluation Data

Evaluation questions are related to the research design, types of impact, outcome data to be collected, and data collection methods. Short-term impact measures often assess knowledge, attitudes, skills, and opinions. Intermediate-term impact measures target behavior change, and longer-term outcome measures address changes in social, economic, and health conditions. In some cases, evaluation data will include program attendance and changes in knowledge, attitudes, values, behaviors, and health outcomes. It is critical to choose impact and outcome indicators that will answer the evaluation questions. **Indicators** are observable and measurable milestones toward an outcome target (Creswell and Creswell, 2018). Occupational therapy outcome indicators include (American Occupational Therapy Association [AOTA], 2014):

- Occupational performance
- Adaptation
- Health and wellness
- Participation
- Prevention
- Quality of life
- Role competence
- Self-advocacy
- Occupational justice

In addition to determining what types of data are needed for the evaluation, the timing of data collection is a consideration. Typically, baseline or pretest data are collected prior to program implementation, posttest data are collected immediately after the intervention has been completed, and follow-up data are collected at intervals following the posttest in order to determine if the program effects are lasting. The bike safety program could offer a bike safety video on its website and collect statistics on how many times that video is viewed as an outcome of dissemination of bike safety knowledge. Figure 7-2 provides an outline for developing the data collection aspect of the evaluation plan (Creswell and Creswell, 2018).

Typically, evaluation data collection falls into two categories: quantitative designs and qualitative designs. These approaches may be combined in a mixed-methods approach, either sequentially or concurrently. Combining the methods can mitigate

Outcome	Indicator(s)	Source of data (program participants, records, census, etc.)	Method of data collection (survey, interviews, observation, etc.)	When data will be collected (baseline, post-intervention, follow-up with dates)	Person responsible for collecting data
1.					
2.					
3.					

Figure 7-2 Evaluation data collection plan.

the weaknesses of each (Creswell and Creswell, 2018).

Quantitative approaches use numbers as raw data in order to test hypotheses and establish cause-effect relationships. Quantitative approaches to program evaluation generally fall into the three broad categories listed here, beginning with the least complex (Creswell and Creswell, 2018):

- Nonexperimental designs (e.g., cross-sectional designs, cohort studies) involve participants serving as their own controls. Evaluation measures are gathered on participants before and after the intervention program. For example, in the bike safety program the number of participants that reported increased bike helmet use after education on proper bike helmet use would be an appropriate pretest-posttest design.
- Quasi-experimental designs (e.g., nonequivalent control group design, interrupted time-series design) compare two groups. The group that is receiving the intervention is matched to a population that is similar demographically but is not receiving the program. Data are collected from both groups at the same time points and compared. In this approach, the evaluation could compare adoption of bike helmet use by children attending two different educational programs to determine which approach is more effective at promoting bike helmet adoption.
- Experimental designs (e.g., randomized controlled trial) randomly assign people to two groups. One group receives an intervention, and the other does not. Data are collected from both groups at the same time points and compared.

Impact evaluations ideally consist of studies that involve experimental designs. These types of evaluations resemble traditional quantitative research studies that test hypotheses and attempt to control for confounding variables that might arise as alternative explanations for the cause-and-effect relationships. Because evaluations occur in the context of the program, evaluators want to minimize any disruption to the normal operation of the program when conducting impact evaluations. These types of evaluations can be difficult to design depending on the contextual constraints of the program (Creswell and Creswell, 2018).

Whereas impact evaluations seek to have the most rigorous design (i.e., randomized, pretest-posttest control group design), in many instances the ability to randomly assign clients to control or experimental groups is not possible. Often, evaluators are faced with selecting the quasi-experimental design that will fit best with the program. Most often this involves the use of a nonequivalent group pretest-posttest design. When employing these designs, evaluators must minimize the threats to internal validity that arise from the selection bias inherent in this design.

Most often evaluators will employ matching techniques or proximity scores as a means of equating the two groups. The main goal of these types of research designs is to measure intervention effects. While evaluators seek the most stringent designs when conducting the impact evaluations, contextual limitations often result in the use of weaker quantitative designs, such as single-group pretest-posttest designs, single-group posttest-only designs, and time-series designs. These designs do not control for many of the threats to internal validity, and as a result, evaluators must address the limitations of these designs when reporting program impact.

These less rigorous designs are better suited for program monitoring because they tend to measure either outcome levels (e.g., the measurement of an outcome at a particular time) or outcome change (e.g., the difference between outcomes measured at two different times) (Creswell and Creswell, 2018). When choosing measurement approaches, the desires and needs of the community remain important considerations. This factor should be prioritized along with the fidelity of the design chosen.

Qualitative approaches use language or narrative as raw data in order to study people's thoughts, experiences, and perspectives. The purpose of qualitative evaluation is "to capture the perspectives of program participants, staff, and others associated with the program" (Patton, 2015, p. 151). A qualitative evaluation approach provides an in-depth perspective on phenomena that are not easily quantifiable. It is especially useful when the evaluator wants to understand not only what worked but also why it worked. Qualitative methods are particularly suited to the analysis and interpretation of the contexts within which programs are operating.

Qualitative assessment can produce a deeper, fuller understanding of the program and its effects. This is done by collecting firsthand, direct observations of naturally occurring situations in naturally occurring settings. Qualitative methods in evaluation use an inductive approach to data gathering and interpretation. It is a holistic, naturalistic orientation, searching for themes in the evaluation data and attempting to understand the lived experience of program participants. A qualitative approach to evaluation can illuminate what happened, to whom, and with what outcomes. There are many benefits to qualitative evaluation, such as providing information about context and meaning (Creswell and Creswell, 2018).

Numerous ways to collect qualitative data exist, including interviews, focus groups, observation, and document review. If the evaluation seeks to understand what the program participants experienced, what they believe, or how they feel, then interviews are a good data collection strategy. Interviews can be conducted individually, face-to-face, over the telephone, online, or with multiple people in a focus group. Semistructured interviews using open-ended questions tend to produce the most useful information. For the bike safety program, focus groups or participant interviews could provide valuable information on the program's perceived impact.

If the evaluation seeks to identify what people do during given time frames, observation is a good data collection strategy to use (Fink, 2015). Observations should be carried out in a variety of contexts and across multiple time periods. Recording observation data in field notes is recommended. For example, the evaluators for the bike safety program may choose to observe and count the number of citizens wearing bike helmets on popular bike paths to determine overall use. If the evaluation seeks to understand the mission, history, and activities of an organization or agency, then document reviews can be a useful data collection approach. Documents to review may include mission statements, policies and procedures, brochures, website content, and meeting minutes (Fink, 2015).

Disseminating Evaluation Results

Evaluation results can and should be disseminated in a variety of ways depending on the information needs of the audience. Reporting evaluation results serves several purposes, including:

- Providing a basis for further program development and quality improvement
- Generating support for continuing or expanding programs
- Enhancing public relations
- Demonstrating good stewardship of funds

There are typically a number of different audiences for evaluation findings. These may include stakeholders, program staff, program participants, funders, collaborating agencies, professional organizations, elected officials, and business groups, among others. The presentation of evaluation results should include the focus of the evaluation, the processes used, and the strengths and limitations of the evaluation. Dissemination involves communicating the procedures and lessons learned from an evaluation in a timely and unbiased way (Fink, 2015). An end-of-year report is one method of dissemination mentioned earlier in this chapter. Another way of disseminating program evaluation results could include publication in a peer-reviewed journal to contribute to the body of research associated with the topic, especially if the program has achieved its objectives, and the stakeholders are supportive of broader dissemination.

Communication may take the form of verbal presentations, written reports, or visuals in the form of graphics or photographs. One particularly effective method for presenting evaluation results for community-based programs is the "success story." A good success story captures the attention of the audience, provides a compelling story, describes specific outcomes, and is based on reliable and valid data. A success story consists of four parts: the situation, the response, the results, and the evidence. The situation refers to the problem, concern, or issue that needed to be addressed. Describe the situation and its impact locally. The response refers to the program characteristics, who participated and benefited, and the services provided. The results section of the success story describes the outcomes, what changed and for whom, and what was learned. For example, in the bike safety program, several champions or success stories for bike helmet use could be described and reported. When choosing champions or role models to publicize, considerations of diversity and appropriate community representation should be a priority. Finally, the evidence component refers to how the program and its outcomes were evaluated and how the results are known to be accurate and credible (University of Wisconsin-Madison, Cooperative Extension, 2009).

Ethical Considerations

Appropriately used evaluation approaches in community-based practice can enhance efficacious community-centered needs assessments, program development, program implementation, and program evaluation. However, inadequate, misused, or incorrectly targeted evaluations can result in community alienation, wasted expenditures of limited resources, and missed opportunities for enhancing quality of life (Johnson and Christensen, 2017). Poorly developed or implemented program evaluations would be in conflict with one or more of the profession's core values and attitudes, which include "altruism, equality, freedom, justice, dignity, truth, and prudence" (AOTA, 2015, p. 2).

In addition, the principles from the AOTA *Occupational Therapy Code of Ethics (2015)* apply to all aspects of the program evaluation process, including:

- Selecting the appropriate evaluation approach and outcome measures (Principle 1, Beneficence)
- Obtaining Institutional Review Board (IRB) approval from all applicable institutions (Principle 1, Beneficence; Principle 3, Autonomy; and Principle 4, Justice)
- Avoiding conflicts of interest (Principle 1, Beneficence; Principle 6, Fidelity)
- Acquiring and using current assessments/ outcome measures and upholding copyright laws (Principle 1, Beneficence)
- Ensuring compliance with established program evaluation protocol and anonymity as appropriate (Principle 1, Beneficence; Principle 3, Autonomy)
- Training program staff and evaluators to ensure competency (Principle 2, Nonmaleficence)
- Reporting accurate results to participants and stakeholders in a timely manner (Principle 1, Beneficence; Principle 5, Veracity)

Additionally, the Joint Committee on Standards for Educational Evaluation and the National Board for Certification in Occupational Therapy (NBCOT, 2016) Candidate/Certificant Code of Conduct can offer guidance regarding the appropriate use of evaluation.

In community-based practice, the client can be an individual, a portion of a community, an entire community, or a population. The same standards that apply when evaluating individuals carry over to working with communities. When the client is a portion of a community, an entire community, or a population, an additional layer of complexity becomes evident due to the involvement of people from a variety of professional backgrounds, along with other numerous stakeholders. All stakeholders may not have the same motives or ethical framework. The AOTA *Occupational Therapy Code of Ethics (2015)* can be used to help support ethical participation in important projects aimed at addressing societal needs.

Performing due diligence to ensure all actions taken support community rights and autonomy is an ethical necessity. Whereas it may be relatively simple to match an assessment to an individual, locating an assessment or developing an outcome measure well suited for a broad array of individuals within a program, community, or population can be complicated. For example, individuals in the community may have significantly differing reading levels, languages and language skills, visual acuity, activity tolerance, and cultural norms. Any of these differences can make it challenging to select an appropriate measure to be part of an evaluation approach for use with all participants. It is essential to avoid selecting approaches that exclude portions of the community or population based on a desire to reduce time, effort, or expense. Program evaluation teams must be open to using multiple methods in order to provide all program participants with the opportunity for inclusion in program development and program evaluation (Johnson and Christensen, 2017).

Evaluation designs should be comprehensive and engage the community to ensure program support and sustainability. While these approaches provide good foundational knowledge for assessment, all evaluations should be program-specific and based on information important to stakeholders, such as the nature of the program being evaluated, the context of the evaluation, the informational needs and intended use of the evaluation results, the programmatic resources, and the specific evaluation questions. It is important to consider all of these factors when determining the program evaluation plan, as the data collected and analyzed during the program evaluation will be disseminated and interpreted by stakeholders and the broader community. By understanding the entire evaluation process sequence and planning appropriately, the evaluator can ensure that all the specific elements to create an ethical, comprehensive assessment of the program are addressed.

Summary

- Program evaluation optimizes the collection of relevant data for various stakeholder groups and then facilitates the use of this information for decision-making and action.
- One main purpose of program evaluation is to assist stakeholders in making changes that will lead to improvements in the program's activities, practices, processes, or operations.
- Programs can be evaluated by either an internal evaluator or by an external evaluator.
- There are four main types of program evaluation approaches that each examine programs differently and demonstrate different evaluation perspectives; they include:
  - Formative evaluation
  - Process evaluation
  - Impact evaluation
  - Outcome evaluation
- The process of program evaluation typically consists of planning an evaluation, identifying an evaluation method, collecting evaluation data, and disseminating the findings to key stakeholders.
- Common ethical considerations when completing program evaluation are choosing the right approach and measures for accurate evaluation, obtaining the necessary IRB approval, maintaining confidentiality, and avoiding conflicts of interest.

CASE STUDIES

CASE STUDY PART 3 Suicide Prevention in a Native American Community

In addition to creating the stress management rooms, the occupational therapist worked with the community to design an evaluation tool to assess the impact of the rooms on the children. Despite exploring evidence-based tools that measure childhood stress, the community wanted to design a tool that was easy to use and appropriate for all ages. The tool developed included a variety of faces that showed different emotions. The children participating in the stress management room circled the face of the emotion felt before the activity and then after. The faces and emotions chosen were representative of literature on stress and based on community input. The tool was pilot tested and edited for cultural aspects. Overall, more than 400 of these were collected to assess the impact of the program.

In addition, other program evaluation approaches used included post-training surveys (see Fig. 7-3) and focus group questions (see Fig. 7-4). To ensure respect and confidentiality, an application to a university institutional review board (IRB) was submitted, and the research was approved.

Post-Training Evaluation

Thank you so much for participating in this training. Please complete this evaluation form to help the trainers improve this session.

1. One thing I learned today that I did not know is:

Please circle your responses to the questions below:

2. I found the training relevant to me and my students.

5	4	3	2	1
Strongly Agree	Agree	Undecided	Disagree	Strongly Disagree

3. I plan to use what I learned today in my classroom.

5	4	3	2	1
Strongly Agree	Agree	Undecided	Disagree	Strongly Disagree

4. I think the stress management room can help my students cope with stress.

5	4	3	2	1
Strongly Agree	Agree	Undecided	Disagree	Strongly Disagree

5. Please list any questions you have that remain unanswered.

Figure 7-3 Post-training evaluation.

CASE STUDY PART 3 Suicide Prevention in a Native American Community

1. What do you like best about the stress management room activities and equipment for your students?
2. Can you describe the way in which you and your students are using the stress management room equipment and activities?
3. What changes have you seen in the students in your classroom following the implementation of the stress management room?
4. What do you view as the most beneficial outcome of the stress management room with the youth following each use?
5. How do you think your training of implementing the stress management room activities could be improved to better facilitate these activities for your students?
6. Do you have any suggestions on ways to improve the use or the implementation of the stress management room activities or equipment?
7. Is there anything else you would like to say regarding the stress management room activities and the impact on the students?

Figure 7-4 Focus group questions.

Discussion Questions and Application

Review the Case Study from Chapters 5 and 6 and answer/discuss the following questions:

1. What types of evaluation approaches were used?
2. What methods for data collection were used?
3. What ethical concerns might be related to program evaluation in this program example?

Learning Activities

1. List at least five school or community health programs in which you or a family member has participated over the years. Who are the stakeholders for each of those programs? How did the programs disseminate program evaluation data to those stakeholders?
2. Design a formative program evaluation plan for a volunteer experience you have completed. Provide one to two objectives to evaluate regarding your role as a volunteer, determine if you would use a quantitative or qualitative measure, and identify to whom you would disseminate the findings.
3. Create an assessment tool to use for outcome evaluation of an occupation-based program designed to enhance the parenting skills of teenage mothers. What outcomes do you plan to measure, and why did you choose these?

REFERENCES

American Occupational Therapy Association. (2014). Occupational therapy practice framework: Domain and process. *American Journal of Occupational Therapy, 68,* S1–S48. doi:10.5014/ajot.2014.682006

American Occupational Therapy Association. (2015). Occupational therapy code of ethics. *American Journal of Occupational Therapy, 69,* 6913410031p1–691340030p8. doi:10.5014/ajot2015.696s03

Barker, C., Pistrang, N., and Elliott, R. (2016). *Research methods in clinical psychology: An introduction for students and practitioners* (3rd ed.). Malden, MA: Wiley.

Bryson, J. M., Patton, M. Q., and Bowman, R. A. (2011). Working with evaluation stakeholders: A rationale, step-wise approach and toolkit. *Evaluation and Program Planning, 34*(1), 1–12.

Centers for Disease Control and Prevention. (1999). Framework for program evaluation in public health. *MMWR, 48*(No. RR-11), 1–42.

Centers for Disease Control and Prevention. (n.d.). *Types of evaluation.* Retrieved from www.cdc.gov/std/program/pupestd/types%20of%20evaluation.pdf

Coghlan, A. T., Preskill, H., and Catsambas, T. T. (2003). An overview of appreciative inquiry in evaluation. *New Directions for Evaluation, 100,* 5–22.

Cooperrider, D. L., Whitney, D., and Stavros, J. M. (2008). *Appreciative inquiry handbook for leaders of change* (2nd ed.). Brunswick, OH: Crown Custom.

Creswell, J. W., and Creswell, J. D. (2018). *Research design: Qualitative, quantitative, and mixed methods approaches.* Thousand Oaks, CA: Sage.

Doll, J. D. (2010). *Program development and grant writing in occupational therapy: Making the connection.* Boston, MA: Jones and Bartlett.

Fink, A. (2015). *Evaluation fundamentals: Guiding health programs, research, and policy* (3rd ed.). Thousand Oaks, CA: Sage.

Fitzpatrick, J. L., Sanders, J. R., and Worthen, B. R. (2011). *Program evaluation: Alternative approaches and practical guidelines* (4th ed.). Upper Saddle River, NJ: Pearson.

Hoefer, R. (2000). Accountability in action?: Program evaluation in nonprofit human service agencies. *Nonprofit Management and Leadership, 11*(2), 167–177.

Johnson, R. B., and Christensen, L. (2017). *Educational research: Quantitative, qualitative, and mixed approaches* (6th ed.). Thousand Oaks, CA: Sage.

Millar, R., and Hall, K. (2013). Social return on investment (SROI) and performance measurement: The opportunities and barriers for social enterprises in health and social care. *Public Management Review, 15*(6), 923–941.

National Board for Certification in Occupational Therapy. (2016). *NBCOT® candidate/certificant code of conduct.* Retrieved from www.nbcot.org/-/media/NBCOT/PDFs/Code_of_Conduct.ashx?la=en

Patton, M. (2007). Process use as a usefulism. *New Directions for Evaluation, 116,* 99–112.

Patton, M. (2015). *Qualitative research and evaluation methods: Integrating theory and practice* (4th ed.). Thousand Oaks, CA: Sage.

Rossi, P., Lipsey, M. W., and Henry, G. T. (2019). *Evaluation: A Systematic Approach* (8th ed.). Thousand Oaks, CA: Sage.

Salabarría-Peña, Y., Apt, B. S., and Walsh, C. M. (2007). *Practical use of program evaluation among sexually transmitted disease (STD) programs.* Atlanta, GA: Centers for Disease Control and Prevention.

University of Wisconsin–Madison, Cooperative Extension. (2019). *Evaluating programs.* Retrieved from https://fyi.extension.wisc.edu/programdevelopment/evaluating-programs/

Yarbrough, D. B., Shulha, L. M., Hopson, R. K., and Caruthers, F. A. (2011). *Evaluation standards: A guide for evaluators and evaluation users* (3rd ed.). Thousand Oaks, CA: Sage.

Chapter 8

Program Support: Innovation, Entrepreneurship, and Business Acumen

Joy D. Doll, OTD, OTR/L, Marjorie E. Scaffa, PhD, OTR/L, FAOTA, and Wendy M. Holmes, PhD, OTR/L

"It always seems impossible until it's done."

—Nelson Mandela

Learning Outcomes

This chapter is designed to enable the reader to:

8-1 Identify the characteristics of innovators and entrepreneurs.

8-2 Describe the process of innovation in the context of community and population health occupational therapy programming.

8-3 List the basic steps in starting a business.

8-4 Compare and contrast for-profit and nonprofit business models.

8-5 Describe the various aspects of developing a business plan.

8-6 Discuss diverse approaches for financial support for a business or program.

Key Terms

Business plan
Change agent
Diffusion
Direct costs
Environmental scan
For-profit company
Grant
Indirect costs
Marketing
Nonprofit organization
Occupational therapy entrepreneur
Social marketing
Strategic planning
SWOT analysis

Introduction

As members of a profession, occupational therapy practitioners possess diverse skill sets that allow for the delivery of varied interventions in many settings. An occupational therapy practitioner who desires to design and implement a new program or business must possess an entrepreneurial spirit and embrace innovation. This is especially true in community and population health programs, where the role of occupational therapy may be even more ambiguous and trailblazing is needed. Additionally, fundamental skills in business, including budgeting and engaging financial resources, are needed, whether starting a for-profit business or nonprofit organization. Topics that will be reviewed in this chapter include innovation, entrepreneurship, setting up a for-profit or nonprofit entity, and budgeting for financial viability. The focus of this chapter is the utilization of these skills in a community or population health occupational therapy program.

Innovation

Any occupational therapy practitioner deciding to start a new program or business must possess the ability to create and innovate. In today's complex healthcare environment, innovation includes elements of novelty, practicality, and scientific soundness (Balas and Chapman, 2018). Innovators typically have a natural ability to understand organizational theory (Suter et al., 2013). Multiple organizational theories are tied to innovation, but the diffusion of innovation theory is probably the most well known (Rogers, 2003). In this approach, innovators are individuals willing to take risks and are open to adventure (Suter et al., 2013). For occupational therapy practitioners in community settings and working in population health, an innovative spirit is critical to success, as a clear road map for implementing an approach will not always exist.

Rogers (2003) defined **diffusion** as "the process by which an innovation is communicated through certain channels over time among the members of a social system" (p. 35). Diffusion of innovation research examines the multiple facets of this process, such as the rate and consequences of trial by others and the factors that affect adoption in a variety of social and cultural settings. The four main elements of the diffusion process Rogers identified include:

- The innovation
- The communication channels
- Time
- The social system

The characteristics of the innovative idea, product, or service itself influence how individuals perceive it when considering its adoption. Customarily, individuals weigh the perceived complexity, usability, and advantages of an innovation before trial. However, a common development during the trial and adoption period is the reinvention or modification of the innovation to better suit the individual's purposes, frequently contributing to the sustainability of the innovation (Rogers, 2003, p. 183). In community settings and population health work, occupational therapy practitioners have many opportunities to engage stakeholders who can provide feedback on the innovation. The communication process and channels by which persons learn about an innovation vary widely and frequently include the mass media and the Internet.

However, research demonstrates that the power of interpersonal communication between individuals with similar interests and values is equally as important to successful diffusion (Balas and Chapman, 2018). An occupational therapy practitioner implementing a new program needs to be aware of the need to thoroughly vet the innovation. Innovation without adoption is truly just an idea. Planning for others to understand the innovation is a critical step toward successful implementation. For example, an occupational therapist wanting to design and implement an innovative community program to address childhood obesity must determine when and where the program will be implemented and garner many stakeholders to successfully implement the innovation.

Next, the element of time considers the speed by which the decision to adopt occurs, along with the characteristics of the persons who adopt the innovation. Rogers (2003) classified these individuals as innovators, early adopters, early majority, late majority, and laggards (p. 22), depending on when each group embraces the innovation. Rogers (2003) suggested that innovativeness is the cornerstone of the diffusion process and associated certain characteristics with each of the adopter categories. "The salient value of the innovator is venturesomeness, due to a desire for the rash, the daring, and the risky" (p. 283). In contrast, the early adopters are more conservative than innovators and yet serve as leaders and role models by embracing the innovation. "In one sense, early adopters put their stamp of approval on a new idea by adopting it" (p. 283). An application of this theory to occupational therapy practice appears in Chapter 3.

Similar to the transtheoretical model of health behavior change, the adoption of and adherence to a program must be considered. For example, in a study exploring adherence to home modifications for fall prevention in older adults, only 50% partially adhered to the recommended home modifications (Cumming et al., 2001). Individuals in this study and similar studies chose to adhere based not on health status or fall history but on subjective reasons like stigma or perception of the impact of the intervention (Cumming et al., 2001). Innovators not only recognize their own excitement for the innovation but realize that others' adoption requires understanding of the impact of the intervention and patience with the subjective reasons for choosing whether to participate. For example, if parents, teachers, and children do not acknowledge childhood obesity as an issue, any innovative approach the occupational therapist may identify most likely will not be effective. Recognizing a readiness for change and adoption to address a community or population health need is important for the occupational therapist to acknowledge in designing and implementing any community-based innovation.

As **change agents,** occupational therapy practitioners frequently promote innovative social changes for the benefit of their clients or service systems. Zaltman and Duncan (1977) suggested that "one of the basic functions performed by a change agent is to establish a link between a perceived need of a client system and a possible means of satisfying that need" (p. 187). Early adopters also function as change agents and, in so doing, demonstrate effective communication of the vision and the ability to motivate and influence others; both entrepreneurs and leaders share similar attributes. However, innovations do not always take hold easily even if important and relevant. Barriers to diffusion of innovation include impulsive adoption of the innovation, misinformation about the innovation, information overload, and poor implementation (Balas and Chapman, 2018). Strategies exist to overcome the challenges of diffusing innovation, including understanding the time and place to disseminate the new program or business to others, recognizing the importance of sharing the evidence behind the proposed program, understanding the interest and demand for the program, and identifying readiness to adopt new approaches or programs (Balas and Chapman, 2018; Dearing and Cox, 2018). Occupational therapy practitioners must be aware of the challenges and strategies of diffusing an innovation as part of planning and implementing a new program or business.

Engage Your Brain 8-1

Typically, occupational therapy students do not think of themselves as change agents in the profession, but innovation requires new ways of thinking. How might you as a student contribute to new ways of thinking that could be viewed as an occupational therapy change agent?

Occupational Therapy Entrepreneurship

Among the multiple skills required of an entrepreneur, the ability to envision, create, transform, and promote a new venture or service effectively is critical to success. Although not discussed extensively in the occupational therapy literature, leaders in the profession have spoken of **occupational therapy entrepreneurs** as "those who tend to perceive themselves simply as allied health practitioners who have discovered and seized opportunities for promulgating the practice of occupational therapy in new directions or perhaps moving it into new venues" (Pattison, 2006, p. 168). An entrepreneur "pursues new or existing opportunities in a market place; however, to do this successfully it is important to employ appropriate planning strategies that take into account these opportunities and how to maximize them" (Pattison, 2006, p. 168).

The delivery of entrepreneurial occupational therapy services often requires the ability to identify an opportunity and address an unmet need through new practice methods (Fazio, 2001; Jacobs, 2002). In addition to the technical skills required to implement the proposed program or business, the occupational therapy entrepreneur must possess strong interpersonal skills, including active listening, and good communication skills to stakeholders outside the field of occupational therapy. All of these skills are critical in community settings, where building relationships with stakeholders and community members is critical to the success of a program.

Flexibility, adaptability, and comfort in working outside the confines of traditional therapy service system are other essential skills of an occupational therapy entrepreneur. Occupational therapy entrepreneurs must explore opportunities to meet gaps in service, understand risk management (financial and liability) when determining an approach to address gaps, accept ambiguity, identify a strong vision for the program or business, and assemble an effective team to support the program or business (Pattison, 2006). These skills may come naturally to some and may be challenging for others. Self-reflection on one's persistence and determination can be a critical factor in determining the design of a new program or business (Verma, Paterson, and Medves, 2006).

Entrepreneurs must be able to engage in creative, critical thinking and complex problem-solving. As stated by Holmes and Scaffa, entrepreneurs "possess the knowledge and skills to recognize and cultivate opportunities, assess risk, communicate convincingly, and manage businesses and organizations" (2009a, p. 86). Alternatively, occupational therapy practitioners may already possess knowledge and skills that, upon self-reflection, are suitable to addressing a cause or social need within their communities. Challenging the status quo may be a natural skill set for some practitioners, providing a foundation for innovation and entrepreneurship encouraging the exploration of the delivery of programs outside traditional settings and payment models (Holmes and Scaffa, 2009b). They may turn their talents and resources to developing an innovative service that best addresses an identified social need (Corner-Doyle and Ho, 2010).

Occupational therapy entrepreneurs create innovative businesses and community-based programs. One occupational therapist developed and implemented a company that provides a catered subscription of monthly toys that are developmentally appropriate for the child. Another opened her own business focused specifically on ergonomics and overall wellness, with a focus on myofascial release and yoga, including both individual and group-based interventions. These two examples are for-profit organizations. Despite being less focused on community-based programs, they demonstrate the innovative and entrepreneurial spirit found among the occupational therapy profession.

Engage Your Brain 8-2

What opportunities and challenges in community or population health practice do you envision for occupational therapy entrepreneurs in the present and future?

Starting a New Business: The Basics

Starting one's own business has many advantages, but not all occupational therapy practitioners have innovative and entrepreneurial characteristics. Most have little, if any, training in business. Therefore, it is critical to identify and utilize experts knowledgeable in business, accounting, and law. In addition, expertise in community organization, population health, and working with community members is important for the design and implementation of community and population health programs. If the business will be marketed as occupational therapy, the services provided must conform to the legal scope of practice in the licensure law of the state in which the business will operate (Glennon, 2007). In addition, understanding the role of occupational therapy in the program or business is critical to ensure an appropriate and thoughtful business plan (Holmes and Scaffa, 2009a). A **business plan** is a road map or blueprint for a business and includes the goals of the business and a description of how the business is going to organize its resources in order to achieve the desired outcomes (Richmond and Powers, 2004). The structure and function of business plans will be discussed later in the chapter.

Types of businesses and legal structures are highly variable. It is important to determine the best organizational structure for the unique needs of one's business. The type of structure may also be influenced by socioeconomic and cultural factors and the population health needs unique to that community. Starting a business can be a daunting process. It is critical to understand all aspects of the business in as much detail as possible. The aim of this chapter is not to provide the reader with a definitive strategy for starting a business, as there are other excellent resources for this purpose. However, some general principles to consider when embarking on a business venture with a community or population health perspective will be presented.

When starting a program or business, deciding how it will be funded and sustained is a critical step toward success. Accessing funding to support a program requires effort and planning. The first step should be to develop a program or business plan. A business plan is especially critical in a for-profit business when applying for a business loan. However, a business plan should be part of any new program development, including nonprofit organizations, to ensure thoughtful implementation and programmatic sustainability.

In regard to financial support, the business plan should include a budget that identifies costs of the program, including personnel, benefits, equipment and supplies, activity costs, travel, insurance, taxes, and more. In addition to cost, income sources need to be considered, including the potential for reimbursable services. If the occupational therapy intervention is not reimbursable, then a revenue stream must be identified. When developing a budget, it is important to be realistic with income and expenses. A projected budget over time can help demonstrate program sustainability.

For-Profit or Nonprofit?

The first decision to be made in starting a business is to determine whether it will be a for-profit or nonprofit organization. There are many differences between these two types, and each has unique benefits and liabilities. First, the purposes are usually different. The purpose of a **for-profit company** is to generate profits for the owner(s) and shareholders. The purpose of a **nonprofit organization** is typically charitable, religious, or educational. An individual or shareholders do not own a nonprofit; it is owned by the public. The board of directors directs and operates the nonprofit but does not own it. Another difference is the source of revenue. For-profit businesses generate income through the sales of products or services. While nonprofit businesses can sell products and services, they are also allowed to solicit donations and apply for grants from the government and private foundations (Fritschner, 2006). A grant is an amount of funding from a private or government organization to support either research or a program. Grants will be discussed in more detail later in the chapter.

The legal structures for incorporation may also be different. A for-profit business can be a sole proprietorship, a partnership, a limited liability company (LLC), or a corporation. A nonprofit can never be a sole proprietorship but can be set up as an LLC, corporation, or trust, depending on state laws. For-profit companies pay federal taxes, state and local income taxes, sales taxes, property taxes, and employment taxes on employees. Nonprofits are often referred to as tax exempt because they do not pay federal taxes and may also be exempt from some state taxes depending on the laws in each state. However, nonprofit companies must pay employment taxes on employees.

In for-profit businesses, profits are usually distributed to the owners or shareholders in the form of dividends. Nonprofit businesses can "make a profit," meaning they can accumulate earnings in excess of their expenses. However, these "profits" must be put back into the nonprofit organization and cannot be distributed as dividends. The excess funds can be used to purchase equipment and supplies, provide staff training, increase salaries and benefits, or be retained for future charitable use. If a for-profit company is dissolved, then the assets are distributed to the owners or creditors. If a nonprofit is dissolved, its assets must be distributed to other nonprofit organizations or to the government (Fritschner, 2006). In either case, both nonprofit organizations and for-profit businesses are incorporated entities.

Incorporation Process

Articles of incorporation provide the legal description of the business or nonprofit organization. Establishing a legal entity protects the board of directors, staff, and volunteers from liabilities such as lawsuits or debts. When the business or nonprofit organization is formalized in this way, it is assigned an employer identification number (EIN), which allows the establishment of a bank account and the ability of the entity to own property. In addition, it allows a nonprofit organization to solicit funds in the form of donations and apply for grants that are often restricted to entities with a 501(c)(3) designation of tax-exempt status. Box 8-1 presents a format for articles of incorporation.

It is important to obtain a copy of the requirements for incorporation from the state in which the business or nonprofit organization will be located. Each state has its own policies and procedures regarding incorporation, and these can usually be obtained from the office of the secretary of state.

Box 8-1 Format for Articles of Incorporation

- Article I: Name of the business or nonprofit organization
- Article II: Street address of the business or nonprofit organization and mailing address of registered agent (usually the president)
- Article III: Name and address of each incorporator or founding board member
- Article IV: Purpose of the business or nonprofit organization and mission statement
- Article V: Membership of the nonprofit organization and mission statement
- Article VI: Meetings of the nonprofit organization membership (if applicable)
- Article VII: Committees
- Article VIII: Board of directors
- Article IX: Officers and duties
- Article X: Amendments to the articles
- Article XI: Dissolution of assets
- Article XII: Limitation on activities (if applicable)

Data from *An Easy, Smart Guide to Starting a Non-profit,* by A. Fritschner, 2006, New York, NY: Barnes and Noble Books.

Box 8-2 Fifteen Steps for Starting a Business

- Perform a self-assessment and identify business opportunities
- Create a vision statement
- Develop a mission statement
- Describe your business concept
- Adopt a legal structure
- Develop an organizational structure
- Research and register your business name
- Write a business plan
- Develop a marketing plan
- Solicit advice from experts
- Complete start-up tasks
- Hire staff
- Implement and manage business operations
- Manage financial operations
- File quarterly and annual reports

Data from *Business Fundamentals for the Rehabilitation Professional,* by T. Richmond and D. Powers, 2004, Thorofare, NJ: SLACK.

Starting a For-Profit Business

Richmond and Powers (2004) outline 15 steps for starting a health-care business (Box 8-2). These steps apply to all types of businesses to some degree and provide a useful framework for planning. Two major factors in the success of a for-profit company are a comprehensive business plan and effective marketing (GALE Small Business Builder, 2018).

The four basic types of legal structures used in for-profit businesses are sole proprietorship, partnership, limited liability company (LLC), and corporation. The simplest for-profit business to develop is a sole proprietorship. This is a business with one owner and no employees. A sole proprietorship is a useful structure for a small private practice, a consulting business, or an independent contractor. The benefits of this type of structure are that it is easy to form, the owner is in total control and receives all of the income, certain business expenses can be deducted from income taxes, and there are few record-keeping requirements. However, the owner assumes all liability risks and legal and operational responsibilities (Richmond and Powers, 2004).

Partnerships have two or more owners and may or may not have employees. Written partnership agreements stating the roles, responsibilities, and liabilities of each partner are essential. This structure is useful for group practices, for joint ventures with separate businesses sharing space and overhead expenses, and for those who prefer to take on a financial partner rather than a loan. The benefits of a partnership are that it is relatively easy to set up, liability risks and operational tasks are shared, and more opportunities for growth exist. The disadvantages are that decision-making is shared, and disagreements between partners can harm the business. In addition, each partner is individually and jointly responsible for the actions of the other (Richmond and Powers, 2004).

The LLC provides owners with the liability protection of a corporation while retaining the operational flexibility of a sole proprietorship or partnership. Each state has specific LLC restrictions, and some states do not permit occupational therapy practitioners and other health-care providers to establish an LLC business structure. Some of the advantages of the LLC are that it is easier to establish than a corporation, there is no personal liability for business debt, there is less record-keeping and paperwork required, and business losses can be used as a tax deduction on personal income taxes.

Corporations are the most complicated business structures, but they also afford the most protection against liability for the owners. Corporations have multiple owners or stockholders. The persons with the largest shares of stock have the most control over business decisions. A corporation has a board of directors and officers, has bylaws and articles of incorporation, and is subject to extensive governmental regulation. There are several types of corporations, such as the C corporation, S corporation, and professional service corporation (PC). Each of these has different tax implications, so an accountant and an attorney should be consulted to determine the most advantageous structure for your business.

Starting a Nonprofit Organization

Nonprofits are often referred to as agencies, foundations, associations, and organizations. The four types of nonprofits are public nonprofits, private foundations, membership-supported nonprofits, and service nonprofits. Funding for public nonprofits comes from the constituencies the nonprofit serves. For example, the American Red Cross and the United Way receive monies from the public to provide services to those in need. Public nonprofits can provide educational, advocacy, community, cultural, and health services. Private foundations exist to distribute money to charities. Three types of foundations exist: community, corporate, and family (Doll, 2010). Community foundations are based in a specific geographic location and raise funds from the community to support community programming. Corporate foundations utilize a portion of a corporation's profits to establish a foundation to support community programs. It is important to keep in mind that the mission of the corporate foundation may differ from the mission of the corporation. A corporate foundation is often named directly after the company. Examples include the Walmart Foundation and the Mutual of Omaha Foundation. Lastly, family foundations are established based on a family's personal wealth. For example, the Bill and Melinda Gates Foundation is a family foundation. Similar to corporate foundations, the mission of family foundations often differs from the focus of wealth propagated by the family who established the foundation.

Membership-supported nonprofits can receive funds from the general public, but what makes them unique is that their members help to financially support them. Environmental groups, labor unions, fraternities, and sororities fit into this category. Service nonprofits provide services to the general public, such as schools and hospitals, and receive their funding from a variety of sources (Fritschner, 2006).

Starting a nonprofit organization is much the same as starting a for-profit business. The tasks for starting a nonprofit organization are listed in Box 8-3. The first stage is the idea phase. It is important to research the services or products one hopes to deliver. Is there a need that is not being met by other

Box 8-3 Tasks Involved in Setting Up a Nonprofit Organization

- Meet with volunteers and discuss what types of services and products the organization will provide and who will be in charge of various operational functions. A board of directors must be established and officers elected. Create a mission statement and choose a name for the organization.
- Develop the organization's articles of incorporation. These describe the nonprofit's legal structure and how it will be operated.
- File the articles of incorporation with the state in order to establish the organization as a legal entity. Be prepared to pay a filing fee.
- Apply to the Internal Revenue Service (IRS) for an Employer Identification Number (EIN). This can be done online. This number identifies the nonprofit and affords the organization the legitimacy to establish a bank account in its name.
- File an application for nonprofit tax-exempt status (referred to as 501(c)(3) status) with the IRS. This allows the organization to receive tax-deductible contributions and avoid paying federal income tax.
- Create a logo and acquire stationery that displays your logo, mailing address, and other contact information.
- Set up a corporate bank account and acquire a mailing permit from the post office for bulk mailings.
- Create a web page to enhance the credibility and visibility of the nonprofit organization. Register your domain name as .org, which is the identifier for a nonprofit, rather than .com.

community agencies? This aspect should be identified in the business plan as well. The second stage is to gather people who share one's vision and commitment. These are people who will become the board of directors, officers, and volunteers. The third stage is determining the form or legal structure for the nonprofit. Considerations at this stage include size of the organization, perceived liabilities, and tax-exempt status. Next is the development of a strategic plan, followed by publicity and a fund-raising campaign. Finally, there must be a plan for growth and the continued development of the organization.

Overall, the decision for a community or population health program to be for-profit or not-for-profit is based on many factors. Reimbursement structures and health-care services vary, meaning communities experience different gaps in services. Although it is typical for most community-based occupational therapy programs to be nonprofit, this model may not be the best choice for all scenarios. Consulting a small-business development office at a local chamber of commerce may be helpful in making these decisions.

Developing a Business Plan

According to entrepreneurs, a business plan can take various forms, depending on the type of business in which one chooses to engage. According to Jaffe and Epstein (1992), "How successful the business's products will be depends on how thoroughly the prospective entrepreneur has researched and analyzed the business plan" (p. 638). A business plan is an evolving document and should be a work in progress that is reviewed and modified on a frequent and routine basis to guide business decisions both large and small. To establish this plan, Richmond and Powers (2004) devised five areas in which the entrepreneur needs to focus. The entrepreneur must:

- Perform a market assessment/analysis
- Develop a mission statement
- Develop a business concept
- Develop business goals
- Develop the plan

Market assessment, also known as market analysis, helps entrepreneurs examine the geographic region of their products, the clientele, and their needs. The Internet has provided occupational therapy entrepreneurs with the world as their market; however, it is wise to develop product lines slowly and create a niche before expanding globally. A market analysis typically contains the proposed impact of the business and explores what already exists to meet the need. The analysis acknowledges gaps in services and describes how the proposed business would fill them. Trends in the area of practice, along with analysis of the customer and competitive bases, are included. In some cases, the occupational therapy practitioner may consult an expert in market analysis to ensure comprehensiveness.

Mission statements are broad ideas of the purpose of the business. "Once a mission statement has been developed, it should serve as a guiding principle for practice. It should meet today's needs and tomorrow's prospects" (Jaffe and Epstein, 1992, p. 639). The development of mission statements is discussed in greater detail in Chapter 6.

A business concept defines specifics of the business. For example, if occupational therapists wished to offer wellness consultation services to underprivileged families, they would describe the specific location of the services, the types of services offered, the times at which services can be offered, and the costs of services. These details are important to focus the business and will later help with marketing those services.

Business goals are those developed initially, and they can change as the business grows. As an entrepreneur, a typical business goal is to be financially stable. Meeting costs versus turning a profit in a specific amount of time can be a goal. Another goal can be one of philanthropy, whereby the business works toward giving to the community. Philanthropic goals and financial goals do not have to be mutually exclusive.

The plan is the organizational structure of the business. This includes the types of people to be employed (if any), bookkeeping practices, and strategies to manage the business financially. In addition, the organizational plan usually contains milestones and a time line for completion. Explaining the business idea to others and establishing a clear road map for implementation helps maintain focus. Many books and other resources are available for entrepreneurs to develop plans that fit their needs. Local chambers of commerce, libraries, the Small Business Administration (SBA), and a local university college of business may also be available to assist with resources.

Even though occupational therapy is a service-oriented profession, developing a clear, focused plan that includes marketing services and products is critical to the success of the business. This is especially true in community and population health programs, in which the role of occupational therapy often differs from clinical delivery models. In addition, occupational therapy as a profession is not widely understood and often requires explanation. Therefore, identifying best practices in marketing an occupational therapy program is especially critical. **Marketing** refers to the "communications activities the organization will undertake in order to attract service users" (Fritschner, 2006, p. 200). The goals of marketing include creating consumer awareness of the product or service, building name recognition, and meeting financial goals. Typically, the goal of commercial marketing is to attract customers in order to generate revenue and make the corporation profitable.

Social marketing has a different focus. **Social marketing** is the adaptation and application of marketing principles, techniques, and processes to create social change. It is designed to influence the behavior of target audiences; these could be individuals, communities, populations, and policymakers, among others. The goal of social marketing is to improve the lives of people, communities, and society as a whole. However, as a consequence of using social marketing, an organization or program may grow and expand. Social marketing has been used to address social issues, such as pollution, sexual harassment, recycling, and smoking (Andreasen, 2006). Occupational therapy entrepreneurs often find the principles of social marketing more compatible with the values of the profession than commercial marketing.

Developing a plan and possessing knowledge of how to implement that plan and market one's services can turn a great idea into a successful practice. Karen Jacobs (1998), a past president of the American Occupational Therapy Association (AOTA), stated that the "use of a marketing approach will allow practitioners to approach the health care environment proactively and be ready to meet the changing needs and wants of the marketplace. In all times of change, there is great opportunity" (p. 620). Part of marketing is taking the time to consider the title of the program and a potential logo to improve community understanding and recognition of the business (Austin and Rust, 2015). Partnering with a graphic artist can be a helpful resource to ensure the logo and business name are unique and appropriate. A budget for the marketing plan should be included in the business plan.

Strategic Planning

Strategic planning is the systematic process of setting short, intermediate, and long-term organizational goals and priorities; identifying organizational activities; and predicting potential outcomes. Strategic planning "is an ongoing, continuous process, which must adapt to environmental changes, both external and internal" (Smith, Bucklin, and Associates, 2000, p. 5). A strategic plan is a realistic agenda for action that operationalizes the organization's mission statement and focuses the organization's energies toward high-yield objectives and activities. A well-designed strategic plan will:

- Establish priorities
- Guide program activities
- Allocate resources
- Establish mechanisms to assess the organization's accomplishments

The steps in the strategic-planning process include:

- Conducting an environmental scan and analysis
- Setting broad organizational goals
- Establishing strategic objectives
- Developing an operational plan

An environmental scan and analysis is the first step in strategic planning. It is important for the planners to understand the trends and issues that have an impact on the organization and how the environment may facilitate or hinder the accomplishment of the organization's mission. An **environmental scan** identifies trends in a variety of spheres, including demographic, economic, technological, political, professional, and educational. An internal scan of the organization's financial and human resources, technological capabilities, and culture is also an important source of information. Sometimes this approach is referred to as a **SWOT analysis**, where *S* refers to strengths and assets, *W* to weaknesses and limitations, *O* to opportunities, and *T* to threats. Once the organization's strengths,

Box 8-4 SWOT Analysis Example: A Senior Center Wishing to Expand and Provide Health Promotion Services

Strengths/Assets	Opportunities
• Stable, experienced staff • Good reputation in the community • Adequate financial resources for current services • Well networked with other nonprofit agencies • Member of the chamber of commerce	• Recent hospital downsizing, producing unused space • Increasing older adult population • University collaboration for potential student training • Lack of local services for older adults with dementia or mental disorders
Weaknesses/Limitations	**Threats**
• Inadequate space to expand • Lack of finances to build a new facility • Limited parking • Location not on public transit routes	• Current economic recession • Inadequate political support • Competition from medically based health services

weaknesses, opportunities, and threats are identified, a strategic plan can be developed to address these factors. An example of a SWOT analysis is provided in Box 8-4.

Trends that have a high probability of occurrence and may potentially have a significant impact on the organization should be considered critical issues to address in the strategic plan (Smith et al., 2000). The second step in strategic planning is setting broad organizational goals. These goals are generally derived from the mission statement and represent the purpose of the organization.

The third step in strategic planning is setting strategic objectives, those "major accomplishments the organization hopes to achieve in a defined time frame," which is usually three to five years (Smith et al., 2000, p. 19). Strategic objectives support the organization's mission and goals, provide direction, and afford a means for measuring outcomes. These objectives should be realistic, meaningful, and measurable. Strategic objectives identify what is to be accomplished.

The next step is to operationalize the strategic objectives; this involves specifying how the objectives will be achieved. An operational plan describes the tasks to be accomplished, who is responsible, what resources are required, when the objectives will be achieved, what results are anticipated, and how these results will be measured. Finally, the strategic plan is implemented, monitored, and adjusted as necessary. To ensure a strategic plan reaches full implementation, a structured and shared plan for reporting progress and reflecting on necessary adjustments is an important ongoing activity.

In summary, a business plan is used to initially structure and start a new business entity, while a strategic plan is used to focus, direct, and implement strategic initiatives for an existing organization. A business start-up plan usually covers the first year of operation, while a strategic plan generally covers a longer time frame, often 3 to 5+ years. These plans are interrelated and both are necessary for the success of a business or organization.

Financing the Business or Program

When beginning a new business or program, the financial aspect is a critical component and an area that not all occupational therapy practitioners feel comfortable navigating. However, an occupational therapy practitioner venturing down this path must develop some business acumen in order to be a successful business owner. In this section, a summary of knowledge related to the business and financial aspect begins the process of ensuring a comprehensive plan for the business or program.

Budgeting

The budget is an important component of program design and implementation. When creating a budget, the occupational therapy practitioner should consider what resources are needed for program implementation. Financial planning and budgeting should be an annual practice for the program, and budgets should be constantly monitored to ensure the program's viability. The operating budget outlines the program's financial plans for revenue, including monies and resources that come into the program as well as operating expenses to be paid out of the program's budget (Weis and Gantt, 2004).

When developing a budget, begin by calculating a thorough analysis of costs and income, often called a cost-benefit analysis. After determining the costs and income, the next step is to consider the balance between the two to ensure that the program at least attains a zero balance or has reserves in place to pay additional expenses (Weis and Gantt, 2004). Budgets, as well as a proposed plan of the income and expenses of the program, are planned for the upcoming year. If a program is new, its expenses and income should be recorded for completing its annual budget in subsequent years. Program budgets should be in constant flux, adjusting to expenses and income. The first few years of a budget will incur more cost as the program gets established, and planning to balance costs with revenue is important for viability and sustainability.

Budgets can be simple or complex, based on the program. A novice in program design and implementation might want to seek external assistance with budgeting. In some organizations, resources for creating a budget are offered. Computer software programs that help organize a budget are also important resources to engage, especially if creating a budget without assistance. Programs often pay auditors to aid them in determining fiscal viability on an annual basis. Financial advisors and accountants are resources for help in developing and managing a program budget. Budget formats differ based on the structure of the business.

Start-Up Costs

When establishing a new program or business, an important consideration is how initial funds, also known as start-up costs, will be acquired (Braveman, 2016; Timmreck, 2003). Depending on the program, start-up costs will vary. It is important to identify what funds are needed to initiate the program and whether these costs will be one-time or ongoing. Costs can comprise overhead to initiate the program, including rental space, phone and Internet services, advertising, new equipment, and supplies. If the program plans on making a profit, then a business loan is an appropriate option to consider to fund start-up costs. On the other hand, if the program plans on simply generating enough funds to cover program costs, then other funding sources, such as a grant or donations, may be more appropriate. The type of business also plays a role here. For-profit businesses are more appropriate for small business loans, whereas nonprofit organizations are eligible for other funding streams like fundraising, grants, donations, and sponsorships.

In some cases, an institution may offer a program and cover the costs in accordance with its mission to serve the community. For a small program, such as a yoga program offered by an outpatient facility, the costs may be minimal, and an institution may be willing to cover the expense of marketing if the occupational therapy practitioners are willing to donate their time. A well-written plan, no matter how small or big the community-based program, is key to successful implementation and sustainability.

Business Loans

Navigating the waters of obtaining a business loan requires some research to ensure the best loan option is acquired. Loans are provided by banks and microlenders. Typically, a bank loan takes longer to acquire and is used when the applicant has good credit. Microlenders are nonprofit organizations that support small business loans. Microlenders may be supported by a foundation like Grameen American, which receives funding from the Grameen Foundation, or exist from private or corporate funding like Lifefund, which has received funding from J. P. Morgan Chase and Company. Banks tend to offer lower-interest loans than microlenders and provide higher loan amounts. Similar to other major purchases, when applying for a loan, shopping around to determine the best fit for interest and repayment options is important. It is also critical to determine the best fit for the business and revenue streams in order to pay back the loan and prevent default or other negative consequences.

When applying for a business loan, a business proposal is a must. The business plan will include a pro forma, which is essentially a budget with predictions over time that will indicate program sustainability (AOTA, 2018). The proforma projects program utilization and revenue. It provides a clear cost-benefit analysis of the projected business plan. In addition, a proforma has a predictive component that identifies revenue and cost, usually over time. A business proposal and proforma will demonstrate to a lender that the business is well planned and presents less risk to the lender. Lenders are more likely to provide loans to well-planned programs with a high likelihood of sustainability.

Grants

Grants, another source of funding, are typically for nonprofit organizations. A **grant** is essentially money donated to an organization to cover the costs of a program (Doll, 2010). The recipient of funds is accountable to the funding agency and has to follow its guidelines, which often include specific accountability and the reporting of program challenges and successes. Grants are typically available only to nonprofit agencies that are categorized with a tax identification of 501(c)(3). Grant funds are available from a variety of sources, including local and federal government agencies and foundations. Grants are also available in various amounts, from very small amounts (e.g., $500) to millions of dollars, depending on the funding agency.

Program development grants are often a source to start a program and are not regarded as a sustainable source of funding to support ongoing program implementation. Grants are often referred to as "soft money," indicating their purpose in helping start or support a program for a short time, typically 1 to 3 years.

Foundations provide nearly 12% of the funds provided to nonprofit organizations. Most foundations require a grant proposal from the organization that is compatible with the mission and purpose of the foundation. There are a number of different types of grants; these are listed in Box 8-5. It is important to identify the type of grant and the appropriate foundation from which to solicit funds before writing a grant proposal (Fritschner, 2006). Information about foundation funding can be obtained from the Foundation Center (www.fdncenter.org) and the Council on Foundations (www.cof.org).

Box 8-5 Types of Grants

- *Start-up grants:* also called "seed money," grants that are used to partially fund new programs or projects in order to attract other donations
- *Program grants:* grants that are used for a specific program within an organization
- *Continuing support grants:* grants that can be renewed for a number of years
- *Consulting grants:* grants that are used to hire consultants for a project
- *Conference grants:* grants that are used to send organization board members or staff to continuing education workshops or to plan and implement conferences or seminars for others
- *Research grants:* grants that provide funding for basic or applied research, usually provided to or through hospitals and universities
- *Challenge or matching grants:* grants that provide partial funding but require other donors to match the funding in order to receive the grant
- *Endowment:* monetary gift, or grant, to be invested, the income from which can be used to fund projects and support the nonprofit organization

Data from *An Easy, Smart Guide to Starting a Non-profit,* by A. Fritschner, 2006, New York, NY: Barnes and Noble Books.

As mentioned previously, there are multiple types of foundations, and finding the right fit for the program is an important step in the grant process.

In addition to foundation sources, funding can be obtained from state and federal government agencies. The *Catalog of Federal Domestic Assistance* is the primary source of information about federal funding opportunities. Government agencies may offer funds in the form of grants or contracts. Grants are funds awarded for a specific purpose based on the submission of an original creative proposal. Contracts are also awarded for a specific purpose, but in this case the government agency has already outlined the scope of services to be provided, and nonprofit organizations are invited to bid competitively on the project (Scaffa, 2001). Multiple federal agencies provide funding that could be a fit for a community or population health occupational therapy program. However, it is important to explore the requirements for eligibility for the program and for the lead person on the grant project, known as the principal investigator (PI). In many federal grants, the PI must have specific credentials and an existing track record of successful funding. Most federal funding is allocated to academic institutions and could be a fit when managing a program through a university. Most community programs will have much more success seeking local funding rather than federal funding. Government funding is available at all levels (i.e., city, county, state, etc.), and local government funding might be a viable option to explore. An excellent starting point for identifying federal funding sources is the Grants.gov website.

Grant proposals are not standardized, and the grant writer should follow the guidelines from the funding agency. Yet grant proposals typically consist of the following components:

- Introduction
- Statement of need
- Goals and objectives
- Program activities
- Program evaluation strategies
- Budget and personnel
- History of organization and prior funding
- Summary or conclusion
- Appendices of supporting materials (Doll, 2010)

Each of these components should be considered prior to writing the grant proposal. In fact, the grant writer should consider the amount of funding needed to support the program prior to searching for funding. These details are important to ensure finding the right funding agency and call for proposal to match the proposed program. When writing a grant, review the grant request for funding, typically called a request for proposal (RFP) but also sometimes known as a request for application (RFA) or a funding opportunity announcement (FOA). Whatever its title, the intent of this document is to outline what the funder wants to know before agreeing to award grant funds. Successful grant writers thoroughly review the RFP and contact the funder to demonstrate interest and seek any clarification regarding the time line or requirements. This means the topics and titles in the RFP act as the foundation for the grant proposal. The grant writer should also use language from the RFP to match with the reviewers' language. Many funders require collaboration among multiple agencies or organizations in the grant application. Therefore, it is important to identify and cultivate partners to participate in the grant proposal early in the writing process.

In addition, the grant writer or team writing the proposal needs to brainstorm each component of the proposal prior to writing. As part of this process, the grant writer and team should identify and describe the following:

- Need for the particular project or service that is being proposed
- Target population for the project
- Population data that are specific to the problem and the geographic area the project is designed to address

Basically, the proposal answers the question "Why is this project important and necessary?" In addition, identifying who the project will serve and benefit is an important priority for the funders, as funding agencies typically desire programming for those currently underserved.

Next, it is important to identify the goals and objectives of the program or project. These define what is to be achieved and how it will be achieved. A goal is a general statement regarding expected outcomes, while an objective is a specific statement that defines the goal in measurable terms. Goals represent the final destination; objectives specify how the goals will be achieved. Examples of goals and related objectives can be found in Box 8-6. The objectives should support the achievement of the goals, and the goals should address the needs identified in the statement of needs. Basically, this section answers the question "What is to be accomplished by this project?" Goals and objectives in grant proposals may be unique to those written in a program plan, and it is best to follow the request-for-proposal guidelines. In Chapter 6, guidelines are provided for writing program and grant goals and objectives.

Describing program activities occurs next in the grant-writing process. These activities are designed to accomplish the specified program objectives. Typically, there are several program activities for each objective. This section of the proposal often includes a time line for completion of the program activities and a list of staff, equipment, and supplies that are necessary to implement the activities. It answers the question "What activities will be done to achieve the objectives?"

Box 8-6 Sample Grant Goals and Objectives

Goal

Increase the ability of teachers, school counselors, clergy, health-care professionals, emergency response personnel, and human resource and personnel directors of local businesses to effectively respond to the mental health needs of persons affected by disaster

Objectives

Workshop participants will demonstrate:

- Increased knowledge of the symptoms of posttraumatic stress disorder (PTSD) and the critical incident stress model
- Improved identification and referral of persons in need of mental health services
- Effective use of appropriate interventions for persons experiencing critical incident stress or PTSD

Goal

Enhance the mental health of individuals affected by disaster

Objectives

Support group participants will demonstrate:

- Reduced symptoms of critical incident stress and PTSD
- Increased use of adaptive coping strategies in response to critical incident stress
- Decreased use of maladaptive coping strategies in response to critical incident stress

Engage Your Brain 8-3

What local foundations in your area offer grants related to community health needs?

Program evaluation, covered in Chapter 7, is an extremely important component of a grant proposal. Funders want to know how program effects will be measured and which program goals and objectives were achieved. The program evaluation describes how and when progress will be measured and what assessment tools will be used. In addition, who completes the evaluation is important to consider. Evaluation can be done either internally by members of the program team or externally by a professional evaluator.

Budgeting and personnel requirements will be dictated by the funding agency. In general, a grant budget answers the question "How will the money be spent?" Funders want to see accurate estimates of the costs of implementing the program. This requires the grant writer to collect cost information for salaries, rent, utilities, equipment, and supplies. Some people speculate that if the costs are underestimated and the total costs are lower, then the grant is more likely to be funded. However, this is typically not true. Funders frequently know the costs of doing business, and proposals that claim to be able to implement programs significantly below market costs are deemed unrealistic and likely to fail. It is useful to have the assistance of an accountant in the preparation of a budget for a grant proposal. When describing personnel by name, mention only those who will play a major role in the project and list their relevant credentials and qualifications. Some grant proposals will require a formal biosketch from each participant on the grant project. The biosketches should be formatted and submitted according to grant requirements. In addition to a budget, grants often require a budget justification, which includes narrative describing why each component of the budget is requested. Like all other components, it is important to follow the grant guidelines. Sample biosketches following the format preferred by the National Institutes of Health (n.d.) can be found on its website (see https://grants.nih.gov/grants/forms/biosketch.htm).

Like each grant proposal, grant budgets are unique to each project, and each has specific criteria. Text from components of the business plan can help when writing a grant proposal. Grant budgets usually consist of two major components: direct costs and indirect costs (Gitlin and Lyons, 2013). **Direct costs** are those items in the budget that will be funded by the program's income. Common direct program costs include salary, benefits, equipment, consultants, and travel. **Indirect costs** are those costs required to implement the program, including overhead and administrative costs (Weis and Gantt, 2004). Funders often limit indirect costs to a certain percentage of the budget. Indirect rates are often negotiated between the funding agency and the organization to whom the funds are distributed.

Discussions about indirect costs should happen early in the process to ensure a proper grant budget is written and matches the funding agency and organizational priorities. Examples of indirect costs include, but are not limited to, overhead such as rent, phone and Internet services, and other institutional costs (Doll, 2010).

Finally, the last step is to write the introduction and the summary or conclusion for the grant application, along with a title for the grant project. These are the first and last impressions the proposal readers will have of the project or program. If the introduction is not well written, clear, and interesting, the readers may choose not to continue or to peruse only superficially. A poorly written introduction is often a death sentence for a grant proposal. The introduction and the conclusion contain basically the same information, and they provide a concise overview of the project as a whole. Fritschner (2006) recommends that the introduction use action words and the conclusion use language that strikes more of an emotional appeal. The introduction and conclusion should include a brief statement of the problem, how the program will address the problem, the nonprofit organization's qualifications, and the amount of money needed. Including the name of the foundation or funding source in both the introduction and conclusion is highly recommended. This personalizes the grant proposal and engages the funding sources as coparticipants.

In addition, certain supporting documents may be requested for the appendices. Supporting material may include letters of support and endorsement from key community stakeholders, newspaper clippings regarding the problem or need to be addressed by the program, resumes of key program staff members, copies of assessments and program evaluation tools, and the Internal Revenue Service (IRS) tax-exempt letter designating the organization as a 501(c)(3) corporation (Fritschner, 2006). As stated previously, following the guidelines outlined in the RFP is critical in all components of the grant proposal. After the grant proposal is submitted, the grant proposal will be reviewed and either awarded funds or rejected for funding. Grant review can take a significant time, from 3 months to 1 year. If accepted, the program should be implemented according to what was proposed in the grant. If rejected, it is recommended that the grant writer seek reviewer feedback in order to determine any modifications for the next grant proposal. Although grants can financially support program activities, grant proposals require significant effort without a guarantee of funding.

Grant writing requires skill, and funding is not guaranteed. In addition, the funder can place very specific requirements on the program, which may help or hinder its implementation. When writing grants, ensuring the requirements are a match is a critical first step in the process. If one is inexperienced in grant writing, hiring a professional grant writer or taking an online course in grant writing might be a wise investment.

Donations

Programs may also benefit from donations, which are appropriate for a nonprofit organization. Donors receive tax benefits when donating to a tax-exempt organization. When soliciting donations, it is important to be very clear about the purpose of the funds and to target individuals or organizations that have a specific interest in the program or participants of the program. Consider donations beyond financial, as donors may be willing to donate equipment or services to support a program. If a donor is willing and able to give a significant amount of funding, the option of "naming" the program or facility where the program occurs can be an incentive. Typically, naming rights are offered for significant donations, but naming can be offered for offices or areas of a clinic, or even large equipment. Thinking proactively about the options for naming rights can influence a donor to make a large donation.

Fundraising

Fundraising is another method for seeking donations for a program. It is important to remember that fund-raising can be time-consuming. If the program exists within an organization, checking with individuals in charge of fundraising is important to avoid conflicting priorities. There is a science and an art to fund-raising. The science is applying fund-raising models and using available data and research to target fund-raising efforts. The art consists of developing and nurturing interpersonal relationships with potential donors and funders. Funding for nonprofit organizations can come from a variety of sources, including individual donors, corporate donors, online donors, and other fund-raising events. The most viable nonprofit organizations bring in dollars, goods, and services from multiple sources. The vast majority of donations, approximately 75%, come from individuals; therefore, it is imperative to cultivate a donor base (Fritschner, 2006).

Developing a donor base occurs in phases. The first phase, prospecting, is when a list of potential donors is developed. These potential donors are then prioritized based on how much they might donate and the probability of successfully soliciting a donation. Prior to engaging a donor, thoroughly explore research on the priorities of the donor and the focus of prior donations. Many significant donors have profiles and can share the organizations and projects they have donated to in the past, especially if making a significant donation. If the donor is a good fit, each potential donor is invited to observe and participate in the activities of the organization, and then a request for a donation can be made. When a donation is solicited, it is important that it is solicited from the right person, for the right amount of money, at the right time, and for the right purpose. This is called the Rule of Rights in fund-raising. In-person solicitation is always more effective than fund-raising through the mail. Thanking the donor, acknowledging the contribution publicly, and informing the donor about how the money was spent will improve the likelihood that the donor will choose to donate again (Fritschner, 2006). The infrastructure of thanking donors and providing appropriate tax forms for donations should be established prior to solicitation.

Corporations are often interested in donating funds to nonprofits that serve the local communities in which their employees live and work. In addition, corporate donations are tax-deductible, often produce publicity, and generate goodwill for the corporation. Typically, corporations are not interested in funding annual operating costs but will provide start-up funds for new projects or programs. In lieu of money, some corporations will provide in-kind donations, often in the form of goods and services, or volunteer hours from their employees. Corporations represent approximately 5% of the dollars, goods, and services donated nationwide (Fritschner, 2006). For example, a homeless shelter needing a vehicle in order to provide transportation to and from health-care appointments and job interviews may receive an in-kind donation of a van from a car dealership. Similar to single donors, research on what the corporation currently supports should be conducted to ensure a match prior to seeking donations.

Online fundraising usually takes the form of selling products to the general public. However, online donation solicitation is also an option. To take advantage of the web as a source of funds, it is necessary for the organization to be able to process credit card payments. Another option is to collaborate with brand name companies that donate a portion of their online sales proceeds to charitable organizations. Fundraising has also evolved with social media, including crowdfunding. Crowdfunding incurs a small fee from the amount donated but can be an easy method to distribute widely when requesting donations. Multiple crowdfunding websites exist and charge varying amounts. Goals for fundraising amounts can be set along with deadlines for raising the funds on crowdfunding sites. The fundraising information can often be shared quickly and easily through digital means and social media. Crowdfunding can reach a large number of people who can each donate a small amount, which may be an effective short-term fundraising approach.

Engage Your Brain 8-4

Name a crowdfunding resource. What are the benefits and limitations of using crowdfunding compared to other forms of funding?

In addition, aligning the organization with others who might assist in fundraising is important. Some cities promote Days of Giving, which provide opportunities for community members to donate to local organizations, along with a website and means for donors to give funds. Being listed and promoting an organization in alignment with one of these events can help raise funds for an organization without a significant investment in time and resources.

Event-based fundraising is an option that typically includes an entertaining event (e.g., a run or dance), and the funds collected support the program or project. These events require significant planning and investment. In addition to raising funds, these events can bring awareness to the organization and program. Special fundraising events may include dinners, concerts, theatrical productions, auctions, and sports outings, with the type of event limited only by the imagination and financial resources. Increased interest can be piqued by offering drawings for door prizes donated by local businesses and items for sale through a silent auction. In addition to garnering revenue from ticket sales, nonprofits may also solicit sponsorships from corporations. Fundraising events are time- and labor-intensive, with costs often approximating 50% of the revenue generated. However, they are useful in publicizing the work of the nonprofit, increasing its visibility, and cultivating new donors (Smith et al., 2000).

For larger organizations, fundraising may be a focused campaign. It usually includes a target for a funding goal and a time line for raising funds. In a campaign, a clear message about the intent of the campaign is developed. Logos and materials about the campaign are developed to distribute. Campaigns often tell "the story" of the organization, identifying a clear purpose and reason for giving to the organization. Donors are then solicited to donate to the campaign.

Most nonprofit organizations pursue multiple strategies to meet fundraising goals. In addition to providing organizational oversight, board members identify clear goals and expectations for fundraising and act as promotors and donors to the organization. The board of directors can be invaluable in developing a clear fundraising strategy and engaging financial supporters.

Sponsorships

Sponsorships are another possibility for garnering funds for a program. Sponsorships are typically monies donated by local corporations that are more willing to sponsor events than programs. When seeking sponsorships, it is important to clearly designate what sponsor monies will cover and how they will benefit the program. Benefits to sponsors should be considered. For example, if a sponsor provides a certain amount of funds, then the sponsor may receive free advertising on the program's website or other organizational materials. Sponsorships may be a useful source for funding a program or program event. Investigating and identifying sponsorship levels before approaching a sponsor is important. Sponsorship levels include the benefits to the sponsor for a specific donated amount. Awareness of the corporation's mission and the types of organizations sponsored in the past can help ensure an appropriate match between a sponsorship and a program.

Establishing Fees-for-Service

Fees-for-service are another method to support a program during implementation and should be properly planned and included in the budget (Braveman, 2001; Grossman and Bortone, 1986). In a fee-structured program, participants are required to pay a fee for services rendered. Fees need to be realistic based on what community members can afford and what services are being offered. The program team will need to complete a careful analysis of costs and develop a fair and reliable fee structure (Braveman, 2016). Another consideration is how to address the differing abilities of program participants to pay for services. In this case, a sliding scale fee may be an appropriate method for addressing the socioeconomic needs across program participants. A sliding scale fee identifies a program payment based on a participant's income. When implementing a sliding scale fee, records of participants' incomes must be maintained, which requires additional recordkeeping and bookkeeping for the program, as well as processes to ensure confidentiality. The community-based health equipment recycling program described in a previous chapter utilized a sliding scale fee for the used equipment. The fees were needed to employ staff and rent the showroom.

Another option is to define a flat fee for program participants that covers program costs. To explore appropriate fees for a program, research should be conducted on what similar programs charge for similar services rendered. This information can be ascertained by contacting similar programs or exploring fees on program websites. If the program offers a service similar to that offered by a local occupational therapy practice, the occupational therapy practitioner may consider charging the same or similar fees. But if the service differs from the local practice, then fees should be competitive with similar programming. Another approach is to consult with an accountant who can provide guidance on appropriate fees to charge.

Fees-for-service should be clearly outlined for program participants. In program planning, the timing and payment requirements should be established. If adjustments in fees-for-service are needed, this must be clearly communicated to program participants with adequate time for participants to determine whether they want to continue to receive program services. A rationale for fee increases is often important to ensure that program participants understand the need for the change. It is important to consider whether fees support the program appropriately. If the fees cannot support at least a balanced budget for the program, supplementing with donations or grants will be necessary.

Reimbursement

In some cases, occupational therapy services may qualify for a reimbursement of services from health insurance companies. Reimbursement rates are set through negotiation with insurance companies. Any organization desiring to bill for reimbursable services should engage a billing and coding expert and a bookkeeper. Taking the time to become aware of all the regulations related to billing for reimbursement is necessary to ensure success. Depending on the services being offered, awareness of federal, state, and private regulations is required. As with all areas of funding a program or business, accessing resources to support and sustain the business must be a top priority.

Summary

- Occupational therapy practitioners are typically creative, adaptive relationship builders. These characteristics provide a solid foundation for developing and successfully implementing one's own program or business.
- In addition to developing creative and meaningful community programs, occupational therapy practitioners need to consider how innovations are supported and their potential to expand.
- Occupational therapy practitioners who aspire to become business owners should develop business acumen, understand basic business principles, and be aware of financial options to support such a business or program.
- Depending on the business model, the occupational therapy practitioner needs to be aware of the multiple approaches to financially supporting a business or program.
- Occupational therapy practitioners must become familiar with the phases of developing and planning a business to ensure the business can achieve its intended outcomes.
- Community programs can be supported through multiple venues by matching the best approach with the community and program.

CASE STUDIES

CASE STUDY PART 4 Suicide Prevention in a Native American Community

The program discussed in this case was grant funded. The grant was received by the Native American community with the occupational therapist actively writing the stress reduction program component of the grant proposal. An excerpt from the grant proposal that the occupational therapist wrote is included here: "The basis of the program will be to develop stress reduction rooms, a curriculum to teach occupation-based stress reduction techniques to Native American youth and teach stress reduction techniques to youth from 10–24 to engage in activities that decrease stress and increase connection and awareness to others and the self. These activities will be based on evidence-based approaches and will utilize a culturally and community-driven approach through the partnership with the community."

The grant funding paid for the time for the occupational therapist to design the program, implement the program, collect program data, and analyze the data. Since the community was located in a rural area some distance from the occupational therapist's home, funding also paid for gas mileage. In addition, grant funding covered stress management equipment costs.

CASE STUDY PART 4 Suicide Prevention in a Native American Community

Discussion Questions and Application

Review the Case Study from Chapters 5 through 7 and answer/discuss the following questions:

- How can you apply concepts of diffusion of innovation theory to replicate the program example?
- The program in this case was grant funded. What other funding models might support such a program?

Learning Activities

1. Identify an entrepreneur in your business or health-care community. Arrange an interview to discover how and why this individual chose to become an entrepreneur, what personal qualities this person brings to the entrepreneurial role, and the challenges and rewards to being an entrepreneur.
2. Visit the Small Business Administration (SBA) website and explore its many resources.
3. With a group of your classmates, identify an unmet need for occupational therapy services in your community. Visit either the Grants.gov or the Foundation Center website to see if you can identify a government agency or foundation with funding criteria that match the proposed new services.

REFERENCES

American Occupational Therapy Association. (2018). *Driving rehabilitation program development toolkit.* Retrieved from www.aota.org/Practice/Productive-Aging/Driving/Practitioners/Develop.aspx

Andreasen, A. R. (2006). *Social marketing in the 21st century.* Thousand Oaks, CA: Sage.

Austin, M. J., and Rust, D. Z. (2015). Developing an experiential learning program: Milestones and challenges. *International Journal of Teaching and Learning in Higher Education, 27*(1), 143–153.

Balas, E. A., and Chapman, W. W. (2018). Road map for diffusion of innovation in health care. *Health Affairs, 37*(2), 198–204.

Braveman, B. (2001). Development of a community-based return to work program for people with AIDS. *Occupational Therapy in Health Care, 13*(3–4), 113–130.

Braveman, B. (2016). *Leading and managing occupational therapy services: An evidence-based approach.* Philadelphia, PA: F. A. Davis.

Corner-Doyle, P., and Ho, M. (2010, July). How opportunities develop in social entrepreneurship. *Entrepreneurship: Theory and Practice,* 635–659.

Cumming, R. G., Thomas, M., Szonyi, G., Frampton, G., Salkeld, G., and Clemson, L. (2001). Adherence to occupational therapist recommendations for home modifications for falls prevention. *American Journal of Occupational Therapy, 55*(6), 641–648.

Dearing, J. W., and Cox, J. G. (2018). Diffusion of innovations theory, principles, and practice. *Health Affairs, 37*(2), 183–190.

Doll, J. D. (2010). *Program development and grant writing in occupational therapy: Making the connection.* Boston, MA: Jones and Bartlett.

Fazio, L. S. (2001). *Developing occupation-centered programs for the community: A workbook for students and professionals.* Upper Saddle River, NJ: Prentice-Hall.

Fritschner, A. (2006). *An easy, smart guide to starting a nonprofit.* New York, NY: Barnes and Noble.

GALE Small Business Builder. (2018). *Small businesses and start-ups.* Retrieved from https://omahalibrary.org/small-business/

Gitlin, L. N., and Lyons, K. J. (2013). *Successful grant writing: Strategies for health and human service professionals.* New York, NY: Springer.

Glennon, T. J. (2007). Putting on your business hat. *OT Practice, 12*(3), 23–25.

Grossman, J., and Bortone, J. (1986). Program development. In S. C. Robertson (Ed.), *Strategies, concepts, and opportunities for program development and evaluation* (pp. 91–99). Bethesda, MD: American Occupational Therapy Association.

Holmes, W. M., and Scaffa, M. E. (2009a). An exploratory study of competencies for emerging practice in occupational therapy. *Journal of Allied Health, 38*(2), 81–90.

Holmes, W. M., and Scaffa, M. E. (2009b). The nature of emerging practice in occupational therapy: A pilot study. *Occupational Therapy in Health Care, 23*(3), 189–206.

Jacobs, K. (1998). Innovation to action: Marketing occupational therapy. *American Journal of Occupational Therapy, 52*(8), 618–620.

Jacobs, K. (2002, June 24). Navigating the road ahead. *OT Practice, 7,* 24–30.

Jaffe, E. G., and Epstein, C. F. (1992). *Occupational therapy consultation: Theory, principles and practice.* St. Louis, MO: Mosby.

National Institutes of Health. (n.d.). *Biosketch format pages, instructions and samples.* Retrieved from https://grants.nih.gov/grants/forms/biosketch.htm

Pattison, M. (2006). OT—Outstanding talent: An entrepreneurial approach to practice. *Australian Occupational Therapy Journal, 53*(3), 166–172.

Richmond, T., and Powers, D. (2004). *Business fundamentals for the rehabilitation professional.* Thorofare, NJ: SLACK.

Rogers, E. M. (2003). *Diffusion of innovations* (5th ed.). New York, NY: Free Press.

Scaffa, M. (2001). *Occupational therapy in community-based practice settings.* Philadelphia, PA: F. A. Davis.

Smith, Bucklin, and Associates. (2000). *The complete guide to nonprofit management* (2nd ed.). New York, NY: Wiley.

Suter, E., Goldman, J., Martimianakis, T., Chatalalsingh, C., DeMatteo, D. J., and Reeves, S. (2013). The use of systems and organizational theories in the interprofessional field: Findings from a scoping review. *Journal of Interprofessional Care, 27*(1), 57–64. doi:10.3109/13561820.2012.739670

Timmreck, T. C. (2003). *Planning, program development, and evaluation: A handbook for health promotion, aging, and health services.* Boston, MA: Jones and Bartlett.

USA TODAY. (2013). *Nelson Mandela's best quotes.* Retrieved from www.usatoday.com/story/news/nation-now/2013/12/05/nelson-mandela-quotes/3775255/

Verma, S., Paterson, M., and Medves, J. (2006). Core competencies for health care professionals: What medicine, nursing, occupational therapy, and physiotherapy share. *Journal of Allied Health, 35*(2), 109–115.

Weis, R. M., and Gantt, V. W. (2004). *Knowledge and skill development in nonprofit organizations.* Eddie Peosta, IA: Bowers.

Zaltman, G., and Duncan, R. (1977). *Strategies for planned change.* New York, NY: Wiley.

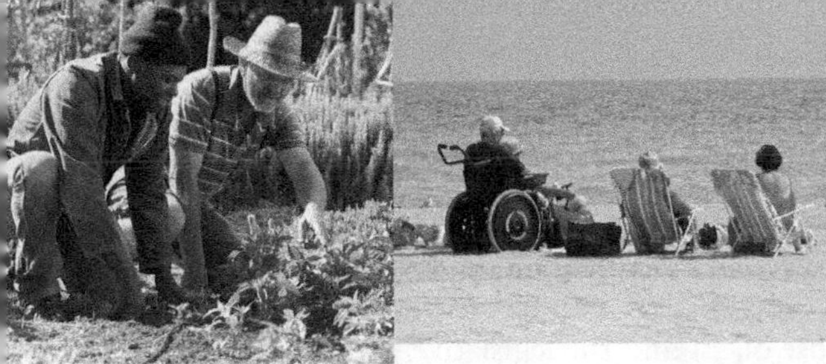
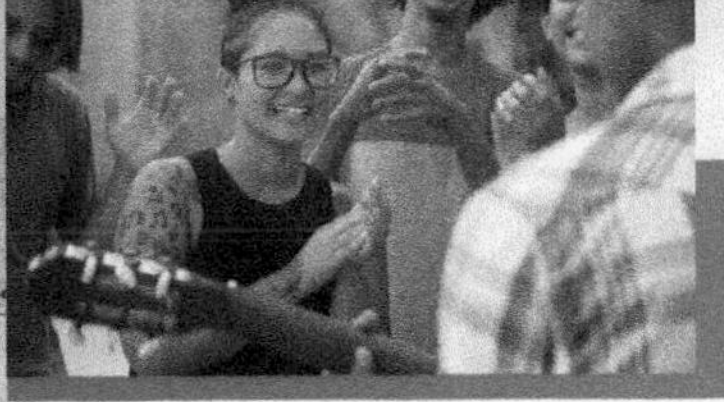

SECTION III

Children and Youth

Chapter 9

Early Intervention Programs

Donna A. Wooster, PhD, OTR/L, BCP and Abigail Baxter, PhD

Children learn as they play. Most importantly, in play children learn how to learn.

—O. Fred Donaldson, National Museum of Play

Learning Outcomes

This chapter is designed to enable the reader to:

9-1 Identify the components of early intervention (EI) programs.

9-2 Discuss the role of the occupational therapy practitioner in EI programs.

9-3 Identify and describe appropriate areas for evaluation and assessment instruments for EI occupational therapy services.

9-4 Discuss the importance of family involvement in EI.

9-5 Identify best practices in occupational therapy EI services.

Key Terms

Amplification
Early intervention
Ecological evaluation
Eligibility
Family-centered
Food neophobia
Individualized family service plan
Joint attention
Natural environments
Service coordinator
Solution-focused questions

Introduction

Early intervention (EI) is a federally supported program implemented by states and territories for infants and toddlers from birth to age 3 years who are experiencing developmental delays or who have diagnosed physical or mental conditions with high probabilities of resultant developmental delays. Birth to age 3 is an especially critical period in a child's development. States and territories that receive federal dollars for EI are mandated to implement a "statewide, comprehensive, coordinated, multidisciplinary, interagency system of EI services for infants and toddlers with disabilities and their families" (Individuals With Disabilities Education Improvement Act [IDEIA], 2004, p. 5). Even though EI is not a federally mandated program, all states and territories have developed an EI system of services based on federal guidelines designed to address its specific needs and resources. Occupational therapy practitioners should seek information specific to the state(s) or territory in which they practice.

The primary purpose of EI services is to identify infants and toddlers who may be eligible for services and to provide the necessary services to promote the family's ability to meet the infant's or toddler's special needs. The aim is to improve the physical, cognitive, communication, adaptive, sensory, and emotional capabilities of these infants and toddlers. The required components of the EI system are detailed in Part C of the IDEIA. Improvements in the legislation have occurred over time. Services for infants and toddlers were first included in the 1986 amendment to the legislation. Subsequent reauthorizations mandated more inclusive environments for infants and toddlers with disabilities. Services are required to be provided in **natural environments** (i.e., places children would normally find themselves, depending on age and activity). These include homes, day-care providers' homes, day-care centers, preschools, and playgrounds. Parents have input guiding the team in the choice of location(s) of service delivery. Service provision is also provided in these inclusive environments. Most recently, the IDEIA 2004 requires that EI services be evidence-based. In addition, the IDEIA emphasizes measurable results. Positive social emotional skills, the acquisition and use of knowledge and skills (including early language and communication), and the use of appropriate behavior to meet needs are mandated indicators for all EI programs.

This chapter discusses the need for, and the purpose of, EI and the legislatively mandated components of EI programs. The chapter also describes the role of the occupational therapy practitioner in EI services, including evaluation, intervention, and family involvement. In addition, two case studies illustrate major points of the chapter.

Engage Your Brain 9-1

If you need to refer a family to early intervention, how would you make the referral? Visit your state's early intervention website and learn about their referral process.

Early Intervention Programs

The number and percentage of children from birth to age 3 being served in EI have increased over the past 20 years (Lazara, Danaher, and Goode, 2017). The quality of neonatal intensive care for premature newborns has improved along with survival rates; however, these premature babies are at high risk for central nervous system disorders. Premature babies are surviving at younger ages and smaller sizes. Estimates suggest that these trends will continue. In the past, parents were urged to place children with disabilities in institutions. Changes in society have contributed to the expectation that families will care for their child at home regardless of the child's disability. Some families need intense intervention and support to competently handle this level of care. Research suggests that professionals can help families by providing information, emotional support, and continuous services (Anderson and Telleen, 1992; Hebbeler et al., 2007).

Medically fragile children now have longer life expectancies than they did in the past (Fitzsimmons, 1993; Strauss, Shavelle, Reynolds, Rosenblum, and Day, 2007). Although the total size of the population of children with disabilities and chronic illness will probably remain stable, the longer life span will result in families with needs that will change over time as the child grows (Wallace, Biehl, MacQueen, and Blackman, 1997).

Societal trends, such as recessions and international crises and conflicts, can also have an impact on the number of families in need. For example, the job relocation and deployment of servicemen and servicewomen are both factors that may result in having fewer family members living close by who could be resources. Research continues to show that low socioeconomic status (SES) is associated with an increased risk of poor health, increased risk of death, and increased risk for hospitalization (Birken and MacArthur, 2004). Poverty is associated with increased risk for disability and increased hospitalizations for problems related to chronic health conditions (Fujiura and Yamaki, 2000), thus placing children with disabilities at greater accumulated risk.

Components of Early Intervention

EI programs have the following three components: identification, eligibility determination, and evaluation.

Identification

Each state must establish a system to identify children who may be eligible for services and refer them to the EI system. Children with suspected developmental delays or disability are identified through a variety of sources, including parents, occupational therapists, physicians, other health providers, and community agencies. Professionals must seek verbal approval from the parents to make a referral to the EI system for an evaluation. A central phone number (usually a toll-free number) is typically available for referrals. Occupational therapy practitioners often participate with other team members in community screenings to identify infants and toddlers who may be behind in their development and who can then receive further evaluation and interventions if needed from EI.

Eligibility Determination

One component of each statewide system is the establishment of a lead agency. This appointed agency varies from state to state and may be part of the state health department, education department, or another department. The lead agency schedules the evaluation with the parents to determine eligibility. **Eligibility** refers to whether or not the child qualifies, under the state's criteria, to receive EI services. States must serve children "who are experiencing developmental delays" in accordance with the state's definition of developmental delay and children with "a diagnosed physical or mental condition that has a high probability of resulting in developmental delay" (IDEIA, 2004, p. 100). States are also given the option to serve infants and toddlers at risk for developmental delay. Once written parental consent is obtained, the evaluation process is initiated. A variety of trained professionals can perform the evaluation. The evaluation scores and other information are used to determine eligibility for services. A specific level of developmental delay (such as 25%) in one or more developmental domains, or two standard deviations below the mean in any two domains, may serve to qualify the infant or toddler for services. Likewise, a diagnosis of a mental or physical condition associated with developmental delays may be used to establish eligibility. In some states, professional opinions of high risk may qualify the child.

Engage Your Brain 9-2

What is the specific eligibility criteria adopted by your state? (Hint: visit the Early Childhood Technical Assistance Center website at http://ectacenter.org, and in the search box type in the state eligibility criteria to locate the eligibility criteria for your state; Early Childhood Technical Assistance Center, 2015).

Evaluation

The IDEIA 2004 includes specific information about the evaluation process. Multidisciplinary evaluations must be done within 45 days of referral and given in the native language or type of communication that suits the family. Best practice research indicates that the evaluation of a child in multiple environments or contexts increases the reliability of the evaluation (Miller, 1994). If possible, occupational therapy practitioners should conduct observations of the child at home and in the community, including day care or nursery school and other natural environments. Factors that may be evaluated include response to different environments, effects of peer role models on performance, solitary versus group function, and social-emotional and communication skills with children as well as adults other than the parents. Gathering information across contexts and environments will help the occupational therapy practitioner to match the child's abilities with the requirements of the occupation and the features of the environment to enhance performance.

A variety of factors, such as the child's age, gender, ethnic background, native language, culture, and information needs of the family and team, influences the selection of assessment tool. However, assessment must cover these five developmental domains:

- Physical (vision, hearing, gross motor, fine motor, sensory processing)
- Cognitive (thinking, learning, problem-solving)
- Social-emotional (play, feeling safe, making friends, being around and interacting with others)
- Communication (expressing self and understating what people are saying)
- Adaptive development (also known as self-help and includes feeding, grooming, toileting, bathing, dressing, and sleeping)

Assessment instruments must not be culturally biased. Many states indicate a specific instrument as the assessment tool of choice and allow other informed clinical opinions to be expressed in writing to support the findings. Parents should be included in the evaluation process to provide information about the abilities of their child. Structured interviews and other informal assessments are used to understand family strengths, needs, and resources.

EI programs primarily apply an educational model, with individuals (i.e., early childhood special educators or others) providing special instruction services as the primary evaluators and providers. EI teams must have many other professionals, including occupational therapists, physical therapists, speech-language pathologists, audiologists, nurses, service coordinators, and others, available. One team member, usually a special instructor, may perform the primary assessment. This person administers assessment tools and then, based on test findings across the five areas, calls in other services, such as speech or occupational therapy. Depending upon state EI personnel standards, special instructors can have varying educational backgrounds. The special instructor is the person on the team who is responsible for:

- Designing learning environments and activities that promote the child's acquisition of skills in a variety of developmental areas, including cognitive processes and social interaction
- Planning curriculum, including the planned interaction of personnel, materials, time, and space, that leads to achieving the outcomes in the child's individualized family service plan (IFSP)
- Providing families with information, skills, and support related to enhancing the skill development of the child
- Working with the child to enhance the child's development (Division for Early Childhood [DEC], 2014, p. 2)

Another evaluation format is the arena-style evaluation. Multiple service providers gather to simultaneously observe the evaluation being conducted by one or two primary evaluators. Each team member records information and discusses the child's abilities. The team members discuss the observations and write a joint evaluation report. A child may be determined eligible for EI services based on

Engage Your Brain 9-3

Compare and contrast the different methods of family assessment found at the Early Childhood Technical Assistance Center website. Once at the website, http://ectacenter.org, go to resources, go to topics, then go to Assessment—DEC RP products, and then scroll down to Assessment Guides for Families at http://ectacenter.org/decrp/topic-assessment.asp (Early Childhood Technical Assistance Center, 2019). What are the strengths and weaknesses of each approach? Select guiding questions that you would use to conduct an assessment of a family's strengths and needs.

the test scores. A report is written following the evaluation, and if the child is eligible for services, an individualized plan is developed based on the assessment information. The results and observations of the evaluation are used to make referrals to appropriate service providers. For example, if the child scored low on adaptive and fine motor skills, then a referral is usually made for occupational therapy services.

Screening

The American Academy of Pediatrics (2018) recommends that all children be screened for developmental delays and disabilities during regular well-child doctor visits at the ages of 9, 18, and 24 or 30 months. Occupational therapy practitioners working in EI are often asked to participate in community events to screen children for possible referrals to EI or to seek further evaluations. Screenings often involve a team approach. A commonly utilized developmental screening tool is Ages and Stages Questionnaires, third edition (ASQ-3, available at Ages and Stages, 2018) because it is highly reliable, valid, and family friendly. It can also be completed in 10 to 15 minutes, relies on parents as experts, and creates the snapshot needed to catch delays and celebrate milestones.

The scores are used to guide the advice given to parents to seek additional evaluations or services either in EI or the school system for those 3 to 5 years of age. Screenings are often completed at events targeted at families, and the families move quickly from station to station, gathering information from various health professionals and community resources. The screening highlights the child's strengths as well as any concerns. The ASQ-3 is available in multiple languages, including Arabic, English, French, Spanish, and Vietnamese (ASQ-3, 2018).

Early Intervention

EI is a system of services for babies and toddlers with developmental delays and disabilities. It is a unique practice setting, with specific eligibility criteria, required documentation, and laws and rules that govern occupational therapy practice. Knowledge of these important aspects helps define the roles and responsibilities of the service providers.

Individualized Family Service Plan

Once eligibility has been established, the team must develop a written plan, or **IFSP**. This process is summarized in Box 9-1 and includes the development of both child and family goals. Only one IFSP is developed despite the involvement of a number of agencies. Family members are key participants in the development of the IFSP. All services needed by the child are documented in the plan, including an indication of the specific community agency that will provide the service. The service providers, the frequency of intervention, the family goals, and the resources that will be involved are specified on the IFSP. Expected measurable outcomes are clearly stated. This process identifies the child's needs, family resources, priorities, concerns, and supports. At the conclusion of the process, which also includes the appointment of a service coordinator and a family meeting, the nature and extent of services will be delineated. The IFSP is reviewed every 6 months (or more frequently if needed) and must be evaluated and revised, if needed, once a year. Outcomes can be modified or changed at any time the parent requests. The IFSP is the primary document in EI; it details how to best serve each family.

Parents or guardians have many rights associated with the IFSP process. The parents may review records at any time and can consent to share medical information with the IFSP team. A parent who is dissatisfied with the service provision or finds that the documented IFSP services are not being provided

Box 9-1 Individualized Family Service Plan Process

The individualized family service plan (IFSP) process gathers information on the following:

- Child's current status
- Family resources, priorities, and concerns
- Major measurable outcomes expected
- Specific services—frequency, duration, provider, and dates to initiate
- Description of natural environment in which services will be provided
- Need for other services—for example, medical
- Name of service coordinator
- Steps to support transition at age 3

has the right to due process. This is a legal proceeding that involves a hearing conducted by an impartial mediator to resolve disputes. This clearly illustrates the rights of the family in planning for the needs of their child who is receiving EI services.

Team Members

Members of an EI team working with a child usually consist of the parents, service coordinator, therapists, and other individuals, including a variety of contracted service providers. There are 14 EI services, as shown in Box 9-2. The occupational therapy practitioner can be one member of this team. The team's primary goal is to provide the needed services to the family as documented in the IFSP. Each team is formed based on the needs of the family. Teams that have a clear, focused statement of purpose, goals, and philosophies function more effectively (Briggs, 1993).

Occupational therapy may be a primary service provider for the infant/toddler, according to the IFSP (Stoffel and Schleis, 2014). Occupational therapy may be the only service provider or may be part of a team of providers. Each plan is customized to the needs of the child and the family. Any child with an identified need for occupational therapy must receive the service. Occupational therapy is one of the "big five" EI services, and more than a third of infants and toddlers receiving EI services receive occupational therapy services (Hebbeler et al., 2007).

Box 9-2 Early Intervention Services

- Assistive technology devices and services
- Early identification, screening, and assessment services
- Family training, counseling, and home visits
- Health services needed to benefit from other early intervention services
- Medical diagnostic or evaluation services
- Occupational therapy
- Physical therapy
- Psychological services
- Service coordination
- Social work
- Special instruction
- Speech/language pathology and audiology
- Transportation-related costs
- Vision services

The **service coordinator** functions as a consultant to the parents and service providers. The service coordinator may be involved in training parents and other family members and professionals, coordinating appointments with professionals, participating in the team IFSP process, and establishing links with service providers. In addition, the service coordinator assists the family in planning for the transition to public school or other settings when the child is 3 years of age. The service coordinator is responsible for implementing the IFSP. An occupational therapy practitioner could also serve in the role of the service coordinator, which would decrease the number of professionals involved.

Transition Planning

Transition planning must be part of any IFSP. In transition planning, families and service providers discuss the possible options for the child after he or she can no longer be served by an EI team at 3 years of age. Possible options include the local school system, a private preschool, a childcare center, a Head Start program, or other community services for young children. The discussion of options should occur early, and referrals to other programs should be made at least 6 months before the child's third birthday. Approximately 60% of children served in EI transition into preschool special education services. If the family wants the child to be considered for such placement, the local education agency will collaborate with the EI provider and families about the nature of the program the student needs. The IFSP team works closely with the family to notify the future placement staff of any special equipment that will be required in the preschool environment. If possible, when given parental permission, the EI occupational therapy practitioner should contact the school occupational therapy practitioner personally to facilitate the transition. This may be helpful to provide pertinent information about techniques and procedures that have worked well, such as positive reinforcers, the amount and course of progress, and the intervention approach. If a mealtime protocol has been developed, providing it to the preschool program staff will improve continuity.

Transitioning into the preschool-based setting is stressful to families. The model changes from a family-friendly model to a special education school-based model. EI teams should assist parents in developing the assertiveness and advocacy skills to request necessary services for their child. If the family is relocating, the occupational therapy practitioner might offer to make a videotape of the current feeding/toileting/dressing programs and routines. This facilitates the carryover of desired techniques. If possible, adaptive equipment should be sent with the child and family. If that is not possible, team members can make a list of specific equipment and purchasing information for the parents and the new team.

Occupational Therapy Services in Early Intervention

Occupational therapy practitioners assume many roles in the EI system. They can be part of the evaluation team, conduct screenings in the community, provide direct services, provide consultation to other team members in a transdisciplinary model, or fulfill any combination of these roles (American Occupational Therapy Association [AOTA], 2015c). The occupational therapist working in EI needs to have good background knowledge of assessment tools for very young children and common therapeutic interventions. Occupational therapy practitioners support and promote the development and engagement of infants, toddlers, and their families or other caregivers in everyday routines that include play, rest and sleep, activities of daily living, education, and social participation. Some best practice guidelines for occupational therapy in EI are listed in Box 9-3.

Box 9-3 Best Practice Guidelines for Occupational Therapy in Early Intervention

- Regard parents as partners in decision-making.
- Use a clear, open, and collaborative communication style with all team members.
- Share responsibilities for service implementation with team members.
- Use knowledge to improve performance and functional outcomes.
- Deliver cost-effective quality intervention.
- View child's abilities in the context of natural environments.
- Incorporate carryover into natural daily routines.
- Use amplification and solution-focused questions.

Occupational Therapy Evaluation

Occupational therapy evaluations are based on analysis of the infant/toddler's performance of occupations and the context for these occupations. Occupational therapy practitioners determine how performance in occupations is influenced by impairment and how the environment hinders or supports performance. Evaluations must be nondiscriminatory; must be performed by qualified and trained personnel; and must include informed professional opinion and a review of the child's pertinent medical records and overall developmental level. Depending on whether or not any other evaluations have been conducted by the EI team members, occupational therapy practitioners must determine the scope of the occupational therapy evaluation process depending on the child's needs, diagnosis, health and medical concerns, and family priorities. Selected assessment instruments should demonstrate high validity and reliability; include comprehensive health, social, behavioral, and environmental components; and involve the family as equal partners with the professionals (DEC, 2007).

Children, especially those between about 6 and 10 months of age, may experience stranger anxiety and therefore need more warm-up or adjustment time with the occupational therapy practitioners before actual testing begins. Allowing the parents to initially remain with the child is important. Also, during this time the child should be approached slowly, with time allowed for gradual interaction and play. Performance will be negatively affected when a child is crying or afraid.

Parent Interview

A parent interview is an essential element of the evaluation process of a young child. The purpose of the interview is to obtain needed information, including:

- Parents' perspectives of their needs for caring for this child
- The child's condition and interventions to date
- An understanding of family daily routines and structure
- Identification of resources available to the family
- The family's story of hopes and wants for the child

Open-ended questions or requests are often better to facilitate retrieval of this information than close-ended questions. Requests such as "Tell me what a typical day is like for you and your child" or "Describe the feeding process for your child" will elicit a much more detailed response. The use of narratives and life stories provides a view that encompasses the child within the family and community context. This interview provides a framework for understanding the child as an occupational being in the context of the family and the physical, social, economic, and cultural worlds.

During the interview with the parent, the message that families are competent and in control of their child's life must be conveyed. One way to do this is to ask solution-focused questions (Andrews and Andrews, 1993). **Solution-focused questions** are worded such that they assume the family is already working toward improving the situation, giving the family credit for their efforts—for example, "I have noticed how carefully you position your child's head and arms when you place him in the infant seat. This is great. Do you do this in any other tasks as well?" Another example is "Turning off the TV during feeding really seemed to help your daughter concentrate on feeding. Have you noticed other things you do that help her pay attention?" Important information, as well as trust building, can be gained from this approach.

Observation

Observation is a key element of the evaluation process that guides interpretation and planning and begins the minute the family is met. The occupational therapy practitioner examines the community and home environments, the parent-child and child-child interactions, and the family caregiving routines and play experiences. Observations are usually made in a variety of areas, including the following:

- Quality of the movement of the infant
- Interactions and communication between the infant/child and others
- Safety, accessibility, and opportunities provided in the home environment
- Daily routines and the amount and types of structure provided
- Caregivers' responsiveness and stress
- Opportunities provided and resources available

The concept of amplification may be a useful strategy for occupational therapy practitioners. **Amplification** is a process of "noticing, describing, and discussing an interactive event between family member and child that is likely to promote child change" (Andrews and Andrews, 1993, p. 42). This means that the occupational therapy practitioner discusses observations with the family regarding any communication attempts the child makes and the responses of the parents that reinforce the child's behavior. This encourages the parents to notice and respond to nonverbal communication attempts. For example, during lunch the occupational therapy practitioner might comment, "I just saw your child look to you and move his head toward the spoon. Try placing the spoon just in front of his mouth again this time and see if he moves that way again." This encourages the parent to attend to nonverbal communication and reinforces the child's efforts. This may be the first recognition of interaction, which can facilitate bonding between the child and parent.

Noting the family's normal daily routine is also important. Families will be better able to implement positioning and exercises if they are taught how to fit them into their established daily routine (Pretti-Frontczak and Bricker, 2001). Examples include suggesting to the parent(s) to:

- Perform range-of-motion exercises during diaper changes
- Plan rough-and-tumble play with one parent or family member while another is cooking dinner
- Incorporate an undressing routine just before bath time
- Implement sensory-calming techniques after dinnertime to promote calming down for sleep

Ecological Evaluation

Ecological evaluation determines the skills needed to be successful in various environments. The home environment will have its own opportunities and obstacles for the child. A child may have the freedom to move about and play in childproofed safe areas, requiring little supervision, while provided with developmentally appropriate toys. In another home environment, the child may be restricted to a very small play area, such as a playpen, for her or his own safety. The opportunities for outdoor play may vary significantly, as may the types of equipment and toys and the presence of other children. The routines at home are often different than those allowed in a childcare center. For example, a childcare setting may require that the child be able to move from his chair to sit in a circle on carpet squares, remove outer clothing and place it on a hanger, request to go to the bathroom, play safely on the playground with other children moving about, and obtain lunch or snacks from a lunch box. These are very different routines than in the home environment. Each environment will require different skills, and therefore task analysis is helpful for determining a child's abilities and needed modifications or adaptations.

Play

Play is assessed by occupational therapy practitioners because it is the primary occupation of children (Fig. 9-1). A variety of assessments are available to assist occupational therapy practitioners in gaining specific information about baseline play performance and skills. Most children are motivated to play and have play preferences. Often, a play history is conducted to find out the child's typical play and preferences (Takata, 1974). This is an interview designed to determine both the quality and quantity of the child's play experiences, interactions, environments, and opportunities across time. There is great diversity in play environments, play opportunities, toys, peers, and the promotion of play skills. Not all children have equal play opportunities. Culture influences adults' views about what is appropriate play for children, what should be provided, and what is the degree of modification of play they will tolerate. Intervention techniques are easily embedded into play routines to improve the skills, participation level, and satisfaction of the child's play experiences.

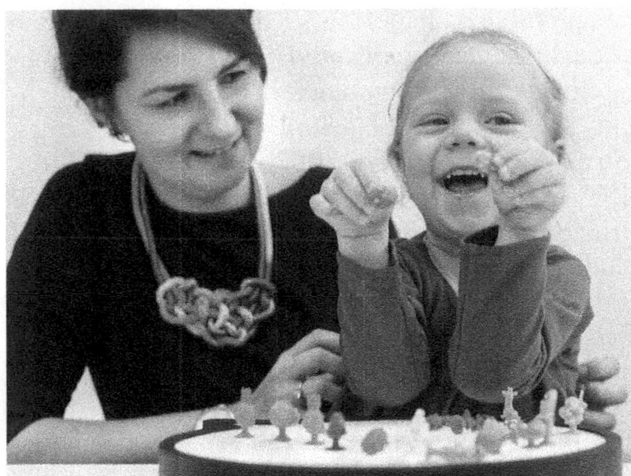

Figure 9-1 Play is an important aspect of occupational therapy EI. *(AndreaObzerova/iStock/Getty Images Plus/Getty Images.)*

Play Assessments

The Transdisciplinary Play Based Assessment, second edition (TPBA2), is an observation-based, transdisciplinary assessment tool (Linder, 2008). The team evaluates the child in normal play in a natural environment. Data are collected on normal developmental sequences of skill acquisition in the areas of cognitive, social-emotional, communication, and sensorimotor skills. Procedures for conducting a transdisciplinary arena-type assessment are included.

The Revised Knox Preschool Play Scale is for children from birth to 6 years of age (Knox, 1997). Four areas of play are examined:

- Space management
- Material management
- Pretense/symbolic
- Participation

The assessment requires play observation both indoors and outdoors in natural environments with peers over a minimum of two 30-minute observations. More detailed descriptions of the evaluation process and the interpretation of play assessments can be found in the work of Parham and Fazio (2008).

The Test of Playfulness (ToP) has been designed specifically to evaluate components of play related to the suspension of reality, source of motivation, and perception of control. This tool can be used with children from 18 months to 18 years old (Skard and Bundy, 2008). Free play is observed and then the test is scored. The test is recommended to evaluate the play skills of children with autism spectrum disorders (ASDs) and those whose delay interferes with their spontaneity and playfulness (Skard and Bundy, 2008). In conjunction with the ToP, the Test of Environmental Supports (TOES) is often administered.

The TOES assesses the environmental support for a child's motivation for play (Bronson and Bundy, 2001). This assessment is helpful for reviewing the relationships between the child's motivation, caregiver supports, playmates, toys and objects, and spaces and the environment (Skard and Bundy, 2008). Scores are only interpreted on a per item basis, and discussion with caregivers can lead to ideas for needed environmental modifications and other adaptations to promote play in that particular environment.

Sensory Processing and Neuromotor Status

Sensory processing and neuromotor status are important components for the occupational therapy practitioner to evaluate. Understanding the body language of premature babies is especially important for practitioners and parents to interpret the behaviors appropriately and avoid under- and overstimulation. Hussey (1988) has developed a helpful manual to consult when working with premature infants. Ayres defined sensory integration as the neurological organization process enabling the effective use of one's body through stimulus from one's body and the environment (Bundy, Lane, and Murray, 2002). An examination of infant states, behaviors, and responses to environmental demands is important for the occupational therapy practitioner to consider. Examination of the infant's behavior includes both environmental and biological factors related to arousal, affect, attention, and action. The Infant-Toddler Symptom Checklist (Degangi, 1995) and the Infant Toddler Sensory Profile-2 (Dunn, 2002) are useful tools to examine the infant's responses to sensory stimulation, including the need for and avoidance of stimulation.

The Newborn Behavioral Observations (NBO) assessment is helpful to practitioners who work with newborn infants up to the age of 4 months (Nugent, Keefer, Minear, Johnson, and Blanchard, 2007). This is an individualized, infant-focused, family-centered assessment for use in examining communication and interactions between infants and parents. This assessment consists of 18 neurobehavioral observations that describe the infant's capacities and behavioral adaptations. It is designed to help parents identify the infant's unique capabilities and vulnerabilities. Occupational therapy practitioners can help parents learn to understand and interpret the infant's behaviors so parents can in turn respond in ways to meet their child's developmental needs.

Additionally, the Infant Neurological International Battery (INFANIB) is useful for infants from birth to 18 months and includes examination items in the categories of spasticity, head and trunk, vestibular functions, legs, and passive movement at a single joint (Ellison, 1994). It is based on observation and includes a rating scale. The scores reflect an infant's neuromotor status and may be useful to the occupational therapy practitioner by identifying specifics about the distribution of abnormal tone and poor-quality motor responses (Ellison, 1994).

Occupational Therapy Interventions

Occupational therapy interventions focus on establishing a variety of family-friendly, customized routines (e.g., morning, mealtime, bedtime, bath time) that address the needs of the infant/toddler and promote social engagement and development. The quality of the care that infants and toddlers experience is predictive of a range of developmental, social-emotional, and health outcomes. Responsive caregiving and parent engagement in healthy behaviors promote biological functions in the child, such as the immune system and the development of neural circuits, that affect multiple body systems throughout life (Bohlin, Hagekull, and Rydell, 2002; Gunnar and Quevedo, 2007; Guyer et al., 2009). Therefore, occupational therapy practitioners will utilize a variety of evidence-based interventions, including parent education to promote the infant/toddler's overall neurodevelopment (Vanderveen, Bassler, Robertson, and Kirpalani, 2009). Some families may also be facing risk factors such as extreme poverty, recurrent physical or emotional abuse, chronic neglect and maltreatment, severe maternal depression, parental substance abuse, and family violence.

Kellegrew (2000) determined that the self-care routines of children with disabilities were often related to the value mothers placed on the routines, the time afforded to conduct them, and the goals established. She also determined that on a daily basis, mothers make small adjustments in their home routines that shape the opportunities for skill development offered to their children. Practices regarding adaptive skills and social-emotional skills are very much dependent on the culture of the family. Views regarding child-rearing vary greatly, including types of foods and the social climate of meals, the involvement of other children in family decisions, hygiene, clothing habits and choices, behavioral expectations, and disciplinary actions and methods. A child's ability to participate in religious ceremonies, cultural activities, and school activities may be especially important for families. In the following section, several activities of daily living (ADL) as well as activities related to sleep and rest will be shared, in addition to potential underlying performance skill deficits and performance patterns (AOTA, 2014).

Activities of Daily Living—Feeding and Swallowing/Eating

Feeding and swallowing are especially important ADL areas to evaluate in infants and toddlers because good nutrition is essential for adequate growth and development. This is one of the key areas in which occupational therapy practitioners must be well versed for EI practice. It is estimated that about 50% of infants and toddlers have feeding problems (Rommel, De Meyer, Feenstra, and Veereman-Wauters, 2003). Infants who have motor delays, immature central nervous systems, or gastrointestinal abnormalities may experience significant difficulties with feeding. Feeding disorders have also been linked to deficits in cognitive development (Reif, Beler, Villa, and Spirer, 1995), behavioral problems, and eating disorders.

Most feeding issues and accompanying interventions fall into one or several of these categories, depending on evaluation-identified needs: (a) mechanical interventions related to establishing normal developmental sequence skills; (b) strategies to improve acceptance of a wide variety of food textures and food categories to promote health; (c) interventions to improve oral-motor skills such as sucking, chewing, propelling, and swallowing; (d) strategies to transition from nonoral to oral independent feeding; (e) behavioral interventions based on operant learning principles (e.g., positive reinforcement, differential attention, physical guidance, extinction, flooding, shaping); and (f) parent-directed educational interventions to increase feeding competence, improve parent-child interactions, and improve overall health and child growth.

Feeding is an experience rich in sensory stimulation that also demands internal processing to coordinate breathing, digestion, postural control, and alignment. Feeding problems are often a result of multiple issues such as anatomical abnormalities, motor dysfunction, sensory dysfunction, medical complications, psychological conditions, growth abnormalities, difficulty with social interactions, or behavioral issues. Some infants who take more than 30 minutes to suck a bottle may actually be burning more calories than they ingest. Morris and Klein (2000) suggest that sensory or medical problems that interfere with feeding develop into more complex emotional and behavioral issues. The occupational therapy practitioner working in EI must have a detailed understanding of normal feeding development, experience with pediatric feeding issues, and knowledge of common interventions.

Most pediatric hospitals have feeding teams available to conduct feeding evaluations. These teams are multidisciplinary and take a holistic view, involve the parents, and typically have the medical resources available for a comprehensive evaluation (Wooster, Brady, Mitchell, Grizzel, and Barnes, 1998). These teams provide the safest environment to evaluate the medically complex and fragile child. Occupational therapy practitioners should develop a link with the nearest feeding team for referrals and consultations. A thorough evaluation must be conducted when an infant is at risk for aspiration. Infants at risk for aspiration often demonstrate apnea, bradycardia, and arching or stiffening of the body during meals. Toddlers may present with coughing, wheezing, congestion, wet burps or wet hiccups, frequent swallowing with negative facial expressions, vomiting, difficulty with sleeping, or hoarse voice. Coughing and gagging during meals that persists for several weeks, repeated bouts of pneumonia, and chronic chest congestion require immediate comprehensive feeding team evaluation (Rudolph and Link, 2002).

Feeding intervention involves establishing safe and appropriate feeding routines that meet a child's nutritional and hydration needs, are competently carried out by family members in a reasonable amount of time, and, whenever possible, are embedded within existing family mealtime customs. Most young infants are fed very frequently, and even preschoolers eat six times a day when both meals and snacks are considered. Interventions with infants often begin with nonnutritive sucking and oral-motor programs to normalize tone, build tolerance for touch in the facial and mouth areas, and promote oral motor skills. Knowledge about positioning options is especially important, as positioning changes as an infant grows and gains head control. Respiratory issues may lead the infant to push into abnormal patterns to protect or increase the size of the airway. The ideal position for the older infant involves a firm base of support with symmetrical and neutral hips, adequate trunk support, feet support, and neutral head and neck with a slight chin tuck. This is often difficult to achieve without additional supports. Howe and Wang (2013) reported that parent-directed and educational interventions for children with feeding problems were moderately to strongly effective at improving children's physical growth and development, increasing the feeding competence of children and their primary caretakers, and improving parent-child interaction.

Most toddlers become somewhat pickier in their eating patterns; however, some children with disabilities will exhibit significant food refusal or selectivity. **Food neophobia** is a fear of new foods. Many children between the ages of 2 and 3 years exhibit this behavior, but it diminishes by age 5 (Ernsperger and Stegen-Hanson, 2004). Howe and Wang (2013) reported that behavioral interventions were effective at leading to the acceptance of a variety of foods, improving mealtime behaviors, increasing weight gain, improving caloric intake, promoting self-feeding skills, and decreasing caregivers' stress. Children with food selectivity accept a very limited number of foods; may avoid entire food groups; may avoid specific textures, temperatures, or flavors; or may refuse to eat foods that are not presented in the same manner, such as the size, shape, or type of plate. Complete evaluation of the sensory system and sensory preferences is warranted to determine if hyper- or hyposensitivities are part of the problem.

Some children are unable to focus on feeding because of distractions in the environment. An observation guide can help identify potential distractions. Wooster (1999) developed a feeding observation guide to assist the occupational therapy practitioner when observing mealtimes with parents and infants. A parent mealtime questionnaire was developed by Morris and Klein (2000). In addition, Wooster (2000) described more specific feeding interventions for children with nonorganic failure to thrive.

Adaptive equipment may include a variety of bottles, nipples, and cups to promote safe nutritional intake and improve sucking skills. As the infant grows older, finger feeding and then feeding with utensils will be introduced. Additionally, more children are able to drink from straws at much earlier ages than previously recorded in the literature (Hunt, Lewis, Reisel, Woldrup, and Wooster, 2000). There are many more pieces of adaptive equipment to consider, which include spoons, cups, bowls, plates, and forks. Morris and Klein (2000) offer guidelines for choosing a variety of pieces of adaptive feeding equipment. Positioning is usually more upright, and a variety of commercial products such as high chairs and booster seats are commonly used and may offer opportunities for adaptation. Some styles of high chair offer a slight tilt, as well as more than one tray size and height adjustment. A more physically involved child may still need to be held or positioned well in a customized seat.

A prefeeding program may be designed to normalize any abnormal tone and promote cheek, lip, and tongue movement and sensory stimulation prior to eating. If adaptive equipment is required, it is set up and ready for the feeding process. Parents should be key members and engage in the decision-making to keep mealtimes manageable. The feeding program and specific techniques should be demonstrated and practiced; the parent should carry this out with the occupational therapy practitioner present and garner feedback for revisions of the process. The feeding program should be documented for the child's record, with copies for the parent and practitioner. Feeding programs should be closely monitored and updated regularly. Effective feeding strategies include:

- Minimizing the negative effects of medical influences
- Improving oral motor function
- Establishing appropriate positioning
- Modifying the environment as needed
- Promoting appetite and a desire to eat
- Promoting eating as a pleasurable and desirable experience
- Providing adaptive equipment as indicated
- Ensuring adequate nutritional and hydration needs are consistently met

Not all children will consume enough calories by mouth; therefore, supplemental feedings may need to continue. The acquisition of skills for oral eating and saliva control are often valued by parents and may allow children to participate in culturally significant events, such as tasting their own birthday cakes or participating in religious events.

Activities of Daily Living—Personal Hygiene and Grooming

Children with developmental disabilities are at high risk for developing dental disease. Many children have dental alterations or malocclusions that make chewing more difficult and increase the risk of decay. Dental decay is related to the presence of bacteria. Children who fall asleep after nursing or drinking a bottle are at great risk. A high, narrow palate may become a place where food particles lodge. The three most important factors for protecting already formed teeth from decay are maintaining good oral hygiene, limiting the ingestion of carbohydrates, and eliminating or reducing cavity-causing bacteria (Acs, Ng, Helpin, Rosenberg, and Canion, 2007).

Young infants can be introduced to a soft baby toothbrush that fits over the adult's finger. This is used for sensory stimulation of the gums and cleaning of the gums and emerging teeth. Next, a NUK brush set is introduced to get the infant used to longer, brush-like instruments being placed in the mouth. This includes a set of three instruments that start out larger and round and end with one resembling a toothbrush. Once this is tolerated well, the child can be transitioned to a regular soft child-sized toothbrush. Most children under the age of 6 do not have the dexterity to adequately brush their teeth. Children should be encouraged to participate by holding and moving the toothbrush; however, an adult needs to go over the entire mouth area to provide adequate cleaning. A child who is willing to use a battery-operated toothbrush may do a more thorough job. Children need to establish dental hygiene routines as part of their daily self-care skills.

Activities of Daily Living—Dressing

Parents will be dressing and undressing children several times daily for diaper changes and cleanliness. Children with specific medical conditions or those who require extensive procedures daily may do best with limited clothing or clothing that has been adapted to allow easy access for parents to get to a gastrostomy tube (G-tube), that is large or flexible enough to go around or over braces or casts, or that has enlarged neckholes to make it easier to get over the child's head. Some infants, especially in colder winter months, may respond negatively to being undressed. Discuss with the parents their comfort level with these procedures and the need for any clothing adaptations to speed up the process and minimize discomfort to the child.

There are multiple opportunities each day for practicing undressing and dressing in the natural context. Going outside in winter often requires putting on a sweater, jacket, or coat and removing these when returning inside. Going to the bathroom necessitates the partial removal of pants and underpants to the knees and then back up. Sometimes parents find it easiest to adapt the clothing by eliminating all fasteners and choosing elastic-waist, loose-fitting clothes that are quickly pulled down. Bath time requires the removal of clothing and putting on sleepwear afterward. A child who wants to go swimming may be motivated to help participate in changing into a swimsuit. Children are encouraged by parents to partially participate in the dressing process as much as time allows. Infants may lift an arm or leg and push it into a sleeve or pants by their first birthday. This process needs to be facilitated and practiced in children with disabilities.

A thorough evaluation and an understanding of the dressing routines will help the occupational therapy practitioner provide the appropriate interventions and expectations for parents. Many evaluations for children under age 3 include adaptive skills as components, such as the Hawaii Early

Learning Profile—Revised (Furuno, O'Reilly, Hosaka, Zeisloft, and Allman, 1997), the Early Learning Accomplishment Profile (Glover, Preminger, and Sanford, 1988), and the Carolina Curriculum for Infants and Toddlers (Johnson-Martin, Attermeier, and Hacker, 2004). The Pediatric Evaluation of Disability Inventory is useful for children 6 months up to age 7 and evaluates self-care, social, and mobility skills (Haley, Coster, Ludlow, Haltiwanger, and Andrellos, 1992). The Wee-Fim includes two versions that evaluate self-care, mobility, and cognition (Hamilton and Granger, 2000)

Activities of Daily Living—Toileting and Toilet Hygiene

Toilet, or "potty," training is a skill often introduced during the second year of life. It is a complex task and involves identification of sensory signals, communication, positioning (usually sitting up), and active control of muscles. Bowel control is usually achieved first. As the infant's bowel or bladder fills, the muscles relax and release automatically, and the infant urinates or defecates. However, as the toddler gains control over these functions, the cerebral cortex sends signals to inhibit the reflexes, and the child takes over control. This skill is often identified as a hallmark of development.

Multiple books about a variety of potty-training programs for parents to consider exist; however, none are targeted specifically for the child with a disability. This process takes fine-tuning and sometimes months to master in a normally developing child with the motor control and cognition to achieve it. A child with a disability may require a medical evaluation to determine if a bladder problem exists and if the bladder is trainable before potty training can begin. A child with a disability to the corticospinal tract or spinal cord may be unable to inhibit the autonomic nervous system, resulting in difficulty in gaining this control.

Positioning is a key component of potty training. The youngest children are often placed on small, stable floor-sitting potty chairs, as standard in-home toilets are too high. Children with motor delays and abnormal tone will need the occupational therapy practitioner to evaluate positioning needs for the potty chair. Adaptations may need to be made to a commercially available chair, or a customized potty chair may be required to promote the correct sitting alignment. Often a tray is helpful to provide some arm stability, which can assist with sitting up, and is useful to place communication cards or devices on to indicate "all done." At times, trays are helpful to restrict the child's access to touching feces.

Tracking success is helpful for both the parent and the child. Often a daily chart with stickers is used to promote success and provide visual reinforcement for the child. The parents may need to track accidents more carefully and determine if the timing of placement on the potty chair needs adjusting. Often when clock changes are made to accommodate daylight savings time, the adults need to remember the child's body is still on the old schedule and will need time to make the adjustments. Parents must want to work on this skill and be committed for success to be achieved.

After toileting, children need to learn the routine of hand washing. Some children can easily move to the sink, use a step stool, and begin to learn the steps of hand washing. Often a hand washing song is used to promote an adequate scrubbing time. Some children may need to clean their hands with anti-bacterial germ products while seated on the toilet. These routines need to be established early on in the process to minimize the risk of infection and help children establish a connection between the two tasks. Shepherd (2005) offers a variety of strategies for improving participation in self-care tasks, including simple picture sequences, task adaptations, environmental modification, clothing adaptation, and task analysis with interventions for toileting skill development.

Engage Your Brain 9-4

Review the resources in Box 9-4 and select one to discuss as a best practice principle with one of your classmates.

Rest and Sleep

Rest and sleep is an occupation that includes rest, sleep preparation, and sleep participation (AOTA, 2014). Many infants have difficulty getting to sleep, staying asleep, and getting enough sleep. Normal, healthy infants spend a majority of their day in

Box 9-4 Resources for Occupational Therapy in Early Intervention

AOTA Tip Sheets

Establishing Bath Time Routines for Children (Doll and Pumerantz, 2013)
www.aota.org/~/media/Corporate/Files/AboutOT/consumers/Youth/BathTimeTipSheet.PDF

Establishing Bedtime Routines for Children (AOTA, 2013)
www.aota.org/~/media/Corporate/Files/AboutOT/consumers/Youth/BedroomRoutineTipSheet.pdf

Establishing Mealtime Routines for Children (Doll, 2014)
www.aota.org/~/media/Corporate/Files/AboutOT/consumers/Youth/Establishing-Mealtime-Routines-for-Children-Tip-Sheet.pdf

Establishing Morning Routines for Children (Doll, 2013)
www.aota.org/~/media/Corporate/Files/AboutOT/consumers/Youth/Morning%20Routine%20Tip%20Sheet.pdf

Establishing Toileting Routines for Children (Doll and Riley, 2014)
www.aota.org/~/media/Corporate/Files/AboutOT/consumers/Youth/Establishing-Toileting-Routines-for-Children-Tip-Sheet.pdf

Other Resources

Children's Sleep Habits Questionnaire—Infant Version
dx.doi.org/10.1016/j.jped.2017.05.012 (Dias, Figueiredo, and Pinto, 2017)

Greenspan Floortime Approach
www.stanleygreenspan.com/ (Greenspan, 2018)

Social and Emotional Development (Public Broadcasting Service, n.d.)
www.pbs.org/wholechild/abc/social.html

Social-Emotional Development Domain (California Department of Education, 2018)
www.cde.ca.gov/sp/cd/re/itf09socemodev.asp

Social and Emotional Development for Infants 0–12 Months (Aussie Childcare Network, 2015)
https://aussiechildcarenetwork.com.au/articles/child-development/social-and-emotional-development-for-infants-0-12-months

Sleep (SleepOT, 2016)
https://sleepot.org/assessment-of-sleep/

Tummy Time (Pathways, n.d.)
https://pathways.org/wp-content/uploads/2014/09/tummytimebrochure_english.pdf

sleepiness and sleep, but infants with immature central nervous systems are often overaroused. Parents report that these infants are difficult to get to sleep and often irritable. Establishing a consistent bedtime routine to help infants and toddlers know that it is time to calm and rest is essential. The sleep preparation component includes the readiness parts such as taking a bath, going potty or getting a fresh diaper, changing into pajamas, brushing teeth, reading books while sitting on a parent's lap in a rocking chair, or whatever routine fits the family and lets everyone know it is time to settle down. Keeping the routine consistent helps establish a predictable pattern to cue the infant/toddler that it is time to settle down and prepare to rest. Some children who use picture communication schedules for other activities during the day will benefit from a bedtime routine with pictures indicating each step in sequence, leading up to getting into bed and sleeping.

Many infants need help with sensory calming to promote sleep. The provision of deep pressure input (i.e., swaddling), slow rhythmical movement (i.e., rocking), and neutral warmth (i.e., infant to parent chest) promotes calming the typical infant. Most often there are changes in the environment related to lighting and sounds that signal a calmer, darker, and quieter home. Occupational therapy practitioners help parents establish the bedtime routine by (a) providing calming sensory strategies to promote calm and sleepiness and infant/toddler self-soothing to return to sleep if awakened, (b) modifying the environment to promote sensory calming to promote both getting to sleep and being able to stay asleep, and (c) utilizing behavioral interventions to promote getting to sleep, staying asleep, staying in the bedroom, staying in the bed, and minimizing getting out of bed. Parents of infants and toddlers with suspected or confirmed autism may benefit from parent education focused on sleep routines and interventions.

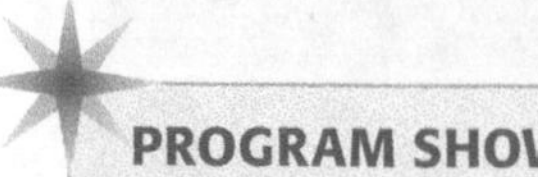

PROGRAM SHOWCASE

Parent Education to Promote Sleep (PEPS)

Wooster et al. (2015) developed the "Parent Education to Promote Sleep" (PEPS program). PEPS is an evidence-based program with emphasis on improving parent education related to improving children's preparation and participation in sleep and rest. The *Occupational Therapy Practice Framework: Domain and Process* (AOTA, 2014) clearly identifies rest and sleep preparation and participation as a part of occupational therapy practice.

Needs assessment: Local pediatricians and therapists reported that parents were asking for information related to improving sleep. A review of the literature indicates that sleep issues are of great concern and a top priority for parents of children with autism (Malow and McGrew, 2008; Sounders et al., 2009), as well as for parents of children with intellectual disability (Cotton and Richdale, 2006). Sleep is needed to maintain our homeostasis and promote overall well-being. A lack of adequate sleep predisposes both the children and the parents to stress, mood disturbances, and behavior changes (Autism Speaks, 2013). Parental knowledge is needed regarding what to change and how to change the home environment and what routines promote sleep.

Goal: The goal of the PEPS program was to improve parental knowledge related to establishing consistent sleep routines, adapting the sleep environment, promoting sensory calming, and enacting behavioral strategies related to improving sleep participation in children.

Population: The population were parents of children attending local pediatric clinics (greater-area Mobile, AL) who identified a need to improve sleep for their child with any disability. Flyers were sent home promoting participation and dates for educational sessions.

Participant's perspectives: "I now know that I can go home and start to make changes to help my child."

"I have been doing so many things wrong, but I know what to do now to make it right."

"We all need more sleep, so things are now going to change at my house. Thank you!"

Evaluation results: Parents participated in a 2-hour educational workshop aimed at promoting knowledge in sleep preparation and participation. A knowledge pretest/posttest design was utilized. Data analysis with a paired t-test demonstrated statistically significant knowledge changes ($P = 0.0003$).

Social Participation

Occupational therapy practitioners provide family-centered interventions to promote social-emotional development. The care provided to each infant lays the groundwork for the development of basic health processes, including attention, self-regulation, and social-emotional functioning (Morris, Silk, Steinberg, Myers, and Robinson, 2007; Patterson, DeBaryshe, and Ramsey, 1989; Scaramella and Leve, 2004). Parent-infant bonding and appropriate responsive interactions can be encouraged by coaching parents to read their infants' cues and to respond sensitively to infants' needs. Responsive parenting is when parents are aware of their children's emotional and physical needs and respond appropriately and consistently. This facilitates the dynamic process between the parent and infant. Later, as infants become toddlers, parents help them become competent in interacting with other children and other adults.

These social interactions are embedded in most activities in which the parent and child will engage. The interventions most often utilized include:

- Some touch-based interventions to enhance physiological stability, calm the child, and reduce disruptive behaviors
- Relationship-based interventions to facilitate caregiver-child interactions in play activities
- Interactional, play-based activities to promote joint attention (e.g., attending to social partners during an activity)
- Naturalistic interventions integrated into the preschool to promote peer-to-peer engagement
- Instruction-based intervention to teach preschool children appropriate social behaviors
- Therapist-selected toys and objects to promote social interaction among preschoolers (AOTA, 2011)

Play

Play is a primary occupation of children and a rich opportunity for social interaction with caregivers, family members, and peers. Developing rich parent-child play-based interactions that provide just the right level of challenge for motor, cognitive, social, and communication skills, yet also include joyous moments for both, is a challenge. Infants and toddlers engage in play at home and in the community.

A recent study showed that all children, regardless of disability or age, who participated in a community playgroup intervention benefited (Fabrizi, Ito, and Winston, 2016). Allowing the caregiver and child to become familiar with play environments in the community also provides further exploration and playful interactions outside the home. Children demonstrated more playful interactions after playgroup participation as noted by increased Test of Playfulness scores in active participation, persistence, and pretending. Increases in playfulness have been linked to improved adaptability and coping, setting the child up for a lifetime of participation, health, and well-being.

The Greenspan Floortime Approach is an intervention method to improve reciprocal social interactions between parents and children, with emphasis on children with autism (Greenspan, 2018). Floortime is an evidence-based intervention that has been shown to strengthen fundamental communication and relationship abilities for children with autism and other special needs (Casenhiser, Binns, McGill, Morderer, and Shanker, 2015). Key components include getting down on the floor to the child's level and meeting the child at his or her developmental level. Parents receive coaching and learn to include these three principles: (a) follow the child's lead so you enter his or her world, (b) challenge the child to be creative and spontaneous, and (c) expand actions and interactions using multisensory preferred toys. Over 100 articles, several books, and web-based resources are available to train professionals and parents in the Greenspan Floortime Approach. Many occupational therapy practitioners working in EI have been trained in this relationship-building approach and incorporate these strategies into play sessions.

Performance Patterns—Motor Skills

A normal, healthy infant will demonstrate significant changes in both gross and fine motor skills during the first year of life. Antigravity strength and postural stability are gained to promote an upright posture in sitting and in preparation for walking. Fine motor skills progress from a visually guided reach (5 months), to a three-jaw chuck grasp (7 to 8 months), to a refined pincer grasp (12 months) that promotes self-feeding finger foods and holding on to a cup. When an infant or toddler demonstrates delays in motor skills, an activity-focused motor intervention based on principles of motor learning and motor development should be considered. These activity-focused motor interventions need to be family focused and fit within the context of daily routines.

Emphasis is placed on the selection of specific motor actions that are embedded into daily routines. For example, "tummy time" is used to help an infant improve head control. To begin, the family identifies times within the day that tummy time opportunities can easily match with what they are doing. During floortime play, parents place the infant prone over their leg (using the leg as a roll) and provide visually stimulating toys or incorporate play with siblings, encouraging the infant to lift their head in peekaboo play. When the parent is helping an older sibling with homework, the infant is placed on the tummy over a rolled towel with visually stimulating toys to look at while visually supervised and intermittently encouraged to lift their head by the parent. Parents may carry an infant football-style, prone and supported by parent's forearm, while they go outside to supervise other siblings playing, and the parent encourages the infant to lift their head and smile at siblings.

These activity-focused motor interventions enhance the development of functional developmental motor skills (Valvano and Rapport, 2006). Interventions that embed behavioral and learning principles with motor skill development appear to show a positive outcome (Case-Smith, Frojek Clark, and Schlabach, 2013). Pathways (n.d.) has an excellent brochure for parents explaining the importance of tummy time and the gradual increase in head control and extension that is gained.

Performance Skills—Cognitive Skills

Occupational therapy practitioners in EI typically partner with family members and caregivers to address cognitive limitations due to their impact on everyday life occupations. The focus is to promote the child's development by recommending specific individual learning opportunities within natural routines and activities (Dunst, Bruder, Trivette, and Hamby, 2006). Executive functioning, which includes self-regulation, behavior sequencing, flexibility, response inhibition, and planning, emerges during the early childhood years. Interventions to enhance cognitive development that were initiated in the neonatal intensive care unit with preterm infants who were at risk for developmental delays led to positive improvements in infancy and at preschool age (Orton, Spittle, Doyle, Anderson, and Boyd, 2009). Effective interventions incorporate parent education such as enhancing child development, promoting parents' sensitivity to their children's needs, and encouraging responsive interactions. Providing parents with information about activities to stimulate infant/toddler cognitive development is particularly effective since cognitive development is related to other areas of development (Orton et al., 2009).

Joint attention is the ability to orient to or attend to other people, including sharing attention on an object, shifting eye gaze, and getting others' attention. Interventions focusing on improving joint attention appear to have positive effects on infants' ability to initiate joint attention. These effective interventions include increasing parents' sensitivity to infant cues, using symbolic play, and incorporating components of Discrete Trial Training (Maurice, Green, and Luce, 1996).

Trauma-Informed Care

It is very likely that within the EI system, occupational therapy practitioners will work with children placed in the foster-care system for their own protection. Foster care was designed to be a temporary service provided by the states for children who cannot live with their families. Children in foster care may live with relatives or with unrelated foster parents. Foster care can also refer to placement settings such as group homes, residential care facilities, emergency shelters, and supervised independent living. It is well known that children in foster care have extensive trauma history. Sometimes, the placement into a new home, often with strangers, is traumatic itself. No other child-serving system encounters a higher percentage of children with a trauma history than the child welfare system. Children served by child welfare have experienced at least one major traumatic event, and many have long and complex trauma histories. Research studies indicate that children in foster care have significant developmental, behavioral, and emotional problems; therefore, services are essential for these children (Pecora, Jensen, Romanelli, Jackson, and Ortiz, 2009).

Trauma and neglect can have significant repercussions on the brain development of the child. Children in the foster care system frequently exhibit behavioral issues, attachment disorders, poor self-regulation, and many other issues associated with their traumatic experiences. Traumatic experiences overwhelm children's natural ability to cope and result in a "flight, fight, fright, or freeze" response that affects children's bodies and brains. Chronic or repeated trauma may result in toxic stress that interferes with normal child development and causes long-term harm to children's physical, social, emotional, or spiritual well-being. These adverse effects can include changes in a child's emotional responses; ability to think, learn, and concentrate; impulse control; self-image; attachments to caregivers; and relationships with others. Across the life span, traumatic experiences have been linked to a wide range of problems, including addiction, depression and anxiety, and risk-taking behavior—and these in turn can lead to a greater likelihood of chronic ill health, including obesity, diabetes, heart disease, cancer, and even early death (ACE Response, 2018).

The trauma-informed care model is the gold standard for education about the complexity of trauma on child development. This model provides information that promotes identification of traumatic events, explains the neuroscience of repetitive trauma, and describes behavioral changes that caregivers and practitioners can make to provide interactions for the children that are sensitive to their needs and therapeutic in their self-development. Children should be treated with compassion, dignity, and acceptance to promote positive changes (U.S. Department of Health and Human Services, n.d.).

The focus of the trauma-informed care model is on healing the impact of the trauma and improving the children's social and emotional well-being, along with the more traditional goals of safety and permanency. EI and foster care programs must learn to collaborate, enhance communication, plan and work toward joint goals, share data about families, and examine ways to blend and utilize all appropriate resources. Focusing more on trauma and collaboration with EI and foster care may help prevent or mitigate some of the long-term effects of trauma.

The occupational therapy practitioner could work directly with the foster family, with the biological family, with extended family members, and with social workers and staff from the foster care system. The unknown family outcomes often mean children are in the system awaiting family compliance with various agencies to determine the longer-term plan. Foster families provide a safe haven while the biological family has a chance to seek needed services. Occupational therapy practitioners can serve important roles because of their knowledge of the cognitive, social and emotional, and sensory components of activity and their impact on behavior (Petrenchik, 2015; Petrenchik and Guarino, 2009). These children need environments that promote safety and predictability while also providing a pleasurable connection to others with some fun activities to promote healing and learning (van der Kolk, 1989). Occupational therapy practitioners can conduct task analysis and recommend environmental modifications to optimize the child-environment-occupation fit to enable successful activity engagement and social participation. Traumatized children have difficulties handling emotions, sensations, stress, and daily routines. They often feel hopeless, worthless, and incompetent (van der Kolk, 2005). Occupational therapy practitioners work with other disciplines to structure environments, teach cognitive strategies, and develop social and emotional skills that promote self-regulation, competence development, trust building and confidence, and resilience through participation (AOTA, 2015b).

Family Involvement in Interventions

A **family-centered** philosophy is based on the assumption that the parents know best. This philosophy is consistent with occupational therapy practice to promote meaningful family engagement (Stoffel et al., 2017). The parents, viewed as partners with the service providers, are expected to be advocates for their child. The role of service providers is to meet the needs of the family by providing the information and instruction designated as important by the parents. Accepting parental reports as reliable information, allowing parents to help define goals, letting parents lead the discussions, and allowing parents to have questions ready for the team to problem-solve together are all aspects of family-centered care. Reynolds and Andelin (2018) discuss caregiver-focused interventions, including coaching, developing home programs, and home modifications, as an integral part of supporting children with difficulties in sensory processing. The AOTA (2017) *Guidelines for Occupational Therapy Services in Early Intervention and Schools* indicates that occupational therapists must apply the principles of family-centered practice to include empowering parents, building relationships, encouraging involvement in decision-making, building on informal community support systems, and being respectful of the family's culture, beliefs, and attitudes. The Centers for Disease Control and Prevention (2018) has developed a website called Learn the Signs. Act Early that provides resources to help both parents and professionals track a child's developmental skills, with an emphasis on the early identification of children who may have autism so families can seek evaluations and interventions sooner.

Simeonsson and Bailey (1990) identified a hierarchy of parental involvement, representing a continuum from passive to active participation, for EI. Families will fluctuate in the levels, depending on the environmental demands and their coping abilities at the time. At the lowest level is *elective noninvolvement,* in which the family chooses not to be involved in the child's care. *Information seeking* is another level of involvement, in which the family focuses on gathering information and developing skills. *Partnership* is when the family views themselves in a reciprocal interaction and decision-making process with the health-care providers. At the highest level, the family assumes the role of *advocacy* for their child. Some families may need the help of the occupational therapy practitioner or other professional to teach them how to be advocates for their own needs and empower them to make decisions for themselves and their child. Identifying the level at which the family is functioning at a given time will assist the occupational therapy practitioner in determining appropriate caregiving roles within the family. Research has indicated that families consistently reported positive perceptions of family-centered and routine-based approaches in EI (Kingsley and Mailloux, 2013).

The nature of the activity can also affect which family members are available to help. Every parent needs time for personal hygiene, meal preparation, and the care of any other children in the family. The occupational therapy practitioner can demonstrate ways the child can be placed in a safe and independent play position when a parent is most likely to be busy. Siblings can be involved by showing them ways to play with and monitor the child. This, of course, depends on the ages and abilities of the siblings.

Parent and Caregiver Instruction

Occupational therapy home programs need to be designed specifically for each child and fit within the family routines and context. Research indicates home programs are important for children with disabilities (Schreiber, Effgen, and Palisano, 1995). A well-designed home program includes therapeutic interventions that are embedded within everyday routine tasks to ease the caregiver strain and to promote the child's functional skills (Anderson and Schoelkopf, 1996; Hinojosa, 1990; Rainforth and Salisbury, 1988). Programs that have assisted parents in their interactions with the child have had better outcomes than services focused exclusively on the child (Bonnier, 2008; Hebbeler et al., 2007).

Caregiver instruction and written directions increase the likelihood of carryover by the caregivers (Simon, 1988). Parent instruction is an ongoing process that includes modeling. Case-Smith and Nastro (1993) found that mothers preferred the use of written handouts with pictures of specific activities. Often, simple, clear diagrams, placed in strategic locations, can be great aids to reinforce these activities. For example, placing pictures near the changing table (and just inside the diaper bag) demonstrating how to relax the child with a high tone, the best position for the child during diaper changing, and some simple range-of-motion exercises may be most effective. Feeding documentation is placed in the appropriate area of the home, such as in the kitchen on the refrigerator. It may include a photograph of the best positioning, the equipment needed, and a bulleted reminder of techniques to promote feeding skills. Practicing techniques with parents and interested family members can provide reassurance.

Parent-training programs with an occupational therapist who has facilitated and provided feedback have been shown to increase positive outcomes in children's behavior, in comparison with group training without the active attendance of a trained therapist (Barlow, Coren, and Stewart-Brown, 2003; Montgomery, Bjornstad, and Dennis, 2006). Parents of children with ASD highly value training that facilitates their skills for improving their child's communication, play, and behavior (Hume, Bellini, and Pratt, 2005). Additionally, evidence suggests that educating parents of preterm infants to be more sensitive to their child's needs and more responsive in interactions improves cognitive and joint attention outcomes (Frolek and Schlabach, 2013).

Summary

- EI programs are comprehensive, with three components—identification, eligibility determination, and evaluation.
- Occupational therapy practitioners meet the comprehensive needs of young children and families for age-appropriate ADL skill development, sensory-appropriate play activities, social skills training, and assistance in navigating resources to promote young children and family participation in everyday routines.
- Occupational therapy practitioners evaluate the home environment, the family's abilities and needs, and the child's performance factors and skills. Comprehensive assessments are often selected that address many areas (gross motor/mobility, fine motor, communication, self-care/adaptive, and social-emotional). Additional assessment tools can then be chosen to address any one area when further evaluation is needed.
- Family-centered care and partnerships are key factors to the establishment of embedded routines that promote a child's occupational participation and performance.
- Best practice in EI involves the application of evidence-based practice to promote infant and toddler participation in culturally relevant and meaningful occupation in natural environments with family members and peers.

CASE STUDIES

CASE STUDY 9-1 Juan

Juan is a 22-month-old toddler with developmental delay. He has just been referred to EI by his pediatrician. Juan lives in a small apartment with his parents. His mother stays at home to care for him, and she is currently 4 months pregnant. The language spoken at home is Spanish; however, both parents know some English. Parental concerns include Juan's lack of eye contact, not eating a wider variety of foods, getting upset with noises, and difficulty with unfamiliar environments. His mother reports that he can finger feed, eats fewer than 10 different foods on a regular basis, and only drinks room-temperature water. Some days he will just play with his food, and his mother then attempts to feed him. He has lots of toys but plays with the same toys each day, mostly dropping them, throwing them, or lining them up in a pattern. He wakes up two to three times per night. His mother has been leaving him in his crib, and sometimes he will go back to sleep. Lately, he is starting to try to climb out, and his parents are concerned he will get hurt. They want to transition him to a bed before their new baby is born but do not want him roaming around the apartment at night. They sometimes bring him into their bed, but he is restless and does not go back to sleep. When outside, he runs around and sometimes spins around. He likes the sandbox and will sit and watch the sand fall through his fingers. He loves television, especially *Diego,* but the volume must be low, and he wants to stand right at the screen. Your observation of his play identifies repetitive play patterns, lining up of toys, lack of eye contact, inconsistent response to his name, and some self-stimulation with hand flapping.

Discussion Questions

1. Which of Juan's behaviors are indicative of possible sensory dysfunction?
2. Which assessment tools could an occupational therapist utilize to further evaluate Juan's occupational performance and developmental level for sensory, motor, self-care, and play skills? Why did you select these tools?
3. Research the "red flag" warning signs of autism in toddlers. Does Juan demonstrate any of these, and if so, which ones?
4. What occupations would you observe as part of your skilled observation?
5. What suggestions might you make to help with Juan's sleeping difficulties and safety?

CASE STUDY 9-2 Community Screening Program

Gertrude, an occupational therapy practitioner and university faculty member, was asked by a local EI program to volunteer to participate in a community screening program targeted at infants and toddlers. She will be working with a large church in the community with many members who are Hispanic, as well as with a speech therapist, physical therapist, and a special education teacher. Gertrude was asked to select at least two tools to be reviewed by the team that have both an English and Spanish version. Gertrude anticipates that about 200 children will be screened during a 4-hour window in one morning.

CASE STUDY 9-2 Community Screening Program

Discussion Questions

1. What additional information might Gertrude ask of the organizer/sponsor?
2. Are there aspects of the *Occupational Therapy Code of Ethics (2015)* (AOTA, 2015a) that Gertrude should consider in completing this work?
3. What additional knowledge or expertise would you need in order to fulfill Gertrude's role?
4. Could Gertrude involve occupational therapy students in this screening program?
5. What resources should Gertrude have on hand to provide to parents to take home to review typical developmental milestones for their child?

Learning Activities

1. Research screening tools for children from birth to age 3 that would review motor (gross and fine), communication, social-emotional, and cognitive areas. Identity which tools come with both an English version and a Spanish version of the form.
2. Students of the local university from occupational therapy, physical therapy, and speech therapy courses are willing to participate in this process with you. Describe how you would set up the screening day.
3. Design a "therapy kit" to keep in your car for children receiving EI services. Name what equipment, supplies, and forms you would include in the kit.
4. Research how to refer a child for EI services in your area.
5. Identify local resources that would be available to help the EI occupational therapy practitioner.

REFERENCES

ACE Response. (2018). *Who are we?* Retrieved from www.aceresponse.org/who_we_are/

Acs, G., Ng, M. W., Helpin, M. L., Rosenberg, H. M., and Canion, S. (2007). Dental care: Promoting health and preventing disease. In M. Batshaw, L. Pellegrino, and N. Roizen (Eds.), *Children with disabilities* (6th ed.). Baltimore, MD: Brookes.

Ages and Stages. (2018). *Ages and stages - 3.* Retrieved from www.agesandstages.com

American Academy of Pediatrics. (2018). *Screening recommendations.* Retrieved from www.aap.org/en-us/advocacy-and-policy/aap-health-initiatives/Screening/Pages/Screening-Recommendations.aspx

American Occupational Therapy Association. (2011). *Early intervention/early childhood—critically appraised topic.* Retrieved from www.aota.org/~/media/corporate/files/secure/practice/ccl/ei/early%20intervention%20social%20emotional.pdf

American Occupational Therapy Association. (2013). *Establishing bedtime routines for children.* Retrieved from www.aota.org/~/media/Corporate/Files/AboutOT/consumers/Youth/BedroomRoutineTipSheet.pdf

American Occupational Therapy Association. (2014). Occupational therapy practice framework: Domain and process (3rd ed.). *American Journal of Occupational Therapy, 68*(Suppl. 1), S1–S48. https://doi.org/10.5014/ajot.2014.682006

American Occupational Therapy Association. (2015a). Occupational therapy code of ethics (2015). *American Journal of Occupational Therapy, 69*(Suppl. 3), 6913410030. http://dx.doi.org/10.5014/ajot.2015.696S03

American Occupational Therapy Association. (2015b). *Occupational therapy's role in mental health promotion, prevention, and intervention with children and youth: Childhood trauma.* Retrieved from www.aota.org/~/media/Corporate/Files/Practice/Children/Childhood-Trauma-Info-Sheet-2015.pdf

American Occupational Therapy Association. (2015c). *The role of occupational therapy with children and youth.* Bethesda, MD: American Occupational Therapy Association.

American Occupational Therapy Association. (2017). Guidelines for occupational therapy services in early intervention and schools. *American Journal of Occupational Therapy, 71*(Suppl. 2), 7112410010. https://doi.org/10.5014/ajot.2017.716S01

Anderson, J., and Schoelkopf, J. (1996). Home-based intervention. In J. Case-Smith, A. S. Allen, and P. N. Pratt (Eds.), *Occupational therapy for children* (3rd ed., pp. 758–765). St. Louis, MO: Mosby-Year Book.

Anderson, P., and Telleen, S. (1992). The relationship between social support and maternal behavior and attitudes: A meta-analytic review. *American Journal of Community Psychology, 20*(6), 753–774.

Andrews, M., and Andrews, J. (1993). Family centered techniques: Integrating enablement into the IFSP process. *Journal of Childhood Communication Disorders, 15,* 41–46.

Aussie Childcare Network. (2015). *Social and emotional development for infants 0–12 months.* Retrieved from https://aussiechildcarenetwork.com.au/articles/child-development/social-and-emotional-development-for-infants-0-12-months

Autism Speaks Inc. (2013). *Treatments for associated medical conditions.* Retrieved from www.autismspeaks.org/family-services/health-and-wellness/sleep

Barlow, J., Coren, E., and Stewart-Brown, S. (2003). Parent training programmes for improving maternal psychosocial health. *Cochrane Database of Systematic Reviews, 2004,* CD002020.

Birken, C. S., and MacArthur, C. (2004). Socioeconomic status and injury risk in children. *Paediatrics and Child Health, 9*(5), 323–325.

Bohlin, G., Hagekull, B., and Rydell, A. (2002). Attachment and social functioning: A longitudinal study from infancy to middle childhood. *Social Development, 9,* 24–39. https://doi.org/10.1111/1467-9507.00109

Bonnier, C. (2008). Evaluation of early stimulation programs for enhancing brain development. *Acta Pediatrica, 97,* 853–858. https://doi.org/10.1111/j.1651-2227.2008.00834.x

Briggs, M. (1993). Team talk: Communication skills for early intervention teams. *Journal of Childhood Communication Disorders, 15,* 33–40.

Bronson, M., and Bundy, A. (2001). A correlational study of the Test of Playfulness and the Test of Environmental Supports. *Occupational Therapy Journal of Research, 21,* 223–240. doi:10.1177/153944920102100403

Bundy, A. C., Lane, S. J., and Murray, E. A. (2002). *Sensory integration theory and practice* (2nd ed.). Philadelphia, PA: F. A. Davis.

California Department of Education. (2018). *Social-emotional development domain.* Retrieved from www.cde.ca.gov/sp/cd/re/itf09socemodev.asp

Casenhiser, D., Binns, A., McGill, F., Morderer, O., and Shanker, S. (2015). Measuring and supporting language function for children with autism: Evidence from a randomized control trial of social-interaction-based therapy. *Journal of Autism and Developmental Disorders, 45*(3), 846–857. https://doi.org/10.1007/s10803-014-2242-3

Case-Smith, J., Frojek Clark, G. J., and Schlabach, T. L. (2013). Systematic review of interventions used in occupational therapy to promote motor performance for children birth–5. *American Journal of Occupational Therapy, 67,* 413–424. http://dx.doi.org/10.5014/ajot.2013.005959

Case-Smith, J., and Nastro, M. (1993). The effect of occupational therapy intervention on mothers of children with cerebral palsy. *American Journal of Occupational Therapy, 46,* 11–817. doi:10.5014/ajot.47.9.811

Centers for Disease Control and Prevention. (2018). *Learn the signs. Act early.* Retrieved from www.cdc.gov/ncbddd/actearly/index.html

Cotton, S., and Richdale, A. (2006). Brief report: Parental descriptions of sleep problems in children with autism, Down syndrome, and Prader-Willi syndrome. *Research in Developmental Disabilities, 27,* 151–161. Retrieved from http://dx.doi.org/10.1016/j.ridd.2004.12.003

Degangi, C. (1995). *Infant toddler symptom checklist.* San Antonio, TX: Therapy Skill Builders/Psychological.

Dias, C. C., Figueiredo, B., and Pinto, T. M. (2017). Children's Sleep Habits Questionnaire—Infant Version. *Journal of Pediatrics, 94,* 146–154. http://dx.doi.org/10.1016/j.jped.2017.05.012

Division for Early Childhood. (2007). *Promoting positive outcomes for children with disabilities: Recommendations for curriculum, assessment and program evaluation.* Retrieved from www.naeyc.org/sites/default/files/globally-shared/downloads/PDFs/resources/position-statements/PrmtgPositiveOutcomes.pdf

Division for Early Childhood. (2014). *DEC position statement: The role of special instruction in early intervention.* Retrieved from file:///C:/Users/coe/Downloads/Position%20Statement%20-%20Role%20of%20Special%20Instruction%20in%20Early%20Intervention%20June%202014.pdf

Doll, J. (2013). *Establishing morning routines for children.* Retrieved from www.aota.org/~/media/Corporate/Files/AboutOT/consumers/Youth/Morning%20Routine%20Tip%20Sheet.pdf

Doll, J. (2014). *Establishing mealtime routines for children.* Retrieved from www.aota.org/~/media/Corporate/Files/AboutOT/consumers/Youth/Establishing-Mealtime-Routines-for-Children-Tip-Sheet.pdf

Doll, J., and Pumerantz, C. (2013). *Establishing bath time routines for children.* Retrieved from www.aota.org/~/media/Corporate/Files/AboutOT/consumers/Youth/BathTimeTipSheet.PDF

Doll, J., and Riley, B. R. W. (2014). *Establishing toileting routines for children.* Retrieved from www.aota.org/~/media/Corporate/Files/AboutOT/consumers/Youth/Establishing-Toileting-Routines-for-Children-Tip-Sheet.pdf

Donaldson, O. F. (2018). *Play quotes. National Museum of Play.* Retrieved from www.museumofplay.org/education/education-and-play-resources/play-quotes

Dunn, W. (2002). *Infant toddler sensory profile.* San Antonio, TX: Therapy Skill Builders/Psychological.

Dunst, C. J., Bruder, M. B., Trivette, C. M., and Hamby, D. W. (2006). Everyday activity settings, natural learning environments, and early intervention practices. *Journal of Policy and Practice in Intellectual Disabilities, 3,* 3–10. http://dx.doi.org/10.1111/j.1741-1130.2006.00047.x

Early Childhood Technical Assistance Center. (2015). *States' and territories definitions of/criteria for IDEA Part C eligibility.* Retrieved from www.nectac.org/~pdfs/topics/earlyid/partc_elig_table.pdf

Early Childhood Technical Assistance Center. (2019). *Family assessment: Gathering information from families.* Retrieved from http://ectacenter.org/decrp/topic-assessment.asp

Ellison, P. H. (1994). *The INFANIB: A reliable method for the neuromotor assessment of infants.* Tucson, AZ: Therapy Skill Builders.

Ernsperger, L., and Stegen-Hanson, T. (2004). *Just take a bite.* Arlington, TX: Future Horizons.

Fabrizi, S. E., Ito, M. A., and Winston, K. (2016). Effect of occupational therapy-led playgroups in early intervention on child playfulness and caregiver responsiveness: A repeated-measures design. *American Journal of Occupational Therapy, 70,* 1–9, 7002220020. http://dx.doi.org/10.5014/ajot.2016.017012

Fitzsimmons, S. (1993). The changing epidemiology of cystic fibrosis. *Journal of Pediatrics, 122,* 1–9.

Frolek Clark, J., and Schlabach, T. L. (2013). Systematic review of occupational therapy interventions to improve cognitive development in children ages birth–5 years. *American Journal of Occupational Therapy, 67*(4), 425–430. doi:10.5014/ajot.2013.006163

Fujiura, G., and Yamaki, K. (2000). Trends in demography of childhood poverty and disability. *Exceptional Children, 66* (2), 187–199.

Furuno, S., O'Reilly, K., Hosaka, C. M., Zeisloft, B., and Allman, T. (1997). *Hawaii Early Learning Profile—Revised.* Palo Alto, CA: Vort.

Glover, M. E., Preminger, J., and Sanford, A. (1988). *The early learning accomplishment profile.* Chapel Hill, NC: Kaplan Press.

Greenspan, S. (2018). *The Greenspan Floortime approach.* Retrieved from www.stanleygreenspan.com/

Gunnar, M., and Quevedo, K. (2007). The neurobiology of stress and development. *Annual Review of Psychology, 58,* 145–173. https://doi.org/10.1146/annurev.psych.58.110405.085605

Guyer, B., Ma, S., Grason, H., Frick, K. D., Perry, D. F., Sharkey, A., and McIntosh, J. (2009). Early childhood health promotion and its life course health consequences. *Academic Pediatrics, 9*(3), 142–148. https://doi.org/10.1016/j.acap.2008.12.007

Haley, S. M., Coster, W. J., Ludlow, L. H., Haltiwanger, J., and Andrellos, P. (1992). *Administration manual for the Pediatric Evaluation of Disabilities Inventory.* San Antonio, TX: Psychological.

Hamilton, B. B., and Granger, C. U. (2000). *Functional Independence Measure for Children (Wee-Fim-II).* Buffalo, NY: Research Foundations for the State University of New York.

Hebbeler, K., Spiker, D., Bailey, D., Scarbourough, A., Mallik, S., Simeonsson, R., Singer, M., and Nelson, L. (2007, January). *Early intervention for infants and toddlers with disabilities and their families: Participants, services, and outcomes. Final report of the National Early Intervention Longitudinal Study (NEILS).* Retrieved from www.sri.com/sites/default/files/publications/neils_finalreport_200702.pdf

Hinojosa, J. (1990). How mothers of preschool children with cerebral palsy perceive occupational and physical therapists and their influence on family life. *Occupational Therapy Journal of Research, 10,* 144–162.

Howe, T.-H., and Wang, T.-N. (2013). Systematic review of interventions used in or relevant to occupational therapy for children with feeding difficulties ages birth–5 years. *American Journal of Occupational Therapy, 67,* 405–412. http://dx.doi.org/10.5014/ajot.2013.004564

Hume, K., Bellini, S., and Pratt, C. (2005). The usage and perceived outcomes of early intervention and early childhood programs for young children with autism spectrum disorder. *Topics in Early Childhood Special Education, 25,* 195–207. http://dx.doi.org/10.1177/02711214050250040101

Hunt, L., Lewis, D., Reisel, S., Woldrup, L., and Wooster, D. (2000). Age norms for straw drinking abilities. *Infant-Toddler Intervention: A Transdisciplinary Journal, 10*(1), 1–8.

Hussey, B. (1988). *Understanding my signals.* Palo Alto, CA: VORT.

Individuals With Disabilities Education Improvement Act of 2004, Pub. L. No. 108–446, §1431 et seq. (2004, December). Retrieved from http://copyright.gov/legislation/pl108–446.pdf

Johnson-Martin, N., Attermeier, S. M., and Hackler, B. (2004). *The Carolina curriculum for infants and toddlers with special needs* (3rd ed.). Baltimore, MD: Brooks.

Kellegrew, D. (2000). Constructing daily routines: A qualitative examination of mothers with young children with disabilities. *American Journal of Occupational Therapy, 54,* 252–259.

Kingsley, K., and Mailloux, Z. (2013). Evidence for the effectiveness of different service delivery models in early intervention services. *American Journal of Occupational Therapy, 67,* 431–436. doi:10.5014/ajot.2013.006171

Knox, S. (1997). Development and current use of the Knox Preschool Play Scale. In L. D. Parham and L. S. Fazio (Eds.), *Play in occupational therapy for children* (pp. 35–51). St. Louis, MO: Mosby/Year Book.

Lazara, A., Danaher, J., and Goode, S. (2017). FPG Child Development Institute, Early Childhood Technical Assistance Center. Chapel Hill, NC: University of North Carolina. Retrieved from http://ectacenter.org/~pdfs/growthcomppartc-2017-04-05.pdf

Linder, T. (2008). *Transdisciplinary play based assessment* (2nd ed.). Baltimore, MD: Brookes.

Malow, B. A., and McGrew, S. G. (2008). Sleep disturbances and autism. *Sleep Medicine Clinics, 3,* 479–488.

Maurice, C., Green, G., and Luce, S. (Eds.). (1996). *Behavioral intervention for young children with autism: A manual for parents and professionals.* Austin, TX: Pro-Ed.

Miller, L. J. (1994). Journey to a desirable future: A value-based model of infant and toddler assessment. *Zero to Three, 14*(6), 23–26.

Montgomery, P., Bjornstad, G. J., and Dennis, J. A. (2006). Media-based behavioral treatments for behavioral disorders in children. *Cochrane Database of Systematic Reviews,* Issue 1. Art. No.: CD002206. DOI: 10.1002/14651858.CD002206.pub3.

Morris, A. S., Silk, J. S., Steinberg, L., Myers, S. S., and Robinson, L. R. (2007). The role of the family context in the development of emotion regulation. *Social Development, 16,* 361–388. doi:10.1111/j.1467-9507.2007.00389.x

Morris, S. E., and Klein, M. D. (2000). *Pre-feeding skills* (2nd ed.). San Antonio, TX: Therapy Skill Builders/Harcourt Health Sciences.

Nugent, J. K., Keefer, C. H., Minear, S., Johnson, L. C., and Blanchard, Y. (2007). *Understanding newborn behavior and early relationships: The Newborn Behavioral Observations (NBO) system handbook.* Baltimore, MD: Brookes.

Orton, J., Spittle, A., Doyle, L., Anderson, P., and Boyd, R. (2009). Do early intervention programmes improve cognitive and motor outcomes for preterm infants after discharge? A systematic review. *Developmental Medicine and Child Neurology, 51,* 851–859. doi:10.1111/ j.1469-8749.2009.03414.x

Parham, L., and Fazio, I. (2008). *Play in occupational therapy for children* (2nd ed.). St. Louis, MO: Mosby.

Pathways.org. (n.d.). *Tummy time: Activities to strengthen baby.* Retrieved from https://pathways.org/tummy-time-brochure/

Patterson, G. R., DeBaryshe, B. D., and Ramsey, E. (1989). A developmental perspective on antisocial behavior. *American Psychologist, 44,* 329–335.

Pecora, P., Jensen, P., Romanelli, L., Jackson, L., and Ortiz, A. (2009). Mental health services for children placed in foster care: An overview of current challenges. NIH Public Access. *Child Welfare, 88* (1), 5–26.

Petrenchik, T. (2015, April). *Developmental trauma and the brain: Understanding and working with children on the arousal regulation continuum.* Workshop presented at the American Occupational Therapy Association Annual Conference and Expo, Nashville, TN.

Petrenchik, T., and Guarino, K. (2009, April). *Understanding traumatic stress and providing trauma-informed care: Applications in occupational therapy.* AOTA-sponsored workshop presented at the American Occupational Therapy Association Annual Conference and Expo, Houston, TX.

Pretti-Frontczak, K., and Bricker, D. (2001). Use of the embedding strategy during daily activities by early childhood education and early childhood special education teachers. *Infant-Toddler Intervention: The Transdisciplinary Journal, 11*(2), 111–128.

Public Broadcasting Service. (n.d.). *Social and emotional development.* Retrieved from www.pbs.org/wholechild/abc/social.html

Rainforth, B., and Salisbury, C. (1988). Functional home programs: A model for therapists. *Topics in Early Childhood Special Education, 7*(4), 33–45.

Reif, S., Beler, B., Villa, Y., and Spirer, Z. (1995). Long-term follow-up and outcome of infants with non-organic failure to thrive. *Israel Journal of Medical Sciences, 31*(8), 483–489.

Reynolds, S., and Andelin, L. (2018). Supporting children with sensory processing differences. *OT Practice, 23*(12), 10–15.

Rommel, N., De Meyer, A. M., Feenstra, L., and Veereman-Wauters, G. (2003). The complexity of feeding problems in 700 infants and young children presenting to a tertiary care institution. *Journal of Pediatric Gastroenterology and Nutrition, 37,* 75–84. http://dx.doi.org/10.1097/00005176-200307000-00014

Rudolph, C., and Link, D. T. (2002). Feeding disorders in infants and children. *Pediatric Clinics of North America: Pediatric Gastroenterology and Nutrition, 49,* 97–112.

Sadeh, A. (2004). A brief screening questionnaire for infant sleep problems: Validation and findings for an Internet sample. *Pediatrics, 113*(6), 570–577.

Scaramella, L. V., and Leve, L. D. (2004). Clarifying parent-child reciprocities during early childhood: The early childhood coercion model. *Clinical Child Family Psychological Review, 7*(2), 89–107. doi:10.1023/B:CCFP.0000030287.13160.a3

Schreiber, J. M., Effgen, S. K., and Palisano, R. J. (1995). Effectiveness of parental collaboration on compliance with a home program. *Pediatric Physical Therapy, 7,* 59–64.

Shepherd, J. (2005). Activities of daily living and adaptations for independent living. In J. Case Smith and J. Clifford O'Brien (Eds.), *Occupational therapy for children* (6th ed., pp. 474–517). St Louis, MO: Elsevier Mosby.

Simeonsson, R. J., and Bailey, D. B. (1990). Family dimensions in early intervention. In S. J. Meisels and J. P. Shonkoff (Eds.), *Handbook of early childhood intervention* (pp. 214–235). Cambridge, United Kingdom: Cambridge University Press.

Simon, G. (1988). Parent errors following physician instruction. *American Journal of Diseases of Children, 142,* 415–416.

Skard, G., and Bundy, A. (2008). Test of playfulness. In L. Parham and L. Fazio (Eds.), *Play in occupational therapy for children* (2nd ed., pp. 71–93). St. Louis, MO: Mosby Elsevier.

SleepOT. (2016). *Assessment of sleep.* Retrieved from https://sleepot.org/assessment-of-sleep/

Sounders, M. C., Mason, T. B., Valladares, O., Bucan, M., Levy, S. E., Mandell, D. S., Weaver, T. E., and Pinto-Martin, J. (2009). Sleep behaviors and sleep quality in children and autism spectrum disorders. *SLEEP, 32,* 1566–1578.

Stoffel, A., Rheim, J., Khetani, M., Pizur-Barnekow, K., James, L., and Schefkind, S. (2017). *Family centered: Occupational therapy's role in promoting meaningful family engagement in early intervention.* Retrieved from www.aota.org/AboutAOTA/Membership/Tools/Periodicals/10-09-17-pediatric-success/Family-Centered-OT-Role-Promoting-Meaningful-Family-Engagement-Early-Intervention.aspx

Stoffel, A., and Schleis, R. (2014). *Frequently asked questions: What is the role of occupational therapy in early intervention?* Bethesda, MD: American Occupational Therapy Association. Retrieved from www.aota.org/~/media/Corporate/Files/Practice/Children/Browse/EI/Role-of-OT_1/Early-Intervention-FAQ.pdf

Strauss, D., Shavelle, R., Reynolds, R., Rosenbloom, L., and Day, S. (2007). Survival in cerebral palsy in the last 20 years: Signs of improvement? *Developmental Medicine and Child Neurology 49,* 86–92. doi:10.1111/j.1469-8749.2007.00086.x

Takata, N. (1974). Play as prescription. In M. Reilly (Ed.), *Play as exploratory learning.* Beverly Hills, CA: Sage.

U.S. Department of Health and Human Services. (n.d.). *Trauma-informed practice.* Retrieved from www.childwelfare.gov/topics/responding/trauma/

Valvano, J., and Rapport, M. J. (2006). Activity-focused motor interventions for infants and young children with neurological conditions. *Infants and Young Children, 19,* 292–307.

van der Kolk, B. A. (1989). The compulsion to repeat the trauma: Re-enactment, re-victimization, and masochism. *Psychiatric Clinics of North America, 12*(2), 389–411. https://doi.org/10.1016/S0193-953X(18)30439-8

van der Kolk, B. A. (2005). Developmental Trauma Disorder: Toward a rational diagnosis for children with complex trauma histories. *Psychiatric Annals, 35*(5), 401–408.

Vanderveen, J. A., Bassler, D., Robertson, C. M., and Kirpalani, H. (2009, January 15). Early interventions involving parents to improve neurodevelopmental outcomes of premature infants: A meta-analysis. *Journal of Perinatology, 29*(5), 343–351. doi:10.1038/jp.2008.229

Wallace, H., Biehl, R., MacQueen, J., and Blackman, J. (1997). *Mosby's resource guide to children with disabilities and chronic illness.* St. Louis, MO: Mosby.

Wooster, D. (1999). Assessment of nonorganic failure to thrive. *Infant-Toddler Intervention, 9*(4), 353–371.

Wooster, D. (2000). Intervention for nonorganic failure to thrive. *Infant-Toddler Intervention, 10*(1), 37–45.

Wooster, D., Brady, N. R., Mitchell, A., Grizzle, M. H., and Barnes, M. (1998). Pediatric feeding: A transdisciplinary team's perspective. *Topics in Language Disorders, 18*(3), 34–51.

Wooster, D., Gwin, H., Gwin, S., Hargis, L, Papania, J., Register, J., and Rood, K. (2015). Efficacy of sleep education for parents with children with autism spectrum disorders. *American Journal of Occupational Therapy, 69*(Suppl. 1): 6911515153p1–6911515153p1. doi:10.5014/ajot.2015.69S1-PO3058

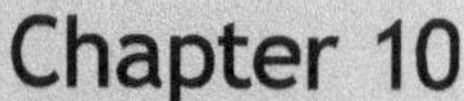

Chapter 10

From School to Community Transition Services

Janet DeLany, DEd, OTR/L, FAOTA, Barbara Demchick, ScD, OTR/L, FAOTA, and Lisa Crabtree, PhD, OTR/L, FAOTA

Let's continue to stand up for those who are vulnerable to being left out or marginalized.

—Hillary Rodham Clinton

Learning Outcomes

This chapter is designed to enable the reader to:

10-1 Substantiate the importance of school-to-community transition planning and programming to support success in adulthood.

10-2 Articulate the scope and challenges of existing legislation and funding systems to support school-to-community transition services.

10-3 Apply an occupation-based and an education-based model to school-to-community transition services.

10-4 Apply evaluation strategies to support occupation-based school-to-community transition.

10-5 Describe best practices to support school-to-community transition.

10-6 Articulate the contributions of occupational therapy to occupation-based school-to-community transition services.

Key Terms

Entitlement
Environmental barriers and supports
Low-intensity support services
Organizational narratives
Person-environment-occupational performance model
Personal narratives
Population narratives
Self-determination
Social relationships
Strengths-based approach
Supported decision-making
Transition services
Universal design for learning

Introduction

Leaving high school can be exciting and daunting for youth with special needs and for those in foster care as they transition to adult roles in their communities. Such transitions can promote or impede participation in post–high school occupations that include community living, productive engagement, or postsecondary education. Federal legislation mandates school to transition planning for youth with special needs as part of the Individuals with Disabilities Education Act (IDEA; U.S. Department of Education [USDE], 2017) and for youth who are in foster care as part of the Fostering Connections to Success and Increasing Adoptions Act (USDE, 2016). IDEA and the Fostering

Connections to Success Act are federal **entitlement** acts that mandate requirements for the provision and funding of services for those youth who meet specified criteria as defined by the USDE (2017).

Transition services require a coordinated set of activities for a student with a disability (or in foster care) within an outcome-oriented process. This process promotes movement from school to postschool activities, such as postsecondary education, and includes vocational training and competitive integrated employment. Active student involvement, family engagement, and cooperative implementation of transition activities, as well as coordination and collaboration between the vocational rehabilitation (VR) agency, the state education association (SEA), and the local education agency (LEA), are essential (USDE,2017, p. iv). The coordinated set of activities is based on each student's needs, taking into account the student's strengths, preferences, and interests, and includes instruction, related services, community experiences, the development of employment and other postschool adult-living objectives, and, if appropriate, the acquisition of daily living skills and the provision of a functional vocational evaluation (p. 49).

Under IDEA, transition services are to be in effect by the time the youth with disabilities turns 16 years of age and may continue through the school year in which the youth turns 21 years old. Students, teachers, parents, and others work to develop a plan for the student's active participation and achievement in the transition process (Cleary, Persch, and Spencer, 2015; USDE, 2017). Under the Fostering Connections Act, youth become eligible for transition services when they turn 14 years old and may continue to receive services until they age out of the foster care system sometime between 18 and 22 years of age, depending on state regulations. The foster care caseworker or other welfare professional is to collaborate with the youth to develop and execute the transition plan (USDE, 2016).

Currently, 6,700,000 public school youth qualify for special education services (National Center for Education Statistics [NCES], 2018a). At least 415,000 youth are in foster care (Sarubbi, Parker, and Sponsler, 2016), with 30% to 40% of these students also qualifying for special education services (Disabled World, 2013). Given that 395,000 special education and foster care students are between the ages of 14 and 21 years (NCES, 2018b), the number who need transition services is substantive.

This chapter highlights the legislation, funding, and best practices for transition planning and services. It also describes the contributions of occupational therapy to occupation-based transition services that are grounded in the aspirations of transition-age youth to live in the community and to engage in educational, productive, and leisure pursuits. Such contributions reflect the core occupational therapy belief about the value of "achieving health, well-being, and participation in life through engagement in occupation" (AOTA, 2014, S2).

Legislation and Funding

Although mandated by IDEA and the Fostering Connections Act, the attainment of successful transition outcomes for transition-age youth with disabilities or in foster care is constrained by legislative challenges, resource limitations, and access barriers. Underemployment, unemployment, housing restrictions, educational barriers, higher dependency levels on public funds for daily life activities, and higher levels of poverty persist despite three decades of legislation (Luecking, Fabian, Contreary, Honeycutt, and Luecking, 2018; Plotner, Oertle, Reed, Tissot, and Kumpiene, 2017; Riesen, Schultz, Morgan, and Kupferman, 2014). In the years following transition, transition-age youth are less likely than other high school graduates to work in paid or well-paying jobs, engage in community activities, and enroll in postsecondary education (USDE, 2016, 2017; Wehman, 2013). For example, only 24% of students with cognitive disabilities are likely to be employed. Those who are often work fewer hours and receive lower wages than those students without disabilities (Migliore, Lyons, Butterworth, Nye-Lengerman, and Bose, 2018). A qualitative study of 198 professionals at centers for independent living (CLI) across 38 states indicated limited to nonexistent collaboration between CLIs and LEAs for postsecondary housing. Currently, 84% of individuals with intellectual disabilities continue to live with family members or in group homes, with only 11.4% eventually leasing or owning their own place of residency (Plotner et al., 2017). Key employment and housing barriers include insufficient educational preparation of transitioning youth related to career awareness, career development, skill training, and independent living; underprepared and underinformed community transition teams; limited interagency collaborations and parental knowledge about resources; few employer incentives and affordable community housing options; inadequate employment and community support services for obtaining and sustaining job placement and housing; and inadequate community transportation options (Migliore et al., 2018; Plotner et al., 2017; Riesen et al., 2014).

Recently, representatives from the USDE, the U.S. Department of Health and Human Services (USDHHS), the U.S. Department of Labor, and the Social Security Administration (SSA) developed the *2020 Federal Youth Transition Plan* to improve transition outcomes for transition-age youth with disabilities or in foster care. Though not a law, the plan outlines how the partnering agencies will advance the transition process by 2020 through interagency identification and coordination of a shared vision, outcome goals, and policy priorities. By creating an integrated system that is easier to navigate, the aspirational aim of the plan is to help transition-age youth, their families, and service providers become more aware of and access health care and integrated work experiences and successfully connect to programs and support for which the youth are eligible (Federal Partners in Transition Workgroup, 2015).

As part of the transition team, occupational therapy practitioners must become familiar with the parameters and constraints of existing laws and funding sources to accurately advise transition-age youth and their families about their legal rights and the available services that support the transition to adult life. This is especially important for those young adults with complex challenges who may not become fully employed or enroll in postsecondary education following secondary school. While some of the laws and funding sources are specific to transition, others provide personal and systemic protection for individuals with disabilities throughout their life span. Legislation that is designed to enhance the participation and integration of those with disabilities is outlined in Table 10-1.

Because funding to support transitioning young adults who are no longer entitled to services provided through IDEA or the Fostering Connections Act is limited, occupational therapy practitioners must consider the implications for young adults as they transition to an adult system of eligibility. Within this system, young adults may meet the criteria to receive but may not be able to access services because there is no mandate that those services be available or funded. Too frequently, the need for services far exceeds their availability and funding opportunities.

Most community-based services for transitioning young adults with disabilities are funded through two state-administered agencies that receive federal funding: VR and DD agencies. The names of the agencies may vary across states. For instance, the VR agency may be called the Department of Rehabilitation or the Department of Rehabilitation Services. State VR programs are time limited and available only if the goal for the transitioning young adult is employment. In contrast, DD agencies assume an ongoing need for intervention. DD agencies generally provide more long-term services, including supported employment, day programming, residential services, and case management (Division of Rehabilitation Services, 2018; Maryland Developmental Disabilities Administration, 2018).

The 2018 federal budget included $103,000,000 in requests for disability programs: $39 million for the Developmental Disabilities Protection and Advocacy Program, $39 million for University Centers for Excellence in Developmental Disabilities, and $45 million for the Partnerships for Innovation, Inclusion, and Independence programs. Monies allocated to states use a statutory formula based on a per capita population and income basis (USDHHS, 2018b). Federal funds for VR are also allocated to states based on statutory formulas based on per capita population and income and are administered in accordance with the Workforce Innovation and Opportunity Act (WIOA) Unified and Combined State Plan Requirements (USDE, 2018b). Federal funds account for 78.7%, and state funds account for 21.3% of the VR budget. WIOA regulations require that states allocate 15% of their federal VR monies to fund transition services (Luecking et al., 2018).

Eligibility for services provided by VR and DD funding varies by state and may impose a minimum age restriction of 21 years. This results in a gap

Table 10-1 Legislation Relevant to Transition

Legislation	Description
Americans With Disabilities Act of 1990 and Revised ADA Regulations Implementing Title II and Title III (U.S. Department of Justice and Civil Rights Division, 2018)	• Promotes community participation for people of all ages • Prohibits discrimination in employment, transportation, public accommodations, public services, and telecommunications • Requires employers to provide reasonable accommodations to workers who are able to perform the essential job functions for them
Rehabilitation Act of 1973 and 1986, 1993, and 1998 amendments (U.S. Department of Labor, 2018a)	• Provides equal access for individuals with disabilities to any program, service, or activity receiving financial assistance from the federal government • Provides money for time-limited job training and employment assistance at the state level and includes transition and transition service language via 1986 amendments
Ticket to Work and Work Incentives Improvement Act of 1999 (Revell and Miller, 2008)	• Provides financial resources to support readiness and employment programs for individuals with disabilities who are receiving Social Security benefits • Includes job readiness and work skills assessment, career counseling, employment placement, internships and apprenticeships, job coaching, and transportation • Removes barriers that require people with disabilities to choose between health-care coverage and work
Workforce Innovation and Opportunity Act (WIOA) of 2014 (U.S. Department of Labor, 2018b)	• Provides quality workforce access for those with disabilities • Requires state vocational rehabilitation (VR) agencies to set aside at least 15% of their funding to provide transition services to youth with disabilities for competitive employment
Achieving a Better Life Experience (ABLE) Act of 2014-H.R. 647, 113th Cong. (2013–2014)	• Allows tax-free savings accounts to help individuals and families finance disability needs such as education, health care, transportation, and housing without risking eligibility for Social Security, Medicaid, and other government programs
Higher Education Opportunity Act of 2008 (U.S. Department of Education, 2018)	• Improves access to postsecondary education for students with intellectual disabilities and allows those students who are accepted at or enrolled in comprehensive transition and postsecondary education programs to be eligible for grants and the Federal Work Study Program • Authorizes the development and expansion of quality inclusive comprehensive transition and postsecondary education programs

between exiting high school and receiving services for many transition-age youth and young adults. However, in some states, VR services can be accessed as early as age 14 years. Many states maintain long waiting lists for services. Those individuals with the most severe needs often take priority, further limiting access to services for others.

> **Engage Your Brain 10-1**
>
> **How would you find the name of the DD agency and the VR agency in your state? What services and funding do they provide for transition-age youth and young adults?**

A small number of states offer **low-intensity support services** (LISS), which may be granted to individuals with developmental disabilities regardless of their priority status. These services provide a small amount of money each year to support the needs of a child, youth, or adult with a developmental disability within the community. LISS funding can be used to purchase items or services and may be administered through the state DD agency (Division of Rehabilitation Services, 2018; Maryland Developmental Disabilities Administration, 2018).

Health and community-based services (HCBS) Medicaid waivers may also provide funds to individuals with disabilities for community-based services as an alternative to long-term care services in institutional settings. State and federal governments fund HCBS waivers jointly. Each state determines which HCBS programs it will provide. In some states, individuals with disabilities may use HCBS waivers for residential and supported employment services (U.S. Centers for Medicare and Medicaid Services [USCMMS], 2018). HCBS waivers generally fund programs and services rather than allocate money directly to a person or family. However, some states offer HCBS waivers with a self-directed option that allows individuals to purchase the services they need to live and work in their communities. HCBS are provided to individuals who traditionally do not qualify for Medicaid services and are only available to a predetermined, limited number of individuals.

Engage Your Brain 10-2

What HCBS Medicaid waivers does your state offer? Do any waivers provide services to transition-age youth and young adults? Does your state offer any kind of LISS?

Transition-age youth with disabilities may qualify for Social Security Supplemental Security Income (SSI) through the SSA. These benefits are based on financial need. Some of these transition-age youths have been eligible for SSI since childhood. Those transition-age youths with previous work experience also may qualify for Social Security Disability Insurance (SSDI) benefits (SSA, 2018). In addition, transition-age youth with disabilities and from foster care programs may be eligible for Medicaid to assist with health-care costs. Eligibility varies across states (USCMMS, 2018). In most states, SSI recipients also receive Medicaid.

Two funded employment programs that benefit youth transitioning from foster care include:

- Job Corps, which provides education and training program for low-income youth who are at least 16 years of age (U.S. Department of Labor [USDL], 2017)
- Registered apprenticeships that combine technical training with paid on-the-job experiences in construction, health care, energy, and homeland security (USDL, 2018b)

Occupational therapy practitioners may also seek funds through insurance companies or community and industry grants to pilot specially designed transition programs tailored to specific populations and needs. By knowing about legislation and funding sources, occupational therapy practitioners can encourage youth and their families to sign up for services while in high school and thus reduce the amount of postsecondary wait time for services that will best meet their needs.

Occupational Therapy Roles and Services

As part of its domain, occupational therapy practice promotes health and participation at the person, institution, and population levels through engagement in occupations (AOTA, 2014, p. S1–48). Consistent with *Healthy 2030* goals (USDHHS, 2018a), this engagement encompasses the array and richness of occupations that give meaning and purpose and that advance the well-being of youth during and after the transition from secondary education. The occupational therapy process requires collaboration with those who are part of the transition process to gather and assess data about the youth, families, institutions, and populations that are part of the transition; develop and implement a transition plan; and measure outcomes of the transition services (AOTA, 2014).

Occupational therapy practitioners work to enhance the capacities of the transition-age youth, adapt contexts to support their occupational engagement, and adjust activities to maximize their occupational performance. They engage collaboratively with youth after they leave the school system to support success within the community, at work sites, and in postsecondary education settings, fostering self-advocacy and autonomy in decision-making. Occupational therapy practitioners need to advocate for their participation on transition teams to support transition-age youth, as only some school districts and community agencies routinely include them (Eismann et al., 2017; Kardos and White, 2005).

Theoretical Models and Frameworks

Theoretical frameworks guide occupational therapy practice by organizing clinical observations; honing critical reasoning about the scope and interdependency of complex factors to consider; and structuring the understanding and analysis of the values, assumptions, research, and priorities that implicitly and explicitly govern decisions. Employing an occupational therapy-based model for school-to-community transition services focuses the assessment, intervention, and outcomes processes within an occupation-based perspective. Applying an education-based model links occupational therapy practice to the educational arena in which school-to-community transitions often occur and strengthens the understanding of the contributions of educational partners in the transition process. Two such models, one of each type, are the person-environment-occupational performance model (PEOP; Christiansen, Baum, and Bass, 2015) and the universal design for learning (UDL; CAST, 2011, 2018). Both models value the family and the transition-age youth as core decision-makers in the planning process; acknowledge transition as an evolving, multiyear learning process; and support the acquisition of transition skills for independent or codependent community living, continuing education systems, and productive voluntary or paid work experiences. Collectively, they guide consideration of the:

- Occupational aspirations, performance capacities, and demonstrated performance skills of the students and their families and of the environments and context that support, constrain, and press these students and their families
- Mission, purpose, and context of the current educational environment and of the community, education, and work to where the students are transitioning
- Instructional approaches that support multiple ways for students to engage in learning and demonstrate mastery of content and skills for transition

Person-Environment-Occupational Performance Model

Originally published by Christiansen and Baum in 1991, the **PEOP model** was revised in 1997 and 2005 and expanded in 2015 to (a) include the personal, organizational, and population narratives and (b) focus the assessment, intervention, and outcome processes of person, environment, and occupation factors toward enhancing occupational performance, participation, and well-being (Christiansen et al., 2015). The model is depicted in Figure 10-1.

The narratives promote the development of the occupational profiles (Christiansen et al., 2015) that are involved in the school-to-community transition process. The **personal narratives** focus on the students' and their family members' perceptions about and meaning of transition from school to the community and their choices, motivations, and responsibilities regarding their transition needs and goals. The **organizational narratives** provide a framework for considering the priorities of the school where the student is currently located and those of the community, educational, and work environments where the student may transition. The **population narratives** address the prevalence of adolescents needing and legally eligible for transition services, the demographic variables and socioeconomic-occupational disparities contributing to the need for and goals of transition services, and the societal and environment factors creating access or barriers to transition services.

The PEOP model highlights the interdependence and complexity of the person, occupation, and environment factors (Christiansen et al., 2015) that are part of the school-to-community transition process. Person factors are intrinsic to the students, their family members, the organizations, and the population and encompass the:

- Meaning, values, and beliefs about the importance of and responsibility for transition

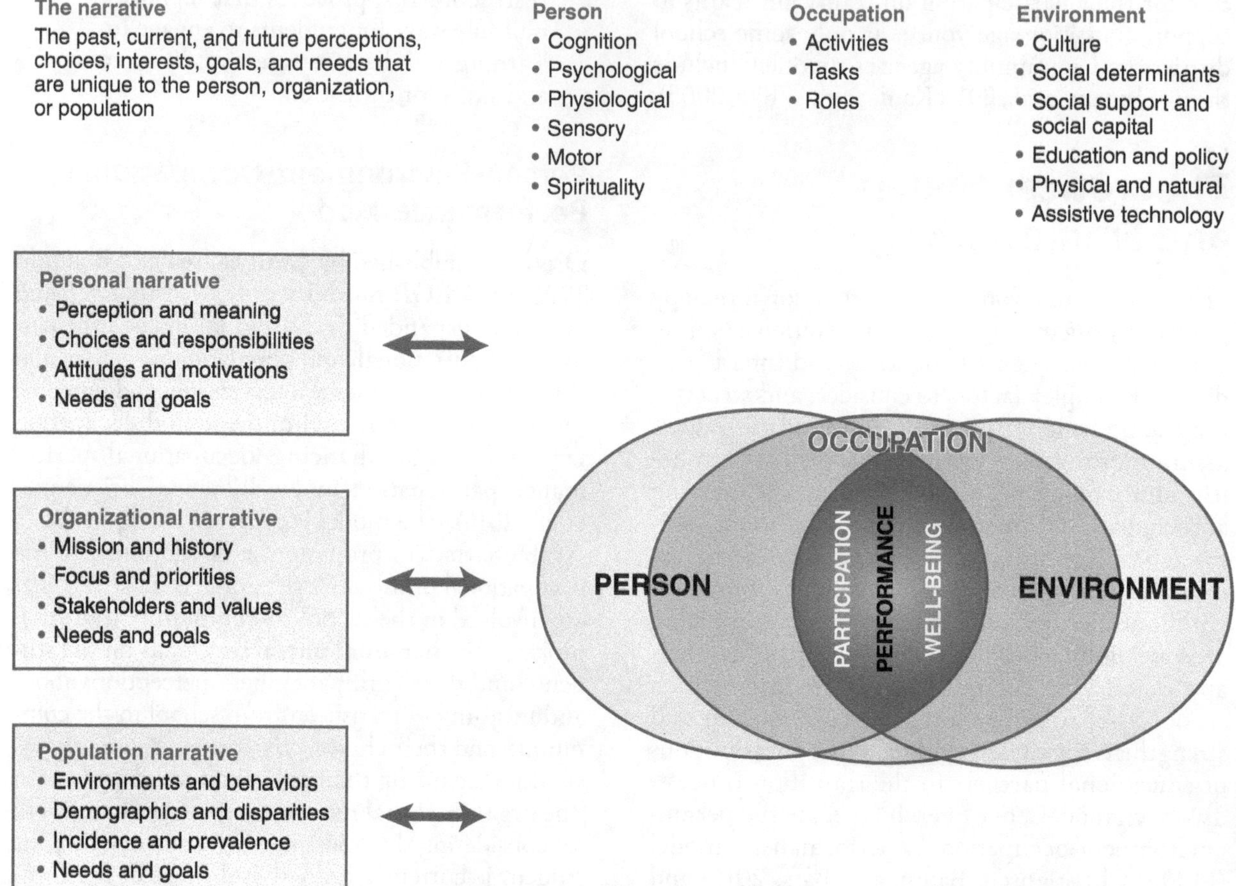

Figure 10-1 PEOP model. Occupational performance (doing) enables participation (engagement) in everyday life that contributes to well-being (health and quality of life). *(Adapted with permission from Figure 4-1, "The Person-Environment-Occupation-Performance [PEOP] Model," in* Occupational Therapy: Performance, Participation, and Well-Being *[4th ed.], by C. M. Baum, C. H. Christiansen, and J. D. Bass, 2015, Thorofare, NJ: SLACK.)*

- Knowledge of and capacity to learn and make decisions about transition services
- Readiness, abilities, and capacities to perform the transition activities, tasks, and roles and to achieve transition goals

Occupation factors incorporate the activities, tasks, and roles performed by students and their families, the organization, and the population (Christiansen et al., 2015) as they engage in or avoid the transition process. Environmental factors are extrinsic to the students and their family members and incorporate:

- Cultural beliefs and behaviors regarding the scope and structure of transition services
- Social determinants, including demographics, economic resources, political influence, and power structures that affect the structure of and commitment to transition services
- Social supports and social capital, including family, professional, educational, and

community norms and resources that coalesce to advocate for the scope and focus of transition services
- Education, social, labor, employment, housing, and other regulatory policies at the local, regional, and national levels that dictate responsibility for and funding of transition services
- Physical and natural environments and assistive technologies that affect the availability of and access to postsecondary community, educational, and work resources (Christiansen et al., 2015)

Rather than bind transition service outcomes to the completion of a series of discrete tasks, the PEOP model connects outcomes to the level of performance, participation, and well-being of the students, their families, the organizations, and the population (Christiansen et al., 2015). These outcomes align with a foundational principle of *Healthy People 2030* that "health and well-being of all people and communities are essential to a thriving, equitable society" (USDHHS, 2018a, para 9).

Universal Design for Learning

As education policy shifts priorities from learning environment access to learning access, **UDL** is emerging as a framework for guiding curricular practices that reduce educational barriers and respect the diversity of learner needs (CAST, 2018; Hehir, 2009; Rose and Meyer, 2002). Grounded in neuroscience, cognitive psychology, and learning research, the three principles of UDL focus on (a) multiple means for learning representation; (b) action and expression; and (c) engagement that is effective, efficient, and motivating for students (CAST, 2011; Hehir, 2009). UDL principles emphasize flexible instructional approaches that are responsive to alternate and individualized methods that students employ to learn, navigate through the learning process, demonstrate what they have learned, and remain invested in learning (CAST, 2011). UDL principles are beneficial for:

- Designing alternative approaches for students, families, organizations, and populations to learn about and indicate their understanding of postsecondary resources
- Developing multiple methods for students to demonstrate mastery of skills for managing their self-care, living in the community, engaging in productive and leisure pursuits, and attending postsecondary education
- Selecting assistive technologies and tools to optimize transition to work or postsecondary education
- Proposing strategies for integrating school-to-community employment

Evaluation Strategies for Transition to Community Participation

As part of a complete evaluation process, occupational therapists assess the skills and abilities of individuals and the related contextual factors that influence community participation. Assessment is a continuous process throughout the transition from secondary school into adulthood and includes the active participation and engagement of youth in the process. Providing opportunities and exposure to a variety of community contexts and assessing each experience during the years prior to transitioning out of secondary school contribute to an understanding of options for postsecondary community involvement (Crabtree and Sherwin, 2011). Information regarding strengths, interests, and daily routines can be gathered through narrative interview; standardized measurement tools can be used to identify patterns of participation and to prioritize goals. Table 10-2 lists measurement tools for practitioners to consider when working with transition-age individuals in community programs.

Person Factors and Skills for Community Participation

Developing an occupational profile and assessing individual strengths and challenges in collaboration with the individual and family members are essential first steps for providing occupational therapy services for transition-age youth. In addition to standardized measurement tools that identify current performance, observations of youth participation in activities within the community context

Table 10-2 Measurement Tools to Evaluate Person and Environment in the Transition to Community

Measurement Tool	Description
Assessment of Life Habits (LIFE-H) (Noreau, Fougeyrollas, and Vincent, 2002)	A measure of activities and social roles within different environments
Canadian Occupational Performance Measure (COPM) (Law et al., 2005)	Individualized outcome measure targeting occupational performance issues
Functional Assessment of Cognitive Transit Skills (Chase, Ratcliff, and Hoesch, 1996)	Performance-based competence scale evaluating community mobility skills in four areas: General Orientation, Community Skills and Safety, Simple Trip, Complex Trip
Goal Attainment Scaling (GAS) (Kiresuk, Smith, and Cardillo, 1994)	A standardized process of personalized goal identification and measurement of achievement
PATH Process (Bunch, Finnegan, and Pearpoint, 2009)	Creative planning tool for transition using a self-directed model, including planning positive and possible actions necessary for goal achievement
Student Transition Questionnaire (STQ) (Collier et al., 2017)	A self-report assessment clustered into five factors: Independent Living Skills; Participation in School, Community, and Work; Planning and Goal Attainment; Disability Awareness and Personal Empowerment; Vocational Rehabilitation
Vineland Adaptive Behavior Scales II (VABS-II) (Sparrow, Cicchetti, and Balla, 2005)	A measure of adaptive behavior for individuals with disabilities. Areas assessed include Communication, Daily Living Skills, Socialization, Motor Skills, and Maladaptive Behavior
Work Behavior Inventory (Bryson, Bell, Lysaker, and Zito, 1997)	A situational measure of onsite work performance, including work habits, work quality, personal presentation, social skills, and cooperativeness
Work Environment Impact Scale (WEIS) (Moore-Corner, Kielhofner, and Olson, 1998)	A semistructured interview to rate individuals' perceptions of the physical, social, and temporal aspects of the work environment

contribute to an understanding of their capacities and occupational preferences. Individual, caregiver, and teacher interviews are effective for identifying the interest and motivation to participate in community activities and for establishing a baseline to begin individualized intervention planning. Interest inventories and a summary of academic and functional skills lay a foundation for exploring options for community participation during the transition years (Hutchinson et al., 2011; Kingsnorth, Healy, and Macarthur, 2007). Consistent with the PEOP model, it is important to facilitate participation of the youth in the evaluation process to assess personal perceptions, attitudes, and motivation (Christiansen et al., 2015).

Environment Factors for Community Participation

When assessing community participation and planning for intervention, **environmental barriers and supports** are also considered. Environmental barriers may include limited opportunities for participation (Bishop-Fitzpatrick, DaWalt, Greenberg, and Mailick, 2017; Chen, Bundy, Cordier, Chien, and Einfeld, 2016), attitudes or perceptions of others that may make participation a negative experience (Anaby et al., 2013), and financial constraints (Memari et al., 2015; Shattuck, Orsmond, Wagner, and Cooper, 2011). Alternatively, social support in the community or workplace can have a positive effect on participation (Rinaldi et al., 2010). Occupational therapy practitioners identify these environmental barriers and supports through skilled observation and interviews, using clinical reasoning skills and collaboration with youth and their family members to identify priorities for intervention (Askari et al., 2015; Crabtree and Sherwin, 2011). As part of the evaluation process, consideration of access to the community (e.g., walkability and the availability of public transportation) and the availability of existing resources to support participation (e.g., family members, friends and coworkers, accommodations, and funding) are critical. As illustrated in Case Study 10-2, contextual factors influence community participation. By including youth in the environmental assessment and collaborative decision-making about available options, an occupational therapy practitioner can evaluate community accessibility and choices for community participation and guide transition-age youth to take more responsibility in the process.

Implementation of Transition Services Using Best Practice Principles

Occupational therapy practitioners working with transition-age youth have a responsibility to move beyond the traditional medical model of service delivery that focuses on the remediation of deficits. Such emphasis on deficit remediation and isolated skill development does not necessarily lead to generalization in everyday settings or to greater community participation. Rather, occupational therapy practitioners should provide services that are guided by best practice principles that emphasize strengths-based approaches (Dunn, 2017; Dunn et al., 2013), foster self-determination, promote social relationships, encourage inclusion, and value family involvement. These foundational principles align with occupational therapy and *Healthy People 2030* goals.

Strengths-Based Approaches

Strengths-based approaches focus on transition-age youths' resources and potential, emphasize their strengths and talents to tailor opportunities for participation within the community, and build capacity for continued development (Stewart, Gorter, and Freeman, 2013). Strengths-based approaches align well with UDL and PEOP frameworks and encompass self-determination, peer mentoring, inclusive opportunities, and environmental supports. When occupational therapy practitioners focus on strengths, they assist families in recognizing the talents of their youth, foster high but realistic expectations, and enhance participation (Hetherington et al., 2010; Stewart et al., 2013). They promote transition-age youths' sense of competency, satisfaction, and capacity to actively engage in their daily life occupations (Dunn, 2017).

Engage Your Brain 10-3

Identify five traits that you or someone you know has that you consider negative. Reframe them as strengths-based characteristics. For example, stubbornness may be viewed as tenacity.

Self-Determination

Activities that encourage and support self-determination are also essential for advancing successful transitions and participation in daily life occupations (Wehmeyer and Abery, 2013). **Self-determination** is the capacity to choose and to act upon the basis of those choices. Self-determined individuals act according to their own preferences, interests, and abilities and are free of undue influences. They have self-awareness and possess the skills necessary to achieve their desired outcomes. Self-determined individuals also can solve problems, advocate for themselves, and self-regulate (Field and Hoffman, 1999, 2012; Wehmeyer and Abery, 2013). Most youth develop self-determination in childhood and adolescence, as they gain greater responsibilities and freedom from their parents and teachers. Theoretically, IDEA and the Fostering Connection Act include opportunities for transition-age youth to become actively involved in planning for the post–high school transition; however, many youth still struggle with self-determination and self-advocacy upon leaving high school (Gennen et al., 2015; Powers et al., 2012, 2018; Webb, Patterson, Syverud, and Seabrooks-Blackmore, 2008). As a result, they may transition to adulthood with limited competency to navigate the challenges they face (Field and Hoffman, 1999, 2012).

Studies suggest that levels of self-determination upon leaving high school predict positive outcomes regarding employment and community access post-school (Shogren, Wehmeyer, Palmer, Rifenback, and Little, 2015; Wehmeyer, 2014). While not all transition-age youth have the capacity to be fully self-determined, most can engage in **supported decision-making,** whereby they get help from a trusted friend, family member, or professional in making decisions but exercise control over who provides the decision-making help and of the ultimate decisions (Jameson et al., 2015; Powers et al., 2012, 2018). Occupational therapy practitioners can facilitate the development of self-determination by offering opportunities for youth to exercise choice and control in daily activities throughout their childhoods (Lough, Rice, and Lough, 2012; Wehmeyer and Abery, 2013), by encouraging them to explore their interests, and by promoting their active participation in IEP meetings and the development of postschool goals.

Social Relationships

Additionally, research has reported that **social relationships** are vital for the development of self-determination (Field and Hoffman, 2012) and successful transitions (Powers et al., 2018). Occupational therapy practitioners can help transition-age youth enhance their ability to form and maintain positive relationships by promoting their self-awareness, implementing social skills training, and fostering naturalistic opportunities to practice social skills. They can also serve as positive role models and facilitate positive student-therapist interactions (Field and Hoffman, 2012; Powers et al., 2012, 2018). Youth who engage in structured social relationships while in school show gains in self-determination and in unstructured social participation in the community following high school exit (Taylor, Adams, and Bishop, 2017) that positively influence their future adult roles (Stewart et al., 2013).

The ability of transition-age youth to generalize daily life skills to a variety of contextual situations is also key to their success in living in the community. Typically developing peers who serve as mentors can aid transition-age youth with generalization and social skill acquisition. These mentors learn how to use explicit interaction strategies, such as modeling, prompting, and reinforcement, within the context of partnered group activities to promote social interaction and generalization (Kamps et al., 2002; Powers et al., 2012, 2018). The mentors change the social context as they encourage those with disabilities or in foster care to strengthen social relationships and discover opportunities for community inclusion (Crabtree, 2014; Powers et al., 2018). Participation in mainstream social activities within the community allows transition-age youth to refine and generalize their social participation skills. For instance, young adults with autism showed improvement in their self-perceptions of task leadership and social competence when engaging in challenge course activities with university student peers (Crabtree and Demchick, 2015). Additionally, the peer mentors develop skills for infusing "more equitable opportunities, resources, privilege, and enablement" (Whiteford and Townsend, 2011, p. 66) when they eventually become peer employees, employers, and community partners of the transition-age youth. The peers' ability to accept and understand youth with disabilities or living in foster care promotes strengths-based, developmentally appropriate relationships and experiences within the community. This potentially leads to the decreased segregation and increased inclusion of transition-age youth in all aspects of community life (Stewart et al., 2013).

Inclusion

Occupational therapy practitioners can promote inclusion through a variety of social preparation activities during school and following transition. During school, occupational therapy practitioners can support transition-age youths' participation in social clubs, sports, and other extracurricular activities that provide structured and accessible community participation opportunities. Those who

Table 10-3 Community Mobility Skills

Skills	Examples
Manual mobility	Walking paths, bicycle and scooter paths, wheelchair routes, animal-assisted mobility
Personal motorized transportation	Driver education; car rental, ownership, safety, maintenance, and insurance; motorized scooter, wheelchair, or golf cart
Public transportation	Transportation schedules, train and bus routes and utilization procedures, paratransit, rideshare services, employer- and agency-sponsored transit
Travel information	Money management, ground positioning systems, map and signage reading, travel brochures and websites, safety procedures, emergency contacts, mobility accessible routes

participate in more inclusive experiences have better postschool outcomes than those who do not (Woodman, Smith, Greenberg, and Malick, 2016). School and community inclusion also incorporates prevocational and work opportunities. However, schools often fail to direct transition-age youth with disabilities or in foster care into meaningful employment opportunities that are appropriate for their strengths and achievements (Collier et al., 2017; Hendricks and Wehman, 2009). It is essential to enhance vocational opportunities for transition-age youth, as their rate of employment compared to typical peers is low (Langi et al., 2017; Sarubbi et al., 2016). Additionally, individuals who are unemployed report lower well-being than their peers.

School-based occupational therapy practitioners have the skills and background to promote valued prevocational and vocational opportunities. The literature suggests that enriching the environment for students with disabilities enhances their vocational success (Eaves and Ho, 2008; Powers et al., 2018). Supportive prevocational activities include instruction in appropriate work behaviors and the facilitation of volunteer and internship experiences (Collier, Griffin, and Wei, 2017; Geller and Greenberg, 2010). Other supportive interventions include teaching organization and self-regulation strategies, facilitating skills to accommodate job routines, crafting sensory accommodations, and recommending appropriate assistive technology. Transition-age youth also benefit from job placements that match their strengths and interests and from job coaching to support performance (Collier et al., 2107; Hillier et al., 2007). Community mobility training is an essential component of successful prevocational and vocational transitions, as it enables the youth to learn how to commute to and from places of employment (see Table 10-3). The order is based on progressive complexity: first, students learn basic skills about community mobility, then learn progressively more complex skills, ending with driver education.

Family Involvement

As part of an overall strengths-based approach, family involvement is essential to successful transition to adulthood. In addition to helping families navigate school-to-community transition services, practitioners can facilitate parents' capacity to advocate for enhanced participation options for their transition-age youth (Hetherington et al., 2010; Stewart et al., 2013). Additionally, practitioners can help families recognize and cultivate their youths' strengths and talents and foster high but realistic parental expectations, as positive parental expectations are associated with better outcomes following transition (Woodman et al., 2016). Practitioners can help parents develop the ability to let go at appropriate times, to enable their youth to try new activities, and to learn from experience (Stewart et al., 2013).

Best Practice Programs

To implement occupation-based, community-focused programs for transition-age youth with disabilities and in foster care requires the integration of current knowledge about legislation, funding, theoretical frameworks, and best practice principles and evaluation processes. Three best practice programs highlight the application of this knowledge, providing examples of methods and strategies that can be replicated in other settings. These programs include the My Life-Self-Determination Model, centers for independent living youth programs, and the College Orientation and Life Activities Program.

PROGRAM SHOWCASE

Best Practices

My Life Self-Determination Model for Foster Youth

The My Life Self-Determination Model is a promising approach that expands upon the traditional focus on the improvement of independent living skills for transitioning foster youth to also enhance self-determination. Developed in collaboration with Portland University, the Portland school district, and the Oregon Department of Human Services Child Welfare, the program lasts 9 to 12 months and includes individual weekly or biweekly meetings with youth and coaches who were previously foster care youth and four peer-mentoring workshops. The coaching sessions focus on "youth-directed relationship support, learning of metacognitive skills . . . partnership development and self-regulation . . . and experiential support . . . to achieve life goals" (Powers et al., 2018, p. 277). Coaches provide support for strategies to address goals selected by foster youth such as obtaining a driver's license, obtaining a diploma, finding housing, and obtaining a job. Coaching fades as the foster youth gain competency and confidence in setting and achieving goals. Mentoring workshops are paired with recreational and networking activities and address employment, postsecondary education, transition steps, and other topics selected by the youth.

The results of three longitudinal randomized control studies involving 310 high school and postsecondary foster care youth indicate significant improvements in self-determination, quality of life, and mental health empowerment (Gennen et al., 2015; Powers et al., 2012, 2018). The foster care youth valued the program's emphasis on empowering their capacity to be self-directed, set goals, take action, be change agents, and generate support systems. The foster care youth also appreciated that the coaches were near their age with lived foster care experiences; facilitated reciprocal, nonjudgmental, and trusting relationships; were transparent and honest in their communications; provided logistical support; and encouraged the development of problem-solving and self-determination skills (Powers et al., 2018).

Centers for Independent Living Youth Program

Centers for independent living (CIL) programs are supported through funding authorized by the Rehabilitation Act of 1973. Programs support community living and independence and are consumer-controlled, nonresidential, and focused on the self-determination and full inclusion of people with disabilities. The IMAGE Center in Towson, Maryland, is a CIL that teamed with occupational therapy students from Towson University to develop youth programs that promote community participation and the development of prevocational skills. Graduate students completed a needs assessment for program development with the CIL youth program director, who also connected students to community agencies that had made inquiries about establishing collaborations with the IMAGE Center. The volunteer coordinator at the local zoo identified a need to include individuals with disabilities in the volunteer pool but had no background in working with individuals with disabilities. Guided by the PEOP model, the occupational therapy students outlined a potential program for transition-age youth that integrated the services of the IMAGE Center with the volunteer-training program at the zoo.

Initial assessment for the program included task analysis of the current and potential volunteer opportunities at the zoo (e.g., grounds work, greeting visitors, animal care); review of the current volunteer-training program materials and schedule; and individual evaluations of youth participants at the IMAGE Center youth program to assess interest, motivation, and skills for inclusion in the volunteer program (see Fig. 10-2). Interviews and standardized measurement tools were used to evaluate the personal skills of potential youth volunteers (e.g., social, cognitive, motor) and to evaluate the skills and attitudes of the trainers for the volunteer-training program (e.g., disability awareness). Students also evaluated the supports and barriers of the zoo environment related to accessibility for youth with disabilities. Ongoing assessment during program implementation monitored participants' skills and motivation so that accommodations could be made that would support success. The final program evaluation included feedback from youth participants, zoo volunteer trainers, supervisors, and the IMAGE Center youth coordinator.

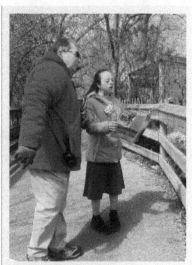

Figure 10-2 Volunteer docents at the zoo successfully guide transition-age interns with disabilities following training sessions conducted by occupational therapy students. *(From The IMAGE Center. Used with permission.)*

Program implementation consisted of 10 weekly meetings with 12 youth participants at the IMAGE Center. Four occupational therapy graduate students planned activities designed to develop community participation skills identified during individual evaluations. Sessions included topics related to social skills, communication, community mobility, budgeting, and self-advocacy. Some sessions included outings in the community to practice skills initially learned at the IMAGE Center. These included shopping, a scavenger hunt at the mall to identify prices and to initiate conversations with store clerks, and eating at a restaurant to integrate social and communication skills. Five participants were selected to participate in volunteer-training sessions at the zoo following the 10-week program. Occupational therapy students worked with the zoo staff to modify training methods and materials using UDL principles and provided staff with informational materials and resources regarding the inclusion of people with disabilities.

College Orientation and Life Activities Program

The number of youth on the autism spectrum who are transitioning from secondary school to college is increasing exponentially. Although they have the academic credentials to enroll in college, many struggle with the transition to a less structured environment with more discretionary time, requiring greater organizational and self-advocacy skills. Many colleges and universities have developed programs to assist them in their transition to college, providing academic and nonacademic supports for the development of time management, organization, personal self-care, social, and leisure skills.

The College Orientation and Life Activities Program (COLA) at Towson University was developed in partnership with occupational therapy graduate students and students with autism at the university. The PEOP model guided conceptualization of the program, and the development of the program structure and activities incorporated concepts of inclusion and self-determination. Before the semester begins, COLA students and their parents meet individually with the program director for an assessment of strengths and needs and the development of individualized goals for the academic year. Each COLA student is partnered with a neurotypical student mentor, with guidance and direction provided by the COLA program director during weekly meetings. Peer support is tailored to each COLA student's self-determined goals in areas of daily living, social experiences, academic success, and work exploration. During meetings with the program director, COLA students discuss progress toward goal attainment and develop a plan of action for the week. The program director also educates student peer mentors about inclusive, supportive relationship strategies that they can integrate into weekly activities with COLA partners. Depending on individualized goals, COLA students participate in a variety of campus activities such as joining study sessions, working out at the gym, attending social or sports events, and sharing meals. Both COLA students and peer mentors benefit from the partnership, with each student learning from the other. Student mentors learn to value the diversity of others, and COLA students develop valuable skills for community participation. For example, through participation in college activities or eating meals in the dining hall with mentors, participants develop social skills that can translate to working on a group project in a course or participating in networking at a job fair. The reduction in loneliness and isolation that COLA participants experience contributes to greater participation in academic courses and overall better mental health.

Summary

- Comprehensive, multiyear school-to-community transition services that integrate the active participation of youth, their families, and education and agency providers in the planning and implementation process promote successful transition to community life, postsecondary education, and productive pursuits.
- The Individuals With Disabilities Act (IDEA) and the Fostering Connections to Success and Increasing Adoptions Act mandate that youth with disabilities and those in foster care are entitled to transition services that encompass their needs and interests and that promote movement from school to postsecondary education, community inclusion, vocational education, and competitive employment.
- Limits to funding and program availability constrain access to adult services for which transition-age youth are eligible after high school.
- Occupation-based models focus services on occupations that are meaningful and purposeful during the transition process to advance the well-being and health of transition-age youth and promote their successful inclusion into adult life.
- Occupation-based assessment occurs at the person, institution, and population levels; it is a continuous process that simultaneously evaluates the interdependence of the person and environmental factors that contribute to successful participation in adult occupations.
- Best practice transition services incorporate strength-based models that facilitate self-determination, social relationships, community inclusion, and family involvement.

CASE STUDIES

CASE STUDY 10-1 Marietta

Marietta is a 17-year-old with spastic quadriplegic cerebral palsy who lives at home with her parents and 13-year-old sister. She is on a regular academic track at her local high school and is enrolled in Honors English courses. She would like to get together with friends and also participate in after-school clubs, but transportation is not always available. She relies on the school bus and her parents to take her to places in the community. Marietta would also like to have a summer job so that she has some money of her own. The occupational therapist interviewed Marietta and her parents and used the COPM to identify current occupational performance issues. The occupational therapist used the Functional Assessment of Cognitive Transit Skills to identify specific issues related to community mobility. With support from the occupational therapist at a transition-planning meeting, Marietta presented a summary of identified contextual barriers and supports and her goals for community inclusion to the school team. The team developed an intervention plan based on assessment results to include the use of public transportation, job application skills, and participation in after-school activities and community outings with friends.

Discussion Questions

1. What three critical components should be included in an initial interview with Marietta that will provide essential information to guide occupational therapy intervention related to goal attainment?
2. What strength-based strategies should the occupational therapist use when discussing score results of the standardized measurement tools with Marietta and her parents? Which scores are relevant to report?
3. What is the unique role of the occupational therapy practitioner on the transition-planning team? What specific occupation-based skills does the occupational therapist contribute to intervention planning?

CASE STUDY 10-2 Foster Care Transition Services from School to Community

The county social service agency has invited you to serve on a task force to investigate the need for transition services from school to the community for students and youth in foster care. In preparation for the first meeting, you conduct a literature review and learn that at least 23,000 students and youth age out of foster care every year (Sarubbi et al., 2016). Students are those who are in a school system; youth are those who may no longer be attending school but are still eligible for transition services (USDE, 2017). The Fostering Connections to Success and Increasing Adoptions Act of 2008 requires foster care agencies to have a defined transition plan 90 days before the youth become 18 years old or age out of the system. Forty-one states have extended foster care beyond 18 years of age, most by 1 additional year. These transition plans are to address housing, life skills, financial management, health insurance and management, health-care proxies, career supports and employment options, social support networks, and educational opportunities. Most states provide educational training vouchers, and 28 states grant some assistance with tuition and fees, but most have caps on the amount of money and the number of recipients (USDE, 2016). Fewer than 46% of foster care youth graduate from high school, and fewer than 3% earn a baccalaureate degree. Many are coping with issues of abuse, neglect, mental health and learning challenges, and food and housing insecurity (Sarubbi et al., 2016).

In preparation for the task force meeting, you choose the PEOP model and UDL to organize your initial thoughts about transition services for foster students and youth. Table 10-4 outlines some of the data to gather for conducting an occupation-based assessment at the person, organization, and population levels.

Table 10-4 Applying PEOP and UDL to Foster Care Transition Services: Data to Gather

	Personal	Organizations	Populations
	Student Family Kinship guardians	School Higher education industry Human service agency Health-care agency	Foster care students Foster care families Community
Narratives	Aspirations Goals Needs Interests	Mission Priorities Value systems Stakeholders	Needs and goals Foster care prevalence Community environments
Person factors	Cognitive Sensory, motor Neurophysiological Psychological Spiritual	Staff number and skills Staff preparation Diversity and motivation Institutional knowledge UDL application	Community demographics Social networks Barriers
Occupation factors	Educational levels Work experiences Self-care responsibilities Community responsibilities Leisure experiences	Institution's tasks Training programs Institutional services Populations served	Occupational access Occupational restrictions Occupational preparation Occupational stability

(*Continued*)

CASE STUDY 10-2 Foster Care Transition Services from School to Community

Table 10-4 Applying PEOP and UDL to Foster Care Transition Services: Data to Gather—cont'd

	Personal	Organizations	Populations
Environmental factors	Social networks Cultural supports Fiscal, legal supports Housing Transportation Health supports Accommodations Technology	Locations Accessibility Policies and regulations Institutional resources Accommodations	Government regulations Economic resources Community location Community systems Community infrastructure Community politics Community culture

Discussion Questions

1. What additional data do you want to gather to assess foster care transition services? Add at least two examples of data to collect for each of the sections in Table 10-4. View the following websites for ideas:
   - Child Trends (Child Trends, 2018)
   - Child Welfare Information Gateway (Child Welfare Information Gate, 2018)
   - Foster Care to Success (Foster Care to Success, 2018)
   - *Foster Youth in Transition* (Michigan Department of Health and Human Services, 2018)
2. What transition services are available for foster care youth in your county and state?
3. How can the domain and process of occupational therapy contribute to services that strengthen the transition outcomes for foster care youth?
4. What additional evidence-based knowledge and skills do you need to acquire to address the complexity of foster care transition issues?

Learning Activities

1. The Functional Assessment of Cognitive Transition Skills includes simple and complex trip planning in a community. Outline how you would facilitate this type of assessment in your own community.
2. Identify at least two resources in your own community that could provide greater mobility access to community activities for youth with disabilities.
3. Design three occupation-based opportunities that promote self-determination as part of the transition plan.
4. Describe socially inclusive activities that prepare a transition-age youth to meet the occupational demands of community living, postsecondary education, and product engagement.
5. Outline steps to include in a community mobility-training program that prepares a transition-age youth to navigate between home and a place of employment.

REFERENCES

American Occupational Therapy Association. (2014). Occupational therapy practice framework: Domain and process (3rd ed.). *American Journal of Occupational Therapy, 68*(Suppl. 1). http://dx.doi.org/10.5014/ajot.2014.682006

Anaby, D., Hand, C., Bradley, L., DiRezze, B., Forhan, M., DiGiacomo, A., and Law, M. (2013). The effect of the environment on participation of children and youth with disabilities: A scoping review. *Disability and Rehabilitation, 35*(19), 1589–1598. doi:10.3109/09638288.2012.748840

Askari, S., Anaby, D., Bergthorson, M., Majnemer, A., Elsabbagh, M., and Zwaigenbaum, L. (2015). Participation of children and youth with autism spectrum disorder: A scoping review. *Review Journal of Autism and Developmental Disorders, 2*(1), 103–114.

Bishop-Fitzpatrick, L., DaWalt, L. S., Greenberg, J. S., and Mailick, M. (2017). Participation in recreational activities buffers the impact of perceived stress on quality of life in adults with autism spectrum disorder. *Autism Research, 10,* 973–982.

Bryson, G., Bell, M. D., Lysaker, P., and Zito, W. (1997). The Work Behavior Inventory: Prediction of future work success of people with schizophrenia. *Psychiatric Rehabilitation Journal, 20*(4), 113–118.

Bunch, G., Finnegan, K., and Pearpoint, J. (2009). *Planning for real life after school: Ways for teachers and families to plan for students experiencing significant challenge.* Toronto, Canada: Inclusion Press.

CAST. (2011). *Universal design for learning guidelines version 2.0.* Retrieved from www.udlcenter.org/research/researchevidence

CAST. (2018). *UDL guidelines.* Retrieved from http://udlguidelines.cast.org

Chase, S., Ratcliff, G., and Hoesch, K. (1996). *Functional Assessment of Cognitive Transit Skills (FACTS).* Pittsburgh, PA: Project ACTION.

Chen, Y., Bundy, A., Cordier, R., Chien, Y., and Einfeld, S. (2016). The experience of social participation in everyday contexts among individuals with autism spectrum disorders: An experience sampling study. *Journal of Autism and Developmental Disorders, 46*(4), 1403–1414. doi:10.1007/s10803-015-2682-4

Child Trends. (2018). *Five things to know about transition from foster care.* Retrieved from www.childtrends.org/child-trends-5/five-things-to-know-about-the-transition-from-foster-care-to-adulthood/

Child Welfare Information Gate. (2018). *Transition to adulthood and independent living programs.* Retrieved from www.childwelfare.gov/topics/outofhome/independent/programs/

Christiansen, C. H., Baum, C. M., and Bass, J. D. (2015). *Occupational therapy: Performance, participation, and well-being* (4th ed.). Thorofare, NJ: SLACK.

Cleary, D. S., Persch, A. C., and Spencer, K. (2015). Transition to adulthood. In J. Case-Smith and J. C. O'Brien (Eds.), *Occupational therapy for children and adolescents* (7th ed., pp. 727–746). St. Louis, MO: Mosby.

Collier, M., Griffin, M., and Wei, Y. (2017). Learning from students about transition needs: Identifying gaps in knowledge and experience. *Journal of National Rehabilitation, 46,* 1–10. doi:10.3233/JVR-16087

Crabtree, L. (2014). The transition years: Adolescents to adults with intellectual and developmental disabilities. In K. Haertl (Ed.), *Adults with intellectual and developmental disabilities* (pp. 83–102). Bethesda, MD: AOTA Press.

Crabtree, L., and Sherwin, A. (2011). Begin with the end in mind: Promoting mental health, social participation, and self-determination in the transition from school to adult life. In S. Bazyk (Ed.), *Mental health promotion, prevention and intervention with children and youth* (pp. 267–286). Bethesda: AOTA Press.

Crabtree, L. A., and Demchick, B. B. (2015). Young adults on the autism spectrum: Perceived effects of participation in a university-based challenge course program in the community. *Occupational Therapy in Mental Health, 31*(3), 253–265.

Disabled World. (2013). *Children with disabilities and foster care.* Retrieved from www.disabled-world.com/disability/children/foster.php

Division of Rehabilitation Services. (2018). *Helping Marylanders with disabilities go to work.* Retrieved from dors.maryland.gov/Pages/default.aspx

Dunn, W. (2017). Strengths based approaches: What if even the "bad" things are good things? *British Journal of Occupational Therapy, 80*(7), 395–396.

Dunn, W., Koenig, K., Cox, J., Sabata, D., Pope, E., Foster, L., and Blackwell, A. L. (2013). Harnessing strengths: Daring to celebrate everyone's unique contributions: Part II. *OT Practice, 36,* 1–3.

Eaves, L. C., and Ho, H. H. (2008). Young adult outcomes of autism spectrum disorders. *Journal of Autism and Developmental Disorders, 38,* 739–747.

Eismann, M. M., Weisshaar, R., Capretta, C., Cleary, D. S., Kirby, A. V., and Persch, A. C. (2017). Centennial topics—characteristics of students receiving occupational therapy services in transition and factors related to postsecondary success. *American Journal of Occupational Therapy, 71,* 7103100010. https://doi.org/10.5014/ajot.2017.024927

Federal Partners in Transition Workgroup. (2015). *The 2020 Federal Youth Transition Plan: A federal interagency strategy.* Retrieved from www.dol.gov/odep/pdf/20150302-fpt.pdf

Field, S. L., and Hoffman, A. S. (1999). The importance of family involvement for promoting self-determination in adolescents with autism and other developmental disabilities. *Focus on Autism and Other Developmental Disabilities, 14,* 36–41.

Field, S. L., and Hoffman, A. S. (2012). Fostering self-determination through building productive relationships in the classroom. *Intervention in School and Clinic, 48*(1), 6–14.

Foster Care to Success. (2018). *America's college fund for foster youth.* Retrieved from www.fc2success.org/our-programs/

Geller, L. L., and Greenberg, M. (2010). Managing the transition process from high school to college and beyond: Challenges for individuals, families, and society. *Social Work in Mental Health, 8,* 92–116.

Gennen, S., Powers, L., Phillips, L., McKenna, I., Winges-Yanez, N., Croskey, A., . . . Research Consortium to Increase Success of Youth in Foster Care. (2015). A randomized field-test of a model for supporting young people in foster care with mental health challenges to participate in higher education. *Journal of Behavioral Health Services Research, 42*(2), 150–171. doi.org/10.1007/s11414-014-9451-6

Hehir, T. (2009). Policy foundations of universal design for learning. In D. T. Gordon, J. W. Gravel, and L. A. Schifter (Eds.), *A policy reader in universal design for learning* (pp. 35–45). Cambridge, MA: Harvard Education Press.

Hendricks, D., and Wehman, P. (2009). Transition from school to adulthood for youth with autism spectrum disorders: Review and recommendations. *Focus on Autism and Other Developmental Disorders, 24,* 77–88.

Hetherington, S. A., Durant-Jones, L., Johnson, K., Nolan, K., Smith, E., Taylor-Brown, S., and Tuttle, J. (2010). The lived experiences of adolescents with disabilities and their families in transition planning. *Focus on Autism and Other Developmental Disabilities, 25,* 163–172.

Hillier, A., Campbell, H., Mastriani, K., Izzo, M. V., Kool-Tucker, A., Cherry, L., and Beversdorf, B. O. (2007). Two year evaluation of a vocational support program for adults on the autism spectrum. *Career Development for Exceptional Individuals, 30*(1), 35–47.

Hutchinson, N. I., Versnel, J., Poth, C., Berg, D., deLugta, J., Daltona, C. J., . . . Munby, H. (2011). They want to come to school: Work-based education programs to prevent the social exclusion of vulnerable youth. *Work, 40*(2), 195–209.

Jameson, J. M., Riesen, T., Polychronis, S., Trader, B., Mizner, S., Martinis, J., and Hoyle, D. (2015). Guardianship and the potential of supported decision making with individuals with disabilities. *Research and Practice for Persons With Severe Disabilities, 40*(1), 36–51.

Kamps, D., Royer, J., Dugan, E., Kravits, T., Gonzalez-Lopez, A., Garcia, J., . . . Morrison, L. (2002). Peer training to facilitate social interaction for elementary students with autism and their peers. *Exceptional Children, 68*(2), 173–187.

Kardos, M., and White, B. P. (2005). The role of the school-based occupational therapist in secondary education transition planning: A pilot survey study. *American Journal of Occupational Therapy, 59,* 173–180.

Kingsnorth, S., Healy, H., and Macarthur, C. (2007). Preparing for adulthood: A systematic review of lifeskill programs for youth with physical disabilities. *Journal of Adolescent Health, 41*(4), 323–332.

Kiresuk, T. J., Smith, A., and Cardillo, J. P. (1994). *Goal attainment scaling: Application, theory, and measurement.* Hillsdale, NJ: Erlbaum.

Langi, F. L., Oberoi, A., Balcazar, F. E., and Awsumb, J. (2017). Vocational rehabilitation of transition-aged youth with disabilities: A propensity-score matched study. *Journal of Occupational Rehabilitation, 27,* 15–23.

Law, M., Baptiste, S., Carswell, A., McColl, M. A., Polatajko, H. J., and Pollock, N. (2005). *Canadian Occupational Performance Measure* (4th ed.). Ottawa, Canada: CAOT Publications Ace.

Lemmon, G. T. (2011, March 6). The Hillary doctrine. *Newsweek.* Retrieved from www.newsweek.com/hillary-doctrine-66105

Lough, C. L., Rice, M. S., and Lough, L. (2012). Choice as a strategy to enhance engagement in a colouring task in children with autism spectrum disorders. *Occupational Therapy International, 19*(4), 204–211.

Luecking, R. G., Fabian, E. S., Contreary, K., Honeycutt, T. C., and Luecking, D. M. (2018). Vocational rehabilitation outcomes for students participating in a model transition program. *Rehabilitation Counseling Bulletin, 61*(3), 154–163. Retrieved from https://doi.org/10.1177/0034355217713167

Maryland Developmental Disabilities Administration. (2018). *Welcome to Maryland Developmental Disabilities Administration.* Retrieved from https://dda.health.maryland.gov/Pages/home.aspx

Memari, A. H., Panahi, N., Ranjbar, E., Moshayedi, P., Shafiei, M., Kordi, R., and Ziaee, V. (2015). Children with autism spectrum disorder and patterns of participation in daily physical and play activities. *Neurology Research International.* doi:10.1155/2015/531906

Michigan Department of Health and Human Services. (2018). *Foster youth in transition: Michigan youth opportunities initiative.* Retrieved from www.michigan.gov/fyit/0,4585,7-240-44524-162619--,00.html

Migliore, A., Lyons, O., Butterworth, J., Nye-Lengerman, K., and Bose, J. (2018). A model of employment supports for job seekers with intellectual disabilities. *Journal of Rehabilitation, 84*(2), 3–13.

Moore-Corner, R. A., Kielhofner, G., and Olson, L. (1998). *A user's manual of work environment impact scale, version 2.0.* Chicago: Model of Human Occupation Clearinghouse, University of Illinois.

National Center for Education Statistics. (2018a). *Children and youth with disabilities.* Washington, DC: U.S. Department of Education. Retrieved from https://nces.ed.gov/programs/coe/indicator_cgg.asp

National Center for Education Statistics. (2018b). *The condition of education: Participation in education—elementary/secondary—children and youth with disabilities indicator.* Washington, DC: U.S. Department of Education. Retrieved from https://nces.ed.gov/programs/coe/indicator_cgg.asp

Noreau, L., Fougeyrollas, P., and Vincent, C. (2002). The LIFE-H: Assessment of the quality of social participation. *Technology and Disability, 14*(3), 113–118.

113th Congress. (2013–2014). *H.R.647—Able Act of 2014.* Retrieved from www.congress.gov/bill/113th-congress/house-bill/647

Plotner, A. J., Oertle, K. M., Reed, G. J., Tissot, K., and Kumpiene, G. (2017). Centers for independent living and their involvement with transition-age youth with disabilities. *Journal of Vocational Rehabilitation, 46*(1), 39–48. doi:10.3233/JVR-160841

Powers, L., Fullerton, A., Schmidt, J., Geenen, S., Oberweiser-Kennedy, M., Dohn, J., . . . Research Consortium to Increase Success of Youth in Foster Care. (2018). Perspectives of youth in foster care on essential ingredients for promoting self-determination and successful transition to adult life: My life model. *Children and Youth Service Review, 8,* 277–286. doi.org/10.1016/j.childyouth.2018.02.007

Powers, L., Geenen, S., Powers, J., Pommier-Satya, S., Turner, A., Dalton, L., . . . Swank, P. (2012). My life: Effects of a longitudinal randomized study of self-determination enhancement on the transition outcomes of youth in foster care and special education. *Children and Youth Services Review, 34*(11), 2179–2187. doi.org/10.1016/j.childyouth.2012.07.018

Revell, G., and Miller, L. A. (2008). Navigating the world of adult services and benefits planning. In P. Wehman, M. Datlow-Smith, and C. Schall (Eds.). *Autism and the transition to adulthood: Success beyond the classroom* (pp. 139–162). Baltimore, MD: Brookes.

Riesen, T., Schultz, J., Morgan, R., and Kupferman, S. (2014). School-to-work barriers as identified by special educators, vocational rehabilitation counselors, and community rehabilitation professionals. *Journal of Rehabilitation, 80*(1), 33–44. Retrieved from www.questia.com/library/p5155/the-journal-of-rehabilitation

Rinaldi, M., Killackey, E., Smith, J., Shepherd, G., Singh, S. P., and Craig, T. (2010). First episode psychosis and employment: A review. *International Review of Psychiatry, 22*(2), 148–162. doi:10.3109/09540261003661825

Rose, D. H., and Meyer, A. (2002). *Teaching every student in the digital age: Universal design for learning.* Alexandria, VA: Association for Supervision and Curriculum Development.

Sarubbi, M., Parker, E., and Sponsler, B. A. (2016). *Strengthening policies for foster youth post-secondary attainment.* Denver, CO: Education Commission of the States. Retrieved from www.ecs.org/strengthening-policies-for-foster-youth-postsecondary-attainment/

Shattuck, P. T., Orsmond, G. I., Wagner, M., and Cooper, B. P. (2011). Participation in social activities among adolescents with an autism spectrum disorder. *PLoS ONE, 6*(11), e27176. doi:10.1371/journal.pone.0027176

Shogren, K. A., Wehmeyer, M. L., Palmer, S. B., Rifenbark, G., and Little, T. (2015). Relationships between self-determination and postschool outcomes for youth with disabilities. *Journal of Special Education, 48*(4), 256–267.

Sparrow, S. S., Cicchetti, D. V., and Balla, D. A. (2005). *Vineland Adaptive Behavior Scales* (2nd ed.). Circle Pines, MN: American Guidance Service.

Stewart, D., Gorter, J. W., and Freeman, M. (2013). Transitions to adulthood for youth with disabilities: Emerging themes for practice and research. *Prevention Researcher, 20*(2), 3–6.

Taylor, J., Adams, R. E., and Bishop, S. L. (2017). Social participation and its relation to internalizing symptoms among youth with autism spectrum disorder as they transition from high school. *Autism Research, 10,* 663–672.

U.S. Centers for Medicare and Medicaid Services. (2018). *Medicaid and CHIP coverage.* Retrieved from www.healthcare.gov/medicaid-chip/getting-medicaid-chip/

U.S. Department of Education. (2016). *Foster care transition toolkit.* Retrieved from www2.ed.gov/about/inits/ed/foster-care/youth-transition-toolkit.pdf

U.S. Department of Education. (2018a). *Higher Education Opportunity Act 2008.* Retrieved from https://ed.gov/policy/highered/leg/hea08/index.html

U.S. Department of Education. (2018b). *Vocational rehabilitation state grants.* Retrieved from www2.ed.gov/programs/rsabvrs/index.html

U.S. Department of Education, Office of Special Education and Rehabilitative Services. (2017, May). *A transition guide to postsecondary education and employment for students and youth with disabilities.* Retrieved from www2.ed.gov/about/offices/list/osers/transition/products/postsecondary-transition-guide-may-2017.pdf?utm_name=

U.S. Department of Health and Human Services. (2018a). *Healthy People 2030 foundational framework.* Retrieved from www.healthypeople.gov/2020/About-Healthy-People/Development-Healthy-People-2030/Proposed-Framework

U.S. Department of Health and Human Services. (2018b). *HHD 2018 budget in brief.* Retrieved from www.hhs.gov/about/budget/fy2018/budget-in-brief/acl/index.html

U.S. Department of Health and Human Services, Administration for Community Living. (n.d.). *Centers for independent living.* Retrieved from www.acl.gov/programs/aging-and-disability-networks/centers-independent-living

U.S. Department of Justice and Civil Rights Division. (2018). *The Americans With Disabilities Act of 1990 and revised ADA regulations implementing Title II and Title III.* Retrieved from www.ada.gov/2010_regs.htm

U.S. Department of Labor. (2017). *Job corps: Careers begin here.* Retrieved from www.jobcorps.gov/

U.S. Department of Labor. (2018a). *Laws and regulations, Rehabilitation Act of 1973.* Retrieved from www.dol.gov/general/topic/disability/laws

U.S. Department of Labor. (2018b). *The Work Innovation and Opportunity Act.* Retrieved from www.doleta.gov/wioa/

Webb, K. W., Patterson, K., Syverud, S. M., and Seabrooks-Blackmore, J. J. (2008). Evidence based practices that promote transition to postsecondary education: Listening to a decade of expert voices. *Exceptionality, 16,* 192–106.

Wehman, P. (2013). *Life beyond the classroom: Transition strategies for young people with disabilities.* Baltimore, MD: Brookes.

Wehmeyer, M., and Abery, B. (2013). Self-determination and choice. *Journal of Intellectual and Developmental Disabilities, 51*(5), 399–411.

Wehmeyer, M. L. (2014). Self-determination: A family affair. *Family Relations: Interdisciplinary Journal of Applied Family Studies, 63*(1), 178–184.

Whiteford, G., and Townsend, E. (2011). Participatory occupational justice framework (POJF 2010): Enabling occupational participation and inclusion. In F. Kronenberg, N. Pollard, and D. Sakellariou (Eds.), *Occupational therapies without borders: Towards an ecology of occupation-based practices* (Vol. 2, pp. 65–84). Philadelphia, PA: Elsevier.

Woodman, A. C., Smith, L. E., Greenberg, J. S., and Malick, M. R. (2016). Contextual factors predict patterns of change in functioning over 10 years among adolescents and adults with autism spectrum disorders. *Journal of Autism and Developmental Disorders, 46,* 176–189.

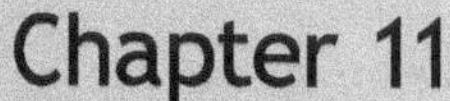

Chapter 11

Promoting Community Inclusion and Integration for Youth

Amanda C. Jozkowski, PhD, OTR/L, and Sarah Anne Hewitt, BA

A deep sense of love and belonging is an irreducible need of all people. We are biologically, cognitively, physically, and spiritually wired to love, to be loved, and to belong. When those needs are not met, we don't function as we were meant to. We break. We fall apart. We numb. We ache. We hurt others. We get sick.

—Brené Brown (2010)

Learning Outcomes

This chapter is designed to enable the reader to:

11-1 Substantiate the importance of community inclusion and integration to support success as a youth and an adult.

11-2 Articulate the contributions of occupational therapy to community inclusion and integration programs and services for youth.

11-3 Describe an occupation-based model and use it to explain and assess the features of community inclusion and integration programs.

11-4 Describe national, regional, and state programs that promote community inclusion and integration programs and services for youth.

11-5 Describe best practices to support community inclusion and integration programs and services for youth.

11-6 Apply evaluation strategies to support occupation-based community inclusion and integration programs and services for youth.

Key Terms

Authentic participation
Community integration
Inclusion
Preventative approach
Strengths-based approach

Introduction

Asserting the importance of community involvement for youth with disabilities and describing ways that occupational therapy practitioners can support this ideal, Ideishi, D'Amico, and Jirikowic (2013) write that "all people, regardless of abilities, should have access to, choice of, and an opportunity to participate in a full range of community activities" (p. 1). Utilizing a life-course perspective, occupational therapy practitioners can support the development of children and youth, regardless of their abilities, through inclusive community programming. Inclusive community programming from a positive development perspective affords opportunities to develop "competence, confidence, character, and connections and making contributions" (Petrenchik and King, 2011, p. 88). Such an inclusive community focus "is often more important than individual skill performance" (Bolton, Plattner, and Faulkner, 2018, p. 17). When young people are included in the community and feel a sense of *belonging* and *purpose* (as Brené Brown so eloquently states in the epigraph), developmental goals can be achieved. In addition, healthy communities are inclusive of all citizens.

As individuals move from childhood to adulthood, occupational opportunities ideally expand, along with their growing access to and engagement with the environment. Initially, children's primary contexts are often in the home and school, but they quickly develop the desire for access to other spaces for participation, such as playground/recreation facilities, natural outdoor spaces, community services and facilities (e.g., transportation, grocery stores, library), and the homes of peers. Depending on the particular affordances of these environments, or those factors that make the space both functional and meaningful (Hadavi, Kaplan, and Hunter, 2015), youth may be integrated into or excluded from aspects of community life. For example, accessible seating areas can be arranged to encourage socialization and allow individuals with varying mobility needs to participate together.

As social work scholar Brené Brown discussed in the 2010 TED Talk quoted above, belonging is desired by all, and a lack of belonging may lead to mental distress and physical pain. Engagement in community occupations is critical to developing a sense of purpose and belonging. By supporting youth in identifying, exploring, and engaging in community occupations, working to develop skills for community participation, and intervening in the community context, the occupational therapy practitioner can prevent or limit disability and isolation.

Community integration is the incorporation of diverse individuals into a group, society, or organization. Typically, individuals thought to be "integrated" retain their labels, so an ethnic group, social class, religion, or other identity marker remains, which can lead to prejudice and isolation, despite all group members ostensibly having the same rights and privileges. **Inclusion,** however, incorporates the core value and principle of *Justice* (American Occupational Therapy Association [AOTA], 2015). In an inclusive model, individuals are offered more than simply the same treatment or conditions as others; they are provided support to access and participate in larger group activities based on their unique needs and interests (Thompson, 2017). Hagiliassis et al. (2014) depict inclusion as a multidimensional construct that includes factors such as social participation, supportive and affirming societal relationships, and access to services, materials, and economic resources. These factors align with two of the social determinants of mental health identified by the World Health Organization (WHO), which include community involvement and social interaction and support (WHO, 2014).

Engage Your Brain 11-1

What other occupational therapy core values and ethical principles support community integration and inclusive program development for children and youth?

To highlight the importance of inclusion, the AOTA (2018) *Vision 2025* statement begins: "As an inclusive profession . . ." The statement then details a vison of occupational therapy practice that includes "working with clients and within systems to produce effective outcomes" and "provide[ing] culturally responsive and customized services" (AOTA, 2018, p. 3). Language concerning working *within systems* in a *culturally responsive* and *customized* manner encourages practitioners to remain person-centered while addressing individual and community-level needs to facilitate occupational participation and maximize health. For youth, inclusion involves access to occupational opportunities in the community, which will lead to new learning (e.g., executive function), social participation, employment possibilities, and other skills for instrumental activities of daily living, facilitating the successful transition to independent adulthood or person-centered supportive services. In this chapter, examples of exemplary community integration and inclusion programming for youth are provided, including discussion of the benefits, challenges, and considerations for the occupational therapy practitioner seeking to develop or implement such programs.

Occupational Therapy Roles and Services

Although occupational therapy practitioners might initially think of those with intellectual and developmental disabilities (IDD) or mobility limitations as the target clients for community inclusion interventions, children and youth with mental health conditions or chronic illness also would benefit. Additionally, those who might otherwise be excluded from community participation, such as immigrants or refugees, speakers of other languages, LGBTQ+ youth, and young people with a wide range of other identity-related differences, should be considered for potential outreach (see Chapter 22 in this text for additional information on these populations).

Roles and Scope of Service

Occupational therapy practitioners may serve in formal and informal advisory or leadership roles in programs and organizations such as those described above, offering their expertise in adapting activities and promoting inclusive practices. Occupational therapy practitioners' professional contributions are different from those provided by community advocates and other professions, such as social work, parks and recreation, and education. Occupational therapy's unique focus on prevention and health promotion, in combination with a nuanced understanding of the complexities of the environment and its effect on participation, results in an occupation-based community practice paradigm (Scaffa, 2001). As the profession moves toward a doctorally prepared workforce, additional opportunities for program development, evaluation, and community-based research abound. Partnering with existing organizations to develop, expand, or refine programming is a good way to initiate collaboration and could potentially lead to the creation of a new position for the occupational therapy practitioner. Inclusive programming can take many forms, as outlined in Box 11-1, and can be achieved through creative community practice

Box 11-1 Occupational Therapy Interventions to Support Community Integration for Individuals With IDD

Occupational therapy services to support community integration may include interventions to:

- Educate caregivers in the best ways to communicate, organize, include, and engage clients in daily home chores and family activities by providing consistency, focusing on skills, and structuring tasks at the level of their differently abled family member
- Provide sensitivity training to public services providers such as local police, fire, and emergency medical personnel on strategies for engaging and communicating with people of different abilities
- Provide community education and training to various business and community members such as store owners, bus drivers, airport personnel, restaurant staff, movie theater staff, and other health-care providers about sensory sensitivities and communication strategies for individuals with diverse learning needs
- Design accessibility and educational programs at public institutions for individuals with different learning needs
- Educate business owners, public policy makers, and community developers about universal design principles, inclusion, and access to services for individuals with IDD
- Foster, support, or develop community-based work experiences in collaboration with existing business owners and service providers in local communities
- Design and implement special training courses for individuals with IDD who live in group homes, focusing on cooking, homemaking, personal care, leisure activities, and other areas of interest
- Design and implement prevocational and vocational training in collaboration with employment services and other rehabilitation service providers
- Provide training and support for the development of inclusive youth services such as child care, community recreational programs, and extracurricular activities

From *Fact Sheet: Supporting Community Integration and Participation for Individuals With Intellectual Disabilities,* by R. Ideishi, M. D'Amico, and T. Jirikowic, 2013, Bethesda, MD: American Occupational Therapy Association. Used with permission.

or connection to local academic institutions, as described below.

Participation in occupation-focused community programs offers two-pronged benefits to adults and youth alike who may be at risk for isolation and disability. In addition to individuals who receive clinic-based services, this may include children who receive early intervention or school-based services, as well as individuals at risk for or marginalized by economic status, immigration status, war, and other issues of occupational injustice. Benefits to community-focused intervention include: (1) continued work on performance components to address personal goals, often filling a gap in the continuum of care once clients have exhausted reimbursable therapy sessions or progress has slowed and (2) increased opportunity to socialize, develop a sense of autonomy and empowerment, and network with like individuals (S. Lawson, personal communication, October 22, 2018).

Many occupational therapy clients are discharged from formal rehabilitation settings and do not immediately resume their prior level of participation. For example, a youth who sustains a head injury while playing football may be allowed to return to school but may still have difficulty concentrating and may not be cleared to return to sports participation. An occupational therapy practitioner might work with the youth and his family to identify safe alternatives that allow him to be physically active and remain part of a social group or team, such as a hip-hop dance class, rowing club, or swim team.

Theoretical Models and Frameworks

The **preventative approach** to community programming also allows practitioners to address potential health concerns before they occur (or reoccur) by connecting participants to additional resources and practice opportunities in the natural environment (S. Lawson, personal communication, October 22, 2018). For children and their families, this may include help locating adaptive equipment and assistive technologies in the community, finding accessible parks and recreation opportunities, and engaging with other families of children with special needs for social interaction, connection, and respite.

The **strengths-based approach**, frequently used by community-based practitioners working with children and youth (Dunn, 2011), emphasizes both physical and psychological inclusion and articulates well with models of positive youth development, which come primarily from mental health disciplines. Petrenchik and King (2011) discuss the adaptive process youth undergo in order to "contribute positively to self, family, community, and civil society" as they mature (p. 72). Their model is unequivocally occupation-based, in that meaningful activity (i.e., occupation), setting (i.e., environment), and experiences (i.e., person or client factors) are central to the development of the senses of self-competence, self-understanding, and belonging. "Positive development," they write, "is fertilized by ongoing participation in *safe, developmentally supportive* life situations in which children and youth enjoy *supportive relationships* with adults and peers, have *meaningful opportunities for involvement* and membership, and *participate actively* in challenging and engaging activities" (Petrenchik and King, 2011, p. 72 [original authors' emphasis]). This assertion encompasses the principles of best practice occupational therapy and can be used to model inclusive community-based programming for youth (Fig. 11-1).

The authors also discuss the restorative and regulatory effects of participation in meaningful or valued places, which, combined with opportunities for social belonging and occupational engagement, can lead to "developmentally favorable" outcomes (Petrenchik and King, 2011, p. 81). **Authentic participation,** also conceptualized as "occupation-in-context" (Gupta and Taff, 2015), aligns with the "most integrated setting" requirements called for in Title II regulations issued under section 504 of the Rehabilitation Act (28 C.F.R. § 35.130, 1991). Therefore, participation in positive "person-in-environment transactions" (in this

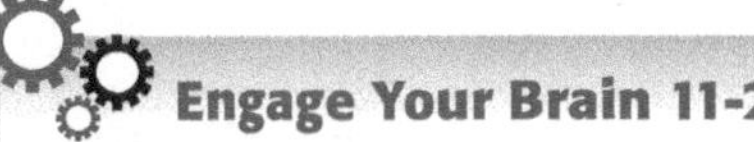

Engage Your Brain 11-2

How can an occupational therapy practitioner promote the inclusion of medically fragile children and youth?

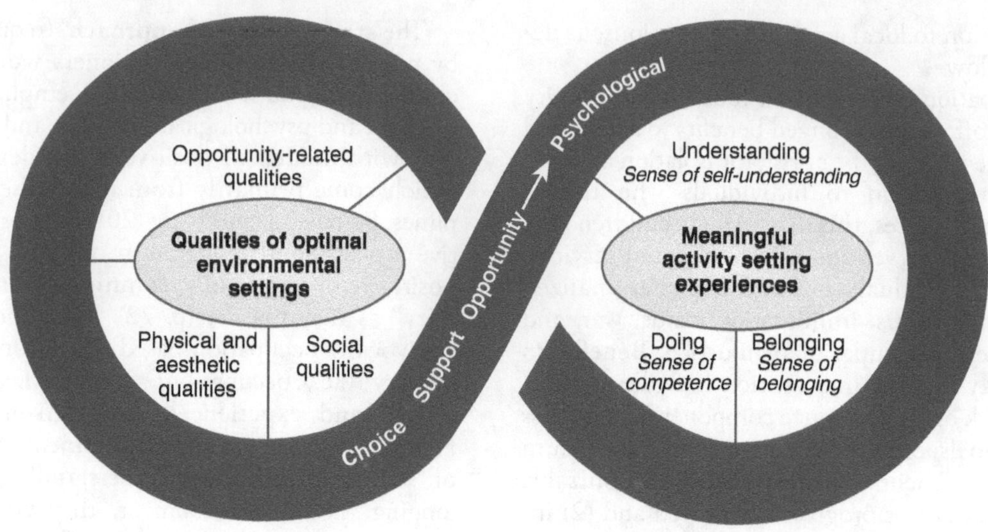

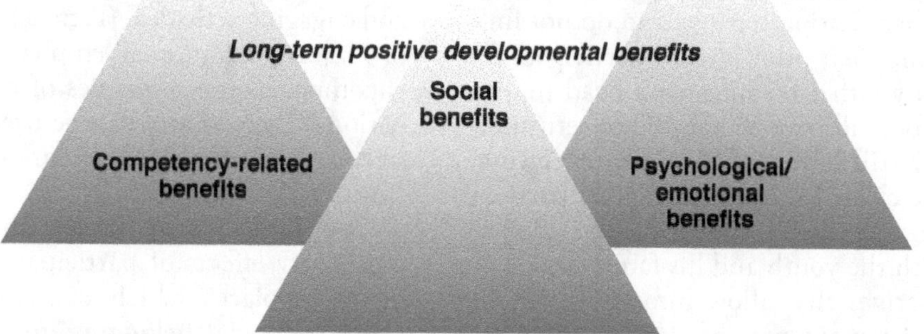

Figure 11-1 A developmental health model of the relationships between environmental qualities and growth-enhancing experiences. Constructs that are important in the derivation of positive benefits from activity participation are embedded within contextual features of optimal environments (Eccles and Templeton, 2002). On the left side, the model incorporates what is known about qualities of optimal environmental settings. The right side of the model is based on work by King, Petrenchik, Law, and Hurley (2009). Meaningful activity-specific experiences arise through doing, belonging, and understanding (King, 2004). *(Adapted from "Pathways to Positive Development: Childhood Participation in Everyday Places and Activities [Figure 4.2, p. 86]," by T. Petrenchik and G. King, in S. Bazyk [Ed.],* Mental Health Promotion, Prevention and Intervention for Children and Youth: A Guiding Framework, *2011, Bethesda, MD: AOTA Press.)*

case, supported community-based occupation) can facilitate healthy outcomes for children and youth (Merryman, Mezei, Bush, and Weinstein, 2012), and programs offered in such contexts are also more likely to be reimbursed by federally funded agencies.

Additionally, models of community integration and inclusion from the fields of community planning and institutional leadership/human resources can be applied to occupational therapy intervention, especially when seeking to conduct larger-scale programming. Salzer and Barron (2006) provide a comprehensive discussion of inclusive practices in the workplace, including useful definitions of terms, identification of eight dimensions of community integration, and strategies for assessing and addressing barriers to these dimensions, such as incident response, the development of a sense of belonging, and a process of inclusive decision-making.

Thompson (2017) describes the difficulty in measuring inclusion and diversity in an organization, given the wide-ranging definitions of these constructs. However, because evidence is critical to implementing best practice interventions, organizations are encouraged to conduct comprehensive and critical self-studies to determine priority areas for enhancing inclusion. These may include general climate, engagement, productivity, recruitment and retention, development and advancement, market impact, and compliance. Some of these factors may be more or less relevant to occupational therapy practitioners, depending on their role (for example, as a program consultant vs. a practice owner). However, all occupational therapy practitioners implementing community-based programs would do well to review materials produced by organizations such as the Employers Network for Equality and Inclusion (2017), which offers workshops, assessment guidelines, and other resources for businesses seeking to improve inclusivity in the workplace and greater community.

Engage Your Brain 11-3

How can an occupational therapy practitioner make a program or space more inclusive when permanent physical changes cannot be made to the property?

Program Exemplars

Many different types of exemplars can be reviewed and used to stimulate the adaptation of existing programs to include an occupation lens or the innovation of new programs to enhance inclusion and occupational engagement for communities and populations; some of these exemplars are described in this section. Programs delivered at national and international levels are described, as are occupation-based programs. In addition, an illustration of how universities can leverage their resources to simultaneously serve the local community while enriching future health professionals' education is detailed.

National and International Programs

Offering nationally recognized exemplars of integration, Easterseals therapeutic programs highlight helping children meet milestones "at their own pace," with a strong emphasis on accessibility for all in their residential and day camps, barrier-free recreation programs, and employment-training opportunities (Easterseals, 2018). Although these programs are geared toward youth with disabilities, they support community integration through the co-participation of youth with and without disabilities in activities such as horseback riding, swimming, and transportation use in the natural setting.

The Girl Scouts of the United States of America and the Boy Scouts of America practice inclusive programming, welcoming youth with disabilities into their troops, providing training and resources for volunteer leaders, and offering merit badges and related honors for Scouts. For example, Girl Scouts can earn the Ability, Awareness, and Inclusion patch, and Boy Scouts can work toward a Disabilities Awareness merit badge and the Special Needs Scouting Service Award (Boy Scouts of America, 2018; Girl Scouts of the United States of America, 2017). The goal of full inclusion is described on the Boy Scouts website: "Every boy wants to participate fully and be respected like every other member of the troop" (Boy Scouts of America, 2018, para. 1). Youth with disabilities are encouraged to enroll in camps, participate in outdoor experiences, and serve in leadership positions within each of these organizations.

Best Buddies International (BBI) promotes friendship, employment, and leadership opportunities for individuals with intellectual and developmental disabilities (IDD). Participants are paired with typically developing peers and helped to form meaningful friendships that may lead to improved self-advocacy, communication skills, social participation, and community involvement. Community integration is achieved by partnering individuals with special needs with those without special needs for social interaction (BBI, 2018).

Very Special Arts is an international organization that seeks to increase access to the arts for all, by integrating people with disabilities into art experiences and education (Kennedy Center, 2018). The programs are offered in schools by art educators trained in inclusion practices. In addition, the organization works to help people with disabilities pursue careers in the arts and access community-based art and culture facilities.

Occupation-Based Programs

The Moco Movement Center (MMC), a pediatric therapy clinic in the Washington, DC, area, is an admirable example of combining outpatient practice with inclusive programming. Therapists at the MMC provide occupational, physical, and speech therapy sessions to children from birth to young adulthood in a sensorimotor gym. However, the clinic also offers a range of inclusion opportunities for children and families. These are composed of integrated summer camps, gymnastics, and music classes for clients and their siblings and child-directed interventions conducted with typically developing peers outside the clinic in public recreation spaces such as playgrounds, a rock-climbing center, and an ice hockey arena. This interdisciplinary method has been deemed *Applied Functional Therapy*™. Founder Andrea Santman states that

> *by taking evidence-based pediatric therapy out of the clinic and integrating it into real life activities, no child misses out on social engagement—we find something for every child to connect with. . . . Children can play and practice real-life skills needed to participate with their community, peers, and family. (A. Santman, personal communication, November 20, 2018)*

Offering birthday parties and social events at the MMC transforms the space from a clinical setting to a community recreation facility available to all community members, where children receiving services have expressed that they do not feel separate or different but rather part of something desirable and fun for all.

Yachad, the National Jewish Council for Disabilities, is an international organization that provides inclusive opportunities for people with disabilities to participate in Jewish life (Yachad, n.d.). New England Yachad, a regional office of the organization, has volunteers who participate in the organization's social and recreational programs so that participants with disabilities have an opportunity to interact with typically developing peers (Fig. 11-2). Activities include an outing to a snow-tubing park, weekend retreats, and bowling. Participants can also receive one-on-one support during an activity from a trained volunteer or staff member, so they receive the attention they need (C. Sandberg, personal communication, December 21, 2018). Chana Sandberg, an occupational therapist who works for the organization, states that task analysis skills and education and training for staff, volunteers, and families are valued skills that occupational therapy practitioners can provide to community programs like Yachad (personal communication, December 21, 2018).

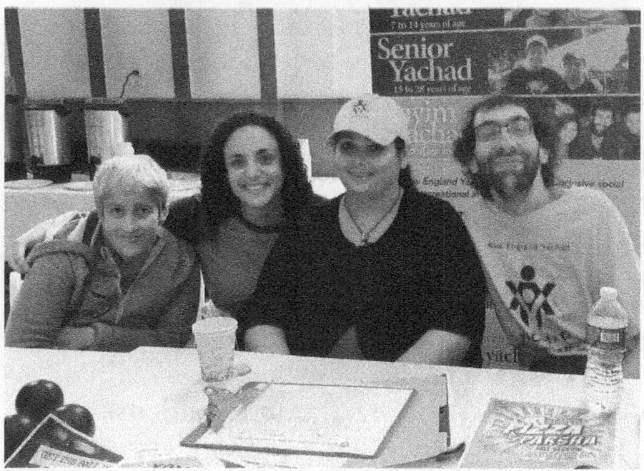

Figure 11-2 Yachad participants and neurotypical peers enjoy learning and socializing during a Pizza and Parsha program session at Cafe Eilat in Brookline, Massachusetts. Pizza and Parsha is a weekly informal Jewish learning program that brings individuals with disabilities and neurotypical peers together for learning and fun over a pizza dinner. *(Used with permission from Orthodox Union.)*

In addressing the needs of youth and their families as they move toward adulthood, transition planning is a critical area for potential occupational therapy intervention. Once students age out of the school system, there may be a gap in services or limited community resources available. Occupational therapists can adopt a strengths-based approach to assessing older students' skills and interests and identifying potential job sites, recreation opportunities, and living situations (Dunn, 2011). The strengths-based approach encourages occupational therapy practitioners to identify characteristics (or client factors) of an individual or group that support participation and to consider these as the foundation for intervention planning and outcomes assessment, as opposed to a focus on deficits (Dunn, 2011). Occupational therapists may provide intervention to an individual, working directly with the client to develop or restore skills, and may also serve in an advocate or case manager role, coordinating team members for planning, as well as researching and communicating with agencies and services, always with a mind toward community participation. Dunn (2011) emphasizes the importance of documenting outcomes related to transition and sharing evidence with the community. As best practices in transition planning are still emerging, processes and outcomes are vital for communities to better understand the needs of young citizens and to develop additional supports as indicated.

As youth and young adults begin to form and maintain friendships and transition to work and/or higher education pursuits, occupational therapy interventions should increasingly move into community spaces. Interventions may include

> *adapting or modifying curricula, the environment, or activities to support participation in educational routines and learning activities; navigating more complex social relationships, including dating; assessing the skills needed to learn to drive or assisting with alternative community mobility options; strengthening self-determination and decision making skills, and enhancing overall independence; helping with vocational planning and transitions, including employer supports; and planning for transition to college, including time management, study habits and routines, and independent living skills (AOTA, 2014, p. 1)*

Several programs addressing sexual health and dating, developed by occupational therapists for youth and young adults with special needs, have recently been described in the literature. One program uses an inclusive approach to evaluate the curriculum by encouraging educators and practitioners to:

- Reflect on whether the learning activities are accessible, developmentally appropriate, and engaging for all
- Consider parent concerns
- Utilize activity analysis to grade the content as necessary (Swanton, 2017)

Swanton (2017) argues that all adolescents and young adults have the right to information about sexual health, and meeting the needs of each student in an individualized manner is meaningful and empowering. Similarly, McCarthy (2018) provides suggestions on how to thoughtfully incorporate occupation into client-centered interventions around dating. The author suggests that practitioners might create an online dating profile with the client, role play, or actually go on a mock date in the community and "browse online social groups to expand . . . opportunities to meet people" (McCarthy, 2018, p. 15). Working with youth and young adults to prepare for the developmental milestones of relationships and sexual encounters, including skills such as grooming and social interaction, is an especially salient and distinctive role for the occupational therapy practitioner. Few other disciplines may have the same level of comfort, resources, or training to assist in this area (Eglseder and Webb, 2017).

Engage Your Brain 11-4

What are ways that technology, including tablets, smart speakers, and virtual and augmented reality, can contribute to the inclusion of young people with disabilities?

Engage Your Brain 11-5

What are the pros and cons of not having medically confirmed diagnoses of individuals in an inclusive program?

University-Community Partnerships

A unique example of the potential of university-community partnerships for inclusive programming can be seen at Towson University, near Baltimore, Maryland. The university-affiliated Institute for Well-Being (IWB), a spacious facility about a mile from the main campus, houses the Occupational Therapy Center, Speech and Language Center, Hearing and Balance Center, Wellness (fitness/recreation) Center, and the Hussman Center for Adults With Autism. Students from several health-professional degree programs assist with programming and complete professional training at the IWB while serving the health and well-being needs of community members. In addition, the βTU—Partnership at Work for Greater Baltimore (n.d.) presidential initiative encourages Towson University faculty and students to collaborate with community partners for service learning, research, health promotion, and community development and provides funding support and other resources to enhance this transactional work. Through the IWB and βTU, opportunities to promote community well-being and support interprofessional education and collaboration are abundant. Occupational therapy professor Marlene Riley, a long-time advocate and initiator of community partnerships, sees such arrangements as "win-win-win." Riley says that as guidelines for service providers and funding regulations shift to require services in the "most integrated setting" (Olmstead 527 U.S. 581, 1999), students at Towson University can plan and implement community-based programs, meet learning goals, and provide a connection for clients to resources and organizations in the community (M. Riley, personal communication, November 7, 2018).

In addition to clinical therapeutic offerings, a wide range of programs designed to engage local community members in new experiences are offered at the campus-affiliated IWB. One example is the Studio One day program for transition-age individuals with IDD and their families, which provides meaningful and integrated involvement in the community for those who have exited high school but may not qualify for additional services until age 21. Occupational therapy graduate students work with Professor Riley to develop relationships with external agencies, conduct a needs assessment in collaboration with potential clients, and implement group programming. In the first year, this resulted in participants working together with occupational therapy students to identify a desired activity and outcome (i.e., creating art and being perceived as artists) and develop a plan for successful performance. Program participants designed, fabricated, and sold beaded crafts in a public space along with typically developing artists, an example of client-centered care (Riley, 2014).

Other community programs at Towson University include the Pre-Driver Readiness Program, which prepares teens and young adults for driving by providing individualized instruction in safe driving practices, along with scaffolding of functional activities by an occupational therapy practitioner, to holistically address cognitive, visual, physical, perceptual, and timing skills (Towson University, 2018). The Cooking 101 Program, run by occupational therapy faculty and students, helps neurodiverse young adults plan a meal and work safely in the kitchen alongside college student peers. Participants build skills (*occupation-as-means*) in planning, organization, decision-making, group interaction, and stress management, but the group is also an opportunity for social participation and friend making, an example of *occupation-as-ends* (C. Exner, personal communication, October 24, 2018).

A seminar course offered every summer through the Towson University Honors College provides an overview of autism across the life span, service delivery models, and community resources for occupational therapy majors and other majors across the university. The course includes a service-learning trip to a surfing camp for children and young adults with autism. University students support participation of the campers in the surfing activities with therapeutic strategies such as individualized coping skills and sensory regulation techniques and interacting with families to understand their lived experiences (Towson University Honors College, 2018). Rather than serve as care providers, the university students learn about being part of the community and improve their comfort with approaching and interacting with individuals with disabilities and special health-care needs.

The above examples highlight the collaborative potential of educational institutions and community organizations to provide inclusive programming. The goals of inclusion and community participation are amplified when programs benefit both community members and university students. For example, preprofessional speech therapy students who completed a portion of their clinical education at the IWB's Hussman Center for Adults With Autism reported that immersive group experiences, such as Friday Night Social Group at the center, resulted in personal and professional growth in a range of areas. These included increased opportunities to interact with neurodiverse individuals, improved collaboration with other students and professionals, and enhanced clinical knowledge and skills, such as increased confidence and openness to working with potential clients on the autism spectrum (Wilson, Chasson, Jozkowski, and Mulhern, 2017). Like the health professions students, Hussman Center members with autism also rated program experiences highly and indicated that the opportunity to interact with students as peers, rather than in a medical/intervention model, was enjoyable, empowering, and destigmatizing (Krutt, Dyer, Arora, Rollman, and Jozkowski, 2018).

Engage Your Brain 11-6

What are the benefits of a community inclusion program that individual clinic-based occupational therapy cannot provide?

Additional Considerations

When planning programs, occupational therapy practitioners should also consider issues such as program location and qualities of the space, as well as needs that may be unique to specific client populations. Practitioners should familiarize themselves with these characteristics within partner organizations, in addition to organizational structure and culture, in order to anticipate challenges and provide recommendations to create the most supportive environment for programming.

Program Location

While university-affiliated programs afford many opportunities for inclusion, programs implemented in traditional academic buildings can be problematic. Because they are not truly in the community *or* the clinic, existing instead in a "third place" (Oldenburg, 1989), a power imbalance may be perceived. For this reason, programs should be offered in neutral locations, such as the Institute for Well-Being described above (which shares space with a local radio station, coffee shop, and other community businesses), rather than in a research lab or classroom. Illustrating the importance of this consideration, neurodiverse participants at the Hussman Center for Adults With Autism expressed satisfaction that programs held at the Institute for Well-Being were "in the heart of the city"—near a large shopping mall, restaurants, public transportation, and other desirable urban amenities that increased the likelihood of access to and participation in community activities (Krutt et al., 2018).

Universal Design and Accessibility

The West Virginia Assistive Technology System, affiliated with the West Virginia University Center for Excellence in Disabilities, publishes a seasonal newsletter with ideas for accessible community engagement. In the summer 2018 newsletter, automated chicken coops/feeders, vertical planters, smart home/automated personal assistant technologies such as the Amazon Echo, and modified bicycles were highlighted. Each of the above can allow better access to community-based occupations across the life span—poultry farming, gardening, self-management/IADL participation, and community mobility, respectively. This approach to thinking "inside" the box (i.e., utilizing existing technologies and universal design to enhance independence and inclusion) is one that occupational therapy practitioners would do well to embrace. Youth, in particular, are acutely aware of differences and desire materials and equipment that do not appear to be "medicalized." They want to fit in and avoid stigmatization. Off-the-shelf items are also often less costly and more familiar to peers, enhancing their acceptability (Jozkowski et al., 2019).

PROGRAM SHOWCASE

Promoting Accessibility in a State Park: An Interview With Gina Kaplanis

Occupational therapist Gina Kaplanis, also a clinical assistant professor at Towson University, is interested in getting children and their families outside in nature and is focusing her recent research on the health benefits of engagement in "blue and green spaces" for individuals with and without disabilities. In the summer of 2017, she met with the volunteer coordinator of a state park local to her university. The coordinator shared that park staff wanted to prioritize inclusivity and accessibility of the park and the programs offered there and invited Professor Kaplanis to partner with them.

The following school year, students in Professor Kaplanis's graduate course OT Health Promotion Initiatives in the Community conducted an accessibility assessment, identifying accessible features and barriers throughout the state park. Students then designed park services, such as an audio tour for children in accessible areas, and identified local resources for renting adaptive recreation equipment such as bikes and kayaks.

Students also surveyed caregivers of children with disabilities in the nearby community. Caregivers indicated that park staff should know how to communicate with their child, understand diagnosis-specific information and expectations, and provide a one-to-one child-to-staff ratio for safety upon request.

Professor Kaplanis then developed and led an educational workshop for park staff. Her work was guided by the transtheoretical (stages of change) model (Prochaska and DiClemente, 1983; Prochaska, DiClemente, and Norcross, 1992) and the person-environment-occupation (PEO) model (Law et al., 1996). She educated park staff about the PEO model, activity adapting and grading, and universal design concepts and highlighted places in the park that were designed for universal access and use. Her goal was to "empower the staff with knowledge and tools they could apply to any program or place in the park." At the end of the workshop, park staff participated in a "rain stick" craft, applying what they had learned about universal design, adapting, and grading to the activity.

Reflecting on the experience, Professor Kaplanis expressed that "building a community program is about being client-centered. Working with a group deeply and continuously means that the program gets what is actually needed. It is not a one-size-fits-all, quick-fix process. It is about building on the strengths that already exist, and working together to build capacity."

Professor Kaplanis noted that park staff are now more likely to ask themselves questions about accessibility when they are designing and implementing programs. At the beginning of the education portion of the program, one staff member shared that he had not even considered that children with learning or behavioral challenges would come to the park. On her next visit, this staff member told Professor Kaplanis that with just a few changes, he felt capable of making programs more inclusive (Fig. 11-3).

Despite the many positive outcomes of this program, navigating the bureaucracy and red tape was a challenge. Professor Kaplanis recalled that working with a state park means many layers of bureaucracy and stated, "You can set everything up for success, but they have to take it to the finish line." In addition, because funding is always a challenge, Professor Kaplanis emphasized the importance of conducting a strong needs assessment. This process allows those planning a program to know what the priorities of the community are, so as not to waste scarce resources.

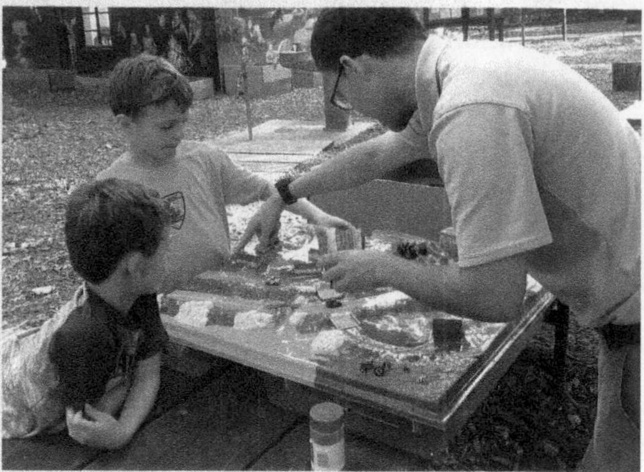

Figure 11-3 A Maryland State Parks ranger works with children on an outdoor activity to promote inclusion at Patapsco Valley State Park. *(Photo courtesy of Gina Kaplanis.)*

Engage Your Brain 11-7

How can the slow growth and progress of community inclusion programs be measured and communicated to stakeholders in a meaningful way?

Working With Community Organizations

Social policy researchers and inclusion educators offer best practice guidelines for all professionals seeking to work with community organizations (Matulewicz and Bayard, 2008). These include:

- Involve program directors, service site supervisors, and other relevant staff at the site throughout the process of program development, implementation, and evaluation.
- Provide opportunities for program clients, including those with and without disabilities, to share their experiences and provide feedback on accessibility and inclusion.

- Consider sharing community resources such as assistive technology across programs and organizations.
- Keep program assessment and improvement a priority but understand that the process is slow, so patience and persistence are key.

Carefully aligning program plans with these strategies enhances the likelihood for success; however, several challenges seem to be common to many programming experiences. Access to funding, as described in more detail below, is a common issue for practitioners seeking to start or continue work in the community. Obtaining accurate information about participants can also be a challenge. Because community organizations often do not collect medical histories on participants and the community model de-emphasizes diagnosis in favor of strengths-based models, occupational therapy practitioners working in community settings may be unaware of participants' functional limitations, difficult behaviors, and other needs (D. Piggott, personal communication, October 16, 2018). Traveling with participants using public transportation may require consent from caregivers, and liability may also be an issue. While regulations may be specific to each state, occupational therapy practitioners should consult with the organization to determine if policies related to transportation and safety exist, and if not, they should work to develop them with legal guidance from their state licensing board, insurance representative, and/or professional organization.

In community programs, occupational therapy practitioners may have less control over what happens than they might have in a controlled clinical space. For example, when people are visiting an actual grocery store, factors such as transportation schedules, inclement weather, and interactions with the public can be unpredictable. Policies and "red tape" must be creatively addressed—ideally, with the support of evidence—to demonstrate the value of community intervention to potential funders and collaborating agencies.

Funding

A lack of funds to secure program materials, appropriate meeting and storage space, compensate staff, and help cover the cost of participation has been consistently raised as a challenge to program growth and sustainability (Van Slyke, 2001) and was echoed by occupational therapists as a considerable limitation to their work in the community (C. Exner; D. Piggott; G. Kaplanis; M. Riley; and S. Lawson, personal communication). One supervisor of an adaptive cooking group, also staffed by graduate occupational therapy students completing fieldwork, stated that while the weekly supply budget did not typically cover all costs, "we like it, so we do it," meaning that clinical supervisors and students often supply a portion of the materials themselves to ensure the session is successful (D. Piggott, personal communication, October 16, 2018). The supervisor also noted that because the group was part of their faculty workload, they did not receive an additional salary or stipend. This represented a cost savings, as an outside clinician would need to be paid separately to run such a group. Financial planning for program development is discussed in detail in Chapter 8.

Evaluation Strategies

Assessing community integration, participation, and group interests is critical to the needs assessment process and to measuring the outcomes of program participation. As with many areas of practice, there are a wealth of options for assessment in community integration and participation, yet many are limited in reliability and validity. For example, Phillips, Olds, Boshoff, and Lane (2013) identified 20 instruments purporting to measure activity and participation in children and youth with disabilities. However, they report that "no single instrument measured extent of involvement, difficulty, and satisfaction/enjoyment in all life areas" (p. 288). Phillips et al. (2013) specifically comment that with fixed-item measures (which require children to report on only those activities listed in the tool) they cannot comment on less common activities that were not included, which is a threat to validity. They suggest that instruments that require youth to recall activity participation over designated time periods may be more accurate and inclusive of all areas of occupation.

In a similar critique, Salter, Foley, Jutai, Bayley, and Teasell (2008) write that the "development of good assessments may be difficult in the absence of agreement regarding the definition of [community integration]. . . . The assessment of community integration is further challenged because it depends on who, or which stakeholder, is defining success" (p. 831). They suggest that "three distinct perspectives, that of the individual, the healthcare system and of society . . . may require a different approach for defining and measuring community integration" (p. 831).

Chien, Rodger, Copley, and Skorka (2014, p. 148) evaluated 16 tools on their ability to "represent broad life areas" and include activities particular to children and determined that the Child and Adolescent Scale of Participation (CASP; Bedell, 2004, 2009), Participation and Environment Measure—Children and Youth (PEM-CY; Coster et al., 2011, 2012), and School Function Assessment—Participation Section (SFA-P; Coster, Deeney, Haltiwanger, and Haley, 1998) came the closest to effectively measuring community participation in youth. Coombs, Nicholas, and Pirkis (2013) compared 10 measures on eight review criteria and determined that the Activity and Participation Questionnaire (APQ-6) (Stewart et al., 2010) and the Social and Community Opportunities Profile (SCOPE)—short form (Huxley et al., 2012) were the most promising for measuring social inclusion.

Community integration and inclusion assessments range from individual inventories of interests and reports of frequency and type of community engagement to comprehensive program evaluation for community agencies and municipalities. Tools and resources that are especially relevant or have excellent psychometric characteristics are summarized in Table 11-1.

Table 11-1 Recommended Assessment Tools for Community Integration and Participation in Youth

Title and Citation	Format/Purpose	Brief Description
Participation in Childhood Occupations Questionnaire ([PICO-Q]; Bar-Shalita, Yochman, Shapiro-Rihtman, Vatine, and Parush 2009)	Parent report of child's occupational participation	22-item instrument to evaluate participation and guide intervention. Includes three rating scales: *performance level, degree of enjoyment of performance,* and *frequency of performance* Age range: primary school age (grade K–6) Diagnoses: none stated
Pediatric Community Participation Questionnaire ([PCPQ]; Washington, Wilson, Engel, and Jensen, 2007)	Child self-report of degree of difficulty performing ADLs, play, and leisure activities	19-item tool; children rate participation restrictions, including physical limitations and self- and society-imposed constraints Age range: 8–20 years Diagnoses: physical disabilities
Child and Adolescent Scale of Participation ([CASP]; Bedell, 2004, 2009)	Parent report of participation in activities, in comparison with same-age peers	20 items rated according to the level of participation expected given the child's age Age range: 3–22 years Diagnoses: none stated
Participation and Environment Measure for Children and Youth ([PEM-CY]; Coster et al., 2011, 2012)	Parent-report questionnaire measures participation and environment of children	25 participation items (*home, school, community*) rated by participation frequency, extent of involvement, and desire for change. Also includes 33 items assessing corresponding environments Age range: 5–17 Diagnoses: none stated
School Function Assessment–Participation Section ([SFA-P]; Coster et al., 1998)	Form completed by school personnel independently via an interview with therapist. Assesses children's participation in school settings.	6 items (*classroom, playground/recess, transportation, bathroom/toileting, transition, mealtime/snack time*), rated on the extent to which the child participates compared to same-grade peers Age range: primary school age (grade K–6) Diagnoses: all students identified as having special needs or referred for evaluation of special needs

Table 11-1 Recommended Assessment Tools for Community Integration and Participation in Youth—cont'd

Title and Citation	Format/Purpose	Brief Description
Child Social Exclusion Index ([CSE]; McNamara and Harding, 2009)	Geographic analysis of children's risk of social exclusion	Measures the degree of disadvantage in five domains (*socioeconomic, education, connectedness, health,* and *housing*) for all children in a given "living area" Age range: 0–15 Diagnoses: all Australian children
Community Integration Questionnaire ([CIQ]; Willer, Rosenthal, Kreutzer, Gordon, and Rempel, 1993)	Self-report or proxy response	15-item questionnaire scored on frequency of participation, with secondary scoring of social interaction during performance (three activity areas include *home integration, social integration,* and *productive activities*) Age range: 18–64 Diagnoses: developed for individuals with traumatic brain injury but frequently used in other adult clinical populations
Activity and Participation Questionnaire ([APQ-6]; Stewart et al., 2010)	Self-report questionnaire (or interview) on employment-related activities, education, and social/community participation	Respondents report actual activity participation, satisfaction, participation goals, and desire to change level of activity on up to 14 items. Age range: "Usual working age range" (Stewart et al., 2010) Diagnoses: adult consumers of ambulatory mental health services (must reside in the community)
Social and Community Opportunities Profile [SCOPE]—short form (Huxley et al., 2012)	Self-report questionnaire (or interview) on opportunities for community participation	48 items in eight areas (*leisure, housing, safety, work, finances, health, education,* and *relationships*), ranked for perceived opportunities, satisfaction with opportunities, and contribution to subjective well-being Age range: adults Diagnoses: none stated
Measuring Inclusion Tool ([MIT]; Alberta Urban Municipalities Association, 2017)	Evaluation completed by an individual or multiple stakeholders to assess level of inclusive culture in a city or town	Community self-assessment of leadership and accountability in inclusive practices. Fourteen "areas of focus" (*Leadership and Accountability; Commitment of Resources; Planning, Implementation and Measurement; Human Resource Policies and Practices; Employee Engagement and Education; Procurement; Municipal Social Services; Economic Development; Infrastructure and Land; Citizen and Community Engagement; Community Areas of Focus; Capacity of Community Organizations; Public Attitudes and Awareness; Responses to Incidents of Discrimination*) Age range: N/A Diagnoses: intended for municipalities, but individual focus areas can be used by organizations

From "Pathways to Positive Development: Childhood Participation in Everyday Places and Activities (Figure 4.2, p. 86)," by T. Petrenchik and G. King, in S. Bazyk (Ed.), *Mental Health Promotion, Prevention and Intervention for Children and Youth: A Guiding Framework,* 2011, Bethesda, MD: AOTA Press. Reprinted with permission.

Summary

- Successful community inclusion and integration influence adaptive function in childhood, leading to better adult outcomes.
- Exemplary international, national, and local programs that promote inclusion and integration can serve as models for occupational therapy practices that connect youth to their communities.
- Occupational therapy practitioners may serve in leadership, consultative, and direct intervention roles relating to community inclusion and integration programs and services for youth.
- The positive youth development model can be applied to community inclusion and integration programs and services for youth, emphasizing a strengths-based orientation to service provision.
- Evaluation practices to support the occupation-based community inclusion and integration of youth should be multimodal and driven by stakeholders. Strategies from organizational management or related fields can be incorporated to address complex issues common to community programming.

CASE STUDIES

CASE STUDY 11-1 Facilitating Inclusive Teen Activities

Matthew, a 15-year-old boy with autism, is one of your clients at an outpatient clinic. He lives at home with his mother, father, and 10-year-old brother. He has expressed interest in joining activities "with more regular kids, so I'm ready for college." His parents have told you he seems to be jealous of his younger brother's activities: Boy Scouts and gymnastics. However, he has not identified specific activities he would like to do. He has also asked questions about dating a few times during the past two sessions.

Matthew and you have been working on goals related to his fine motor and social interaction skills. Matthew states that he'd like to learn to use a mobile tablet to complete homework assignments more efficiently and be able to play the Fortnite video game (Epic Games, 2017) with peers. He is making progress on his fine motor skills but is reluctant to participate in your social interaction sessions because "it's not real." Your sessions have included role-playing and cotreating with another client, an 11-year-old girl, and her occupational therapist.

You want to suggest inclusive programs to Matthew and his family and help him engage in more activities. His parents told you they are nervous about him being included in programs "outside our safe bubble" at home and in the clinic. They worry about him being teased or left out, as well as not having the needed skills to be included.

You develop an intervention plan to help Matthew identify and use his interests to help discover inclusive experiences for Matthew.

Discussion Questions

1. Describe an intervention plan in which you can help Matthew identify and explore the performance skills he will need to be successful in his stated goals.
2. When researching possible community programs with Matthew, you encounter language such as "Everyone is welcome!" and other nondiscrimination language. How can you assess if the programs are truly *inclusive*?
3. Matthew's parents are reluctant to have him engage in activities outside of the home or therapy setting. How would you explain to them the importance of the setting and context of the activity being in the community?
4. Matthew's parents have indicated that they want to help their son understand dating and relationships but that they "don't think that's something that occupational therapy does." What would you say to Matthew's parents? What kinds of client-centered and appropriate interventions would you develop to address dating?

CASE STUDY 11-2 Collaborating With an Inclusive Community Organization

Nancy is an occupational therapist who volunteers at her synagogue, caring for young children during weekly services. The leadership has approached her about developing programs for children with intellectual and developmental disabilities so that they and their families can feel more connected to the community. Synagogue leaders have indicated that they "don't really know what these families need" and have concerns about the medical needs of the children, including what kind of documentation about the children's diagnoses is required. The leadership also indicated they were concerned about how to handle issues such as feeding, self-care, and communication. They also want to know what kind of special training synagogue staff will need to work with children with disabilities and how to help fellow congregants feel more comfortable interacting with children with disabilities.

Nancy conducted a literature review and found that children with disabilities are less likely to attend religious services than children without disabilities (Whitehead, 2018). From her own observations, families with children who have disabilities often do not go to synagogue events, or they leave that child at home with a parent while the rest of the family attends the event. Nancy also created a survey to assess the needs of these families and recruited three parents of children with disabilities to join an Inclusion Committee.

Discussion Questions

1. Nancy would like to use an occupation-based model to show the committee what occupational engagement in the community looks like. Which models should she consider sharing with the committee and why?
2. Parents on the committee have experience with occupational therapy in a clinical setting. How should Nancy describe what occupational therapy offers in a community setting?
3. After 6 months, Nancy wants to assess the effectiveness of the inclusion initiative. How should she assess how effective it is?
4. The parents on the committee tell Nancy that they are not comfortable sharing all of their child's medical information with the synagogue. The leadership insists that they need to know for liability reasons. How much about the medical diagnoses should be shared with the organization? What resources would you use to help you advocate for the parents' wishes?
5. Nancy wants to work with the director of educational programs at the synagogue to develop additional programs, but the director says that he does not know enough about disabilities and is concerned that it will cost too much to make programs inclusive. How can Nancy describe a mutually beneficial partnership?

Learning Activities

1. Visit the Dance Without Limits website (http://dancewithoutlimitsfoundation.org/). Is there a similar organization in your community? If you wanted to replicate the program, who would you partner with? What ethical principles would you need to consider when replicating such a program?
2. Brainstorm a community program idea to enhance inclusion for youth in your community, paying particular consideration to the financial context. Review the potential partner organization's website and conduct a search for small local grant opportunities. Are there funds available to support new programs and/or training initiatives? How could public support be generated to subsidize new programming? Adapted from Salzer and Baron (2006).

REFERENCES

Alberta Urban Municipalities Association. (2017). *Measuring inclusion tool.* Retrieved from https://auma.ca/sites/default/files/Advocacy/Programs_Initiatives/WIC/measuring_inclusion_tool_-_paper_user_0.pdf

American Occupational Therapy Association. (2014). *Fact sheet: The role of occupational therapy with children and youth.* Retrieved from www.aota.org/~/media/Corporate/Files/AboutOT/Professionals/WhatIsOT/CY/Fact-Sheets/Children%20and%20Youth%20fact%20sheet.pdf

American Occupational Therapy Association. (2015). Occupational therapy code of ethics (2015). *American Journal of Occupational Therapy, 69*(Suppl. 3), 6913410030. http://dx.doi.org/10.5014/ajot.2015.696S03

American Occupational Therapy Association. (2018). *Vision 2025.* Retrieved from www.aota.org/AboutAOTA/vision-2025.aspx

Bar-Shalita, T., Yochman, A., Shapiro-Rihtman, T., Vatine, J., and Parush, S. (2009). The Participation in Childhood Occupations Questionnaire (PICO-Q): A pilot study. *Physical and Occupational Therapy in Pediatrics, 29*(3), 295–310. doi:10.1080/01942630903028440

Bedell, G. (2009). Further validation of the Child and Adolescent Scale of Participation (CASP). *Developmental Neurorehabilitation, 12*(5), 342–351. https://doi.org/10.3109/17518420903087277

Bedell, G. M. (2004). Developing a follow-up survey focused on participation of children and youth with acquired brain injuries after discharge from inpatient rehabilitation. *NeuroRehabilitation, 19*(3), 191–205.

Best Buddies International. (2018). *Mission.* Retrieved from www.bestbuddies.org/what-we-do/mission-vision-goals/

Bolton, T., Plattner, L., and Faulkner, K. (2018). Play ball! A story about authentic participation. *OT Practice, 22*(19), 16–18.

Boy Scouts of America. (2018). *Disabilities awareness—serving scouts with disabilities.* Retrieved from www.scouting.org/programs/boy-scouts/disabilities/

Brown, B. (2010, October). *Brené Brown: The power of vulnerability* [Video file]. Retrieved from www.ted.com/talks/brene_brown_on_vulnerability?language=en

βTU—Partnership at Work for Greater Baltimore. (n.d.). *About βTU.* Retrieved from www.towson.edu/campus/community/about/

Chien, C-W., Rodger, S., Copley, J., and Skorka, K. (2014). Comparative content review of children's participation measures using the International Classification of Functioning, Disability and Health—Children and Youth. *Archives of Physical Medicine and Rehabilitation, 95*(1), 141–152.

Coombs, T., Nicholas, A., and Pirkis, J. (2013). A review of social inclusion measures. *Australian and New Zealand Journal of Psychiatry, 47*(10), 906–919. doi:10.1177/0004867413491161

Coster, W., Bedell, G., Law, M., Khetani, M. A., Teplicky, R., Liljenquist, K., . . . Kao, Y. (2011). Psychometric evaluation of the Participation and Environment Measure for Children and Youth. *Developmental Medicine and Child Neurology, 53*(11), 1030–1037.

Coster, W., Deeney, T. A., Haltiwanger, J. T., and Haley, S. M. (1998). *School function assessment user's manual.* San Antonio, TX: Therapy Skill Builders.

Coster, W., Khetani, M., Law, M. Cousins, M., Teplicky, R., and Bedell, G. (2012). Development of the Participation and Environment Measure for Children and Youth: Conceptual basis. *Disability and Rehabilitation, 34*(3), 238–246.

Dunn, W. (2011). Developing intervention plans that reflect best practice. In W. Dunn, (Ed.), *Best practice occupational therapy for children and families in community settings* (2nd ed., pp. 125–156). Thorofare, NJ: SLACK.

Easterseals. (2018). *Our programs.* Retrieved from www.easterseals.com/our-programs/live.html

Eccles, J. S., and Templeton, J. (2002). Extracurricular and other after-school activities for youth. *Review of Research in Education, 26,* 113–180.

Eglseder, K., and Webb, S. (2017). Sexuality education and implications for quality of care for individuals with adult onset disability: A Review of current literature. *American Journal of Sexuality Education, 12*(4), 409–422.

Employers Network for Equality and Inclusion. (2017). *Your diversity journey.* Retrieved from www.enei.org.uk/

Epic Games. (2017). *Fortnite Battle Royale* [Computer software]. Cary, NC: Epic Games.

Girl Scouts of the United States of America. (2017). *GSSD ability and awareness and inclusion patch.* Retrieved from www.girlscoutshop.com/GSSD-ABILITY-AWARENESS-INCLUSION-PATCH

Gupta, J., and Taff, S. D. (2015). The illusion of client-centered practice. *Scandinavian Journal of Occupational Therapy, 22*(4), 244–251.

Hadavi, S., Kaplan, R., and Hunter, M. C. R. (2015). Environmental affordances: A practical approach for design of nearby outdoor settings in urban residential areas. *Landscape and Urban Planning, 134,* 19–32.

Hagiliassis, N., Wilson, E., Campain, R., McGillivray, J., Caldwell, M., Graffam, J., . . . Koritsas, S. (2014, November 5). *Measuring social inclusion of people with intellectual disability in Australia: Initial evidence about a new tool.* Presented at the Australasian Society for Intellectual Disability Conference, Freemantle, Western Australia.

Huxley, P., Evans, S., Madge, S., Webber, M., Burchardt, T., McDaid, D., and Knapp, M. (2012). Development of a social inclusion index to capture subjective and objective life domains (phase II): Psychometric development study. *Health Technology Assessment, 16*(1), 1–248. doi:10.3310/hta16010

Ideishi, R., D'Amico, M., and Jirikowic, T. (2013). *Fact sheet: Supporting community integration and participation for individuals with intellectual disabilities.* Bethesda, MD: American Occupational Therapy Association. Retrieved from www.aota.org/~/media/Corporate/Files/AboutOT/Professionals/WhatIsOT/RDP/Facts/Intellectual-Disabilities.pdf

Jozkowski, A. C., Abbott, C., Brunermer, S., Del Franco, D., Gosnell, T., Maguffin, A., and Capulong, A. (2019, February 2). *Testing yCAT with typically developing children: A user study.* Presented at the Assistive Technology Industry Association Conference, Orlando, FL.

King, G., Petrenchik, T., Law, M., and Hurley, P. (2009). The enjoyment of formal and informal recreation and leisure activities: A comparison of school-aged children with and without physical disabilities. *International Journal of Disability, Development and Education, 56*(2), 109–130.

King, G. A. (2004). The meaning of life experiences: Application of a meta-model to rehabilitation sciences and services. *American Journal of Orthopsychiatry, 74*(1), 72–88.

Kennedy Center. (2018). *About VSA.* Retrieved from http://education.kennedy-center.org/education/vsa/

Krutt H., Dyer, L., Arora, A., Rollman, J., and Jozkowski, A. C. (2018). PhotoVoice is a feasible method of program evaluation at a center serving adults with autism. *Evaluation and Program Planning, 68,* 74–80. 10.1016/j.evalprogplan.2018.02.003

Law, M., Cooper, B., Strong, S., Stewart, D., Rigby, P., and Letts, L. (1996). The person-environment-occupation model: A transactive approach to occupational performance. *Canadian Journal of Occupational Therapy, 63*(1), 9–23.

Matulewicz, H., and Bayard, L. (2008, October 17). *Inclusion outcomes and indicators of success.* Presented at the National Conference on Disability and Inclusion National Service, Alexandria, VA. Retrieved from www.serviceandinclusion.org/conf_08/E5%20Outcomes.ppt

McCarthy, K. (2018). Dating as an occupation: Swipe right for occupational therapy. *OT Practice, 23*(4), 12–15.

McNamara, J., and Harding, H. (2009, July 9). *Child social exclusion: An updated index from the 2006 census.* Paper presented at the 10th Australian Institute of Family Studies Conference, Melbourne, Australia.

Merryman, M., Mezei, A., Bush, J. A., and Weinstein, M. (2012). The effects of a summer camp experience on factors of resilience in at-risk youth. *Open Journal of Occupational Therapy, 1*(1), 1–33.

Oldenburg, R. (1989). *The great good place: Cafes, coffee shops, community centers, beauty parlors, general stores, bars, hangouts, and how they get you through the day.* New York, NY: Paragon House.

Olmstead v. L.C. ex rel. Zimring. 527 U.S. 581 (1999).

Petrenchik, T., and King, G. (2011). Pathways to positive development: Childhood participation in everyday places and activities. In S. Bazyk (Ed.), *Mental health promotion, prevention and intervention for children and youth: A guiding framework.* Bethesda, MD: AOTA Press.

Phillips, R. L., Olds, T., Boshoff, K., and Lane, A. E. (2013). Measuring activity and participation in children and adolescents with disabilities: A literature review of available instruments. *Australian Journal of Occupational Therapy, 60*(4), 288–300.

Prochaska, J. O., and DiClemente, C. C. (1983). Stages and processes of self-change in smoking: Toward an integrative model of change. *Journal of Consulting and Clinical Psychology, 51*(3), 390–395.

Prochaska, J. O., DiClemente, C. C., and Norcross, J. C. (1992). In search of how people change: Applications to the addictive behaviors. *American Psychologist, 47*(9), 1102–1114.

Riley, M. (2014). *Studio One.* Retrieved from https://issuu.com/otosnewsletter/docs/february_newsletter

Salter, K., Foley, N., Jutai, J., Bayley, M., and Teasell, R. (2008). Assessment of community integration following traumatic brain injury. *Brain Injury, 22*(11), 820–835. doi:10.1080/02699050802425428

Salzer, M. S., and Baron, R. C. (2006). *Promoting community integration: Increasing the presence and participation of people with psychiatric and developmental disabilities in community life.* Philadelphia, PA: University of Pennsylvania Collaborative on Community Integration. Retrieved from http://tucollaborative.org/wp-content/uploads/2017/05/Increasing-the-Community-Presence-and-Participation-of-People-with-MH-and-DD-Disabilities.pdf

Scaffa, M. E. (2001). Paradigm shift: From the medical model to the community model. In M. E. Scaffa (Ed.), *Occupational therapy in community-based practice settings* (pp. 19–34). Philadelphia, PA: F. A. Davis.

Stewart, G., Grant, S., Harris, M., Waghorn. G., Hall. A., Sivarajasingam, S., Gladman, B., and Mowry, B. (2010). Brief measure of vocational activity and community participation: Development and reliability of the Activity and Participation Questionnaire. *Australian and New Zealand Journal of Psychiatry, 44,* 258–266. doi:10.3109/00048670903487175

Swanton, J. (2017). Sexual health education: Developing and implementing a curriculum for adolescents and young adults with intellectual disabilities. *OT Practice, 22*(19), 14–17.

Thompson, S. (2017). Defining and measuring "inclusion" within an organisation. In *K4D Helpdesk Report.* Brighton, United Kingdom: Institute of Development Studies.

Towson University. (2018). *Youth and young adult programs.* Retrieved from www.towson.edu/iwb/centers/occutherapy/programs/youngadult.html

Towson University Honors College. (2018). *Fall 2018 seminars and courses.* Retrieved from www.towson.edu/honors/academics/documents/fall-summer-2018-courses.pdf

Van Slyke, N. (2001). Legislation and policy issues. In M. E. Scaffa (Ed.), *Occupational therapy in community-based practice settings* (pp. 85–94). Philadelphia, PA: F. A. Davis.

Washington, L. A., Wilson, S., Engel, J. M., and Jensen, M. P. (2007). Development and preliminary evaluation of a pediatric measure of community integration: The Pediatric Community Participation Questionnaire (PCPQ). *Rehabilitation Psychology, 52*(2), 241–245. http://dx.doi.org/10.1037/0090-5550.52.2.241

Whitehead, A. L. (2018). Religion and disability: Variation in religious service attendance rates for children with chronic health conditions. *Journal for the Scientific Study of Religion, 57*(2), 377–395. https://doi.org/10.1111/jssr.12521

Willer, B., Rosenthal, M., Kreutzer, J. S., Gordon, W. A., and Rempel, R. (1993). Assessment of community integration following rehabilitation for traumatic brain injury. *Journal of Head Trauma Rehabilitation, 8*(2), 75.

Wilson, K. P., Chasson, G. S., Jozkowski, A. C., and Mulhern, M. V. (2017). Impact of a pre-professional clinical education experience with adults with autism spectrum disorder: Preparation of future speech-language pathologists. *Teaching and Learning in Communication Sciences and Disorders, 1*(1), 1–23.

World Health Organization, and Calouste Gulbenkian Foundation. (2014). *Social determinants of mental health.* Geneva, Switzerland: World Health Organization.

Yachad. (n.d.). *About Yachad.* Retrieved from www.yachad.org/about-yachad

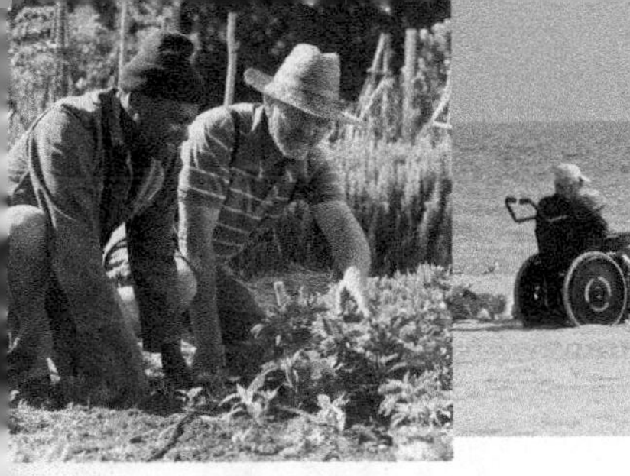
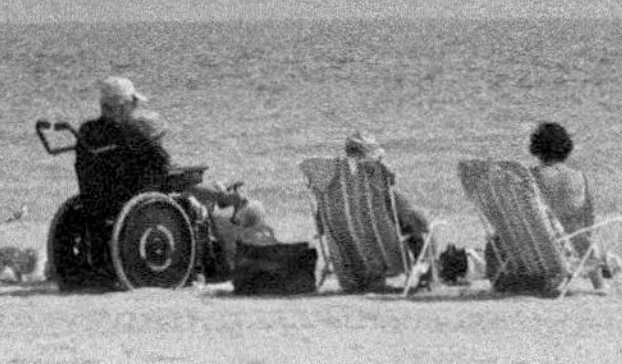
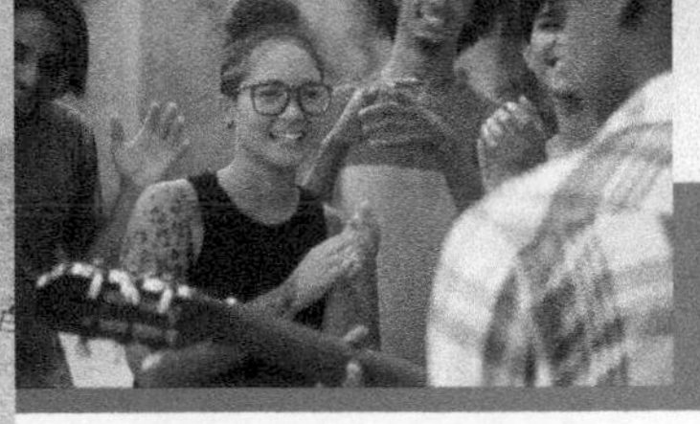

SECTION IV

Productive Aging

Chapter 12

Aging in Place and Home Modifications

Janie B. Scott, MA, OT/L, FAOTA, and Trish H. Foley, MOT, OT/L, CAPS

I could not, at any age, be content to take my place by the fireside and simply look on. . . . One must never, for whatever reason, turn his back on life.

—Eleanor Roosevelt

Learning Outcomes

This chapter is designed to enable the reader to:

12-1 Define the meaning of home as it pertains to older adults who wish to age in place.
12-2 Explain how home modifications can support an individual's desire to age in place.
12-3 Describe community living options for older adults.
12-4 Identify features of communities that support aging in place.
12-5 Identify roles and opportunities for occupational therapy practitioners to assist clients during the aging-in-place process.
12-6 Describe the occupational therapy process for assessing the need for home modifications.
12-7 Apply ethical principles and related standards of conduct to potential ethical dilemmas encountered in community-based practice.

Key Terms

55-plus communities
Advocacy
Age-restricted communities
Aging in place
Americans With Disabilities Act
Assisted living
Cohousing
Continuing care retirement communities
Home modifications
Independent living communities

Livable community
Naturally occurring retirement communities
Productive aging
Universal design
Villages

Introduction[1]

The population of older adults is growing, and people are living longer. The population of people 60 and older in 2017 in the United States was 38,730,000 women and 32,130,000 men (U.S. Census Bureau [USCB], 2018b). Census data revealed that 87.9% of people aged 60 and older lived with a householder or spouse, and the majority, 77.8%, lived in owner-occupied housing units (USCB, 2017). By 2100, the number of people globally who are at least 80 years old is expected to reach 909,000,000, "nearly seven times its value in 2017" (United Nations Department of Economic and Social Affairs, 2017, para. 4). While countries and cultures may have different social norms in regard to housing the elderly, public health experts agree about the health benefits of providing age-friendly community living options for this population. "Adults aged 65 and over had the highest rate of health insurance coverage in 2017 (98.7 percent), with 93.7 percent covered by a government plan (primarily Medicare) and 51.1 percent covered by a private plan, which may have supplemented their government coverage" (USCD, 2018a, p. 8).

Aging in place is a universally recognized concept with various definitions. The World Health Organization (WHO) emphasizes age-friendly environments and reflects a global view of aging in place:

> *Cities and communities around the world are working towards becoming more age-friendly. . . . Creating environments that are truly age-friendly requires action in many sectors: health, long-term care, transport, housing, labour, social protection, information and communication, and by many actors—government, service providers, civil society, older people and their organizations, families and friends. It also requires action at multiple levels of government. (2018, para. 3–4)*

The Centers for Disease Control and Prevention (CDC, 2009) defines aging in place as "the ability to live in one's own home and community safely, independently, and comfortably, regardless of age, income, or ability level" (para. 7). The National Aging in Place Council (n.d.) also addresses the importance of "living in a familiar environment, and being able to participate in family and other community activities." Intrinsic to the concept of aging in place is the individual's right to self-determination by making choices and decisions for one's self. The majority of people who opt to age in place do so to maintain connections to their families, their social networks, their health-care providers, and the systems integral to their lives and well-being. They also value their independence and their ability to manage their financial resources (University of Southern California Leonard Davis School of Gerontology, n.d.).

Social connectedness with family and friends is important to a sense of well-being. As older adults age, their circle of friends often diminishes due to relocations and death. This constriction of relationships may lead to social isolation. Social isolation has negative impacts on an individual's physical and mental health, as well as quality of life (Landeiro, Barrows, Musson, Gray, and Leal, 2016; Nicholson, 2012). The reduction in social isolation is discussed throughout this chapter, particularly in the "Community Living Options for Older Adults" section, and should be a consideration for occupational therapy interventions.

The American Occupational Therapy Association (AOTA, 2017) document *Vision 2025* focuses the practice of occupational therapy more fully into people's homes and communities. "Occupational therapy maximizes health, well-being, and quality of life for all people, populations, and communities through effective solutions that facilitate participation in everyday living" (AOTA, 2017, p. 1). Occupational therapy practitioners and other professionals

1. The term *occupational therapy practitioner* will be used throughout this chapter to refer to the occupational therapist and occupational therapy assistant. The use of the term *therapist* is primarily seen in the discussion of the ecology of human performance and the occupational therapist's roles.

may potentially expand their service delivery into the community, providing supportive services for those who wish to age in place. This will help to meet the anticipated needs of the growing aging population (Neufeld, 2014).

Vision 2025 (AOTA, 2017) has great relevance to aging in place and **home modifications,** as will be described in this chapter. *Vision 2025* provides context for the belief that if one is able to live in one's own community with access to transportation, health care, and socialization opportunities, one's health and well-being will likely be more positive. Promoting access to individuals and communities enables greater participation in daily occupations by older adults. The four Guideposts identified in *Vision 2025* include "accessible," "collaborative," "effective," and "leaders" and will be referred to throughout this chapter.

The meaning of *home* is a relevant consideration in the decision-making process related to aging in place. Home has physical, cultural, and emotional meanings. Some older adults become attached to the familiar physical structure that they have lived in for years and often decades. People know where things are in their homes and, over time, have developed ways of adapting to the physical environment. Cultural and family norms (e.g., favored occupations, frequency of moving, size and proximity of extended family, celebratory gatherings) may influence the meaning of home (Fig. 12-1). Emotional connections to home involve memories within the physical structure and surrounding community. Aging in place is often thought of as making the necessary modifications to the existing home environment to make it safe and comfortable for extended living. An alternate view of this concept includes moving from the known home to a new dwelling that contains features to support long-term living in a safe and accessible home and community that captures as much of the meaning of home as possible (Beck, 2011).

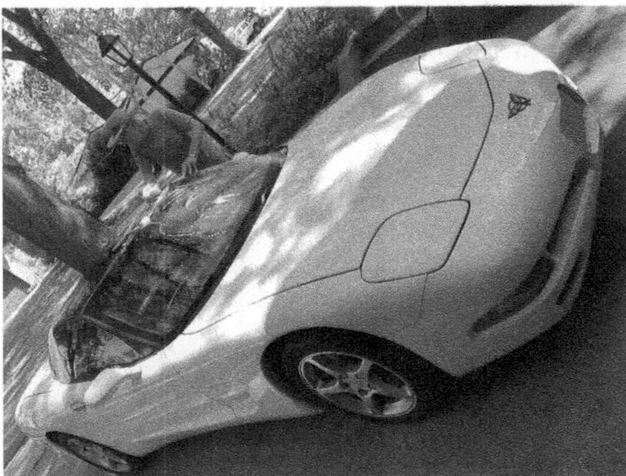

Figure 12-1 People who choose to age in place do so engaging in occupations that are meaningful and pleasurable. *(Photo courtesy of Janie B. Scott.)*

Community Living Options for Older Adults

The aging population is growing globally. This expansion is anticipated for people 60 years and older in decades to come, with a slower growth rate for older adults living on the African Continent (United Nations Department of Economic and Social Affairs, 2017a, 2017b). People are living longer. In the United States the majority would prefer remaining in their communities, as opposed to within institutions (U.S. Department of Housing and Urban Development [HUD], 2013), and many older adults have an expanding number of community-based living options to support their desires to age in place.

Decisions surrounding where to age in place can involve consideration of these different living options. The following examples describe some of the community living options for older adults. Selection of the "right" community is a personal and financial choice. Those who wish to stay in their current homes are also making a choice to age in place. Table 12-1 summarizes features of community living options for older adults.

55-Plus Communities

The options for individuals who wish to live in communities designated primarily for active older adults include **55-plus communities,** or **age-restricted communities.** Typically, when an age-restricted community is selected, at least one resident of the household is age 55 or older and interested in taking advantage of the recreational and social activities sponsored by the community.

Table 12-1 Community Living Options for Older Adults

	Age Restrictions	Recreation/ Social Activities	Health Care	ADL Services Provided	IADL Services Provided	Housing Options
55-plus communities	•					•
Assisted living	•	•	•	•	•	
Cohousing						•
Continuing Care Retirement Communities	•	•	•	•		•
Livable communities		•				•
Independent living communities	•	•				•
Naturally occurring retirement communities		•				•
Villages		•			•	•

Settings range from luxury communities with higher-priced homes and more amenities, college-town and university communities that can offer work and learning opportunities, and active senior communities planned to foster an active lifestyle to recreational vehicle (RV) retirement parks for individuals who want to travel and live with others who share similar interests and ages for as long as they like. Other options can include golf and resort communities, religion-specific communities, and singles-only communities.

Assisted Living

Assisted living residences provide a home and support services to meet the needs of residents who are unable to perform, or who need help with performing, the activities of daily living (Maryland Health Care Commission, n.d.). The residents are usually unable to live alone but have fewer health and personal needs than those living in nursing facilities. This option offers a more home-like setting that promotes independence. Assisted living facilities can be "board and care," "personal care" homes, or part of a multilevel senior living community.

Cohousing

"**Cohousing** is an intentional community of private homes clustered around shared space" (Cohousing Association of the United States, 2015, para. 1). These communities do not have age restrictions; people of all ages—from children to older adults—can share living and/or communal spaces. Cohousing living spaces can take a variety of forms, which include a single room, apartment, or house. A key feature is that there is shared space where congregate meals and activities may occur (Scott, 2018). These homes may be purchased or rented. Due to the philosophy of cohousing, older adults who may experience social isolation in other types of communities are less likely to do so here. Community members feel comfort in these living situations as people work together and try to help one another without reducing individual autonomy (Jayson, 2017).

Continuing Care Retirement Communities

Continuing care retirement communities (CCRCs) offer a variety of housing options (e.g., individual homes, apartments, assisted living, and nursing homes) and health-care services. Social and recreational opportunities vary and are dependent on resources and resident interests. The resident pays an entrance fee, and monthly charges depend on the resident's utilization of services (e.g., health-care services).

Government Housing Programs

The U.S. Department of Housing and Urban Development (HUD) funds programs for rent assistance, homeownership, and assistive services for older adults and individuals with disabilities who have limited financial resources, thereby creating affordable housing. The three types of affordable rent programs are public housing, which is owned and run by local public housing agencies (PHAs); multifamily subsidized housing, which is privately owned and subsidized by HUD; and voucher housing programs, which provide rental assistance to individuals and families for housing in the private market (Hawkins, n.d.).

Independent Living Communities

Independent living communities are designed for active, independent, healthy individuals over age 55 who are able to live alone or as couples. Grandchildren and relatives are allowed to visit for short stays in many of these communities. Housing options include houses, condominiums, townhouses, and mobile homes that can be owned, rented, or obtained as part of a cooperative. Benefits can include meals in a restaurant setting, housekeeping, transportation, and social activities. Wellness programs may be available, but typically, there are no medical-care options.

Naturally Occurring Retirement Communities

Naturally occurring retirement communities (NORCs) form when people continue to live in neighborhoods (or move to them) where the residents have lived for a long period of time. The residents are older, but not exclusively so. The neighborhoods may be composed of single-family homes or a combination of homes, apartments, and condominiums (Masotti, Fick, Johnson-Masotti, and MacLeod, 2006). An example of a NORC is one where homes were built in a new community, and the majority of the residents continue to live there as they age. People of any age can move into the community; however, the majority of households are composed of older adults.

Livable Community

Some people seek, or naturally find themselves residing in, a **livable community.** These settings incorporate environmental features that promote accessibility in housing, workplaces, community services, and public buildings. Environmental adaptations make getting around the community by walking or biking easier, increasing the feasibility of enabling residents to become less dependent on cars. A livable community does not have age restrictions and is designed for all ages.

A livable community is one that is safe and secure, has affordable and appropriate housing and transportation options, and offers supportive community features and services. Once in place, those resources enhance personal independence; allow residents to age in place; and foster residents' engagement in the community's civic, economic, and social life (AARP [formerly the American Association of Retired Persons], 2017, para. 1).

Villages

Villages are nonprofit member organizations with few staff and many volunteers. They provide services to those who wish to age in place. Services vary from village to village but typically include transportation and home repair, as well as social, educational, and wellness activities and supports. The outcomes of these community organizations often result in reduced social isolation and an increased ability of the residents to remain in their own homes (Village to Village Network, 2018).

Community Living Features for Aging in Place

Many aspects of communities facilitate the quality of living for all, including older adults. Community mobility via a variety of transportation options, employment and volunteer opportunities, exercise and recreation facilities, entertainment venues, and access to grocery stores, restaurants, entertainment venues, health-care sites, social contexts, and support services are integral to aging in place.

Community Mobility

When the decision is made to retire from driving, alternate options (e.g., public transportation) need to be found. If one is unable to drive to doctor appointments, the grocery store, and social and other activities, the quality of living is jeopardized. "Seniors must have access to adequate transportation alternatives in order to successfully age in place" (AARP, n.d., p. 8). This situation is discussed in depth in Chapter 14.

The **Americans With Disabilities Act** (ADA), a civil rights law enacted in 1990 with amendments added in 2009, prohibits discrimination against individuals with disabilities in all areas of public life. In order to ensure that all individuals have access to employment, transportation, and public buildings and services, accommodations have been mandated. These include features such as curb cuts, wider doorways, ramps or vertical lifts at building entrances, and modified public bathrooms. These environmental adaptations have benefited the community at large, including individuals who are aging in place.

Access to transportation alternatives such as accessible taxis and buses, which have been instituted for people with disabilities, are available to those aging in place. Title II of the ADA addresses all public entities that provide public transportation, whether or not they receive federal financial assistance. In addition to mandatory modifications to make fixed-route transportation (e.g., buses, subways, and trains) more accessible, paratransit was instituted. Paratransit is available for trips with origins and destinations within three-fourths of a mile of a route or station and for those individuals who cannot use fixed-route public transportation. The service must be available at the same hours and days as fixed-route services, and the cost must be no more than twice the regular fixed-route fare. Riders must also meet eligibility guidelines and be evaluated before they can avail themselves of paratransit. These transportation options may include curb-to-curb dial-a-ride service with discounted cabs and door-to-door, or door-through-door, assisted transportation for individuals who require an escort to provide assistance between the car and the door or to stay throughout the trip. Funding for these programs is typically via a combination of federal, state, and local monies (National Rural Transit Assistance Program, 2016).

Curb cuts, or curb ramps, as mandated by Title III of the ADA and the United States Access Board, an independent agency of the U.S. government devoted to accessibility for people with disabilities, are required along accessible routes when changes in level are greater than one-half inch. They are designed with wheelchairs in mind, but individuals who ambulate in their community with walkers or canes and have difficulty stepping up or down also benefit from curb cuts in intersections or parking lots. People propelling strollers or shopping carts have also found curb cuts to be enormously helpful to their community mobility.

Employment and Volunteer Opportunities

Older adults who wish to age in place typically want to do so productively. "**Productive aging** is the continued participation of older adults in self-care, work, volunteering, informal caregiving, civic participation, and engagement in leisure and social activities as they grow older" (Scott, 2017c, p. 134). A number of programs exist that focus on helping older adults gain and sustain employment or volunteer roles.

The Senior Community Service Employment Program (SCSEP) is the only federal program to assist individuals aged 55 plus who are unemployed or have low income find work. Found in nearly every county in the nation, the SCSEP is operated by a network of national, state, and local organizations. SCSEP funding is administered by the U.S. Department of Labor under Title V of the Older Americans Act (National Council on Aging, 2017).

In its report, the U.S. Senate Special Committee on Aging acknowledges that the transition from work to retirement has changed. Rather than moving directly from work to retirement, an increasing number of people transition "from full-time work into bridge jobs, second careers, and encore careers, or decide to become self-employed" (Collins and Casey, 2017, p. 5). The report concludes, "Supportive policies can help workers leverage benefits and overcome the challenges in ways that benefit not only workers and their families, but their employers, their communities, and the nation overall" (Collins and Casey, 2017, p. 53). The committee suggests that policies should promote flexibility, respect, and financial stability for older workers.

One of the goals of the AARP Foundation is to help connect older job seekers with employers who are looking to benefit from mature, experienced employees. Workers who wish to remain in or return to the workforce have access to a number of programs, including Work for Yourself at 50+ (AARP, n.d.c) and Back to Work 50+ (AARP Foundation, n.d.a).

The AARP Foundation also sponsors Experience Corps, which "is an intergenerational volunteer-based tutoring program that is proven to help children who aren't reading at grade level become great readers by the end of third grade" (AARP Foundation, n.d.b, para. 1). Each of the 20 sites participating in this program uses one of three tutoring models: one-to-one, small group, or literacy assistance, in which the volunteers help teachers with classroom-wide activities.

Retired Brains is an online job and information resource for retirees and people planning their retirement years. Their "Jobs and Work" section offers "to help boomers, seniors and retirees find the perfect part time, seasonal, temporary or work at home job to help supplement retirement income, or to help stay social and active in retirement" (Retired Brains, 2018, para. 1).

Similar to the resources and services available to help older adults obtain employment, many community groups also provide assistance to this population who wish to remain in, or return to, the workforce. They can work for pay or as volunteers with the youth of their community, help other seniors, or volunteer with a nonprofit charity. Occupational therapy practitioners can assist older adults identify their work skills, build resumes, and review interview techniques to assist in their searches. Older adults and occupational therapy practitioners working with them can find additional information about opportunities through local school systems, nonprofit tutoring organizations, and senior centers that offer intergenerational programs. Grocery, department, and big-box stores often hire older adults for full- or part-time work. These positions can be found at individual stores and through community newspapers. Local papers often publish listings of volunteer opportunities (e.g., "handyman"). A sampling of organizations that may offer employment and volunteer connections includes Volunteers of America, Senior Corps, Meals on Wheels, Foster Grandparents, and food banks. Participation in meaningful, productive activities such as volunteering may lower the risk of health problems, including dementia, and can improve longevity.

Exercise and Recreation Facilities

Older adults may wish to participate in exercise or recreational programs. Endurance, flexibility, and muscle mass decrease as one ages. This then affects balance and the risk of falls. There are many different strategies to mitigate the effects of aging on the body. Aerobic exercises such as walking, dancing, biking, and swimming are good options. Older adults who wish to exercise at home can find exercises online, at local public libraries in the form of DVDs, or through downloadable apps for smartphones or some watches. Additionally, the National Institute on Aging (NIA, 2009) Go4Life program offers online materials as well as publications to help people 50 and older remain active and fit. Aerobic exercise or resistance exercise classes also may be available at local senior centers, recreation centers, or fitness studios.

Exercise and recreational activities are also important for cognitive and emotional well-being. Evidence from both animal and human studies supports the role of physical exercise in modifying metabolic, structural, and functional dimensions of the brain and preserving cognitive performance in older adults (Kirk-Sanchez and McGough, 2014).

Stores and Restaurants

Some grocery stores such as Whole Foods have taken their senior shoppers into account when designing their layout. Wider aisles, nonskid floors with less glare, magnifiers to assist with reading small print, and easy-to-use utensils at the food bar are a few of the accommodations employed. More attention is also being paid to the tempo and volume of overhead music, the height of shelves (Milne-Tyte, 2011), and the size and color of the information shown on displays.

Many restaurants offer senior discounts on meals. Some offer "senior menu" choices, which have smaller portions. Larger restaurants may provide large-print menus, magnifiers, and lighting to help make menu reading easier for their customers.

Entertainment Venues

Community entertainment, travel businesses, television stations, and streaming services are expanding their focus to include older adults. In addition, entertainment-related businesses such as movie theaters offer discounts for "seniors" (After 55, n.d.). These businesses often promote matinees and generational programming to appeal to the elderly.

Health-Care Sites

Many health-care facilities have narrow hallways or doorways, examination tables that are not height adjustable, and check-in counters and restrooms that are inaccessible to wheelchair users. The U.S. Access Board is developing accessibility standards for medical diagnostic equipment under the Patient Protection and Affordable Care Act. This is an important policy step to assist older adults in maintaining their health and lives in the community.

For those patients who are homebound, many communities have instituted home-based primary care. These programs improve the quality of care and lower health-care costs (Warshaw, 2018). Information about doctors, physician assistants, and others who offer home visits can be found for each state through the American Academy of Homecare Physicians. As telehealth and telemedicine expands, people who are homebound may have greater access to in-home services.

Easy-to-reach sites to access health-care services, such as pharmacies, 24-hour urgent-care centers, respite services, and home health services, are all important features of a community that supports aging in place. Pharmacy chains are becoming more "senior friendly" by offering senior discount days, easy-opening caps on prescription bottles, mail delivery services, and in-store magnifiers to help customers read labels more easily.

Social Contexts

As people age and retire, they may have fewer opportunities to socialize. The social interactions gained from going about daily routines are necessary to keep one alert and healthy and may protect against dementia. A study at Northwestern University found a link between brain health and positive relationships when studying men and women over the age of 80 with exceptional memories. The researchers identified distinctive brain features such as thicker cortexes, a resistance to age-related atrophy, and a larger left anterior cingulate, a part of the brain important to attention and working memory. These "Super Agers," as they were called, also reported that they had warm and trusting relationships. The researchers concluded that social relationships are important and may play a significant role in preserving cognition (Graham, 2017).

Support Services

Every state's department of human services has an aging services division that focuses on providing seniors with home- and community-based services so they can continue living in their own homes. State assistance programs, including access to home health aides and skilled nursing care, home-delivered meals, help with household chores, and transportation to shopping and medical appointments, as well as counseling, advocacy, and legal aid, are generally available to eligible seniors.

Eligible seniors who need a level of care that would ordinarily require admission into a nursing home may receive in-home care services paid for by the Medicaid waiver program. The goal of this program is to prevent or delay nursing home admissions and provide frail seniors with the necessary medical and support services to enable them to continue living safely and comfortably at home with their families for as long as possible.

The State Health Insurance Assistance Program (SHIP) is staffed with trained insurance counselors who provide accurate, objective information and guidance with regard to available public and private health insurance options for older adults in their state. These options include Medicare and Medicaid benefits, Medicare Advantage and Supplement Plans, and state-sponsored prescription assistance programs for older adults (Eldercare Directory, n.d.).

The Older Americans Act funds services at the state and county levels through the Area Agencies on Aging (AAA) and state departments of aging. The mission of the AAA is to provide personal care, chore services, meals, money management assistance, transportation, and respite care (National Association of Area Agencies on Aging, 2016).

Many communities have senior support services that offer a range of assistance, from personalized financial assessments for long-term care placement, the sale of a home, legal documents, long-term care insurance, investment strategies, and geriatric placement (Philadelphia Corporation for Aging, n.d.) to medical day-care centers for seniors that provide meals, food and clothing banks, computer and Internet access, transportation, housing benefits, and medical care (Senior Support Services, n.d.). These support services also offer information about a variety of art, fitness, and continuing education classes and equipment loan closets (Howard County Government, n.d.). Additionally, there are programs that provide online, searchable resource directories to serve the public and professionals in identifying, connecting, and accessing private and public resources (Maryland Access Point, n.d.)

Engage Your Brain 12-1

How would access to these services vary by geography (e.g., Indian reservations, rural areas, postdisaster areas, suburban or urban places)?

Occupational Therapy and Aging in Place

Occupational therapy practitioners are in unique positions to meet the upcoming challenges of helping older adults age in place by expanding their services to address the needs for health care, support and social services, consultation, and case management through direct and indirect services to individuals and communities. Preparation to meet these needs requires occupational therapy practitioners to understand and contribute to the base of evidence surrounding this practice area.

Roles and Opportunities

The *Occupational Therapy Practice Framework* (AOTA, 2014c) supports the multiple roles that occupational therapy practitioners fill relative to aging in place. The framework articulates that interventions with clients promote "achieving health, well-being and participation in life through engagement in occupation" (AOTA, 2014c, p. S4).

Whenever an occupational therapy practitioner engages with a client who establishes goals aimed at aging in place, the framework "can be used to analyze their living situations and supports and to make recommendations that promote function, safety, independent living, and quality of life. The . . . *Framework* identifies the domains of occupational therapy as occupation, client factors, performance skills, performance patterns, and context and environment" (Scott, 2017a). The framework guides the way occupational therapy assesses, plans for, and collaborates with individuals and communities to support aging in place.

Occupational therapy practitioners' assessments of individuals and communities can lead to multiple leadership opportunities within agencies, communities, organizations, and government. The notions of collaboration and effective leadership are consistent with the Guideposts identified in *Vision 2025*. Effective leadership requires the use of advocacy for and with individuals and communities.

Occupational therapy practitioners may have roles as direct-care providers, consultants, or case managers. Occupational therapy practitioners can contact their local AAA to explore the potential for collaboration. The role of the occupational therapy practitioner may be through the provision of direct services to AAA clients, providing consultation for population-based policy development, or helping train agency personnel to provide effective services.

The role of case manager is a good fit for the occupational therapy practitioner. Use of the occupational profile and activity analysis helps the occupational therapy case manager identify and coordinate needed services with individuals who wish to age in place. The occupational therapist helps to establish goals with clients and uses interagency and interprofessional collaboration to ensure that clients obtain needed services.

In addition to the case manager role, occupational therapy practitioners can provide direct services to the individual and community as well as fulfill organization and agency needs as volunteers on boards and commissions. The expertise and viewpoints that are often unique to occupational therapy are invaluable to organizations in the community that serve the aging population. Opportunities for this leadership are consistent with the Guideposts identified in *Vision 2025*. Leadership opportunities exist on boards and commissions that can have an impact on local, state, and national policies focused on aging in place.

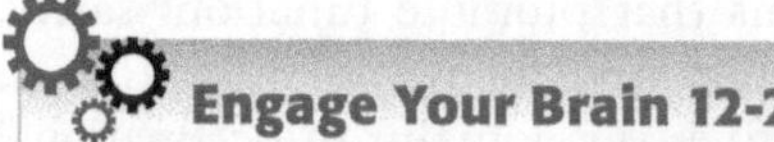

Engage Your Brain 12-2

Consider your home or your family's home. Would it support aging in place?

Home Evaluator

Occupational therapy practitioners have access to a variety of assessment tools to determine a client's ability to safely age in place. Some of these tools are explained in this section. A number of home assessment tools consider functional safety in the home. The In-Home Occupational Performance Evaluation (I-HOPE; Stark, Somerville, and Morris, 2010) consists of a card-sorting activity targeting 44 activities that are essential for aging in place. Using a 5-point scale, it measures activity participation, the individual's rating of and satisfaction with her or his performance, and the severity of environmental barriers.

The Safety Assessment of Function and the Environment for Rehabilitation—Health Outcome Measurement and Evaluation (SAFER-HOME v3; Breeden, 2016) assesses the environment and the individual's ability to safely carry out functional activities in the home. The level of safety of 74 items is rated on a 4-point scale. The Home Falls and Accidents Screening Tool (HOME FAST; Mackenzie, Byles, and Higginbotham, 2000) is designed to identify individuals at risk of falling due to hazards within their home environment. The tool consists of 25 items with a yes/no rating, with a higher score indicating a greater risk of falling.

Role of Advocacy

According to the AOTA, **advocacy** includes "efforts directed toward promoting occupational justice and empowering clients to seek and obtain resources to fully participate in their daily life occupations" (AOTA, 2014d, p. S36). Advocacy related to aging in place is the "promotion of or support for a client, program, or policy" (Scott, Reitz, and Harcum, 2017, p. 89). Achieving these objectives often involves interprofessional collaboration. The role of advocacy as stated in the *Occupational Therapy Code of Ethics* (2015; hereafter referred to as the *Code*) follows.

Principle 4, Justice, of the *Code* states, "Occupational therapy personnel shall promote fairness and objectivity in the provision of occupation therapy services" (AOTA, 2015, p. 5). Under the related standards of conduct for this principle, the following are relevant to the discussion of aging in place and home modifications.

> *Occupational Therapy Personnel Shall*
>
> *B. Assist those in need of occupational therapy services in securing access through available means.*
>
> *C. Address barriers in access to occupational therapy services by offering or referring clients to financial aid, charity care, or* pro bono *services within the parameters of organizational policies.*
>
> *D. Advocate for changes to systems and policies that are discriminatory or unfairly limit or prevent access to occupational therapy services. (AOTA, 2015, p. 5)*

Occupational therapy practitioners can fulfill these obligations under the *Code* by teaching clients self-advocacy skills and working with organizations, agencies, and governments to identify where barriers to services exist and propose changes to policies and legislation to help overcome them. This may also require the occupational therapy practitioner to defend and promote the need for occupational therapy services to payers. Case Study 12.2 provides an example of steps to maintain ethical integrity in occupational therapy practice focused on aging in place.

Theories/Models[2]

A variety of theories and models are applicable to this practice arena, including those described in Chapter 3. According to Reitz, Scaffa, and Merryman (2014), another model readily applicable to occupational therapy community-based practice is the ecology of human performance (EHP). This model provides "five alternatives for therapeutic intervention" (Dunn, Brown, and McGuigan, 1994, p. 603). The first of these five levels is identified as the establish/restore level. For example, this level would include interventions that seek to restore function via the development and improvement of skills and abilities that would enhance a person's or couple's efforts to age in place.

Another level of intervention is that of adapt. At this level, the therapist adapts "the contextual features and task demands to support performance in context" (p. 604). This level of intervention would include home modifications. Yet another intervention level is the alter level, wherein the therapist changes the actual context rather than adapting the current one. An example of such an intervention would be supporting a person's or couple's choice to move into a single-level home from a townhouse as they age to avoid climbing stairs. The prevent level of intervention seeks to "prevent the occurrence or evolution of maladaptive performance in context" (p. 604). Recommending the removal of scatter rugs as part of a home evaluation to support aging in place would be an example of this level of intervention. The last level of intervention in the EHP is the create level. This level has great potential for community-based practice since its goal is to create "circumstances that promote more adaptable or complex performance in context" (p. 604). Policy initiatives, program development, community development, and community empowerment are all activities at this level of intervention.

When using the EHP model, regardless of the level of intervention chosen, intervention should always be guided by the culture of the individual or the community. Tasks that an individual or community selects to pursue are determined by its skills and abilities, as well as personal choices, priorities, and values that are often guided by both life experience and cultural values.

Engage Your Brain 12-3

What occupational therapy theories other than those identified in Chapter 3 could support aging-in-place practice?

Evidence-Based Practice

Occupational therapy practitioners become effective and competent in their practice through the use of evidence-based practice. Understanding the research and incorporating it into areas of clinical, academic, leadership, and further research is an aspirational goal of the profession. A number of evidence-based research articles and their relevance to occupational therapy practitioners interested in aging in place appear in Box 12-1. This clearly is not an exhaustive list but one that exemplifies how research can influence practice. An AOTA (2014b) critically appraised topic (CAT) summarizes the evidence for occupational therapy's role in home modifications (see Box 12-2).

Occupational Therapy Process for Home Modifications

Home modifications are defined as alterations to the home environment in order to make living functional and safe while promoting independence (Estes, Lowrey, and Baxter, 2014). These modifications often include ramps or vertical lifts for entry and exit to the home, stair lifts for access to the second floor or basement, grab bars throughout the house for support and safety, and other customized adaptations. Homeowners may need to consult with their neighborhood homeowners' association (HOA) before modifying the outside of their home for greater access. Renters may need to consult with their landlord before changing any aspect of the rental property. The Fair Housing Law Act prohibits

2. Portions of this section first appeared in Reitz, S. M., Scaffa, M. E., Campbell, R. M., and Rhynders, P. A. (2010). Health behavior frameworks for health promotion practice. In M. E. Scaffa, S. M. Reitz, and M. A. Pizzi, *Occupational therapy in community-based practice settings* (pp. 46–69). Philadelphia, PA: F. A. Davis.

Box 12-1 Systematic Reviews of Occupational Therapy's Role With Community-Dwelling Older Adults

Liu, C.-J. (2018). Guest editorial—functional ability in the changing demographic landscape: Evidence and opportunities for occupational therapy. *American Journal of Occupational Therapy, 72,* 7204170010. https://doi.org/10.5014/ajot.2018.724002

# of studies: N/A
Ages: older adults
Focus: "Health care spending for high-need, high-cost beneficiaries is three times higher for beneficiaries who have multiple chronic conditions but do not have ADL difficulty" (7204170010p1).
Results: "Preserving functional ability is fundamental to support autonomy, quality of life, and aging in place" (7204170010p2).
"The profession of occupational therapy can help older people live independently, safely, and comfortably in their own home by promoting functional ability" (7204170010p1).

Berger, S., Escher, A., Mengle, E., and Sullivan, N. (2018). Effectiveness of health promotion, management, and maintenance interventions within the scope of occupational therapy for community-dwelling older adults: A systematic review. *American Journal of Occupational Therapy, 72,* 7204190010. https://doi.org/10.5014/ajot.2018.030346

# of studies: 36
Ages: average age greater than or equal to 65
Focus: Do occupational therapy interventions "improve occupational performance and quality of life (QOL) and decrease health care utilization in community-dwelling older adults" (7204190010p1)?
Results: "This systematic review provides strong support for occupational therapy practitioners to consider using health promotion, management, and maintenance interventions when working with older adults living in the community" (7204190010p7).
"Strong evidence supports the use of group and individual interventions to improve occupational performance" (7204190010p1).

Smallfield, S., and Lucas Molitor, W. (2018). Occupational therapy interventions supporting social participation and leisure engagement for community-dwelling older adults: A systemic review. *American Journal of Occupational Therapy, 72,* 7204190020. https://doi.org/10.5014/ajot.2018.030627

# of studies: 14 articles
Ages: average age greater than or equal to 65
Focus: Loneliness and social isolation. "Because health and wellness risks are associated with social isolation and loneliness in older adults, mitigating these health risks may improve not only mental health but also physical health and quality of life (QOL) in this population" (7204190020p1).
Results: "Strong evidence supports leisure education programs and moderate evidence supports chronic disease self-management programs to enhance leisure engagement. Mixed evidence exists for community-based group programs and electronic gaming interventions to promote social participation" 7204190020p7.

Elliott, S., and Leland, N. E. (2018). Occupational therapy fall prevention interventions for community-dwelling older adults: A systematic review. *American Journal of Occupational Therapy, 72,* 7204190040. https://doi.org/10.5014/ajot.2018.030494

studies: 50 articles
Ages: mean age greater than or equal to 65
Focus: Fall prevention interventions. "What is the evidence for the effect of fall prevention interventions on fall-related outcomes, occupational performance, quality of life (QOL), and health care facility readmissions for community-dwelling older adults?" (7204190040p2).
Results: "Because all multi-factorial intervention studies with positive results included home assessment, modification, or hazard abatement, practitioners should consider these vital fall prevention components for community-dwelling older adults" (7204190040p6).
"Addressing older adults' fall risk during postacute care stays and in the community is essential for minimizing future risk and facilitating safe care transitions and aging in place" (7204190040p7).

Hunter, E. G., and Kearney, P. J. (2018). Occupational therapy interventions to improve performance of instrumental activities of daily living for community-dwelling older adults: A systematic review. *American Journal of Occupational Therapy, 72,* 7204190050. https://doi.org/10.5014/ajot.2018.031062

Box 12-1 Systematic Reviews of Occupational Therapy's Role With Community-Dwelling Older Adults—cont'd

studies: 14 articles
Ages: 65 and older
Focus: Occupational therapy interventions to improve IADL performance of community-dwelling older adults.
Results: "This systematic review identified four areas of intervention that have been shown to have a positive impact on either improving IADL performance or slowing decline in performance: cognitive, self-management, prevention, and home-based multidisciplinary rehabilitation interventions" (7204190050p6).

Liu, C.-J., Chang, W.-P., and Chang, M. C. (2018). Occupational therapy interventions to improve activities of daily living for community-dwelling older adults: A systematic review. *American Journal of Occupational Therapy, 72,* 7204190060. https://doi.org/10.5014/ajot.2018.031252

# of studies: 43 studies
Ages: average age greater than or equal to 65
Focus: Occupational therapy interventions to improve ADLs.
Results: "A high benefit was identified for the home visits or home-based interventions for older adults with ADL difficulty" (7204190060p7).
"The review found moderate benefit of using an exercise approach, particularly for frail older adults. The review also found a high benefit of using home visits or home-based intervention, particularly for older adults with ADL difficulty; such high-benefit interventions often include home modifications, highlighting the importance of including older adults' living environments in the treatment plan to promote ADL independence" (7204190060p7).

Ruiz, S., Snyder, L. P., Rotondo, C., Cross-Barnet, C., Colligan, E. M., and Giuriceo, K. (2017). Innovative home visit models associated with reductions in costs, hospitalizations, and emergency department use. *Health Affairs, 36*(3), 425–432. doi:10.1377/hlthaff.2016.1305

# of studies: 281 adults
Ages: greater than or equal to 65
Focus: Teams include a nurse, an occupational therapist, and a handyman to address both the home environment and uses the strengths of the older adults themselves to improve safety and independence.
Result: "Community Aging in Place—Advancing Better Living for Elders (CAPABLE) addresses both function and cost. Roughly $3,000 in program costs yielded more than $30,000 in savings in medical costs driven by reductions in both inpatient and outpatient expenditures.

Participants had difficulty with an average of 3.9 out of 8.0 Activities of Daily Living (ADLs) at baseline, compared to 2.0 after five months.

Symptoms of depression, as well as the ability to grocery shop and manage medications also improved.

The change in physical environment further motivates the participant. Addressing both the people and the environment in which they live allows the person to thrive."

housing discrimination and makes it illegal for HOAs or landlords to deny requests for reasonable modifications. The person requesting the modification is responsible for the expense, and the landlord can require that the modification be removed once the tenant leaves.

Occupational therapy leverages knowledge regarding interaction of the triad of person, activity, and environment to enhance a client's performance of an occupation. If the person and/or the environment interfere with satisfactory performance, then something must be modified. The occupational therapy process, consisting of the evaluation, intervention, and documentation of outcomes, relates to the home modification process in that the occupational therapist assesses the client's needs, identifies the solution, and then evaluates the outcome.

A home-building contractor or the person needing the modifications usually contacts the occupational therapy practitioner for a home evaluation. The occupational therapist, in collaboration with the client, develops the individual's occupational profile (AOTA, 2014c), evaluating the needs, problems, risks, and concerns. The profile should include the individual's occupational history, interests, and priorities. The occupational therapist then will assess the client's performance patterns and skills, considering the stability of skills. The framework will

Box 12-2 Evidence That Supports Occupational Therapy's Roles in Home Modification

- Strong evidence supports the efficacy of home modifications as an effective prevention treatment for reducing the rate and risk of falls among older adults, especially when delivered by occupational therapists. The effect is strongest for older adults at high risk of falling (previous fall, age 70 or older). The intervention is effectively delivered as either a single- or multicomponent intervention. The benefit has been measured at 12 months.
- Home modifications can reduce the decline associated with aging with chronic conditions.
- Strong evidence demonstrates that home modifications can improve caregivers' ability to provide care for individuals with dementia.

From *Home Modifications: Critically Appraised Topic (CAT)* (p. 9), by the American Occupational Therapy Association, 2014b.

help the occupational therapy practitioner define these areas and apply them to client interactions.

The occupational therapy practitioner must remember to acknowledge and respect the meaning of home. When evaluating the home or the individual's ability to carry out the daily routines required to maintain one's self and home, the occupational therapy practitioner must take the personal, cultural, and emotional factors and the home's physical environment into account. One part of the evaluation process is asking open-ended questions regarding the individual's different needs. These include the following types of questions:

- Physical: "Where do you spend the most/least amount of time?"
- Social: "How often do friends or family visit, and what do you typically do?"
- Personal: "What is most important about your home?" "Do you feel free to move about in your home?"
- Temporal: "How long have you lived in your home?"
- Occupational: "What do you most enjoy doing in your home?" "Where and how do you complete most of your personal activities?" (Lipman, 2015 p. 12).

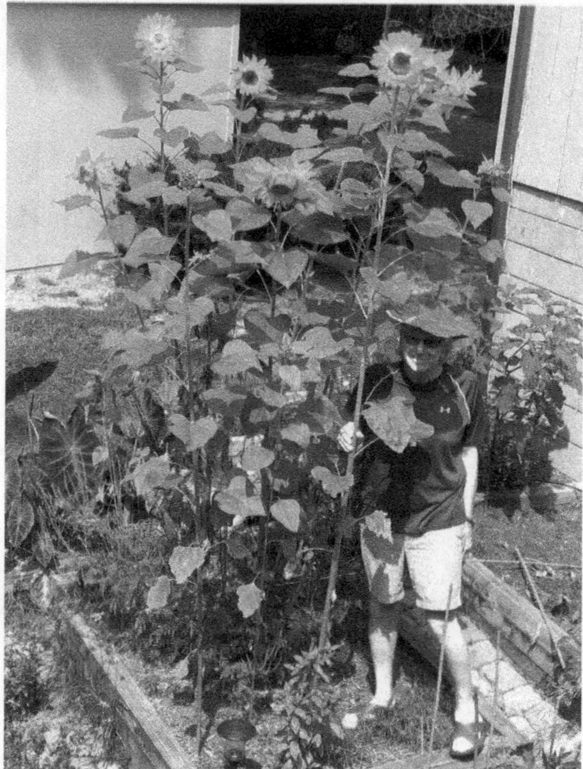

Figure 12-2 All parts of the home should be considered in any aging-in-place or home modification consultation. *(Photo courtesy of Janie B. Scott.)*

Open-ended questions help the occupational therapist elicit and appreciate the thoughts and emotions of older adults regarding how the proposed home modifications or alterations might have an impact on their sense of security and control.

Whenever possible, it is important to assess the individual interacting in his or her home environment. In this way, the occupational therapist can analyze how the home's physical environment affects the individual's performance. This environmental scan should include any outdoor spaces (Fig. 12-2).

Following the assessment of the home and the individual's performance of needed skills, the occupational therapy practitioner develops an intervention plan and goals with the client and family members. The goals should take into account the individual's potential benefit from the modification based on the individual's definitions of independence, safety, and autonomy. Reducing the risk that may be associated with a given activity, for both the individual and the caregiver, may be the desired outcome of the intervention. In contrast to only evaluating the home's physical space, the person-environment approach identifies interventions that are based on their relevance to the individual. Addressing occupations that are important to the individual directs interventions. In this way the abilities and preferences of the individual and his or her desired activities are considered rather than focusing on the environment alone.

Typical Home Modifications

According to an *Aging in Place Survey Report,*

> *grab bars and entrance ramps are the most commonly completed projects representing the needs both of people in wheelchairs (ramps and wider doorways) and those with balance, strength or mobility concerns (grab bars, levers and softer flooring). In fact, these projects represented 76 percent and 64 percent of completed projects, respectively. (Cusato, 2015, p. 3)*

Replacing round doorknobs with levers makes gripping easier on arthritic hands. In the kitchen, opening the area below the sink and countertops enables people to sit while working. The addition of pull-down shelves above and/or pull-out shelves below eases reaching and bending. Other modifications may include adding a bathroom or moving the master bedroom to the ground floor. When this is not feasible, adding a stair lift to the stairway to access the upper floor may suffice. As with any intervention, the client's interests, needs, and priorities must lead the intervention. The client should agree to any modification and demonstrate an ability to safely move through the modified environment.

Funding for Home Modifications

Funding for home modifications can be challenging. Medicare, Medicaid, and most insurance do not cover modifications and assistive devices, as they are often seen as "luxury items." AARP (Salomon, 2010) reported that about 80% of homeowners pay the full cost of home modifications. If the homeowner is eligible, banks may lend money through a home equity loan or second mortgage, or, if at least one of the owners is 62, a reverse mortgage may be possible. This funding may be a stronger option when a more expensive modification, such as a ramp or changing a tub to a roll-in shower, is needed.

A reverse mortgage may be available to homeowners aged 62 and older who wish to remain in their homes (age in place) for the rest of their lives. The tax-free money can be used to pay for home health care, monthly bills, the self-funding of long-term care policies, and home modifications (e.g., ramps, kitchen or bathroom remodels). The homeowners are not required to pay monthly mortgage payments; however, they continue to be responsible for property taxes, insurance, utilities, and other expenses. In addition, they still own their home and are able to pass the equity down to their heirs (Federal Trade Commission, 2015; J. Eichmiller, personal communication, December 10, 2018).

Cities, towns, or counties often have special programs for housing repairs. Programs for low-income families who are renters or homeowners may include kitchen or bathroom modification or ramp installation. Certain private nonprofit organizations such as the American Cancer Society, National Multiple Sclerosis Society, National Muscular Dystrophy Association, and National United Cerebral Palsy Association may provide partial funding for those who meet their need-based criteria. Rebuilding Together is a national organization that implements free home repairs and services for older adult homeowners who are at risk and have low income. Local chapters can be contacted for information regarding eligibility requirements.

Since it is difficult to locate funding, many homeowners pay for their own modifications. However, if the modification meets certain criteria, it may be tax deductible. For example, part of the expense of a modification may be deductible if the resale value of the property is increased and the modification was prescribed as medically necessary. Additional information may be obtained via consultation with a tax professional and a review of Internal Revenue Service (IRS, 2018) Publication 502. Some financial institutions offer low-income loans to seniors. The local Office on Aging is a good source to learn if such programs are available.

Some home modifications and assistive equipment, as well as medical expenses, can be claimed on personal taxes if the amount exceeds a set percentage of the adjusted gross income (e.g., 7.5% if over 65 years of age, 10% if under 65). When requesting a tax deduction, the individual should obtain a letter of medical necessity from a medical professional stating that accessible equipment or home modifications are necessary for safe and independent functioning. Individuals should also contact a tax advisor to learn which tax credits or deductions they are eligible to receive.

The Veterans Health Administration (VA) offers medical, rehabilitation, and behavioral health services to veterans. The VA may pay for eligible veterans' home modifications, car/van modifications, and assistive technologies. The VA's website and veterans' service organizations (e.g., Disabled American Veterans) offer specific details about how to access these funds (Scott, 2017b).

Occupational Therapy Considerations and Interventions

It is of prime importance for occupational therapy practitioners working in this area to be knowledgeable of and understand existing laws (e.g., ADA, Fair Housing Act), building codes, and guidelines; however, these are not mandatory for private homes. Within the ADA, the 2010 ADA Standards for Accessible Design (ADA-SAD) covers the construction requirements for both public and private facilities that are sites of public accommodations and commercial facilities. The following standards are often used as guidelines for private accommodations.

International Code Counsel/American National Standards Institute A117.1-2009 Accessible and Usable Building and Facilities

This is the primary standard and current model for most accessibility laws and codes. It focuses on minimum design requirements for persons with physical disabilities and serves as the foremost industry standard and valuable guideline for nonregulated residential construction and modifications.

Uniform Federal Accessibility Standards

These commercial standards are useful for dimensions, standards of construction, clearances, and construction details. Though not binding in residential buildings, these clearly defined standards can be used in meeting accessibility goals.

Fair Housing Accessibility Guidelines

These nonmandatory guidelines for state and local agencies help to properly implement the requirements of the Fair Housing Act.

State and Local Codes

State and local codes apply to home modifications such as ramps and grab bars since most construction is regulated by state and local buildings codes.

Universal Design

Universal design (UD) is the design of environments and products in a way that is usable by all people, without the need for alteration. When applied, the seven principles of universal design (see Box 12-3) provide convenience and function while making the environment or product safer and easier to use. These principles are compatible with the

Box 12-3 The Seven Principles of Universal Design

Principle 1. Equitable Use—useful for people with diverse abilities.
Principle 2. Flexibility in Use—accommodates a wide range of preferences and abilities.
Principle 3. Simple and Intuitive Use—use is easy to understand, regardless of experience, knowledge, language skills, and concentration level.
Principle 4. Perceptible Information—communicates necessary information effectively, regardless of ambient conditions or the user's sensory abilities.
Principle 5. Tolerance for Error—minimizes hazards and adverse consequences of accidental or unintended actions.
Principle 6. Low Physical Effort—can be used efficiently and comfortably and with a minimum of fatigue.
Principle 7. Size and Space for Approach and Use—appropriate size and space are provided for approach, reach, manipulation, and use regardless of user's body size, posture, or mobility.

From *The Universal Design File: Designing for People of All Ages and Abilities* (pp. 34–35), by M. F. Story, J. L. Mueller, and R. L. Mace, 1998, Raleigh: Center for Universal Design, North Carolina State University. Reprinted with permission.

occupational therapy process as outlined in the framework, as well as with the guidelines of other professions with whom occupational therapy practitioners collaborate.

Interprofessional Collaboration

The National Association of Home Builders (NAHB), in collaboration with AARP and other experts, developed a multicourse educational program designed to facilitate individuals desiring to become a certified aging-in-place specialist (CAPS; AARP, 2015). Following a course of training and testing, a CAPS understands the unique needs of the older adult population, aging-in-place home modifications, common remodeling projects, and the solutions to common barriers. CAPS designees are often remodelers, although designers, occupational therapy practitioners, architects, and others frequently achieve this designation as well. The CAPS program divides aging-in-place clients into three distinct categories:

- Those without urgent needs who want to age in place and are addressing the need before they experience significant health issues
- Those with progressive conditions who require home modifications that allow them to continue to live in their homes
- Those with a traumatic change who need immediate accommodations to allow them to continue to live in their homes (Bawden, 2017, p. 18)

Many occupational therapists have become CAPS certified and collaborate with architects, contractors, and designers. For example, architects may design and coordinate with the contractor when modifications involve changes to the home. Designers specialize in enhancing the aesthetics of the home environment while designing modifications. Contractors work with the designer, the occupational therapist, and the client to ensure accessibility of the home modifications. The contractor is often the team member responsible for securing building permits and meeting local codes and regulations. Home modifications can involve tradespeople specializing in carpentry, plumbing, and electrical work.

Another area for collaboration is in disaster preparedness for older adults aging in place. Occupational therapy practitioners can collaborate with clients, the Red Cross, first responders, and others to help develop evacuation plans for individuals and agencies. The Federal Emergency Management Agency (FEMA) provides information on its ready .gov website specific to the needs of older adults and people with disabilities who may need to evacuate during a disaster such as a fire, flood, or earthquake. This includes suggestions on creating emergency kits and where to place them at home, at work, or in a vehicle. A kit should contain extra medicine, keys to the house, a radio, a flashlight, a first aid kit, batteries, trash bags, a whistle, a manual can opener, and other items. Recommendations about the plans and emergency kits needed for pets and service animals are also available (FEMA, n.d.a; FEMA, n.d.b).

Summary

- Home is more than a physical space. Residents' preferences and needs, cultural experiences, and resources influence the meaning of home.
- A variety of living options are available for older adults to consider as they age.
- Occupational therapy practitioners should be aware of the need for and advocate for the presence of features that support aging in place.
- Aging in place will occur more successfully if occupational therapy practitioners are prepared to evaluate the environment and make recommendations based on the needs of the individual and community.
- Home modifications are best completed through a process that evaluates persons in their environment based on their goals.
- Occupational therapy practitioners are uniquely qualified to help people anticipate age-related changes and prepare for them through the use of home modifications and assistive devices. The *Code* (AOTA, 2015) provides guidance to the ethical practice of these efforts.

CASE STUDIES

CASE STUDY 12-1 Client-Centered Approach to Modifications

Ms. K. lives alone in a single-story, one-bedroom home. Her son lives a half-hour drive away and is often out of town on business. Her sister lives in the next state. Ms. K. has recently returned home following a hospitalization and rehabilitation due to a left cerebrovascular accident (CVA), which left her with increased tone in her right leg, ataxia in her right arm, and a slight speech deficit.

The front porch has four steps, and the back porch has five steps. The house also has a side entrance, which has five steps to the sidewalk leading to her driveway. Her home is accessible throughout the interior, with wide doorways and hallways. Her bathroom is small but accessible.

Ms. K. contacted the occupational therapist at her local center for independent living, asking for assistance with obtaining a ramp for either her front door or backdoor. She needed to be able to leave her home independently for doctor's appointments. At the time of evaluation, Ms. K. had been receiving physical and occupational therapy in her home and was able to ambulate short distances in the home with a walker. When traveling longer distances, she used a wheelchair.

An evaluation of Ms. K. showed that she had functional strength on her left side, but due to the increased tone and ataxia, her right side was not functional for wheelchair propulsion for any distance or on an incline.

An evaluation of the house revealed that a ramp at the front door at the ADA-recommended 1:12 ratio would be 30 ft after the 5 × 5 platform at her door. If the ratio is 1:20, which is often used for outside ramps, the ramp would be 50 ft long, in addition to two 5 × 5 platforms. Neither of these options were reasonable or affordable. Ms. K. did not have the strength or endurance for such a long a ramp. In addition, a ramp on the front of her home might lessen her safety while in the home or while traveling on the ramp.

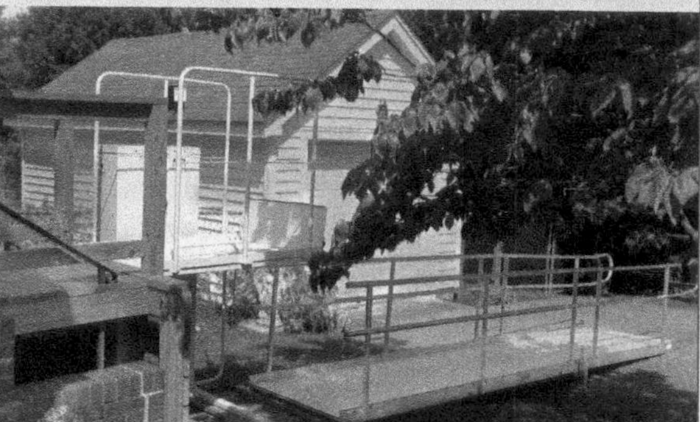

Figure 12-3 Access to the backdoor requires a wooden frame over existing brick steps, a vertical lift, and a 20-ft ramp. *(Photo courtesy of Trish H. Foley.)*

The backdoor ramp would need to be 38 ft with two platforms or 63 ft with three platforms. There was not enough room at the side entrance for this length of ramping.

The occupational therapist met with a contractor who had an aging-in-place specialist certification to discuss the options. They then met with Ms. K. and offered a third option—a vertical lift over the side entrance stairs with a short ramp over the existing sidewalk to the driveway. This would make the side entrance accessible only by using the lift, but it would take up less room in the yard, and Ms. K would be expending less energy when entering or exiting the home (Fig. 12-3).

The contractor installed the lift and the ramp. A grant paid for the majority of the work. The contractor offered a discount, and family members contributed to the renovation. The occupational therapist conducted follow-up visits to ensure that Ms. K. could use the technology safely and independently.

Discussion Questions

1. What safety considerations should be made when adding a ramp to the front of a house?
2. How might Ms. K.'s ataxia and increased muscle tone affect her ability to maneuver a manual wheelchair on a ramp?
3. The case study mentioned that the bathroom was accessible. What areas of the bathroom needed to be assessed to come to this conclusion? What other areas of the home should be evaluated?

CASE STUDY 12-2 Ethical Challenges Faced by Occupational Therapy Practitioners

Selena, an occupational therapist, and Desmond, an occupational therapy assistant, have worked together in a long-term care facility since their graduation 5 years ago. They enjoy their work with older adults. Often eating lunch together and participating in an occasional happy hour, they have many opportunities to explore their professional hopes and dreams. A subject that frequently arises is their desire to work in the community helping people who wish to age in place. Selena and Desmond begin to plan for a time when they can leave institutional care and move to the community.

They want to plan their transition to ensure their competent and ethical practice. They want to make sure they do not provide inferior care, as other occupational therapy practitioners did when they switched practice areas without engaging in an appropriate level of education and research to ensure competent and ethical practice. Above all, Desmond and Selena want to protect future clients from potential harm by adhering to the principles in the *Code* (AOTA, 2015). These occupational therapy practitioners want to make sure their career changes will be aligned with best practices so that they will retain their standing in the community. Desmond proposes that they research the occupational therapy literature, institutional rules, and applicable regulations to ensure they will not violate standards of practice. Selena suggests that they also identify potential barriers to their transition to a practice focused on aging in place.

Discussion Questions

1. Would Desmond, as an occupational therapy assistant, have limits to the range of services he could provide in the community?
2. What would Selena's responsibility as an occupational therapist be for supervising Desmond?
3. How would they be paid for their services? What local, state, federal, and AOTA resources provide information or funding for aging-in-place services?
4. If they gradually transitioned from the long-term care facility, would they encounter any conflicts of commitment with their current employer? If so, how could they be avoided?
5. What evidence exists to support occupational therapy's role in aging in place?
6. What professional and legal resources would need to be reviewed in order to answer their questions and determine if a change to this practice area is feasible?

Learning Activities

1. Review Case Study 12-2. Questions have been posed and guidance provided to help Selena and Desmond decide if changing their practice to an aging-in-place focus is feasible. Identify the ethical principles and their related standards of conduct from the *Code* that will help in answering their questions. Review the AOTA *Scope of Practice* (AOTA, 2014c) and the *Guidelines for Supervision, Roles, and Responsibilities During the Delivery of Occupational Therapy Services* (AOTA, 2014a) for answers to questions 1, 2, and 6.
2. Are there any NORCs in your area? What recommendations could be made to assist aging residents with the challenges of aging in place? Consider the different levels of need that people present at different stages of aging.

REFERENCES

AARP. (n.d.). Waiting for a ride: Transit access and America's aging population. *AARP Livable Communities.* Retrieved from www.aarp.org/ppi/issues/livable-communities/transportation/future-of-transportation/

AARP. (2015). How an OT or CAPS can make a home a good fit. *AARP Livable Communities.* Retrieved from www.aarp.org/livable-communities/info-2014/using-an-OT-or-CAPS.html

AARP. (2017). What is a livable community? *AARP Livable Communities.* Retrieved from www.aarp.org/livable-communities/about/info-2014/what-is-a-livable-community.html

AARP Foundation. (n.d.a). *Back to work 50+*. Retrieved from www.aarp.org/aarp-foundation/our-work/income/back-to-work-50-plus/

AARP Foundation. (n.d.b). *Experience corp*. Retrieved from www.aarp.org/experience-corps/

AARP Foundation. (n.d.c). *Working for yourself at 50+*. Retrieved from https://workforyourself.aarpfoundation.org/?intcmp=AE-FOU-R2-C2

After 55. (n.d.). *Senior discount guide*. Retrieved from www.after55.com/blog/wp-content/uploads/2017/12/Senior-Discount-Guide-After55.pdf

American Occupational Therapy Association. (2014a). Guidelines for supervision, roles, and responsibilities during the delivery of occupational therapy services. *American Journal of Occupational Therapy, 68*(Suppl. 3), S16–22. doi.5014/ajot.2014.686503

American Occupational Therapy Association. (2014b). *Home modifications: Critically appraised topic (CAT)*. Retrieved from www.aota.org/~/media/corporate/files/secure/practice/ccl/occupation/homemodificationscat.pdf

American Occupational Therapy Association. (2014c). Occupational therapy practice framework: Domain and process (3rd ed.). *American Journal of Occupational Therapy, 68*(Suppl. 1), S1–S48. http://dx.doi.org/10.5014/ajot.2014.682.006

American Occupational Therapy Association. (2014d). Scope of practice. *American Journal of Occupational Therapy, 68*(Suppl. 3), S34–S40. doi:10.5014/ajot.2014.686504

American Occupational Therapy Association. (2015). Occupational therapy code of ethics (2015). *American Journal of Occupational Therapy, 69*(Suppl. 3), 6913410030. http://dx.doi.org/10.5014/ajot.2015.696S03

American Occupational Therapy Association. (2017). Vision 2025. *American Journal of Occupational Therapy, 71*, 7103420010. doi:10.5014/ajot.2017.713002

Bawden, D. (2017). *Marketing and communicating with the aging in place client (CAPS I)*. Washington, DC: National Association of Home Builders.

Beck, J. (2011, December 30). *The psychology of home: Why where you live means so much*. Retrieved from www.theatlantic.com/health/archive/2011/12/the-psychology-of-home-why-where-you-live-means-so-much/249800/

Breeden L. E. (2016). Occupational therapy home safety intervention via telehealth. *International Journal of Telerehabilitation, 8*(1), 29–40. doi:10.5195/ijt.2016.6183

Centers for Disease Control and Prevention. (2009). *Healthy places terminology*. Retrieved from www.cdc.gov/healthyplaces/terminology.htm

Cohousing Association of the United States. (2015). *What is cohousing?* Retrieved from www.cohousing.org/book/export/html/165

Collins, S. M., and Casey, R. P. (2017). *America's aging workforce: Opportunities and challenges*. Washington, DC: U.S. Senate Special Committee on Aging.

Cusato, M. (2015). Aging in place survey report. *Home matters: Preparing for America's aging population*. Retrieved from www.homeadvisor.com/r/wp-content/uploads/2015/10/HomeAdvisor-Aging-in-Place.pdf

Dunn, W., Brown, C., and McGuigan, A. (1994). The ecology of human performance: A framework for considering the effect of context. *American Journal of Occupational Therapy, 48*, 595–607.

Eldercare Directory. (n.d.). *Essential resources for senior citizens and their caregivers*. Retrieved from www.eldercaredirectory.org/

Elliott, S., and Leland, N. E. (2018). Occupational therapy fall prevention interventions for community dwelling adults: A systematic review. *American Journal of Occupational Therapy, 72*, 7204190040. https://doi.org/10.5014/ajot.208.030494

Estes, R. I., Lowery, P., and Baxter, M. F. (2014). Technology and environmental interventions in community based practice. In M. E. Scaffa and S. M. Reitz, *Occupational therapy in community based practice settings* (2nd ed.). Philadelphia, PA: F. A. Davis.

Federal Emergency Management Agency. (n.d.a). *Individuals with disabilities: Get informed*. Retrieved from www.ready.gov/individuals-access-functional-needs

Federal Emergency Management Agency. (n.d.b). *Seniors: Get informed*. Retrieved from www.ready.gov/seniors

Federal Trade Commission. (2015, June). *Consumer information: Reverse mortgages*. Retrieved from www.consumer.ftc.gov/articles/0192-reverse-mortgages

Graham, J. (2017). *Good friends might be your best brain booster as you age*. Retrieved from https://khn.org/news/good-friends-might-be-your-best-brain-booster-as-you-age/

Hawkins, C. (n.d.). *HUD-sponsored senior housing programs*. Retrieved from www.seniorliving.org/lifestyles/hud-senior-housing-programs/

Howard County Government. (n.d.). *Office on aging and independence*. Retrieved from www.howardcountymd.gov/Departments/Community-Resources-and-Services/Office-on-Aging-and-Independence

Internal Revenue Service. (2018). *About publication 502, medical and dental expenses*. Retrieved from www.irs.gov/forms-pubs/about-publication-502

Jayson, S. (2017, November 8). For active seniors, cohousing offers a cozier alternative to downsizing. *Kaiser Health News*. Retrieved from https://khn.org/news/for-active-seniors-cohousing-offers-a-cozier-alternative-to-downsizing/

Kirk-Sanchez, N. J., and McGough, E. L. (2014). Physical exercise and cognitive performance in the elderly: Current perspectives. *Clinical Interventions in Aging, 9*, 51–62.

Keep Inspiring Me. (2018). *Strong women quotes—inspirational quotes for women: Eleanor Roosevelt*. Retrieved from www.keepinspiring.me/inspirational-quotes-for-women/

Landeiro, F., Barrows, P., Musson, E. N., Gray, A. M., and Leal, J. (2016). Reducing social isolation and loneliness in older people: A systematic review protocol. *BMJ Journals, 7*(5). Retrieved from https://bmjopen.bmj.com/content/715/e013778#article-bottom

Lipman, S. (2015). *Modifications for aging in place guide for occupational therapy practitioners in home health*. Philadelphia, PA: Thomas Jefferson University.

Mackenzie, L., Byles, J., and Higginbotham, N. (2000). Designing the Home Falls and Accidents Screening Tool (HOME FAST): Selecting the items. *British Journal of Occupational Therapy, 63*(6), 260–269, doi.org/10.1177/030802260006300604

Maryland Access Point. (n.d.). *Your link to health and support services*. Retrieved from http://aging.maryland.gov/accesspoint/Pages/default.aspx

Maryland Health Care Commission. (n.d.). *Consumer guide to long-term care: Assisted living*. Retrieved from http://mhcc.maryland.gov/consumerinfo/longtermcare/assistedliving.aspx

Masotti, P. J., Fick, R., Johnson-Masotti, A., and MacLeod, S. (2006). Healthy naturally occurring retirement communities: A low-cost approach to facilitating healthy aging. *American Journal of Public Health, 96*(7), 1164–1170. http://doi.org/10.2105/AJPH.2005.068262

Milne-Tyte, A. (2011). In an aging nation, making stores senior-friendly. *NPR Morning Edition.* Retrieved from www.npr.org/2011/05/10/135773106/in-an-aging-nation-making-stores-senior-friendly

National Aging in Place Council. (n.d.). *Glossary of terms.* Retrieved from www.ageinplace.org/Practical-Advice/article/Glossary-of-Terms

National Association of Area Agencies on Aging. (2016). *Mission, vision and work.* Retrieved from www.n4a.org/ourmission

National Association of Home Builders. (n.d.). *Marketing and communicating with the aging in place clients (CAPS I): Who should take this course.* Retrieved from www.nahb.org/en/learn/course-overviews/marketing-communication-strategies-for-aging-accessibility-caps-1.aspx

National Council on Aging. (2017, July 27). *SCSEP: Providing jobs and economic impact across the country.* [Blog post]. Retrieved from www.ncoa.org/blog/scsep-providing-jobs-economic-impact-across-country/

National Institute on Aging. (January, 2009). *Your everyday guide: Fitness and physical activity.* Bethesda, MD: National Institute on Aging.

National Rural Transit Assistance Program. (2016). *ADA Toolkit.* Retrieved from http://nationalrtp.org.

Neufeld, P. S. (2014). Aging in place and naturally occurring retirement communities. In M. E. Scaffa and S. M. Reitz (Eds.), *Occupational therapy in community-based practice settings* (pp. 210–221). Philadelphia, PA: F. A. Davis.

Nicholson, N. R. (2012). A review of social isolation: An important but underassessed condition in older adults. *Journal of Primary Prevention, 33*(2–3), pp. 137–152. Retrieved from https://link.springer.com/article/10.1007/s10935-012-0271-2

Philadelphia Corporation for Aging. (n.d.) *Senior services.* Retrieved from www.pcacares.org/services-for-seniors/

Reitz, S. M., Scaffa, M. E., and Merryman, M. B. (2014). Theoretical frameworks for community-based practice. In M. E. Scaffa and S. M. Reitz (Eds.), *Occupational therapy in community-based practice settings* (pp. 31–50). Philadelphia, PA: F. A. Davis.

Retired Brains. (2018). *Jobs and work for boomers and retirees.* Retrieved from www.retiredbrains.com/jobs--work.html

Ruiz, S., Snyder, L. P., Rotondo, C., Cross-Barnet, C., Colligan, E. M., and Giuriceo, K. (2017). Innovative home visit models associated with reductions in costs, hospitalizations, and emergency department use. *Health Affairs, 36*(3), 425–432.

Salomon, E. (2010). *AARP Public Policy Institute fact sheet 168—Home modifications to promote independent living.* Retrieved from https://assets.aarp.org/rgcenter/ppi/liv-com/fs168-home-modifications.pdf

Scott, J. B. (2017a). *OT 07 Aging in place: Part 1. OnCourse learning.* Retrieved from https://ce.todayinot.com/bundle/bot05/geriatrics-bundle/

Scott, J. B. (2017b). *OT 08 Aging in place: Part 2. OnCourse learning.* Retrieved from https://ce.todayinot.com/bundle/bot05/geriatrics-bundle/

Scott, J. B. (2017c). Productive aging: Ethics from community to supportive living. In J. B. Scott and S. M. Reitz (Eds.), *Practical applications for the Occupational Therapy Code of Ethics* (2015). Bethesda, MD: American Occupational Therapy Association.

Scott, J. B., Reitz, S. M., and Harcum, S. (2017). Principle 4: Justice. In J. B. Scott and S. M. Reitz (Eds.), *Practical applications for the Occupational Therapy Code of Ethics (2015).* Bethesda, MD: American Occupational Therapy Association.

Scott, P. S. (2018, August 12). The new American neighborhood (pp. 8–14). *Parade.*

Senior Support Services. (n.d.). *Senior support services.* Retrieved from http://www.seniorsupportservices.org/

Stark, S. L., Somerville, E. K., and Morris, J. C. (2010). In-Home Occupational Performance Evaluation (I–HOPE). *American Journal of Occupational Therapy, 64*(4), 580–589. doi: 10.5014/ajot.2010.08065

Story, M. F., Mueller, J. L., and Mace, R. L. (1998). *The universal design file: Designing for people of all ages and abilities* (pp. 34–35). Raleigh, NC: Center for Universal Design, North Carolina State University.

United Nations Department of Economic and Social Affairs. (2017a). *World population prospects: The 2017 revision, key findings and advance tables.* Working Paper No. ESA/P/WP/248. Retrieved from https://esa.un.org/unpd/wpp/Publications/Files/WPP2017_KeyFindings.pdf

United Nations Department of Economic and Social Affairs. (2017b). *World population prospects: The 2017 revision: Lower fertility leads to ageing populations.* Retrieved from www.un.org/development/desa/publications/world-population-prospects-the-2017-revision.html

University of Southern California Leonard Davis School of Gerontology. (n.d.). *The value of aging in place.* Retrieved from https://gerontology.usc.edu/resources/articles/the-value-of-aging-in-place/

U.S. Census Bureau. (2017). *Population 60 years and over in the United States. 201 American Community Survey 1-year estimates.* Retrieved from https://factfinder.census.gov/faces/tableservices/jsf/pages/productview.xhtml?pid=ACS_17_1YR_S0102&prodType=table

U.S. Census Bureau. (2018a). *Percentage of people by type of health insurance coverage by age: 2016 and 2017.* Retrieved from www.census.gov/content/dam/Census/library/publications/2018/demo/p60-264.pdf

U.S. Census Bureau. (2018b). Resident population of the United States by sex and age as of July 1, 2017 (in millions). *Statista.* Retrieved from www.statista.com/statistics/241488/population-of-the-us-by-sex-and-age/

U.S. Department of Housing and Urban Development. (2013, Fall). Measuring the costs and savings of aging in place. *Evidence matters: Transforming knowledge into housing and community development policy.* Retrieved from www.huduser.gov/portal/periodicals/em/fall13/highlight2.html

Village to Village Network. (2018). *What is a village?* Retrieved from www.vtnetwork.org/content.aspx?page_id=22&club_id=691012&module_id=248578

Warshaw, R. (2018, February). House call medicine makes a comeback. *Association of American Medical Colleges News.* Retrieved from https://news.aamc.org/patient-care/article/house-calls-make-comeback/

World Health Organization. (2018). *Age-friendly environments.* Retrieved from www.who.int/ageing/age-friendly-environments/en/

Chapter 13

Driving and Community Mobility

Anne E. Dickerson, PhD, OTR/L, SCDCM, FAOTA, FGSA

Being mobile is important in maintaining community, through attendance at community events and activities. The car is often seen as vital for this role, especially in rural settings and especially for older people who could not otherwise engage in such activity.

—Musselwhite (2011, p. 24)

Learning Outcomes

This chapter is designed to enable the reader to:

13-1 Discuss driving as an occupation for older adults.

13-2 Describe the role of the community-based occupational therapist in addressing the complex instrumental activities of daily living (IADLs) of driving and community mobility.

13-3 Differentiate the diverse roles of stakeholders in older drivers' services and driving rehabilitation programs.

13-4 Use the model of OT-DRIVE to appropriately refer clients to the right services at the right time.

13-5 Utilize the functional observation of complex IADLs to determine risk level for the activity of driving.

13-6 Discuss the potential for vehicle technology as an intervention for improving older driver safety.

Key Terms

Advanced driver assistance system
Comprehensive driving evaluation
Crash avoidance system
Driving and community mobility
Driving rehabilitation
Driver rehabilitation specialist
Medically at-risk driver
Occupational Therapy Performance Analysis of Driving
OT-DRIVE
Transportation network companies

Introduction

Occupational therapy practitioners who choose to work in community practice with older adults have the opportunity to focus on client needs and desires. For most older adults that is *aging in place* (Rosenbloom, 2012), in terms of both their home and going beyond their "door" to engage with their community. For the fortunate older adults who live in walkable communities and planned retirement communities, or who have reasonable and safe public transportation, these options extend opportunities for productive aging. However, for most older adults the personal vehicle is needed to get to where they need and want to go. In fact, driving is the most common form of community mobility in the United States (Womack and Silverstein, 2012). Furthermore, **driving and community mobility** as an instrumental activity of daily living (IADL) is recognized as critical for participating in all other occupations (Dickerson, 2012) and as such is considered an *occupation enabler* (Stav and Lieberman, 2008). Thus, older adults who cannot drive or who refrain from driving may have difficulty engaging in many of the fundamental activities for achieving productive aging.

Driving is one of the most valued IADLs (Dickerson, Reistetter, and Gaudy, 2013). This is highlighted by the change in wording from community mobility to driving and community mobility as the identified IADL in the revision of *Occupational Therapy Framework: Domain and Process* (American Occupational Therapy Association [AOTA], 2014). The definition of this IADL remains the same; driving is one means of community mobility along with walking, biking, and other transportation systems. However, specifying driving in naming the IADL reflects the importance of driving to clients, as well as a recognition that the majority of older adults use their personal motor vehicles as their means of community mobility and will continue to do so in the foreseeable future (Coughlin, D'Ambrosio, Pratt, and Mohyde, 2012). Thus, as a profession, occupational therapy has an opportunity to be nationally recognized in meeting the driving needs of older adults. Moreover, if this need goes unmet, other stakeholders or professions will fill the gap and, in fact, are beginning to do so.

Driving as an Occupation

The baby boomers, the generation born between 1945 and 1964, will continue to have an impact on occupational therapy practice, especially community practice, for the next generation of practitioners. Just in terms of sheer numbers, the baby boomers will dominate health-care services. In 2021, the oldest of this generation will be turning 75, the age at which fragility issues begin to affect persons in greater ways (Federal Interagency Forum on Aging-Related Statistics, 2008). But more importantly, the boomers are not the silent generation of their parents but individuals who will insist on services that meet their unique needs. For example, they will want adaptive equipment that is not only useful but also attractive and fits their lifestyle. They will demand that occupational therapy practitioners find effective ways to modify home and work environments before paying for services. And, they will want to be able to do occupations beyond the basic ADLs of dressing, eating, and bathing. Most importantly, the boomers expect to live in their own homes in order to remain independent. For this generation, nothing means *independence* more than having a car outside their door to take them where they want and need to go at any given moment.

To understand the boomers' attachment to the motor vehicle, this generation grew up during a time when cars had just become readily available for most families. While only the wealthy had cars before World War II, in the 1950s and 1960s mass production made vehicles affordable, allowing families to move into the suburbs and expanding their social and physical environments. Every teenager counted the days to get a driver's license because the "car" was the *social networking* tool of this generation. In other words, the car was the equivalent of the smartphone today! Driving down the main street of any town in the "right" vehicle was comparable to posting the latest on Facebook or Twitter—making sure to connect with peers as well as seeing who everyone was with or who had the best "wheels." Although telephones were available to communicate, they were often shared on party lines, and teens had little privacy. The popular method of socialization was driving to local gathering places, whether it was a high school sports game, drugstore, diner, concert, swimming pool, or a drive-in movie theater. With the expansion of the interstate highway system, families explored beyond their immediate communities, going on road trips (e.g., Route 66); taking vacations to the beach, mountains, or lake; traveling to extended family gatherings; or simply enjoying Sunday drives. Thus, driving for the boomers is not just about community mobility (i.e., getting to where they want and need to go) but about the occupation of driving. Regardless of available alternative transportation, an older adult at risk of losing his or her ability to drive may not be losing just an option of community mobility. The older adult will be losing the highly valued occupation of driving "my car"—possibly equivalent to a younger person losing phone privileges. Moreover, it is recognized that driving is crucial to engaging in other occupations, including work, education, play, leisure, and social participation, as well as most other IADLs (e.g., shopping, health management, money management, and caregiving; Schold Davis, Dickerson, Dellinger, and Chodrow, 2016).

Finally, it is important to recognize that older adults are generally safe drivers, overall having the lowest risk of collisions. Part of the reason for fewer crashes is the lower exposure to risk factors. Older adults tend to avoid driving during rush hour, at night, or on high-speed interstates. Additionally, research has clearly demonstrated that it is not "age" that leads to declines in driving but the functional impairments associated with medical conditions that put older drivers at risk (Coughlin and D'Ambrosio, 2012; Dickerson et al., 2017).

Demographics Affecting Driving and Community Mobility

With normal aging, a person has slower information processing and motor responses. As with most activities, older adults compensate by driving more slowly and conservatively. It is really not until drivers are over the age of 70 years that crash risk increases—for example, when intersections require quick information processing and immediate decisions (e.g., yield signs, flashing signals; Dickerson et al., 2007). Moreover, the frailty and fragility of some older adults puts them at more risk of dying from a crash than younger or middle-aged adults (Sifrit, Stutts, Staplin, and Martell, 2010), which is why driver safety is so important. The issue to understand about age and driving is that the number and implications of medical conditions increase as one ages (Kent and Transportation Resarch Board, 2010). Thus, the older adults who are at risk are typically clients who have medical conditions with functional impairments that affect driving skills.

Roles of Occupational Therapy Practitioners in Driving and Community Mobility

The role of occupational therapy practitioners in community-based services differs widely by setting, disability, and the environment in which the client resides. However, at the core the unique value of community-based services is the opportunity to be truly client centered—that is, meeting client needs within the environment in which individuals live their lives. While the value of distinct occupations is different for each individual, in the initial therapeutic process interventions generally start with basic ADLs to ensure the individual is able to perform the daily tasks of self-care or develop compensation strategies to meet those needs. As the client improves, attention moves to the valued IADLs (e.g., cooking, medication management, shopping). Unfortunately, sometimes the IADL of driving and community mobility is not addressed. However, unless the client wants to remain homebound or has an impairment that severely limits mobility, this highly valued IADL (Dickerson et al., 2013) is essential to the recovery of function and quality of life for clients. While the occupational therapy practitioner may not expect driving to be a viable option based on the client's condition/diagnosis, if driving is a valued goal for the client, the practitioner should make every effort to engage the client in appropriate therapy for the increasing capacities needed for driving and, if not possible, work on other methods of community mobility.

Driving and Community Mobility as an Instrumental Activity of Daily Living

Although driving is a privilege granted by the state, community mobility is a right for everyone. It is critical to understand that many of the ADLs and most of the IADLs are affected by whether someone is able to be mobile in their community. Table 13-1 outlines aspects of occupations, as identified by the practice framework (AOTA, 2014), that warrant consideration when addressing driving and community mobility of the client (Dickerson, 2016).

During the occupational therapy process, when the question of driving arises from the client or family members, the occupational therapy practitioner must acknowledge and respond without hesitation. This does not mean the practitioner is making an immediate decision about a client's licensure to drive. However, by working with the client in the client's familiar environment, the community-based therapist probably has the best perspective in terms of the client's true functional abilities and deficits and thus can easily identify functional deficits that will affect the activity of driving. Identifying potential risk when considering driving is the same as identifying risk with other complex tasks. If a client has difficulty independently organizing a meal or

Table 13-1 Occupations and Considerations for Driving and Community Mobility

Occupations as Identified by Framework	Considerations in Planning for Driving and Community Mobility
ADLs: bathing or showering, toileting and toilet hygiene, dressing, swallowing or eating, feeding, functional mobility, personal device care, personal hygiene and grooming, and sexual activity	• Incontinence management to be able to use transportation • Secure and store mobility devices in the vehicle • Ingress and egress from the vehicle
IADLs: care of others, care of pets, child-rearing, communication management, driving and community mobility, financial management, health management and maintenance, home establishment and management, meal preparation and cleanup, religious and spiritual activities and expression, safety and emergency maintenance, and shopping	• Transporting family member who does not drive • Transporting grandchildren to school, day care, or from family home • Going to the bank, post office, and pharmacy • Medical and/or therapy appointments • Health club, exercise group, yoga, trainer • Grocery stores and restaurants • Religious activities • Managing a second home or vacation spot • Support groups such as Alcoholics Anonymous
Rest and sleep: sleep preparation, sleep participation, and rest	• Fatigue increases crash risk
Education: formal education participation, informal personal education needs or interests exploration, and informal personal education participation	• Attending community college classes to learn new skills (e.g., computer skills, retirement planning, estate planning) • Attending formal educational classes • Attending community recreational activities such as senior sports, painting, quilting, or plays
Work: employment interests and pursuits, employment seeking and acquisition, job performance, retirement preparation and adjustment, and volunteer exploration and participation	• If working outside the home, must be able to use some mode of transportation • Volunteering in community, especially understanding that older adults are the largest age group of volunteers
Play or leisure: exploration and participation	• Access to play or leisure any day or time • Sports, fishing, golf, quilting bee, yard sales, boating, walking, hiking
Social participation: community, family, peer, or friend	• Access to social participation any day or time • Visiting friends and family • Lunch/coffee with colleagues, family, and friends • Social events such as graduations, movies, concerts, birthday parties, reunions, and other celebrations • Vacations with family or friends

using the stove, determining how to put on garments, or managing the household budget, there is clear risk with the IADL of driving and community mobility.

When considering the IADL of driving, the identification process is not more complex, but it is more complicated. With driving, the potential risk is not just to the client and maybe the caregivers. It is likely to affect the general public, as the negative result is a crash that often involves more than one person. While the fear of making a decision about driving is often the reason occupational therapy practitioners do not have the confidence to address driving (Dickerson, Schold Davis, and Chew, 2011), driving and community mobility is within the scope of occupational therapy practice and the ethical obligation of the practitioner to identify risk (Slater, 2012). In fact, practitioners cannot make decisions about driving *licensing,* as only the state licensing agencies grant licenses. However, because occupational therapy practitioners observe functional performance and identify risk, they have been identified as the "go to" profession for driver evaluation and rehabilitation (Society and Pomidor, 2016). Furthermore, unless occupational therapy practitioners step up to address this IADL with all clients, it could be another practice area lost to other less-qualified service providers (who are without or have less medical training or education), who are already devising certificate programs that purport to be able to evaluate older adults effectively (Dickerson, 2012; Dickerson, 2014).

Unlike the older adult driver experiencing normal age changes, a **medically at-risk driver** may have specific visual, perceptual, motor, and cognitive issues that are best addressed by professionals with medical training (Dickerson and Schold Davis, 2012). Without the appropriate medical knowledge, a medically at-risk driver may be inaccurately evaluated, offered inappropriate recommendations concerning vehicle modification, and/or told that driving is no longer an option when that may be inaccurate. In order to preserve this highly valued IADL, the potential to return to driving must be considered by those who understand activity analysis and the occupation of driving. Thus, the goals for this chapter are to review driving and community within the context of occupational therapy practitioners working in community practice through a review of the IADL of driving and community mobility, the process and importance of identifying risk, and ways to address this IADL through appropriate interventions.

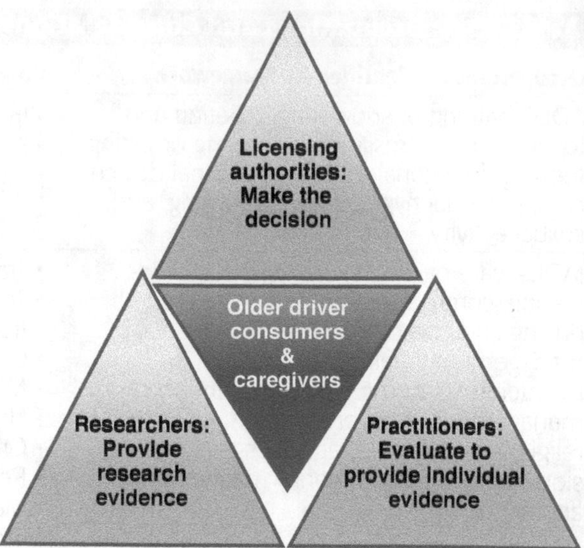

Figure 13-1 Four stakeholder groups with essential functions related to driving. *(Adapted from "Can Clinicians, Researchers, and Driver Licensing Officials Build a Shared Vocabulary?" [p. 189], by A. Dickerson and E. S. Davis, 2014,* Occupational Therapy in Health Care, 28*[2], 188–193. Used with permission.)*

Stakeholders in Driving

Dickerson and Schold Davis (2014) identified four categories of stakeholders and their essential functions when considering driving, which include state licensing authorities, researchers, practitioners, and consumers (i.e., drivers, caregivers, family members; see Fig. 13-1). Each stakeholder comes from a different perspective to play an essential role in the determination of driving privileges for older drivers.

State licensing agencies make the legal determinations about the status of all drivers. While federal guidelines influence state laws and practices, each individual state in the United States develops its own policies. Under ideal conditions, to determine an appropriate licensing decision licensing authorities use recommendations from practitioners, who evaluate the individual client using evidence from researchers.

Researchers provide the evidence for making decisions about fitness to drive, particularly when related to screening and assessment. With provided evidence concerning the validity and reliability of assessment tools, researchers assist in the establishment of appropriate constraints, limitations, and potential "cutoff" scores to be used by practitioners and/or licensing authorities. In best practice, researchers translate the research outcomes into practical criteria for an objective decision about fitness to drive. Researchers may be psychologists, occupational therapists, physicians, or other professionals with research degrees.

Practitioners provide the professional screening and evaluation of individual drivers and provide recommendations to the licensing authorities. Occupational therapy practitioners are uniquely qualified to use their skilled observation and clinical reasoning to provide the most accurate picture of older adults performing complex IADLs, which includes driving. In some cases, driving decisions are the responsibility of the primary physician. However, it is clear that physicians are not always comfortable with this decision-making process (Brooks et al., 2011) and often look to other professionals for insight into the client's level of risk. This "other" professional group has traditionally been the **driver rehabilitation specialist** (DRS), who can provide an expert evaluation and recommendation. However, significant research evidence and work has been done to promote general practice occupational therapists as the first line of evaluation for the IADL of driving and community mobility (Dickerson and Bédard, 2014; Dickerson, Schold Davis, and Carr, 2018; Society and Pomidor, 2016). This will be the topic of the next sections.

Finally, the essential category of stakeholder groups are consumers, who are the drivers, caregivers, or family members at the center of the issue. In order to retain driving privileges, consumers attempt to understand and manage the complexities of the evaluation and licensing process. Consumers seek services that will assist them in this process and, conversely, will avoid services that do not offer a desired outcome or appear not to be worth the investment of time, money, or effort.

In an ideal world, this framework illustrates a process that is integrated between stakeholder groups in order to be responsive to the consumer as the beneficiary of services. This process depends on communication and cooperation among stakeholder groups. As such, communication is built on common knowledge and language. Unfortunately, each profession has its own language, including occupational therapy. So referring an older adult to get "a driving evaluation" would likely be interpreted by the consumer as meaning he or she should go to the licensing agency or a driving school, not to an occupational therapist or a driver rehabilitation specialist for a skilled, medically based evaluation. Although progress has been made in this process (Transportation Research Board [TRB], 2016), continued work is needed to facilitate a common nomenclature in order to benefit clients. Box 13-1 provides definitions for important terms in driver rehabilitation. Since this was recognized as an issue, the goal of a unified taxonomy for use by practitioners, licensing authorities, and researchers has been developed by leaders in the transportation field (TRB, 2016).

Driving Rehabilitation and the Driver Rehabilitation Specialist

Driving rehabilitation is a form of therapy—traditionally compensatory—that plans, develops, and implements services for individuals with disabilities in order for the individual to drive. A DRS is a general term that encompasses a diverse group of providers. The requirements for the certification and education of a DRS are not based on being a member of a specific medical profession, and there is no consistency between states. Providers who use the initials *DRS* have diverse backgrounds, including engineers, driving instructors, and health-care professionals. The reason is based on the history of driving rehabilitation.

The field of driving rehabilitation developed after the proliferation of the automobile (Pellerito, 2006). In the 1920s, adaptations to vehicles were created to allow individuals to return to driving despite physical impairments (Hyde, 2006). Occupational therapists, driver educators, and engineers collaborated to provide driver rehabilitation based on medical and vocational rehabilitation service models (Pellerito, 2006). The focus was on *compensatory* rehabilitation through vehicle modification and adaptive equipment for individuals with very specific *physical* impairments (e.g., spinal cord injuries, amputations, spina bifida, and dwarfism). One example is determining the most appropriate type of vehicle hand controls for a specific driver with a spinal cord injury. In this case, a DRS with an engineering or driver instructor background may be more practical.

With the medical advancements of the later 20th century and the technology advances in vehicles, individuals with acquired brain injury and/or progressive diseases are able to return to driving. Thus, current DRSs need an advanced education to be able to evaluate fitness to drive from a cognitive perspective, not just adjust the vehicle to physical deficits. From this historical perspective, the complementary roles of a diverse group of DRS skill sets functioned well and continue to be best practice in some cases.

In addition, with the advent of technology such as driving simulators, as well as the deeper understanding of recovery from conditions, driving rehabilitation is no longer just compensatory but also

Box 13-1 Select Definitions From the 2016 Transportation Research Board's *Taxonomy and Terms for Stakeholders in Senior Mobility*

Driving assessment: use of an on-road test to measure and qualify driving skills and abilities, which may be triggered by a screening outcome indicating increased risk for driving impairment crash involvement.

Driving evaluation: obtaining and interpreting data and documenting results to inform an individualized mobility plan based on an individual's driving abilities or potential to be an independent driver or inform a determination of fitness to drive.

Clinical driving evaluation: a health-care professional obtains and interprets data and documents results to determine fitness to drive through assessment of sensory-perceptual, cognitive, or psychomotor functional abilities using specific tools or instruments.

Comprehensive driving evaluation: a complete evaluation of an individual's driving knowledge, skills, and abilities by a health-care professional that includes:

1. Medical and driving history
2. Clinical assessment of sensory-perceptual, cognitive, or psychomotor functional abilities
3. On-road assessment, as appropriate
4. An outcome summary
5. Recommendations for an inclusive mobility plan, including transportation options

Driving mobility equipment evaluation: obtaining and interpreting data and documenting results to inform an individualized mobility plan based on an individual's abilities or potential to be an independent driver using mobility equipment, including wheelchair seating, that may include:

1. Screening or assessment of sensory-perceptual, cognitive, and psychomotor functioning
2. Wheelchair seating or mobility equipment as they pertain to the functional skills necessary to safely operate a motor vehicle
3. On-road assessment of the individual using equipment similar to that which will be recommended

Fitness to drive: a driver characteristic or a description of a driver, defined by the absence of any functional (sensory-perceptual, cognitive, or psychomotor) deficit or medical condition that significantly impairs an individual's ability to fully control the vehicle while conforming to the rules of the road and obeying traffic laws or that significantly increases crash risk.

Standardized road test: a road test with specific components (e.g., right turns, highways, intersections) that are always performed to establish a score that is comparable across individuals. [Note: Standardized road tests may only be standardized for a specific city, evaluator, or research study.]

Road test: an examination of driving maneuvers and knowledge of rules of the road performed in a motor vehicle on a public highway or street.

Driving test: an examination including specified driving maneuvers performed in a motor vehicle.

Data from "Taxonomy and Terms for Stakeholders in Senior Mobility," by Transportation Research Board, 2016, *Transportation Research Circular, Number E-C211.*

restorative. In other words, driving rehabilitation has become a more comprehensive service. Accordingly, the field needs more differentiation of services into both professionals with more general skills and professionals with specialized skills. However, when an individual has a neurological issue or cognitive impairment, such as dementia, it is essential that the practitioner doing driving rehabilitation has a medical background. Determining the profession with the appropriate qualifications can be complicated by a number of factors, including the type of driving evaluation to be conducted, compensation or rehabilitation strategies needed, and the anticipated progression of the medical condition.

A DRS who is also an occupational therapist typically performs a comprehensive driving evaluation to determine an individual's fitness to drive. The **comprehensive driving evaluation** is defined as

> *a complete assessment of an individual's driving knowledge, skills, and abilities by a health care professional that includes: 1) medical and driving history, 2) clinical assessment of physical, cognitive, vision, and/or perception abilities, 3) on road assessment, as appropriate, 4) an outcome summary, and 5) goals and recommendations for an inclusive mobility plan including transportation options. (TRB, 2016)*

Once completed, the outcomes of the evaluation may include one or a combination of the following implementation plans:

- Rehabilitation of underlying human components (e.g., increase scanning abilities through specifically designed intervention)
- Compensation through training (e.g., driving simulator training, avoiding left turns)
- Compensation through adaptation of the vehicle (e.g., using hand controls or a steering knob for one-handed turning)
- Cessation of driving counseling and planning

Because of advances in technology, a wide range of options and innovations are available to compensate for specific physical impairments. For example, bioptic telescope systems compensate for low vision, hand controls can compensate for lower-limb amputations, or a joystick can be used to steer by an individual with spinal cord injury. These are all examples of vehicular modification that allow for independent driving. However, the individual must have the capacity for new learning and skill development. Technological advances are not yet able to compensate for deficits in executive functioning, a key determinant of driver strategies, tactics, and safety (Dickerson, 2014). Additionally, individuals with decreased insight or poor cognitive abilities, in addition to their physical impairments, no longer have the ability to voluntarily limit or adapt their behaviors to be deemed fit to drive. This is where the observations of the occupational therapist, especially in the home environment, are critical in the identification process. As the therapist works with a client and observes whether new learning is possible or difficult, the practitioner considers the activity analysis of driving and the client's learning outcomes and then informs team members about the client's observed potential or risk.

Levels of Driving Programs

The field of driving rehabilitation is changing with differing needs of clients, advanced vehicle technology, and 50 different state licensing authorities trying to meet the ever-growing numbers of drivers. To complicate matters, physicians are frequently asked about driving by their patients and/or family members and may not know about the services of either DRSs or the role of occupational therapy in addressing the IADL of driving and community mobility. Similarly, consumers (e.g., clients, caregivers, and family members) are also confused by the concept and cost of a medically based comprehensive driving evaluation because they do not understand the level of service needed. Consumers typically do not understand that licensing authorities can simply withdraw a license based on a diagnosis, and they are also unaware of where to go for help if this happens.

In an effort to clarify services, the two professional associations most closely related to driving rehabilitation, the Association for Driver Rehabilitation Specialists (ADED) and the AOTA, created and adopted the *Spectrum of Driver Services,* a document describing the range and diversity of driver services (Lane et al., 2014). This seminal document illustrates the diverse types of services related to driving (Lane et al., 2014).

The *Spectrum of Driver Services* has two sections. The first section illustrates the range of available services, from community awareness to specific services of driver rehabilitation (see Fig. 13-2). The second section breaks driver rehabilitation programs into three general groupings according to the level and complexity of services (see Fig. 13-3). The significant features include:

1. The differentiation between community-based education; medically based assessment, education, and referral; and specialized evaluation and intervention with driving rehabilitation programs.
2. For each of the five different program types (driver safety programs, driving schools, driver screening, clinical IADL evaluations, and DR [driver rehab] programs), the typical providers and credentials are described. This helps differentiate which programs use providers with a medical/professional licensing background.
3. For each program, the required providers' knowledge and typical services illustrate the difference between preventative services (i.e., updating driving skills or acquiring a driver's license) from the medically based assessments. These sections also articulate the differences between screening at a

Spectrum of Driver Services: Right Services for the Right People at the Right Time

A description consumers and health-care providers can use to distinguish the type of services needed for an older adult.

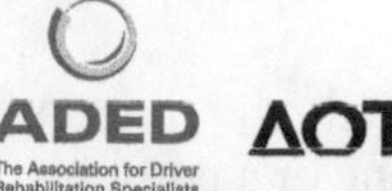

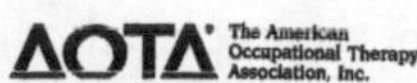

	Community-based education		Medically-based assessment, education and referral		Specialized evaluation and training
Program type	**Driver safety programs**	**Driving school**	**Driver screen**	**Clinical IADL evaluation**	**Driver rehabilitation programs (Includes driver evaluation)**
Typical providers and credentials	Program-specific credentials (e.g., AARP and AAA Driver Improvement Program).	Licensed Driving Instructor (LDI) certified by state licensing agency or Dept. of Education.	Health-care professional (e.g., physician, social worker, and neuropsychologist).	Occupational Therapy Practitioner (Generalist or Driver Rehabilitation Specialist#). Other health professional degree with expertise in Instrumental Activities of Daily Living (IADL).	Driver Rehabilitation Specialist,# Certified Driver Rehabilitation Specialist,* Occupational Therapist with Specialty Certification in Driving and Community Mobility.+
Required provider's knowledge	Program-specific knowledge. Trained in course content and delivery.	Instructs novice or relocated drivers, excluding medical or aging conditions that might interfere with driving, for purposes of teaching/training/refreshing/updating driving skills.	Knowledge of relevant medical conditions, assessment, referral, and/or intervention processes. Understand the limits and value of assessment tools, including simulation as a measurement of fitness to drive.	Knowledge of medical conditions and the implication for community mobility including driving. Assess the cognitive, visual, perceptual, behavioral, and physical limitations that may impact driving performance. Knowledge of available services. Understands the limits and value of assessment tools, including simulation as a measurement of fitness to drive.	Applies knowledge of medical conditions with implications to driving. Assesses the cognitive, visual, perceptual, behavioral, and physical limitations that may impact driving performance. Integrates the clinical findings with assessment of on-road performance. Synthesizes client and caregiver needs, and assists in decisions about equipment and vehicle modification options available. Coordinates multidisciplinary providers and resources, including driver education, health-care team, vehicle choice and modifications, community services, funding/payers, driver licensing agencies, training and education, and caregiver support.
Typical services provided	1) Classroom- or computer-based refresher for licensed drivers: review of rules of the road, driving techniques, driving strategies, state laws, etc. 2) Enhanced self-awareness, choices, and capability to self-limit.	1) Enhance driving performance. 2) Acquire drivers permit or license. 3) Counsel with family members for student driver skill development. 4) Recommend continued training and/ or undergoing licensing test. 5) Remedial Programs (e.g., license reinstatement course for teens/adults, license point reduction courses).	1) Counsel on risks associated with specific conditions (e.g., medications, fractures, post-surgery). 2) Investigate driving risks associated with changes in vision, cognition, and sensory-motor function. 3) Determine actions for the at-risk driver: • Refer to IADL evaluation, driver rehabilitation program, and/or other services. • Discuss driving cessation; provide access to counseling and education for alternative transportation options. 4) Follow reporting/referral structure for licensing recommendations.	1) Evaluate and interpret risks associated with changes in vision, cognition, and sensory-motor functions due to acute or chronic conditions. 2) Facilitate remediation of deficits to advance client readiness for driver rehabilitation services. 3) Develop an individualized transportation plan considering client diagnosis and risks, family, caregiver, environmental and community options and limitations: • Discuss resources for vehicle adaptations (e.g., scooter lift). • Facilitate client training on community transportation options (e.g., mobility managers, dementia-friendly transportation). • Discuss driving cessation. For clients with poor self-awareness, collaborate with caregivers on cessation strategies. • Refer to driver rehabilitation program. 4) Document driver safety risk and recommended intervention plan to guide further action. 5) Follow professional ethics on referrals to the driver licensing authority.	Programs are distinguished by complexity of evaluations, types of equipment, vehicles, and expertise of provider. 1) Navigate driver license compliance and basic eligibility through intake of driving and medical history. 2) Evaluate and interpret risks associated with changes in vision, cognition, and sensory-motor functions in the driving context by the medically trained provider. 3) Perform a comprehensive driving evaluation (clinical and on road). 4) Advise client and caregivers about evaluation results, and provide resources, counseling, education, and/or intervention plan. 5) Intervention may include training with compensatory strategies, skills, and vehicle adaptations or modifications for drivers and passengers. 6) Advocate for clients in terms of access to funding resources and/or reimbursement. 7) Provide documentation about fitness to drive to the physician and/or driver-licensing agency in compliance with regulations. 8) Prescribe equipment in compliance with state regulations and collaborate with Mobility Equipment Dealer^ for fitting and training. 9) Present resources and options for continued community mobility if recommending driving cessation or transition from driving. Recommendations may include (but not restricted to): 1) drive unrestricted; 2) drive with restrictions; 3) cessation of driving pending rehabilitation or training; 4) planned re-evaluation for progressive disorders; 5) driving cessation; 6) referral to another program.
Outcome	Provides education and awareness.	Enhances skills for healthy drivers.	Indicates risk or need for follow-up for medically at-risk drivers.		Determines fitness to drive and provides rehabilitative services.

#DRS – Health professional degree with specialty training in driver evaluation and rehabilitation. *CDRS – Certified Driver Rehabilitation Specialist-Credentialed by ADED (Association for Driver Rehabilitation Specialists). +SCDCM – Specialty Certified in Driving and Community Mobility by AOTA (American Occupational Therapy Association).
^Quality Approved Provider by NMEDA (National Mobility Equipment Dealers Association).

Driver Rehabilitation Programs: Defining Program Models, Services, and Expertise.
Occupational Therapy In Health Care, 28(2):177–187, 2014

Figure 13-2 *Spectrum of Driver Services:* A list of the diverse types of driving services with a description of how to differentiate their services. Provides information and/or service to older adults. *(Taken from "Driver Rehabilitation Programs: Defining Program Models, Services, and Expertise," by A. Lane, E. Green, A. E. Dickerson, E. S. Davis, B. Rolland, and J. T. Stohler, 2014,* Occupational Therapy in Health Care, *28[2], 177–187.)*

Spectrum of Driver Rehabilitation Program Services

A description consumers and health care providers can use to distinguish the services provided by driver rehabilitation programs which best fits a client's need.

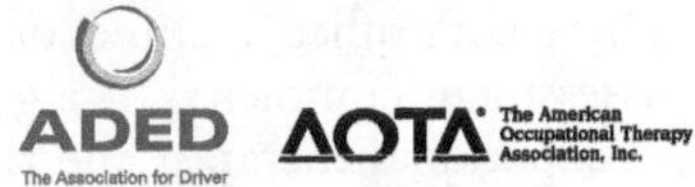

Program Type	Driver Rehabilitation Programs Determine fitness to drive and/or provide rehabilitative services .		
Levels of program and typical provider credentials	**Basic** Provider is a Driver Rehabilitation Specialist (DRS)# with professional background in occupational therapy, other allied health field, driver education, or a professional team of CDRS or SCDCM with LDI.**	**Low tech** Driver Rehabilitation Specialist,# Certified Driver Rehabilitation Specialist,* Occupational Therapist with Specialty Certification in Driving and Community Mobility,+ or in combination with LDI. Certification in Driver Rehabilitation is recommended as the provider for comprehensive driving evaluation and training.	**High tech** Driver Rehabilitation Specialist,# Certified Driver Rehabilitation Specialist,* Occupational Therapist with Specialty Certification in Driving and Community Mobility.+ Certification in Driver Rehabilitation is recommended as the provider for comprehensive driving evaluation and training with advanced skills and expertise to complete complex client and vehicle evaluation and training.
Program service	Offers driver evaluation, training and education. May include use of adaptive driving aids that do not affect operation of primary or secondary controls (e.g., seat cushions or additional mirrors). May include transportation planning (transition and options), cessation planning, and recommendations for clients as passengers.	Offers comprehensive driving evaluation, training, and education, with or without adaptive driving aids that affect the operation of primary or secondary controls, vehicle ingress/egress, and mobility device storage/securement. May include use of adaptive driving aids such as seat cushions or additional mirrors. At the Low Tech level, adaptive equipment for primary control is typically mechanical. Secondary controls may include wireless or remote access. May include transportation planning (transition and options), cessation planning, and recommendations for clients who plan to ride as passengers only.	Offers a wide variety of adaptive equipment and vehicle options for comprehensive driving evaluation, training and education, including all services available in Low Tech and Basic programs. At this level, providers have the ability to alter positioning of primary and secondary controls based on client's need or ability level. High Tech adaptive equipment for primary and secondary controls includes devices that meet the following conditions: 1) capable of controlling vehicle functions or driving controls, and 2) consists of a programmable computerized system that interfaces/integrates with an electronic system in the vehicle.
Access to driver's position	Requires independent transfer into OEM^ driver's seat in vehicle.	Addresses transfers, seating, and position into OEM^ driver's seat. May make recommendations for assistive devices to access driver's seat, improved positioning, wheelchair securement systems, and/or mechanical wheelchair loading devices.	Access to the vehicle typically requires ramp or lift and may require adaptation to OEM driver's seat. Access to driver position may be dependent on use of a transfer seat base, or clients may drive from their wheelchair. Provider evaluates and recommends vehicle structural modifications to accommodate products such as ramps, lifts, wheelchair and scooter hoists, transfer seat bases, wheelchairs suitable to utilize as a driver seat, and/or wheelchair securement systems.
Typical vehicle modification: primary controls: gas, brake, steering	Uses OEM^ controls.	Primary driving control examples: A) mechanical gas/brake hand control; B) left foot accelerator pedal; C) pedal extensions; D) park brake lever or electronic park brake; E) steering device (spinner knob, tri-pin, C-cuff).	Primary driving control examples (in addition to Low Tech options): A) powered gas/brake systems; B) power park brake integrated with a powered gas/brake system; C) variable effort steering systems; D) reduced diameter steering wheel, horizontal steering, steering wheel extension, joystick controls; E) reduced effort brake systems.
Typical vehicle modification: secondary controls	Uses OEM^ controls.	Secondary driving control examples: A) remote horn button; B) turn signal modification (remote, crossover lever); C) remote wiper controls; D) gear selector modification; E) key/ignition adaptions.	Electronic systems to access secondary and accessory controls. Secondary driving control examples (in addition to Low Tech options): A) remote panels, touch pads or switch arrays that interface with OEM^ electronics; B) wiring extension for OEM^ electronics; C) powered transmission shifter.

#DRS - Health professional degree with specialty training in driver evaluation and rehabilitation, *CDRS – Certified Driver Rehabilitation Specialist – Credentialed by ADED (Association for Driver Rehabilitation Specialists). +SCDCM – Specialty Certified in Driving and Community Mobility by AOTA (American Occupational Therapy Association) ^OEM – Original Equipment installed by Manufacturer.
**LDI-licensed driving instructor.

Driver Rehabilitation Programs: Defining Program Models, Services, and Expertise.
Occupational Therapy In Health Care, 28(2):177–187, 2014

Figure 13-3 A comparison of the three levels of driving rehabilitation services. *(Taken from "Driver Rehabilitation Programs: Defining Program Models, Services, and Expertise," by A. Lane, E. Green, A. E. Dickerson, E. S. Davis, B. Rolland, and J. T. Stohler, 2014,* Occupational Therapy in Health Care, 28*[2], 177–187.)*

physician's office, a clinic, or an IADL assessment completed by a generalist occupational therapist and the specialized services provided by the DRS.

4. The outcome of each program type is succinctly stated. Driver safety programs provide education and awareness, and driving schools enhance skills for healthy drivers. As such, these two categories should not be the intervention resource for individuals with medical conditions affecting driving. These individuals should be referred to the programs that provide medically based assessment, evaluation, and/or specialized programs.

Figure 13-3 illustrates the different levels of driver rehabilitation programs. This document marks the first time that driving rehabilitation programs began the process of describing the different types and levels of service. For example, if clients have any upper- or lower-extremity paresis, they should be referred to a *Low Tech* program because adaptive equipment may be needed to compensate for the operation of the primary or secondary controls of the vehicles. The *Basic* program would not be appropriate since the typical evaluation vehicle does not have any modification, and therefore, the most effective and efficient evaluation could not be completed. However, for older adults with a cognitive issue, the Basic program provides a lower-cost service, since the evaluation vehicle does not need an extensive amount of enhancement. Finally, those who will need the high-tech modification required for driving from a wheelchair, for example, should seek the services of a DRS in a *High Tech* program.

Screening and Evaluation of Driving and Community Mobility

In the process of addressing driving and community mobility, it is critical to differentiate screening versus evaluation. Screening is the process of obtaining and reviewing data to determine the needs for evaluation, while evaluation is obtaining and interpreting data to document results, inform, and, if appropriate, formulate a treatment plan (TRB, 2016). In the case of driving and community mobility, the process of screening might be done by training, skilled, or highly skilled individuals, while evaluations are done by highly trained/skilled professionals.

Levels of Risk

One of the barriers to community practice occupational therapists addressing driving and community mobility may be their level of confidence (Dickerson et al., 2011). Experienced therapists may be hesitant to make recommendations concerning driving because they may mistakenly believe their recommendation about the IADL of driving and community mobility is the same as a recommendation from an occupational therapy practitioner with the expertise of driving rehabilitation (Schold Davis and Dickerson, 2017). A practitioner who is observing a client struggling to prepare a meal or manage a budget or medication is confident addressing observed deficits and making recommendations about living alone or needing supervision because the therapist *is* an expert in activity analysis. This reasoning also applies to the complex task of driving. Community practice occupational therapists can competently make recommendations about the IADL of driving and community mobility, especially since the context of their observations are within the client's familiar home environment. If the client is unable to be left alone for 2 hours, manage medication or finances, or cook unsupervised due to cognitive deficits, the client is not competent to drive. Thus, if the client has observed difficulties with complex IADL tasks, a recommendation for ceasing driving, refraining from driving during intervention, or scheduling a comprehensive driving evaluation is justified and can and should be made to be in compliance with the AOTA (2015) *Occupational Therapy Code of Ethics (2015).*

Engage Your Brain 13-1

What theoretical framework can support your justification for making a recommendation about fitness to drive?

Research demonstrating that fitness to drive can be determined through evaluating IADL tasks was used to design an algorithm (Dickerson et al., 2011). More recently, using the logical steps of the algorithm, a model for general practice occupational therapy practitioners—which would include community practice occupational therapists—was developed to describe and support the clinical judgment for determining older adults' risk factors based on evidence from observing occupational performance (Schold Davis and Dickerson, 2017). Figure 13-4 illustrates this conceptual model.

This model can be used to describe the current status of patients in terms of risk for safe driving and the interventions that are most appropriate. The *red* zone (i.e., top light) proposes that there is strong evidence through evaluation that driving risk is high; visual, motor, perceptual, and/or cognitive impairments exceed the threshold for safe driving. Clients in the red zone include individuals with moderate/severe dementia or those who have neurological issues that impair insight and judgment. Referral to a specialist is unwarranted, as it would result in duplication of services since many of the same assessments would be utilized, with the DRS likely choosing not to go forward with the on-road component. The intervention for mobility should include driving retirement if driving was a goal and focus on mobility preservation through the exploration of supportive transportation.

Engage Your Brain 13-2

Based on the AOTA (2015) *Code of Ethics,* what are some ethical considerations when a patient who has significant cognitive issues is being discharged and you know he or she is planning to drive?

The *green* zone (i.e., bottom light) describes clients with temporary health issues that preclude them from driving for a period of time. These clients will likely return to a level of recovery without evidence of impaired fitness to drive. Examples would be clients recovering from hip or knee replacement. With these clients, physical impairments may limit current driving options, but the expertise of the DRS is again not needed because these clients have an intact cognitive capacity to self-restrict during this interval. However, the occupational therapist should ensure that short-term mobility options are addressed during the period of nondriving. In addition, the therapist should pursue the health promotion/prevention objectives of encouraging physical exercise, promote driver safety programs, and discuss the warning signs of driving risks for the future.

When there is no clear evidence (not red or green), determining the degree to which impairments affect the fitness to drive is categorized as *yellow* (i.e., middle light). That is, the occupational therapist does not have enough information or evidence from evaluations/observations to make a recommendation. However, using evidence from evaluations and clinical judgment, the practitioner can determine if it is best to:

- Optimize subskills for driving through interventions
- Consider other services to improve fitness to drive
- Determine readiness for a comprehensive driving evaluation by a DRS, scheduled at the "right time" (Lane et al., 2014; Schold Davis and Dickerson, 2017)

In order to use the model, a translational tool was developed to help occupational therapy practitioners understand how to apply their clinical knowledge and reasoning skills to the IADL of driving and community mobility for older adult clients (Schold Davis and Dickerson, 2017). This tool, called **OT-DRIVE,** is intended to guide practitioners to ethically address driving as an IADL and to develop a plan that will prioritize the health and safety of the client and community. It is of prime importance for community practice occupational therapists to understand that driving is the primary means for older adults to meet social and personal needs. Using this model, practitioners can broaden their conceptualization of driving and community mobility, understand the importance of community access to the individual, and develop a plan for driving and community mobility to address clients' goals beyond their home to achieve productive aging.

OT-DRIVE Model for Community Practice

Occupational therapy evaluations begin with the occupational therapy profile to determine the client's desires and goals. In addition to other occupations, including ADLs and other IADLs, the

SPECTRUM OF DECISION INDICATORS FOR DRIVING & COMMUNITY MOBILITY

Risk Determination Based on Evidence and Clinical Judgment

Normal aging

Medical issues with increasing complexity

Occupational profile:

Higher Risk: Evidence is **Strong**; Above thresholds of impairment in most areas.

Risk: Degree to which impairment affects fitness-to-drive must be addressed.

- Determine driving potential now and in the future
- Consider need for Comprehensive Driving Evaluation

Lower Risk: Evidence is **weak**; below threshold for impairment that would affect Fitness to Drive.

NON-DRIVER

Impairments exceed threshold for safe driving.

DRIVER

No impairment indicators to report restriction on driving.

Occupational therapy intervention with individualized plan for mobility includes:

- Promote driving retirement
- Mobility preservation through supportive transportation

- Rehab: To optimize subskills
- Assess readiness for comprehensive driving evaluation "at the right time"
- Consider need for services to improve Fitness to Drive

- Encourage fitness, strength, flexibility
- Promote driver safety programs & CarFit
- Discuss warning signs

From: Schold Davis, E., & Dickerson, A. (2017). OT-DRIVE: Integrating the IADL of driving and community mobility into routine practice. *OT Practice, 22*(13), 8–14. Copyright American Occupational Therapy Association, 2017.

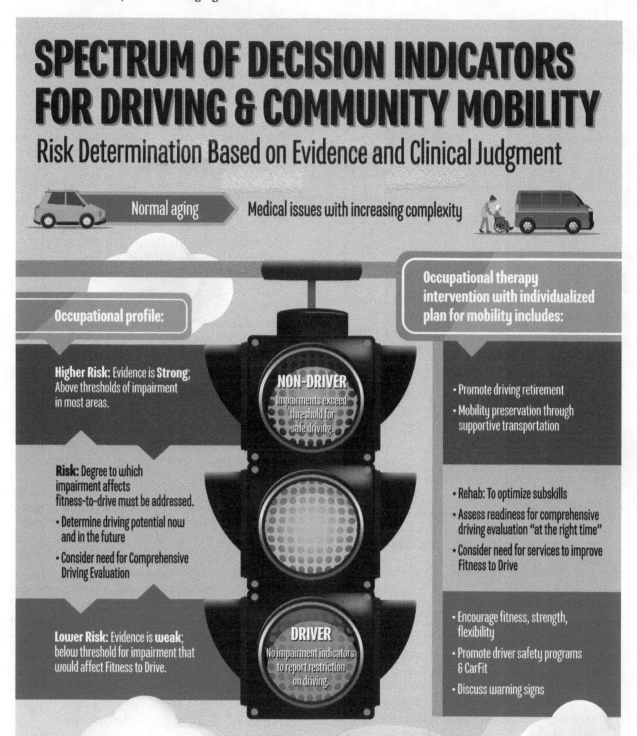

Figure 13-4 The model of decision indicators for determining the degree of driving risk for older drivers, as well as guidelines for intervention. *(Adapted from "OT-DRIVE: Integrating the IADL of Driving and Community Mobility Into Routine Practice," by A. Schold Davis and A. Dickerson, 2017,* OT Practice, *22[13], 8–14. Copyright American Occupational Therapy Association, 2017.)*

occupational therapist explores if and how the client attains community mobility (i.e., self-driver, ride with family or friends, public transit). The profile would also include determining if driving is a goal. The next step in the framework is the observation of performance; the occupational therapist evaluates the client's visual, sensory, motor, and cognition function through the performance skills evaluation (AOTA, 2014). A common misperception is that addressing the IADL of driving and community mobility requires a different process. Although the comprehensive driving evaluation includes the on-road assessment, the broader IADL of driving and community mobility evaluation begins with the same client factors underlying performance (e.g., vision, motor, cognition). The outcome of this evaluation is the first step in the OT-DRIVE model; the *OT* represents the process of an occupational therapist determining whether driving is important to this client and whether driving will be a risk (Schold Davis and Dickerson, 2017).

As the practitioner completes a typical occupational therapy evaluation, clinical reasoning is used to consider the client's level of risk for driving at this moment. As with all other ADLs/IADLs, this is not a final outcome but a current status based on evidence. In this case, the client is rated at great safety risk for driving (i.e., red) or low risk (i.e., green), or there may not be enough information (yellow). This is the first step—the *D* in OT-DRIVE—and will be used in determining the next steps based on this initial assessment.

R is for readiness; the occupational therapist determines the intervention plan considering the client's impairments on the potential for driving. *I* is for intervention. For each of the risk areas (i.e., red, green, or yellow) guidance has been identified for specific interventions that address driving. *V* represents verification. Since driving is a complex IADL, verification with the client, family, primary care provider, and other team members is important. Finally, *E* is for evaluation. Does the client need the comprehensive driving evaluation? The key to a successful outcome is the timing and readiness of the client for the comprehensive driving evaluation. The OT-DRIVE model is summarized in Table 13-2.

> **Engage Your Brain 13-3**
> What additional competencies should an occupational therapy practitioner have in order to use the OT-DRIVE framework to address the issue of driving as a therapist in the community?

Using Functional Observation

While occupational therapists are educated to observe, analyze, and describe functional performance using clinical reasoning, it is in community practice that practitioners use this skill consistently. In the recent "accounting" study, it was found that occupational therapy was the only spending category where additional spending has a statistically significant association with lower readmission rates (Rogers, Bai, Lavin, and Anderson, 2017). The authors suggested this is true because occupational therapy places a unique and immediate focus on patients' functional and social needs, important factors in the prevention of readmission. This was an important study for all occupational therapy but especially for community practice therapists—first, because addressing clients in the community is focused on functional and social needs and second, because the skill set of the occupational therapist to observe and critically analyze (i.e., in an activity analysis) functional tasks is a very unique contribution of the occupational therapy profession.

Since driving is an IADL using the same client factors, performance patterns, and performance skills (AOTA, 2014) as other complex IADLs, performance can be extrapolated from observing everyday activities such as meal preparation, medication management, and household maintenance. Dickerson et al. (2011) and Dickerson and Bédard (2014) developed an evidence-based decision tool for identifying driving risk, as well as the potential to return to driving, called the **Occupational Therapy Performance Analysis of Driving** (OT-PAD). Utilizing activity analysis skills, any occupational therapy practitioner can extrapolate from the client skills needed for cooking or cleaning the skills needed for driving.

The framework is based on Michon's three levels of driving behavior: strategic, tactical, and operational (TRB, 2016). The highest and overarching level, the strategic level, is the decision-making

Table 13-2 Summary of the Framework OT-DRIVE to Address the IADL of Driving and Community Mobility

Summary of the OT-DRIVE		
OT	Occupational therapist	Use of professional clinical observation, activity analysis, and clinical reasoning at the "top of our license"
D for *develop*	Develop the occupational profile and do performance evaluation	Is driving a goal? Complete performance evaluation to determine client's readiness for driving or other forms of transportation
R for *readiness*	Based on impairments (identified by evaluation), use clinical reasoning to determine level of *readiness* or level of risk to drive	Red: clear risk for driving; ethical responsibility to address driving with client, family, team Green: expected to heal; projected outcome is to premorbid status. Temporary transportation options may be needed; no need for a specialized driving evaluation Yellow: mix of strengths and impairments in IADLs. May need remediation/compensation and, when ready, a referral for a CDE
I for *intervention*	Plan intervention based on readiness	Red: focus on transportation plan, not driving; develop with client and family in terms of timing and options Green: cautionary guidance for temporary cessation; strategies for health promotion and prevention Yellow: restoring or optimizing the critical abilities for safe driving (domains of vision, cognition, and physical ability); knowledge of spectrum of services to guide recommendation for CDE
V for *verification*	Discuss plan with client and verify with the physician and team	Red: discuss recommendation of driving cessation with physician and team prior to client and the family Green: return to driving verified with physician after resolution of acute condition Yellow: verify the referral recommendations with the physician and team and, ideally, a collaborating driving rehabilitation specialist
E for *evaluation*	Referral for the CDE—the right service, at the right time for the right person	Red: although there is no clinical justification for a CDE, families may demand a specialized evaluation and can make an informed decision, understanding the consequences and associated costs, both monetary and emotional, with a likely failed CDE Green: sometimes clients or families want to be sure the person is safe to drive after an extended period Yellow: the key for a successful outcome is the timing and readiness of the client of the CDE

Summarized from "OT-DRIVE: Integrating the IADL of Driving and Community Mobility Into Routine Practice," by E. Schold Davis and A. E. Dickerson, 2017, *OT Practice, 22,* 8–14.

process of planning trip goals, deciding on a mode of transport (e.g., vehicle, walking, biking), and following the directions to get to the destination. The driving behavior skill at the strategic level is also needed during the driving process—for example, when a driver comes upon an accident and has to decide how to find an alternative route. Unexpected route changes are often the cause of older adults with cognitive impairment getting lost in familiar areas, and this indicates that education in skills that improve problem-solving is needed (Dickerson, Stressel, Justice, and Luther-Krug, 2012).

The second level of driving behavior consists of tactical behaviors, the behaviors related to decisions made during driving maneuvers. These include deciding when to slow down for weather and road changes, whether to stop for a yellow light, when to make a turn or use a turn signal, and other routine maneuvers. These tactical decisions are governed by traffic rules and roadways (e.g., protected turns) and well-learned and practiced habits. The lowest level, operational behaviors, are the overlearned human-machine interactions necessary to control the vehicle. These include using the brake, turning the steering wheel, and pressing the accelerator. These are the skills one does automatically—for example, driving a familiar route every morning so that the memory of actually driving the route is forgotten.

Describing the person factors needed for safe driving (i.e., physical/sensory, cognitive, emotional regulation, insight), Dickerson and Bédard (2014) link these factors under each of the three levels of driving behaviors (see Table 13-3). Then, using examples of clinical observation questions for each level of behavior (see Table 13-4), the practitioner

Table 13-3 Examples of Client Factors for Each of the Levels of Driving Behaviors

Levels	Client Factors and Examples
Strategic	Physical/sensory—awareness of physical limitations and is able to plan for successful compensation (e.g., if in a wheelchair, demonstrates ability to plan time and/or assistance for transfer)
	Cognitive—demonstrates ability to plan in advance using appropriate decisions to meet the goals of the task; self-regulates with insight into decisions; organizes steps to complete task
	Emotional regulation—can plan with appreciation of the emotional state (e.g., does not drive if experiencing excessive anxiety, depression, or anger)
	Insight—has accurate awareness of the skills and abilities he or she possesses to meet the demands of the task (e.g., to clean the windows, skills/abilities to use a ladder safely? Can make modified decisions based on driving experience and/or training)
Tactical	Physical/sensory—is aware of his or her physical limitations and adjusts as required (e.g., if floors are wet, walks more slowly)
	Cognitive—can evaluate a complex, dynamic context and adjust or accommodate through appropriate actions
	Emotional regulation—can recognize and manage emotions that arise in challenging situations
	Insight—can accurately gauge the risk and skills/abilities needed to meet the demands of a task requiring immediate decisions
Operational	Physical/sensory—meets the minimum requirements (e.g., vision) or is able to compensate for limitation (e.g., with training, will be able to use hand controls to compensate for a lower extremity amputation)
	Cognitive—awareness and flexibility to use the appropriate actions to achieve desired results
	Emotional regulation—emotional state does not negatively affect performance of automatic tasks
	Insight—not applicable

Adapted from "Decision Tool for Clients With Medical Issues: A Framework for Identifying Driving Risk and Potential to Return to Driving," by A. Dickerson and M. Bédard, 2014, *Occupational Therapy in Health Care, 28*(2), 194–202.

Table 13-4 Clinical Observation Questions for Other IADLs at Each Level of Behavior

Examples of IADL Applications for Each of the Three Levels

Strategic: ***Does the client have the cognitive ability to make decisions at the strategic level?***

- Does the client know whether he or she has the information to make an appropriate decision? Does the client initiate seeking additional or clarifying information?
- If the client were to make a meal, would he or she be able to plan it correctly (as with competence similar to what existed prior to his or her medical condition)?
- Can the client recognize, organize, reorder from the pharmacy, and remember to take medication accurately and safely?
- Can the client plan a meeting with a friend or family member or make an appointment and appropriately follow through without instructions from others?
- Is the client able to calm down and perform tasks after being surprised, flustered, or annoyed by any incidents or other people?
- Does the client plan how to manage his or her physical mobility within the immediate environment without significant assistance (i.e., how to plan to get his or her wheelchair in and out of a vehicle as well as in and out of the home)?

Tactical: ***Does the client have the performance skills to perform actions at this level?***

- Does the client immediately slow down when there is a wet floor or pavement?
- Does the client acknowledge others passing by in the hallway or on the sidewalk to say hello in recognition?
- Does the client adjust or accommodate immediately and appropriately when problems occur, such as when disconnected on a phone call, when coffee is spilled, when a pet jumps up and down, when a family member does not show up, when a household item breaks, or when food burns on the stove?
- Is the client able to multitask (i.e., one task being automatic), like walk and talk, read and drink, wash dishes and talk on the phone, tell a story and exercise, give instructions and make coffee?

Operational: ***Does the client have the performance skills to perform actions at this level?***

- Does the client perform normal daily tasks efficiently and automatically without cues (e.g., brushing teeth, eating, dressing)?
- Does the client have difficulty manipulating tools like cutlery?
- Does the client bump into doorways or walls?
- If the client loses balance, is his or her recovery effective?
- How is the client's reaction to environmental changes?
- How fast does the client recognize change in the environment? For example:
  - Does the client immediately see when someone enters the room?
  - Does the client recognize sounds and the sources of the sound?

Adapted from "Decision Tool for Clients With Medical issues: A Framework for Identifying Driving Risk and Potential to Return to Driving," by A. Dickerson and M. Bédard, 2014, *Occupational Therapy in Health Care, 28*(2), 194–202.

can use the questions to complete the designed checklist (see Table 13-5). Using this decision tool to extrapolate from the client's performance of tasks identifying fitness to drive, the therapist can identify the risk and the degree of impairment (i.e., none, mild, moderate, severe). As this is a new tool, there is no research to identify how many "flags" warrant a recommendation, but the community practice occupational therapist can decide to:

- Perform a further or specified evaluation
- Change intervention strategies to address the performance skills underlying driving and community mobility
- Make a referral to a DRS for a specialized evaluation

The OT-PAD can be used on paper or can be accessed by contacting the author of this chapter.

Table 13-5 OT-PAD's Clinical Decision-Making Tool Matrix

Levels	Descriptors of How to Consider Each Factor Under Each Level: Physical/Sensory, Cognitive, Emotional Regulation, and Insight	Degree of Impairment			
		None	Mild	Moderate	Severe
Strategic: *Does the client have the cognitive ability to make decisions?*	Physical/sensory—aware of physical limitations and is able to plan for successful compensation (e.g., if in a wheelchair, demonstrates ability to plan time and/or assistance for transfer) Cognitive—demonstrates ability to plan in advance using appropriate decisions to meet the goals of the task; self-regulates with insight into decisions; organizes steps to complete task Emotional regulation—can plan with appreciation of the emotional state (e.g., does not drive if experiencing excessive anxiety, depression, or anger) Insight—has accurate awareness of the skills and abilities he or she possesses to meet the demands of the task (e.g., to clean the windows, skills/abilities to use a ladder safely? Can make modified decisions based on driving experience and/or training)				
Tactical: *Does the client have the performance skills to perform actions at this level?*	Physical/sensory—is aware of his or her physical limitations and adjusts as required (e.g., if floors are wet, walks more slowly) Cognitive—can evaluate a complex, dynamic context and adjust or accommodate through appropriate actions Emotional regulation—can recognize and manage emotions that arise in challenging situations Insight—can accurately gauge the risk and skills/abilities needed to meet the demands of a task requiring immediate decisions				
Operational: *Does the client have the performance skills to perform actions at this level?*	Physical/sensory—meets the minimum requirements (e.g., vision) or is able to compensate for limitations (e.g., with training, will be able to use hand controls to compensate for a lower extremity amputation) Cognitive—awareness and flexibility to use the appropriate actions to achieve desired results Emotional regulation—emotional state does not negatively affect performance of automatic tasks Insight—not applicable				

Adapted from "Decision Tool for Clients With Medical Issues: A Framework for Identifying Driving Risk and Potential to Return to Driving," by A. Dickerson and M. Bédard, 2014, *Occupational Therapy in Health Care, 28*(2), 194–202. Used with permission.

Driving and Community Intervention

The profession of occupational therapy is predicated on using occupation as "means and ends" through skilled evaluation and intervention. In the practice of driving rehabilitation with older adults, the emphasis has been on evaluating fitness to drive, often leaving the consumers to figure out the next steps (Dickerson, 2012). As with all areas of practice, occupational therapy practitioners must move beyond just evaluation and provide options in terms of appropriate interventions, resources, and/or referrals.

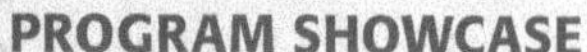

PROGRAM SHOWCASE

Community Educational Event to Celebrate Older Driver Safety: CarFit

Contributed by Susan Touchinsky, OTR/L, SCDCM, CDRS

Since 2009, the first full week in December has been designated Older Driver Safety Awareness Week (ODSAW). First started by the AOTA, ODSAW is now endorsed by a range of organizations, including AARP, AAA, and the Hartford Insurance Company, with the aim of increasing awareness for older driver safety (Elin Schold Davis, personal communication, October 5, 2018). In an effort to increase awareness of driving safety, especially for the aging adult, a community practice occupational therapist developed an annual CarFit event to take advantage of the activities offered during ODSAW.

What Is CarFit?

"CarFit is an educational program that offers older adult drivers the opportunity to check how well their personal vehicles 'fit' them" (CarFit, 2018, para. 1). "At a CarFit event, a team of trained technicians and/or health professionals work with each participant to ensure they 'fit' their vehicle properly for maximum comfort and safety. A CarFit check takes approximately 20 minutes to complete" (CarFit, 2018, para. 5).

Events are held in community settings with the driver, their parked car, and trained CarFit technicians. A CarFit event is not designed to address a person's driving ability; instead, the event focuses on person-vehicle fit. The goal of CarFit is to increase safety by improving a driver's fit with a vehicle's safety features.

What Happens at a CarFit Event?

On arrival, drivers enter the check-in station, where they receive an event overview. Next, drivers proceed to the checkup station, the main event of CarFit, where they meet pairs of trained CarFit technicians who provide education on a 12-safety-points checklist. These points include measuring the space between the driver and the airbag, the mirror position to improve side views, the seat positioning, and the safety belts, as well as others. During the checkup, the CarFit technicians circle any areas of concern (red flags) that indicate questions about the driver's understanding or areas of difficulty. Examples of red flags may be a lack of space between the driver and the airbag, difficulty with vision over the steering wheel, or slowness in turning their heads.

After completing the 12-point checklist, the driver moves to the checkout. Here an occupational therapy practitioner meets with the driver to address any identified red flags. For example, if it is painful for the driver to reach up and across to grasp the safety belt (red flag), the occupational therapy practitioner might review the pros and cons of a seat belt pull. In most cases, there are no red flags, and the occupational therapy practitioner reviews helpful gadgets and resources to improve general driving fitness. Lastly, the occupational therapy practitioner typically gives the driver a "goodie bag" that includes donations from local vendors (e.g., car wash coupons, free coffee coupons, eyeglass repair kits) and information on local resources such as driver rehabilitation specialists, therapy, and/or alternative modes of transportation.

In the rare case of a driver who needs additional help, the occupational therapy practitioner can provide information about driving evaluations for fitness to drive. Fitness to drive evaluations are completed by skilled driver rehabilitation specialists and involve an in-vehicle driving evaluation in a specialized driving rehabilitation vehicle.

CarFit Training Roles

Within CarFit, the four primary roles are untrained volunteer, technician, event coordinator, and instructor. Untrained volunteers may assist with traffic flow, answer phones, organize paperwork, or simply lend a hand. They have not completed the training needed to work at checkup or checkout stations.

Trained volunteers who have completed a technician training course with a CarFit event coordinator and then participated in an event to become a CarFit technician manage the checkup stations. CarFit technicians are trained on the 12-point checklist and understand the flow of CarFit events.

CarFit event coordinators are CarFit technicians who have volunteered at three events and then participated in the next level of training, a four-hour course taught by CarFit instructors. CarFit event coordinators are trained to host and run CarFit events, using the CarFit marketing and planning resources. In order to plan an event, occupational therapy practitioners must first become CarFit event coordinators. CarFit event coordinators are also trained to train CarFit technicians. CarFit instructors can train both technicians and event coordinators.

Plan the Materials

Prior to the event, the occupational therapy practitioner prepares resources and uses a CarFit promotional kit to advertise. The practitioner connects with the local AAA and AARP chapters for volunteers and for support for securing CarFit resources, such as the 12-point checklist and CarFit brochure. The practitioner also uses the CarFit resources to send out media releases to local newspapers, radio stations, and news channels and publishes the event on social media and through the CarFit website (www.car-fit.org).

Plan for Volunteers

The occupational therapy practitioner event coordinator spends time recruiting and training local occupational therapy practitioners. The event coordinator registers practitioners for an online technician training course. Practitioners receive an e-mail invitation to log on to the CarFit website and visit the "OT Training Module" section, where they are asked to carefully read all information, review the training video, and come to the event with their certificate of completion. Typically, on the day before or morning of the event, the event coordinator also provides a hands-on lab to ensure the newly trained CarFit technicians are prepared to complete the 12-point checklist at the CarFit event. The hands-on practice ensures the technicians are ready, fully understand all 12 points, and are oriented to the flow of the CarFit event.

The Day of the Event

The occupational therapy practitioner works with volunteers to prepare the designated parking lot for the event. The CarFit technicians arrive an hour early to set up any additional resources, become oriented to the flow, and be ready for the first car.

A CarFit event is typically scheduled from 9 a.m. to 12 p.m. CarFit events range in times and size from one-on-one events to a couple of hours to 4-hour events. One-on-one events are individual CarFit checks completed by one CarFit technician and a driver. One-on-one CarFit checks are a great way to provide individual checks outside of a CarFit event.

Benefits

Drivers who participate in CarFit events report feeling empowered to have learned so much about the fit and safety features of their own cars. They love the information gained about their car's safety features and strategies for improving their views out the front and sides of the car with mirror positioning (Fran Carlin Rogers, personal communication, October 26, 2018). While CarFit was initially geared toward aging adults, participants often find so much value in participating that they encourage their adult children and grandchildren to complete a CarFit checkup.

CarFit volunteers report a range of benefits as well. The AAA and AARP volunteers have reflected that CarFit is an excellent way to connect with both drivers and a range of resources in the community, including occupational therapy practitioners.

Occupational therapy practitioners report that CarFit technician training has given them more insight into safety features to help improve seating and positioning for both the passengers and the drivers that they see for rehabilitation. They also benefit from an increased understanding of AAA and AARP and many times meet local driver rehabilitation specialists who become resources for their clients' driving needs. CarFit events are a great opportunity to connect adult drivers in the community with local resources in a fun, nonthreatening manner and facilitate direct interaction between CarFit technicians and occupational therapy practitioners.

Interventions to Facilitate Returning to Driving

As driving is such an important occupation for older adult clients, they may not ask about driving in order to avoid the answer of "no driving." Family members may not recognize driving as an issue or may want to avoid responsibility for the spouse, parent, or sibling who will need assistance with transportation. Thus, it is important for the practitioner to bring up the issue of community mobility with the client and/or primary caregiver. This is especially true if the client is expected to recover function and gain independence. As an IADL, driving and community mobility is essential to maintain quality of life and connections to the community and therefore is a part of the occupational therapist's ethical obligation (Slater, 2012).

If the client does ask about returning to driving, the obvious question regards what interventions improve the functional abilities needed for driving. Since driving is a complex task requiring the integration of sensory, motor, visual, and perceptual skills with good executive functioning, it is not a simple answer with "cookbook" activities to use. Client skill sets for driving can be improved by doing exercises on paper to improve scanning skills, block sorting for facilitating perceptual skills, and computer rehabilitation. *Using* actual complex activities is best to build the underlying component skills and to practice functional tasks. The main dynamic is that the occupation of driving uses the same underlying processes as other complex IADLs. Therefore, until the client is needing vehicular modifications or training in a vehicle, therapeutic interventions to assist the client in regaining driving skills and abilities are no different than other ADL or IADL interventions. Making a meal in the kitchen requires using the same component skill set as driving. The key to success is using all occupation-based therapeutic interventions possible to ensure that the client has recovered functionally and has the potential to pass the on-road assessment before sending the client for a comprehensive driving evaluation or driving test.

Vehicle Technology as an Intervention

According to some sources, there soon will be no need to address driving, as driverless cars will be the norm! The idea that fully automated motor vehicles are ready to roll out and take away our transportation problems is simply not true. While some functioning "driverless" vehicles exist, their range, speed, and abilities are limited at this point. Often overlooked is that the *environment* also needs to have the technology to communicate with a driverless car, and at this point, perfect weather conditions are required. Driving in snow, in rain, or in rural areas is unsafe. Other issues yet to be resolved include:

- The legal ramifications of who is responsible if there is a crash
- Situational awareness if and when a driver needs to immediately take over control
- Determining the criteria for a "license" to use an automated vehicle

Finally, it is important to understand that even if the perfect driverless vehicle were available tomorrow, it will take years to make the transition. Presently, it takes at least 20 years for new technology to be included on most registered vehicles (Highway Loss Data Institute [HLDI], 2012). For example, an antilock braking system (ABS) is an important safety feature that has decreased crashes. In 1990, only 1% of all registered vehicles had an ABS as a standard feature, and they were optional on 5%. Twenty years later in 2010, the ABS was standard or optional on 88% of all registered vehicles (HLDI, 2012). In 2013, the National Highway Traffic Safety Administration (NHTSA) mandated an ABS on all new passenger vehicles. As of 2014, rearview cameras and video displays are required on new vehicles. However, the HLDI predicts that it will not be until 2039 that 95% of registered vehicles will have rear cameras (Cicchino, 2018; HLDI, 2012).

Great strides have been made in automating aspects of driving to improve driver safety and comfort. There are two general categories: the **crash avoidance system** (CAS) and the **advanced driver assistance system** (ADAS). A CAS provides warnings, such as lane departure warnings, forward collision warnings, and blind spot warnings, to prevent potential crashes. Current research has found that both blind spot-monitoring systems (Cicchino, 2017a) and rearview cameras (Cicchino, 2017b) are effective in preventing police-reported lane change crashes regardless of severity. For older adults, rear cameras are cutting crashes 40% for drivers 70 and older, compared to 15% for younger drivers (Cicchino, 2017b).

An ADAS provides timely information to assist drivers in the driving task, such as night vision enhancement, navigational assistance, adaptive cruise control, and adaptive headlights. Many of these systems can be turned on and off. Thus, while they may be helpful for older adults, they only work if they are used. Research from manufacturers on the status of systems being on or off reported that while front crash prevention systems tend to remain "on," lane maintenance systems are more frequently considered annoying and are turned "off" in from 25% to 79% of equipped vehicles, depending on the vehicle type (Cicchino, 2017c).

There are barriers to the adoption of the ADAS technology by older adults (Trubswetter and Bengler, 2013). First, older adults do not necessarily perceive the systems as useful and demonstrate a lack of trust. This is likely because older drivers do not fully understand the operations of the technology and may actually incorrectly use it (Dickerson et al., 2017). For example, they may incorrectly attribute collision prevention features to the adaptive cruise control. Additionally, when training older adults on use of the in-vehicle information systems (e.g., hands-free commands), the workload of the driver was moderate to high, and practice did not eliminate interference with driving (Strayer, Cooper Turrill, Coleman, Ortiz, and Hopman, 2015). Other barriers include the undesired system feedback, risk of inattentiveness/distraction because of the feedback, functional limitations of the systems, and cost of the systems. Therefore, more research is needed to understand older adults' use of the technology, including their unique needs and learning styles and behavioral adaptations (e.g., less use of turn signals with blind spot detection), as well as the real-world safety benefits and, most importantly, the effect on situational awareness or the ability to take over when using automation (e.g., adaptive cruise control; Dickerson et al., 2017).

Community-based occupational therapists working with clients and family members in their homes and communities know whether their clients have the capacity to understand and learn new systems. However, if the spouse needs to take over the role of household driver, would an updated vehicle decrease the risk of crash or serious injury? There is no easy answer as to whether vehicle technology can and should be an intervention for older adults. Certainly, for healthy community living for older adults, the newest systems have been shown to have real-world benefits (Cicchino, 2018). However, most of these systems are only found in the top models of manufacturers and even then are considered options. Nevertheless, for the older drivers who can afford them and have the cognitive ability to learn and understand their use, the new systems may prolong the driving life of these drivers. The knowledgeable therapist can offer meaningful information.

GPS Use for Wayfinding

Still, one potential option to improve safety is an electronic navigational system, or what is commonly known as a global positioning system (GPS) device. A recent study comparing the performance of drivers familiar and unfamiliar with GPS examined whether GPS units improved older drivers' safety on unfamiliar routes and whether training with GPS devices had an impact on performance for those who were unfamiliar (Thomas et al., 2018). Results demonstrated that when traveling in unfamiliar areas, all drivers made fewer driving errors when using GPS units compared to using written directions, and those familiar with the system did better. Results also showed that drivers in their 60s exhibited safer behaviors than those in their 70s. In terms of programming a GPS unit, drivers who were familiar with GPS did much better than those unfamiliar with it. These findings, supporting previous studies results (Dickerson et al., 2019), suggest that age is an important factor in using GPS systems to drive safely.

In a follow-up study, the use of video training and hands-on training found that older adults who had both forms of training performed significantly better than controls. The group who had hands-on training did better than those learning only by video, but the difference was not significant (Coleman, 2018). The results of these studies have important implications for practitioners. Practitioners should encourage their clients to use a GPS unit, especially for unfamiliar areas. If they do not know how to use and/or program the GPS unit, providing information on how to use one is helpful. While other vehicle technology is vehicle-specific (including manufacturer-installed navigational systems), a GPS device purchased separately from the vehicle is inexpensive and can easily be installed in a vehicle of any age or type or used on a smartphone. However, as with all tasks, occupational therapy practitioners must use their clinical judgment. Using a GPS device may not be appropriate with cognitively impaired drivers, as GPS technology is sometimes wrong or cannot predict a closed roadway or street under construction. Cognitively impaired drivers may blindly follow the GPS instead of being able to make a judgment that technology has made an error. Therefore, a GPS should not be recommended when driving cessation should be the ultimate outcome. The following are excellent resources for practitioners to use and share with clients:

1. In a research synthesis of advanced in-vehicle technologies, the systems rated as high value for older adults included the following: forward collision, parking assist: rearview display, parking assist: cross-traffic warning, parking assist: semiautonomous, navigational assistance, automatic crash notification, adaptive headlights, and blind spot warnings (Eby et al., 2015).
2. What My Car Does.org is an excellent website developed by the University of Iowa and the National Safety Council that demonstrates and describes the safety features of vehicles in entertaining videos.
3. The Hartford and Massachusetts Institute of Technology (MIT) Aging Lab researched the technologies and offers its version of the top 10 technologies for mature drivers in a free downloadable handout.

Transitioning to Nondriving

Unfortunately, for many older adults there may not be functional recovery from a medical event due to deficits in perceptual or cognitive functions or due to the aging process slowing processing speed so significantly that self-driving is not realistic. Because this is often very difficult for an older adult to accept (Patomella, Johansson, and Tham, 2009), many individuals continue to drive regardless of the medical recommendation (Dobbs, Carr, and Morris, 2002). The loss of driving independence changes a person's life dramatically. The person may no longer be able to live alone and will need to depend on others for transportation. If there are no family members or friends available, the client may be further isolated. Typically, if driving is not possible due to medical impairments, public transportation is not an option for the same functional reasons (Kerschner and Silverstein, 2018). This will further eliminate many social activities that are important to maintain contact with others. Although **transportation network companies** (TNCs; e.g., taxis, Uber, Lyft) may be seen as expensive, one strategy is to work out a budget with the client to show that these services may be cheaper than owning a car and paying for maintenance, gas, parking, and insurance. An unique service called GoGoGrandparent can provide services that do not require the senior to use technology. The program is set up by linking the cost to an account, and the senior "talks to a live person" to order a ride (using services like Uber or Lyft). There is an additional surcharge for this "real-person" service, but it does include alerts to an adult child, for example, who can monitor the senior's transportation needs.

With clients who must retire from driving, the occupational therapy practitioner needs to address their community mobility needs through transportation planning beyond just offering the client and family information and a list of resources. Analyzing the actual transportation needs of the client—that is, where the individual needs and wants to go—with family and friends not only assists with planning but helps the therapist address the client's anxiety of not knowing what to do. Because each community is unique, community practice occupational therapists should establish relationships and work with local agencies (e.g., local councils on aging, Area Agencies on Aging, public transport) as well as national agencies (e.g., AARP, Veterans Health Administration) to build informed options to guide clients and caregivers.

Finally, as discussed previously, driving is a valued occupation for older adults who grew up with their "car." The occupation of driving is and will continue to be an activity that defines many baby boomers in terms of success and independence. Sometimes it is not just about getting where they need and want to go. It may be the feeling of independence, choice, and power to make their own decisions. Some older adults do not actually drive, but they like seeing their vehicle in its spot "just in case." It is important to respect that losing their ability to drive is a significant loss—just like losing one's pet, walking ability, or home. It is not always about needing to find the answer but respecting their feelings and demonstrating understanding and empathy.

Although websites and resources may have good information, as with anything, there may be competing agendas and opinions. An informed occupational therapy practitioner can ensure evidenced-based information, using resources and websites that are medically based or research-based, without trying to "sell" something.

Summary

- Community mobility, regardless of the method (e.g., walking, biking, driving, public transit) is critical for older adult clients. It is the means by which they participate in community life.
- Addressing the IADL of driving and community mobility requires the collaboration of multiple stakeholders, including general practice occupational therapists, DRSs, state licensing agencies, and other service providers.
- Community-based practitioners have the opportunity to use their skilled observation of performance as the key to identifying risk, make appropriate referrals to DRSs, and offer intervention to assist with community mobility options.
- Many new tools and resources are available for the occupational therapy practitioner to use, including a framework—OT-DRIVE—that can guide community-based practice.
- An occupational therapy practitioner working with adult clients has an obligation to address driving and community mobility as an IADL.
- Emerging vehicle technologies have the potential to enhance the driving capabilities of older adults, but more research is needed to determine the best uses of this technology with this population.

CASE STUDIES

CASE STUDY 13-1 Jeanne Dobson

Mrs. Jeanne Dobson is an 87-year-old female who lives in a one-bedroom, fixed-income apartment at a large continuing care facility in Allentown, Pennsylvania. She has five children; three live nearby and two live out of state. Jeanne has lived in the apartment for over 15 years and has an older-model sedan and pays for a parking slot at the apartment complex. When Jeanne moved to the apartment, she walked without a cane and typically drove daily, just to get out of the apartment. Over the last 5 years, she has limited her night driving and stopped driving any distances longer than 45 minutes. The last time one of her daughters visited from out of town, the social worker discussed some concerns about Jeanne with her. While Jeanne was once the treasurer of a social group, she was now having difficulty handling the money. The social worker was also concerned that Jeanne remained friends with a former resident who was expelled from the apartment for abusive language. Jeanne felt sorry for the former resident and did not understand why he could not continue to visit her. The social worker explained to Jeanne that the individual was not allowed in the building, and Jeanne was at risk of losing her ability to stay if she continued to admit him. The daughter spoke to her mother about this issue and quickly became aware of the cognitive impairment that Jeanne was demonstrating. The daughter scheduled an appointment with Jeanne's physician, during which time she asked the physician about her mother's ability to drive. The physician indicated that Jeanne had passed the Mini-Mental State Exam (MMSE) and drives very safely but does have difficulty getting in and out of her bathtub. The physician referred Jeanne to an occupational therapist for an evaluation of her IADLs.

Discussion Questions

1. What would the priorities be for occupational therapy evaluation and intervention?
2. Using the OT-DRIVE model, what should the occupational therapist consider doing about the IADL of driving?
3. What would the intervention be if Jeanne was a red or yellow?

CASE STUDY 13-2 Greenville Medical Center

Greenville Medical Center is a medium-size city medical center with over 500 beds, including a rehabilitation unit covering over 10 counties in the Midwest. The occupational therapy department sees patients in the acute care, rehabilitation, and outpatient unit. While the center is located in a city, the vast majority of its patients come from rural areas where there is little or no public transportation. Recently, the lead occupational therapist, Sarah, attended an occupational therapy conference that included a presentation on the OT-DRIVE model. Sarah attended the session, as she was interested in how to refer to a DRS when physicians asked about a patient's ability to drive. Sarah was surprised about two things: First, that it was her ethical duty to address driving as an IADL. She had avoided addressing the topic of driving with her clients because, without formal training, she felt unable to discuss it. The second surprise was that she realized she could use the OT-DRIVE model to develop her and her colleagues' skills at addressing driving and to collaborate with either the driving school in town or connect with an OT/DRS in a nearby city.

Discussion Questions

1. What should Sarah do first to prepare for meeting her clients' needs?
2. How would Sarah best communicate with the stakeholders around driving?
3. What is Sarah's role in transportation planning?

Learning Activities

1. Start making a list of all the methods of alternative transportation in your area, in conjunction with social services and/or case managers, to understand the options for individuals who may need to retire from driving. Include the types of service, criteria, cost, and availability.
2. Interview a DRS in your area and determine what services he or she offers (e.g., basic, low tech, high tech) and the degree of collaboration with occupational therapy generalists.
3. Analyze what screening and/or assessment tools you know could offer information about the IADL of driving and write a brief justification for your practice or fieldwork setting.
4. Identify one occupation-based theory and one health behavior change theory that would support a driving rehabilitation program. Hint: review Chapter 3.

REFERENCES

American Occupational Therapy Association. (2014). Occupational therapy practice framework: Domain and process. *American Journal of Occupational Therapy, 68,* S1–S48.

American Occupational Therapy Association. (2015). Occupational therapy code of ethics (2015). *American Journal of Occupational Therapy, 69*(Suppl. 3), 6913410030. http://dx.doi.org/10.5014/ajot.2015.696S03

Brooks, J. O., Dickerson, A., Crisler, M. C., Logan, W. C., Beeco, R. W., and Witte, J. C. (2011). Physician knowledge, assessment, and reporting of older driver fitness. *Occupational Therapy in Health Care, 25*(4), 213–224. doi:10.3109/07380577.2011.607227

CarFit. (2018). *Program goals and outcomes.* Retrieved from https://car-fit.org/

Cicchino, J. B. (2017a, August). *Effects of blind spot monitoring systems of police-reported lane-change crashes.* Retrieved from www.iihs.org/frontend/iihs/documents/masterfiledocs.ashx?id=2143

Cicchino, J. B. (2017b, October). *Effects of rearview cameras and rear parking sensors on police-reported crashes.* Retrieved from www.iihs.org/bibliography/topic/2130

Cicchino, J. B. (2017c, August 8). *What do (older) drviers need to know about ADAS technologies?* Paper presented at the TRB Safe Mobility of Older Persons Midyear Meeting, Woods Hole, MA.

Cicchino, J. B. (2018, February). *Real-world benefits of rear cross-traffic alert on police-reported backing crashes.* Retrieved from www.iihs.org/frontend/iihs/documents/masterfiledocs.ashx?id=2151

Coleman, M. C. (2018). *Comparing the effectiveness of video training alone versus hands-on training for older adults using GPS technology.* The Scholarship: East Carolina University's Institutional Repository, East Carolina University, Greenville, NC. Retrieved from http://thescholarship.ecu.edu/handle/10342/112/discover

Coughlin, J. F., and D'Ambrosio, L. A. (2012). Purpose of this volume. In J. F. Coughlin and L. A. D'Ambrosio (Eds.), *Aging in America and transportation: Personal choices and public policy.* New York, NY: Springer.

Coughlin, J. F., D'Ambrosio, L. A., Pratt, M. R., and Mohyde, M. (2012). The continued and growing importance of mobility. In J. F. Coughlin and L. A. D'Ambrosio (Eds.), *Aging America and transportation: Personal choices and public policy* (pp. 11–26). New York, NY: Springer.

Dickerson, A. E. (2012). Driving as a valued occupation. In M. J. Maguire and E. S. Davis (Eds.), *Driving and community mobility: Occupational therapy strategies across the lifespan* (pp. 417–422). Bethesda, MD: AOTA Press.

Dickerson, A. E. (2014). Driving with dementia: Evaluation, referral, and resources. *Occupational Therapy in Health Care, 28*(1), 62–76. doi:10.3109/07380577.2013.867091

Dickerson, A. E. (2016). Driving and community mobility as an instrumental activity of daily living. In G. Gillen (Ed.), *Stroke rehabilitation* (4th ed., pp. 237–264). St. Louis, MO: Elsevier.

Dickerson, A. E., and Bédard, M. (2014). Decision tool for clients with medical issues: A framework for identifying driving risk and potential to return to driving. *Occupational Therapy in Health Care, 28*(2), 194–202. doi:10.3109/07380577.2014.903357

Dickerson, A.E., Molnar, L.J., Bédard, M., Eby, D. W., Berg-Weger, M., Choi, M., Greigg, J., Horowitz, A., Meuser, T., Myers, A. O'Connor, M., and Silverstein, N. (2019). Transportation and aging: An updated research agenda for advancing safety mobility among older adults transitioning from driving to non-driving. *The Gerontologist, 59*(2), 215-221, *doi.org/10.1093/geront/gnx120*

Dickerson, A. E., Molnar, L., Bédard, M., Eby, D. W., Classen, S., and Polgar, J. (2017). Transportation and aging: An updated research agenda for advancing safe mobility. *Journal of Applied Gerontology,* 733464817739154. doi:10.1177/0733464817739154

Dickerson, A. E., Molnar, L. J., Eby, D. W., Adler, G., Bédard, M., Berg-Weger, M., . . . Trujillo, L. (2007). Transportation and aging: A research agenda for advancing safe mobility. *Gerontologist, 47*(5), 578–590.

Dickerson, A. E., Reistetter, T., and Gaudy, J. R. (2013). The perception of meaningfulness and performance of instrumental activities of daily living from the perspectives of the medically at-risk older adults and their caregivers. *Journal of Applied Gerontology, 32*(6), 749–764. doi:10.1177/0733464811432455

Dickerson, A. E., and Schold Davis, E. (2012). Welcome to the team! Who are the stakeholders? In M. Maguire and E. Schold Davis (Eds.), *Driving and community mobility: Occupational therapy strategies across the lifespan* (pp. 44–79). Bethesda, MD: American Occupational Therapy Association.

Dickerson, A. E., and Schold Davis, E. (2014). Driving experts address expanding access through pathways to older driver rehabilitation services: Expert meeting results and implications. *Occupational Therapy in Health Care, 28*(2), 122–126. doi:10.3109/07380577.2014.901591

Dickerson, A. E., Schold Davis, E., and Carr, D. B. (2018). Driving decisions: Distinguishing evaluations, providers and outcomes. *Geriatrics, 3*(2). https://doi.org/10.3390/geriatrics3020025

Dickerson, A. E., Schold Davis, E., and Chew, F. (2011). Driving as an instrumental activity of daily living in the medical setting: A model for intervention and referral. *Transportation Research Board: Emerging issues in safe and sustainable mobility for older people.* Washington, DC: The National Academies of Sciences, Engineering, and Medicine.

Dickerson, A. E., Stressel, D., Justice, M., and Luther-Krug, M. (2012). Behind the wheel: Driver rehabilitation intervention. In M. Maguire and E. Schold Davis (Eds.), *Driving and community mobility: Occupational therapy strategies across the lifespan* (pp. 345–382). Bethesda, MD: American Occupational Therapy Association.

Dobbs, B., Carr, D. B., and Morris, J. C. (2002). Management and assessment of the demented driver. *Neurologist, 8*(3), 61–70.

Eby, D., Molnar, L., Zhang, L., St. Louis, R., Zanier, N., and Kostyniuk, L. (2015, December). *Keeping older adults driving safely: A research synthesis of advanced in-vehicle technologies.* AAA Foundation for Traffic Safety. https://aaafoundation.org/keeping-older-adults-driving-safely-research-synthesis-advanced-vehicle-technologies/

Federal Interagency Forum on Aging-Related Statistics. (2008). *Older Americans 2008: Key indicators of well-being.* Washington, DC: U.S. Government Printing Office.

Highway Loss Data Institute. (2012, April). Predicted availability of safety features on registered vehicles. *Bulletin, 28.*

Hyde, C. (2006). History of the automobile. In J. M. Pellerito Jr. (Ed.), *Driver rehabilitation and community mobility: Principles and practice* (pp. 23–31). St. Louis, MO: Elsevier, Mosby.

Kent, R. W., and Transportation Research Board. (2010). *The biomechanics of aging.* Paper presented at the NTSB Forum on Safety, Mobility, and Aging Drivers, Washington, DC.

Kerschner, H. K., and Silverstein, N. M. (2018). *Introduction to senior transportation: Enhancing community mobility and transportation services.* New York, NY: Routledge.

Lane, A., Green, E., Dickerson, A. E., Davis, E. S., Rolland, B., and Stohler, J. T. (2014). Driver rehabilitation programs: Defining program models, services, and expertise. *Occupational Therapy in Health Care, 28*(2), 177–187. doi:10.3109/07380577.2014.903582

Musselwhite, C. (2011). The importance of driving for older people and how the pain of driving cessation can be reduced. *Signpost: Journal of Dementia and Mental Health, 15*(3), 22–26.

Patomella, A. H., Johansson, K., and Tham, K. (2009). Lived experience of driving ability following stroke. *Disabiility and Rehabilitation, 31*(9), 726–733.

Pellerito, J. M. (2006). Pioneers in driving rehabilitation. In J. M. Pellerito Jr. (Ed.), *Driver rehabilitation and community mobility: Principles and practice* (pp. 32–34). St. Louis, MO: Elsevier, Mosby.

Rogers, A. T., Bai, G., Lavin, R. A., and Anderson, G. F. (2017). Higher hospital spending on occupational therapy is associated with lower readmission rates. *Medical Care Research and Review, 74*(6), 668–686. doi:10.1177/1077558716666981

Rosenbloom, S. (2012). The travel and mobility needs of older persons now and in the future. In J. D. A. Coughlin (Ed.), *Aging America and transportation* (pp. 39–54). New York, NY: Springer.

Schold Davis, E., and Dickerson, A. E. (2017). OT-DRIVE: Integrating the IADL of driving and community mobility into routine practice. *OT Practice, 22*(13), 8–14.

Schold Davis, E., Dickerson, A. E., Dellinger, A., and Chodrow, B. (2016). *Older driver initiative update: Translation of developed pathways to service providers in home and primary care—the older driver initiative expanded.* Paper presented at the Annual Conference and Expo of the American Occupational Therapy Association, Chicago, IL.

Sifrit, K. J., Stutts, J., Staplin, L., and Martell, C. (2010). *Intersection crashes among drivers in their 60s, 70s and 80s.* Paper presented at the Human Factors and Ergonomics Society Annual Meeting, San Francisco, CA.

Slater, D. Y. (2012). Consensus statements on occupational therapy ethics related to driving. *Occupational Therapy in Health Care, 28*(2), 163–168.

Society, A. G., and Pomidor, A. (2016). *Clinician's guide to assessing and counseling older drivers* (3rd ed.). Report No. DOT HS 812 228. Washington, DC: American Geriatrics Society.

Stav, W. B., and Lieberman, D. (2008). From the desk of the editor. *American Journal of Occupational Therapy, 62*(2), 127–129.

Strayer, D. L., Cooper, J. M., Turrill, J., Coleman, J. R., Ortiz, E. V., and Hopman, R. J. (2015, October). *Measuring cognitive distraction in the automobile III: A comparison of the ten 2015 in-vehicle information systems.* Retrieved from http://newsroom.aaa.com/wp-content/uploads/2015/10/Phase-III-Research-Report.pdf

Thomas, F. D., Dickerson, A. E., Blomberg, R. D., Graham, L. A., Wright, T. J., Finstad, K. A., and Romoser, M. E. (2018). *Older drivers and navigation devices.* Washington, DC: National Highway Traffic Safety Administration.

Transportation Research Board. (2016). *Taxonomy and terms for stakeholders in senior mobility.* No. E-C211 2016. Washington, DC: Transportation Research Board.

Trubswetter, N., and Bengler, K. (2013). *Why should I use ADAD? Advanced driver assistance systems and the elderly: Knowledge, experience, and usage barriers.* Paper presented at the 7th International Driving Symposium on Human Factors in Driver Assessment, Training, and Vehicle Design: Driving Assessment, Bolton Landing, NY.

Womack, J., and Silverstein, N. (2012). The big picture: Comprehensive community mobility options. In M. Maguire and E. S. Davis (Eds.), *Driving and community mobility: Occupational therapy strategies across the lifespan* (pp. 19–48). Bethesda, MD: AOTA Press.

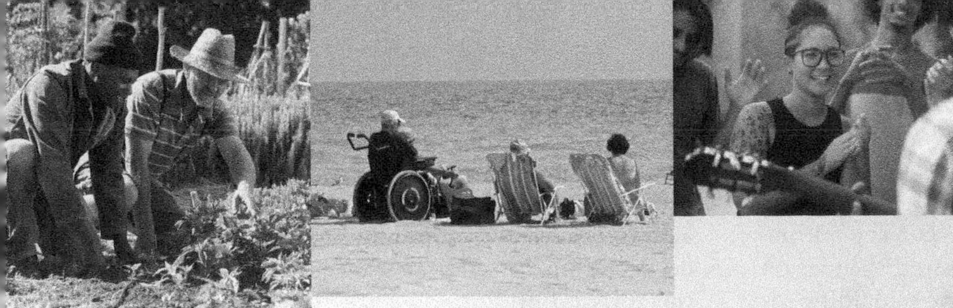

Chapter 14

Low Vision Services in the Community

Theresa M. Smith, PhD, OTR, CLVT

It's not what you look at that matters, it's what you see.

—Henry David Thoreau

Learning Outcomes

This chapter is designed to enable the reader to:

14-1 Articulate the reasons for the growing population of persons with low vision.
14-2 Identify the four major causes of low vision and the available medical treatments.
14-3 Describe how low vision affects occupational performance.
14-4 Recognize low vision team members and the services provided for this population.
14-5 Explain occupational therapy services for clients with low vision.
14-6 Discuss the psychosocial aspects of low vision.
14-7 Describe community support.
14-8 Identify billing and funding issues.

Key Terms

Age-related macular degeneration
Cataract
Certified low vision therapist
Diabetic retinopathy
Eccentric viewing
Glaucoma
Low vision
Ophthalmologist
Optometrist
Orientation and mobility specialist
Specialty certification in low vision

Introduction

In the United States, approximately 3,220,000 people had low vision in 2015, and this number is expected to increase to 6,950,000 by 2050 (Varma et al., 2016). One in every 28 persons in the United States age 40 and above have low vision, and the prevalence of visual impairment increases with age (Vision Council, 2015). In 2011 the oldest baby boomers turned 65, and by 2030 the baby boomers will make up 18% of the U.S. population (Heimlich, 2010). The most common eye diseases for those age 40 and over include cataract, glaucoma, diabetic retinopathy, and macular degeneration.

Etiology, prevalence, and medical treatment for the common eye diseases vary. **Cataract,** or clouding of the eye lens, is the most frequently reported condition in persons with low vision; the prevalence of this diagnosis ranges from 11.8% to 18.8% for African American, Caucasian, and Hispanic individuals (National Eye Institute [NEI], n.d.). Cataracts cause low vision, but there is a surgical procedure that can correct this problem. Cataract removal surgery has an estimated 90% chance of improving vision, with a rare incidence of issues occurring postsurgery (NEI, 2015b). **Glaucoma,** damage to the optic nerve, occurs when the normal fluid pressure inside the eyes rises, resulting in vision loss and blindness. Treatment to save remaining vision may include eye drops, laser trabeculoplasty, and/or conventional surgery (NEI, 2015d). **Diabetic retinopathy** develops secondary to diabetes and results from a change in the blood vessels of the retina. From 40% to 45% of persons diagnosed with diabetes have some stage of diabetic retinopathy, and many are unaware of this fact (NEI, 2015c). Diabetic retinopathy can occur as nonproliferative or proliferative retinopathy. Proliferative retinopathy is treated with laser surgery or with a vitrectomy (Johns Hopkins Medicine, n.d.). Lastly, **age-related macular degeneration** (AMD), damage to the central part of the retina, occurs in one of two forms, dry or wet. It is the leading cause of vision loss in the United States for persons age 50 and older (NEI, 2015a). There is no medical treatment for dry macular degeneration; however, some patients are advised to take Age-Related Eye Disease Study (AREDS) or AREDS2 formula eye vitamins (Age-Related Eye Disease Study Research Group, 2001; Age-Related Eye Disease Study 2 [AREDS2] Research Group, 2013). Treatment for wet macular degeneration includes laser surgery, photodynamic therapy, and eye injections (NEI, 2015a). Eye injections are used to stop the growth of excessive blood vessels, and there are three types of medicines used: Avastin, Eylea, and Lucentis (Mogk, n.d.).

Low Vision and Occupational Performance

Vision provides approximately 80% of what individuals perceive through their senses (Protect-your-sight.com, 2008). Using the *ICD-10-CM* threshold criteria, people are considered to have **low vision** if they have an impairment of visual functioning even after treatment and refractive correction and have visual acuity of less than 20/70 or a visual field of less than 10° (World Health Organization [WHO], 2016). Levels of visual impairment are allocated to categories (see Table 14-1). Low vision is irreversible and may be hereditary, congenital, or acquired.

Table 14-1 *ICD-10-CM* Visual Impairment Categories

Category	Worse Than	Equal to or Better Than
0 Mild or no visual impairment		6/18 3/10 (0.3) 20/70
1 Moderate visual impairment	6/18 3/10 (0.3) 20/706/18 3/10 (0.3) 20/70	6/60 1/10 (0.1) 20/200
2 Severe visual impairment	6/60 1/10 (0.1) 20/200	6/60 1/20 (0.05) 20/400
3 Blindness	1/60* 1/50 (0.02)	1/60* 1/50 (0.02) 5/300 (20/1,200)
4 Blindness	5/300 (20/1200)	Light perception
5 Blindness	No light perception	No light perception

* *Note:* Or count fingers at 1 m.
Patients with a visual field of the better eye no greater than 10° are placed under category 3.
From *International Statistical Classification of Diseases and Related Health Problems 10th Revision (ICD-10)*, section H54.9, by World Health Organization, 2016. Reprinted with permission.

Low vision adversely affects an individual's ability to perform everyday activities (American Academy of Ophthalmology Vision Rehabilitation Committee, 2001). Compared to individuals without disabilities (Burmedi, Becker, Heyl, Wahl, and Himmelsbach, 2002), individuals with low vision demonstrate a 15% to 30% higher dependence on others to perform activities of daily living (ADLs). Despite their decreased ability to perform ADLs and instrumental activities of daily living (IADLs), persons with low vision still have the need and desire to perform everyday activities that support their life roles (Crews and Campbell, 2001; Horowitz, 2004; Raina, Wong, and Massfeller, 2004; Travis, Boerner, Reinhardt, and Horowitz, 2004).

The eye diseases that result in low vision affect different areas of occupational performance. Clients with cataracts may have difficulty with taking care of themselves, recognizing faces, reading or watching television, doing their job, or leaving their home (Nordqvist, 2017). Ramulu (2009) found that the most frequent complaints of those with glaucoma were difficulties with extremes in lighting, such as walking out of a darkened theater to a sunlit parking lot, and those with bilateral glaucoma reported difficulty with reading, walking, and driving. Diabetic retinopathy at all levels of severity results in difficulty in reading and driving (Coyne et al., 2004). Persons more severely affected have difficulty with diabetic care routines and mobility issues and have an increased fear of accidents, leading to decreased social participation. AMD adversely affects the individual's ability to read standard print and can limit independence in preparing meals, using a telephone, taking care of finances, traveling, shopping, taking medications, and washing laundry (Ryan, Anas, Beamer, and Bajorek, 2003).

Low Vision Rehabilitation Team

A number of team members, in addition to occupational therapy practitioners, work with clients with low vision (see Table 14-2). **Ophthalmologists** are medical doctors (MDs) who diagnose and treat

Table 14-2 Low Vision Rehabilitation Team Members

Team Member	Referral Source	Team Function
Ophthalmologists	Self, physician	Diagnose and treat disease, prescribe medications, and perform eye surgery
Low vision optometrists	Self, physician, and/or ophthalmologist	Diagnose and treat refractive errors with optical devices
Occupational therapy practitioner	Physician and in some states optometrists and nonprofit agencies	Teach optical and nonoptical device use, visual skills, and adaptive techniques and modify the environment
Certified low vision therapist	Optometrists and nonprofit agencies	Teach optical device use and visual skills
Vision rehabilitation therapists	State or nonprofit agencies	Train in the home for adaptive techniques to perform everyday activities and modify the environment
Orientation and mobility specialists	State or nonprofit agencies	Train in safe travel using canes, guide dogs, and/or electronic devices and public transportation
Psychiatrists, psychologists, and/or social workers	Physician, self, other team members	Assist with difficulties coping and adjusting
Family members	Not applicable	Transport the client to appointments, perform home modifications, and assist in home program

eye diseases, prescribe medications, and perform surgery. **Optometrists** are doctors of optometry (ODs) who treat refractive errors with glasses, contacts, and magnifiers. Vision rehabilitation therapists receive referrals from state or nonprofit agencies to provide training in the home for adaptive techniques to perform everyday activities and modify the environment. **Orientation and mobility (O&M) specialists** are consulted for difficulties in mobility and provide training for people to travel safely using devices such as canes, guide dogs, and/or electronic devices. They teach people to take public transportation on their own and also receive referrals through the state or a nonprofit agency. Mental health service providers such as psychiatrists, psychologists, and/or social workers may be consulted to assist with psychosocial difficulties in coping and adjusting to low vision. They may address such issues as anxiety, frustration, fear, anger, and depression. Finally, family members often transport the client to appointments, may perform home modifications for the client, and assist in follow-through with home programs. Family members of the visually impaired are often more involved than are family members of other populations with functional deficits.

Engage Your Brain 14-1

Other disciplines have historically and currently treated clients with low vision. What knowledge and skills do occupational therapy practitioners possess to make them a valuable member of the low vision rehabilitation team?

Occupational Therapy for Clients With Low Vision

Occupational therapists are uniquely qualified to address the psychosocial and physical rehabilitation needs of persons with low vision through the provision of meaningful engagement in occupations. Research has shown that "occupational therapists working in low vision can support clients by facilitating development of a social network, acting as liaisons between clients and other health practitioners, especially ophthalmologists, and encouraging policy development that supports barrier-free LVAD (low vision assistive device) acquisition and use" (Copolillo and Teitelman, 2005, p. 305).

Participating in occupational therapy may help people with low vision enhance their independence and functional ability (American Occupational Therapy Association [AOTA], 2013). Although occupational therapy practitioners have worked with persons with low vision for decades, it was not until 1990 that physicians could refer clients for occupational therapy with a sole diagnosis of low vision. At that time the Health Care Financing Administration expanded the meaning of *physical impairment* to include low vision (Warren, 1995). In 2002, Congress created a program memorandum to enforce Medicare coverage for beneficiaries with low vision for rehabilitation services (U.S. Department of Health and Human Services Centers for Medicare and Medicaid Services, 2002). The AOTA considers low vision services important for productive aging and provides evidence-based practice resources on its website (AOTA, n.d.b).

Two low vision certifications are available for occupational therapists. In 2000, the Academy for Certification of Vision Rehabilitation and Education Professionals (ACVREP) developed several certifications for low vision providers, including the **certified low vision therapist** (CLVT; Watson, Qillman, Flax, and Gerritsen, 1999). To better meet the growing need for occupational therapy services, in 2006 the AOTA established a **specialty certification in low vision** (SCLV). The SCLV credential provides a formal recognition to occupational therapists and occupational therapy assistants for their specialized knowledge and practice expertise with the low vision population. There are currently 43 occupational therapists who have obtained the SCLV certification (AOTA spokesperson, personal communication, August 31, 2018).

Low Vision Practice Settings

Occupational therapy practitioners may provide services for clients with low vision in a variety of settings, using different business models, and on vision rehabilitation teams with various service members (see Table 14-2). Familiar settings for occupational therapy practitioners to provide these types of service include outpatient clinics, low vision centers associated with universities, or private practices. In these settings, clients with low vision are scheduled and billed for their care in a manner consistent with clients seen for other diagnoses. Occupational therapy practitioners working in physicians' offices or eye clinics may need to see clients on the same day they see the physician. The Veterans Health Administration (VA) offers outpatient services and inpatient services for blind and low vision veterans (Vets.gov, n.d.). Veterans are placed in the program most consistent with their needs. In the VA system, veterans receive the technology they need to become independent at no cost, counseling to adjust to blindness, orientation and mobility training, and training in new visual skills.

Occupational therapy practitioners also work in community agencies serving the blind and visually impaired. In this type of setting, clients are considered consumers of the agency's services. Their care may be covered through grant funding or reimbursed by the state. In this model, funding may be available not only for therapy but also for some assistive devices. Community agencies frequently provide a continuum of care for their consumers. They usually offer services that include diagnosis, instruction in visual efficiency skills and optical device use, classes in ADLs and IADLs, support groups for coping with and adjusting to visual impairments, referrals for O&M specialists, and home safety evaluations and modifications. Occupational therapy practitioners can provide many of these services for the community agency.

Referrals for Occupational Therapy

As in any other area of occupational therapy practice, a referral for occupational therapy is required for reimbursement from Medicare or private insurance companies. Exactly what type of low vision professional (e.g., physician, optometrist) is able to refer a client for occupational therapy depends on state law. Because best practice requires specialized skills by all team members and occupational therapy requires a referral source, an occupational therapist should try to partner with an existing low vision provider. The low vision referral for occupational therapy should state that an evaluation is required and what areas of occupation are affected by the client's low vision.

Interventions for Clients With Low Vision

Occupational therapy service needs are determined by a comprehensive evaluation. Relevant background information to collect includes the client's diagnosis and treatment received, prior level of function, living situation, and social support system. The evaluation should then focus on the client's current level of function. The occupational therapist should determine which areas of occupation are affected by low vision. This may be accomplished with a self-report questionnaire developed by occupational therapists, such as the Smith's Low Vision Independence Measure (LVIM; Smith, 2013) or the Self-Report Assessment of Functional Vision Performance (SRAFVP; Velozo, Warren, Hicks, and Berger, 2013) supplemented with observational assessments. Specific skills may be assessed, such as reading with the Pepper Visual Skills for Reading Test (Watson, Whittaker, Steciw, Baldasare, and Miller-Shaffer, 1995) and the MNREAD Test (Legge, Ross, Luebker, and LaMay, 1989). Writing skills can be evaluated with the Low Vision Writing Assessment (Watson, Wright, Wyse, and De l'Aune, 2004). Depending on test results provided by the referral source, the occupational therapy practitioner may also assess visual acuity, tracking, and visual fields. Once the client's current level of function is determined, the occupational therapist works with the client to develop an intervention plan to prioritize and establish goals. Intervention for clients with low vision generally involves improving affected client factors and training the person to use assistive devices, providing environmental modifications to facilitate safe participation in desired occupations, and completing task modification to maximize occupational performance.

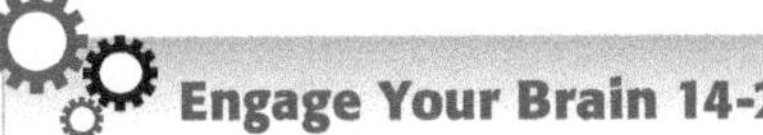

Engage Your Brain 14-2

Which occupational therapy theories would be appropriate for a client who has recently been diagnosed with low vision?

Engage Your Brain 14-3

Which occupational therapy theories would be appropriate for a client who has long-standing low vision?

Person

First, clients need to improve their visual efficiency skills, including eccentric viewing and visual scanning. Clients with macular diseases affecting their central vision need to be taught **eccentric viewing,** or how to use the area of the retina that has not been damaged (Stelmack, Massof, and Stelmack, 2004). Eccentric viewing is particularly useful in reading and writing tasks and for viewing people's faces. Visual scanning, eye movements designed to locate an object of interest in the environment, is needed to complete most tasks (Warren, 1990). Clients with low vision need to be taught efficient visual-scanning skills to compensate for their decreased visual fields. As with all new skills, eccentric viewing and visual scanning need to be incorporated into the performance of preferred occupations by clients as a means of adaptation.

When clients' vision cannot be improved, they can learn to use their residual vision more efficiently and adopt the use of optical devices to help in task completion. As in the selection of any type of assistive device, it is important to know the client's abilities, heed client preferences, work within any financial constraints, understand the purpose of the device, and have extensive knowledge of optics. Due to the various variables affecting assistive device use by persons with low vision, many low vision clinics allow clients the opportunity to test different types of equipment before purchasing.

Several optical devices can aid near-vision tasks. Head-mounted devices such as spectacles free both hands for bilateral activities. However, learning the working distance or focal distance for spectacles can be difficult for the client. Handheld magnifiers can have the added advantage of a built-in light. However, one hand is required to hold the magnifier, and finding and maintaining the focal distance with handheld magnifiers may also be difficult. Stand magnifiers provide the correct focal distance for the client, but handheld magnifiers are easier to manipulate and transport. In addition, electronic devices such as closed-circuit televisions (CCTVs) or computer programs can enlarge print so that it is legible to the client. Some newer models of CCTV feature detachable tablets and vertical scrolling. However, CCTVs and computers with low vision software are expensive.

Other optical devices are available for distance viewing and driving. Clients who need devices for distance viewing, such as watching sports, can use telescopes. Although telescopes provide greater acuity, they significantly limit the size of the visual field. Clients with visual field deficits may be prescribed field enhancement devices, although these devices may be difficult for some to use due to the perceptual adjustment. Bioptic telescopes that are used for driving require training, and their use is dependent on state laws.

In addition to optical devices that allow clients to participate in their preferred occupations, many nonoptical devices are available. Some of these devices are dependent on the client's use of other senses, such as auditory. Examples include talking clocks and watches, liquid indicators, books on tape, and talking blood glucose meters and scales. Clients can use their tactile sense by marking personal-care products with rubber bands and different-colored clothing with safety pins.

Other devices utilize the concept of enlargement, such as large-print address books, calendars, datebooks, or fonts on computers. Some personal-care devices have large print, including pillboxes and syringes. Grooming activities, such as applying makeup or shaving, are much easier to perform using a lighted magnification mirror. Devices with large print to aid in cooking include kitchen timers and measuring cups and spoons. Clients can participate in leisure activities by using large-print playing cards, bingo cards, or a big-button television remote control.

Still other devices improve occupational performance by using high contrast (Fig. 14-1). Print is much easier to read if a client uses a black felt pen on bold-lined paper. Signature guides provide an outlined area within which to sign, as check templates do to fill out a check.

Computers, cell phones, and tablets now come with accessibility options for the visually impaired. Numerous apps are available for easily portable cell phones and tablets to facilitate participation in

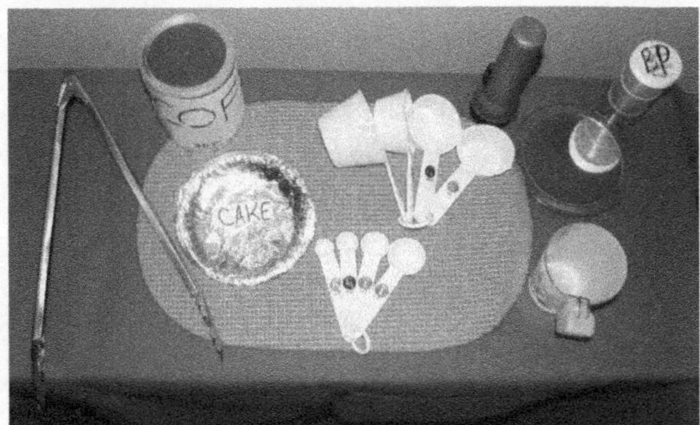

Figure 14-1 *From left to right,* the items are long-handled tongs; the top row is a coffee can labeled with enlarged print on a note card, enlarged-print measuring cups, a flashlight, an enlargement mirror, and blood pressure medicine with enlarged print on the pill top. The bottom row contains a single-portion food item with enlarged print on aluminum foil, enlarged-print measuring spoons, and a liquid indicator. *(Courtesy of Theresa Smith.)*

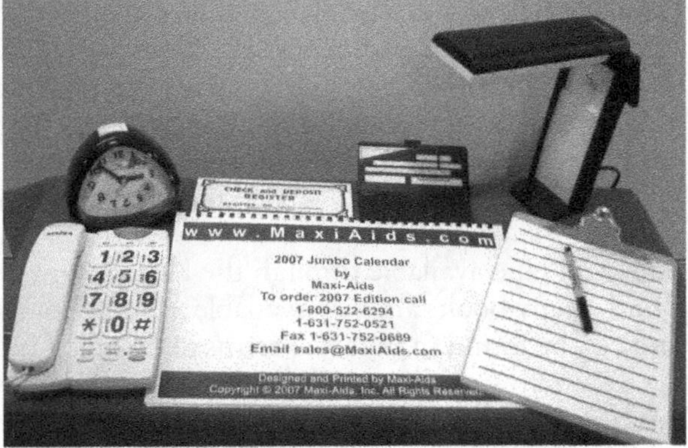

Figure 14-2 *From left to right,* the top row contains a clock with enlarged and bold numbers, enlarged check register, check-writing template, and task lamp. In the bottom row is a telephone with enlarged numbers and a bump dot on #5, a jumbo calendar, and a bold-lined yellow paper with a fine-point Sharpie. *(Courtesy of Theresa Smith.)*

preferred occupations. Examples include, but are not limited to, audio clocks, global positioning systems, enlarged keyboards, flashlights, scanners, text-to-audio readers, and color identifiers (AppleVis, n.d.; Brisbin, 2016).

Environment

In general, an older person needs two to three times more light to see than a younger person, but people with some eye diseases may be sensitive to glare (Watson, 2001). Therefore, it is important to increase lighting without causing glare, which can be accomplished with lighting placement, choice of lighting, and glare elimination. Light can be aimed to illuminate the task at hand by using a gooseneck lamp. The type of lighting used is important. Incandescent light is commonly used in desk lamps but may not provide good contrast or color perception. Halogen provides a bright white light but generates a lot of heat. Fluorescent light is energy efficient but may be harsh and flicker annoyingly (Watson, 2001). Full-spectrum lighting is the closest to sunlight but is high on the blue light spectrum, which may result in glare. Glare can be controlled by covering high-glare surfaces such as tabletops with tablecloths and windows with sheer drapes (Cole, 2003).

Tactile markings, utilization of enlargement and contrast, and organization are all useful adaptations. Tactile markings on appliances can be very effective in facilitating occupational performance. For example, frequently used settings on the microwave, dishwasher, and washer and dryer can be marked with bump dots. The concepts of enlargement and/or contrast can also be utilized in modifying the environment (Fig. 14-2). Those with low vision can select clocks with large numbers on sharp contrast backgrounds. Dark bath mats can be placed over white tub edges or contrasting placemats chosen for the table. To improve contrast throughout the home, walls can be painted a lighter color and dark furniture selected. Creating a system of organization can be very helpful for those with low vision. Inexpensive high-contrast baskets can be used to store like items, including cleaning supplies, personal-care items, medications, and/or leisure activity equipment.

Occupation

Many tasks may need modification for a person with low vision to be able to complete them in a timely and efficient manner. For example, instead of attempting to apply low-contrast toothpaste to a white toothbrush, a more efficient means is to put the toothpaste in a small cup and drag the brush in the cup, or to simply put the toothpaste in the mouth.

Locating one's food on a plate can be difficult, but if food is always placed using the clock method, it is easy to find. Writing can be problematic, but writing a short message on or signing a greeting card can be more easily accomplished. Reading, a leisure activity enjoyed by many, may become too difficult for those with low vision. In addition to books on tape available through the Library for the Blind, many books are now available as audiobooks and can be found in library systems or downloaded via Internet streaming. Clients can "read" while performing other activities, like doing the dishes or taking a bath.

Social participation is an important area of occupation (AOTA, 2014). Unfortunately, people with low vision often become socially isolated secondary to difficulties with transportation. People can and do engage socially through virtual means. In a study by Smith, Ludwig, Andersen, and Copolillo (2009), several participants mentioned that social participation was achieved on the telephone. Today even more virtual means exist, such as communicating via e-mail or with webcams. The results of a systematic review by Berger, McAteer, Schreier, and Kaldenberg (2013) yielded four themes related to interventions for social participation and leisure for older adults with low vision. The authors concluded that best practices to increase social participation and leisure for older visually impaired adults include:

- Using a problem-solving approach to achieve goals
- Including a blend of services for "education, skills training, social support, guide training and home visit" from appropriate disciplines (Berger et al., 2013, pp. 307–308)
- Improving all lighting, with special attention to task lighting

PROGRAM SHOWCASE

Submitted by Linda D. Moon, OTR/L

Needs assessment: A 3-month assessment period was utilized to identify the need for occupational therapy at the Eye Center of North Florida, located in the Florida panhandle. The practicing optometrist struggled to provide services beyond in-clinic patient education and introductory low vision aid demonstration. The following needs were identified: training in the use of eccentric fixation, visual field awareness, and adaptation to visual field loss; low vision device introduction with follow-through training on multiple occasions prior to prescription of device(s); education regarding disease process/prognosis/expectations; behavior modifications to reduce risk factors/disease progression; low vision adaptation basics such as lighting and nonoptical devices; and in-home occupational therapy visits for modifications and carryover of low vision training.

Specific groups with identified needs for low vision examination, training, and device use included:

- Older adults with transportation limitations (75% of patients did not meet the visual acuity requirements to possess a valid Florida driver's license and/or had limited availability of family or caregivers to provide transportation)
- Veterans in the community who were eligible for low vision devices and nonoptical aids but could not travel to the nearest Veterans Affairs facility
- Clients in the Independent Living Program and Vocational Rehabilitation Program associated with the Florida Division of Blind Services
- Students who were registered with the Florida Division of Blind Services via the Transitional Program (K–12)

Goal of the program: Through the use of evaluation, education, and skilled interventions, equip visually impaired clients with the means to regain and maintain their highest level of safety and independence with all aspects of basic self-care, instrumental activities of daily living, functional mobility in the home and community, and leisure pursuits. For those services not within the scope of occupational therapy, make referrals to other professionals who could best meet their need(s): orientation and mobility specialists, physical therapists, grief counselors, council on aging, public transportation services, and other caregiving agencies/organizations.

Population: client age demographics: 85% 65 years of age and older, 10% 20 to 64-year-olds, 5% children and youth

Participant's perspective: "I had no idea services like this were available. When I began losing my vision, I just thought that I would have to give up everything, because that is what my doctors and family kept telling me. All I've heard up to this visit are things like, 'You can't drive anymore,' 'You can't cook on the stove,' 'You can't take care of your mail, bills, and medicines.' But here you are telling me how I CAN DO a lot of these things again, though I will have to learn to do them differently."

Evaluation results: Before this program began, most patients who were referred for low vision services presented with visual acuities that qualified them as legally blind (less than or equal to 20/200). In contrast, this comprehensive program allowed for intervention with patients in the early stage(s) of their eye disease (less than 20/60), providing extensive education, making adaptations, and setting realistic expectations for the future. Clients were then followed throughout the disease process, provided with more in-depth interventions along the way, and connected to more community resources, thus leading to less anger and frustration as clients progressed to advanced disease. These clients had a greater level of satisfaction, with positive functional outcomes, despite their loss of vision, and it was determined that this program was instrumental in assisting clients through the stages of grief associated with vision loss.

The primary limiting factor with this program was associated with the change in health-care coverage options, as more Medicare Advantage/Replacement plans entered the market. As a result, reimbursement was significantly reduced, not allowing for the support of a full-time position in this setting. The occupational therapist transitioned to PRN (i.e., as needed) status prior to further changes in clinic management that led to an integration of this program into the traditional home care setting (see details below).

Funding: Traditional Medicare, Medicare Advantage Plans with pre-authorization (some, not all), private insurance with pre-authorization, Tricare with pre-authorization, Florida Blind Services with pre-authorization, private pay

Other information: Due to changes in the ownership of the eye clinic and health-care marketplace, the occupational therapist transitioned out of the clinic and into the home care setting. A referral network was created for optometrists to communicate the need for low vision occupational therapy services (after completion of their low vision examination in the clinic) to a retinal specialist, neurologist, or cardiologist. The referral would then be sent to the home care agency. The occupational therapist would follow the recommendations for optical device trial/use based on reports provided by all eye medical service providers involved. Upon completion of occupational therapy interventions, the occupational therapist would then communicate which device(s) were most appropriate for the person in order to have prescriptions provided for aids requiring such documentation. For nonoptical aids (e.g., talking devices, large-button phones, tactile markings, lighting devices, etc.), the occupational therapist provided the person with information on how to obtain them through a public vendor.

Psychosocial Issues Associated With Low Vision

Psychosocial issues are inherent for those diagnosed with low vision due to the loss of independence and relinquishing of desired occupations. In a study of adults ages 65 and older with vision impairment, 63.4% also experienced mild to moderate or severe depressive symptoms (Crews, Jones, and Kim, 2006). Persons who experience activity limitations or functional impairments because of AMD, the most common cause of visual impairment in the older adult, are at significant risk for depression (Casten and Rovner, 2013). It is important for occupational therapy practitioners to be vigilant for the signs of depression, as it may reduce the effectiveness of low vision rehabilitation interventions (Discovery Eye Foundation, 2015). In a low vision depression prevention trial with participants with AMD, Rovner et al. (2014) determined that the combination of low vision rehabilitation by occupational therapists and behavior activation by supportive therapy therapists enabled participants to remain socially engaged and improved their functional vision. The researchers concluded that depression may be prevented in patients with AMD if interactions between ophthalmology, optometry, rehabilitation, psychiatry, and behavioral psychology are promoted.

In interviews of persons with visual impairments, Teitelman and Copolillo (2005) noted three main themes related to the psychosocial aspects of low vision: emotional challenges, negative emotional outcomes, and indicators of emotional adaptation. Some of the emotional challenges identified by interviewees were lost independence, relinquishing of desired activities, lost spontaneity, and impact on social interactions. In addition, the participants reported distressing emotional reactions such as depression, stigma and embarrassment, frustration, and resignation. The most commonly used emotional adaptation strategies were cognitive restructuring, social support, contributions to family and friends, and faith. The greater the number of favorite activities that could be retained, even with adaptations, the easier the emotional adjustment appeared to be. Attending to the psychosocial issues related to low vision is an important aspect of occupational therapy services.

Low vision rehabilitation services are important in combating the psychological effects of visual disability. Horowitz, Reinhardt, and Boerner (2005) found that counseling services, low vision clinical services, and participants' use of optical devices were significant contributors in reducing participants' depressive symptoms. Unfortunately, people with AMD tend to underutilize the available rehabilitation services shown to improve their visual function and quality of life (Casten, Maloney, and Rovner, 2005).

Low Vision Community Support

It is important for occupational therapy practitioners to be aware of community resources available for their clients with visual impairments. Is there a radio station that reads the daily newspaper or offers other interesting programming? What are the public and private transportation options? Is there a low vision support group? Are there organizations that provide social support, reading to the visually impaired, or light housekeeping duties? Where can low vision nonoptical devices be obtained? Knowing where to refer clients who need these services is imperative. Keeping on hand forms qualifying clients for services and catalogs featuring low vision assistive devices can facilitate acquisition of these resources.

Funding and Billing Issues for Low Vision Occupational Therapy Services

The primary funder for occupational therapy services in low vision is Medicare Part B unless clients are seen through a home health agency. However, low vision services are also covered by many private insurance companies and some state or nonprofit agencies serving the blind and visually impaired. When billing Medicare for clients with low vision, practitioners must follow the same regulations as for any client receiving Medicare services (AOTA, n.d.a; U.S. Department of Health and Human Services, n.d.). Medicare Part B currently pays 80% of total occupational therapy outpatient charges, and clients must make up the 20% difference unless they have a Medicare Part B supplement policy.

Necessary optical and nonoptical devices for clients with low vision are not covered by Medicare or private insurance companies. Most state or nonprofit agencies serving the blind and visually impaired are able to provide some optical and nonoptical devices. They may have loaner programs for CCTVs or used CCTVs for resale. These agencies may also have donated equipment that can be distributed.

Summary

- The population of persons with low vision is growing and will increase dramatically with the aging population.
- The most common eye diseases for those age 40 and over include cataract, glaucoma, diabetic retinopathy, and macular degeneration. Etiology, prevalence, and medical treatment for the common eye diseases vary. Low vision is irreversible and may be hereditary, congenital, or acquired.
- Low vision adversely affects an individual's ability to perform everyday activities. The eye diseases that result in low vision affect different areas of occupational performance.
- A number of team members work with clients with low vision, including, but not limited to, ophthalmologists, optometrists, certified low vision therapists, and orientation and mobility specialists. Occupational therapy is one of the disciplines identified as a low vision provider by Medicare and by optometrists and ophthalmologists.
- Occupational therapy practitioners have the skills to facilitate participation in all areas of occupation and maintain independence and health for this expanding population. Most of these services are provided in the community, and there is ample opportunity for occupational therapists to expand low vision services through the development of new programs.
- Emotional challenges experienced by persons with low vision include lost independence, relinquishing of desired activities, lost

spontaneity, depression, stigma, embarrassment, frustration, and resignation.

- Communities have different types of support for persons with visual impairment. Some examples of support might be a radio station that reads the newspaper, inexpensive transportation services, volunteer readers, and/or volunteers who do light housekeeping duties.
- Rehabilitation services are covered by Medicare and some private insurance companies for the visually impaired. Clients seen through a home health agency are covered by Medicare Part A. If not, then their care is most likely billed through Medicare Part B and requires a copayment. Medicare and insurance companies do not pay for any optical or nonoptical equipment the client may need, but state or nonprofit agencies are able to provide some equipment needs.

CASE STUDIES

CASE STUDY 14-1 Mrs. Drew

Mrs. Drew is a 75-year-old widow who has bilateral dry macular degeneration with right-eye visual acuity of 20/200 and left-eye visual acuity of 20/100. She lives in her own apartment in an assisted living facility. The building has an elevator and is within 2 miles of her daughter, Rachel. Mrs. Drew is a grandmother to Rachel and her husband's child, Melissa, who is a junior in college. Although Mrs. Drew spends most major holidays with Rachel and her family, she maintains an active social calendar with other residents at the assisted living facility.

During an occupational therapy evaluation, Mrs. Drew reports difficulties in a number of areas that she would like to address. Self-care issues for Mrs. Drew include moderate difficulty keeping her fingernails and toenails trimmed. Mrs. Drew uses only a microwave for food preparation, primarily to heat up frozen entrees. However, she has moderate difficulty reading the meal preparation instructions and minimum difficulty operating the microwave controls. She also would like to be able to communicate via e-mail with her granddaughter and text her daughter. Rachel has managed Mrs. Drew's finances for some time, and both women are happy with this arrangement. However, Mrs. Drew would like to be able to sign her name independently and is self-conscious about the level of legibility of her current signature. Mrs. Drew's problems with reading small print have adversely affected participation in her leisure activities in a number of ways. Every 2 weeks, she goes out to dinner with a small group of friends to different restaurants. Transportation is not an issue, as several members of the group still drive. However, she has great difficulty reading the menu and would prefer not to constantly have to ask that a friend read the menu to her. Mrs. Drew is a petite lady interested in maintaining her weight, as well as staying within a monthly budget. She also loves to read and wants to keep up with current releases by her favorite authors. The occupational therapist reports to Mrs. Drew's insurance carrier that she has good potential for rehabilitation and would benefit from occupational therapy services.

Discussion Questions

1. What areas of occupation are affected by Mrs. Drew's low vision?
2. How might you improve her occupational performance in those areas?
3. What optical and nonoptical devices would you suggest to Mrs. Drew to improve her occupational performance?
4. Using the ecology of performance model, reflect upon the best intervention approaches to use at this time with Mrs. Drew.

CASE STUDY 14-2 Low Vision Service Provision in an Assisted Care Facility

You have been providing low vision rehabilitation to clients in a nearby assisted living facility. Several of your low vision clients have told their friends about the therapeutic interventions and environmental modifications you have recommended. All agree these changes have improved their occupational performance. You believe these changes have been so beneficial that some residents may have remained in their individual apartments for longer periods of time versus moving to a greater level of assistance. In addition, you are aware of the high percentage of persons with visual impairment that have depression. You approach the director of the assisted living facility with a plan to conduct educational sessions for residents with visual deficits and/or depressive symptoms secondary to vision loss.

Discussion Questions

1. What type of evidence will you need to present to the director that supports your program?
2. What are some vision-dependent ADLs and IADLs in which a majority of the residents with vision deficits may be having problems?
3. What are some possible environmental changes that could be recommended to facilitate a better fit in the residents' apartments?
4. What topics should you include in your depression prevention sessions?
5. How would you negotiate payment for the development and implementation of your program? How would the AOTA (2015) *Occupational Therapy Code of Ethics (2015)* guide your decision-making?

Learning Activities

1. Develop a resource list of transportation sources available in your community that serve the blind or visually impaired.
2. What are some virtual means that people with low vision might use to engage in social participation? What accommodations might you anticipate to facilitate social engagement through virtual means?
3. Choose one room or work area in a home and design and depict environmental modifications for a client with low vision.

REFERENCES

Age-Related Eye Disease Study Research Group. (2001). A randomized, placebo-controlled, clinical trial of high-dose supplementation with vitamins C and E, beta carotene, and zinc for age-related cataract and vision loss: AREDS Report No. 9. *Archives of Ophthalmology, 119*(10), 1439–1452.

Age-Related Eye Disease Study 2 Research Group. (2013). Lutein + zeaxanthin and omega-3 fatty acids for age-related macular degeneration: The Age-Related Eye Disease Study 2 (AREDS2) randomized clinical trial. *Journal of the American Medical Association, 309*(19), 2005–2015.

American Academy of Ophthalmology Vision Rehabilitation Committee. (2001). *Preferred practice pattern: Visual rehabilitation for adults.* San Francisco, CA: American Academy of Ophthalmology.

American Occupational Therapy Association. (n.d.a). *Medicare.* Retrieved from www.aota.org/Advocacy-Policy/Federal-Reg-Affairs/Medicare.aspx

American Occupational Therapy Association. (n.d.b). *Productive aging evidence-based practice resources.* Retrieved from www.aota.org/Practice/Productive-Aging/Evidence-based.aspx#Low

American Occupational Therapy Association. (2006). *AOTA Board Certification and Specialty Certification.* Retrieved from http://aota.org/nonmembers/area15/index.asp

American Occupational Therapy Association. (2013). *Tips for living life to its fullest: Living with low vision.* Retrieved from www.aota.org/~/media/Corporate/Files/AboutOT/consumers/Adults/LowVision/Low%20Vision%20Tip%20Sheet.pdf

American Occupational Therapy Association. (2014). Occupational therapy practice framework: Domain and process (3rd ed.). *American Journal of Occupational Therapy, 68*(Suppl. 1), S1–S48.

American Occupational Therapy Association. (2015). Occupational therapy code of ethics (2015). *American Journal of Occupational Therapy, 69*(Suppl. 3), 6913410030. http://dx.doi.org/10.5014/ajot.2015.696S03

AppleVis. (n.d.). *Empowering blind and low-vision users of Apple products and related applications: Find, share and recommend accessible iOS, Mac, Apple Watch and Apple TV apps.* Retrieved from www.applevis.com/apps/ios-apps-for-blind-and-vision-impaired

Berger, S., McAteer, J., Schreier, K., and Kaldenberg, J. (2013). Occupational therapy interventions to improve leisure and social participation for older adults with low vision: A systematic review. *American Journal of Occupational Therapy, 68,* 303–311.

Brisbin, S. (2016). Best Android apps for people with low vision. *Access World Magazine, 17*(2). Retrieved from www.afb.org/afbpress/pubnew.asp?DocID=aw170208

Burmedi, D., Becker, S., Heyl, V., Wahl, H., and Himmelsbach, I. (2002). Behavioral consequences of age-related low vision: A narrative review. *Visual Impairment Research, 4*(1), 15–45.

Casten, R. J., Maloney, E. K., and Rovner, B. W. (2005). Knowledge and use of low vision services among persons with age-related macular degeneration. *Journal of Visual Impairment and Blindness, 99*(11), 720–724.

Casten, R. J., and Rovner, B. W. (2013). Update on depression and age-related macular degeneration. *Current Opinion in Ophthalmology, 24*(3), 239–243.

Cole, R. (2003). *Lighting for low vision.* Retrieved from http://mdsupport.org/library/lighting.html

Copolillo, A., and Teitelman, J. L. (2005). Acquisition and integration of low vision assistive devices: Understanding the decision-making process of older adults with low vision. *American Journal of Occupational Therapy, 59*(3), 305–313.

Coyne, K. S., Margolis, M. K., Kennedy-Martin, T., Baker, T. M., Klein, R., Paul, M. D., and Revicki, D. A. (2004). The impact of diabetic retinopathy: Perspectives from patient focus groups. *Family Practice, 21*(4), 447–453.

Crews, J. E., and Campbell, V. (2001). Health conditions, activity limitations, and participation restrictions among older people with visual impairments. *Journal of Visual Impairment and Blindness, 95,* 453–467.

Crews, J. E., Jones, G. C., and Kim, J. H. (2006). Double jeopardy: The effects of comorbid conditions among older people with vision loss. *Journal of Visual Impairment and Blindness, 100,* 824–848.

Discovery Eye Foundation. (2015). *Vision loss and depression.* Retrieved from https://discoveryeye.org/vision-loss-and-depression/

Heimlich, R. (2010). *Baby boomers retire.* Retrieved from www.pewresearch.org/fact-tank/2010/12/29/baby-boomers-retire/

Horowitz, A. (2004). The prevalence and consequences of vision impairment in later life. *Topics in Geriatric Rehabilitation, 20,* 185–195.

Horowitz, A., Reinhardt, J. P., and Boerner, K. (2005). The effect of rehabilitation on depression among visually disabled older adults. *Aging Mental Health, 9,* 563–570.

Johns Hopkins Medicine. (n.d.). *Diabetic retinopathy.* Retrieved from http://hopkinsmedicine.org/wilmer/Conditions/diabetic_retinopathy.html

Legge, G. E., Ross, J. A., Luebker, A., and LaMay, J. M. (1989). Psychophysics of reading (Vol. 8). The Minnesota Low-Vision Reading Test. *Optometry and Vision Science, 66,* 843–853.

Mogk, L. G. (n.d.). *What treatments are available for wet macular degeneration?* Retrieved from www.visionaware.org/info/your-eye-condition/age-related-macular-degeneration-amd/treatments-for-wet-macular-degeneration/125

National Eye Institute (n.d.). *Cataracts.* Retrieved from https://nei.nih.gov/eyedata/cataract#2

National Eye Institute (2015a). *Facts about age-related macular degeneration.* Retrieved from https://nei.nih.gov/health/maculardegen

National Eye Institute (2015b). *Facts about cataract.* Retrieved from https://nei.nih.gov/health/cataract

National Eye Institute (2015c). *Facts about diabetic eye disease.* Retrieved from https://nei.nih.gov/health/diabetic

National Eye Institute (2015d). *Facts about glaucoma.* Retrieved from https://nei.nih.gov/health/glaucoma

Nordqvist, C. (2017). What you need to know about cataracts. *Medical News Today.* Retrieved from www.medicalnewstoday.com/articles/157510.php#

Protect-your-sight.com. (2008). *Do you know how to protect your eyesight?* Retrieved from http://protect-your-eyesight.com/

Raina, P., Wong, M., and Massfeller, H. (2004). The relationship between sensory impairment and functional independence among elderly. *BMC Geriatrics, 4,* 3.

Ramulu, P. (2009). Glaucoma and disability: Which tasks are affected, and at what stage of disease? *Current Opinion in Ophthalmology, 20*(2), 92–98.

Rovner, B. W., Casten, R. J., Hegel, M. T., Massof, R. W., Leiby, B. E., Ho, A. C., and Tasman, W. S. (2014). Low Vision Depression Trial in age-related macular degeneration: A randomized clinical trial. *Ophthalmology, 121*(11), 2204–2211.

Ryan, E. B., Anas, A. P., Beamer, M., and Bajorek, S. (2003). Coping with age-related vision loss in everyday reading activities. *Educational Gerontology, 29*(1), 37–54.

Smith, T. M. (2013). Refinement of the Low Vision Independence Measure: A qualitative study. *Physical and Occupational Therapy in Geriatrics, 31*(3), 182–196.

Smith, T. M., Ludwig, F., Andersen, L., and Copolillo, A. (2009). Engagement in occupation and adaptation to low vision. *Occupational Therapy in Healthcare, 23*(2), 119–133.

Stelmack, J. A., Massof, R. W., and Stelmack, T. R. (2004). Is there a standard of care for eccentric viewing? *Journal of Rehabilitation Research and Development, 41*(5), 729–738.

Teitelman, J., and Copolillo, A. (2005). Psychosocial issues in older adults' adjustment to vision loss: Findings from qualitative interviews and focus groups. *American Journal of Occupational Therapy, 59*(4), 409–417.

Travis, L. A., Boerner, K., Reinhardt, J. P., and Horowitz, A. (2004). Exploring functional disability in older adults with low vision. *Journal of Visual Impairment and Blindness, 98*(9), 534–546.

U.S. Department of Health and Human Services. (n.d.). *Centers for Medicare and Medicaid Services.* Retrieved from http://cms.gov/default.asp

U.S. Department of Health and Human Services Centers for Medicare and Medicaid Services. (2002). *Program memorandum intermediaries/carriers.* Transmittal AB-02078. Baltimore, MD: Centers for Medicare and Medicare Services.

Varma, R., Vajaranant, T. S., Burkemper, B., Wu, S., Torres, M., Hsu, C., . . . McKean-Cowdin, R. (2016). Visual impairment and blindness in adults in the United States: Demographic and geographic variations from 2015 to 2050. *JAMA Ophthalmology, 134*(7), 802–809.

Velozo, C. A., Warren, M., Hicks, E., and Berger, K. A. (2013). Generating clinical outputs for self-reports of visual functioning. *Optometry and Vision Science, 90*(8), 765–775.

Vets.gov. (n.d.). *Vision care for blind and low vision veterans.* Retrieved from www.vets.gov/health-care/about-va-health-care/vision-care/blind-and-low-vision-veterans/

Vision Council. (2015). *Vision loss in America: Aging and low vision.* Retrieved from www.thevisioncouncil.org/sites/default/files/VC_LowVision_Report2015.pdf

Warren, M. (1990). Identification of visual scanning deficits in adults after cerebrovascular accident. *American Journal of Occupational Therapy, 44*(5), 391–399.

Warren, M. (1995). Including occupational therapy in low vision rehabilitation. *American Journal of Occupational Therapy, 49*(9), 857–860.

Watson, G. R. (2001). Low vision in the geriatric population. *Journal of American Geriatrics Society, 49*(3), 317–330.

Watson, G. R., Quillman, R. D., Flax, M., and Gerritsen, B. (1999). The development of low vision therapist certification. *Journal of Visual Impairment and Blindness, 93*, 451–456.

Watson, G. R., Whittaker, S. G., Steciw, M., Baldasare, J., and Miller-Shapper, H. (1995). *Pepper test instruction manual.* Elkins Park, PA: Pennsylvania College of Optometry.

Watson, G. R., Wright, V., Wyse, E., and De l'Aune, W. (2004). A writing assessment for persons with age-related vision loss. *Journal of Visual Impairment and Blindness, 98*(3), 160–167.

World Health Organization. (2016). *International statistical classification of diseases and related health problems 10th revision (ICD-10).* Retrieved from http://apps.who.int/classifications/icd10/browse/2016/en

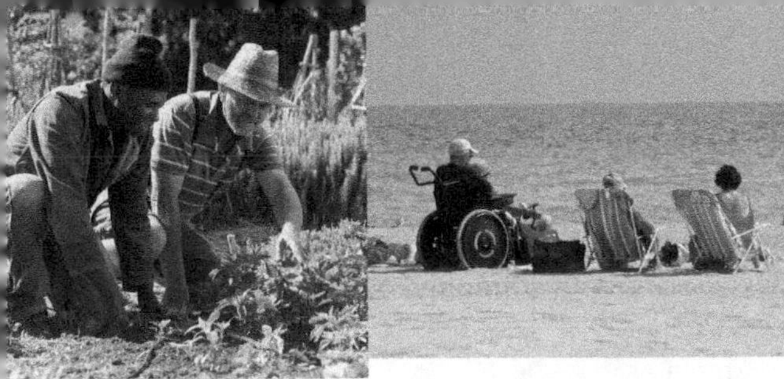
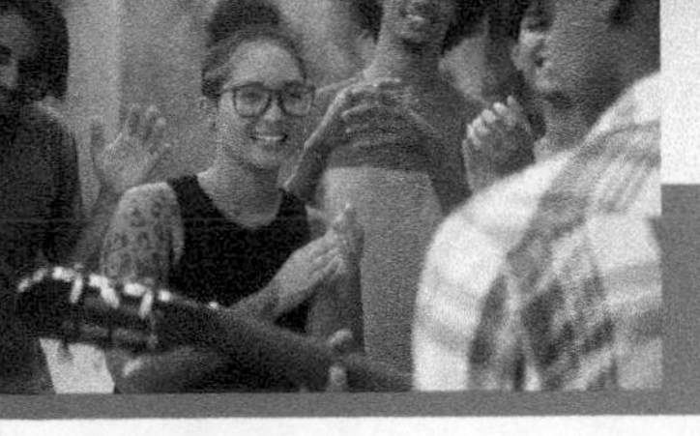

SECTION V

Work and Industry

Chapter 15

Community Ergonomics and Prevention of Work-Related Injuries

Lynne Murphy, EdD, OTR/L, and Peter Bowman, OTD, MHS, OTR/L, OT(C), Dip COT

More than 3.5 million non-fatal injuries and illnesses were recorded in private, state and local government jobs in 2016.

—U.S. Bureau of Labor Statistics, *2017c*

Although injury prevention efforts continue to influence a downward trend in workplace injuries, there is clearly still work to do.

Learning Outcomes

This chapter is designed to enable the reader to:

15-1 Understand the evolution of ergonomics and current terminology.

15-2 Describe the components of the physical demands, cognitive workload, and psychosocial factors inherent in ergonomic assessment.

15-3 Differentiate among common ergonomic interventions in home, recreational, educational, and work settings.

15-4 Apply the seven concepts of universal design.

15-5 Discuss the potential ergonomic risks and controls relevant for work injury prevention and the role of occupational therapy practice.

15-6 Discuss the issues involved in the provision of ergonomic intervention in community settings and the role of occupational therapy practitioners in providing community ergonomic services.

Key Terms

Administrative controls
Cognitive workload
Community ergonomics
Engineering controls
Ergonomic controls
Ergonomics
Physical demands
Psychosocial factors
Universal design
Workplace
Work practice controls

Introduction

The practice of ergonomics in occupational therapy continues to evolve. During entry-level education, occupational therapy practitioners gain foundational skills in the analysis of client factors; an understanding of the principles of biomechanics and ergonomics; and the ability to assess and modify home, work, and community contexts (Accreditation Council for Occupational Therapy Education [ACOTE], 2018). In addition, entry-level education aims to prepare occupational therapy practitioners to enhance safety, health, and well-being in many different occupations and contexts for our clients (ACOTE, 2018). The intent of the chapter is to build on this foundational knowledge and these skills to explore the components of ergonomic principles in the community as they apply to the remediation and prevention of musculoskeletal injuries. Clients for this service may include individuals, groups, agencies, governments, businesses, organizations, and communities. Community ergonomic assessment is specialized, and continued education is required to develop and maintain the expertise required to deliver community-based services.

This chapter defines the term **ergonomics** and provides a brief history and then outlines areas of ergonomic consideration. This is followed by an exploration of occupational therapy's role in community ergonomics in the home, at recreational or public sites, in educational settings, and at the workplace, with consideration of universal design concepts. The chapter concludes with information about work-related practice in injury prevention, ergonomic controls, and ergonomic programs for injured workers.

Ergonomics Terminology and History

Ergonomics is generally understood to be the interaction between a worker and his or her work, undertaken to enhance safety for the worker while optimizing work productivity (Sanders and Wright, 2016). Ergonomics is based on human factors, the body of knowledge about human abilities and limitations that is relevant to performance in a number of environments. However, the field of ergonomics extends beyond the human factors required to complete a task and encompasses the design of tools, machines, systems, and tasks required to complete a job and an understanding of safety in the environments in which the work occurs (Chapanis, 1991; Jacobs, 2008; Sanders and Wright, 2016). Ideally, professionals from different disciplines are included in completing ergonomic assessments and making related recommendations for change to determine whether those changes should be to the worker, work demands, environment, or tools and equipment. These professionals may have education and training in engineering, industrial safety or hygiene, industrial design, psychology, or health and medicine, among others. The role of the occupational therapist is typically to address the risk or presence of musculoskeletal injury to the worker within the relevant context, consider the cognitive and social demands of occupational performance, and make recommendations to prevent or manage these injuries (Jacobs, 2008).

Bernardino Ramazzini, considered to be the father of occupational medicine, was an Italian physician in the early 1700s who had an interest in occupational health. He observed workers primarily in foundries and tanneries and made connections between their work tasks, postures, work behaviors, and the musculoskeletal pain and disorders that they developed (Franco, 1999; Sanders and Wright, 2016).

During the Industrial Revolution (1750–1830), machines and equipment were modernized as manufacturing became both more sophisticated and more efficient. At this stage of industrial development, the primary goal was to increase production, not improve working conditions. Frederick Taylor, a mechanical engineer, pioneered a method called scientific management, used to determine the best method to complete a job and all its component tasks. Known as Taylorism, this became a very popular method to improve worker efficiency. Taylor also addressed the issues of human capabilities and limitations relative to the demands of work (Internet Center for Management and Business Administration, 2010). The current practice of requiring screening tests after job offers was influenced by Taylorism. In 1857, Wojciech Jastrzebowski, a Polish philosopher and scientist, created the term *ergonomics* from the Greek words *ergos,* or work, and *nomos,* meaning law (Ergoweb, 2012).

The Second World War prompted greater interest in human factors and ergonomics. Military equipment, such as aircraft, required redesign to ensure the best fit to the size of the soldiers operating the machine, as well as to ensure that controls were logical and understandable (Ergoweb, 2017; Jacobs, 2008). After the Second World War, the focus of ergonomics expanded to include worker safety and productivity. Professional and research organizations were created to further explore and disseminate information to improve productivity, with a focus on worker safety. Areas of research included muscle forces, low back forces, and cardiovascular requirements for a variety of manual labor tasks. One of the most widely known is a safe lifting calculation developed by the National Institute for Occupational Safety and Health (NIOSH) in 1981, which has been updated, expanded, and revised several times since its inception (Waters, Putz-Anderson, Garg, and Fine, 1993).

In the 1980s and 1990s, federal agencies attempted to mandate ergonomic programs in various workplace settings. The Occupational Safety and Health Administration (OSHA, n.d.d) identified repetition, force, awkward postures, contact stress, and vibration as risk factors that contributed to work-related musculoskeletal disorders. Employers were expected to educate workers about these risks and provide job hazard analysis, reduction, and control for workers who may encounter them in the workplace (Siegel, 2001). In addition, in 1993 NIOSH expanded and revised the lifting standards and recommendations that intended to ensure worker safety (Waters, Putz-Anderson, and Garg, 1994). Although OSHA issued mandated ergonomics rules for all business and industry in 2000, Senate Joint Resolution 6 was passed in 2001, which rescinded the ergonomics rule. Instead, employer-run ergonomics programs were made voluntary, due to the potential employer cost to implement the standards. OSHA and NIOSH continue to provide industry-specific guidelines to the public and to employers to promote worker safety (OSHA, n.d.c; Sanders and Wright, 2016).

As the workplace continues to change, the role of workers and the potential demands on them evolve in many different types of work. Advancements in information and communication technologies, and the rise of virtual interaction between and among humans, have increased the repetitive nature of work conducted through technology. As economies become increasingly global, the field of ergonomics must include the health and safety of more diverse users (Dul et al., 2012). Rather than consideration of only the physical factors of work, the cognitive, psychological, and organizational factors must be considered to prevent work-related injury (International Ergonomics Association [IEA], 2018). Two main strategic directions identified by the IEA for the future of ergonomics include strengthening the demand for ergonomics by communicating with stakeholders (i.e., designers of tools or systems and the decision-makers regarding the systems and personnel) and strengthening the application of ergonomics by promoting education and research of providers of ergonomic services (Dul et al., 2012). Clearly, the field of ergonomics will never be static, and the need for professionals to remain invested in human safety and productivity will continue to change and advance.

Areas of Ergonomic Consideration

When assessing the ergonomic risk of any activity, the primary categories or factors to consider must include motor or physical demands, cognitive workload, and psychosocial factors. The traditional consideration of physical demands alone has not been able to address ergonomic difficulties in a comprehensive way.

Physical Demands

The **physical demands** of an activity may include posture, working position, lifting, materials handling, and considerations related to hand use. These factors are important to consider in intensity, duration, and biomechanical positioning. Generally, using the body to its best advantage, with the ability to move periodically between postures and physical demands, is optimal for both productivity and safety. Joints that are maintained in neutral or mid-range positions will allow both safety and efficiency for the individual and decrease the risk of injury. Rest breaks, variations in tasks and positions, and performing work tasks with variations in the length and intensity of physical demand are generally useful for reducing risk of injury in the workplace (Canadian Center for Occupational Health and Safety [CCOHS], 2018; Cohen, Gjessing, Fine, Bernard, and McGlothlin, 1997).

More specific guidelines have been generated based on anthropometric data, or specific measurements of the human body. There are clearly challenges to this approach due to the variability of human shape and size according to gender, ethnicity, age, and cultural considerations (Baker, 2008). However, this type of data has provided some direction in making recommendations for workstation design to facilitate the appropriate physical demands of work, including horizontal and vertical reach, clearance around workstations, working postures, and strength demands (Baker, 2008; OSHA, n.d.a.; Sanders and Wright, 2016). Widely accepted standards based on human measurements include standing workstations that are above elbow height for precision work, just below elbow height for light work, and several inches below elbow height for heavy work (Baker, 2008; CCOHS, 2018; Cohen et al., 1997).

Prolonged standing has been associated with a number of risks, including back and leg pain, cardiovascular problems, venous insufficiency, fatigue, and other musculoskeletal pain. Potential supports to address these risks includes compression types of hosiery, floor mats, supportive shoes, and shoe inserts. Sit-to-stand workstations, pelvic tilt task-related chairs, and other mechanisms to alter postures have also been used to address the risk associated with prolonged standing. All of these interventions tend to decrease subjective pain, although they do not address all of the negative effects of prolonged standing (Waters and Dick, 2014). The ability to change positions between sitting and standing can increase worker comfort. Examples of alternate postures for sit-to-stand desks are shown in Figure 15-1.

Prolonged sitting is a considerable challenge, especially for those with back injuries, as sitting places more strain on the back than standing (Chaffin, Andersson, and Martin, 1984). In addition, prolonged sitting can have negative effects on cardiac, vascular, and metabolic health and can result in fatigue, muscular aches, and sensory complications (CCOHS, 2016). Although sitting positions increase disc pressure, utilizing a chair that fits the person and the task and that can be easily adjusted from the sitting posture can reduce these negative effects. Ideally, a chair should have adjustability in height, tilt, seat depth, lumbar support and armrests; the seat pan and armrests should have a rounded waterfall edge; and supports such as footrests should be available to ensure optimal human positioning (CCOHS, 2014; OSHA, n.d.a). Tables should have adequate size, clearance, and space for the placement of equipment or supplies that are necessary for the job (OSHA, n.d.b). Computer equipment and accessories should be placed so the person can look directly ahead without awkward positioning of the head or neck and maintain the wrists in a neutral position with elbows at a right angle. When other types of specialized equipment are used for seated work tasks, or when individuals engage in home or recreational activities performed while sitting, the optimal positioning for the individual includes an upright seated posture, with avoidance of prolonged static positioning, and the ability to move periodically.

Whether a person is seated at a computer workstation or engaged in other tool use, OSHA (n.d.d) guidelines have identified the following risk factors for musculoskeletal disorders for any work setting: exerting excessive force in any position, performing repetitive tasks, working in awkward or sustained positions, being exposed to cold temperatures, placing localized pressure on a body part, or

A

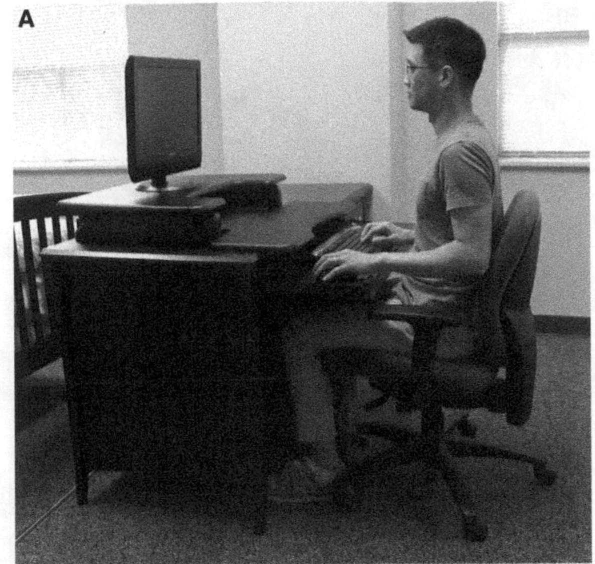

B

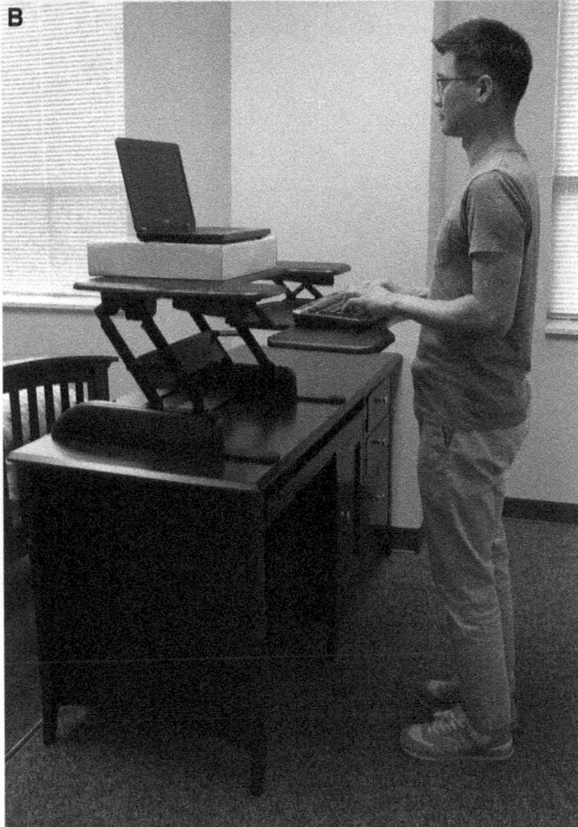

Figure 15-1 A. Sitting posture at sit-to-stand workstation. **B.** Standing posture at sit-to-stand workstation. *(Photos courtesy of Alyssa DeSantis, University Program Associate, College of Allied Health Sciences, East Carolina University.)*

exposing the body or the upper extremity to vibration. When any of these risk factors occur in combination, it increases the risk of musculoskeletal disorders to the individual.

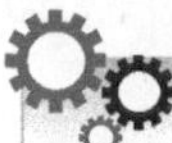

Engage Your Brain 15-1

Consider your sitting habits for computer activities. Are you following these recommendations? If not, what can you do to enhance your safety?

Lifting too much weight or improper positioning during lifting at home, work, and sites of recreation is also associated with risk of injury. The official lifting limitation set by NIOSH for the workplace is 51 pounds in the revised lifting equation, when the conditions of the lift are ideal (Waters et al., 1994). Waters (2007) reports a 35-pound limitation for patient-handling tasks due to the complex nature of manual handling when applied to health-care settings.

Considerations for calculating the recommended lifting limit include the location of the object lifted related to the floor and the handler, the distance the item is moved, the asymmetry angle or twisting requirement, the frequency and duration of lifting, and the ways in which the objects can be held or gripped (Waters et al., 1994). In any situation, when weight exceeds the recommended weight limit (the product of the lifting calculations), assistive devices should be used. Proper lifting technique is clearly important in preventing injury. Good posture should be maintained with the spine held in alignment and while avoiding twisting, and the large muscles of the legs should be used to raise objects from the floor to other levels. The ease with which an object can be grasped and held with the hands must also be considered. Examples of preferred and problematic lifting are shown in Figures 15-2 and 15-3.

Cognitive Workload

While the field of ergonomics has traditionally included assessment of the musculoskeletal risks of activities, the cognitive demands of tasks cannot be underestimated and must also be considered in community ergonomics. Occupational therapy

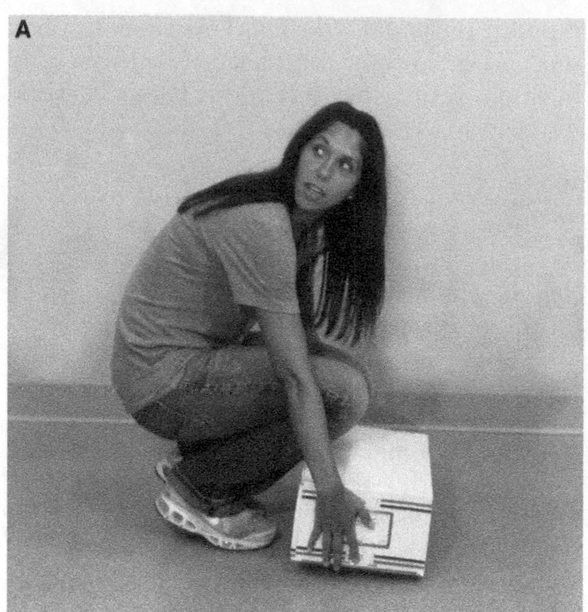

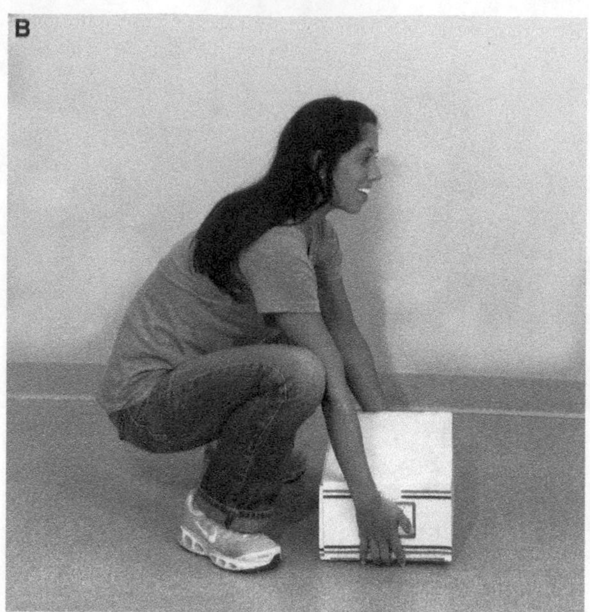

Figure 15-2 A. Poor lift from floor. **B.** Improved lift from floor. *(Photos courtesy of Gary Melancon, Audio Visual Production Manager, College of Health Professions, Information and Educational Technology Team at the Medical University of South Carolina.)*

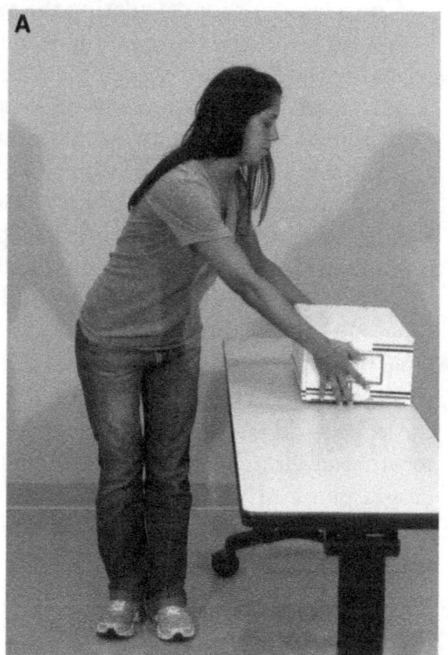

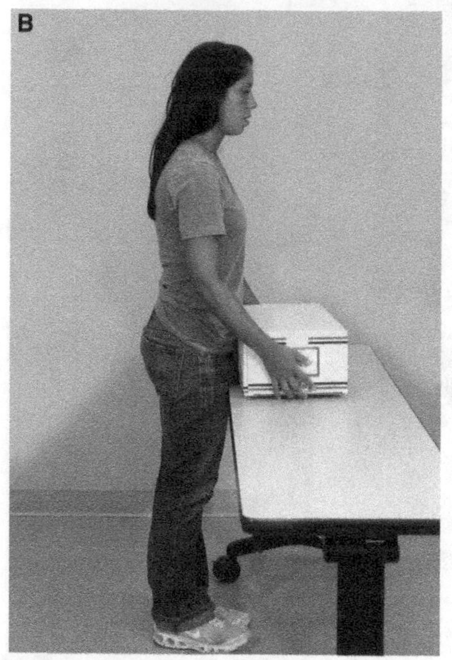

Figure 15-3 A. Poor lift/positioning at workstation. **B.** Improved lift/positioning at workstation. *(Photos courtesy of Gary Melancon, Audio Visual Production Manager, College of Health Professions, Information and Educational Technology Team at the Medical University of South Carolina.)*

practitioners typically consider the cognitive skills of an individual when evaluating occupational performance, which may include factors such as memory, problem-solving, visual information processing, and executive functions, among others. When conducting ergonomic assessments, it becomes necessary to determine the cognitive requirements of a task or activity as it is situated in the workplace, home, or community. Those cognitive demands must be a good fit for the individual performing that activity to ensure the person's sustained health and safety (Shaw and Lysaght, 2008).

The measurement of **cognitive workload** in a workplace setting involves assessing how much mental effort is used to accomplish a task, based on that worker's perception of work performance, work difficulty, and associated psychological stress. Information that may contribute to understanding this stress includes time pressure or how busy the individual appears, the complexity of work tasks and the contribution of technology to this complexity, the attention demands of the task, and the supports or resources available to the worker. If the cognitive demands of work exceed the cognitive abilities of the worker, cognitive overload can occur. Conversely, if the work is routine and automatic, the worker may experience underload. In either case, errors in work performance or incidents that can be harmful to the worker may occur. Therefore, it is important to balance the cognitive task demands and the cognitive skills of the worker for optimal health and work performance. Understanding the cognitive stress of work, and its resulting worker strain, cannot be ignored in a thorough ergonomic analysis (Young, Brookhuis, Wickens, and Hancock, 2015).

When determining the cognitive workload of a job, information can be gathered from a job description, a job observation or on-site analysis, or cognitive task assessments and surveys (Shaw and Lysaght, 2008; Wei and Salvendy, 2003). The U.S. Department of Labor Occupational Information Network (O*NET) offers a comprehensive online source of job descriptions that include not only physical demands but the knowledge, skills, and abilities often categorized as cognitive tasks. When employee or employer job descriptions do not provide details related to cognitive factors, this resource may prove valuable for the practitioner engaged in community ergonomic practice (O*NET, 2017).

Cognitive workload is influenced by intellectual and genetic endowment, learned knowledge, social status, and emotional regulation, as well as social and behavioral factors (Shaw and Lysaght, 2008). These vary from person to person; therefore, the occupational therapy practitioner must assess these factors for each individual in order to maximize full engagement in occupation. To address cognitive workload in all other settings, such as home, education, and leisure pursuits, the same principles of cognitive activity analysis that have been described in the workplace must be applied. Optimizing the fit between the cognitive demands of the activity and the cognitive skills of the individual will increase occupational engagement and decrease the negative influences of cognitive overload or underload that may result in fatigue, stress, errors in performance, or injury. Typical approaches to address a poor fit that are consistent with other areas of occupational therapy practice may include modifying or adapting the cognitive demands of the task or, conversely, establishing or restoring the cognitive skills of the person. From an ergonomic perspective in fitting the demands of the tasks to the individual, the adaptive approach is usually undertaken. In educational settings, accommodations for learning may be explored. In the case of a leisure activity, adaptations may be recommended to the complexity of the task. To ensure a maximum level of achievement in occupations in all community settings, the occupational therapy practitioner needs to observe and measure the actual and perceived client workload; offer strategies that enable the client to eliminate, reduce, or ignore extraneous factors; and move the worker from a negative, overwhelmed state to one of balance and efficiency.

Psychosocial Factors

NIOSH (1997) reports three main categories of **psychosocial factors** that may influence how workers perceive their jobs and that can ultimately have an impact on a worker's physical health. These include factors associated with the work environment, factors associated with the extrawork environment, and personal characteristics. Work environment factors may include interpersonal relationships at work, perceived individual control of the job tasks, the level of interest or engagement in the work tasks, financial or other benefits of the job, and organizational structure as it supports or inhibits the individual. The extrawork environment refers to factors that occur outside of work but may have an impact on the job, such as work-life balance and roles within the family or community. Finally, the individual's personal characteristics that may influence health include personality and disposition, gender, education, cultural factors, and social class (Erez, 2008). Although these categories were initially described by NIOSH, the inclusion of factors outside of the work environment provides a useful framework for the occupational therapist to consider psychosocial factors in the community.

Low levels of job satisfaction, the perception of an intensified workload, and work that is viewed as monotonous have been linked to a variety of work-related musculoskeletal disorders (Erez, 2008). However, the two psychosocial factors that are most consistently linked to poor health symptoms are a lack of job control and poor social supports. Wahlstedt, Norback, Wieslander, Skoglund, and Runeson (2010) found that workers who had a strained or passive work situation, in which they perceived high work demands and low control over their work environment, had an increased incidence of neck, shoulder, and upper-back symptoms. In addition, women exhibited more of these symptoms than their male counterparts in the workforce. Low-back symptoms were found to be statistically more common in workers who had low social supports when this was combined with passive work situations. Finally, health-care workers who identified low job control, effort-reward imbalance, and low social supports demonstrated higher rates of musculoskeletal pain (Bernal et al., 2015). Although it is unclear exactly how psychosocial factors contribute to physical dysfunction, some theories include a resultant increase in muscle tension related to the mental stress, changes in postures and sustained positions related to workload and perceived deadlines, and generalized worry or fatigue (Erez, 2008).

Considerations of psychosocial factors are a part of ergonomic assessments that may be documented through client interviews, observations within the context of occupational performance, or assessments that specifically address the psychosocial factors. Understanding the mental health status of individuals is important to gain the understanding of the physical symptoms that is necessary to client-centered practice.

Engage Your Brain 15-2

Consider a job or activity in your past that you have enjoyed and another that you did not enjoy. How did the cognitive workload and your personal characteristics contribute to your opinions? What questions could you develop to discern this type of information from a client?

Universal Design

The purposeful design of products and environments to promote use by the greatest number of people to the greatest extent possible is called **universal design** (R. L. Mace Universal Design Institute [RLMUDI], 2019b). This concept, although not unique to community ergonomics, is particularly relevant when trying to ensure that people with a wide variety of abilities will be able to access environments and participate in occupations without barriers or the need for retroactive adaptations. As occupational therapy practitioners consider ergonomic factors in a variety of settings, universal design principles become part of the assessment process and can be included in advocacy efforts. The seven principles of universal design (RLMUDI, 2019a), which are the gold standard for ensuring maximum access for all, appear in Table 15-1.

Occupational Therapy Role in Community Ergonomics

Historically, ergonomic considerations and assessments have been conducted in the workplace by practitioners of occupational therapy as well as other professional disciplines. However, occupational performance occurs within a variety of settings, contexts, and occupational roles. Therefore, injury prevention and consideration of the fit between the task and individual should not be limited only to work environments and activities. **Community ergonomics** describes the fit of the person or group to the activities performed in the broader context of

Table 15-1 Principles of Universal Design

Principle	Guidelines
PRINCIPLE ONE: Equitable Use The design is useful and marketable to people with diverse abilities.	1a. Provide the same means of use for all users: identical whenever possible, equivalent when not. 1b. Avoid segregating or stigmatizing any users. 1c. Provisions for privacy, security, and safety should be equally available to all users. 1d. Make the design appealing to all users.
PRINCIPLE TWO: Flexibility in Use The design accommodates a wide range of individual preferences and abilities.	2a. Provide choice in methods of use. 2b. Accommodate right- or left-handed access and use. 2c. Facilitate the user's accuracy and precision. 2d. Provide adaptability to the user's pace.
PRINCIPLE THREE: Simple and Intuitive Use Use of the design is easy to understand, regardless of the user's experience, knowledge, language skills, or current concentration level.	3a. Eliminate unnecessary complexity. 3b. Be consistent with user expectations and intuition. 3c. Accommodate a wide range of literacy and language skills. 3d. Arrange information consistent with its importance. 3e. Provide effective prompting and feedback during and after task completion.
PRINCIPLE FOUR: Perceptible Information The design communicates necessary information effectively to the user, regardless of ambient conditions or the user's sensory abilities.	4a. Use different modes (pictorial, verbal, tactile) for redundant presentation of essential information. 4b. Provide adequate contrast between essential information and its surroundings. 4c. Maximize "legibility" of essential information. 4d. Differentiate elements in ways that can be described (i.e., make it easy to give instructions or directions). 4e. Provide compatibility with a variety of techniques or devices used by people with sensory limitations.
PRINCIPLE FIVE: Tolerance for Error The design minimizes hazards and the adverse consequences of accidental or unintended actions.	5a. Arrange elements to minimize hazards and errors: most used elements, most accessible; hazardous elements eliminated, isolated, or shielded. 5b. Provide warnings of hazards and errors. 5c. Provide fail safe features. 5d. Discourage unconscious action in tasks that require vigilance.
PRINCIPLE SIX: Low Physical Effort The design can be used efficiently and comfortably and with a minimum of fatigue.	6a. Allow user to maintain a neutral body position. 6b. Use reasonable operating forces. 6c. Minimize repetitive actions. 6d. Minimize sustained physical effort.
PRINCIPLE SEVEN: Size and Space for Approach and Use Appropriate size and space is provided for approach, reach, manipulation, and use regardless of user's body size, posture, or mobility.	7a. Provide a clear line of sight to important elements for any seated or standing user. 7b. Make reach to all components comfortable for any seated or standing user. 7c. Accommodate variations in hand and grip size. 7d. Provide adequate space for the use of assistive devices or personal assistance.

Data from *Principles of Universal Design,* by B. R. Connell, M. Jones, R. Mace, J. Mueller, J. Mullick, E. Ostroff, J. Sanford, J. Steinfeld, E. Story, and G. Vanderheiden, 1997, The Principles of Universal Design, Version 2.0, Raleigh, NC: North Carolina State University.

The Principles of Universal Design were conceived and developed by The Center for Universal Design at North Carolina State University. Use or application of the Principles in any form by an individual or organization is separate and distinct from the Principles and does not constitute or imply acceptance or endorsement by The Center for Universal Design of the use or application.

the community, which may include the home, public sites, recreational facilities, and other locations within the community. Ensuring this fit allows that person or group to perform occupations safely and effectively, to prevent injury, and to promote health and well-being.

This view of community ergonomics is consistent with the person-environment-occupation-performance (PEOP) model developed by Baum and Christiansen in 1991 and the subsequent updates of this model, which support the practice and process of occupational therapy. It is a transactional systems model, in which the relationships between the person or population, the environment, and the occupations that are performed should be optimized in order to enhance and support effective occupational performance and well-being (Baum, Christiansen, and Bass, 2015). Factors of the person or population considered in this model include physiological, psychological, neurobehavioral, and cognitive abilities that provide a specific set of skills of the individual or the group of people performing tasks and roles. The environment includes not only the built physical environment but also the social, cultural, and societal environment that may act as a barrier or enabler to the person or group so that they can participate in desired occupations. It is the relationship or fit of the person, environment, and occupation, which interact in order to facilitate the performance and well-being of the person or population (Baum et al., 2015). This model allows the occupational therapy practitioner to frame the ergonomic analysis in considering the skills and abilities of the person, the community environment, and the occupations performed by the person in the environment to optimize safety, health, and well-being. And this view of occupational performance is not limited to the workplace; rather, it should be applied to all of the community environments and occupations in which a person engages.

Occupational therapy community ergonomics involves the analysis of a person's occupational performance in many areas to understand how that individual's abilities can best be matched to the activities in which the person engages. Rather than traditional considerations of the interaction of the work and worker, this view of community ergonomics directs practitioners to consider the interaction of the human and the occupation, to enhance safety and optimize performance, and to expand potential ergonomic interventions to broader contexts. These community interventions may include direct observations of the ergonomic aspects of the client's activities of daily living (ADLs), instrumental activities of daily living (IADLs), education, leisure activities, and work, as well as the contexts in which these occupations are performed. During the initial evaluation of a client, occupational therapists must ascertain the future needs and goals of the client in carrying out ADLs, IADLs, education, work, and leisure activities.

In general, there are two types of community ergonomic practice. One focuses on individual work with clients; the other type addresses program development through consultation with a business, agency, or other entity. The knowledge of and skills in ergonomics necessary to perform either role are similar, however, and rely on the occupational therapist's skills in client assessment, activity and occupation analysis, and clinical reasoning to develop appropriate interventions to achieve desired outcomes.

When working in the community, occupational therapy practitioners must be prepared to work with clients from several types of referring sources and agencies, including but not limited to physicians; workers' compensation and insurance companies; home health agencies; attorneys; individual clients; family members; federal, state, and local government agencies; and manufacturing and industrial companies. Funding sources for community-based ergonomic practice vary tremendously and potentially can include health insurance, fee-for-service, workers' compensation, legal settlements, Medicare, Medicaid, nonprofit organizations, foundations, government agencies, and private agencies.

Community-based practice for the occupational therapist, specifically considering ergonomic interventions, is consistent with the broad outcomes of occupational therapy services identified in *Occupational Therapy Practice Framework: Domain and Process* (American Occupational Therapy Association [AOTA], 2014). These include occupational performance, prevention, health and wellness, quality of life, participation, role competence, and well-being. These outcomes have implications for groups and populations in addition to individuals, according to both occupational therapy practice and community ergonomics. Similarly, interventions identified in the framework (AOTA, 2014) focusing on advocacy and education and training promote the occupational performance of clients, client groups, and populations that is consistent with the goals of community ergonomics practice by occupational therapy practitioners. The collaborative and client-centered nature of community ergonomics empowers individuals and groups to remain or regain safety and productivity in a wide variety of occupations.

Occupational Therapy Applications in Community Ergonomics

When considering how community ergonomics interventions can be designed and implemented for occupations of ADLs, IADLs, education, work, and leisure, it is helpful to discuss each of these in the locations or environments where it typically occurs. Therefore, ergonomics in the home, educational setting, recreational or public settings, and the workplace is undertaken with a focus on the primary occupations that occur in each setting.

PROGRAM SHOWCASE

Although many occupational therapy practitioners begin their practice working in traditional medically based settings, those who become skilled in ergonomics and community-based programs have wider practice opportunities to explore. A consultative approach for individuals, groups, and populations can facilitate injury prevention, health, and well-being before medical care is necessary. To become an independent practitioner, a business model may be useful in establishing a community ergonomic practice. This Program Showcase describes an ergonomic practice established by an occupational therapist.

In an effort to increase her flexibility in work hours and establish a community-based practice in ergonomics, Erin, an occupational therapist, resigned from her job in an industrial rehabilitation facility and began strategic planning for her own business. Based on her experience in performing job analysis, ergonomic consultations, comprehensive assessments, and work-hardening programs for injured workers, she developed a mission statement for a new venture. Her vision was to provide a wide range of consultative ergonomic services in diverse contexts and environments to improve access for all and facilitate health and well-being in the local and regional community.

Strategic planning was the first step. This involved conducting an analysis of the strengths and weaknesses of the business, as well as the opportunities and threats in the community. Some of her strengths included a network of professionals, including engineers, safety managers, vocational evaluators, physical therapists, building contractors, and assistive technology professionals who may be available for contracting. She had space in her home to make an office and some savings to establish the business. Finally, she was able to contract the services of a lawyer to ensure that she was able to set up the business as a limited liability company. Weaknesses of the business included the lack of evaluation space, limited assessment equipment, and initially limited clients. Erin had had little experience in seeking out funding opportunities that were not linked to medical reimbursement models. She would need to learn about alternate funding opportunities, such as grants and governmental resources. External to the ergonomic consulting business were several key opportunities. These included recent efforts in the local government to renovate recreational and common spaces to improve access and boost the economy. In addition, some of the managers of local businesses had expressed an interest in injury prevention-training programs for employees when Erin had facilitated the return of injured workers to those companies. The only threat Erin was able to identify was the availability of online resources that some employers could access without significant cost; she would have to demonstrate the unique skills she brought to these settings that facilitated custom-tailored ergonomic programs.

Based on the strengths, weaknesses, opportunities, and threats (SWOT) analysis, Erin decided to start with two very specific services. Initial contacts were made with employers and managers that she knew to provide an on-site analysis, which would be followed by injury prevention programs that were specific to the setting. She would provide the injury prevention-training programs or produce the materials so that managers could deliver the programs. The second service was to consult with the city council members to provide a review of their community recreation programs and spaces considering the principles of universal design. Each of these services required minimal up-front costs without the need for contracting with other professionals, to maximize the profit margin.

Over time, Erin was able to provide these services and grow the business. She became more well known in the community, purchased additional equipment and marketing materials, and consulted with other professionals for a number of community projects. Some of the projects included collaboration with other professionals to design the common spaces in a senior housing co-op, to design educational spaces for a transportation company in the community, and to consult with local high school administrators to facilitate accommodations for students regarding both physical and psychosocial needs.

Home

All occupations may occur in the home, to varying degrees. Social participation is also relevant in this setting, depending on how many people live together in the home and what social roles each person assumes. Computer and technology use may also be prevalent in the home for social participation, work, education, or leisure tasks. However, the primary areas of ADLs, IADLs, and leisure will be explored in this section related to ergonomic considerations in the home. With the utilization of good biomechanical positioning, occupational therapy practitioners enable clients to be independent in their daily activities and routines while accounting for psychosocial and cognitive factors.

ADLs include basic self-care skills and functional mobility concerns. Storage of items used for basic self-care should be easily accessible and allow for safe lifting and carrying demands. Furniture should allow safe and comfortable sitting postures and room to move freely throughout the space. Safe and appropriate use of stairs and bathtubs can be adapted with grab bars, elevated toilet seats, ramps, and other modifications as needed to match the physical needs of the user. Occupational therapists are skilled in home assessments and can make recommendations for safe access to ADL supplies and materials. When significant modifications to the home are needed to match the person's skills and abilities, contractors and/or architects may be consulted. Ideally, a partnership with these professionals can allow the occupational therapist to advocate for client needs, while the construction professionals are well versed in what is possible given the physical layout and constraints of the home.

IADLs are unique to the environments in which they occur and the responsibilities assumed by the individual within social and cultural contexts. Ergonomic considerations are relevant in the IADL of cooking. This may include the positioning of kitchen equipment, food storage, and basic items used for cooking. The use of electrical kitchen devices, such as can openers and carving knives, can decrease stress on joints in the hands and wrists. Knives with large and/or ergonomically shaped handles and protective blade guards are very useful. Food processors can be used to reduce the pressure on hands for intensive chopping, shredding, slicing, and dicing. Universally designed kitchen implements that have large cushioned handles to minimize the strain on the hands may be used for preparing foods. Keeping frequently used items within easy reach and avoiding heavy lifting are commonly accepted principles. Simple hints—for instance, sliding heavy pots and pans along the kitchen counter surface—can reduce lifting. Successful transfers of tools and food from one surface to another are an obvious practical concern for many occupational therapy clients to avoid slips and falls.

Home management tasks, such as cleaning inside the home or yard and outdoor maintenance, should be considered related to the use of tools and equipment available to the client. For example, the weight of vacuum cleaners may be influenced by client strength. Snow shovels with bent handles may support lifting and carrying movements that are safe for the user, and gardening equipment may be designed to support the upper extremity in neutral postures. It is incumbent on the occupational therapist to assess the client's needs and activities performed in the home to determine the best fit for the client's physical abilities.

Some leisure activities are performed in and around the home, with sewing, crafting, playing video games, recreational computer use, gardening, and musical pursuits as examples. Two primary areas for the occupational therapy practitioner to address are the sustained amounts of time in which individuals engage in the activity, as well as the postures they assume to perform them. Crafting and sewing, for example, are often performed at tables or desks, and participants may be positioned with seated, flexed postures, exposing them to the risk factors of sustained grasp and awkward positions of the hands, arms, and shoulders. These positions may contribute to pain and musculoskeletal dysfunction in the hands, arms, shoulders, neck, and back. Adaptations such as tilt tables or adjustable work chairs may improve positioning and reduce discomfort and ergonomic risks. Education in improved body positioning, regular breaks and stretching, and joint protection may also have a positive effect. Adaptive tools, such as rotary or spring-loaded scissors for quilters, ergonomic gardening tools, or built-up-handle crochet hooks, are more routinely available for leisure pursuits and may also reduce the risk of pain and injury (Baxter, 2008).

Cognitive and psychosocial factors that are relevant in the home for ADLs and IADLs often include the person's ability to adapt routines and to control when and how activities are performed. If a person has suffered an illness or injury that necessitates a different way of accomplishing an ADL or IADL, the occupational therapist is skilled in making these adaptations. As a person ages, adaptations for cognitive and/or physical changes may also allow a person to remain safe, productive, and efficient in ADLs and IADLs. Assistive technologies are available that may address either the cognitive or physical changes that can occur as individuals remain in their homes after their skills and abilities change.

Recreation and Public Sites

Recreational and public IADL activities may include spiritual or religious pursuits, meeting with others in community settings, and shopping, which is still often performed outside of the home even with the increasing trend of shopping online. Some of the concerns associated with access to these activities are addressed from the perspective of universal design. Community access is also addressed through the Americans With Disabilities Act regarding access to public buildings and services. This legislation supports engagement in leisure pursuits, such as being a spectator at community sporting, performing arts, or cultural events. Ergonomics in the community is often about safe access for all, regardless of physical ability, social class, ethnicity, or need for assistive devices. Many sports and recreational activities can be adapted to allow full participation. Because occupational justice is a desirable outcome of occupational therapy interventions (AOTA, 2014), occupational therapists should advocate for clients' abilities to fully integrate in every environment in their communities, including recreation sites.

Community playgrounds promote opportunities for physical, social, and emotional growth in children. While many are being designed to be accessible to children with disabilities, this does not make them usable by all. For example, some accessibility features remove children with mobility impairments from their freely mobile peers and limit their ability to feel included and social with other children by offering them separate accessible features (Ripat and Becker, 2012). The occupational therapist may help children and their families to utilize the features of the playground with biomechanics in mind; however, the psychosocial factors of social interaction with peers and emotional engagement in the activities should be considered. When occupational therapy practitioners discover community locations designed for leisure and recreation to be lacking access, inclusion, and adaptability, advocacy within the community should be considered an opportunity to take action.

Engage Your Brain 15-3

Think of a space in your community that is identified as common or public access. What principles of universal design could improve the design of these spaces? What ergonomic changes could make the space more usable by individuals with differing abilities?

Education

Initially, the focus of ergonomics in schools was on anthropometric data about students at different ages and stages of development, since students spend the majority of their school day seated in chairs, at desks, or at tables. A mismatch of student fit to the seated workspace results in musculoskeletal discomfort in many students (Erez, Shenkar, Jacobs, and Gillespie, 2008). Initiatives have followed in many schools to provide classroom furniture that is ergonomically designed and to incorporate different sizes of furniture into classrooms to allow a better fit among varied-sized children in the same grade. Since children and youth also spend time every day at a computer in both home and school environments, the design of computer labs in schools has improved to address proper seated and computer positioning.

A focus on backpack weight followed, as improper wear or carrying heavy weights can negatively affect posture, balance, and spinal alignment and result in back and shoulder pain. Initiatives by the professional organizations of occupational therapists, physical therapists, and pediatricians have attempted to educate children and families to reduce the backpack load and wear backpacks correctly (Erez et al., 2008).

The next influence of ergonomics in schools affected the learning environment. Cognitive and psychosocial factors were considered in pedagogy, timing and duration of learning activities, and school policies (Legg and Jacobs, 2008). Research followed to understand how educational ergonomics influence student learning. The changes to the physical design of learning environments that support cooperative or collaborative learning, physical and emotional student health and well-being, and school-community integration have all been associated with student academic success (Smith, 2012). This supports how ergonomic considerations in the community should focus not only on the physical demands but also on the cognitive and psychosocial factors of ergonomics.

Workplace

A **workplace** can be any number of environments in which work activities occur, including both paid and volunteer endeavors. These workplace settings are as varied as the work that is conducted. Common to most workplace settings, however, is the ergonomic focus on the physical demands of the job. A primary goal in the workplace is matching the capabilities of the person to work demands through the understanding and use of occupational biomechanics to decrease the risks to the worker of musculoskeletal dysfunction. Additionally, an understanding of the cognitive workload and psychosocial factors should be included in workplace ergonomics to ensure that the occupational therapy practitioner is utilizing a client-centered and comprehensive approach to worker safety and productivity.

A variety of occupational therapy interventions are appropriate for workplace ergonomics in the community. Those focused on an individual client may include jobsite observation and analysis, identification of ergonomic risk factors, education and training in injury prevention or management of prior injuries, and the development of recommendations for workplace changes to enhance worker safety. These interventions are often conducted following a model of participatory ergonomics involving collaboration with the worker and administrative personnel at the worksite. This promotes solutions that are reasonable for both the employer and employee. Occupational therapy interventions focused on groups often include consultation with employers to identify comprehensive ergonomic risk factors, to develop programs to promote injury prevention, and, potentially, to implement education and training programs for groups of employees. Finally, occupational therapy practitioners often work with individual clients who have been injured on the job in clinical settings to evaluate and possibly remediate function related to work demands, identify ergonomic risk factors in all occupational roles, and collaboratively develop solutions to reduce those risk factors. When conducted in outpatient settings, interventions provided to an injured worker may include functional capacity evaluations and work-conditioning and/or work-hardening programs. These are typically conducted with the goal of facilitating a return to work or assisting with the development of other vocational goals.

Occupational Risks and Injury Prevention

A review of injury statistics can assist in recognizing where both prevention and rehabilitation efforts have been successful and where continued efforts still need to be targeted. The U.S. Department of Labor's Bureau of Labor Statistics (BLS, 2017b) reports that the 2016 injury rate was 2.9 per 100 full-time workers, a decrease from 3.7 per 100 in 2009 and 5 per 100 in 2003. The total number of incidents requiring days away from work decreased from 1,238,490 in 2009 to 892,270 in 2016 (BLS, 2017b). One way to determine the severity of injury or illness, median days away from work, has remained unchanged. Median days away from work has held steady at 8 days from 2008 to 2016 (BLS, 2017b).

Positive findings are noted in the decreasing injury and incident rates over time. In 2016, however, workers with carpal tunnel syndrome (CTS) reportedly missed a median of 25 days of work, and workers with tendonitis missed a median of 16 days of work, both higher than the average of 8 days (BLS, 2017a). In addition, workers reporting strains, sprains, and tears had the highest incidence rate of any nonfatal injury type, at 36.3 per 10,000 workers (BLS, 2017a). All of these injury types have the potential to be reduced through effective ergonomic programs. Occupational therapy practitioners continue to be valuable members of interprofessional teams to improve workstation design to decrease these incidents.

It is useful to understand in what industries injuries are occurring to target ergonomic interventions and injury prevention programs to these workers. In private industry for 2016, workers in health care and social assistance had the highest number of reported occupational injuries (552,600), followed by workers in manufacturing (410,500) and retail workers (386,700). These three industries combined to have about half of all the injuries reported in the private sector (BLS, 2017a). See Table 15-2 for additional data. Higher incidence rates (injuries per 100 workers) were noted in agriculture, forestry, fishing, and hunting (6.1 per 100 workers) and transportation and warehousing (4.6 per 100 workers; BLS, 2017a). Understanding both the type of work and the types of injuries in each category can assist the ergonomic professionals in developing the most effective and relevant ergonomics programs for work injury prevention. When employers are able to identify high-risk jobs and are willing to address ergonomic considerations proactively, injury can be prevented for the larger workforce, and insurance and disability costs may be reduced.

NIOSH has developed a Total Worker Health program to guide participatory ergonomics programs and promote worker safety (Lee et al., 2016). The primary directions of this document include establishing an organizational leadership commitment, designing work to promote worker safety and well-being, engaging workers in the design and implementation of the program, and integrating systems to advance worker well-being. Included in the guidelines for workplace assessment is a focus on the social determinants of health, which include many of the cognitive and psychosocial factors often considered in community ergonomics. Collaboration with other health and ergonomic professionals is encouraged (Lee et al., 2016). These types of initiatives provide an excellent opportunity for occupational therapy practitioners to become involved in injury

Table 15-2 Distribution of Nonfatal Occupational Injuries by Private Industry, 2016

Industry Type	Number of Cases in Thousands
Health care and social assistance	552.6
Manufacturing	410.5
Retail trade	386.7
Accommodation and food services	272.3
Transportation and warehousing	202.2
Construction	197.7
Wholesale trade	152.7
Administrative and waste services	113.8
Other services (except public administration)	70.9
Professional and technical services	67.8
Arts, entertainment, and recreation	55.6
Agriculture, forestry, fishing, and hunting	54.2
Real estate and rental and leasing	49.0
Educational services	35.6

Data from *Chart 2: Distribution of Nonfatal Occupational Injuries and Illnesses by Private Industry Sector, 2016*, by U.S. Bureau of Labor Statistics, Table Summary 2, 2017.

prevention programs in collaboration with workers and employers and in developing and implementing education and training programs at various levels within an organization. The occupational therapy practitioner brings the knowledge of biomechanical principles, extensive occupational analysis skills, and a client-centered focus to this interprofessional team.

Types of educational programs for workers that utilize the occupational therapy practitioner's expertise include appropriate working postures and joint positions, arrangement of the workspace for human safety, avoidance of injury risk factors, use of breaks or stretching during work breaks, moving between work positions, and optimal materials-handling processes. In addition, occupational therapy practitioners are able to identify work tools or tasks that may put the workforce at risk and discuss recommendations for alternate tools or equipment with managers or leaders within an organization. Finding or developing those tools is an opportunity for collaboration with engineers or professionals within the industry who have expertise in the functions of the tools used on the job. Not all existing tools that are labeled as ergonomic are in fact useful in preventing injury in specific settings; assessment of the worker using these tools is essential for success.

Types of Ergonomic Controls

Ergonomic solutions that are designed to facilitate the fit between the worker's capabilities and the demands of the job, ultimately improving worker health, can be categorized according to whether they change the dimensions of the job, the way that job tasks are administered, or the way in which the worker performs the job. These **ergonomic controls** are known, respectively, as engineering controls, administrative controls, or work practice controls (OSHA, n.d.e; Sanders and Wright, 2016).

Engineering Controls

The design of tools and equipment, the workstation, the workstation layout, materials handling tools, or mechanical lifts and other changes to the design of a job are considered **engineering controls.** Implementing these physical changes to a job is promoted by OSHA (n.d.e) as the most effective means to eliminate hazards in the workplace and facilitate worker safety. An example of administrative controls includes a nurse using a mechanical lift to move patients who are unable to safely transfer on their own. Similarly, installing a sit-to-stand desk to vary working positions for a worker who spends much of the workday utilizing a computer reduces the risk of repetitive strain injuries. The use of a pneumatic tool with a handle that can move between horizontal or vertical orientation according to the position of the work task for neutral joint positioning also reduces the risk of musculoskeletal dysfunction. Although these are considered most effective in ensuring worker safety, they have the potential to be costly and may require significant changes to the worksite. This solution is often selected by an employer when making changes for multiple workers or groups; however, if changes are necessitated for individual workers, the cost and ease of implementation could make engineering controls more problematic to institute.

Administrative Controls

Management approaches to work processes are classified as **administrative controls.** This requires a focus not just on productivity but on ensuring worker safety. Some examples of administrative controls may include scheduling the rotation of workers between job tasks, giving workers a larger variety of tasks to complete to avoid sustained postures or repetition, implementing regular rest breaks, or monitoring symptoms for all employees. Implementing requirements for two-person lifting or regularly and routinely maintaining equipment used by workers are also types of administrative controls. These are recommended by OSHA (n.d.e) when engineering controls are not possible or not effective to manage risk alone.

Work Practice Controls

The worker is responsible for implementing **work practice controls,** which are methods of carrying out the work by the individual. Some examples of work practice controls include performing proper lifting techniques according to sound biomechanics, consistently using personal protective equipment when it is warranted, performing regular stretches during breaks, or wearing antivibration gloves when using power tools. If a worker feels pressure to complete a task quickly or becomes complacent in a hazardous job and does not follow these procedures, injury prevention may be difficult. Both administrative and work practice controls rely on human adherence to procedures and therefore are not as reliable as engineering controls. However, the cost of work practice controls is typically less than engineering controls and can be effective if consistently used. It is up to the occupational therapist and ergonomic team to determine which approach or combination of these approaches will most effectively ensure the best fit between worker capabilities and work tasks.

Engage Your Brain 15-4

What barriers might the occupational therapy practitioner need to overcome to engage in jobsite analysis or implementing an on-site ergonomic program? Why might an employer be hesitant to bring in a consultant to engage in these assessments?

Ergonomic Programs for Injured Workers

So far, the discussion of work-related ergonomic practice has focused on the prevention of injury and disability. However, health professionals often provide evaluation and intervention services to people who have been injured at work. Following diagnosis and medical management, injured workers may participate in rehabilitation programs that are designed to facilitate the return to work process when possible.

Client Evaluation

The accurate assessment of the client's functional abilities is critical to support decision-making about returning to work. First in this process for the occupational therapist is to create the client's occupational profile (AOTA, 2014). Consideration should be given to all areas of occupation as well as the physical, cognitive, and psychosocial factors that may support or inhibit a return to work. In the evaluation process, attention should be given to the body functions and structures and the client factors that were affected by the injury necessitating the referral to occupational therapy, as they are needed for occupational and job performance.

In addition to the assessments typically used to determine physical, cognitive, and psychosocial abilities and limitations, the evaluation of the injured worker must include gathering data about the job demands and measuring the injured worker's abilities in those areas. The job demands that may need to be considered include materials handling, such as lifting, carrying, pushing, or pulling; sustained standing, sitting, or walking; and cardiorespiratory and muscular endurance. Finally, activities to simulate work activities may be included in the evaluation process to gain a better ability to predict work performance in context. This often takes the form of a functional capacity evaluation. A variety of commercially available systems provide functional capacity evaluations systems, including the Blankenship System Functional Capacity Evaluation©, Ergo Science Physical Work Performance Evaluation©, ERGOS Work Simulator©, Isernhagen Functional Capacity Assessment©, LIDO WorkSET Work Simulator©, and Matheson Work Capacity Evaluation©, among others. Several ergonomic assessment tools are also available that may contribute to the decision-making process of the client, the occupational therapist, and the interprofessional ergonomic team. These include, but are not limited to, the Rapid Upper Limb Assessment (RULA), Rapid Entire Body Assessment (REBA), Strain Index (SI), Occupational Repetitive Actions Index (OCRA), and the Cumulative Trauma Disorders (CTD) Risk Index. It is incumbent on the practitioner to determine which assessment tools best meet the client and team needs.

Jobsite Assessment

Job demands must be explored to set appropriate goals and to make return to work decisions. This information can be gathered from several sources. Clients may describe their physical job duties, work environment considerations, cognitive workload, and psychosocial factors. Employers may provide job descriptions and similar information. The O*NET database can be used as a starting point to review with the injured worker. Finally, the occupational therapy practitioner can visit the jobsite to measure the physical duties of the job and observe the work environment. Pertinent data may include the layout and dimensions of the workspace(s), seating, equipment and controls for that equipment, climate, lighting, noise, potential risks, and safeguards in place for worker safety. The potential physical demands include standing, walking, sitting, lifting, carrying, pushing, pulling, climbing, balancing, stooping, crouching, kneeling, twisting, turning, crawling, handling/manipulating, and reaching to a variety of heights. Task factors include the required postures, required mobility, frequency of activity, duration of activity, workload, work/rest pattern, range-of-motion requirements, and force requirements. The perceptual requirements may include vision, sensation, audition, balance, smell, and taste. The cognitive demands may include information processing, decision-making, maintaining or enhancing knowledge and skills, inductive or deductive reasoning, comprehension and expression, and attention.

Work-Related Intervention

When a determination is made that an individual is not currently able to meet job demands but has the potential to return to work, the occupational therapy practitioner can plan and implement several interventions in collaboration with the injured worker, which are functionally based, rather than medically based.

Work hardening and work conditioning are typically based in outpatient settings, with the goal of increasing the muscular strength and cardiovascular endurance required for work. Work hardening builds on the strength and conditioning components of work conditioning by adding job simulations and work tasks that are required for the job, which are based on careful occupational analysis. Work-hardening programs require the injured worker to attend for 6 to 8 hours a day in order to build endurance for specific job skills. There is strong evidence that workers who have been out of work for less than 12 weeks due to a musculoskeletal disorder have reduced pain and an increased likelihood of returning to work when participating in appropriate exercise, resistive training, and therapy that promotes reengagement in daily activities (AOTA, n.d.)

Some employers are able to provide work-hardening programs that are situated in the workplace (Fig. 15-4). These often include rehabilitation services combined with modified work demands, such as light duty or altered materials-handling demands. Some employers are able to offer alternate job placements in order to return the injured worker to employment, although job tasks will be different to accommodate for activity restrictions or limitations. Ergonomic consultations can be conducted on-site and changes implemented in combinations of engineering, administrative, and work practice controls as appropriate. Hoosain, de Klerk, and Burger (2018) determined that while exercise programs were typically best at reducing symptoms, the implementation of ergonomic controls, ergonomic training, and workstation adjustments generally facilitated a return to work for people with upper-limb conditions. While methods such as case management and work hardening appear to have positive effects, research on these outcomes is limited. However, on-site work rehabilitation programs, when coordinated among the worker, supervisor, and on-site health and safety professionals, have been shown to decrease work absenteeism and increase productivity (AOTA, n.d.).

According to Basich, Driscoll, and Wickstrom (2007), the transitional model of return to work has significant advantages over the traditional medical or clinical model of return to work programs. This job-specific intervention approach increases the worker's functional capacities, teaches safe work methods to prevent reinjury, and provides and modifies job accommodations as needed. Services are provided at the jobsite instead of in medical facilities. The transitional return to work model involves a job analysis and thorough evaluation of the worker. Job tasks are then assigned based on what the worker is capable of performing safely and productively. Safe performance means that the work will not cause reinjury, so work activities are assessed in light of the specific injury. Productive work duties are those that contribute to the needs of the employer and the purpose of the job position. Some job tasks are also therapeutic and may improve strength, endurance, and flexibility. Identification of the job tasks that the worker is not capable of performing is also important. This information can be used to guide intervention planning. An effective intervention usually consists of three elements: therapy services provided at the jobsite, participation in

Work Hardening Program Example: Job: Bridge Tender for Railroad Co.

Target Heart Rate:______/______ BP:______/______

5 minutes	Debrief with therapist/pain sheet
15 minutes	Warm up stretches
20 minutes	Bike at 2.5–3.0 mph (5 minute intervals)
20 minutes	Arm bike: switching direction every 60 seconds
60 minutes	Repetitive lifting: 1. Squat lift 40 lb from the floor, carry 25 feet to OH height, then carry back 1 x 60 seconds for 20 minutes 2. 5 minutes standing: push/pull BTE lever with 200 lb of force with both hands x 10, then 140 lb of force 1 x 5 seconds for 5 minutes 3. Squat lift 50 lb from the floor, carry 25 feet to waist height then carry back 1 x 60 seconds for 20 minutes 4. 3 minutes kneeling push/pull BTE lever with 120 lb of force directly in front of him, like cranking a jack. 5. Climb stairs carrying 40 lb, repeat x 10 once each minute switching hands
10 minutes	Break
10 minutes	Lifting assessment: 1. Floor–OH 40 lb x 2 2. Floor–W 50 lb x 2 3. B-B carry 50 lb x 2 4. Swing 16 lb sledge hammer x 15, rest 1 minute and repeat.
60 minutes	Treadmill at 3.5 mph Reassess grip strength: R _____ _____ _____ _____ _____ L _____ _____ _____ _____ _____
20 minutes	BTE ladder pull/push: Resistance 350 in lb standing 1 minute in each direction. Use a small block to put one foot on while standing
20 minutes	Brick shelving unit. Place 15 lb object from the Floor–Waist–Shoulder–Overhead (all positions) within one minute. Repeat for 20 minutes.
30 minutes	Lunch
15 minutes	Warm up stretches
15 minutes	Crawl under 4-foot high structure, begin threading chain with rope at eye level for 10 minutes (squatting/kneeling/sitting on heels), every 2 minutes, lift and hold 5 lb object at eye level for 10 seconds x 2, climb out and perform 2 back extensions. Lift and carry 15 lb tools up/down 3 flights of stairs.
20 minutes	Squat lift 40 lb from the floor, carry 25 feet to OH height then carry back 1 x 60 seconds for 20 minutes
20 minutes	Seated ladder pull with 350 lb 1 minute in each direction (place one foot on 6" block)
10 minutes	Break
20 minutes	Push/Pull sled with 120 lb force for 10 feet 1 x 60 seconds
30 minutes	Squat lift 50 lb from the floor, carry 25 feet to waist then carry back 1 x 60 seconds for 20 minutes. Then perform BTE seated with right hand 120 lb 1 x 5 seconds for 5 minutes, then repeat with left hand.
15 minutes	Standing: Push/Pull BTE lever with 200 lb of force with both hands x 10
20 minutes	Multi assembly working from floor to overhead.
20 minutes	P/P sled with 120 lb force 1 x 60 seconds
10 minutes	Standing: P/P BTE lever with 200 lb of force (position 4) with both hands x 10, then 140 lb (560 in lb on pos. 4) of force 1 x 5 seconds for 2 minutes. Then kneeling P/P BTE lever with 120 lb of force directly in front of him, like cranking a jack for 3 minutes. Then performing light hand activity on bus bench at floor level for 5 minutes (kneeling/squatting/sitting on his heels)
15 minutes	Cooldown stretches/pain sheet BP:______/______

Figure 15-4 Sample work-hardening plan. *(From* Adult Physical Conditions: Intervention Strategies for Occupational Therapy Assistants, *by Amy J. Mahle and Amber L. Ward, 2019, Philadelphia, PA: F. A. Davis, Philadelphia.)*

work tasks that have therapeutic benefit, and job accommodations.

Generally, returning to the job should be done as soon as possible for the injured worker. After 12 weeks of disability, only 50% of workers return to the job; after 1 year of disability, 85% do not return to work (Basich et al., 2007). Ergonomic intervention and worksite accommodations make it possible for a worker to return to the job sooner and be productive.

Program Development and Business Consultation

As noted earlier in this chapter, community ergonomic practice is situated in the community. It can include interventions with individuals and consultations with groups, agencies, governments, businesses, organizations, and communities. Whereas occupational therapy ergonomic practice often focuses on the individual worker, growing numbers of practitioners are using this expertise to provide services at the community level. Examples include providing ergonomic consultative services at a university (Scaffa et al., 2010) and for an engineering firm (Goodman et al., 2005). Knowledge of the specific mission and needs of a community business (or other institution) is needed to develop these programs, as well as current and sufficient expertise in ergonomics. In fact, workers who are able to remain at work when discomfort has been identified have decreased days off from work and decreased pain intensity and prevalence when consultation or participatory ergonomic programs are implemented on the job (AOTA, n.d.). It is crucial for occupational therapy practitioners to develop programs that are mutually beneficial to the business, its employees, and relevant community groups.

Summary

- The industrialization of work and the scientists who studied work productivity contributed to the development of ergonomics, the interaction between workers and their work demands, within the environments in which the work is conducted to enhance both productivity and worker safety.
- An ergonomic assessment must include considerations of the physical demands, cognitive workload, and psychosocial factors involved in task completion. Physical demands include intensity and duration of the body positions, hand use, and strength demands. Cognitive workload refers to the fit between the cognitive skills of the person and cognitive task factors such as sustained attention, engagement in the task, and perceived difficulty of the task. Psychosocial factors include control and relationships in the work environment, family and community roles, and personal characteristics.
- Community ergonomics includes analysis of ADLs, IADLs, and leisure activities in the home; access and impact of universal design in public and recreational sites; seating and appropriate equipment in schools, consideration of cognitive and psychosocial factors in learning environments, and ergonomic risk and remediation in workplace settings.
- Principles of universal design, when applied to community ergonomics, can ensure appropriate access to spaces and safe and effective design of products for all individuals, regardless of individual abilities and limitations. These principles include equitable use, flexibility in use, simple and intuitive use, perceptible information, tolerance for error, low physical effort, and size and space for approach and use.
- Although workplace injury rates are gradually declining, injury prevention remains a concern of occupational therapy practice in workplace ergonomics. This includes working with both employers and employees to implement engineering, administrative, and work practice controls. This addresses changes to work tools or equipment, improving the management of work tasks, and ensuring that workers optimize their health and safety in the ways they perform work tasks. Occupational therapy practitioners utilize client assessments focused on work performance, as well as jobsite analysis, to recommend specialized rehabilitation programs or ergonomic changes to facilitate the safe return to work of injured workers.
- Using an ergonomic perspective to analyze community settings that include homes,

public areas, and educational and workplace settings allows these practitioners to facilitate changes to the people, environments, and tasks in the community to promote health and safety. When practicing within a community, the skilled occupational therapy practitioner can utilize this ergonomic approach to promote the well-being of individuals, groups, and populations.

CASE STUDIES

CASE STUDY 15-1 Mary

Mary, a 58-year-old woman, is an executive administrative assistant at a large corporation. Her job duties require sustained computer use, and she is often given work to do by several different people, with short deadlines. She is currently using a traditional desktop computer workstation in a common area of a large office. She is married and shares the responsibilities of maintaining her home with her husband, who also works full-time. Her adult children live nearby, and she enjoys spending time with her grandchildren, who range from infancy to age 8. Mary enjoys knitting, playing the piano, and walking her two small dogs. Socializing with a small friend group and keeping up with her family over social media rounds out her leisure time.

Over time, Mary has noticed weakness and paresthesia in the median nerve distribution of her dominant right hand and reports generalized hand and wrist pain. She was recently evaluated by a hand specialist, who made the diagnosis of carpal tunnel syndrome (CTS). The physician recommended conservative treatment first, so a cortisone shot was administered, and she has been referred to outpatient occupational therapy, in a facility that often works with people who are being supported by worker's compensation.

June, the occupational therapist, has initiated the evaluation process. This has included the development of an occupational profile and a hand evaluation. Active and passive range of motion are normal throughout both upper extremities. Grip and pinch tests are below average in the right hand but within average ranges in the left hand. Tinel's test is positive in the right hand. The use of Semmes-Weinstein monofilaments has identified diminished light touch in the index and middle fingertips. Performance on both the blocks and box test and the Purdue Pegboard have identified bilateral dexterity to be within average ranges, although the right hand performance is decreased when compared to the left hand. Volumetric tests have identified no significant differences in volume or edema of the right hand compared to the left or in changes between pretesting and posttesting during the hand evaluation. Initial intervention has included a thermoplastic wrist cock-up splint for night use and an elastic support for the right wrist during daytime wear. Although Mary reports that these are helping, she also feels restricted when wearing the splints and does not like the way the splint looks while she is at work. She is continuing to work full-time.

Discussion Questions

1. What other assessments would be relevant and important to perform in light of the many activities that Mary performs both at work and in the community? What barriers might exist to conducting these assessments?
2. What ergonomic risk factors is Mary currently exposed to at work, at home, and in the community? What recommendations could prevent worsening injury in each of these settings?
3. How do cognitive and psychosocial factors influence the consideration of this case and the development of interventions for Mary?
4. Consider the AOTA (2015) Occupational Therapy Code of Ethics. Which principles would apply to Mary's situation and the services you plan on providing?

CASE STUDY 15-2 Job Analysis

A clothing manufacturer has noted rising numbers of missed days from work and associated workers' compensation costs. The managers are very motivated to make changes to decrease these problems. They contact you to act as a consultant to give them an assessment of the workplace, make recommendations for change, and possibly provide education for the workers regarding injury prevention. However, they are concerned about the type of information that you might give their workers. They ask you not to discuss specific conditions or possible mechanisms of injury because they are concerned this will give workers the ability to "fake new injuries," miss days of work, or file new workers' compensation claims.

Your first step is to analyze the worksite. A manager takes you through the plant and describes the jobs. The primary products of this manufacturer are jackets, raincoats, and trench coats. Along the way, he asks workers to briefly stop and explain their jobs to you. There are several key job classifications. The majority of workers are using sewing machines to repeatedly perform a small set of motions to complete only one part of a jacket or coat. Other workers then bundle these pieces and carry them to another station for final assembly. Finally, the completed jackets or coats are taken to an inventory room, where they are sorted, packed, and shipped. You learn that all of the workers belong to a union, and they are paid according to the amount of items they sew or produce, or piecework. Because of the repetition of the small sets of skills, you notice that workers are moving very quickly and are using repetitive motions.

After the tour, you ask the manager what types of injuries are prevalent and what efforts have already been made to reduce injuries. The sewing-machine operators typically have experienced various types of repetitive strain injuries. The workers who bundle and transport materials, as well as the shippers, tend to have more back and shoulder injuries. Management has considered job rotation in the past, in which the sewing machine operators change to different workstations or sew different parts of the jackets to change the motions used, but the union has been resistant to this idea, stating that it would slow the workers down and reduce their pay, since they are paid according to piecework. You ask if there has even been consideration of a different pay structure and are told that management is concerned about slowing production.

Discussion Questions

1. How will you measure the job demands, considering the physical demands, cognitive workload, and psychosocial factors?
2. Apply the PEOP model to this worksite. How could you improve the fit among the people, the environment, and the occupation to facilitate optimal occupational performance?
3. What recommendations could you make regarding ergonomic controls? Consider engineering, administrative, and work practice controls.
4. If you were to design an injury prevention educational program at this jobsite, what would you include? How could you avoid describing possible injuries to address management's concerns that this could allow workers to falsify injuries? How could you facilitate attendance, as workers would not be productive during this time?

Learning Activities

1. Identify an area of your university or institution that could benefit from an ergonomic consultation. Develop a plan to address the possible barriers for this consultation.
2. Compare and contrast the ergonomic considerations for each area of occupation described in the occupational therapy practice framework (AOTA, 2014). Describe the outcomes or benefits of ergonomic improvements to each of these occupations.
3. Perform an ergonomic consultation of a colleague's work space and discuss recommendations to prevent injury.

REFERENCES

Accreditation Council for Occupational Therapy Education. (2018). 2011 *Accreditation Council for Occupational Therapy Education (ACOTE®) standards and interpretative guidelines: June 2018 interpretive guide version.* Retrieved from www.aota.org/~/media/Corporate/Files/EducationCareers/Accredit/Standards/2011-Standards-and-Interpretive-Guide.pdf

American Occupational Therapy Association. (n.d.). *Critically appraised topic: Evidence for the effectiveness of exercise and work-related interventions.* Retrieved from www.aota.org/practice/rehabilitation-disability/evidence-based/cat-musculo-work.aspx

American Occupational Therapy Association. (2014). Occupational therapy practice framework: Domain and process (3rd ed.). *American Journal of Occupational Therapy,* 68(Suppl.1) S1–S48. doi:10/5014/ajot.2014.682006

American Occupational Therapy Association. (2015). Occupational therapy code of ethics (2015). *American Journal of Occupational Therapy, 69*(*6* Suppl. 3), 6913410030. http://dx.doi.org/10.5014/ajot.2015.696S03

Baker, N. A. (2008). Anthropometry. In K. Jacobs (Ed.), *Ergonomics for therapists* (3rd ed., pp. 73–93). St. Louis, MO: Mosby Elsevier.

Basich, M., Driscoll, T., and Wickstrom, R. (2007). Transitional work therapy on site: Work is therapy. *Professional Case Management, 12*(6), 351–355.

Baum, C. M., Christiansen, C. H., and Bass, J. D. (2015). The person-environment-occupation-performance (PEOP) model. In C. M. Baum, C. H. Christiansen, and J. D. Bass (Eds.), *Occupational therapy: Performance, participation and well-being* (4th ed., pp. 49–55). Thorofare, NJ: SLACK.

Baxter, M. F. (2008). Ergonomics of play and leisure. In K. Jacobs (Ed.), *Ergonomics for therapists* (3rd ed., pp. 313–328). St. Louis, MO: Mosby Elsevier.

Bernal, D., Compos-Serna, J., Tobias, A., Vargas-Prada, S., Benavides, G., and Serra, C. (2015). Work-related psychosocial risk factors and musculoskeletal disorders in hospital nurses and nursing aides: A systematic review and meta-analysis. *International Journal of Nursing Studies, 52*(2), 635–648. doi:10.1016/j.ijnurstu.2014.11.003

Canadian Center for Occupational Health and Safety. (2014). *Ergonomic chair.* Retrieved from www.ccohs.ca/oshanswers/ergonomics/office/chair.html

Canadian Center for Occupational Health and Safety. (2016). *Working in a sitting position: Overview.* Retrieved from http://ccohs.ca/oshanswers/ergonomics/sitting/sitting_overview.html

Canadian Center for Occupational Health and Safety. (2018). *Working from a standing position: Basic information.* Retrieved from http://ccohs.ca/oshanswers/ergonomics/standing/standing_basic.html

Chaffin, D. B., Andersson, G., and Martin, B. J. (1984). *Occupational biomechanics* (4th ed.). New York, NY: Wiley.

Chapanis, A. (1991). To communicate the human factors message, you have to know what the message is and how to communicate it. *Human Factors Society Bulletin, 34*(11), 1–4.

Cohen, A. L., Gjessing, C. C., Fine, L. J., Bernard, B. P., and McGlothlin, J. D. (1997). *Elements of ergonomics programs: A primer based on workplace evaluations of musculoskeletal disorders.* Atlanta, GA: National Institute for Occupational Safety and Health. Retrieved from http://cdc.gov/niosh/docs/97–117/eptbtr6a.html

Dul, J., Bruder, R., Buckle P., Carayon, P., Falzon, P., Marras, W. S., . . . van der Doelen, B. (2012). A strategy for human factors/ergonomics: Developing the discipline and profession. *Ergonomics, 55*(4), 377–395. doi:10.10080/00140139.2012.661087

Erez, A. B. H. (2008). Psychosocial factors in work-related musculoskeletal disorders. In K. Jacobs (Ed.), *Ergonomics for therapists* (3rd ed., pp. 123–136). St. Louis, MO: Mosby Elsevier.

Erez, A. B. H., Shenkar, O., Jacobs, K., and Gillespie, R. M. (2008). Ergonomics for children and youth in the educational environment. In K. Jacobs (Ed.), *Ergonomics for therapists* (3rd ed., pp. 246–264). St. Louis, MO: Mosby Elsevier.

Ergoweb. (2012). *Revisiting the roots of ergonomics.* Retrieved from https://ergoweb.com/revisiting-the-roots-of-ergonomics/

Ergoweb. (2017). *History of ergonomics.* Retrieved from https://ergoweb.com/history-of-ergonomics/

Franco, G. (1999). Ramazzini and workers' health. *Lancet, 354,* 858–861.

Goodman, G., Landis, J., George, C., McGuire, S., Shorter, C., Sieminski, M., and Wilson, T. (2005). Effectiveness of computer ergonomics interventions for an engineering company: A program evaluation. *Work, 24,* 53–62.

Hoosain, M., de Klerk, S., and Burger, M. (2018). Workplace-based rehabilitation of upper limb conditions: A systematic review. *Journal of Occupational Rehabilitation,* 1–19. doi:10.1007/s10926-018-9777-7

International Ergonomics Association. (2018). *Definition and domains of ergonomics.* Retrieved from www.iea.cc/whats/index.html

Internet Center for Management and Business Administration. (2010). *Frederick Taylor and scientific management.* Retrieved from http://netmba.com/mgmt/scientific/

Jacobs, K. (2008). *Ergonomics for therapists* (3rd ed.). St. Louis, MO: Mosby Elsevier.

Lee, M. P., Hudson, H., Richards, R., Chang, C. C., Chosewood, L. C., and Schill, A. L. (2016). *Fundamentals of total worker health approaches: Essential elements for advancing worker safety, health, and well-being.* Publication 2017-112. Cincinnati, OH: National Institute for Occupational Safety and Health.

Legg, S., and Jacobs, K. (2008). Ergonomics for schools. *Work, 31,* 489–493.

National Institute for Occupational Safety and Health. (1997). *Chapter 7: Work-related musculoskeletal disorders and psychosocial factors.* Retrieved from http://cdc.gov/niosh/docs/97–141/

Occupational Safety and Health Administration. (n.d.a). *Computer workstations eTool: Good working positions.* Retrieved from http://osha.gov/SLTC/etools/computerworkstations/positions.html

Occupational Safety and Health Administration. (n.d.b). *Computer workstations eTool: Workstation components.* Retrieved from www.osha.gov/SLTC/etools/computerworkstations/components.html

Occupational Safety and Health Administration. (n.d.c). *Ergonomics.* Retrieved from www.osha.gov/SLTC/ergonomics/

Occupational Safety and Health Administration. (n.d.d). *Identify problems.* Retrieved from www.osha.gov/SLTC/ergonomics/identifyprobls.html#RiskFactors

Occupational Safety and Health Administration. (n.d.e). *Solutions to control hazards.* Retrieved from www.osha.gov/SLTC/ergonomics/controlhazards.html

Ripat, J., and Becker, P. (2012). Playground usability: What do playground users say? *Occupational Therapy International, 19,* 144–153. doi:10.1002/oti.1331

R. L. Mace Universal Design Institute. (2019a). *Universal design principles.* Retrieved from https://www.udinstitute.org/principles

R. L. Mace Universal Design Institute. (2019b). *What is universal design?* Retrieved from https://www.udinstitute.org/what-is-ud

Sanders, M. J., and Wright, R. (2016). Work. In C. Meriano and D. Latella (Eds.), *Occupational therapy interventions: Function and Occupations* (pp. 325–361). Thorofare, NJ: SLACK.

Scaffa, M. E., Chromiak, S. B., Reitz, S. M., Blair-Newton, A., Murphy, L., and Wallis, C. B. (2010). Unintentional injury and violence prevention. In M. E. Scaffa, S. M. Reitz, and M. A. Pizzi (Eds.), *Occupational therapy in the promotion of health and wellness* (pp. 350–375). Philadelphia, PA: F. A. Davis.

Shaw, L., and Lysaght, R. (2008). Cognitive and behavioral demands of work. In K. Jacobs (Ed.), *Ergonomics for therapists* (3rd ed., pp. 103–122). St. Louis, MO: Mosby Elsevier.

Siegel, P. (2001). *Expert commentary: The new OSHA ergonomics program standard.* International Risk Management Institute Inc. Retrieved from www.irmi.com/articles/expert-commentary/new-osha-ergonomics-program-standard

Smith, T. J. (2012). Integrating community ergonomics with educational ergonomics—Designing community systems to support classroom learning. *Work, 41,* 3676–3684. doi:10.3233/WOR-2012-0009-3676

U.S. Bureau of Labor Statistics. (2017a). *2016 Survey of occupational injuries and illnesses charts package.* Retrieved from www.bls.gov/iif/osch0060.pdf

U.S. Bureau of Labor Statistics. (2017b). *Employer-reported workplace injuries and illnesses, 2016* [News release]. Retrieved from www.bls.gov/news.release/archives/osh_11092017.pdf

U.S. Bureau of Labor Statistics. (2017c). *Numbers of nonfatal occupational injuries and illnesses by industry and case types, 2016* [Summary Table 2]. Retrieved from www.bls.gov/iif/oshsum.htm#16Summary_News_Release

U.S. Department of Labor Occupational Information Network. (2017). *Browse by O*NET Data Abilities.* Retrieved from www.onetonline.org/find/descriptor/browse/Abilities/1.A.1/

Wahlstedt, K., Norbäck, D., Wieslander, G., Skoglund, L., and Runeson, R. (2010). Psychosocial and ergonomic factors and their relation to musculoskeletal complaints in the Swedish workforce. *International Journal of Occupational Safety and Ergonomics, 16*(3), 311–321. doi:10.1080/10803548.2010.11076848

Waters, T. R. (2007). When is it safe to manually lift a patient? *American Journal of Nursing, 107*(8), 53–58.

Waters, T. R., and Dick, R. B. (2014). Evidence of health risks associated with prolonged standing at work and intervention effectiveness. *Rehabilitation Nursing, 40*(3), 148–165. doi:10.1002/rnj.166

Waters, T. R., Putz-Anderson, V., and Garg, A. (1994). *Application manual for revised NIOSH lifting equation.* Retrieved from http://cdc.gov/niosh/docs/94-110/pdfs/94-110.pdf

Waters, T. R., Putz-Anderson, V., Garg, A., and Fine, L. J. (1993). Rapid communication: Revised NIOSH equation for the design and evaluation of manual lifting tasks. *Ergonomics, 36*(7), 749–776.

Wei, J., and Salvendy, G. (2003). The utilization of the Purdue cognitive job analysis. *Human Factors and Ergonomics in Manufacturing, 13*(1), 59–84. doi:10.1002/hfm.10028

Young, M. S., Brookhuis, K. A., Wickens, C. D., and Hancock, P. A. (2015). State of science: Mental workload in ergonomics. *Ergonomics, 58*(1), 1–17. doi:10.1080/00140739.2014.956151

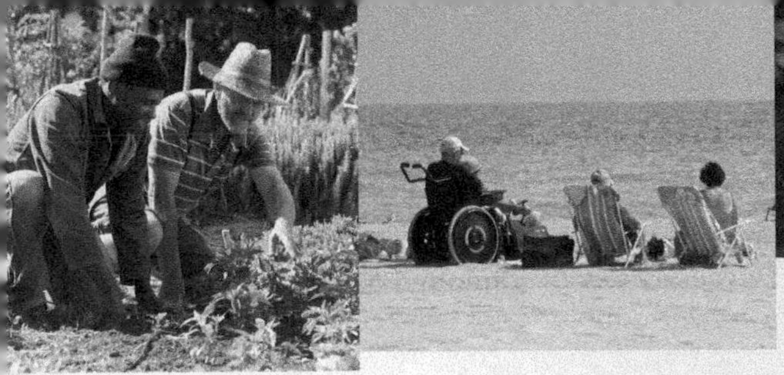

Chapter 16

Work and Career Transitions

Marjorie E. Scaffa, PhD, OTR/L, FAOTA, and S. Maggie Reitz, PhD, OTR/L, FAOTA

Real success is finding your lifework in the work that you love.
—David McCullough

Learning Outcomes

This chapter is designed to enable the reader to:

16-1 Describe the importance of work as an occupation.
16-2 Identify the types of work transitions a person may experience in a lifetime.
16-3 Discuss issues related to returning to work after disability.
16-4 Describe the options available for transitioning from full-time employment into retirement.
16-5 Identify the benefits of volunteer participation.
16-6 Describe the roles of occupational therapy practitioners in various aspects of work transition and work transition programs.

Key Terms

Bridge employment
Encore career
Engaging occupations
Job accommodation network
Legacy planning
Occupational adaptation
Occupational transition
Retirement
Transition
Unemployed person
Volunteerism
Volunteer participation
Warrior transition units
Work

Introduction

Work has diverse meanings for different people at various times in their lives. Within occupational therapy practice, work and volunteer participation can be both a means and an end. In the American Occupational Therapy Association (AOTA, 2014, p. S20) *Occupational Therapy Practice Framework,* **work** is defined as "labor or exertion; to make, construct, manufacture, form, fashion, or shape objects; to organize, plan, or evaluate services or processes of living or governing; committed occupations that are performed with or without financial reward" (Christiansen and Townsend, 2010, p. 423). The occupation of work is divided into six components:

- Employment interests and pursuits
- Employment seeking and acquisition
- Job performance
- Retirement preparation and adjustment
- Volunteer exploration
- Volunteer participation (AOTA, 2014)

Satisfying work contributes to mental and physical health, while unemployment and underemployed are linked to poor health (Fouad and Bynner,

2008). Work, paid or unpaid, can provide a sense of mastery, competence, productivity, and achievement (Siporin, 1999). Work provides a sense of purpose and structures time. In addition, work is often a source of identity and self-worth. Identity consists of how people think about themselves, the characteristics that define them, and how they are perceived by others. When meeting someone new socially, the first question one is asked is "What do you do?" (meaning what is your job or work?). This question is understandable considering how much time the average adult in the United States spends on the job. In 2015, the average number of hours worked per week was 38.7, and the average number of weeks worked per year was 46.8 (Pew Research Center, 2016). Work is also a source of relationships, social networks, and social participation. Therefore, it is not surprising that when someone experiences a change in work status or setting, that person may also experience losses not only in income but also in roles, relationships, and identity.

Whether focusing on a school-to-work transition, transition into employment, or transition into partial or complete retirement, occupational therapy practitioners can play an important role in facilitating positive outcomes. Increasing the visibility of the profession in the provision of occupational therapy transitional work services and programs is supported by the profession's commitment to social and occupational justice and the prevention of occupational imbalance (AOTA, 2014, 2015; Scaffa, Van Slyke, and Brownson, 2008). Increasing access to transitional work services, collecting data on the results of these services, and disseminating outcome data from such efforts are very important steps along the road to fulfilling the AOTA (2017) *Vision 2025*.

In this chapter, the concept of work transitions is introduced, and several specific transitions are described in detail. The relevance and connection to occupational therapy services in community and population health practice are provided.

Work Transitions

All individuals experience transitions in a variety of areas throughout their life spans. **Transition** can be described as a process of change or movement from one place, situation, or context to another (Schlossberg, 2004). Work and career transitions include transitioning into and out of the workplace. It can include the transition of youth with disabilities from school to employment or the transition of people returning to or starting work following a disability, injury, or illness. Other types of work transition include wounded warriors returning to civilian employment; high school, college, and professional athletes retiring from a sport; parents returning to work after maternity or paternity leave; family caregivers returning after a prolonged period of caring for a family member; and older adults transitioning from the workforce into retirement. Some work transitions are made voluntarily and driven by a desire for change; others are involuntary, caused by environmental demands beyond one's control. Voluntary work transitions, typically self-initiated, provide time to consider options and prepare for the necessary changes. Involuntary transitions are frequently characterized by insufficient time and resources to prepare for, complete, and adjust to the necessary changes (Fouad and Bynner, 2008).

Work and career transitions can be exciting or troubling but are almost always stressful and typically require adaptation. **Occupational adaptation** refers to "the extent to which persons are able to develop, change in response to challenges, or otherwise achieve a state of well-being through what they do" (Kielhofner, 2008, p. 106). A person may experience a number of work transitions throughout the life span, requiring career adaptability and a wide range of occupational competencies. It is important to recognize that work transitions not only affect the worker but also the worker's family (Fouad and Bynner, 2008).

Work transitions cannot easily be separated from transitions in other life domains—for example, facing changes in relationships, becoming a parent, or moving to a new home. Often, job changes result from, or precipitate, other life transitions, meaning a person experiencing a work transition is likely experiencing transitions in other areas of life as well. According to Fouad and Bynner (2008), "how effective an individual is in making a transition and adjusting to its consequences depends on a number of personal factors, including the emotional, personal, social and financial resources he or she brings to that transition" (p. 244).

Transitioning From School to Employment

For adolescents and young adults, the transition from high school to employment or postsecondary education is very significant (Orentlicher and Michaels, 2000). However, for students with disabilities, transitioning from secondary schools to adult roles can be problematic, and school-to-work transitioning has been far from optimal for many of these students. Statistics indicate that students with disabilities have significantly less successful outcomes related to employment rates and retention, advancement in employment, independent living, and community participation than students without disabilities (Kohler and Field, 2003; Wagner and Davis, 2006; Wagner, Newman, Cameto, Levine, and Garza, 2006). Growing numbers of students with disabilities are exiting the public school system without the occupational skills needed to succeed in entry-level jobs. Due to an increase in high-performance businesses across the nation, there is also an increasing demand for employees with a combination of academic and occupational skills, making employment for persons with disabilities even more challenging (Benz, Yovanoff, and Doren, 1997). According to a U.S. Department of Labor report on employment statistics in the United States, the unemployment rate has decreased; nevertheless, "the unemployment rate of people living with disabilities is more than double that of the rate attributed to those living without any disabilities" (Disabled World: Towards Tomorrow, 2019, para. 2).

Quality of life, participation, prevention, and other outcomes of the occupational therapy process (AOTA, 2014) are well matched to the outcomes of transitional work programs. However, the services of occupational therapy practitioners are often not utilized to their fullest potential, especially in school systems where occupational therapy practitioners are already present. Transition services for students with disabilities are described in more detail in Chapter 10.

Returning to Work Following a Disability

The transition of persons with disabilities into or out of community employment is an important societal issue that can be addressed by occupational therapy. Data indicate that approximately 78% of adults between 18 and 64 years of age are employed, compared with only 37% of adults with disabilities; employment rates are even lower for individuals with severe disabilities (Long-Bellil and Henry, 2009; Wehman, 2001).

Similar to school-to-work transition, federal legislation has been enacted in an effort to facilitate and enable persons with disabilities to return to work. The Americans With Disabilities Act (ADA) of 1990 and its 2008 amendments and the Ticket to Work and Work Incentives Improvement Act (TWWIIA) of 1999 have important implications for individuals transitioning to work following a disability.

Stapleton and Burkhauser (2003) view the ADA of 1990 as a driving force in changing disability policy so that individuals with disabilities can become competitively employed rather than rely on various types of disability benefits. The ADA and its reauthorizations in 2008 and 2010 protect the civil rights of, and prohibit discrimination against, workers with disabilities. The ADA also mandates the provision of reasonable accommodations to enable workers with disabilities to be successful in the workplace. The 2010 amendment also clarifies the use of service animals; wheelchairs; manual mobility devices, which include canes, crutches, and walkers; and other types of power-driven mobility devices, such as Segways, which are not designed for the exclusive use of persons with disabilities (Resource Centers on Independent Living, n.d.).

Although the purpose of the ADA was well intended, research has suggested that the employment rates of persons with disabilities did not significantly increase after the passage of this legislation. One possible reason for the lack of marked change in employment rates was that many persons with disabilities were concerned about the loss of benefits, particularly health benefits. Many persons with disabilities, because of the nature of their disability, are able to work only on a part-time basis. However,

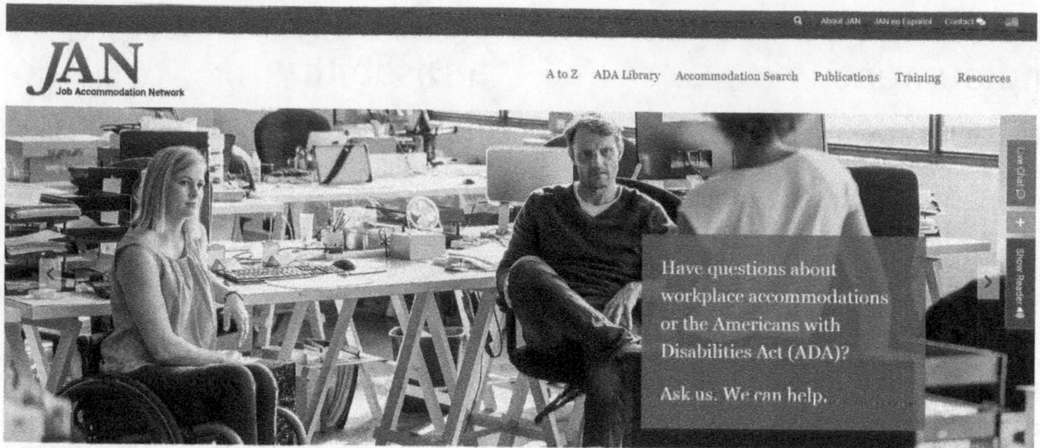

Figure 16-1 Job Accommodation Network website. *(Photo courtesy of JAN.)*

in many situations a person must be employed full time in order to be covered by health insurance plans offered by their employer. The TWWIIA legislation enables persons with disabilities to return to work and continue to receive health-care coverage from programs such as Medicaid.

In community and population health practice focusing on the transition to work by persons with disabilities, there are numerous roles for occupational therapy practitioners, including:

- Completing ergonomic evaluations and interventions in the workplace
- Consulting on community and transportation accessibility
- Making recommendations for reasonable accommodations
- Providing individualized direct service focusing on the occupational performance areas of activities of daily living (ADLs) and instrumental activities of daily living (IADLs)

An increasing number of occupational therapy practitioners are involved in workplace ergonomic evaluations and interventions (AOTA, 2004), which are described in detail in Chapter 15. Evaluations might include the identification and minimization of factors that contribute to accidents or injury in the workplace. Interventions might focus on the modification of tools and equipment and the provision of education and training on injury prevention.

An accessible community and transportation are necessary in order for a person with a disability to return to work. Although still relatively uncommon, consulting on community and transportation accessibility is an emerging role for occupational therapy practitioners (Iwarsson, Stahl, and Carlsson, 2003).

Occupational therapy practitioners are frequently called upon to make recommendations for workplace accommodations. The **Job Accommodation Network** (JAN, 2009) is a program under the auspices of the Office of Disability Employment Policy in the U.S. Department of Labor whose major purpose is to facilitate the employment and retention of workers with disabilities. Through its website, the JAN addresses physical, cognitive, sensory, and mental conditions and disabilities, including etiology, symptoms, and treatment. Whether or not the disability or condition is covered under the ADA, numerous examples of accommodations for a variety of disabilities or conditions are also included. The JAN provides a valuable resource that can be used by occupational therapy practitioners for their own information or to share with persons with disabilities and employers (see Fig. 16-1).

Occupational therapy practitioners continue to have a crucial role in providing direct service to persons with disabilities in order to enable their return to work. Depending on the nature of their disability, people may need assistance or suggestions for ADLs related to getting ready for work or IADLs related to getting to work. They might also need assistance with assertiveness and self-advocacy in asking for reasonable accommodations or information on what accommodations might be reasonable to request.

Becoming Unemployed

Becoming unemployed is an **occupational transition,** "a major change in the occupational repertoire of a person in which one or several occupations change, disappear, and/or are replaced by others" (Jonsson, 2010, p. 212). The U.S. Bureau of Labor Statistics (2015) defines an **unemployed person** as one who does not have a job, is currently available for work, and has actively tried to find work in the past 4 weeks. Becoming unemployed, whether by being fired, downsized, or laid off, is usually a traumatic experience, and these involuntary work transitions may occur several times during a lifetime (Fouad and Bynner, 2008). Older workers, those over the age of 55, are disproportionately represented among the unemployed and are more adversely affected (Voss et al., 2018).

Unemployment may be brief, temporary, or long term, depending on the circumstances, and may also be challenging to an individual's adaptive capacity. Lost income is not the only consequence of unemployment. Job loss also has adverse psychological effects and has been linked to depression, alcohol and drug use, suicide, and violence. Underemployment or economically inadequate employment can have similar consequences (Dooley, 2003). If a person becomes unemployed by choice—for example, for maternity leave, family caregiving, or the pursuit of education—these negative mental health effects are mitigated (Voss and Chen, 2015).

Daily routines are significantly altered, and there is a dramatic shift in time use when a person becomes unemployed. Research has shown that after becoming unemployed, people tend to spend more time sleeping and watching television and little time in goal-directed pursuits (Voss and Chen, 2015). The structured use of time during unemployment is correlated with improved coping, and engagement in purposeful activity is associated with better mental health (Van Hoye and Lootens, 2013). From an occupational therapy perspective, unemployment can be construed as occupational disruption, imbalance, marginalization, and/or deprivation.

Job searching is a transitional occupation that occurs when a person is unemployed and desires employment. Occupational therapy practitioners are able to assist job seekers to realistically assess themselves, identify types of work for which they are suitable, and enact job search strategies. Historically, this work has been carried out with persons with disabilities, but programs built on these strategies could be developed for other populations experiencing unemployment. A useful resource for job seekers is the O*NET website, which provides job descriptions for more than 1,000 occupations in a wide variety of work categories (O*NET Resource Center, 2019).

Engage Your Brain 16-1

What are strategies an occupational therapist could use to assess a client's interests and aptitudes for employment in preparation for a job search?

Transitioning From Active Duty to Civilian Employment

Occupational therapy has been actively involved in providing services to military personnel since the early years of the profession (McDaniel, 1968). Beginning in World War I, its practitioners have responded to the reconstruction and rehabilitation needs of injured soldiers, both stateside and abroad. The goal of the reconstruction work in World War I was to enable soldiers to return to either active service or paid employment following discharge from the military.

Increasing attention is being placed on facilitating the transition of military service personnel into civilian life, including employment. Based on the results of a congressionally mandated review of care for "warriors in transition," 35 **warrior transition units** (WTUs) were developed by the army to better meet the rehabilitation and vocational training needs of injured soldiers. The WTUs were designed for soldiers who required more than 6 months of medical care and were located close to medical treatment facilities across the United States and in a few international locations. The philosophy of the WTUs was to band together soldiers with the same duties in units, a traditional organizational structure in the military, and then train them to return to active military duty or to gain civilian employment (Erickson, Secrest, and Gray, 2008). Active and reserve duty troops, whether they are deployed in areas of conflict or are based within the United States, are eligible for services provided through WTUs. Updates regarding programs are posted on the WTU section of the U.S. Army (n.d.) website.

Although occupational therapy interventions for wounded warriors, regardless of their diagnoses, may be similar to those for their civilian counterparts, these individuals also need access to specialized transitional services. Occupational therapy practitioners who wish to seek funding and support for developing such programs in their own community must ensure they understand the military lifestyle and culture as well as resources such as Pets for Vets (Hendrix, 2011). Pets for Vets is an organization that trains and matches animals in need of a home with Veterans in need of companionship (Pets for Vets, 2017; see Fig. 16-2). This knowledge can be gained through a variety of ways, including:

- Communicating via e-mail (e.g., Johnson, n.d.) or social media with occupational therapists in the military
- Seeking evidence-based articles on interventions with military personnel
- Reviewing military websites, such as www.army.mil

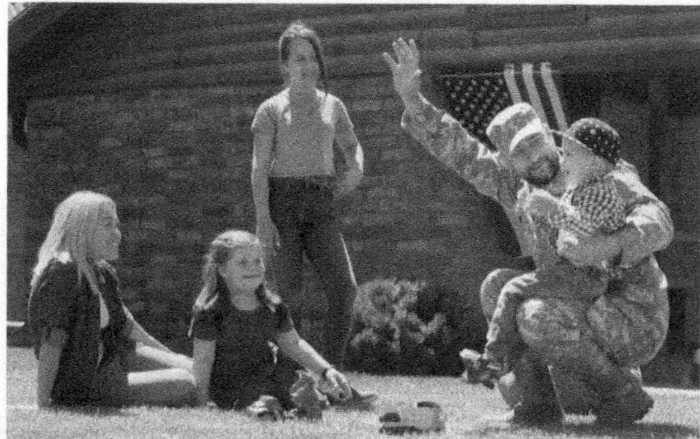

Figure 16-2 Warriors in transition: the homecoming. *(Evgeniy Shkolenko/Stock/Getty Images Plus/Getty Images.)*

- Reading current related literature
- Attending state and national conferences and sessions on this population
- Volunteering with organizations that provide services for Veterans

A variety of initiatives are being developed to meet the needs of wounded warriors. The potential to facilitate transitions of military personnel to civilian paid work or volunteer positions is being partially realized but requires expansion; occupational therapy practitioners are well equipped to meet this growing need. Transition services for Veterans are described in more detail in Chapter 21.

Changing Careers

In the past, it was possible to choose a preferred career path in high school or college and pursue it in a predictable and sustained fashion. Due to the fast pace of changes in technology, a turbulent labor market, and a shift in the types of jobs available, a single career path is not always feasible. Unpredictable and unavoidable events require workers to continually adapt to new demands and evolving work contexts. According to the U.S. Bureau of Labor Statistics (2017), the average worker will have had at least 10 different jobs before the age of 50.

Some people choose to change careers, while others are forced into new careers out of necessity. A career change is typically described as a change in both job function and industry. Interviews of career changers indicated a desire for assistance with identifying transferable skills and the skills needing to be acquired through additional training and mentors who have been successful in their career transitions (Phan, 2018). The variables that appear to facilitate adaptive responses to career changes are an internal locus of control, generalized self-efficacy, and trait curiosity (Van der Horst, Klehe, and Van der Heijden, 2017).

Phan (2018) identified two types of career changers: (1) the explorers who do not have a specific career in mind and are willing to explore different options and paths and (2) the targeted searchers who know exactly what they want their next job function and industry to be and need to learn the necessary steps to achieve their career transition. The career changers in the study experienced similar stages in the career change process. First, there was a trigger for change—for example, being laid off, feeling bored or not challenged at work, and/or overworked. This was followed by a time of self-reflecting, researching potential careers, evaluating options, selecting a direction, and planning a strategy to achieve the career change goal. Community-based programs for career changers could easily be developed by occupational therapy practitioners.

Transitioning to Retirement

Retirement refers to permanently leaving the workforce, usually after midlife. Many older adults, when given the choice, choose to transition into retirement gradually, rather than abruptly. The average length of retirement is 17.2 years for men and 20.6 years for women (Organization for Economic Cooperation and Development, 2017). More than half of U.S. adults retire earlier than planned, often due to health problems, disability, unexpected job loss, or the need to provide care for a family member. This indicates a need for retirement-planning education that includes an occupational engagement focus. An analysis of research studies on 11 retirement programs indicates that such programs result in positive impacts on knowledge, attitudes, and planning activities; 2 of the 11 studies were based on the transtheoretical model (Leandro-França, Murta, Hershey, and Martins, 2016). While the programs involved in the study do not appear to include an occupational science perspective, it is believed that including an occupation-based theoretical model for program design, and occupational participation as part of the program curriculum, would further enhance outcomes.

According to Gallup (2013, 2018) the average retirement age has increased to 61 from 59 in 2003 and 57 in 1993. However, nonretired adults expect to continue working until at least age 66. Delaying retirement appears to have its advantages. Those who continue to work in their 60s have slightly better emotional health than those who are not working (Gallup, 2013). Many baby boomers, although officially retired, continue to work part-time (20% of women, 39% of men) or provide 10 or more hours of volunteer service to community organizations (62% of women, 45% of men; Moen and Fields, 2002). As U.S. demographics continue to change with increasing numbers of older adults entering the retirement transition, occupational therapy practitioners will be challenged to address the needs of this population.

Retirement Transition

According to Schlossberg (2004), retirement is not one but many transitions. A transition can be an event (e.g., moving, getting married) or nonevent, something you would reasonably expect to happen but does not (e.g., having grandchildren). These events and nonevents change one's life by altering relationships, roles, and assumptions. Transitions are turning points between periods of relative stability and are opportunities for growth and change.

The retirement transition can be expected and planned, unexpected and unplanned, or desirable or undesirable. Retirement is not simply leaving a job; it is also a change in identity, routine, relationships, roles, and lifestyle. There are several styles people use when approaching retirement (Schlossberg, 2004; see Box 16-1). The findings of a systematic review by Barbosa, Monteiro, and Murta (2016) identified factors that predicted a positive adjustment to retirement. These factors included physical health, financial security, involvement in leisure activities, social participation, psychological health, and personality characteristics such as optimism, an internal locus of control, and humor. For persons who must retire earlier than expected due to a chronic

Box 16-1 Retirement Styles

- Continuers, those who maintain their use of existing skills and interests in new ways
- Adventurers, those who seek out new experiences and initiate new endeavors
- Searchers, those who explore new opportunities through trial and error, trying to find where they best fit
- Easy gliders, those who are content to go with the flow and see what each day brings
- Retreaters, those who disengage from life and relationships

Data from *Retire Smart, Retire Happy: Finding Your True Path in Life*, by N. Schlossberg, 2004, Washington, DC: American Psychological Association.

health condition or disability, the challenges to a positive adjustment are greater. If their retirement is involuntary, the transition is more difficult and can result in significant economic disadvantage and limited opportunities for productive participation in society. Occupational therapy practitioners are "well positioned to ensure success with planning and carrying out transition plans because of our unique skills in tailoring education and support to the individual needs of people with illness or disability" (Brown, 2018, p. 3).

Through qualitative interviews of retirees, Jonsson, Josephsson, and Kielhofner (2001) identified an important determinant of retirement adjustment and satisfaction: engaging occupations. **Engaging occupations** "are those that evoke a depth of passion or feeling" and "are done with great commitment, enthusiasm, perseverance, and passion" (p. 428). Frequently, these are activities connected to a person's former work or long-term leisure interest. Engaging occupations appear to have six characteristics in common (see Box 16-2).

The examination of professional and collegiate athletes' retirement planning and experiences is a recent area of research. While this retirement process happens at an earlier age than in most careers, many of the same challenges exist. A cross-cultural study of European elite athletes found that while the impact of individual characteristics was similar across the three countries studied, differences in cultural contexts influenced the transition (Kuettel, Boyle, and Schmid, 2017). The results of a study of transitioning collegiate athletes through an occupation lens led the researchers to identify the "need for occupational therapists to develop interventions aimed at improving quality of life for postcareer athletes" (Smoot and Marterella, 2017, para. 5). Similar themes emerged from the semistructured interviews:

- Initial relief
- Struggling with identity
- Missing the support of a team
- Lost connection to the sport
- An enduring search for other meaningful occupations (Smoot and Marterella, 2017, para. 5)

Box 16-2 Characteristics of Engaging Occupations

Engaging occupations are:

- Infused with positive meaning, enjoyable, interesting, and challenging
- A coherent set of related activities, not a single activity
- Analogs to work—similar to work in that they are done with the same level of commitment and seriousness
- Participated in with intensity and a regularity of involvement
- Activities that go beyond personal pleasure and evoke a sense of commitment and responsibility
- A shared, common interest that provides an occupational community

Data from "Narratives and Experience in an Occupational Transition: A Longitudinal Study of the Retirement Process," by H. Jonsson, S. Josephsson, and G. Kielhofner, 2001, *American Journal of Occupational Therapy, 55*, 424–432.

The need for comprehensive preretirement (Cantor, 1981) and retirement planning (Broderick and Glazer, 1983), beyond solely financial planning, has been appreciated by occupational therapists for some time. While financial planning is essential for a quality retirement, an activity or occupation engagement plan is also needed. However, the financial planning portion of retirement planning must occur first, as occupation planning will be constrained by the projected financial resources for retirement. Preparation for retirement may include consideration of an encore career, bridge employment, legacy planning, and volunteerism.

Engage Your Brain 16-2

What theory or model might you use to facilitate the transition to retirement? How would you operationalize the theory or model for this purpose?

Encore Careers

An **encore career** is "continued work in the second half of life that combines social impact, purpose, and often, continued income" (Freedman, n.d., para. 2). Encore careers are transitions typically made in the mid- to late stages of an individual's career and are chosen in lieu of retirement. Many working adults are choosing to reinvent their careers at midlife and later, becoming fully engaged in a new occupation and exploring new passions motivated by a desire for work that has personal meaning and impact.

Encore careers can be found in a variety of fields, but they tend to cluster into five areas: health care, the environment, government, education, and nonprofit organizations. A wonderful example of encore careers is the story of three 60-plus individuals who began second careers as personal trainers. Not only did they find joy from their new careers; their clients appreciated having a trainer of the same age (Korchok, 2008). Encore careers provide an opportunity for engaged aging, social participation, generativity, and lifelong learning. Encore careers attract a diverse group of older adults, including all levels of education, blue-collar and white-collar workers, and urban, suburban, and rural residents (Schaefers, 2012).

The transition to an encore career may take months to years and may require retraining, the cost of which may be a significant obstacle. However, in the long term there is usually a financial payoff in the form of postponed access to social security and the associated increase in benefits, the delayed need for drawing on retirement savings, and an extended work life. In addition to income during the retirement years, older adults are often looking for flexible hours and opportunities for social contact.

Murphy and Volpe (2014) identified five factors motivating individuals to leave their current careers in pursuit of encore careers. Three of the motivating factors are personal: the desire for meaningful work, fun, and novelty. Two of the motivating factors are structural: the desire for increased work flexibility and more attractive work characteristics. Attractive work characteristics include more autonomy, fewer physical demands, decreased travel requirements, and less stress. Outcomes associated with an encore career transition included a new professional identity, a revived career and life satisfaction, and an improved work-life balance.

Encore careers can provide high-quality workers to tackle societal needs while providing satisfying work for older adults (Schaefers, 2012). Freedman (2007) believes the encore career movement is "one of the most significant social trends of the new century and the biggest transformation of the American workforce since the women's movement" (p. 2).

PROGRAM SHOWCASE

Submitted by Lisa Carson, OTD, OTR/L, and Ryan Risley, MPM, Washington University in St. Louis

Program Name: Life Transitions

City/State: Saint Louis, Missouri, metro region

Needs assessment: An informal needs assessment was conducted through literature review (Carson, 2014) and meetings with representatives from human resources departments and wellness programs. Results indicated a gap in services in which people going through a significant life transition, such as retirement or a new health diagnosis, were lacking support to successfully make that transition while managing their health, environment, and occupations.

Goal: To promote purposeful, meaningful, and active lifestyles during all phases of life and to promote long-term independent and healthy living. The program encourages use of meaning, motivation, and action to establish and maintain healthy and productive habits, roles, and routines.

Population: middle-age to elderly adults living in the community

Program description: The Life Transitions program is based on an occupational therapy practice model (Carson, 2014) influenced by the person-environment-occupational performance (PEOP) model (Baum, Christiansen, and Bass, 2015), the competence press model (Nahemow and Lawson, 1973), the ecological systems model (Howe and Briggs, 1982), and the transtheoretical model of change. Life Transitions begins with a comprehensive health and wellness assessment followed by individual coaching sessions to create and monitor action plans. Action plans are client-centered and geared toward increasing self-management, health education, and healthy behaviors, building social networks, pursuing productive activities, utilizing systems and services, and using modifications and technology in the home and community. The program is customizable to fit the needs of various populations, such as those undergoing a role transition, health transition, career transition, or transition to retirement. Clients are encouraged to reflect on their current occupations and discover what they might want to change about their daily roles, habits, and routines both at their jobs and in their personal lives.

Participant's perspective: A program participant stated, "It actually made me think about myself, what I do with my day, what my plans are, how to age better, such as staying active and involved."

Evaluation results: Results are not yet available. Outcomes are being measured using PROMIS-57 Profile v2.1 and self-efficacy measures.

Funding: The Life Transitions program is part of Washington University Occupational Therapy Clinical Services (otservices.wustl.edu) and is a self-pay program.

Bridge Employment

A phased or graded approach to retirement, known as bridge employment, can aid in the transition to the retirement role. **Bridge employment** is less than full-time employment in which people engage prior to their full retirement (Feldman, 1994). Zhan, Wang, Liu, and Shultz (2009) found that bridge employees had improved mental health if they continued their employment in the same career and decreased functional limitations if they worked either in their original career or a new career. An occupational therapist may recommend a graded approach to bridge employment, in which a person progressively decreases his or her work hours until full retirement. Bridge employment can be a planned reduction in both work hours and responsibility in order to provide for increased time for family, volunteer activities, or other desired occupations.

Individuals may wish to retire but due to unplanned circumstances, such as a disadvantageous financial situation, need to continue bridge employment or full-time work. Employees often find themselves continuing to work beyond their planned retirement date due to the impact on retirement savings from financial downturns or the illness or loss of a partner or spouse. While these are painful possibilities, they need to be addressed in both financial and occupational retirement planning. In reality, more than one plan is needed. The first plan is based on the individual or the individual and his or her partner remaining healthy and able to work until their desired time frame for full retirement or bridge employment. The second is a plan that accounts for the possibility that one or both become ill and need care.

Engage Your Brain 16-3

Identify ethical considerations when proposing the participation of an occupational therapist in a company's bridge or other retirement program. Refer to the AOTA (2015) *Occupational Therapy Code of Ethics* to formulate your response.

Legacy Planning in Employment and Volunteer Settings

Legacy planning refers to projecting when one no longer wants to be responsible for specific roles or tasks and then working with the appropriate people in the organization proactively to ensure a smooth transition. In many ways, legacy planning is a type of phased retirement. The eventual transition can be eased by ensuring that the individuals who will be assigned the work tasks in the future are oriented to them while the expert is still available for questions and guidance. This type of planning may make it easier for individuals to leave roles and not feel obligated to stay to protect the work or volunteer unit. Erickson's developmental stage of older adults referred to as generativity has been shown to be met through bridge employment (Dendinger, Adams, and Jacobson, 2005); legacy planning might be fashioned in a manner that also meets this developmental task.

With the projected workforce needs in the near future, individuals, including occupational therapy practitioners, will have many options regarding when and how they choose to transition to retirement. Community- and population-based retirement programs can be developed that focus on individuals with similar financial and occupational plans. While individuals with upper-middle incomes and above may have funds to pay for these services, others may not. Seeking grant funding to ensure that people in other economic brackets can also benefit from such planning and support programs would be an important contribution of the profession to occupational justice.

Volunteer Exploration and Participation

Volunteer participation is a form of community engagement that can provide physical and mental health benefits for the volunteers, as well as positive

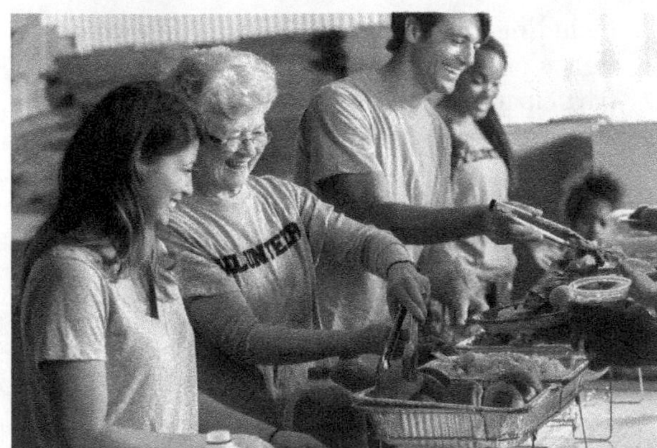

Figure 16-3 Volunteer participation. *(Steve Debenport/E+/Getty Images.)*

outcomes for the organizations for which they work and the community (see Fig. 16-3). The United Nations Volunteers (2018) describe **volunteerism** as "a wide range of activities undertaken of free will, for the general public good, for which monetary reward is not the principal motivating factor" with "volunteers making an ongoing or sustained commitment to an organization and contributing their time on a regular basis" (p. 101). Volunteering can be done formally within the context of organizations and associations or informally on one's own or directly between persons.

People are more likely to initiate and maintain volunteer activity if the volunteer experience coincides with their motivations and satisfies their goals. There are a variety of motivations for volunteer participation (see Box 16-3). Other-oriented, altruistic motives (values, social, and understanding) tend to sustain volunteer participation longer and provide more health benefits than self-oriented motives (enhancement, protective, and career) for volunteerism (Stukas, Hoye, Nicholson, Brown, and Aisbett, 2016).

In the framework, **volunteer participation** is defined as "performing unpaid work activities for the benefit of selected causes, organizations, or facilities" (AOTA, 2014, p. S21). Volunteer participation, although typically unpaid, has social and economic value as well as many of the same personal benefits as paid work. It can provide a sense of identity and purpose, an opportunity for social interaction, and a productive and satisfying daily structure. Volunteerism can be a precursor or training ground for paid employment, but it is also a socially valuable and desirable occupation itself, with many

Box 16-3 Motivations for Volunteer Participation

- Values—a desire to express and actively demonstrate prosocial and humanitarian values
- Understanding—a desire to learn more about the world and other people
- Enhancement—a desire to feel needed and enhance one's self-esteem
- Protective—a desire to distract oneself from one's own problems or reduce guilt about one's own good fortune
- Social—a desire to reinforce bonds with friends and family members who also volunteer
- Career—a desire to obtain skills and experience that will assist one in gaining paid employment

Data from "Motivations to Volunteer and Their Associations With Volunteers' Well-Being," by A. A. Stukas, R. Hoye, M. Nicholson, K. M. Brown, and L. Aisbett, 2016, *Nonprofit and Voluntary Sector Quarterly, 45*(1), 112–132.

associated benefits. People of all ages and abilities volunteer; however, retirees and unemployed adults with disabilities are likely to provide more volunteer hours than other age groups and identify more strongly with the volunteer role as a result. Role identity provides a sense of meaning and purpose in life that in turn improves psychological well-being (van Ingen and Wilson, 2017).

A systematic review of studies on older adult volunteers suggests time spent in volunteer participation positively affects psychological, physical, and social quality of life. Other benefits noted included reduced depression, increased social integration and connectedness, diminished levels of loneliness, and decreased risk of mortality. Although no ideal amount of volunteer activity was identified, it appears that benefits accrue with as little as 100 hours per year, or approximately 2 hours per week (Milbourn, Saraswati, and Buchanan, 2018).

Summary

- The occupation of work is important, as it contributes to mental and physical health, quality of life, and a sense of purpose and self-worth. Work is a source of identity and structures the use of time.
- Individuals may experience a variety of work-related transitions in their lifetimes,

including school to work, career change, bridge employment, retirement, and volunteer participation.
- Returning to work after disability may require retraining, identifying accommodations, and self-advocacy. The Job Accommodation Network is an excellent source of information for occupational therapy practitioners who are assisting persons with disabilities in job seeking, acquisition, and performance.
- A number of options exist for transitioning from full-time employment into retirement, including encore careers, bridge employment, legacy planning, and volunteer participation.
- Volunteer participation provides many of the same benefits as paid employment and contributes to mental and physical health and well-being.
- Occupational therapy practitioners can enact a variety of roles in the work transition process, including advocacy, ergonomics assessment, identification of reasonable accommodations, and retirement planning.

CASE STUDIES

CASE STUDY 16-1 Ted: Planning for Retirement

Ted worked as a contractor for an environmental science company, enjoying the work, the impact of the work on the environment, and the socialization at work with like-minded people. Recently, however, he became frustrated with the increasing demands of the government liaison and not getting paid during the 5-week partial U.S. government shut down. This frustration, coupled with increasing family demands, resulted in Ted deciding to retire and move to a part-time casual employment status. Four months later, he is enjoying working from home on specific work projects, returning to playing the trumpet, and being available to pick his granddaughter up from preschool as needed. His wife, Lily, seeing Ted's happiness, is considering having a conversation with her supervisor about developing a legacy plan so that she can join him in retirement from full-time work. Lily also plans to contact the Pre-Retirement Resource Group at the educational institution at which she works. The Pre-Retirement Resource Group includes an occupational therapist, a benefits specialist from human resources, and a long-term retiree.

Discussion Questions

1. As a member of the Pre-Retirement Resource Group, describe the role you would envision for interactions with Lily.
2. As a member of the Pre-Retirement Resource Group, what theoretical framework(s) and tools would you use to support your interaction with Lily?
3. Would you suggest the addition of any other members to the Pre-Retirement Resource Group?

CASE STUDY 16-2 The Ivy Center for Older Adults

The Ivy Center is a social club that provides hot meals, transportation, recreational activities, field trips, and educational sessions for older adults. Anyone age 55 and older is eligible to join. The fees are minimal, and "scholarships" are available for persons with limited financial resources. Currently, there are approximately 150 club members. The center is open Monday through Saturday from 7 a.m. to 7 p.m. and Sunday from noon to 5 p.m. The members were surveyed

CASE STUDY 16-2 The Ivy Center for Older Adults

regarding desired topics for educational sessions, and one of the most popular suggestions was "making the most of your retirement."

The executive director of the Ivy Center contacted an occupational therapy program at a local university and requested assistance. A faculty member in collaboration with a small group of students developed and implemented a four-session group protocol based on the principles of Lifestyle Redesign®. The session topics included: (1) planning the retirement transition, (2) encore careers, (3) bridge employment, and (4) volunteer participation. Each session included a didactic presentation, a group discussion, a topic-related experiential activity, and suggestions for personal exploration. The group sessions were held once per week on a weekday from 3 p.m. to 5 p.m.

Discussion Questions

1. If you were to expand the number of sessions, what topics might you add?
2. What strategies would you use to evaluate the effectiveness of this intervention?
3. What other services might an occupational therapy practitioner provide in this setting?

Learning Activities

1. Investigate your community or county and determine what work transition programs are available for youth, high school and collegiate athletes, returning warriors, parents reentering the workforce, and retirees exiting the workforce. Summarize your findings in a table.
2. Develop an interview protocol and then conduct an interview with a manager or director of one of the programs. Based on the interview, develop an outline for a potential proposal to describe occupational therapy's contribution to the program.
3. Visit the AARP (aarp.org) website and read about the mission of the organization. How does AARP carry out its mission? What resources does it provide?
4. Visit the Job Accommodation Network (askjan.org) website, choose a disability, and conduct a search for reasonable accommodations for work.

REFERENCES

American Occupational Therapy Association. (2004). *Ergonomics: Occupational therapy in the workplace.* Retrieved from http://promoteot.org/docs/Ergonomics.pdf

American Occupational Therapy Association. (2014). Occupational therapy practice framework: Domain and process (3rd ed.). *American Journal of Occupational Therapy, 68*(Suppl. 1), S1–S51.

American Occupational Therapy Association. (2015). Occupational therapy code of ethics (2015). *American Journal of Occupational Therapy, 69*(Suppl. 3), 6913410030. http://dx.doi.org/10.5014/ajot.2015.696S03

American Occupational Therapy Association. (2017). Vision 2025. *American Journal of Occupational Therapy, 71,* 7103420010. doi:10.5014/ajot.2017.713002

Americans With Disabilities Act of 1990, PL 101–336, 42 U.S.C. §§12101 *et seq.*

Americans With Disabilities Amendments Act (ADAA) of 2008, PL 110–325.

Barbosa, L. M., Monteiro, B., and Murta, S. G. (2016). Retirement adjustment predictors—a systematic review. *Work, Aging, and Retirement, 2,* 262–280. https://doi.org/10.1093/workar/waw008

Baum, C., Christiansen, C., and Bass, J. (2015). Person-environment-occupational performance (PEOP) model. In C. Christiansen, C. Baum, and J. Bass (Eds.), *Occupational therapy: Performance, participation, well-being* (4th ed., pp. 49–56). Thorofare, NJ: Slack.

Benz, M. R., Yovanoff, P., and Doren, B. (1997). School-to-work components that predict post-school success for students with and without disabilities. *Exceptional Children, 63*(2), 151–165.

Broderick, T., and Glazer, B. (1983). Leisure participation and the retirement process. *American Journal of Occupational Therapy, 37*(1), 15–22.

Brown, C. L. (2018). Expanding the occupational therapy role to support transitions from work to retirement for people with progressive health conditions. *American Journal of Occupational Therapy, 72,* 7206347010. https://doi.org/10.5014/ajot.2018.028407

Cantor, S. G. (1981). Occupational therapists as members of pre-retirement resource teams. *American Journal of Occupational Therapy, 35*(10), 638–643.

Carson, L. G. (2014). *Keeping your gears in motion: The self-maintained, OT-facilitated occupational plan for productive aging (OPPA) model.* Unpublished manuscript.

Christiansen, C. H., and Townsend, E. A. (2010). *Introduction to occupation: The art and science of living* (2nd ed.). Cranbury, NJ: Pearson Education.

Dendinger, V. M., Adams, G. A., and Jacobson, J. D. (2005). Reasons for working and their relationship to retirement attitudes, job satisfaction and occupational self-efficacy of bridge employees. *Aging and Human Development, 61*(1), 21–35.

Disabled World: Towards Tomorrow. (2019). *Employment rate remains low for people with disabilities.* Retrieved from www.disabled-world.com/disability/employment/usa/job-rate.php

Dooley, D. (2003). Unemployment, underemployment, and mental health: Conceptualizing employment status as a continuum. *American Journal of Community Psychology, 32*(1/2), 9–20.

Erickson, M. W., Secrest, D. S., and Gray, A. L. (2008, July 28). Army occupational therapy in the warrior transition unit. *OT Practice, 13*(13), pp. 10–14.

Feldman, D. C. (1994). The decision to retire early: A review and conceptualization. *Academy of Management Review, 19,* 285–311.

Fouad, N. A., and Bynner, J. (2008). Work transitions. *American Psychologist, 63*(4), 241–251.

Freedman, M. (n.d.). *Questions about Encore.org and the encore movement.* Retrieved from https://encore.org/faq/

Freedman, M. (2007). *Encore: Finding work that matters in the second half of life.* New York, NY: Public Affairs.

Gallup Inc. (2013). *In U.S., average retirement age up to 61.* Retrieved from www.gallup.com/poll/162560/average-retirement-age.aspx

Gallup Inc. (2018). *Snapshot: Average American predicts retirement age of 66.* Retrieved from https://news.gallup.com/poll/234302/snapshot-americans-project-average-retirement-age.aspx

Hendrix, S. (2011, June 23). Dogs' devotion helps heal vets' inner wounds. *Washington Post,* B1, B10.

Howe, M. C., and Briggs, A. K. (1982). Ecological systems model for occupational therapy. *American Journal of Occupational Therapy, 36*(5), 322–327.

Iwarsson, S., Stahl, A., and Carlsson, G. (2003). Accessible transportation: Novel occupational therapy perspectives. In L. Letts, P. Rigby, and D. Stewart (Eds.), *Using environments to enable occupational performance* (pp. 235–251). Thorofare, NJ: SLACK.

Job Accommodation Network. (2009). *A to Z of disabilities and accommodations.* Retrieved from http://jan.wvu.edu/media/atoz.htm

Johnson, E. (n.d.). *About me.* Retrieved from http://web.me.com/johnsonvillemelee/armyOTguy.com/About_Me.html

Jonsson, H. (2010). Occupational transitions: Work to retirement. In C. H. Christiansen and E. A. Townsend (Eds.), *Introduction to occupation: The art and science of living* (2nd ed., pp. 211–230). Upper Saddle, NJ: Pearson Education.

Jonsson, H., Josephsson, S., and Kielhofner, G. (2001). Narratives and experience in an occupational transition: A longitudinal study of the retirement process. *American Journal of Occupational Therapy, 55,* 424–432.

Kielhofner, G. (2008). *Model of human occupation: Theory and application* (4th ed.). Baltimore, MD: Lippincott, Williams and Wilkins.

Kohler, P. D., and Field, S. (2003). Transition-focused education: Foundation for the future. *Journal of Special Education, 37*(3), 174–183.

Korchok, K. (2008). Encore careers: How three 60-plus retirees swap retirement for flourishing fitness careers. *Fitness Trainer Canada,* 46–49.

Kuettel, A., Boyle, E., and Schmid, J. (2017). Factors contributing to the quality of the transition out of elite sports in Swiss, Danish, and Polish athletes. *Psychology of Sport, 29,* 27–39.

Leandro-França, C., Murta, S. G., Hershey, D. A., and Martins, L. B. (2016). Evaluation of retirement planning programs: A qualitative analysis of methodologies and efficacy. *Educational Gerontology, 42*(7), 497–512.

Long-Bellil, L., and Henry, A. D. (2009). Promoting employment for people with disabilities. *OT Practice, 14*(7), CE1–CE8.

McDaniel, M. L. (1968). Occupational therapists before World War II (1917–40). In H. S. Lee and M. L. McDaniel (Eds.), *Army Medical Specialist Corps* (pp. 69–97). Washington, DC: Office of the Surgeon General, Department of the Army. Retrieved from http://history.amedd.army.mil/corps/medical_spec/chapteriv.html

Milbourn, B., Saraswati, J., and Buchanan, A. (2018). The relationship between time spent in volunteering activities and quality of life in adults over the age of 50 years: A systematic review. *British Journal of Occupational Therapy, 81*(11), 613–623.

Moen, P., and Fields, V. (2002). Midcourse in the United States: Does unpaid community participation replace paid work? *Aging International, 27*(3), 21–48.

Murphy, W. M., and Volpe, E. H. (2014). Encore careers: Motivating factors for career exit and rebirth. In A. M. Broadbridge and S. L. Fielden, *Handbook of gendered careers in management* (pp. 425–444). Northampton, MA: Edward Elgar.

Nahemow, L. and Lawson, M. O. (1973). Toward an ecological theory of adaptation and aging. In W. Preiser (Ed.). *Environmental design research* (pp. 24–32). Stoudsburg, PA: Dowden, Huckison and Ross.

O*NET Resource Center. (2019). *O*NET Resource Center.* Retrieved from www.onetcenter.org

Orentlicher, M., and Michaels, C. (2000). Some thoughts on the role of occupational therapy in the transition from school to adult life: Part I. *American Occupational Therapy Association: School System Special Interest Section Quarterly, 7*(2), 1–4.

Organization for Economic Cooperation and Development. (2017). *Employment: Expected number of years in retirement by sex.* Retrieved from https://stats.oecd.org/index.aspx?queryid=54758

Pets for Vets. (2017). *Helping Veterans and pets create new beginnings together.* Retrieved from www.petsforvets.com/

Pew Research Center. (2016). *The state of American jobs: Changes in the American workplace.* Retrieved from www.pewsocialtrends.org/2016/10/06/1-changes-in-the-american-workplace/

Phan, A. M. (2018). *A study of the challenges of nonlinear career changers and a new service to ease the transition.* Retrieved from https://dspace.mit.edu/bitstream/handle/1721.1/118529/1054924928-MIT.pdf?sequence=1

Resource Centers on Independent Living. (n.d.). *Highlights of the final rule to amend the Department of Justice's regulation implementing Title II of the ADA.* Retrieved from http://reachcils.org/home/disability_info/2011-ada-changes.php4

Scaffa, M. E., Van Slyke, N., and Brownson, C. A. (2008). Occupational therapy in the promotion of health and the prevention of disease and disability. *American Journal of Occupational Therapy, 62*(6), 694–703.

Schaefers, K. G. (2012). Working for good: The encore career movement. *Career Planning and Adult Development Journal, 28*(2), 84–95.

Schlossberg, N. (2004). *Retire smart, retire happy: Finding your true path in life.* Washington, DC: American Psychological Association.

Siporin, S. (1999). Help wanted: Supporting workers with developmental disabilities. *OT Practice, 4,* 19–24.

Smoot, M., and Marterella, A. (2017). The occupational transition of athletic retirement: An emerging area of practice for the occupational therapy profession. *American Journal of Occupational Therapy, 71,* 7111505097p1. doi:10.5014/ajot.2017.71S1-PO2071

Stapleton, D. C., and Burkhauser, R. V. (Eds). (2003). *The decline in employment of people with disabilities: A policy puzzle.* Kalamazoo, MI: W. E. Upjohn Institute for Employment Research.

Stukas, A. A., Hoye, R., Nicholson, M., Brown, K. M., and Aisbett, L. (2016). Motivations to volunteer and their associations with volunteers' well-being. *Nonprofit and Voluntary Sector Quarterly, 45*(1), 112–132.

Ticket to Work and Work Incentive Improvement Act (TWWIIA) of 1999, PL 106–170, 42 U.S.C. §§1305 *et seq.*

United Nations Volunteers. (2018). *2018 state of the world's volunteerism report: The thread that binds, volunteerism and community resilience.* Retrieved from unv-swvr2018.org/files/51692_UNV_SWVR_2018_WEB.pdf

U.S. Army. (n.d.). *Warrior transition units.* Retrieved from www.army.mil/article/10671/warrior_transition_units

U.S. Bureau of Labor Statistics. (2015). *Labor force statistics from the current population survey.* Retrieved from www.bls.gov/cps/faq.htm#Ques5

U.S. Bureau of Labor Statistics. (2017). *Number of jobs, labor market experience, and earnings growth among Americans at 50: Results from a longitudinal survey.* Retrieved from www.bls.gov/news.release/pdf/nlsoy.pdf

Van der Horst, A. C., Klehe, U. C., and Van der Heijden, B. (2017). Adapting to a looming career transition: How age and core individual differences interact. *Journal of Vocational Behavior, 99,* 32–145.

Van Hoye, G., and Lootens, H. (2013). Coping with unemployment: Personality, role demands, and time structure. *Journal of Vocational Behavior, 82,* 85–95.

van Ingen, E., and Wilson, J. (2017). I volunteer, therefore I am? Factors affecting volunteer role identity. *Nonprofit and Voluntary Sector Quarterly, 46*(1), 29–46.

Voss, M., and Chen, J. (2015). Health status after job loss: Does the reason for job change matter? *Journal of Occupational and Environmental Medicine, 57*(12), 1319–1324.

Voss, M. W., Merryman, M. B., Crabtree, L., Subasic, K., Birmingham, W., Wadsworth, L., and Hung, M. (2018). Late career unemployment has mixed effects in retirement. *Journal of Occupational Science.* https://doi.org/10.1080/14427591.2018.1514645

Wagner, M., and Davis, R. (2006). How are we preparing students with emotional disturbances for the transition to young adulthood? Findings from the National Longitudinal Transition Study—2. *Journal of Emotional and Behavioral Disorders, 14*(2), 86–98.

Wagner, M., Newman, L., Cameto, R., Levine, P., and Garza, N. (2006). An overview of findings from wave 2 of the National Longitudinal Transition Study—2. Menlo Park, CA: SRI International. Retrieved from http://nlts2.org/reports/2006_08/

Wehman, P. (2001). *Life beyond the classroom: Transition strategies for young people with disabilities.* Baltimore, MD: Brookes.

Zhan, Y., Wang, M., Liu, S., and Shultz, K. S. (2009). Bridge employment and retirees' health: A longitudinal investigation. *Journal of Occupational Health Psychology, 14*(4), 374–389.

Chapter 17

Health Professional Well-Being

S. Maggie Reitz, PhD, OTR/L, FAOTA, Marjorie E. Scaffa, PhD, OTR/L, FAOTA, and S. Blaise Chromiak, MD

Our future depends on our ability to take care of ourselves both personally and professionally. Taking care of ourselves is the positive force that promotes the ability to seize opportunities for the future.

—Gilfoyle (1986, p. 387)

Learning Outcomes

This chapter is designed to enable the reader to:

17-1 Describe the characteristics of health professional well-being.

17-2 Describe health-care worksite risks to well-being with potential risk-reduction strategies.

17-3 Identify stressors common to all health professionals, as well as those unique to occupational therapy.

17-4 Discuss evidence-based microlevel, mesolevel, and macrolevel strategies to enhance resilience.

17-5 Identify theoretical frameworks that support occupation-based approaches to health professional well-being program development and evaluation.

Key Terms

Burnout
Compassion fatigue
Compassion satisfaction
Coping
Emotional intelligence
Gratitude
Hazard
Injury
Job engagement
Mindfulness
Moral distress
Professional self-care
Resilience
Risk factor
Self-compassion
Well-being

Introduction[1]

Professional codes of ethics guide and direct attention to the care, safety, and well-being of those served, including clients and students. Less visible in these professional documents is a description of the employer's responsibility for the well-being of its employees. The American Occupational Therapy Association (AOTA) *Occupational Therapy Code of Ethics (2015)* addresses employee well-being within Principle 2, nonmaleficence—prevention of harm—and Principle 6, fidelity—collegiality and safety (AOTA, 2015b). However, it does not

1. Portions of this chapter first appeared in Scaffa, M. E., Chromiak, S. B., Reitz, S. M., Blair-Newton, A., Murphy, L., and Wallis, C. B. (2010). Unintentional injury and violence. In M. E. Scaffa, S. M. Reitz, and M. A. Pizzi (Eds.), *Occupational therapy in the promotion of health and wellness* (pp. 350–375). Philadelphia, PA: F. A. Davis.

address the proactive support of employees' overall well-being.

Well-being is described by the World Health Organization (WHO, 2001) as a state "in which the individual realizes his or her own abilities, can cope with the normal stresses of life, can work productively and fruitfully, and is able to make a contribution to his or her community" (para. 3). The markers of well-being for health-care professionals are no different than those of the general population. Often-cited characteristics of well-being include, but are not limited to, building and maintaining positive and fulfilling relationships, receiving and providing emotional support, experiencing positive emotions, pursuing personal growth, engagement, and accomplishment, and participating in spiritual or other activities that provide meaning (Picco et al., 2017; Seligman, 2011).

The Triple Aim proposes that health-care systems pursue three aims: improving the health of populations, enhancing the patient experience of care, and reducing the per capita cost of health care (Berwick, Nolan, and Whittington, 2008). Burnout negatively affects patient care, satisfaction, and clinical outcomes and may contribute to higher costs due to the overuse of resources. As a result, some health-care providers are advocating that the Triple Aim become the Quadruple Aim. The fourth aim would be improving the work life and well-being of health-care professionals and staff (Bodenheimer and Sinsky, 2014). This fourth aim is supported by findings from a recent Gallup Poll that concluded, "Health-care workers who don't feel connected to their community or who are struggling with debt may find it difficult to focus on their patients or model healthy behaviors to them while they are at work" (Wood and Riffkin, 2015, p. 4).

Burnout, defined by Maslach and Leiter (2008), "is a psychological syndrome that involves a prolonged response to chronic interpersonal stressors on the job" that results in "feelings of being overextended and depleted of one's emotional and physical resources" (Maslach and Leiter, 2008, p. 498). The burnout syndrome consists of emotional exhaustion, depersonalization, cynicism, and a reduced sense of personal accomplishment (Maslach, 1982). Emotional exhaustion is characterized by feeling overextended and overwhelmed by job demands. Depersonalization is exemplified by detachment, indifference, and cynicism. A reduced sense of personal accomplishment is manifest by feelings of inadequacy, perceptions of failure, and decreased confidence (Maslach, 2003).

According to the National Academy of Medicine (NAM, 2016), physicians have double the suicide rate of the general public and twice the rate of burnout compared to workers in other fields. However, physicians are not the only health-care professionals at risk, as 24% of intensive care nurses reported symptoms of posttraumatic stress disorder related to their work. Although there is little data on other health-care professions, given the intense and continuous nature of contact with patients and the demands and pressures of health-care delivery, there is little reason to think that other professionals are not similarly affected (NAM, 2016). In one study of health-care professionals in Canada, 47% of occupational therapists rated their work as quite to extremely stressful. Occupational therapists in that study were ranked as the seventh most stressed health-care profession, behind family physicians, nurses, and medical lab technicians (Wilkins, 2007). Workplace fatigue in occupational therapists has been identified as an unrecognized threat to their health and well-being. There is a need to develop assessments and interventions to address this concern (Brown, Schell, and Pashniak, 2017).

Attention to the well-being of health-care professionals is important because emotional exhaustion negatively affects the quality and safety of health-care delivery. For example, research has shown emotional exhaustion to be an independent predictor of medical error (Shanafelt et al., 2010) and health care–associated infections (Cimiotti, Aiken, Sloane, and Wu, 2012). In addition, emotional exhaustion results in higher health-care costs due to staff turnover and lower job productivity. Burnout also produces significant personal suffering for health-care providers in the form of broken relationships, alcohol and substance abuse, depression, and suicide (Dyrbye et al., 2017).

The focus of this chapter is on health professional well-being—specifically, the risks to employee health and potential strategies to minimize risks and maximize well-being. Paying attention to the needs of health professionals improves retention and work performance and ultimately enhances client care, outcomes, and satisfaction.

Engage Your Brain 17-1

How can you enhance your well-being at school/work?

Health-Care Worksite Risks and Risk-Reduction Strategies

According to the National Institute for Occupational Safety and Health (NIOSH), "healthcare is the fastest-growing sector of the U.S. economy, employing over 18 million workers" (2018, para. 1). This large group of health-care workers, including occupational therapy practitioners, face risks that include injuries, allergies, infectious diseases, violence, and stress. Women are vastly overrepresented in this employment category, accounting for as much as 80% of the workforce (NIOSH, 2018); similarly, women make up the overwhelming majority of occupational therapy practitioners (AOTA, 2015a). This is important to note, as women tend to have more caregiving responsibilities for either aging parents, children, or both, further compounding the impact of an injury or infection.

In 2011, the NIOSH instituted the Total Worker Health® program in order to provide employers with needed resources to address the overall well-being of their employees through sharing evidence-based workplace strategies. These strategies include the development and implementation of policies and programs with the goal of positively affecting employees at the workplace, with secondary benefits reaped by families, communities, employers, and the nation through an enhanced economy (NIOSH, 2017b). Specifically, the trademarked program Total Worker Health® is defined as "policies, programs, and practices that integrate protection from work-related safety and health hazards with promotion of injury and illness prevention efforts to advance worker well-being" (NIOSH, 2017b, para. 1). There are numerous potential issues that can be addressed through this approach (see Fig. 17-1). The next section of this chapter will focus on the risks associated with working in a health-care setting, specifically injuries, infectious disease, and stress.

Engage Your Brain 17-2

Review Figure 17-1. Which of these issues are faced by occupational therapy practitioners in their workplace? Which of these issues can occupational therapy practitioners be viable partners with in crafting solutions?

Injuries

The prevention of employee injuries was a catalyst for the development of the Total Worker Health® program for health-care employees, as these employees are subject to a variety of potential injuries. An **injury** is defined as "unintentional or intentional damage to the body resulting from acute exposure to thermal, mechanical, electrical, or chemical energy or from the absence of such essentials as heat or oxygen" (U.S. Department of Health and Human Services, 2000, pp. 15–55). Injuries are a central factor in the health profile of the United States and a major threat to well-being and quality of life. They are clearly a public health concern and a highly preventable source of morbidity and mortality. Millions of people are temporarily incapacitated or permanently disabled due to unintentional injury—among them health-care workers, including occupational therapy practitioners. In fact, according to NIOSH (2018, para. 1.), "cases of nonfatal occupational injury and illness with healthcare workers are among the highest of any industry sector."

In 2013, the U.S. Department of Labor's Occupational Safety and Health Administration (OSHA) reported the top five causes of injury that resulted in hospital employees being absent from work (see Fig. 17-2). These include, in descending order of frequency:

- Overexertion and bodily reaction
- Slips, trips, and falls
- Contact with objects
- Violence
- Exposure to substances

OSHA also reported injury rates by health-care occupations, including the category "therapist." For this category, the frequency rates for missed work

Issues Relevant to Advancing Worker Well-being Through Total Worker Health®

Control of Hazards and Exposures
- Chemicals
- Physical Agents
- Biological Agents
- Psychosocial Factors
- Human Factors
- Risk Assessment and Risk Management

Organization of Work
- Fatigue and Stress Prevention
- Work Intensification Prevention
- Safe Staffing
- Overtime Management
- Healthier Shift Work
- Reduction of Risks from Long Work Hours
- Flexible Work Arrangements
- Adequate Meal and Rest Breaks

Built Environment Supports
- Healthy Air Quality
- Access to Healthy, Affordable Food Options
- Safe and Clean Restroom Facilities
- Safe, Clean and Equipped Eating Facilities
- Safe Access to the Workplace
- Environments Designed to Accommodate Worker Diversity

Leadership
- Shared Commitment to Safety, Health, and Well-Being
- Supportive Managers, Supervisors, and Executives
- Responsible Business Decision-Making
- Meaningful Work and Engagement
- Worker Recognition and Respect

Compensation and Benefits
- Adequate Wages and Prevention of Wage Theft
- Equitable Performance Appraisals and Promotion
- Work-Life Programs
- Paid Time Off (Sick, Vacation, Caregiving)
- Disability Insurance (Short- & Long-Term)
- Workers' Compensation Benefits
- Affordable, Comprehensive Healthcare and Life Insurance
- Prevention of Cost Shifting between Payers (Workers' Compensation, Health Insurance)
- Retirement Planning and Benefits
- Chronic Disease Prevention and Disease Management
- Access to Confidential, Quality Healthcare Services
- Career and Skills Development

Community Supports
- Healthy Community Design
- Safe, Healthy and Affordable Housing Options
- Safe and Clean Environment (Air and Water Quality, Noise Levels, Tobacco-Free Policies)
- Access to Safe Green Spaces and Non-Motorized Pathways
- Access to Affordable, Quality Healthcare and Well-Being Resources

Changing Workforce Demographics
- Multigenerational and Diverse Workforce
- Aging Workforce and Older Workers
- Vulnerable Worker Populations
- Workers with Disabilities
- Occupational Health Disparities
- Increasing Number of Small Employers
- Global and Multinational Workforce

Policy Issues
- Health Information Privacy
- Reasonable Accommodations
- Return-to-Work
- Equal Employment Opportunity
- Family and Medical Leave
- Elimination of Bullying, Violence, Harassment, and Discrimination
- Prevention of Stressful Job Monitoring Practices
- Worker-Centered Organizational Policies
- Promoting Productive Aging

New Employment Patterns
- Contracting and Subcontracting
- Precarious and Contingent Employment
- Multi-Employer Worksites
- Organizational Restructuring, Downsizing and Mergers
- Financial and Job Security

CDC NIOSH TOTAL WORKER HEALTH™

November 2015

Total Worker Health® is a registered trademark of the US Department of Health and Human Services

Figure 17-1 Issues relevant to advancing worker well-being through Total Worker Health®. *(From* Total Worker Health *[p. 1], by National Institute for Occupational Safety and Health, 2015.)*

were similar to all hospital employees, with the addition of transportation incidents, which were slightly less prevalent than "contact with objects" injuries, and a reduced exposure to violence.

According to the AOTA Salary and Workforce Survey (2015a), the primary work setting for 25.8% of occupational therapy practitioners is in long-term care (LTC) or skilled nursing facilities (SNFs). The two next most common employment sites are hospital settings (23.9%) and schools (19%). While it may seem obvious that occupational therapy practitioners working in LTC or SNF settings face similar risks as those employed by a hospital, it may be less apparent that occupational therapy practitioners working in schools also face these same types of injuries.

In California, school employees "have a higher-than-average rate of job-related injuries and illnesses when compared to all industries in California" (California Department of Industrial Relations Commission on Health and Safety Workers' Compensation, n.d., p. 2). School employees in California were reported to be at risk for injury from hazards such as:

- Chemical spills
- Ergonomics
- Infectious disease

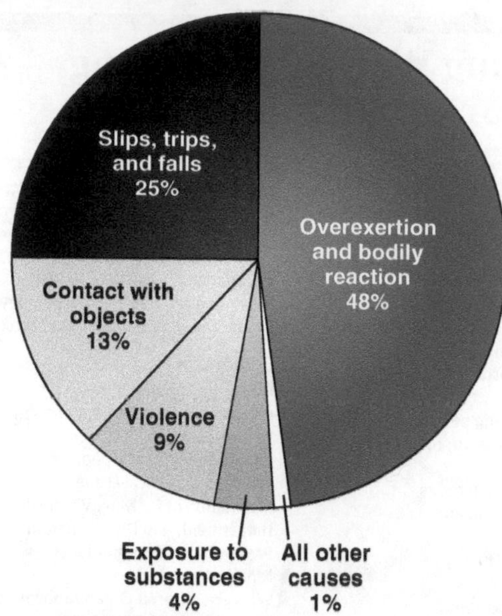

Data source: Bureau of Labor Statistics, 2011 data

Figure 17-2 Hospital workers' injuries resulting in days away from work, by event or exposure, 2011. *(From* Caring for Our Caregivers: Facts About Hospital Worker Safety *[p. 6], by Occupational Safety and Health Administration, 2013.)*

- Poor indoor air quality
- Trips, slips, and falls

Based on the Workforce Survey data (AOTA, 2015a) previously discussed, it is projected that nearly 69% of occupational therapy practitioners are at risk for similar injuries, with musculoskeletal injury a common risk across these three practice settings.

Risk-Reduction Strategies

Traditionally, injuries have been viewed as accidental and thus not preventable. This perspective allowed injuries to be seen as isolated problems of individual victims instead of as a public health concern. However, prevention is now viewed as the best strategy to address this problem. The consideration of risk factors should be part of planning a comprehensive prevention program initiative.

The WHO (2018, para. 1) defines a **risk factor** as

> *any attribute, characteristic or exposure of an individual that increases the likelihood of developing a disease or injury. Some examples of the more important risk factors are underweight, unsafe sex, high blood pressure, tobacco and alcohol consumption, and unsafe water, sanitation and hygiene.*

Haddon's matrix, developed by William Haddon Jr., a physician and engineer, is a matrix that conceptualizes injury as occurring in three phases: preinjury event, injury event, and postinjury event, in interaction with human factors, an agent or vehicle, and physical and sociocultural environments. A Haddon's matrix for health-care workers appears as Table 17-1. Levels of prevention correspond to the phases of the matrix. In the preinjury event phase, primary prevention efforts are appropriate—for example, speed limit enforcement to reduce motor vehicle crashes. During the injury event phase, secondary prevention is the focus—for instance, airbag deployment to reduce injury. In the postinjury event phase, tertiary prevention approaches are most relevant—for example, shortening emergency response times and improving the efficacy of rehabilitation (Christoffel and Gallagher, 2006). Haddon identified 10 categories of injury prevention strategies focused on addressing hazards.

A **hazard** is defined as the potential to cause harm, or a condition or activity that if not controlled could result in illness or injury (OSHA, 2002). Hazards typically fall into four broad categories: physical, chemical, biological, and psychological. Physical hazards include such things as radiation, noise, and poor working conditions. Chemical hazards may be naturally occurring or human-made, such as vapors and gases from industry and tobacco smoke. Biological hazards take the form of allergens, blood, bacteria, viruses, and other microbiological organisms. Psychological hazards are typically occurrences that induce unreasonably high levels of stress, such as exposure to violence (Agius, 2007).

Haddon's categories of injury prevention strategies, known as the Haddon Ten, include:

- Preventing the initial creation of a hazard
- Reducing the amount of energy a hazard contains
- Preventing the release of existing hazards
- Modifying the rate or distribution of a hazard
- Separating the hazard, by time or space, from the person

Table 17-1 Haddon's Matrix for Health-Care Workers

Phase	Health-Care Worker	Agent (cause of injury)	Physical Environment	Social/Economic Environment
Pre-event (Prepare)	Is the person predisposed or overexposed to risk? What is the person's level of experience working with the hazard? Worker's ability to use safety equipment and procedures effectively?	Is the agent hazardous? In what ways? Can the agent be modified?	What hazards are in the environment? Is it possible to reduce the hazards?	Does the environment encourage/discourage risk-taking? What are the workers' and administrators' attitudes toward risk? Record of safety policy and procedure enforcement? Use of safety incentives?
Intervention (Primary prevention)	Training in risk reduction, safety procedures, etc.	Modify the agent to enhance safety.	Modify the environment to enhance safety.	Social norming to reduce risk. Enforcement of safety policies and procedures. Incentivize safety.
Event (React/respond)	What is the person's overall health at the time of the incident? Severity of injury? Response time to the incident?	Does the agent provide protection? (e.g., syringe with safety shield) Functioning of safety equipment?	Does the physical environment contribute to injury during the event? Access to safety equipment?	Does the social environment contribute to injury during the event?
Intervention (Secondary prevention)	Provide fast, adequate emergency medical care to the staff person in the event of hazard exposure.	Ensure safety equipment is functional and staff are properly trained in use.	Ensure safety equipment is accessible with good signage in multiple languages as appropriate.	Train all staff in CPR and basic first aid to be able to respond effectively to injury of a coworker.
Postevent (Mitigate)	How severe is the trauma, injury, or harm to the person? Timely access to medical care?	Does the agent contribute to the trauma?	Does the physical environment contribute to recovery or add to the trauma after the event?	Does the social environment contribute to recovery or add to the trauma after the event?
Intervention (Tertiary prevention)	Medical treatment ASAP and follow-up to reduce potential secondary complications.	Containment of the hazard to prevent further injury.	Ensure that supplies for hazard containment are readily available.	Debriefing of all involved to determine what aspects of the response were effective and what changes should be made in advance of future incidents.

- Using material barriers to prevent exposure to a hazard
- Modifying qualities of a hazard to reduce its impact
- Increasing the person's resistance to damage from a hazard
- Countering the damage already done as quickly as possible
- Stabilizing, repairing, and rehabilitating the damage produced by a hazard (Christoffel and Gallagher, 2006, p. 158)

The most effective unintentional injury and violence prevention programs address all three phases (i.e., pre-event, event, and postevent) and components that could be changed (i.e., human factors, agent or vehicle, physical environment, and sociocultural environment) of the Haddon matrix and use a combination of education, engineering/environmental modification, and enforcement strategies (Christoffel and Gallagher, 2006).

Occupational therapists also can provide risk-reduction education and train persons to engage in activities in the safest manner possible. These strategies can be used as primary prevention (prior to the occurrence of any injury) and as secondary prevention to reduce the likelihood of reinjury.

As in most areas of prevention, the identification of risk and protective factors is critical. In injury prevention, occupational therapists are uniquely equipped to analyze daily activities in work, leisure, and self-care; to identify potential risk and protective factors; and to then design strategies to reduce the risk of injury. These strategies may include modifying environmental, equipment, and activity variables to increase safety in the workplace, decreasing individual risk factors for injury, and increasing protective factors. For example, in falls prevention, environmental and activity modifications and improving an individual's protective factors (motor strength and balance) decrease the risk of falls.

Reducing the risk of musculoskeletal injury is well within the scope of occupational therapy practice (AOTA, 2014, 2016). In addition, occupational therapy practitioners with expertise in ergonomics have the responsibility to provide preventative ergonomic education and strategies to all coworkers, including themselves and other occupational therapy practitioners. This self-responsibility is supported by the opening quote from Gilfoyle—to be able to heal others, time must be invested in one's own well-being.

Ergonomic consulting is especially needed in health-care settings. These work settings are anything but typical and may include a wide variety of jobs in addition to health-care providers—for example, office, food service, housekeeping, and security staff, among others. Workers of all types in health-care settings can benefit from an occupational therapist's ergonomic consultation by learning to reduce their risk of cumulative trauma disorders, especially those associated with ways to transfer clients safely and the rapid and repetitive pace of data entry on computer systems and keyboarding functions on other portable devices.

Occupational therapy students could offer ergonomic education and individual worksite evaluations to local health-care facilities and/or on their own campuses. Evidence-based literature such as the *AOTA Critically Appraised Topic (CAT) on Musculoskeletal Disorders* (AOTA, 2016) provides specific guidance for these types of interventions (see Box 17-1). Funding for injury prevention activities can be justified on the basis of the evidence and state and federal worksite health regulations.

BOX 17-1 Evidence-Based Workplace Interventions

- Ergonomic interventions (training, rest breaks, forearm supports, specially designed glasses, workstation redesign) increase work comfort.
- Ergonomic workstation redesign and training reduce days lost, pain prevalence and intensity, and injury rate among health-care workers.
- Changes in the workplace design, equipment, and organization reduce sickness absence in several occupational classifications.
- Participatory ergonomics reduces pain among workers.
- Web-based monitoring at work only may not be better than no intervention to reduce pain. Adding strengthening and relaxation exercises to a web-based monitoring program may have a positive effect on pain and on stress.

From *AOTA critically appraised topic (CAT) on musculoskeletal disorders* (p. 3), by American Occupational Therapy Association, 2016.

Infectious Diseases

When a previously unknown disease agent emerges, those who provide care are the ones most affected. According to the WHO, close to 10% of those who died from severe acute respiratory syndrome (SARS) were health-care workers, and over half of those sickened were health-care workers or students (Sepkowitz and Eisenburg, 2005). While the public, or parents of future health-care workers, might appreciate or be concerned about the risk health-care workers face when epidemics like Ebola or unknown diseases such as SARS strike, they might not consider the risks that a multitude of health-care workers face on a daily basis from a host of more common infectious agents, such as hepatitis B, multidrug-resistant tuberculosis (MDR-TB), and methicillin-resistant *Staphylococcus aureus* (MRSA). Infectious agents include bacteria, fungi, viruses, and parasites that have the ability to spread an infection or infectious disease. According to the NIOSH (2017a), health-care workers are at risk from the following infectious agents:

- Blood-borne pathogens (BBPs)
- Ebola
- Influenza
- Middle East respiratory syndrome (MERS)
- MRSA
- SARS
- TB

Sharps injuries, which include needlesticks, can transmit BBPs such as HIV, hepatitis B virus, and hepatitis C virus. The reported incident rates for this type of injury vary from 1.4 to 9.5 per 100 health-care workers; however, there is concern regarding possible underreporting of these types of incidents (Elseviers, Ariias-Guillén, Gorke, and Arens, 2014). The impact on a worker's well-being following a sharps injury includes the stress of undergoing immediate and long-term testing, waiting for results, and being treated if infected. The health-care system faces financial impacts from sharps injuries, including additional staffing to cover missed work, testing expenses, preventative or curative treatment regimens, and the time and cost of injury investigation and documentation (Elseviers et al., 2014).

Health-care workers are at risk of contracting infectious diseases from sharps injuries and other methods of disease transmission. TB continues to be a public health concern in the United States, with 9,272 cases reported by the Centers for Disease Control and Prevention (CDC) in 2016, for a total cost of $451,000,000 (CDC, 2017c). While health-care workers were found to be at higher risk than the general population for developing TB, following infection control measures when patients are suspected of having TB helps decrease the risk for health-care workers (Baussano et al., 2011). The good news is that there have only been two documented cases of MERS in the United States (CDC, 2017b), and cases of MRSA are decreasing (CDC, 2018a). Health-care workers have a major role to play in protecting themselves as well as other colleagues and patients in the prevention of infectious disease. While it may be impossible to prevent all infectious disease transmission, efforts can be taken to substantially decrease risk.

Risk-Reduction Strategies

Regardless of the infectious agent, the primary prevention strategy is education regarding specific risk-reduction techniques and the appropriate use of safety supplies and equipment. A less obvious primary prevention strategy is the consistent reporting and reviewing of data on infection rates at the institution or in the community, as well as at state, national, and global levels. While there is a goal of 100% prevention of the transmission of infectious diseases, an awareness of how an institution, community, or state compares to national and global norms is important in continuing to be vigilant and up to date on solutions. If there is an indication of exposure, then the secondary prevention technique of containment to avoid transmitting infection to a patient or professional colleague is of paramount concern. The CDC provides guidelines for isolation procedures, including a list of which infections require isolation (Siegel, Rhinehart, Jackson, Chiarello, and Healthcare Infection Control Practices Advisory Committee, 2007). While the cited document was written in 2007, it is updated electronically as needed to maintain currency, including immunization recommendations.

Occupational therapy practitioners in hospitals, skilled nursing facilities, home health settings, and school practice are all at risk of exposure to infectious

BOX 17-2 Workers' Rights

Workers have the right to:

- Working conditions that do not pose a risk of serious harm
- Receive information and training (in a language and vocabulary the worker understands) about workplace hazards, methods to prevent them, and the OSHA standards that apply to their workplace
- Review records of work-related injuries and illnesses
- File a complaint asking OSHA to inspect their workplace if they believe there is a serious hazard or that their employer is not following OSHA's rules. OSHA will keep all identities confidential.
- Exercise their rights under the law without retaliation, including reporting an injury or raising health and safety concerns with their employer or OSHA. If a worker has been retaliated against for using his or her rights, the worker must file a complaint with OSHA as soon as possible but no later than 30 days.

From *Bloodborne Pathogens and Needlestick Prevention,* by Occupational Safety and Health Administration (n.d.a, para. 6).

Figure 17-3 Clean Hands Count campaign. *(Courtesy of the* Clean Hands Campaign: Promotional Materials, *by Centers for Disease Control and Prevention, 2017.)*

diseases and are responsible for educating themselves and staff on the prevention and containment of infectious disease. There are many federal governmental organizations responsible for assisting with these efforts (e.g., NIOSH, OSHA). CDC guidelines (OSHA, n.d.c) address the isolation procedures referred to previously (Siegel et al., 2007), hand hygiene, and eye protection, among others. These guidelines provide guidance regarding actions that can be taken to minimize risk to health-care professionals. In addition to providing education and information on workers' risks, OSHA communicates workers' rights (OSHA, n.d.a), which can be found in Box 17-2.

Hand hygiene is a simple but very effective prevention strategy to decrease the transmission of infectious agents (CDC, 2018b), but "studies show that some healthcare providers practice hand hygiene less than half of the times they should" (CDC, 2016a, para. 9). The CDC, through its Clean Hands Count campaign materials, provides assistance to occupational therapy practitioners in educating themselves and colleagues about the importance of hand hygiene at work. One potential strategy is the annual celebration and acknowledgement of World Hand Hygiene Day, which is held at the beginning of May. The CDC provides free posters, stickers (see Fig. 17-3), and brochures to support these types of preventive educational activities (CDC, 2017a). Funding for infection control and prevention activities can be justified on the basis of state and federal worksite health regulations and the Workers' Rights outlined by OSHA.

Stress

Another threat to the well-being of health-care workers is stress. The source of this stress can include exposure to infectious diseases, productivity demands, insufficient staffing, role ambiguity, complex authoritarian management systems (CDC, 2008; OSHA, n.d.b), ethical dilemmas and moral distress that arise from being involved in decisions that have an impact on people's health and well-being, and burnout, which will be discussed in a later section of this chapter. In addition, stress can lead workers to leave their respective professions, which is of concern given the current workforce shortage of health-care professionals and the projected increased need in the future. According to the U.S. Bureau of Labor Statistics (BLS; 2018), "employment of occupational therapists is projected to grow 24 percent from 2016 to 2026, much faster than the average for all occupations" (para. 5).

The adverse effects of occupational stress can appear as psychological (e.g., irritability), behavioral (e.g., difficulty sleeping, attendance issues), and physical (e.g., headache; CDC, 2008). Stress takes a toll on the health of workers and their professional engagement in the workplace. "Some frequently reported consequences of stress among hospital workers are difficulties in communicating with very ill patients, maintaining pleasant relations with co-workers, and judging the seriousness of a potential emergency" (OSHA, n.d.b, para. 2). This can lead to compromised ethics and moral distress, which exacerbate stress. "**Moral distress** is tension that arises when a moral agent (e.g., a practitioner) is unsure of the best course of action to take or encounters a barrier that prohibits doing what" is known to be right (Erler, 2016).

A recent study of occupational therapy practitioners working in skilled nursing facilities examined the relationship between productivity demands and incidents of perceived moral distress (Smith-Gabal, Kuzminski, and Eldridge, 2018). No difference was found between occupational therapists and occupational therapy assistants in levels of moral distress. While the researchers did not find a statistically significant relationship between productivity demands and perceived level of moral distress, the average score indicated a minimal to moderate level of moral distress. Expectations that were linked to the highest level of moral distress include (Smith-Gabal et al., 2018, p. 25):

- "Being expected to obtain as many billable units as possible per client regardless of individual client needs"
- "Being unable to provide optimal therapy services because of limited insurance coverage or insurance cutoffs reported"
- "Being expected to treat and/or write documentation for more clients than time allows"

In addition, they found a statistically significant relationship in levels of moral distress between those who were planning on leaving their position versus those who were staying. Smith-Gabal et al. (2018) recommend that moral distress be recognized and addressed through strategies to improve communication, increase professional development opportunities, and enhance coping skills. Additional risk-reduction strategies are discussed in the next section.

Risk-Reduction Strategies

Recommended risk-reduction strategies for health-care workers include organizational change interventions and stress management interventions (CDC, 2016b). Organizational change interventions recommended by the CDC (2016b) include:

- Involvement of employees in all aspects of planning and evaluating the intervention with a focus on team processes
- Use of interdisciplinary health-care teams
- Multipronged interventions that include risk assessment

OSHA (n.d.b, para. 3) suggestions that would fall under this category include:

- "Address work-related stressors such as inadequate work space, unreasonable work load, lack of readily available resources, inadequate and unsafe equipment"
- "Recognize and take action on legitimate concerns regarding overbearing physicians and supervisors"
- Establish employee assistance programs and organizational change programs
- Provide greater flexibility with job assignment, hours, and alternative job arrangements

The case studies at the end of this chapter discuss the use of walking meetings, which could be an organizational strategy to decrease the occupational stress of health-care workers. Providing ethics training and ethics rounds (Erler, 2016) and developing and implementing training for supervisors on techniques to reduce worker stress (NIOSH, 2017b) are other examples of organizational strategies.

Suggestions from OSHA (n.d.b, para. 3) that would fall under the second category of risk-reduction strategies, stress management interventions, include:

- "Educate employees . . . about job stress"
- Establish and maintain stress-management programs
- "Provide readily available counseling from a nonjudgmental source"
- Provide group therapy for specific job-related stressors (e.g., death of patients)
- Use of relaxation exercises and biofeedback until stress source is identified

The AOTA (2018) has articulated the profession's role in addressing stress, trauma, and posttraumatic stress disorder. Occupational therapy practitioners would be an integral part of any interdisciplinary team effort to address workplace stress within the health-care or school setting in which they work. In addition, occupational therapy practitioners can apply stress-reduction techniques, including occupation-based strategies, to enhance their own professional well-being. The next section explores professional self-care, a broader technique to decrease work stress and maintain well-being as an occupational therapy practitioner or other health-care professional.

Improving the Well-Being of Health-Care Professionals

In addition to the worksite risks for injury and infectious diseases, health-care professionals are also at risk for compassion fatigue and burnout due to the stress they experience in their daily work. The impact of burnout on individual health-care professionals includes increases in instances of anxiety, depression, disrupted sleep, substance abuse, marital discord, early retirement, and, as mentioned earlier, suicide rates. Patients and coworkers are also affected by working with physicians and other health-care professionals who are burned out. Medical errors, team disruptions, and angry interactions with patients have been reported (Kumar, 2016). Stressors in the health-care work environment that lead to burnout include, but are not limited to, new payment and health-care delivery approaches, electronic health records, publicly reported quality of care metrics, excessive workloads, inadequate staffing, and decreased autonomy and lack of control over work processes (Dyrbye et al., 2017). Specific stressors related to occupational therapy reported by Lloyd and King (2001) include staff shortages, work overload, role ambiguity, lack of recognition and support from colleagues, and low visibility of the occupational therapy profession.

Resilience is protective against compassion fatigue and burnout. **Resilience** refers to "patterns of positive adaptation during or following significant adversity or risk" (Masten, Cutuli, Herbers, and Reed, 2009, p. 118). Resilience is not an intrinsic enduring trait of an individual but rather a dynamic, adaptive process throughout the life span that can be learned. Factors that contribute to resilience can be internal and/or external. Internal factors include personality traits such as optimism, beliefs such as self-efficacy, and skills such as adaptive coping. External factors refer to environmental resources (material and energy) and the access to and stability of those resources over time (Chmitorz et al., 2018). Social factors also contribute to resilience and include feelings of connectedness to the people around us. For health-care workers, mutual trust and connectedness to colleagues has a significant impact on resilience and protects against burnout (McKenna, Hashimoto, Maguire, and Bynum, 2016).

A resilient health-care professional is one who has "the ability to maintain personal and professional well-being in the face of ongoing work stress and adversity" (McCann et al., 2013, p. 61). Resilience consists of two complementary types of behaviors: preventive and corrective. Preventive behaviors are those activities someone engages in that protect from burnout and help the person resist adversity. Corrective behaviors are those activities a person engages in that help the individual cope effectively with stressful conditions (Beresin et al., 2016). Resilience enhances the practitioner's likelihood of experiencing **compassion satisfaction,** defined as the joy and fulfillment a person derives from helping other people (Rossi et al., 2012). In general, when levels of compassion satisfaction are high, there is less risk of burnout (Smart et al., 2014).

Compassion fatigue (CF), the opposite of compassion satisfaction, is defined as "an emotional state with negative psychological and physical consequences that emanate from acute or prolonged caregiving of people stricken by intense trauma, suffering, or misfortune" (Bush, 2009, p. 28). CF is a direct result of a caregiver ignoring the symptoms of personal stress combined with inattention to personal emotions over time. One of the most insidious features of CF is its attack on a key element of occupational therapy practice, the practitioner's empathy and the ability to show compassion (Mathieu, 2007).

CF presents with signs that are similar to common, everyday difficulties such as stress. It is important for the practitioner to be able to recognize the following signs and symptoms (Mathieu, 2007; Negash and Sahin, 2011):

- Trouble sleeping/exhaustion
- Increased emotional reactivity/hypersensitivity to emotional material
- Hypervigilance or heightened sensitivity to potential threats to self
- Diminished interest in regular activities
- Reduced ability to feel empathy
- Anger and irritability
- Absenteeism (work, family event, social events) or poor work skills
- Difficulty separating work life from personal life

Emotional exhaustion is known to be the primary product of CF and can lead to difficulties with creating a genuine empathic relationship with clients, which in turn can negatively affect the delivery of services (Negash and Sahin, 2011). Furthermore, loss of empathy can have a negative impact on the development of therapeutic relationships. These symptoms not only affect the practitioner at work but also carry over to other contexts, such as home and family. CF, if unaddressed, can become burnout.

Burnout is conceptualized as a transaction between the characteristics of the work environment and the characteristics of the health-care worker. Burnout develops when the cumulative stress of the job overcomes the person's ability to cope and problem-solve effectively. This process can produce a variety of negative consequences for the individual and the worksite. Physical symptoms may include chronic fatigue, headaches, muscle pain, insomnia, hypertension, and gastrointestinal disorders. Psychological manifestations may include feelings of helplessness, anxiety, and depression, as well as difficulties with concentration, memory, and decision-making (Gonzalez-Gutierrez et al., 2004). Behavioral manifestations may include absenteeism, poor work performance, aggression, defensiveness, social withdrawal, substance use, and risk-taking behavior (Costa, 2018). The stages of burnout development are presented in Box 17-3.

Gupta, Paterson, Lysaght, and von Zweck (2012) examined burnout experiences and coping strategies used by occupational therapists. They reported high levels of emotional exhaustion (34.8%), high levels of cynicism (43.5%), and low professional efficacy (24.6%) among Canadian occupational therapists. The coping strategies used by occupational therapists included self-awareness and self-monitoring, spending time with family and friends, striving for a personal and work-life balance, and maintaining a sense of humor. In a study on burnout by Painter, Akroyd, Elliot, and Adams (2003), occupational therapists reported higher levels of emotional

BOX 17-3 Stages of Burnout

Stage 1: A compulsion to prove oneself
Stage 2: Working harder to meet one's own high expectations
Stage 3: Neglecting basic personal self-care needs
Stage 4: Displacement and the inability to recognize and deal with the source of one's distress
Stage 5: Revision of values and the dismissal of once-important relationships and activities
Stage 6: Denial of emerging problems, intolerance, cynicism, and aggression
Stage 7: Withdrawal, isolation, loss of hope or direction, escape through alcohol or drug use
Stage 8: Behavioral changes obvious to family and friends and increasing feelings of worthlessness
Stage 9: Depersonalization and a loss of emotional connectedness to self and others
Stage 10: Pervasive feeling of inner emptiness that may lead to addictive behaviors, such as gambling, overeating, compulsive sexual behavior, and drug and alcohol abuse
Stage 11: Depression, loss of meaning, apathy, and hopelessness
Stage 12: Burnout, total mental and physical collapse, potential for suicide, a need for immediate medical and psychological attention

Adapted from "The Burnout Cycle," by H. J. Freudenberger and G. North, 2006, *Scientific American MIND, 17*(3), 31.

exhaustion, lower levels of depersonalization, and higher levels of personal accomplishment that were statistically significant when compared to the Maslach Burnout Inventory norms. Levels of emotional exhaustion varied by work settings, with occupational therapists working in chronic care (long-term care, rehabilitation, and psychiatric settings) reporting the highest levels as compared to occupational therapists working in acute care hospitals, outpatient clinics, schools, and home health settings.

Professional identity appears to be protective against burnout. In a study of occupational therapists, Edwards and Dirette (2010) found that practitioners who had a strong professional identity exhibited lower levels of burnout than those who were not confident in their ability to define the role of occupational therapy at their worksite. Luken and Sammons (2016) advocate that occupational therapy practitioners be aware of their own risk factors and susceptibility to burnout and use objective measures to assess their own levels of burnout. Interventions are different for each of the three components of burnout, and therefore interventions need to be tailored to the specific component of burnout being addressed. This is an opportunity for "occupational therapy practitioners to heed their own advice to monitor and maintain occupational balance and well-being" (Luken and Sammons, 2016, p. 7).

The antithesis of burnout is job engagement. **Job engagement** is conceptualized as an "energetic state of involvement with personally fulfilling activities that enhance one's sense of professional efficacy" (Maslach and Leiter, 2008, p. 498). Characteristics of engagement include pleasurable engrossment with work tasks (similar to the concept of flow), enthusiasm, persistence, and a sense of professional efficacy, satisfaction, and success with work. Both burnout and engagement are affected by both individual and organizational factors. According to a model developed by Schaufeli and Bakker (2004), overwhelming job demands combined with inadequate resources can produce burnout, which can cause mental and physical health problems and lead to employee turnover. However, job resources facilitate engagement and decreased turnover. The authors suggest that different intervention strategies should be used to reduce burnout and enhance job engagement.

Health-Care Provider Well-Being Models

In 2017, the National Academy of Medicine (NAM) initiated the Action Collaborative on Clinician Well-Being and Resilience, designed to address health-care provider well-being and prevent burnout. The project is a collaboration of more than 60 organizations and has the following goals:

1. Improve baseline understanding of challenges to clinician well-being
2. Raise the visibility of clinician stress and burnout
3. Elevate evidence-based, multidisciplinary solutions that will improve patient care by caring for the caregiver (NAM, 2018, para. 6)

The NAM created a model that can be applied to a variety of health-care professionals, work settings, and career stages. The model depicts the individual and organizational/environmental factors that affect clinician well-being and resilience (see Fig. 17-4). This holistic model captures the relationship between the patient and the clinician and the complex interaction of factors that affect professional well-being and thereby have an impact on patient care. The three concentric circles in the center of the diagram form the nucleus and represent (from the inside outward) patient well-being, the clinician-patient relationship, and clinician well-being. Individual and external factors that affect clinician well-being and resilience encircle the nucleus. Individual factors include health-care role, personal factors, and skills and abilities. Environmental factors include sociocultural factors; regulatory, business, and payer environment; organizational factors; and learning/practice environment. The factors are not listed in any hierarchy, as the intent is for users to determine the salience of these features for each specific situation. The purpose of the model is to guide research on clinician well-being and the development of effective intervention strategies at individual, organizational, and systems levels (Brigham et al., 2018).

The Stanford (University) Physician Wellness Model identifies personal resilience, efficiency of practice, and a culture of wellness as determinants of well-being, the interaction of which promotes

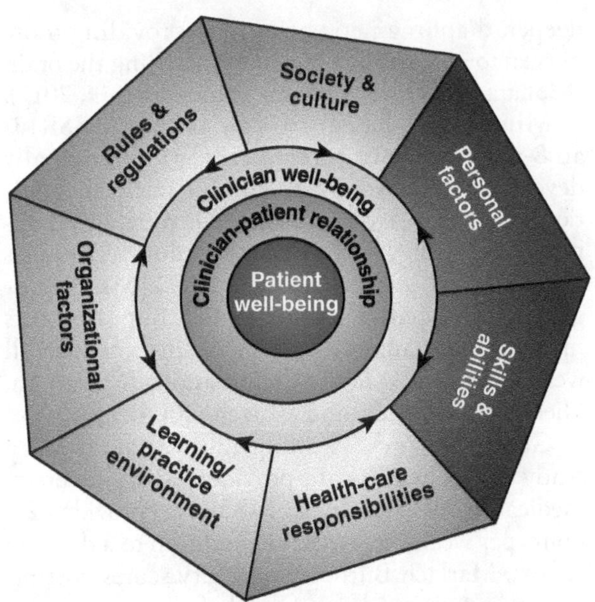

Figure 17-4 Clinician well-being model: factors affecting clinician well-being and resilience. *(Adapted from the National Academy of Medicine Collaboration on Clinician Well-Being and Resilience, cited in "A Journey to Construct an All-Encompassing Conceptual Model of Factors Affecting Clinician Well-Being and Resilience" [p. 3], by Brigham et al., 2018, Washington, DC. Reproduced with permission.)*

professional fulfillment. Professional fulfillment in this model refers to "happiness or meaningfulness, self-worth, self-efficacy, and satisfaction at work" (Trockel, Hamidi, Murphy, Purpur de Vries, and Bohman, 2017, p. 2). This model is similar to the NAM model in that it emphasizes the interaction of internal (personal resilience) and external factors (efficiency of practice and culture of wellness) that affect clinician well-being. A culture of wellness is exemplified by an organizational and work environment that promotes values and behaviors consistent with "self-care, personal and professional growth, and compassion for ourselves, our colleagues, and our patients" (Trockel et al., 2017, p. 2).

Prevention and Intervention Strategies

Prevention and intervention programs to reduce burnout and enhance resilience can be directed at the individual, the worksite or organization, the community or system, or some combination of these. The causes of professional burnout are multifactorial, and therefore, single interventions are not likely to be successful. Multidimensional, multilevel approaches are more apt to be effective. Best practice dictates that interventions to prevent and reduce burnout and enhance resilience simultaneously occur at the micro- (individual), meso- (worksite), and macro- (socio-cultural-political) levels.

Salazar and Beaton (2000) propose an ecological approach that addresses the context in which occupational stress occurs. The context consists of four levels, each generating unique occupational stressors and providing opportunities for intervention:

- The microsystem, consisting of the individual and immediate work environment
- The organizational system, including the physical structures, organizational culture, and policies and procedures
- The periorganizational system or societal influences on the worker and the organization
- The extraorganizational system, including customs, cultures, traditions, and government policies that affect the worker and the organization

These levels are not discrete entities; their boundaries are blurred, and they are in constant dynamic interaction, influencing each other. Improving health-care outcomes for patients and providers requires attention to each level (WHO, 2002).

Most of the research to date has focused on individual or microsystem resilience, with less attention given to the organizational system and even less to the socio-cultural-political context (periorganizational and extraorganizational systems) in which the health-care practitioner is working (Montgomery, 2014).

Microsystem Individual-Level Strategies

Professionals who care for their mind, body, and spirit generally will provide better care for clients, thereby increasing both client and practitioner satisfaction. Attending to one's own health and wellness needs is often referred to as professional self-care.

In its most basic form, **professional self-care** means engaging in behaviors and activities that increase energy, lower stress, and contribute to health and well-being. The exact combination of behaviors and activities may vary from person to person, but there are some basic recommendations that are universal. These include restful sleep, good nutrition, and adequate physical activity. In addition, social support enhances resilience and is an important contributor to emotional well-being (Ozbay et al., 2007). People who have positive, fulfilling relationships live longer, healthier lives (Seligman, 2011). There are a variety of evidence-based strategies for preventing burnout and building personal and professional resilience, including active coping, mindfulness, yoga, gratitude, and self-compassion. Through the exploration and practice of professional self-care strategies, occupational therapy students can prevent burnout and increase resilience before entering the health-care workforce.

Coping can be described as "conscious, volitional efforts to regulate emotion, cognition, behavior, physiology, and the environment in response to stressful events or circumstances" (Compas, Connor-Smith, Saltzman, Thomsen, and Wadsworth, 2001, p. 89). Coping strategies can be problem-focused or emotion-focused. Problem-focused coping involves planning and engaging in specific behaviors to overcome or solve the problem causing the distress. Emotion-focused coping addresses the feelings associated with stressful situations and can be active or avoidant. Examples of active emotion-focused coping strategies include positive reappraisal, relaxation techniques, emotional support from others, use of humor, and prayer or meditation. Avoidant emotion-focused coping involves avoiding distress through denial, distraction, behavioral disengagement, or escape (i.e., use of substances). The behaviors will vary depending on the nature of the problem, but soliciting instrumental support from others is a strategy that is often employed (Carver and Scheier, 1994).

Mindfulness is "the awareness that emerges through paying attention, on purpose, and nonjudgmentally to the unfolding of experience moment by moment" (Kabat-Zinn, 2003, p. 145). Mindfulness practices include sitting and walking meditations, breath training, and body scans. Breath training modifies shallow or quick breathing into deeper, diaphragmatic breathing, providing more oxygen to all tissues of the body, including the brain (Moharana, Lipika, Moharana, and Pattnaik, 2017).

Mindfulness-based stress reduction (MBSR) is an 8-week evidence-based intervention, originally developed for persons with chronic medical conditions, that teaches mindfulness meditation, diaphragmatic breathing, and other relaxation techniques (Kabat-Zinn, 1990). In a meta-analysis, MBSR programs consistently demonstrated improvements in depression, anxiety, quality of life, and overall well-being in a variety of populations (Grossman, Niemann, Schmidt, and Walach, 2004).

Goodman and Schorling (2012) conducted a study of 93 health-care providers at a university medical center. Training in MBSR was provided 2.5 hours per week for 8 weeks in addition to a daylong retreat. Maslach Burnout Inventory scores postintervention improved significantly from preintervention scores on the emotional exhaustion (p less than 0.03), personal accomplishment (p less than 0.001), and depersonalization (p less than 0.04) scales. In addition, mental well-being scores on the SF12v2 also improved significantly (p less than 0.001).

In an effort to reduce the in-person time spent in MBSR and to make the training more accessible off-site, Bazarko, Cate, Azocar, and Kreitzer (2013) evaluated the effectiveness of an alternative hybrid format with nurses. The intervention consisted of two full-day retreats, one at the beginning of the intervention and the other at the end, augmented by six group teleconference calls in between. Statistically significant improvements were noted in perceived stress, mindfulness, empathy, mental health, vitality, social functioning, self-compassion, and burnout. The improvements were either sustained or continuing to improve at a 4-month postintervention follow-up, demonstrating the effectiveness of this scalable, affordable, and sustainable novel format (Bazarko et al., 2013). Based on the evidence to date, it is recommended that occupational therapy students, educators, and practitioners consider the use of mindfulness training as a preventive intervention for burnout (Luken and Sammons, 2016).

Yoga is an ancient practice that originated in India. Derived from Sanskrit word roots, *yoga* means unity and refers to the union of mind and body and the union of individual and universal consciousness. This union is achieved through the practice of asana

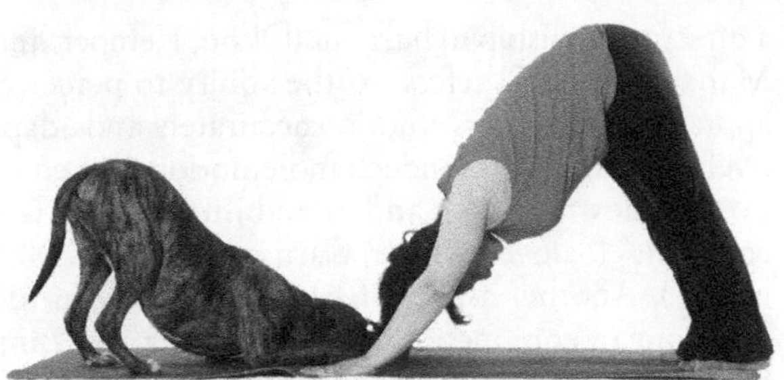

Figure 17-5 Yoga Downward Dog pose. *(Photo courtesy of ErharYaksaa and Wikimedia Commons.)*

(physical postures) and pranayama (breath control). The ultimate aim of yoga is self-awareness. The practice of yoga reduces stress levels and prevents autonomic dysregulation. Participants in yoga report decreased mental and emotional distress, improved quality and duration of sleep, and an enhanced sense of well-being (Moharana et al., 2017; Simard and Henry, 2009).

Yoga has been shown to increase parasympathetic activity and the sedating effects of the neurotransmitter GABA in the brain, producing a relaxation response and feelings of calmness and tranquility (see Fig. 17-5). Yogis believe that "through a flexible body we gain a flexible mind. This helps people become more patient, forgiving, less prone to anger and sadness" (Shroff and Asgarpour, 2017, p. 132). Other benefits of yoga include:

- A more positive outlook on life
- Increased efficiency at work and job satisfaction
- Enhanced self-confidence, self-sufficiency, and sociability
- Healthier interpersonal relationships
- More effective responses to life challenges (Shankar, 2007)

In a randomized, controlled trial of university personnel, Hartfiel, Havenhand, Khalsa, Clarke, and Krayer (2011) assessed the effectiveness of a 6-week yoga intervention for moderating workplace stress. Yoga instruction was provided 1 hour per week during the workday at no charge. In comparison to the wait-list control group, yoga participants reported increased self-confidence during stressful situations and a greater sense of life purpose and satisfaction. Significant improvements were also noted in emotional well-being and resilience. Hartfiel et al. (2011) suggested that employers consider offering yoga classes on-site to reduce workplace stress and build resilience in employees. Similar results were found for nurses who participated in an 8-week workplace yoga intervention. Yoga participants reported higher levels of health-promoting lifestyle behaviors and mindfulness and less emotional exhaustion and depersonalization than those in the control group (Alexander, Rollins, Walker, Wong, and Pennings, 2015).

Gratitude is an emotional response based on the recognition that one has received an unexpected and unmerited benefit due not to one's own efforts but to the good intentions of another person (Emmons and McCullough, 2003). Gratitude is both a state or temporary reaction and a trait or enduring characteristic. State gratitude is an emotional response to a specific situation; trait gratitude is a predisposition toward the experience of gratefulness (Watkins, Van Gelder, and Frias, 2009).

Higher levels of gratitude are protective against stress and depression and contribute to resilience and well-being (Wood, Maltby, Gillett, Linley, and Joseph, 2008). Gratitude improves sleep (Emmons and McCullough, 2003; Wood, Joseph, Lloyd, and Atkins, 2009), enhances adaptive coping (Wood, Joseph, and Linley, 2007), and strengthens relationships (Algoe, 2012). Positive emotions like gratitude are also associated with improved immune system function, lower cortisol levels in response to stress, decreased risk of cerebrovascular accidents, and cardiovascular benefits (Fredrickson and Losada, 2005).

Gratitude can be cultivated through a variety of evidence-based practices, including keeping a gratitude journal, writing and delivering a letter of gratitude to someone you had not previously thanked, mindfulness, and meditation. Mindfulness helps focus attention, thereby increasing appreciation for the simple blessings in life. Putting gratitude in writing magnifies and sustains the positive emotions that promote resilience and well-being. Gratitude is a practice that requires discipline. It is "systematically paying attention to what is going right in one's life, to see the contributions that others make in these good things, and then expressing gratitude verbally and behaviorally" (Emmons and Stern, 2013, p. 853).

Self-compassion is treating oneself with the same care, concern, and acceptance you would show a family member or good friend. **Self-compassion** is "being kind and understanding toward oneself in instances of pain or failure rather than being harshly self-critical" (Neff, Kirkpatrick, and Rude, 2007, p. 139). Self-compassion consists of three components:

- Self-kindness versus self-judgment
- Common humanity versus isolation
- Mindfulness versus overidentification

Self-kindness refers to the ability to provide warm, nonjudgmental understanding to oneself when confronting feelings of inadequacy or failure rather than berating oneself for perceived personal shortcomings. Self-compassion also requires the recognition that humans are imperfect, all people make mistakes, and imperfection is part of a common humanity. Finally, this process also involves a balanced mindful objectivity toward one's painful emotions, so the feelings are neither repressed and unacknowledged nor amplified and exaggerated (Neff et al., 2007).

According to Gilbert (2005), self-compassion deactivates the neurophysiological threat system in response to feelings of insecurity and defensiveness and activates the self-soothing system to generate feelings of safety and secure attachment. Research has demonstrated that brief self-compassion training, when compared to placebo, dampens sympathetic nervous system reactivity and produces adaptive parasympathetic cardiac activity, reducing the damaging psychobiological responses to stress (Arch et al., 2014).

Self-compassion also positively correlates with life satisfaction, healthy relationships, adaptive psychological functioning, and resilience. Mindfulness-based stress-reduction training and loving-kindness meditation have been shown to increase self-compassion in health-care professionals (Raab, 2014). A study of first-year residents in pediatric and combined medicine-pediatric residencies demonstrated that self-compassion and mindfulness were positively associated with resilience and inversely related to the emotional exhaustion component of burnout.

Emotional intelligence (EI) was also positively correlated with resilience but did not appear to have a direct relationship to burnout (Olson, Kemper, and Mahan, 2015). EI refers to "the ability to perceive, appraise, and express emotion accurately and adaptively; the ability to understand emotion and emotional knowledge . . . and the ability to regulate emotions" (Salovey, Mayer, Caruso, and Yoo, 2009, p. 237). Another aspect of EI is the ability to use emotions in conjunction with cognitive processing for problem-solving and creativity. In addition to resilience, EI is also positively correlated with higher-quality personal relationships, social competence, and subjective happiness (Salovey et al., 2009).

Mesosystem Worksite/ Organizational-Level Strategies

Employers are responsible for providing a safe and hazard-free worksite; however, there is much more to a healthy work environment. The CDC promotes workplace health programs that are "a coordinated

PROGRAM SHOWCASE

Although this program was developed by and for medical students, it can be used as a model for other health professional students. The following description was provided by Tyler Kaelin, third-year medical student.

The Wellness Program in the College of Medicine at the University of South Alabama is a student-led initiative to enhance all aspects of health and well-being among our medical students and to cultivate a community of comradery and resiliency. With physician burnout at an all-time high, it is crucial for medical students to develop healthy and sustainable habits while in medical school that they can carry with them into the workplace.

Competent and compassionate physicians keep patient well-being at the center of their practice. With this in mind, a major contributor to patient well-being is a clinician's understanding and mastery of their own personal well-being. We strive to place medical students at the center of our efforts, to promote self-awareness, and to teach strategies for enhancing well-being so students can provide competent and compassionate care in the future.

Although medical school is a stressful time with a variety of challenges, students can lead full and well-balanced lives during their education and develop resiliency through maintaining personal priorities and embracing challenges with optimism. We hope that the resources and events we provide for our students will not only support them during their time in medical school but also serve them well into their futures as thriving medical professionals.

The Wellness Program has several components, including Wellness Houses, a mentorship program, the Wellness Council, and health and wellness counseling.

Wellness Houses and House Mentors

During orientation, each incoming student is assigned to one of five virtual Wellness Houses, which they will remain in for the duration of medical school. Each house bears the name of a river that empties into Mobile Bay—for example, Blakeley, a tribute to our institution's mission of providing "the highest quality healthcare for the citizens of Alabama and the Central Gulf Coast region." Each Wellness House has house mentors, faculty members who are committed to seeing students excel both in and outside the classroom. House mentors serve not only as career and academic mentors for their house but also as "house parents" who play an integral role in cultivating an encouraging and uplifting home away from home. Throughout the year, Wellness Houses compete against one another in various drives and events, gather for dinners and socials, and help foster comradery among classmates.

Mentorship Program

Shortly after arriving to the College of Medicine, each incoming student will be matched with a student mentor from the preceding class. This matching process is based on personality and mutual interests, both personal and professional. Mentors act as a point of contact for practical information such as recommended academic resources, study habits, transitioning to life in Mobile, Alabama, and more.

Wellness Council and Student Leadership

The Wellness Council is the guiding body for the Wellness Program. Consisting of medical students and faculty advisors, the Wellness Council advocates for medical student wellness by creating initiatives and events for students, overseeing the Wellness Houses, and increasing awareness of barriers to wellness. The Wellness Council sends student representatives to serve on other College of Medicine committees (e.g., Student Affairs Committee, Curriculum Committee) to keep student wellness in mind while making fundamental and formative decisions for the College of Medicine.

Health and Wellness Counseling

The health and wellness counselor for the College of Medicine provides the following services:

- Confidential counseling—individual, couples, and group. Students do not need to have an identified mental health problem to be seen by the counselor, although these clinical mental health services are offered. Students come to counseling for a variety of reasons, including improving their health and wellness and increasing resiliency.
- Monthly wellness forums covering topics such as managing the transition to medical school, emotional well-being, healthy relationships, and mindfulness.
- Mental health first aid training for medical students to enhance their ability to identify and respond to mental health concerns and emergencies.

Examples of Wellness-Sponsored Events

Below are examples of events and initiatives that have been sponsored by the Wellness Program during the past academic year:

- Annual College-Wide Fall Cookout
- Wellness House dinners
- Bowling and laser tag nights
- Mentor/mentee lunches
- Breakfast and coffee before lectures
- Biweekly book club
- Yoga classes
- Self-Care Month

and comprehensive set of strategies which include programs, policies, benefits, environmental supports, and links to the surrounding community designed to meet the health and safety needs of all employees" (CDC, 2016b, para. 6). The CDC workplace health model, depicted in Figure 17-6, consists of four steps—assessment, planning and management, implementation, and evaluation—and emphasizes the need for individual, organizational, and community evaluation and intervention.

The Mayo Clinic may be the best example of organizational leadership engaged in efforts to reduce burnout and promote job engagement. Although the strategies used by the Mayo Clinic were directed at physician well-being, there is no reason to believe they could not be generalized to other health professionals.

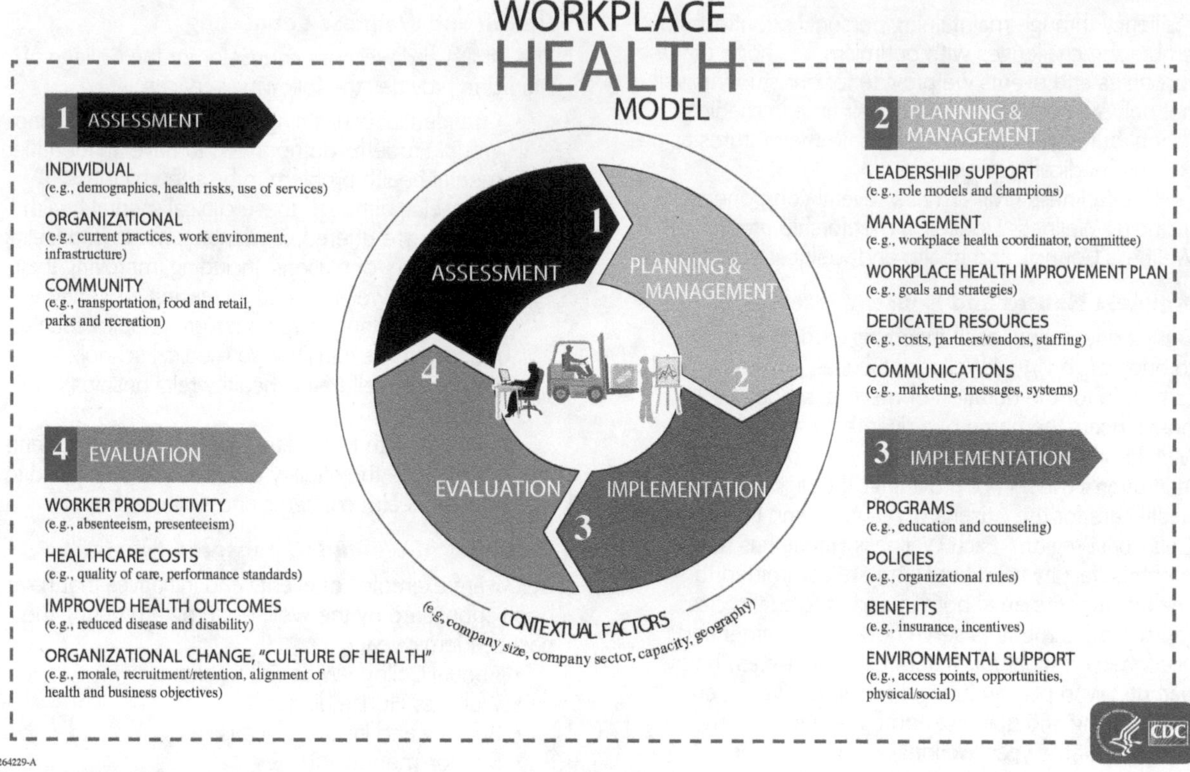

Figure 17-6 Workplace health model. *(From* Workplace Health Model *[para. 4], by Centers for Disease Control and Prevention, 2016.)*

Organizational strategies implemented by the Mayo Clinic that demonstrated significant impact included targeting interventions to each specific work group based on needs, cultivating community at work, promoting flexibility and work-life integration, and providing resources to promote professional self-care and resilience. Funding was provided to routinely measure changes in burnout, engagement, professional fulfillment, emotional health, and quality of life. The data are compared to national benchmarks and used to set goals and design interventions for identified work units. Cultivating community at work facilitates peer support. Toward this end, the Mayo Clinic created spaces and protected time for physicians to meet with colleagues and engage in semistructured and unstructured discussions. A variety of options for work schedules were adopted to encourage work-life balance while still meeting the labor needs of the organization (Shanafelt and Noseworthy, 2017).

The Healthy Work Place (HWP) Study, a cluster randomized controlled trial, was designed to assess whether improvements in work conditions reduced clinician burnout. Participants in the study consisted of 34 primary care clinics and 166 primary care clinicians (i.e., physicians, physician assistants, nurse practitioners). Baseline data were collected on clinicians' perceptions of work conditions (i.e., organizational structure, workflow, job characteristics, leadership, policies and procedures) and clinician stress, burnout, job satisfaction, and intent to leave the practice. Interventions were tailored to each specific primary care setting based on the data collected. Results indicated that burnout decreased among clinicians in the intervention group but increased among clinicians in the control group. In addition, there was a statistically significant improvement in clinician satisfaction in the intervention group. The three interventions that had the largest impact were workflow redesign,

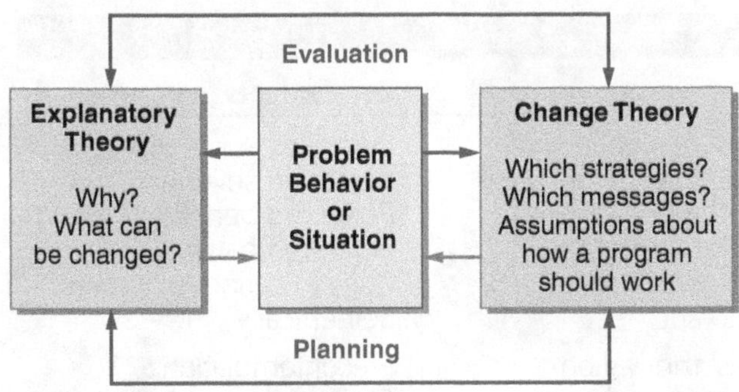

Figure 17-7 Using explanatory theory and change theory to plan and evaluate programs. *(From Figure 1 in* Theory at a Glance *[2nd ed., p. 6], by National Cancer Institute, 2005.)*

improved communication among clinicians and staff, and quality improvement projects addressing clinician concerns. This research demonstrates that organizational change can reduce stress, decrease burnout, and increase health-care professional satisfaction (Linzer et al., 2015).

Macrosystems Periorganizational- and Extraorganizational-Level Strategies

The macrosystem of health care consists of federal and state agencies, legislatures, accreditation organizations, and third-party payers, among others. These entities create policies, procedures, and regulations that directly affect health-care providers. This is the level at which overall values, principles, and strategies for health-care develop and where decisions concerning resource allocation occur (WHO, 2002, pp. 34–35). As such, this level has significant impacts on both the mesosystem (organizational) and microsystem (individual) levels in health care.

Macrosystems-level strategies to prevent burnout and build resilience are rarely addressed in the literature yet may be the most important of all. Productivity expectations, certification requirements, reduced practitioner autonomy, regulatory requirements, quality metrics, documentation requirements, and electronic health records are examples of occupational stressors at the macrosystem or periorganizational and extraorganizational levels. The demands of increased documentation, increased patient loads, evening and weekend intakes, progress evaluations, and discharges have added stress to occupational therapy practitioners' professional role and lifestyle. More research on macrosystems-level strategies for burnout prevention is clearly needed.

Development of Theory-Based Health Professional Well-Being Programs[2]

The *Occupational Therapy Practice Framework* (AOTA, 2014) supports engagement in health promotion activities by occupational therapy practitioners. The description of the occupational therapy process and specific interventions such as advocacy, self-advocacy, and group interventions are particularly relevant for developing programming to enhance the well-being of health-care professionals. The framework is an excellent starting point but is not entirely sufficient to guide the development of intervention programs for health-care workers. In addition to the framework's language and occupational therapy process description, a theory-based foundation is also required to support the development and implementation of evidence-based interventions for this population.

In addition to occupational therapy theoretical frameworks, those from other disciplines can also be useful tools in occupational therapy health promotion at the worksite or population level. Health behavior theories are particularly relevant and can be divided into two major types: explanatory and change (National Cancer Institute [NCI], 2005). Figure 17-7 shows the relationship between these types of health behavior theories. Explanatory theory, also referred to as *theory of the problem,* seeks to discover why a health condition exists and to

2. Portions of this section first appeared in Reitz, S. M., Scaffa, M. E., Campbell, R. M., and Rhynders, P. A. (2010). Occupational therapy conceptual models for health promotion practice. In M. E. Scaffa, S. M. Reitz, and M. A. Pizzi (Eds.), *Occupational therapy in the promotion of health and wellness* (pp. 22–45). Philadelphia, PA: F. A. Davis.

Table 17-2 Summary of Theories

	Theory	Focus	Key Concepts
Individual Level	Health Belief Model	Individuals' perceptions of the threat posed by a health problem, the benefits of avoiding the threat, and factors influencing the decision to act	Perceived susceptibility Perceived severity Perceived benefits Perceived barriers Cues to action Self-efficacy
	Stages of Change Model	Individuals' motivation and readiness to change a problem behavior	Precontemplation Contemplation Decision Action Maintenance
	Theory of Planned Behavior	Individuals' attitudes toward a behavior, perceptions of norms, and beliefs about the ease or difficulty of changing	Behavioral intention Attitude Subjective norm Perceived behavioral control
	Precaution Adoption Process Model	Individuals' journey from lack of awareness to action and maintenance	Unaware of issue Unengaged by issue Deciding about acting Deciding not to act Deciding to act Acting Maintenance
Interpersonal Level	Social Cognitive Theory	Personal factors, environmental factors, and human behavior exert influence on each other	Reciprocal determinism Behavioral capability Expectations Self-efficacy Observational learning Reinforcements
Community Level	Community Organization	Community-driven approaches to assessing and solving health and social problems	Empowerment Community capacity Participation Relevance Issue selection Critical consciousness
	Diffusion of Innovations	How new ideas, products, and practices spread within a society or from one society to another	Relative advantage Compatibility Complexity Trialability Observability
	Communication Theory	How different types of communication affect health behavior	Example: *Agenda Setting* Media agenda setting Public agenda setting Policy agenda setting Problem identification, definition Framing

From Table 11 in *Theory at a Glance* (2nd ed., p. 45), by National Cancer Institute, 2005, Bethesda, MD: National Institutes of Health.

identify modifiable factors (e.g., access to resources, attitudes, knowledge, self-efficacy). The health belief model, discussed in Chapter 3, is an example of an explanatory theory. Change theory, also known as *theory of action,* is useful to direct the decision-making around program interventions. Diffusion of innovation, which is also described in Chapter 3, is an example of this type of theory. Health behavior theories can also be classified according to their potential target: individuals, groups, or communities. Table 17-2 identifies and classifies the most prominent health behavior models currently applied in the United States (NCI, 2005). They are categorized as addressing health issues at the individual level, the interpersonal level, or the community level.

An occupational therapy theoretical framework that may be particularly useful for developing an individual-level professional self-care plan is the Kawa model. The Kawa model was developed by a Japanese Canadian occupational therapist, working with a group of Japanese occupational therapists, with the goal of designing an Eastern-influenced model for occupational therapy practice (Iwama, 2005b). *Kawa* is the Japanese word for *river.* In the model, a free-flowing river represents the ideal life (i.e., maximal life flow). The names of the constructs—for example, *mizu* (water), *iwa* (rocks), *ryboku* (driftwood)—reflect an East Asian philosophical perspective, including beliefs from Buddhist, Confucian, and Taoist philosophical orientations (Iwama, 2005a, 2006b, 2006c).

The Kawa model was developed within a social structure that values interdependence and the collective more than independence and the self. Within this context, both self and occupation are imbedded in nature in a manner that precludes separation. The three-dimensional aspects of the model can assist with visually identifying assets and liabilities through nontraditional techniques such as drawing and sculpting.

The Kawa model has been used at the individual level to promote the well-being and decision-making of an occupational therapy practitioner in her continuing professional development planning (Tripathi and Middleton, 2018). The Kawa model was used to assist in a self-assessment process of the barriers to continuing education and the practitioner's readiness to take on additional leadership responsibilities. Maintaining a sense of professional competence and professional growth is part of a professional self-care plan, which was discussed earlier. The Kawa model has shown promise as a professional and personal tool for self- and team development (Tripathi and Middleton, 2018).

Based on the use of the Kawa model reported by Tripathi and Middleton (2018) and the substantial work of the Kawa model's developer (Iwama, 2006), the authors of this chapter developed the *Self-Care Worksheet for Personal Planning and Accountability Based on the Kawa Model.* This worksheet is displayed in Figure 17-8. The premise is that users would utilize this worksheet to review their past (i.e., the 2-year period prior to starting their current position), current, and projected river or life flow on a routine basis as a mechanism to plan for personal growth and to hold themselves accountable for those plans. Contextual features such as policies (i.e., the river walls and the river bottom) that can adversely influence the best of plans need to be considered and appreciated. The review-pattern timing (e.g., quarterly, annually) should be established the first time the worksheet is completed. Ideally, the completed worksheet would lead to a drawing, painting, or sculpture of the river, which can then be photographed and stored digitally for future reference and comparison. This depiction of the model's constructs helps illuminate the interrelationship between the river's features and reenvision potentials. It is recommended that prior to using the model, either the seminal work (Iwama, 2006) or the website (Kawa model, 2016) developed to archive research on the model be explored.

Summary

- The characteristics of well-being for health-care professionals are no different than those of the general population. Aspects of well-being include building and maintaining positive and fulfilling relationships, receiving and providing emotional support, experiencing positive emotions, pursuing personal growth, engagement, and accomplishment, and participating in activities that provide meaning.
- Health-care workers face many risks to their well-being, including injuries, exposure to infectious disease, and high levels of stress. Risk-reduction strategies include education,

Past River Flow (Consider the two-year period prior to starting your current position)				
Water (life flow)				
Driftwood (attributes and resources)				
Rocks (challenges)				
Spaces and gaps (potential places to leverage driftwood to disrupt rocks and increase life flow)				
River walls and bottom (environmental structures embedded or surrounding other elements)				
Assess the past flow of your river (highlight the box that corresponds to your self-assessment)				
Very strong, unencumbered	Strong, with a few barriers	Moderate, with significant barriers	Weak and slow	Very weak, barely moving at all
Self-reflection				

Figure 17-8 Self-care worksheet for personal planning and accountability based on the Kawa model.

monitoring and surveillance, and employee input into risk-reduction programming.

- Stressors in the health-care work environment that lead to burnout include, but are not limited to, new payment and health-care delivery approaches, electronic health records, publicly reported quality of care metrics, excessive workloads, inadequate staffing, and decreased autonomy and control over work processes. Additional stressors specifically related to occupational therapy include staff shortages, work overload, role ambiguity, lack of recognition, and low visibility of the profession.
- Causes of professional burnout are multifactorial, and therefore multidimensional, multilevel approaches are most effective. Best practice dictates that interventions to prevent and reduce burnout and enhance resilience simultaneously occur at the micro- (individual), meso- (worksite) and macro- (socio-cultural-political) levels.
- A variety of explanatory theories and change theories combined with occupation-based approaches can support the development and evaluation of interdisciplinary health professional well-being programs.

<table>
<tr><th colspan="5">Current River Flow</th></tr>
<tr><td colspan="2">Water (life flow)</td><td colspan="3"></td></tr>
<tr><td colspan="2">Driftwood (attributes and resources)</td><td colspan="3"></td></tr>
<tr><td colspan="2">Rocks (challenges)</td><td colspan="3"></td></tr>
<tr><td colspan="2">Spaces and gaps (potential places to leverage driftwood to disrupt rocks and increase life flow)</td><td colspan="3"></td></tr>
<tr><td colspan="2">River walls and bottom (environmental structures embedded or surrounding other elements)</td><td colspan="3"></td></tr>
<tr><td colspan="5">Assess the current flow of your river (highlight the box that corresponds to your self-assessment)</td></tr>
<tr><td>Very strong, unencumbered</td><td>Strong, with a few barriers</td><td>Moderate, with significant barriers</td><td>Weak and slow</td><td>Very weak, barely moving at all</td></tr>
<tr><td colspan="5">Self-reflection</td></tr>
<tr><td colspan="2">Action Steps—What changes can you make to increase the free flow of your river?
(At time of the next review, reflect on planned action steps and incorporate as driftwood or rocks.)</td><td colspan="3"></td></tr>
</table>

Continued

Future River Flow	
Water (life flow)	
Driftwood—What future attributes or resources do you anticipate (additional degree, certification, pay cut, promotion)?	
Rocks—What future new challenges do you anticipate (company downsizing, planned joint replacement surgery)?	
Spaces and gaps (potential places to leverage driftwood to disrupt rocks and increase life flow)	
River walls and bottom (environmental structures embedded or surrounding other elements)	
Self-reflection	

Figure 17-8 *cont'd*

CASE STUDIES

CASE STUDY 17-1 Walking Meetings: Multitasking for Health

Veronica was recently promoted from an occupational therapy floor supervisor to the administrative head of the rehabilitation department in a large suburban hospital. At lunch Veronica was bemoaning the fact that she was having difficulty achieving her daily 10,000 steps goal since she was no longer actively engaged in providing care and supervising students and junior occupational therapy personnel on four different floors. Veronica also expressed concern that she did not have sufficient time to get to know Jill, the administrative assistant responsible for managing the clerical and transportation staff of the department and overseeing the budget. Veronica was overheard by Stacy, an occupational therapist and the director of the hospital's community health outreach programs. In addition to her master's degree in occupational therapy, Stacy had a degree in health education and was well versed in health behavior change theories (see Chapter 3). During Stacy's next monthly supervision meeting with Veronica, she mentioned that she had overheard her lunch conversation and suggested that Veronica might want to consider

CASE STUDY 17-1 **Walking Meetings: Multitasking for Health**

Table 17-3 Walking Meetings

Positives/Benefits	Negatives/Barriers
Stimulates creativity (University of California, Riverside [UCR], n.d.)	Meeting size must be small, two to four people (UCR, n.d.)
Fresh air and light improve physical/mental well-being (UCR, n.d.)	Requires planning for appropriate footwear and clothing (UCR, n.d.)
Allows mind to become more flexible (UCR, n.d.)	If there are mobility issues, walking meetings could be a challenge (UCR, n.d.)
Increases confidentiality/privacy (UCR, n.d.)	Inclement weather (UCR, n.d.)
Provides chance to incorporate movement during the day (UCR, n.d.)	Walking is bad for convergent thinking (Ward, 2017)
Physical activity energizes and increases alertness (UCR, n.d.)	Preset course could hinder benefits (Ward, 2017)
Benefits collaborative performance (Ward, 2017)	Time pressure of busy working day (Gilson, McKenna, and Cooke, 2008)
Increases communication between coworkers (Chelik, 2017)	Hard to integrate if there is a large volume of desk-based work (Gilson et al., 2008)
Decreases risk of diseases (Chelik, 2017)	Not considered the "norm" or an accepted practice (Gilson et al., 2008)
Improves cardiovascular health (Chelik, 2017)	Management culture (Gilson et al., 2008)
Promotes higher levels of engagement (Clayton, Thomas, and Smothers, 2017)	Avoid high-calorie destinations that can negatively affect health benefits from walking (Clayton et al., 2017)
Fosters more honest exchanges with employees (Clayton et al., 2017)	
More productive than traditional sit-down meetings (Clayton et al., 2017)	
Resolves interpersonal tensions (Gilson, McKenna, and Cooke, 2008)	
Better coping with low or sad feelings (Gilson et al., 2008)	

starting weekly walking meetings with Jill. Stacy shared the pros and cons of walking meetings and strategies to maximize the benefits from this type of meeting format with Veronica (see Table 17-3).

The following week, on a fine fall day, Stacy saw Veronica and Jill walking the perimeter of the hospital complex. She noted both were wearing sensible shoes, sunglasses, and sun hats and seemed to be smiling while they conversed. Jill used her phone to take notes while Veronica made sure that Jill was looking when they approached a crosswalk. Stacy pondered whether the hospital would be interested in her providing a hospital-wide service on the health benefits of walking meetings and tips for successful walking meetings.

CASE STUDY 17-1 Walking Meetings: Multitasking for Health

Discussion Questions

1. Review the theoretical frameworks presented in Chapter 3. Which occupational therapy and which non–occupational therapy framework do you think best supports the walking meeting suggestion offered by Stacy to Veronica?
2. Would this be the same framework you would use for establishing a hospital-wide walking meeting program? Why or why not?
3. What additional work would you need to complete before proposing a hospital-wide walking meeting program?

CASE STUDY 17-2 Interdisciplinary Approach to Health Promotion for Health Professionals

In her new role, Veronica was expected to attend the hospital board of directors' meetings. At the first meeting she attended, the hospital's current and past annual report using *OSHA Form 300A: Summary of Work-Related Injuries and Illnesses* was shared. This summary reports "number of cases, number of days away from work/transferred/restricted, and number of each type of injury and illness" (OSHA, 2013, p. 23). Veronica was surprised at the escalating incident rate of musculoskeletal injuries and the fact that they were higher than state and national rates. The following week Veronica met with Joe, the vice president of Finance, who was responsible for risk management and human resources, to further review the data shared with the directors and to address their request to establish a task force to review current employee training regarding body mechanics and slip, trip, and fall prevention strategies and compare to best practices.

Engage Your Brain 17-3

Who would you include in the Task Force and why?

Veronica thought that Stacy would be an excellent member of the task force based on her knowledge of body mechanics, patient education, and health behavior change theories. Joe agreed and suggested that Langston, the head of Human Resources, cochair the task force with Veronica.

Other members appointed to the task force included:

- Amy, a nurse who had recently returned to work following a back strain
- Jerri, the human resources benefits and training specialist
- Jerome, a senior physical therapist
- Bethany, the public relations and communications director
- Sharon, the housekeeping supervisor
- Bart, the employee health and safety manager

The task force was given 6 months to issue a report with recommendations to address the following specific charge from the hospital's Board of Directors:

> *The Injury Reduction Task Force is charged to review the Hospital's annual report and trend data on employee musculoskeletal injuries and current employee training regarding body mechanics, with a focus on patient transfers and environmental causes for slips, trips, and falls. In addition, the Task Force should evaluate the pros and cons for investing in contracting a third-party vendor to develop preventive programming and procedures or to utilize the expertise of current hospital personnel to complete this work. A list of recommendations and accompanying rationale should be presented to the Hospital Board within 6 months.*

Prior to the first meeting, Stacy and Joe met to select a theoretical framework, establish the agenda for the first meeting, and identify reading

CASE STUDY 17-2 Interdisciplinary Approach to Health Promotion for Health Professionals

assignments to be completed prior to that meeting. Stacy and Joe selected the PRECEDE-PROCEED framework (Green and Kreuter, 2005) and the model of human occupation (MOHO, Taylor, 2017) as potential theoretical models to guide the review and structure of the recommendations. Reading assignments included the hospital's annual report, trend data on employee musculoskeletal injuries and current employee training regarding body mechanics, an introductory reading about the PRECEDE-PROCEED framework (Wasilewski, Mateo, and Sidorovsky, 2007), an OSHA (2013) report on hospital worker safety titled *Caring for Our Caregivers: Facts About Hospital Worker Safety,* and articles about the success of zero lift programs (Black, Shah, Busch, Metcalfe, and Lim, 2011; Charney, Simmons, Lary, and Metz, 2006; Chhokar et al., 2005).

Discussion Questions

1. If the Injury Reduction Task Force was given a broader charge that included overall employee safety and well-being, who else would you suggest to add to the task force?
2. Would the same combination of theoretical approaches work to address this new broader charge?
3. What other theoretical frameworks could be used to guide the support of either the original charge or the expanded charge?
4. Are there any ethical principles for Jill and Joe to consider if the hospital wanted to offer health promotion programming to other health-care providers in the region?

Learning Activities

1. Create a list of people, places, things, and activities that energize you and a list of people, places, things, and activities that exhaust you. The more energizers you have access to, the less likely you are to experience burnout. The goal is to increase your number of energizers and decrease your exhausters to the fullest extent possible.
2. Go to the Substance Abuse and Mental Health Services Administration (SAMHSA) website (www.integration.samhsa.gov/about-us/MaslachScoringAbbreviated.pdf) and download a copy of the Abbreviated Maslach Burnout Inventory. Take the assessment (substituting the word *occupational therapist* for *doctor*) to determine your level of burnout and develop a personal prevention or intervention plan as appropriate.
3. Reflective exercise from Costa (2018): "Each day, try to identify at least one positive event that you could classify as a joy of practice. Write it down in a journal and you will find that, over time, the cumulative effect will be to focus more on the positive than on the negative" (p. 14).
4. Review the health and well-being benefits offered by your employer or a potential future employer. Are there any benefits missing that are important to you? If so, consider what actions are available to either thank the employer or advocate for change.

REFERENCES

Agius, R. (2007). *Stress and work: Introduction to occupational stress.* Retrieved from www.agius.com/hew/resource/stress.htm

Alexander, G. K., Rollins, K., Walker, D., Wong, L., and Pennings, J. (2015). Yoga for self-care and burnout prevention among nurses. *Workplace Health and Safety, 63*(10), 462–470.

Algoe, S. B. (2012). Find, remind, and bind: The functions of gratitude in everyday relationships. *Social and Personality Psychology Compass, 6,* 455–469.

American Occupational Therapy Association. (2014). Occupational therapy practice framework: Domain and process (3rd ed.). *American Journal of Occupational Therapy, 68*(Suppl. 1), S1–S48. doi:10.5014/ajot.2014.682006. doi:10.5014/ajot.2014.682006

American Occupational Therapy Association. (2015a). *2015 AOTA Salary and Workforce Survey.* Bethesda, MD: AOTA Press.

American Occupational Therapy Association. (2015b). Occupational therapy code of ethics (2015). *American Journal of Occupational Therapy, 69*(Suppl. 3), 6913410030. http://dx.doi.org/10.5014/ajot.2015.696S03

American Occupational Therapy Association. (2016). *AOTA critically appraised topic (CAT) on musculoskeletal disorders.* Retrieved from www.aota.org/~/media/Corporate/Files/Secure/Practice/CCL/MSD/CAT_MSD_Worker_Pain.pdf

American Occupational Therapy Association. (2018). AOTA's societal statement on stress, trauma, and posttraumatic stress disorder. *American Journal of Occupational Therapy, 72*(Suppl. 2), 7212410080. https://doi. org/10.5014/ajot.2018.72S208

Arch, J. J., Warren-Brown, K., Dean, D. J., Landy, L. N., Brown, K., and Laudenslager, M. L. (2014). Self-compassion training modulates alpha-amylase, heart rate variability, and subjective responses to social evaluative threat in women. *Psychoneuroendocrinology, 42,* 49–58. http://doi.org/10.1016/j.psyneuen.2013.12.018

Baussano, I., Nunn, P., Williams, B., Pivetta, E., Bugiani, M., and Scano, F. (2011). Tuberculosis among health care workers. *Emerging Infectious Diseases, 17*(3), 488–494.

Bazarko, D., Cate, R. A., Azocar, F., and Kreitzer, M. J. (2013). The impact of an innovative mindfulness-based stress reduction program on the health and well-being of nurses employed in a corporate setting. *Journal of Workplace Behavioral Health, 28*(2), 107–133. http://doi.org/10.1080/15555240.2013.779518

Beresin, E. V., Milligan, T. A., Balon, R., Coverdale, J. H., Louie, A. K., and Roberts, L. W. (2016). Physician well-being: A critical deficiency in resilience education and training. *Academic Psychiatry, 40*(1), 9–12. https://doi.org/10.1007/s40596-015-0475-x

Berwick, D. M., Nolan, T. W., and Whittington, J. (2008). The Triple Aim: Care, health, and cost. *Health Affairs, 27,* 759–769. http://dx.doi.org/10.1377/hlthaff.27.3.759

Black, T. R., Shah, S. M., Busch, A. J., Metcalfe, J., and Lim, H. J. (2011). Effect of transfer, lifting, and reposition (TLR) injury prevention program on musculoskeletal injury among direct care workers. *Journal of Occupational and Environmental Hygiene, 8,* 226–235.

Bodenheimer, T., and Sinsky, C. (2014). From triple to quadruple aim: Care of the patient requires care of the provider. *Annals of Family Medicine, 12*(6), 573–576.

Brigham, T., Barden, C., Dopp, A. L., Hengerer, A., Kaplan, J., Malone, B., . . . Nora, L. M. (2018). A journey to construct an all-encompassing conceptual model of factors affecting clinician well-being and resilience. *NAM Perspectives.* Discussion Paper. Washington, DC: National Academy of Medicine. doi:10.31478/201801b

Brown, C. A., Schell, J., and Pashniak, L. M. (2017). Occupational therapists' experience of workplace fatigue: Issues and actions. *Work, 57,* 517–527.

Bush, N. J. (2009). Compassion fatigue: Are you at risk? *Oncology Nursing Forum, 36*(1), 24–28. doi:10.1188/09.ONF.24–28.

California Department of Industrial Relations Commission on Health and Safety Workers' Compensation. (n.d.). *SASH School Action for Safety and Health: Promoting safe and healthy workplaces for California's school employees.* Retrieved from www.dir.ca.gov/chswc/SASH/Publications/SASH_brochure.pdf

Carver, C. S., and Scheier, M. F. (1994). Situational coping and coping dispositions in a stressful transaction. *Journal of Personality and Social Psychology, 66,* 184–195.

Centers for Disease Control and Prevention. (2008). *Exposure due to stress: Occupational hazards in hospitals.* Retrieved from www.cdc.gov/niosh/docs/2008–136/pdfs/2008–136.pdf

Centers for Disease Control and Prevention. (2016a). *Hand hygiene in healthcare settings: Show me the science.* Retrieved from www.cdc.gov/handhygiene/science/index.html

Centers for Disease Control and Prevention. (2016b). *Workplace health model.* Retrieved from www.cdc.gov/workplacehealthpromotion/model/index.html

Centers for Disease Control and Prevention. (2017a). *Clean Hands Campaign: Promotional materials.* Retrieved from www.cdc.gov/handhygiene/campaign/promotional.html

Centers for Disease Control and Prevention. (2017b). *MERS in the U.S.* Retrieved from www.cdc.gov/coronavirus/mers/us.html

Centers for Disease Control and Prevention. (2017c). *Take on TB.* Retrieved from www.cdc.gov/tb/publications/infographic/pdf/take-on-tuberculosis-infographic.pdf

Centers for Disease Control and Prevention. (2018a). *General information about MRSA in healthcare settings.* Retrieved from www.cdc.gov/mrsa/healthcare/index.html

Centers for Disease Control and Prevention. (2018b). *Hand hygiene in healthcare settings.* Retrieved from www.cdc.gov/handhygiene/index.html

Charney, W., Simmons, B., Lary, M., and Metz, S. (2006). Zero lift programs in small rural hospitals in Washington state: Reducing back injuries among health care workers. *American Association of Occupational Health Nursing Journal, 54*(8), 355–358.

Chelik, A. (2017, March). *How walking meetings improve productivity.* American Council on Exercise. Retrieved from www.acefitness.org/education-and-resources/professional/expert-articles/6348/how-walking-meetings-improve-productivity

Chhokar, R., Engst, C., Miller, A., Robinson, D., Tate, R. B., and Yassi, A. (2005). The three-year economic benefits of a ceiling lift intervention aimed to reduce healthcare workers injuries. *Applied Ergonomics, 36,* 223–229.

Chmitorz, A., Kunzler, A., Helmreich, I., Tuscher, O., Kalisch, R., Kubiak, T., . . . Lieb, K. (2018). Intervention studies to foster resilience—a systematic review and proposal for a resilience framework in future intervention studies. *Clinical Psychology Review, 59,* 78–100.

Christoffel, T., and Gallagher, S. S. (2006). *Injury prevention and public health: Practical knowledge, skills and strategies* (2nd ed.). Gaithersburg, MD: Jones and Bartlett.

Cimiotti, J. P., Aiken, L. H., Sloane, D. M., and Wu, E. S. (2012). Nurse staffing, burnout, and health care-associated infection. *American Journal of Infection Control, 40,* 486.

Clayton, R., Thomas, C., and Smothers, J. (2017, September 27). *How to do walking meetings right.* Retrieved from https://hbr.org/2015/08/how-to-do-walking-meetings-right

Compas, B. E., Connor-Smith, J. K., Saltzman, H., Thomsen, A. H., and Wadsworth, M. E. (2001). Coping with stress during childhood and adolescence: Problems, progress, and potential in theory and research. *Psychological Bulletin, 127*(1), 87–127.

Costa, D. (2018). Better days at work: Identifying, preventing burnout in occupational therapy practice. *OT Practice, 23*(6), 10–15.

Dyrbye, L. N., Shanafelt, T. D., Sinsky, C. A., Cipriano, P. F., Bhatt, J., Ommaya, A., . . . Meyers, D. (2017). Burnout among health care professionals: A call to explore and address this underrecognized threat to safe, high-quality care. *NAM Perspectives.* Discussion Paper. Washington, DC: National Academy of Medicine. Retrieved from https://nam.edu/burnout-among-health-care-professionals-a-call-to-explore-and-address-this-underrecognized-threat-to-safe-high-quality-care

Edwards, H., and Dirette, D. (2010). The relationship between professional identity and burnout among occupational therapists. *Occupational Therapy in Health Care, 24,* 119–129.

Elseviers, M. M., Ariias-Guillén, M., Gorke, A., and Arens, H.-J. (2014). Sharps injuries amongst healthcare workers: Review of incidence, transmissions and costs. *Journal of Renal Care, 40*(3), 150–156.

Emmons, R. A., and McCullough, M. E. (2003). Counting blessings versus burdens: Experimental studies of gratitude and subjective well-being in daily life. *Journal of Personality and Social Psychology, 84,* 377–389.

Emmons, R. A., and Stern, R. (2013). Gratitude as a psychotherapeutic intervention. *Journal of Clinical Psychology: In Session, 69*(8), 846–855.

Erler, K. S. (2016). *The American Occupational Therapy Association advisory opinion for the Ethics Commission: Role of occupational therapy ethics rounds in practice.* Retrieved from www.aota.org/~/media/Corporate/Files/Practice/Ethics/Advisory/Role-of-Occupational-Therapy-Ethics-Rounds-in-Practice.pdf

Fredrickson, B. L., and Losada, M. F. (2005). Positive affect and the complex dynamics of human flourishing. *American Psychologist, 60*(7), 678–686.

Freudenberger, H. J., and North, G. (2006). The burnout cycle. *Scientific American MIND, 17*(3), 31.

Gilbert, P. (2005). Compassion and cruelty: A biopsychosocial approach. In P. Gilbert (Ed.), *Compassion: Conceptualisations, research and use in psychotherapy* (pp. 9–74). London: Routledge.

Gilfoyle, E. M. (1986). Taking care of ourselves as health care providers. *American Journal of Occupational Therapy, 40,* 387–389. doi:10.5014/ajot.40.6.387

Gilson, N., McKenna, J., and Cooke, C. (2008). Experiences of route and task-based walking in a university community: Qualitative perspectives in a randomized control trial. *Journal of Physical Activity and Health, 5,* S176–S182.

Gonzalez-Gutierrez, J. L. G., Rodriguez, R. M., Puente, C. P., Costa, N. A., Recio, L. A., Cerro, P. D., and Cuadros, J. A. (2004). Burnout in occupational therapy: An analysis focused on the level of individual and organizational consequences. *Psychology in Spain, 8*(1), 98–105.

Goodman, M. J., and Schorling, J. B. (2012). A mindfulness course decreases burnout and improves well-being among healthcare providers. *International Journal of Psychiatry in Medicine, 43*(2), 119–128.

Green, L. W., and Kreuter, M. W. (2005). *Health promotion planning: An educational and ecological approach* (4th ed.). New York, NY: McGraw Hill.

Grossman P., Niemann L., Schmidt S., and Walach H. (2004). Mindfulness-based stress reduction and health benefits: A meta-analysis. *Journal of Psychosomatic Research, 57,* 35–43.

Gupta, S., Paterson, M. L., Lysaght, R. M., and von Zweck, C. M. (2012). Experiences of burnout and coping strategies utilized by occupational therapists. *Canadian Journal of Occupational Therapy, 79,* 86–95. doi:10.2182/cjot.2012.79.2.4

Hartfiel, N., Havenhand, J., Khalsa, S. B., Clarke, G., and Krayer, A. (2011). The effectiveness of yoga for the improvement of well-being and resilience to stress in the workplace. *Scandinavian Journal of Work Environment and Health, 37*(1), 70–76.

Iwama, M. K. (2005a). Situated meaning: An issue of culture, inclusion, and occupational therapy. In F. Kronenberg, S. S. Algado, and N. Pollard (Eds.), *Occupational therapy without borders: Learning from the spirit of survivors* (pp. 127–39). London: Elsevier.

Iwama, M. K. (2005b). The Kawa (river) model: Nature, life flow, and the power of culturally relevant occupational therapy. In F. Kronenberg, S. S. Algado, and N. Pollard (Eds.), *Occupational therapy without borders: Learning from the spirit of survivors* (pp. 213–27). London: Elsevier Limited.

Iwama, M. K. (2006a). *The Kawa model: Culturally relevant occupational therapy.* Philadelphia, PA: Elsevier.

Iwama, M. K. (2006b). *The* KAWA model discussion forum: How does your river flow?: Index. Retrieved November 29, 2006, from http://kawamodel.phpbbnow.com/.

Iwama, M. K. (2006c). *The Kawa model website: Concepts and structures.* Philadelphia, PA: Elsevier. Retrieved November 29, 2006, from http://www.kawamodel.com/.

Kabat-Zinn, J. (1990). *Full catastrophe living: Using the wisdom of your body and mind to face stress, pain, and illness.* New York, NY: Bantam Dell.

Kabat-Zinn, J. (2003). Mindfulness-based interventions in context: Past, present, and future. *Clinical Psychology: Science and Practice, 10,* 144–156. http://doi.dx.org/10.1093/ clipsy.bpg016

Kawa Model. (2016). *About.* Retrieved from www.kawamodel.com/v1/about/

Kumar, S. (2016). Burnout and doctors: Prevalence, prevention, and interventions. *Healthcare, 4*(3), 37–47.

Linzer, M., Poplau, S., Grossman, E., Varkey, A., Yale, S., Williams, E., . . . Barbouche, M. (2015). A cluster randomized trial of interventions to improve work conditions and clinician burnout in primary care: Results from the Health Work Place (HWP) Study. *Journal of General Internal Medicine, 30*(8), 1105–1111.

Lloyd, C., and King, R. (2001). Work-related stress and occupational therapy. *Occupational Therapy International, 8*(4), 227–243.

Luken, M., and Sammons, A. (2016). Systematic review of mindfulness practice for reducing job burnout. *American Journal of Occupational Therapy, 70*(2), 1–10.

Maslach, C. (1982). *Burnout: The cost of caring.* Englewood Cliffs, NJ: Prentice-Hall.

Maslach, C. (2003). *Burnout: The cost of caring.* Los Altos, CA: Malor Books.

Maslach, C., and Leiter, M. (2008). Early predictors of job burnout and engagement. *Journal of Applied Psychology, 93,* 498–512.

Masten, A. S., Cutuli, J. J., Herbers, J. E., and Reed, M. J. (2009). Resilience in development. In S. J. Lopez and C. R. Snyder (Eds.), *The Oxford Handbook of Positive Psychology* (2nd ed.). New York, NY: Oxford University Press.

Mathieu, F. (2007). Running on empty: Compassion fatigue in health professionals. *Rehab and Community Care Medicine.* Retrieved from www.compassionfatigue.org/pages/RunningOnEmpty.pdf

McCann, C. M., Beddoe, E., McCormick, K., Huggard, P., Kedge, S., Adamson, C., and Huggard, J. (2013). Resilience in health professions: A review of recent literature. *International Journal of Well-being, 3*(1), 60–81.

McKenna, K. M., Hashimoto, D. A., Maguire, M. S., and Bynum, W. E. (2016). The missing link: Connection is the key to resilience in medical education. *Academic Medicine, 91*(9), 1197–1199.

Moharana, S., Lipika, M., Moharana, D. N., and Pattnaik, S. S. (2017). Yoga as a health promotion lifestyle tool: A study on medical students from a tertiary care centre. *International Journal of Scientific Study, 5*(3), 275–279.

Montgomery, A. (2014). The inevitability of physician burnout: Implications for interventions. *Burnout Research, 1,* 50–56.

National Academy of Medicine. (2016). *National Academy of Medicine launches "Action Collaborative" to promote clinician well-being and combat burnout, depression, and suicide among health care workers.* Retrieved from https://nam.edu/national-academy-of-medicine-launches-action-collaborative-to-promote-clinician-well-being-and-combat-burnout-depression-and-suicide-among-health-care-workers/

National Academy of Medicine. (2018). *Action collaborative on clinician well-being and resilience.* Retrieved from https://nam.edu/initiatives/clinician-resilience-and-well-being/

National Cancer Institute. (2005). *Theory at a glance* (2nd ed.). Bethesda, MD: National Institutes of Health. Retrieved from https://sbccimplementationkits.org/demandrmnch/ikitresources/theory-at-a-glance-a-guide-for-health-promotion-practice-second-edition/

National Institute for Occupational Safety and Health. (2015). *Issues relevant to advancing worker well-being through total worker health®*. Retrieved from www.cdc.gov/niosh/twh/pdfs/TWH-Issues-4x3_10282015_final.pdf

National Institute for Occupational Safety and Health. (2017a). *Healthcare workers*. Retrieved from www.cdc.gov/niosh/topics/healthcare/infectious.html

National Institute for Occupational Safety and Health. (2017b). *Total worker health*. Retrieved from www.cdc.gov/niosh/twh/totalhealth.html

National Institute for Occupational Safety and Health. (2018). *Healthcare workers*. Retrieved from www.cdc.gov/niosh/topics/healthcare/

Neff, K. D., Kirkpatrick, K. L., and Rude, S. S. (2007). Self-compassion and adaptive psychological functioning. *Journal of Research in Personality, 41,* 139–154.

Negash, S., and Sahin, S. (2011). Compassion fatigue in marriage and family therapy: Implications for therapists and clients. *Journal of Marital and Family Therapy, 37*(1), 1–13. doi:10.1111/j.1752–0606.2009.00147.x

Occupational Safety and Health Administration. (n.d.a). *Bloodborne pathogens and needlestick prevention*. Retrieved from www.osha.gov/SLTC/bloodbornepathogens/index.html

Occupational Safety and Health Administration. (n.d.b). *Healthcare wide hazards: Stress*. Retrieved from www.osha.gov/SLTC/etools/hospital/hazards/stress/stress.html

Occupational Safety and Health Administration. (n.d.c). *Infectious diseases*. Retrieved from www.osha.gov/SLTC/healthcarefacilities/infectious_diseases.html

Occupational Safety and Health Administration. (2002). *Job hazard analysis*. Retrieved from www.osha.gov/Publications/osha3071.pdf

Occupational Safety and Health Administration. (2013). *Caring for our caregivers: Facts about hospital worker safety*. Retrieved from http://mtpinnacle.com/pdfs/OSHA-1.2_Factbook_508.pdf

Olson, K., Kemper, K. J., and Mahan, J. D. (2015). What factors promote resilience and protect against burnout in first-year pediatric and medicine-pediatric residents? *Journal of Evidence-Based Complementary and Alternative Medicine, 20*(3), 192–198.

Ozbay, F., Johnson, D. C., Dimoulas, E., Morgan, C. A., Charney, D., and Southwick, S. (2007). Social support and resilience to stress: From neurobiology to clinical practice. *Psychiatry (Edgemont), 4*(5), 35–40.

Painter, P., Akroyd, D., Elliot, S., and Adams, R. D. (2003). Burnout among occupational therapists. *Occupational Therapy in Health Care, 17*(1), 63–78. doi:10.1080/ J003v17n01_06

Picco, L., Yuan, Q., Vaingankar, J. A., Chang, S., Abdin, E., Chua, H. C., Chong, S. A., . . . Subramaniam, M. (2017). Positive mental health among health professionals working at a psychiatric hospital. *PloS One, 12*(6), e0178359. doi:10.1371/journal.pone.0178359

Raab, K. (2014). Mindfulness, self-compassion, and empathy among health care professionals: A review of the literature. *Journal of Health Care Chaplaincy, 20*(3), 95–108.

Rossi, A., Cetrano, G., Pertile, R., Rabbi, L., Donsi, V., Grigoletti, L., . . . Amaddeo, F. (2012). Burnout, compassion fatigue, and compassion satisfaction among staff in community-based mental health services. *Psychiatry Research, 200*(2–3), 933–938.

Salazar, M. K., and Beaton, R. (2000). Ecological model of occupational stress. Application to urban firefighters. *Official Journal of the American Association of Occupational Health Nurses, 48*(10), 470–479.

Salovey, P., Mayer, J. D., Caruso, D., Yoo, S. H. (2009). The positive psychology of emotional intelligence. In S. J. Lopez and C. R. Snyder (Eds.), *The Oxford Handbook of Positive Psychology* (2nd ed.). New York, NY: Oxford University Press.

Schaufeli, W. B., and Bakker, A. B. (2004). Job demands, job resources, and their relationship with burnout and engagement: A multi-sample study. *Journal of Organizational Behavior, 25,* 293–315.

Seligman, M. E. (2011). *Flourish*. New York, NY: Free Press.

Sepkowitz, K. A., and Eisenburg, L. (2005). Occupational deaths among health care workers. *Emerging Infectious Diseases, 11*(7), 1003–1008.

Shanafelt, T. D., Balch, C. M., Bechamps, G., Russell, T., Dyrbye, L., Satele, D., . . . Freischlag, J. (2010). Burnout and medical errors among American surgeons. *Annals of Surgery, 251,* 995–1000.

Shanafelt, T. D., and Noseworthy, J. H. (2017). Executive leadership and physician well-being: Nine organizational strategies to promote engagement and reduce burnout. *Mayo Clinical Proceedings, 92*(1), 129–146.

Shankar, G. (2007). *Yoga psychotherapy and its applications*. New Delhi, India: Satyam.

Shroff, F. M., and Asgarpour, M. (2017). Yoga and mental health: A review. *Journal of Physiotherapy and Physical Rehabilitation, 2*(1), 132–134.

Siegel, J. D., Rhinehart, E., Jackson, M., Chiarello, L., and the Healthcare Infection Control Practices Advisory Committee. (2007). *2007 guideline for isolation precautions: Preventing transmission of infectious agents in healthcare settings*. Retrieved from www.cdc.gov/infectioncontrol/guidelines/isolation/index

Simard, A. A., and Henry, M. (2009). Impact of a short yoga intervention on medical students' health: A pilot study. *Medical Teacher, 31,* 950–952.

Smart, D., English, A., James, J., Wilson, M., Daratha, K. B., Childers, B., and Magera, C. (2014). Compassion fatigue and satisfaction: A cross-sectional survey among US healthcare workers. *Nursing and Health Satisfaction, 16*(1), 3–10. doi:10.1111/nhs.12068

Smith-Gabal, H., Kuzminski, S., and Eldridge, E. (2018, October). Surveying moral distress among skilled nursing facility practitioners. *OT Practice, 23*(18), 24–25.

Taylor, R. R. (Ed.). (2017). *Kielhofner's model of human occupation* (5th ed.). Philadelphia, PA: Wolters Kluwer.

Tripathi, N. S., and Middleton, C. (2018, September). Using the Kawa's model for self-assessment in continuing education. *OT Practice, 23*(17), 12–16.

Trockel, M., Hamidi, M., Murphy, M. L., Purpur de Vries, P., and Bohman, B. (2017). *2016 Physician wellness survey: Full report*. Palo Alto, CA: Stanford Medicine. Retrieved from https://wellmd.stanford.edu/content/dam/sm/wellmd/documents/Full-2016-Physician-Wellness-Survey-Report-16-Aug-2017-Final-rd.pdf

University of California, Riverside. (n.d.). *Walking Meetings 101* [Pamphlet].

U.S. Bureau of Labor Statistics. (2018). Occupational therapists. *Occupational Outlook Handbook*. Retrieved from www.bls.gov/ooh/healthcare/occupational-therapists.htm

U.S. Department of Health and Human Services. (2000). *Healthy People 2010: Understanding and improving health* (2nd ed.). Washington, DC: U.S. Government Printing Office.

Ward, T. (2017, March 13). *Walking meetings? Proceed with caution*. Retrieved from www.psychologytoday.com/us/blog/creativity-you/201703/walking-meetings-proceed-caution

Wasilewski, R. M., Mateo, P., and Sidorovsky, P. (2007). Preventing work-related musculoskeletal disorders within supermarket cashiers: An ergonomic training program based on the theoretical framework of the PRECEDE-PROCEED model. *WORK: A Journal of Prevention, Assessment and Rehabilitation, 28*(1), 23–31.

Watkins, P. C., Van Gelder, M., and Frias, A. (2009). Furthering the science of gratitude. In S. J. Lopez and C. R. Snyder (Eds.), *The Oxford Handbook of Positive Psychology* (2nd ed.). New York, NY: Oxford University Press.

Wilkins, K. (2007). Work stress among health care providers. *Health Reports, 18*(4), 33–36.

Wood, A. M., Joseph, S., and Linley, P. A. (2007). Coping style as a psychological resource of grateful people. *Journal of Social and Clinical Psychology, 26,* 1076–1109.

Wood, A. M., Joseph, S., Lloyd, J., and Atkins, S. (2009). Gratitude influences sleep through the mechanism of pre-sleep cognitions. *Journal of Psychosomatic Research, 66,* 43–48.

Wood, A. M., Maltby, J., Gillett, R., Linley, P. A., and Joseph, S. (2008). The role of gratitude in the development of social support, stress, and depression: Two longitudinal studies. *Journal of Research in Personality, 42,* 854–871.

Wood, J., and Riffkin, R. (2015). *Often ignored: Healthcare employees' well-being.* Retrieved from www.thefreelibrary.com/Often+Ignored%3a+Healthcare+Employees%27+Well-Being.-a0432112088

World Health Organization. (2001). *Mental health: Strengthening our response.* Retrieved from www.who.int/news-room/fact-sheets/detail/mental-health-strengthening-our-response

World Health Organization. (2002). *Innovative care for chronic conditions: Building blocks for action.* Retrieved from www.who.int/diabetes/publications/icccreport/en/

World Health Organization. (2018). *Health topics: Risk factors.* Retrieved from www.who.int/topics/risk_factors/en/

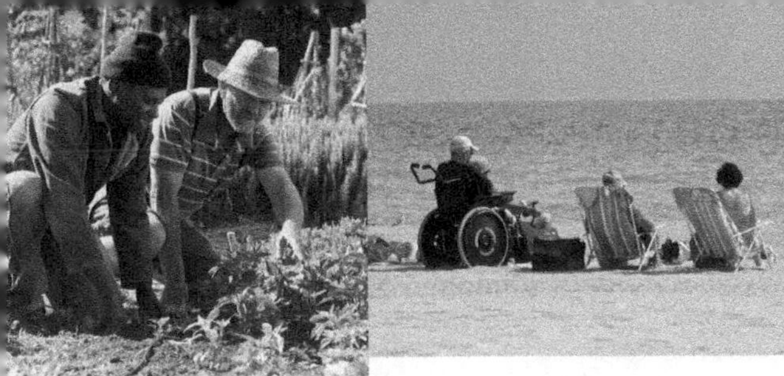
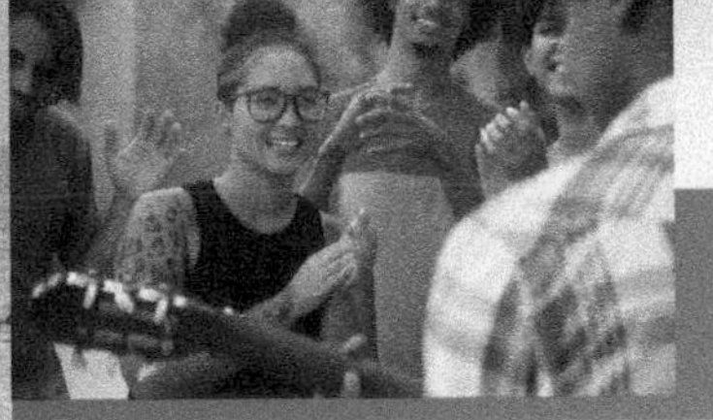

SECTION VI

Mental Health

Chapter 18

Community Mental Health Programs

Rita P. Fleming-Castaldy, PhD, OTR/L, FAOTA

Recovery is a process, a way of life, an attitude, and a way of approaching the day's challenges. . . . The need is to meet the challenge of the disability and to re-establish a new and valued sense of integrity and purpose within and beyond the limits of the disability; the aspiration is to live, work, and love in a community in which one makes a significant contribution.

—Deegan (1988, p. 11)

Learning Outcomes

This chapter is designed to enable the reader to:

18-1 Describe how major sociopolitical and professional paradigm shifts influenced the evolution of community mental health services.

18-2 Articulate the relevance of mental health practice models to community-based occupational therapy.

18-3 Describe how community mental health programs and services enable the recovery and participation of persons with serious mental illness.

18-4 Discuss the role of occupational therapy practitioners in community-based mental health settings.

18-5 Describe key resources that can guide evidence-based practice and fund community mental health services.

Acknowledgments: I thank Emily Dineen, MS, OTR/L, AY 2017–2018 University of Scranton work study student, and Victoria Crociata, AY 2018–2019 University of Scranton work study student, for their research and production assistance.

18-6 Articulate challenges, opportunities, and future directions for occupational therapy in community mental health practice.

Key Terms

Assertive community treatment
Case management
Certified community behavioral health center
Clubhouses
Peer support services
Permanent supported housing
Personal assistance in community existence
Resilience
Serious mental illness
Supported education
Supported employment
Supportive transitional housing
Transitional employment
Wellness
Wellness Recovery Action Plan

Introduction

Community-based occupational therapy practitioners work with persons with mental health disorders across the life span (American Occupational Therapy Association [AOTA], 2016a). This chapter focuses on services and programs for adults with **serious mental illness** (SMI). An SMI is "a mental, behavioral, or emotional disorder resulting in serious functional impairment, which substantially interferes with or limits one or more major life activities" (National Institute of Mental Health [NIMH], 2017, para. 4). Conditions meeting these criteria include psychotic, schizophrenia, schizoaffective, bipolar, major depressive, and borderline personality disorders. Developmental and substance use disorders, dementias, and mental disorders due to medical conditions are not included in this definition (Substance Abuse and Mental Health Services Administration [SAMHSA], 2010a).

Persons with SMI were previously and inaccurately called chronically mentally ill and seriously and persistently mentally ill. SMI is not always chronic or persistent. People with SMI can attain and maintain health and wellness (SAMHSA, 2010a). However, the need for effective programs that enable recovery is great. In the United States, nearly one in five adults (44,700,000 people) are living with a mental health disorder. Over 10,000,000 adults live with an SMI (NIMH, 2017). The personal impact of mental illness ranges from no impairment to severe. Comorbidities (e.g., physical and/or intellectual disorders) and maladaptive coping strategies (e.g., self-harm, substance use) can significantly influence the effect of mental illness on people's lives (NIMH, 2017).

As noted in the chapter's opening quote, the realities of living with SMI can be challenging and disabling. According to the World Health Organization (WHO, 2002), disability results from an interaction between a person with a health condition and that person's contexts. Thus, having a mental illness is not inherently disabling. Impairments (e.g., cognitive deficits), activity limitations (e.g., difficulty performing tasks), and/or participation restrictions (e.g., stigmatizing attitudes, marginalizing policies) cause disability (WHO, 2002). Because the social determinants of health place people at risk for disabilities and chronic health conditions, it is important to recognize the epidemiological factors that have an impact on public health and welfare (Accreditation Council for Occupational Therapy Education [ACOTE®], 2017). The mortality rate of people with SMI is two to three times higher than the general population, and their life expectancy is shortened by 10 to 20 years (Van Camp et al., 2015). Their rates of smoking, substance use, obesity, and diabetes are also higher (National Alliance on Mental Illness [NAMI], 2018a). As a result of antipsychotic medications used to manage symptoms, over 32% of people with SMI have metabolic syndrome (MetS). MetS is a combination of conditions (e.g., hypertension, obesity, diabetes) that are strongly related to cardiovascular diseases (Van Camp et al., 2015). Modifiable risk factors (e.g., smoking), the impact of psychiatric symptoms on health management and maintenance activities, and poor access to, and utilization of, health-care services increase mortality and morbidity rates (NAMI, 2018a; Van Camp et al., 2015).

Systemic service gaps contribute to unacceptable social outcomes for people with SMI. They have significantly higher rates of poverty, incarceration, and homelessness than the general population. These factors further limit their health-care access (NAMI, 2018a). Because the effect of social policies on health cannot be ignored, this chapter highlights the major social movements, paradigm shifts, and legislation that have affected U.S. mental health care and occupational therapy practice since the profession's inception. Community-based practice models, programs, and services and occupational therapy practitioner roles, evaluation tools, and intervention approaches are described. Evidence-based practice (EBP) resources are integrated throughout the chapter. A discussion of community mental health (CMH) challenges, opportunities, funding, and future directions concludes the chapter.

Historical Overview

Occupational therapy practice with persons with SMI began with the profession's founding in 1917 and was strongly influenced by the moral treatment and settlement house movements (Reed and Anderson, 2017). Early occupational therapists used habit training and purposeful activities (e.g., crafts, gardening, and work) "to arouse interest, courage, and confidence; to exercise mind and body in health activity; to overcome functional disability; and to re-establish capacity for industrial and social usefulness" (Dunton, 1919, pp. 71–72). While these purposes are clearly relevant to community-based practice, mental health occupational therapy was predominantly institution-based until the 1980s. The dominance of the medical model sustained the yearslong and often lifetime hospitalization of persons with SMI (Gutman, 2011).

CMH programs emerged in the 1950s, but it was not until the 1960s that the locus and focus of psychiatric care was critically assessed. At this time, widespread institutional abuses were exposed, and medications that effectively managed psychiatric symptoms became available. These developments and the civil rights movement impelled mental health activists to reject institution-based custodial/maintenance care and demand community-based recovery-oriented treatment (Swarbrick, 2009).

In 1963, the Community Mental Health Act (CMHA) mandated that services be provided in the least restrictive environment and primarily focus on community integration. Some CMHA initiatives (i.e., emergency, acute inpatient, outpatient, consultation, and education services) positively affected mental health care. However, these services predominantly benefited persons with less serious conditions (Torrey, 2013). Consequently, patients with SMI were discharged to ill-prepared and often resistant communities with scant to nil services. This mass deinstitutionalization was a debacle (Turner and TenHoo, 1978).

The creation of the Medicare and Medicaid programs in 1965 and the Supplemental Security Income benefit in 1972 accelerated the deinstitutionalization movement (Turner and TenHoo, 1978). Having federal funding to support community living was a major fiscal incentive for states to transfer thousands of people with SMI from state-financed institutions into the community. Because funding for the integrated medical, rehabilitative, and supportive services required for successful community integration never materialized, deinstitutionalized persons often became homeless or lived in deplorable conditions that were "as stultifying and disabling as mental institutions" (Turner and TenHoo, 1978, p. 322).

In 1977, the NIMH attempted to rectify this systemic neglect by creating community support programs (CSPs) to serve people with SMI. CSPs included crisis stabilization, psychosocial rehabilitation, case management, employment, and housing services; medical and mental health care; and support to families, friends, and the community (Turner and TenHoo, 1978). Many CSPs were successfully established, but due to inadequate funding, their potential was never realized. In 2003, the president's New Freedom Commission on Mental Health addressed this failure and made numerous recommendations to transform the mental health-care system and enable the recovery and full community participation of persons with SMI (Cottrell, 2007). The subsequent Federal Mental Health Action Agenda articulated concrete steps for building a recovery-oriented, evidence-based, and consumer- and family-driven system. Funded actions have been successful. However, services for people with SMI still vary greatly between states. Some have model programs; most provide inadequate care (NAMI, 2015).

The CMHA's ideals and the CSP's approaches were highly compatible with occupational therapy. Yet the profession did not respond dynamically to this paradigm shift (Kielhofner, 2009). Although occupational therapy had a prominent role in psychiatric institutions, few practitioners successfully transitioned into the community (Gutman, 2011). The dramatically reduced number of mental health occupational therapists has been attributed to their difficulty transitioning from structured hospitals with predictable expectations into fluid community settings with numerous complexities, the assumption of occupational therapy roles by others, and pay disparities (Dasler, 1984; Gutman, 2011). During the 1970s and 1980s, the passage of federal legislation that mandated and funded school-based, nursing home, and home-care services and the growth of specializations (e.g., hand therapy) greatly expanded practice opportunities (Gutman, 2011; Reed and Anderson, 2017). Despite diminished practitioner numbers, mental health occupational therapy prevailed. A robust practice is documented in the peer-reviewed journal *Occupational Therapy in Mental Health* (first published in 1984) and in the *AOTA Mental Health Special Interest Section* (founded in 1977) publications and presentations.

The viability of mental health occupational therapy is evident in the AOTA's effective articulation of the profession's distinct value and its successful advocacy for occupational therapists to be recognized as qualified mental health professionals (AOTA, 2016a, 2016b, 2017). Most recently, occupational therapy was included in federally funded **certified community behavioral health center** (CCBHC) staff recommendations. CCBHCs "are coordinated, fully integrated comprehensive community-based providers serving people with behavioral health challenges across the lifespan, while focusing on the needs of those with serious mental illness and chronic substance use disorders facing life transitions" (Swarbrick, 2016, p.11). These developments and the paradigm shift to recovery-oriented models afford multiple opportunities for occupational therapy practitioners to revitalize their role as primary mental health providers.

Practice Models

Occupational therapy practitioners use practice models "to guide and inform interventions for persons, groups, and populations in a variety of practice contexts and environments" (ACOTE®, 2017, p. 26). In CMH, psychiatric rehabilitation, recovery/wellness, stress-vulnerability/coping-competence, and occupation-based models are commonly used. The following describes these models' origins, major concepts, and practice applications.

Psychiatric Rehabilitation Model

The psychiatric rehabilitation model was developed in the 1970s to help people with SMI acquire the skills and resources needed to live self-determined and satisfying lives in their environments of choice (Liberman, 1988). Often called psychosocial rehabilitation, this model integrates concepts and principles from the physical rehabilitation and community integration movements. The collaborative, individualized, person-directed, and evidence-based approaches used in psychiatric rehabilitation are designed to promote recovery, enable community integration, and improve quality of life (Krupa, Fossey, Anthony, Brown, and Pitts, 2009). This model has much in common with the occupational therapy principles that contributed to its development. Similarities include the belief that health is attained and human potential is optimized when people engage in meaningful occupation; a conviction that change is achieved through personal choice and empowerment; and a commitment to providing interventions that enable doing in people's chosen environments (Krupa et al., 2009).

Psychiatric rehabilitation approaches parallel occupational therapy processes: comprehensive evaluation, personalized goal setting, individualized interventions to resolve underlying performance difficulties and restore/build capabilities, and the provision of activity adaptations, environmental modifications, and supports to enable engagement in desired social roles (Krupa et al., 2009). The psychiatric rehabilitation model is widely used to inform the programs and services described in this chapter. Chapter sections on occupational therapy evaluation and intervention further highlight psychiatric rehabilitation's congruence with occupational therapy.

Recovery/Wellness Models

In the 1990s, the application of recovery and wellness concepts to the lived experiences of persons with SMI challenged the mental health-care system's status quo, which primarily focused on ameliorating symptoms and preventing hospitalization (Merryman and Riegel, 2007). Recovery/wellness models recognize that people desire more than stability and that aspirations and ambition do not end with illness (Wollenberg, 2002). Recovery-oriented services are person-driven and continuously evolving to enable the attainment of, and engagement in, a desired life. Recovery is "a process of change through which individuals improve their health and wellness, live a self-directed life, and strive to reach their full potential" (SAMHSA, 2012, para. 5). It is a nonlinear journey that can occur with active symptoms and without professional intervention (Wollenberg, 2002). Box 18-1

Box 18-1 Implementation of the Recovery Model by Occupational Therapy Practitioners

Recovery Component	Representative Occupational Therapy Practitioner Actions
Individualized and Person-centered	Intervention plans are based on collaboration with service recipients, address the individual's unique concerns, and enable engagement in self-identified, personally desired occupational roles.
Self-direction	The person's voice is actively solicited to establish self-determined goals and design interventions that reflect the person's priorities and support autonomy, control, and choice.
Hope	Hope for recovery is raised by increasing occupational performance skills, expanding social resources, improving self-efficacy, promoting health and well-being, and improving quality of life.
Responsibility	Interventions that integrate personal choice, expect active participation, respect risk-taking, and facilitate external support foster the individual's ownership of illness management and recovery.
Empowerment	Practitioners empower people with SMI by teaching them the self-advocacy skills to confront the sociopolitical contexts that limit occupational engagement and social participation.
Respect	Services that support and accept people with SMI, value and protect their civil liberties, and are designed *with* a person and not provided *to* a person convey respect.
Peer support	Peer support and a sense of belonging and community are fostered when opportunities for sharing encouragement, knowledge, occupational engagement, and participation are provided.
Strengths-based	The occupational profile and occupation-based assessments provide information about a person's roles, abilities, aspirations, and resources to support the construction of a strengths-based intervention plan.
Nonlinear	A continuous, dynamic, transactional relationship is established that recognizes progress can include setbacks; learning to make meaning from them can foster personal growth and positive change.
Holistic	Occupation-based practice models describe the interrelationships among people's aspirations, capabilities, roles, and contexts to address the multiple, complex dimensions of occupational engagement.

Adapted from "Shared Principles: The Recovery Model and Occupational Therapy," by P. Clay, 2013, *Mental Health Special Interest Section Quarterly, 36*(4), 1–3.

outlines how the key components of recovery are actualized in occupational therapy.

Because unrelenting symptoms can compromise recovery, effective recovery-oriented services use a self-management approach for wellness. **Wellness** is "a conscious, deliberate process whereby a person is aware of and makes choices for a more satisfying lifestyle" (Swarbrick, 2013, p. 2). To self-direct their health management, people with SMI often use a **Wellness Recovery Action Plan** (WRAP®). A WRAP "is a structured system for monitoring uncomfortable and distressing symptoms and, through planned responses, reducing, modifying or eliminating those symptoms" (Copeland, 2001, p. 129). To create a WRAP, a person develops a "wellness toolbox" comprising strategies and skills for maintaining daily wellness, dealing with symptom triggers, managing early warning signs, and addressing worsening symptoms. A desired action plan to be implemented if a crisis impedes the ability to self-manage, make decisions, and/or be safe is formulated (Copeland, 2001). Occupational therapy practitioners can support the development and implementation of individualized WRAPs by applying the recovery principles and actions outlined in Box 18-1.

To help implement recovery-oriented interventions, SAMHSA's (2010a) free illness management and recovery (IMR) evidence-based curriculum includes information about mental illness, the stress-vulnerability model, and strategies for reducing relapses, effectively using medications, building social support, accessing the mental health-care system, and coping with symptoms, stress, and daily problems. Motivational, educational, and cognitive-behavioral techniques are described to facilitate the implementation of individualized recovery-oriented approaches (SAMHSA, 2010a). Consistent with a psychoeducation approach, participants are assigned "homework" to practice IMR strategies at home and in the community. This action-oriented approach is congruent with the knowledge, skills, and philosophy of occupational therapy practitioners (Bjørkedal, Torsting, and Møller, 2016). Merryman and Riegel (2007) describe a four-stage recovery model by which people with SMI move from occupational dependence to successful occupational performance (see Table 18-1).

Stress-Vulnerability/Coping-Competence Model

The stress-vulnerability/coping-competence model was proposed in the 1980s to explain the occurrence and reoccurrence of psychiatric symptoms (Liberman, 1988). According to this model, increased stress in susceptible individuals can intensify symptoms and trigger a crisis (Liberman, 1988). Unfortunately, the singular application of the model's stress-vulnerability dimension resulted in people with SMI being advised by service providers to avoid engaging in activities that could potentially challenge their adaptive capabilities (Krupa et al., 2009). The pervasive disregard of this model's coping-competence dimension erroneously classified persons with SMI as fragile. This myopic perspective and the resulting harmful advice dissuaded many from pursuing meaningful activities and desired occupations, contributing to occupational disruption and deprivation (Krupa et al., 2009).

Multiple factors can contribute to a person's vulnerability. These include genetics and trauma; neurological, biological, and cognitive impairments; and physical, developmental, and substance use disorders (SAMHSA, 2010a). A lack of opportunities during childhood and adolescence to develop psychosocial skills and performance competencies can increase susceptibility to stress-related exacerbations in adulthood (Russo, Murrough, Han, Charney, and Nestle, 2012). Conversely, when stress-inducing situations are encountered and overcome during development, people acquire proresilience capabilities, perceived internal control, and a sense of mastery (Russo et al., 2012). The coping-competence dimension of this model recognizes the influence that development has on promoting adaptive responses to adult stress. Because this process does not always occur, the balanced application of the stress-vulnerability/coping-competence model emphasizes the development of coping skills and functional competencies throughout life. These capacities serve as protective factors to prevent symptom exacerbation and promote future resilience (Liberman, 1988; Ventura, Nuechterlein, Subotnik, Green, and Gitlin, 2004).

Resilience is the personal capacity to avoid the negative consequences of stress that compromise physical and/or psychological well-being (Pitts,

Table 18-1 Four-Stage Occupation-Based Recovery Model

	Stage 1: Occupational Dependence Due to illness and consumer label; occupational decisions by health-care professionals	**Stage 2: Supported Occupational Performance Provided through structure of mental health programs**	**Stage 3: Active Engagement in Meaningful Occupations Facilitated by ongoing support from mental health professionals**	**Stage 4: Successful Occupational Performance Community participation**
Self-determination	Professionals make major decisions = dependent	Person plays role in decision-making; decisions largely made by mental health providers	Person's decisions influenced by mental health programs	Capable of making decisions for oneself = self-determining
Social support	Mental health system provides social supports	Person relies on mental health system for social supports but maintains relationships with family or other consumers within program	Person has developed network of friends and family but still uses mental health system for some social support	Network beyond care providers as social supports
Social role/identity	Consumer role predominates identity	Primary role is consumer; other roles play minor part in life	Person identifies self as client but actively engages in other meaningful life roles	Person who is a worker, parent, student, or other role
Illness management and coping skills	Medication understanding and compliance primary issue/lack of illness awareness	Medication plays major role but individual acknowledges the role of other factors in recovery	Person actively participates in mental health programs and other structured wellness activities	Medication is one tool among many freely chosen by the individual

From "Recovery Process and People With Serious Mental Illness Living in the Community," by M. B. Merryman and S. K. Riegel, 2007, *Occupational Therapy in Mental Health, 23*(2), 60. Reprinted with permission.

2004). Resilience is not just the absence of a maladaptive response in vulnerable people; it is the outcome of an active, selective, adaptive process (Russo et al., 2012). Thus, instead of advising persons with SMI to avoid potentially challenging activities and stressful situations, multiple opportunities to develop protective factors that can prevent or diminish the intensity of symptoms, avert or end a negative cycle of relapse and rehospitalization, and enable engaged and productive lives should be provided (Edward, Welch, and Chater, 2009; Russo et al., 2012).

The SAMHSA (2010a) IMR evidence-based kit includes a module on the stress-vulnerability model, but it does not describe its coping-competence dimension. However, the kit's recovery-oriented strategies for reducing stress, managing problems and persistent symptoms, building social supports, and selecting treatment options can be used to develop coping skills and functional competencies. SAMHSA (2010a) emphasizes that meaningful activities and a healthy lifestyle are needed to decrease vulnerability and attain well-being. Occupational therapy practitioners are well equipped to provide interventions that effectively address the coping-competence goals of this model and facilitate resilience (Krupa et al., 2009; Pitts, 2004).

Occupation-Based Models

Research and contemporary first-person accounts of people living with SMI underscore the importance of engaging in occupation to enable recovery, wellness, and quality of life (Bjørkedal Torsting, and Møller, 2016; Doroud, Fossey, and Fortune, 2015; Hohl, Moll, and Pfeiffer, 2017; Roby, Goldstein, Rose, and Kerman, 2018). The therapeutic relevance of occupation-based models is supported by a meta-analysis that concluded that "interventions based on theoretical conceptual practice models may lead to improvement in occupational performance and well-being among people with a mental health diagnosis" (Ikiugu, Nissen, Bellar, Maassen, and Van Peursem, 2017, p. 6). Ikiugu et al. (2017) found that the most common models used to inform practice were the Canadian model of occupational performance and engagement, the behavioral/cognitive-behavioral model, and the model of human occupation. Occupation-based models describe the interaction between the person, the environment, and the occupation (Kielhofner, 2009). When applying these models, practitioners use person-focused interventions that increase self-awareness, skills, and self-efficacy; occupation-focused interventions that adapt, grade, and/or modify characteristics of tasks to enable participation in meaningful and desired activities; and environment-focused interventions that modify, adapt, and/or engage the environment to support community participation (see Fig. 18-1; AOTA, 2014; Krupa et al., 2009).

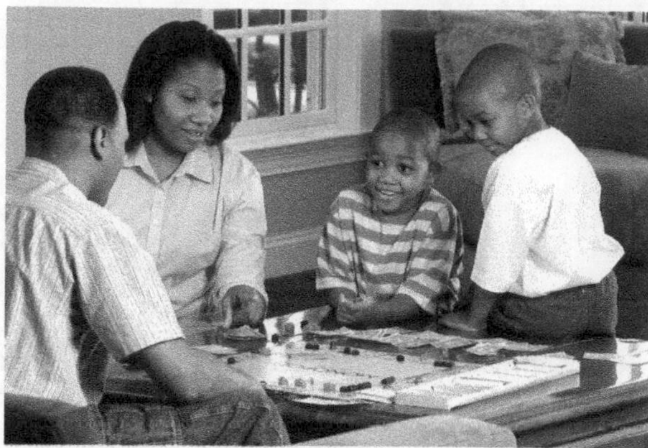

Figure 18-1 The use of occupation-based models with persons with SMI can enable their engagement in desired and valued occupational role activities, such as family game nights. *(Photo courtesy of the National Institutes of Health.)*

Community-Based Programs and Services for People With Serious Mental Illness

Programs to help people with SMI attain their goals include partial hospitalization, intensive outpatient, assertive community treatment, home health, housing, supported education, and work programs. Case management, peer-delivered, and family services are integrated into most programs. The following describes these programs and services and highlights occupational therapy's contribution to each.

Partial Hospitalization and Intensive Outpatient Programs

Partial hospitalization programs (PHPs) and intensive outpatient programs (IOPs) were developed as cost-effective alternatives to inpatient hospitalization for people with psychiatric symptoms that significantly impair function but do not raise safety concerns (Mahaffey and Holmquist, 2011). These outpatient services typically use a medical model to address presenting symptoms and are provided in a hospital or health-care center (Association for Ambulatory Behavioral Healthcare [AABS], 2010). PHPs are full-time (an average of 6 hours per day) and at least 4 days per week; IOPs average 3 hours per day for fewer days. An IOP can serve as a post-PHP "step-down" (AABS, 2010). Insurance coverage may determine PHP versus IOP participation (Mahaffey and Holmquist, 2011).

PHPs and IOPs provide more intense treatment than psychosocial rehabilitation or general outpatient programs. Services incorporate personal strengths, utilize existing resources, and engage family/community supports. Both programs provide coordinated multidisciplinary interventions based on a comprehensive evaluation

(AABS, 2010). Occupational therapy is covered by Medicare and significantly contributes to PHP and IOP outcomes (Roby et al., 2018). Because program participants live at home, practitioners can directly address the person's lived experience. Targeted interventions develop needed skills, attain desired goals, and enable participation (Mahaffey and Holmquist, 2011). Potential postdischarge challenges should be directly addressed by providing predischarge interventions that develop time management and organization skills and the ability to successfully access resources (Roby et al., 2018).

The in situ PHP and IOP approach to skill acquisition is a significant advantage over hospital-based programs. Research comparing the outcomes of PHP and inpatient hospitalization found equivalent results in symptom reduction, suicide risk, readmissions, social functioning, unemployment, family burden, and service utilization. PHP participant and family satisfaction were greater (Horvitz-Lennon, Normand, Gaccione, and Frank, 2001; Schene, 2004). Roby et al. (2018) found that postdischarge, PHP participants reported an improved sense of wellness, a more active use of resources, a greater engagement in productive occupations and leisure activities, and increased social support.

Assertive Community Treatment

Programs for **assertive community treatment** (ACT) provide intensive case management, crisis intervention, continuous support, and rehabilitative services to persons with SMI who have difficulty accessing or engaging with community-based services, have poor and/or erratic community functioning, and/or have frequent relapses (Rossen, Mueser, and Teesson, 2007). These programs began when researchers found that access to intensive and uninterrupted postdischarge interventions were more critical to community integration than the presence or absence of psychiatric symptoms (Pitts, 2001). Assertive community treatment (ACT) is provided by a transdisciplinary professional team who are cross-trained in each other's areas of expertise (Rossen et al., 2007). Rather than refer consumers to other services, team members provide direct services with no time limits. As a mobile mental health agency, they are available 24 hours a day year-round (SAMHSA, 2008). ACT teams collaboratively complete comprehensive evaluations, plan treatment, and implement interventions to provide highly individualized in situ services. Team members are jointly responsible for all persons served and share a professional/consumer caseload ratio of 1 to 10 or fewer (Rossen et al., 2007).

As designated ACT providers, occupational therapists provide general mental health services (e.g., illness management) and discipline-specific services (e.g., instrumental activities of daily living [IADLs] skills training). A focus on occupational health and well-being informs their generalist and specialist roles (Krupa, Radloff-Gabriel, Whippey, and Kirsh, 2002). Occupational therapists can apply their occupational lens at the individual, program, and community level of ACT (Krupa et al., 2002). Working with individuals, they assess strengths and difficulties, establish client-centered goals, and implement interventions that enable occupational health. They also consult with other team members to address the occupational needs of all ACT service recipients. Programmatically, occupational therapists can help the team recognize the value of prioritizing and assessing program participants' community integration, occupational well-being, and quality of life outcomes. Community-wise, they can assess the barriers to and supports for occupational health and develop resources and opportunities for occupational engagement (Krupa et al., 2002). Occupational therapists can also facilitate the team's understanding of the need to consider participants' daily life routines and how health is promoted through activity (Krupa, McLean, Eastabrook, Bonham, and Baksh, 2003).

SAMHSA's (2008) evidence-based ACT kit has comprehensive guidelines for structuring PACTs and integrating them into mental health-care systems. The NAMI and the Commission on Accreditation of Rehabilitation Facilities (CARF®) also provide ACT standards (Pitts, 2001). Research supports ACT's efficacy and cost-effectiveness. Multiple studies found ACT participants had fewer and shorter hospitalizations, greater employment and higher earnings, more independent living and housing stability, increased treatment compliance and decreased symptoms, greater life satisfaction, and increased social functioning (Rossen et al., 2007; SAMHSA, 2008). To determine if services adhere to established ACT principles, the Dartmouth ACT

Fidelity Scale can be used in program evaluation and research (Pitts, 2001).

Although PACTs are recovery-oriented, fiscal constraints have placed more emphasis on the biomedical aspects of treatment (e.g., symptom management; Krupa et al., 2002). A primary focus on compliance contributes to paternalistic and coercive practices (Ahern and Fisher, 2001). The "round-the-clock," all-inclusive nature of ACT can be invasive (e.g., an evening call inquiring about a missed appointment). When ACT is a court-mandated service for persons committed to involuntary community treatment, its recovery focus is diminished (Ahern and Fisher, 2001; Rossen et al., 2007). SAMHSA reports that "most team members have never examined their own attitudes and behaviors about consumer recovery and, therefore, uncritically accept many social control functions without paying attention to how disempowering these practices are for consumers" (2008, p. 19). The prevalence of intrusive and coercive practices prompted the National Empowerment Center to develop the **personal assistance in community existence** (PACE) model (Ahern and Fisher, 2001). PACE programs offer people with SMI a noncoercive service option. PACE development teams provide system-wide training to redesign existing services based on provider-consumer collaboration and the principles of recovery, empowerment, self-help, and peer support. Occupational therapy's philosophical base matches the PACE philosophy; thus, its practitioners are well suited to serve on PACE teams (Ahern and Fisher, 2001).

Home Health

The movement to treat illnesses and manage chronic conditions in the community rather than hospitals and institutions has increased demand for home-based services (Craig, 2012). Home health for people with SMI is primarily covered by Medicare. To receive Medicare-covered services, a person must be "confined" to the home and, typically, not able to leave without the assistance of others or considerable effort (Centers for Medicare and Medicaid Services [CMS], n.d.). Refusing to leave the home due to agoraphobia, paranoia, and/or anxiety and the presence of acute depression, cognitive impairments, positive symptoms, and/or thought disorders that impair judgment and safety meet these criteria (Azok and Tomlinson, 1994; Earle, 1999). Although "homebound," the person can attend adult day care, religious services, medical appointments, and infrequent, short-term, nonmedical appointments or events (CMS, n.d.). Persons with physical or medical conditions who have psychiatric symptoms that interfere with occupational performance may also receive mental health occupational therapy (Chapleau and Tessel, 2010). Given the prevalence of occupational performance problems among home health service recipients, practice opportunities are substantial.

Medicare-covered occupational therapy includes patient and caregiver education and training and direct services to remediate limitations, restore cognition and functional capabilities, slow decline, maintain a person's current condition or functional level, improve safety, and enable independence and self-sufficiency in daily activities (CMS, n.d.; Earle, 1999). Individualized task-oriented therapeutic activities, activity adaptations, and environmental modifications are skilled occupational therapy services that can attain improvement and maintenance goals. Home health practitioners work with people in the actual environments in which daily activities are performed. Collaboration with the person and family to assess needs and plan and implement intervention occurs in situ (Azok and Tomlinson, 1994; Gray, Haertl, Bowman, Leonard, and Leslie, 2018). Subsequent sections on family support and education and occupational therapy evaluation and intervention further describe methods that can be used in home health.

Engage Your Brain 18-1

Based on the AOTA *Occupational Therapy Code of Ethics (2015)*, what are important ethical considerations for providing psychiatric home health occupational therapy?

Housing Programs

Having a safe and stable place to live is key to recovery (SAMHSA, 2010b). However, when people with SMI were deinstitutionalized, housing options were scant. Consequently, most became homeless or were placed in custodial settings (e.g., shelters, foster homes, group homes, nursing homes, and for-profit board-and-care or single-room occupancy facilities). These settings provided no mental health services to support community integration (Nelson, 2010; Turner and TenHoo, 1978). When housing was unavailable, people remained institutionalized. In 1999, the U.S. Supreme Court's Olmstead decision ruled that the forced institutionalization and segregation of persons with mental illness was a violation of the Americans With Disabilities Act (ADA; Cottrell, 2005). Despite this ruling, many people with SMI continue to live in inadequate and/or segregated housing. Market rate housing in the United States is out of reach for the vast majority of people with SMI. If housing is found, most pay 50% (or more) of their income for housing that is often substandard (SAMHSA, 2010b).

Interventions are frequently needed to help people acquire the resources and competencies needed to establish and manage a home (AOTA, 2014). Because SMI typically develops during adolescence and young adulthood, opportunities to develop and/or retain independent living skills may be limited due to a primary focus on illness management (SAMHSA, 2010a). Transitional and permanent housing programs provide varying levels of skills training and support to enable independent living. The following describes these programs and housing resources. Chapter 20 addresses the needs of people who are homeless.

Supportive transitional housing provides "active rehabilitation programs with a focus on the promotion of life and social skills, independence, and work" (Nelson, 2010, p. 126). Program staff provide support and skills training that decreases in intensity along a residential continuum of quarterway houses, halfway houses, and shared or clustered apartments. Residents are expected to move along the continuum as competencies are acquired (e.g., from a halfway house to a supervised apartment). Upon completion of these time-limited programs, they must find permanent housing (Nelson, 2010). When available, supportive transitional housing enables independent living and community integration. However, communities often lack the facilities needed for this residential continuum. When post-discharge resources to enable autonomous living are unavailable, the loss of a supportive residence is often disruptive (Nelson, 2010). Consequently, contemporary housing approaches focus on services that support permanent homes for people with SMI.

Permanent supported housing programs respect participants' personal housing preference, use mainstream housing, and provide individualized, flexible, and consistent support (Swarbrick, 2016). Case management, employment assistance, family services, and independent living and community integration skills training are provided. Participants are educated about leases, tenant rights and responsibilities, and the Fair Housing Act, which prohibits housing discrimination (e.g., refusing tenancy to people with SMIs). As tenants, residents can remain in their homes as long as they meet lease requirements or choose to end the lease. Landlord and roommate education and support are provided to resolve conflicts and maintain tenancy (SAMHSA, 2010b; Swarbrick, 2016). Although some service providers and nonprofit agencies offer affordable permanent housing, most people with SMI rely on public project-based rental assistance and Section 8/811 vouchers to afford housing. Apartments available through these programs are often limited and have yearslong wait lists. Hence, there is a pressing need for more permanent housing (SAMHSA, 2010b).

SAMHSA provides a system-wide method for developing and implementing permanent supported housing programs. This evidence-based tool kit outlines action steps to expand community-based housing options; describes services to help people with SMI choose, obtain, and maintain housing; and provides program exemplars (SAMHSA, 2010b). Permanent supported housing is a cost-effective, evidence-based approach that increases housing tenure and reduces emergency room and crisis service use, hospitalizations, homelessness, and incarceration (Rog et al., 2014; SAMHSA, 2010b).

Occupational therapy practitioners can provide vital services to housing programs as supervisors, team leaders, activities of daily living (ADLs) specialists, and program consultants (SAMHSA, 2010b; Swarbrick, 2016). Lindström, Sjöström, and Lindberg (2012) integrated individualized, recovery-oriented, in vivo occupation-based training into housing programs to help persons with SMI (who often live alone and have sedentary lifestyles) attain self-identified goals for occupational engagement. They found significant improvements in participants' symptoms, goal attainment, occupational performance, and occupational engagement. Occupational therapy's contributions to independent living and community integration are further described in this chapter's evaluation and intervention sections.

Supported Education

Postsecondary education for adults is a socially valued developmental norm in the United States (Gutman, Kerner, Zombek, Dulek, and Ramsey, 2009). Sharing this value, adults with mental illness often initiate postsecondary education. However, they withdraw from college at almost double the rate of the general student population (Salzer, 2012). Because postsecondary education helps people acquire viable employment, become financially independent, and fully participate in society, abandoning it can negatively affect people's lives (Gutman et al., 2009; SAMHSA, 2011). **Supported education** (SEd) helps people with mental illness effectively access and engage in postsecondary education by confronting attitudinal barriers (i.e., discrimination, stigma) and providing support, resources, and services as needed to enable student success (Chandler, 2008; SAMHSA, 2011). Programs are provided in postsecondary institutions (i.e., 2- and 4-year colleges, universities, technical schools, and adult education programs) or by mental health agencies or programs (e.g., clubhouses) that have affiliations with education providers (Chandler, 2008; Ringeisen et al., 2017). Participants, called students, typically receive services that use a psychoeducation approach and a college semester format (Chandler, 2008).

SEd services include educational and vocational exploration, assessment, and goal planning; assistance in securing financial aid, tutors, and reasonable accommodations; individual and group instruction in study strategies, interpersonal skills, and stress and time management; academic advising, professional counseling, and peer mentoring to address concerns, develop solutions, and support engagement; and collaboration with campus and community resources to obtain essential services (e.g., childcare, transportation; Chandler, 2008; Ringeisen et al., 2017). An integral component of SEd is educating and training administrators, faculty, and staff about the capabilities and needs of students with mental illness and how they can positively contribute to student success (SAMHSA, 2011). Some SEd programs offer specialized training in marketable skills (e.g., computer literacy) or specific vocations (e.g., peer counseling; Chandler, 2008). All SEd programs support recovery by enabling participants to assume the socially recognized student role and discard a personal identity defined by illness (Chandler, 2008; Gutman et al., 2009). SAMHSA's (2011) EBP kit on SEd provides comprehensive information and concrete resources for program development and individualized service delivery.

Occupational therapy practitioners are well qualified to provide SEd services, and the evidence supporting the profession's efficacy in SEd programs is growing (Ringeisen et al., 2017; Schindler, 2010, 2018; Spencer, Sherman, Nielsen, and Thormodson, 2018). Schindler and Sauerwald (2013) and Gutman et al. (2009) provide an exemplary example of an occupational therapy SEd program that successfully enabled participants to acquire the skills, habits, and routines needed to assume and maintain the desired role of adult student. A systemic review of occupational therapy postsecondary SEd programs found that a group or classroom format that incorporated mentoring, setting goals, developing basic education knowledge and skills, and learning to manage available postsecondary resources resulted in increased postprogram enrollment in academic or vocational education (Arbesman and Logsdon, 2011).

PROGRAM SHOWCASE

Skills for Success

Population served: Stockton University undergraduate students with *DSM-5* diagnoses including attention deficit/hyperactivity, learning, autism spectrum, anxiety, depressive, and bipolar disorders.

Needs assessment: Prior to program initiation, a survey determined the need for a SEd program for individuals with *DSM-5* diagnoses. A questionnaire about SEd program availability, support for program development, and recommended program components was distributed to administrators of the University Office of Disabilities and local CMH service providers. Follow-up in-person or telephone meetings obtained additional information. All participants supported the development of an SEd program.

Goal(s): The program's goal is to facilitate undergraduate student success. If factors (e.g., academic deficiencies, symptom exacerbation, homesickness) impede goal attainment, an alternative plan is developed with the student (e.g., transferring to a community college close to home, obtaining a job). Participant goals are based on the results of an occupational profile and the Canadian Occupational Performance Measure (COPM) (AOTA, 2016b). The resulting self-identified occupational performance goals relate to the student role (e.g., study, writing, presentation, and social skills). Residential life and leisure goals are also common.

Services provided: The Skills for Success program is offered as a university general education curriculum course and is conducted twice per week for 2-hour sessions during the fall and spring semesters. Graduate occupational therapy students, supervised by occupational therapy faculty, provide weekly one-to-one SEd mentoring to systematically address participant goals. Client-centered and occupation-based interventions are strategically used to address participants' academic (e.g., current course demands) and social realities (e.g., residential life and extracurricular activities). Uniform written procedures address common participant goals and guide interventions.

Participant perspective: Jenna is a 35-year-old mother, home maintainer, worker, and student whose chronic anxiety and depression interfered with her ability to complete college. In the Skills for Success course, she learned organizational strategies and time-management skills to successfully complete her many role-related tasks. The specific study (e.g., Quizlet) and stress management (e.g., square breathing) techniques she learned were beneficial "because at college there is every type of stress you can imagine, and these techniques help me both inside and outside of the classroom."

Program outcomes: Beginning in 2005 and continuing yearly, the Skills for Success program has served both community members and university undergraduate students. When the number of undergraduates interested in the program exceeded the enrollment limit, it evolved to serve only these students. In 2012, the program became a credit-bearing undergraduate course. The analysis of the COPM reevaluations conducted at the end of each semester found that COPM satisfaction, performance, and total scores increased significantly ($p = 0.001–0.000$). Outcome studies also found that of the 83 students who started the program, 80 (96%) completed at least one semester. Of these, 62 continued at the university, for a retention rate of 77.5%, and 43 of the 62 had graduated as of 2018. These positive outcomes contrast with national data, which report that 86% of students with mental illness withdraw from college before completing their degree (Salzer, 2012) and that their graduation rates are lower than the general student population ([NAMI], 2012).

Funding: No funding is required because the program is embedded in credit-bearing courses.

Victoria P. Schindler, PhD, OTR, BCMH, FAOTA, provided this Program Showcase. See Schindler (2010, 2018) for more information.

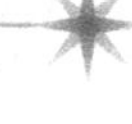

Postsecondary education institutions can also provide a setting for the implementation of enhanced SEd programs that use person-centered, occupation-based approaches to help students attain their academic objectives and work, leisure, and/or life skills goals (Schindler, 2010). Because the desired outcome of postsecondary education is for graduates to attain employment, SEd programs often integrate supported employment (Schindler, 2018). Supported employment is described in the next section.

Work Programs

Persons with SMI identify work as important to recovery (Doroud et al., 2015). Paid and unpaid work encourages occupational engagement, fosters a positive identity, develops personal responsibility, and increases self-worth (Doroud et al., 2015; Iannelli and Wilding, 2007). Volunteer work is a productive occupation that can be used to develop skills for paid work, or it can be a final work outcome. Volunteering enables people for whom paid employment is not viable to make altruistic societal contributions doing activities they choose for self-selected causes, facilities, and/or organizations (e.g., animal shelters, senior centers) according to their personal schedules (AOTA, 2014).

While volunteering has many benefits, paid employment has been found to contribute to improved economic, psychosocial, and clinical outcomes for people with SMI (Luciano and Meara, 2014; Noyes, Sokolov, and Arbesman, 2018). These benefits are well recognized, with 70% of people with SMI identifying a desire to work. However, 80% of persons receiving public mental health services are unemployed (NAMI, 2014). This gap between aspiration and reality must be addressed. When persons with SMI receive evidence-based services, their employment rates double (Luciano and Meara, 2014).

Engage Your Brain 18-2

Based on the AOTA (2014) *Practice Framework*, what are the similarities and differences between the activities and occupational demands of volunteer work versus competitive employment?

Historically, segregated "sheltered" workshops were typically the only work option for many with SMI. These provided rote and repetitive work with pay at a subminimum piecework rate. In the 1950s, **transitional employment** (TE) programs were initiated by Fountain House to help members acquire the skills needed for competitive employment (Dulay and Steichen, 1982; McKay, Nugent, Johnsen, Eaton, and Lidz, 2018). In communities without TE, workshops often remained the only vocational program. Recently, consumer advocacy for competitive work opportunities and evidence supporting integrated employment has led to a paradigm shift away from isolating workshops and to the defunding of these programs (Luciano and Meara, 2014). Contemporary programs enable mainstream employment at prevailing wages (McKay et al., 2018). **Supported employment** (SE) is an evidence-based approach for people with SMI that "emphasizes helping them obtain competitive work in the community and providing the supports necessary to ensure their success in the workplace" (SAMHSA, 2009, p. 9). Both SE and TE apply principles of recovery and promote community integration through the attainment of competitive employment that matches people's capabilities. SE and TE are provided by psychosocial rehabilitation and peer-delivered programs and state mental health and vocational rehabilitation agencies (SAMHSA, 2009). SE has no time limits, while TE programs are time limited (usually, 6 to 9 months). The SAMHSA (2009) SE evidence-based kit is a primary resource on how to build, implement, evaluate, and sustain an SE program.

Systemic reviews have found strong evidence that occupational therapy employment programs that use the individual placement and support (IPS) approach increase participants' competitive employment (Arbesman and Logsdon, 2011; Noyes et al., 2018; Smith, Atmatzidis, Capogreco, Lloyd-Randolfi, and Seman, 2017). Outcomes improved when cognitive or social skills training was provided along with IPS (Arbesman and Logsdon, 2011). Incorporating additional training and supports increased employment (Smith et al., 2017).

While SE is regarded as the gold standard for enabling the competitive employment of people with SMI, fewer than 2% of those who receive public mental health services in the United States receive state-provided SE (NAMI, 2014). The number of people able to access private SE programs is determined by funding and job availability; both are limited. Thus, the need for more meaningful work opportunities is great. Consumer-run businesses (e.g., coffee or thrift shops) offer viable work-training options (Herron, Gioia, and Dohrn, 2009). Individuals with SMI can start a business or attain other employment goals through the federal Plan to Achieve Self-Support (PASS) and Ticket to Work (TTW) programs and state one-stop centers (Social Security Administration [SSA], 2018).

The social enterprise model provides another alternative to agency-sponsored work programs and the open job market for people with SMI (Herron et al., 2009; Lancto, Durand, and Corbiere, 2012). Also called affirmative businesses, social firms, and work collectives, social enterprise businesses have two missions:

- To use economic enterprise to provide a service or product that generates income
- To employ marginalized people and meet a social need for the betterment of their lives (Lancto et al., 2012)

Social enterprise employees are permanent and receive competitive salaries and benefits, peer and supervisor support, work accommodations, and acceptance of relapses (Herron et al., 2009; Lancto et al., 2012). Social enterprise is highly congruent with occupational therapy's mission to attain occupational justice by enabling full participation in meaningful occupations and opportunities for social inclusion (AOTA, 2014).

The passage of the ADA in 1990 resulted in many opportunities for occupational therapy. These included determining essential and marginal job functions, assessing work environments, educating employers, advocating for reasonable accommodations, implementing programs that develop work readiness and self-advocacy, and serving as a liaison between employees and employers (Crist and Stoffel, 1992).

Case Management

Case management, a core mental health service since the 1970s, is

> *a collaborative process of assessment, planning, facilitation, care coordination, evaluation and advocacy for options and services to meet an individual's and family's comprehensive health needs through communication and available resources to promote patient safety, quality of care, and cost-effective outcomes. (Case Management Society of America [CMSA], 2016, p. 11)*

In 2011, the AOTA Model Practice Act identified case management as an occupational therapy intervention (AOTA, 2011). Recently, the AOTA (2018) asserted "that occupational therapy practitioners are well prepared and qualified to be case managers for persons with conditions that interfere with occupational performance" (p. 1). However, this declaration only described an indirect service model in which the case manager connects people to needed services and resources, makes recommendations, and oversees their implementation but does not provide direct services (AOTA, 2018; Dallas, 2011). In contrast, clinical case management includes direct services (e.g., in vivo life skills training) and indirect services (e.g., referrals to social services; Chapleau, Seroczynski, Meyers, Lamb, and Buchino, 2012; Dallas, 2011). Box 18-2 outlines case management's main components and tasks, including person-centered, environmental, and person-environment interventions. Because many administrators and payers emphasize cost containment, the use of a strengths- and competency-based model is needed to guide service provision and attain case management goals (Treiger and Fink-Samnick, 2014).

Case management is not a distinct field; it is a specialized health and human services practice modality (Commission for Case Management Certification [CCMC], 2018). While many case managers have professional degrees, not all do (Chapleau et al., 2012). Because this education and training diversity

Box 18-2 Case Management Components and Tasks

Initial Phase

Engagement to form a therapeutic relationship; build rapport and trust
Assessment to determine a person's strengths, needs, concerns, and aspirations
Planning to determine an individualized person-directed plan

Intervention Phase

Person-Centered Interventions

Counseling and support
Training in independent living skills
Assistance with daily tasks and their complexities
Psychoeducation and wellness promotion
Evaluation of functional and social participation outcomes

Environmental Interventions

Linkage with community resources and services
Consultation with families and other caregivers
Maintenance and expansion of social networks
Collaboration with service providers
Advocacy to acquire needed resources and services

Person-Environment Interventions

Crisis prevention and intervention
In vivo life skills and community participation training
Monitoring daily functioning and social participation

Intervention Review Phase

Reevaluation of outcomes, service utilization, goals, and options
Collaboration to modify and revise the individualized, person-directed plan

From "Clinical Case Management: Definition, Principles, Components," by J. Kanter, 1989, *Hospital and Community Psychiatry, 40*, 361–368. Reprinted and adapted with permission.

cannot assure a qualified workforce, the CCMC has established certification standards. Certified case managers (CCM®) must demonstrate knowledge about case management and the ability to complete essential service activities. Occupational therapists' education and professional license meet the CCMC examination eligibility requirements, enabling them to become CCMs® (CCMC, 2018). The profession's emphasis on functional outcomes that enable occupational performance and community participation and practitioners' evaluation and intervention skills are highly applicable to clinical case management. The CCMC and CMSA provide multiple resources for practitioners to further develop case management competencies.

The literature supporting the efficacy of case management is limited and largely focused on services provided to persons who are homeless or at risk for homelessness and those with substance abuse disorders (Chapleau et al., 2012; SAMHSA, 2016). Throckmorton and Windle (2009a, 2009b) advocate for the use of systematic reviews and meta-analyses to develop case management's evidence base.

Peer-Delivered Services

Peer-delivered services are designed, developed, and implemented by persons who share the lived experience of mental illness. They include self-help groups, drop-in centers, peer support services, and consumer-operated services and businesses (Rogers and Swarbrick, 2016; Swarbrick and Pratt, 2006). **Peer support services** "assist in developing coping and problem-solving strategies for illness self-management; draw on lived experiences and empathy to promote hope, insights, skills; help engage in treatment, and access community supports (to) establish a satisfying life" (Chinman et al., 2014, p. 430). Peer support services in the United States became available in 1938 when Recovery Incorporated (RI) was established to help discharged patients with mental illness adjust to community living (Myrick and del Vecchi, 2016). Now called Recovery International, RI's peer-to-peer, structured cognitive-behavioral training system is used globally in self-help groups to help members manage distressful symptoms and gain skills to lead healthy, productive lives (Myrick and del Vecchi, 2016).

Peer-directed services were significantly advanced in 1948 when former psychiatric patients established Fountain House, a "clubhouse" where persons with mental illness could support each other, destigmatize mental illness, and promote recovery (McKay et al., 2018). "**Clubhouses** are intentionally formed, non-clinical, integrated therapeutic working communities composed of adults and young adults diagnosed with SMI (members) and staff who are active in all Clubhouse activities" (McKay et al., 2018, p. 29). Membership is voluntary, open, and ongoing. It confers personal ownership and responsibility for program success. Using a strengths-based approach, members and staff work as colleagues to complete day-to-day operations. Clubhouses typically provide case management, social activities, skills-building groups, employment programs, community outreach, and assistance with accessing housing, entitlement programs, and health-care services (Clubhouse International, 2016). Evidence supports the efficacy of clubhouses in decreasing hospitalization(s), enabling employment, promoting social relationships, and improving quality of life (McKay et al., 2018).

Over the past 40 years, the consumer advocacy movement has contributed to the recognition that "people in recovery can bring sensitive understanding, unique skills, knowledge, and support to facilitate long-term recovery" (Rogers and Swarbrick, 2016, p. 193). Thus, peer-delivered services are now an integral component of behavioral health care and are widely used to supplement and/or replace traditional psychiatric services (Chinman et al., 2014; Myrick and del Vecchi, 2016; Rogers and Swarbrick, 2016). As paid employees and key members of multidisciplinary teams, peers can work in traditional clinical settings (e.g., PHP), fill existing clinical roles (e.g., case manager), and provide specific structured curricula (e.g., IMR; Chinman et al., 2014). Peer support specialists develop one-to-one relationships and provide individualized support to enable recovery. They can be specifically trained to address health-care disparities and provide wellness interventions that increase health, enhance quality of life, and extend life span (Swarbrick, Tunner, Miller, Werner, and Tiegreen, 2016).

Peer support services have been recognized by the CMS as an evidence-based care model (SAMHSA, 2018). Research on the efficacy of peer-delivered services is nascent, but promising (Swarbrick et al., 2016; Swarbrick and Pratt, 2006). Chinman et al. (2014) found that peer support services reduced hospitalization, improved consumer-provider relationships, and increased consumer engagement, empowerment, self-efficacy, and hope. SAMHSA Consumer Network Grants fund training, education, and resources to develop public peer-directed services (Myrick and del Vecchi, 2016). For those who do not have access to public or agency peer-directed programs, the NAMI (2018b) peer-to-peer psychoeducational recovery course and online discussion groups are valuable free resources.

Occupational therapy practitioners can collaborate with consumers and peer service providers to develop, implement, promote, and evaluate peer-directed programs (Swarbrick and Pratt, 2006). They can provide direct, consultative, and administrative services using their discipline-specific expertise when participation complexities and challenges to recovery are beyond the experience and knowledge of these providers (Stoffel, 2013).

Family Support and Education

The medical model's historical dominance in psychiatry perpetuated a conceptualization of SMI as a condition to be cured. Focused on eliminating symptoms, psychiatric practitioners disregarded the lived experiences of persons with SMI and their families (Ragins, 2011). This paternalistic and disempowering approach resulted in frustrating, unsupportive, and, at times, adversarial relationships between mental health professionals and families (Ragins, 2011).

Deinstitutionalization and the precipitous decline in the number of inpatient psychiatric beds contributed to a reconceptualization of the family's role in treatment (Liberman, 1988). With families having increased responsibilities for the care of their members with SMI, the need for family support services became critical (Goldman, 1988). Over 18% of adults in the United States live with mental illness; thus, having a family member with a mental illness is not uncommon. Yet few are prepared for this role (Bourke, Sanders, Allchin, Lentin, and Lang, 2015). Families often need help to cope with the complex emotional responses (e.g., guilt, fear, anger, loss, frustration, embarrassment, and bewilderment) that often accompany a psychiatric diagnosis and the resulting behavorial and functional changes (Liberman, 1988; Urish and Jacobs, 2011). They must learn how to navigate an oft fragmented system of care to help their family member receive essential services and respond adaptively to changed capabilities (Urish and Jacobs, 2011). The long-term and often unpredictable course of SMI can have a substantial impact on a family's well-being, with many experiencing a physical, emotional, and financial strain that can become burdensome if not relieved (Bourke et al., 2015).

In the 1980s, psychoeducation programs were developed to decrease family burden and support recovery by teaching persons with SMI and their relatives how to effectively communicate and solve daily problems (Liberman, 1988). The efficacy of family psychoeducation (FPE) is well established. FPE increases family knowledge about and understanding of SMI, improves family well-being, decreases isolation and stress, and reduces the occurrence of medical illnesses and medical-care use. For the person with SMI, FPE results in fewer relapses and hospitalizations and increases participation in vocational rehabilitation programs (SAMHSA, 2010c). The NAMI Family-to-Family course is a SAMHSA-designated evidence-based program and an invaluable free resource to help families better understand mental illness, improve coping skills, and become empowered mental health advocates (NAMI, 2018b). The SAMHSA (2010c) free evidence-based tool kit can be used to develop FPE programs.

Occupational therapy practitioners can lead FPE groups on symptom, medication, and stress management and cognitive-behavioral strategies to manage the impact of mental illness on family life (Urish and Jacobs, 2011). They can provide home-based services to enable occupational performance and help maintain the familial role(s) of the person with SMI. Caregivers' need to maintain their personal well-being can also be addressed. Bourke et al. (2015) describe a peer support program that embedded occupational therapy into a mental health service to enable families and others who provide care to persons with SMI attain and maintain occupational balance. This program has provided an occupationally focused service model since 1999 and has been replicated throughout Australia (Bourke et al., 2015).

Being a parent is a significant family role that many people living with a mental illness share (Goodyear et al., 2015). Occupational therapy to develop effective parenting skills can help persons with SMI continue their involvement in this valued role (Bassett, Lampe, and Lloyd, 2001; Urish and Jacobs, 2011). A family-focused approach that supports internal and external protective factors (e.g., self-efficacy, community resources) and reduces risk factors (e.g., symptom exacerbation) can promote parent, child, and family resilience and well-being (Foster, O'Brien, and Korhonen, 2012). Established family-inclusive practice standards can be integrated into the continuum of care and support recovery for parents of dependent children with SMI (Goodyear et al., 2015).

Role of Occupational Therapy

Occupational therapy practitioners contribute significantly to the recovery of persons with SMI by collaborating with interdisciplinary team members, including psychiatrists, psychologists, psychiatric nurses, social workers, vocational rehabilitation counselors, family therapists, paraprofessionals, and peer specialists to provide person-directed recovery-oriented services across the mental health continuum of care (AOTA, 2016a; Wollenberg, 2002). They ensure that barriers to recovery that are often overlooked by other disciplines (e.g., cognitive impairments, sensory-processing disorders) are identified during evaluation and addressed in treatment (Swarbrick and Noyes, 2018). Occupational therapy practitioners can work as direct service providers, supervisors, administrators, case managers, employment specialists, and consultants in all of the CMH programs described in this chapter (AOTA, 2016a) They can also provide services as sole proprietors of private practices (Gray et al., 2018), work as consultants to mental health-care systems (AOTA, 2016a), and operate freestanding CMH occupational therapy clinics (Haertl, Behrens, Houtujec, Rue, and Ten Haken, 2009).

Evaluation

The evaluation process begins with a screening to obtain a preliminary understanding of a person's priorities and identify the client factors, areas of occupation, and performance skills, patterns, and/or contexts that require further evaluation (AOTA, 2014). This information determines the evaluation foci and ensures that chosen assessments are relevant to a person's unique situation and desired outcomes. Ascertaining an individual's personal stage of recovery (see Table 18-2) can also inform evaluation foci.

Practice models and the evidence supporting a measure's rigor (e.g., reliability, validity) and its

Table 18-2 Personal Stages of Recovery

Overcoming Stuckness	Returning to Basic Functioning	Discovering Self-Empowerment	Learning and Self-Redefinition	Improving Quality of Life
• Acknowledging and accepting illness • Desire and motivation to change • Finding/having source of hope/inspiration	• Taking care of basic needs: eating, hygiene, basic physical health • Being active: exercising, leisure activities • Connecting with others	• Taking responsibility for own recovery • Taking responsibility for behaviors • Determined and hardworking • Courage to challenge self and take risks	• Recapturing parts of old self and discovering new aspects of self • Learning there is more to self than illness	• Striving to attain overall sense of well-being • Striving for ideals often associated with stable mental health • Serving as a recovery role model for others

From "Recovery and Occupational Therapy in the Community Mental Health Setting," by J. L. Wallace, 2002, *Occupational Therapy in Mental Health, 17*(3–4), 103. Reprinted with permission.

value (e.g., intended purposes) should inform assessment selection (Hinojosa and Kramer, 2014). Multiple publications describe measures commonly used in occupational therapy (AOTA, 2016b). Box 18-3 identifies several. These assessments obtain people's perspectives and determine their capabilities, but they do not consider systemic barriers or resources.

Box 18-3 Assessments Commonly Used in Community Mental Health Practice

ADL/IADL Assessments

Assessment of Motor and Process Skills
Performance Assessment of Self-Care Skills
Test of Grocery Shopping Skills

Cognitive Performance-Based Measures

Lowenstein Occupational Therapy Cognitive Assessment
Executive Function Performance Test

Self-Assessments and Interviews

Goal Attainment Scaling
Canadian Occupational Performance Measure
Modified Interest Checklist
Occupational Circumstances Assessment Interview Rating Scale
Occupational Self-Assessment
Role Checklist

Social Interaction Measures

Assessment of Communication and Interaction Skills
Assessment of Social Interaction

Sensory-Processing Assessment

Adult/Adolescent Sensory Profile

Work Assessments

McCarron-Dial Evaluation System
Work Environment Impact Scale
Worker Role Interview

Developed from *Occupational Therapy Service Outcome Measures for Certified Community Behavioral Health Centers (CCBHCS): Framework for Occupational Therapy Service With Rationale for Outcome Measures Selection and Listing of Occupational Therapy Outcome Measure Tools,* by American Occupational Therapy Association, 2016, Rockville, MD: American Occupational Therapy Association; *An Annotated Index of Occupational Therapy Evaluation Tools* (3rd ed.), by I. E. Asher, 2007, Bethesda, MD: AOTA Press; "Stories of Rediscovering Agency: Home Based Occupational Therapy Interventions Among People With Severe Psychiatric Disability," by M. Lindström, S. Sjöström, and M. Lindberg, 2012, *Occupation, Participation and Health, 32*(2), 5–12.

Thus, the person's contextual and environmental supports and obstacles must also be evaluated (Fleming-Castaldy, 2015). The ccupational profile provides targeted questions in order to acquire a more complete understanding of people and their contexts (AOTA, 2014). Initial and ongoing in situ observations of occupational performance in the person's natural environment provide valuable information to guide interventions (Gray et al., 2018).

Intervention

Occupational therapy interventions are designed to help people with SMI attain self-determined goals. Practitioners use activity analyses, activity adaptations and gradations, compensatory strategies, environmental modifications, and explicit skills training to enable occupational performance; time-use planning to foster satisfying routines and balanced lifestyles; and education to promote personal empowerment (Gray et al., 2018; Hohl et al., 2017; Krupa et al., 2009; Leufstadius and Eklund, 2008; Swarbrick and Noyes, 2018). Services are provided in the natural environment (e.g., completing self-care in a person's home, shopping at a neighborhood store). Occupational therapy practitioners educate and train multidisciplinary staff, community workers, and people in the person's routine environments (e.g., home, work, school) on methods and strategies to support the person's autonomy, optimal performance, independence, and recovery (Gray et al., 2018). They provide illness management, health, and wellness services (e.g., WRAP development, smoking cessation, weight loss, diabetes management) to address existing conditions, prevent the occurrence of comorbidities, and reduce the health impact of MetS (Brown, Gelszer, Lewis, and Arbesman, 2018; Swarbrick and Pratt, 2006). Table 18-3 identifies occupational therapy intervention approaches used to promote health, establish and restore skills, maintain capabilities, compensate for limitations, and prevent occupational performance problems.

The evidence supporting the efficacy of occupational therapy for persons with SMI is strong. A systemic review of interventions to maintain and improve the participation and occupational performance of people with SMI examined ADL, IADL, social participation, leisure, rest, and sleep outcomes (D'Amico, Jaffe, and Gardner, 2018). Evidence

Table 18-3 Occupational Therapy Intervention Approaches in Community Mental Health

Intervention Approach	Practice Example
Health promotion - Disability and performance deficits are not assumed. - Interventions are designed to enhance activity performance in natural contexts.	An illness management group is designed to help clubhouse members acquire knowledge about the positive impact medication(s) can have on occupational performance and develop self-advocacy skills to address any negative impact medication(s) may have on function.
Remediation/restoration - Used when skills and abilities were not developed or were lost due to incurred illness and/or disability. - Interventions address client impairments and variables that limit performance and are designed to develop and/or restore performance skills.	Life skills and parenting psychoeducation modules are provided in a PHP to help parents with SMI acquire the skills needed to implement a structured daily routine that is self-determined, manageable, and balanced to complete ADLs and IADLs, effectively meet their needs and those of their children, and enable satisfactory performance of valued occupational roles.
Maintenance - Recognizes that capabilities, well-being, and health can be lost or diminished without intervention. - Strategies and supports are provided to preserve acquired abilities, meet occupational needs, and maintain health, wellness, and quality of life.	An occupational therapy consultant to a peer-run program provides ongoing individualized interventions to members with SMI and their families to support the continued use of environmental modifications, activity adaptations, and cognitive-behavioral strategies that can preserve acquired competencies, sustain participation in desired occupations, and maintain familial wellness and occupational balance.
Compensation/adaptation - Used when people cannot complete desired activities or engage in valued roles in a "typical" manner. - An analysis of activity demands and contexts is used to determine activity adaptations, compensatory techniques, and environmental modifications that can enable occupational engagement.	In a transitional employment program, the analysis of the activity demands of a job's essential and marginal functions and provision of environmental modification and work simplification recommendations (e.g., remove work station clutter to decrease distractibility, break down large work tasks into smaller components) allow the successful completion of work tasks within a person's capabilities to enable successful engagement in the role of employee.
Disability prevention - Addresses the reality that all people can be at risk for developing problems with occupational performance. - Interventions to prevent personal and/or contextual barriers to satisfactory and effective performance from occurring or escalating are provided.	Advising persons who hum and move in response to auditory hallucinations to wear unconnected headphones/earbuds in public can prevent the occurrence of stigmatizing reactions that can hinder social participation and limit occupational performance. Many people hum and move while wearing these socially acceptable devices; thus, a person with SMI using these will fit in with this norm.

Adapted from "Approaches to Intervention" (Table 8) in "Occupational Therapy Practice Framework: Domain and Process" (3rd ed.), by American Occupational Therapy Association, 2014, *American Journal of Occupational Therapy, 68*(Suppl. 1), S3. Reprinted with permission.

supporting the efficacy of psychoeducation and occupation- and cognitive-based interventions was strong. Evidence for occupation-based interventions that addressed individualized, client-centered ADL, IADL, and social participation goals was particularly strong. The evidence for skills-based intervention was moderate (D'Amico et al., 2018). An earlier systemic review of recovery-oriented occupational therapy interventions that focused on the normative life roles and community reintegration of people with SMI found moderate to strong evidence for the effectiveness of social skills training and moderate evidence for life skills, IADL, and neurocognitive training (Gibson, D'Amico, Jaffe, and Arbesman, 2011). These findings can be used to guide occupational therapy interventions, program development, and practice-based research.

Practice Challenges and Opportunities

The limited number of CMH occupational therapy practitioners often results in one being the sole representative of the profession on the multidisciplinary team (O'Connell and McKay, 2010). Consequently, workloads can be heavy (Haertl et al., 2009). This singular status and increased demands for autonomy can be challenging for entry-level practitioners and those acclimated to working in well-defined occupational therapy departments (Fox, 2013; Lloyd, King, and Ryan, 2007; O'Connell and McKay, 2010; Ramsey, 2011). CMH teams expect all members to perform generic tasks along with their discipline-specific ones. This role blurring can lead to a decline in specialized skills, a diminished professional identity, and the lack of recognition of occupational therapy's unique contributions (Haertl et al., 2009; Lloyd et al., 2007; Michetti and Dieleman, 2014; O'Connell and McKay, 2010). These practice realities can be effectively mediated by participating in supervision, mentorship, continuing and/or postgraduate education, and local, state, and national association professional development and networking opportunities (O'Connell and McKay, 2010; Ramsey, 2011; Reeves and Mann, 2004).

Occupational therapy practitioners can develop and maintain strong professional identities by embedding occupation-based models and research into their daily practice and routinely using occupational performance and participation assessments and interventions (Haertl et al., 2009; Michetti and Dieleman, 2014; Pettican and Bryant, 2007; Reeves and Mann, 2004). An enhanced role identity contributes to increased perceptions of self-efficacy and greater job satisfaction (Haertl et al., 2009). CMH occupational therapy practitioners report satisfaction with their workplace autonomy, job diversity, opportunities for learning and creativity, and interdisciplinary communication, cooperation, and support (Haertl et al., 2009; Holmes and Scaffa 2009; O'Connell and McKay, 2010). Additional reported rewards of community-based practice include being able to promote the profession, act as change agents, serve underserved communities, and provide individualized in situ occupation-based interventions that enable goal attainment (see Fig. 18-2; Haertl et al., 2009; Holmes and Scaffa, 2009; Ramsey, 2011).

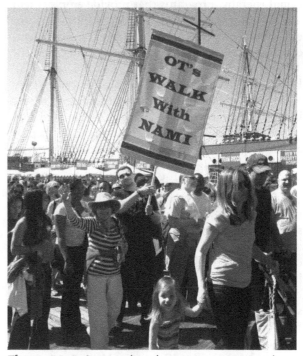

Figure 18-2 Partnerships between occupational therapy practitioners and mental health advocacy groups provide opportunities to promote the profession and provide health and wellness programs that support recovery and confront stigma. *(Photo courtesy of SUNY Downstate Medical Center. Visit www.downstate.edu/chrp/ot/outreach/nami/index.html.)*

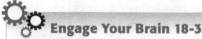

Engage Your Brain 18-3

Actively reflect on your personal attributes and competencies. How can you use these to meet the challenges and seize the opportunities of community-based mental health occupational therapy practice? How can you use the resources identified in this chapter and its references to support your personal and professional development?

Funding and Advocacy for Community Mental Health

Funding for CMH includes private insurance, Medicare, and Medicaid; state-, city-, and local government-budgeted allocations; and private and federal grants. All can include payment for occupational therapy. Programs that provide employment and training services (i.e., supported education, vocational rehabilitation, and supported employment) can also receive funds from one-stop centers and the TTW program (Ringeisen et al., 2017; SSA, 2018). Home-based and PHP occupational therapy is covered by Medicare and third-party payers; private insurance coverage varies (Craig, 2012). Medicare home health coverage excludes occupational therapy as an initial qualifying service. This constraint and limited knowledge about the profession's role in home health may contribute to its underutilization (Craig, 2012). Medicare PHP benefits specify occupational therapy as an included, but not mandated, service. Since 2000, a prospective payment system has reimbursed PHPs according to a daily rate based on an average of all patients. Occupational therapy is bundled into this rate (CMS, 2012).

Medicaid CMH coverage varies greatly from state to state. The use of managed-care companies to administer Medicaid has resulted in the "carving out" of mental health benefits, coverage gaps, and state inconsistencies (Palanker, Volk, Lucia, and Thomas, 2018). Regulations for private insurance also differ significantly. Twenty-eight states do not require any coverage for mental health services, while five states mandate comprehensive coverage (Palanker et al., 2018). Over the past decade, federal legislation has sought to remediate these inequities. The 2008 Mental Health Parity and Addiction Equity Act required group health insurance plans that offered mental health and substance use disorder benefits to provide this coverage at the same cost and level as their medical/surgical benefits. Because this law only applied to group plans, individual plans continued to deny and/or limit coverage for mental health and substance use disorders (Palanker et al., 2018). In 2010, Congress passed the Patient Protection and Affordable Care Act (ACA), which addressed these inequities by establishing federal regulations for private insurance. These regulations mandated parity in mental health and substance abuse treatment and required comprehensive coverage equivalent to other medical coverage (Palanker et al., 2018). Current proposed federal regulatory changes and/or future legislation may roll back some of these parity advances and limit mandated coverage for mental health services (Palanker et al., 2018).

The heavy reliance of CMH programs on public funding can significantly limit services if legislative bodies do not recognize their value (Palanker et al., 2018). Similarly, a lack of understanding about occupational therapy's role in CMH can constrain practice opportunities. Thus, practitioners must recognize the "dynamic nature of contemporary health and human services delivery systems . . . to advocate for the profession and the consumer" (ACOTE®, 2017, p. 1). Practitioners in states who receive SAMHSA Block Grants can volunteer to serve on their state-mandated mental health advisory planning council, which gives input on how grant money is spent (SAMHSA, 2017). These councils provide a forum for promoting occupational therapy's cost-effectiveness and efficacy and advocating for its inclusion in CMH programs. All can support the advocacy efforts of the NAMI and other mental health rights organizations to obtain funding to increase the availability and quality of CMH services.

Membership in the AOTA and state occupational therapy associations can help practitioners remain informed about federal and state policies that have an impact on the profession's ability to provide services. For example, few states specifically identify occupational therapists as qualified mental health professionals (Gray et al., 2018). However, recent federal actions have recognized the profession's importance to the provision of quality recovery-oriented CMH services (AOTA, 2017).

The Future of Community Mental Health Practice

The mental health-care system has been irrevocably changed by the decades-long demands of people with SMI and their advocates for services that enable wellness, occupational engagement, and social participation in environments of choice (Cottrell, 2007; Swarbrick, 2009). Reformative legislation and policies now support community-based prevention, health promotion, and recovery-oriented services (Stoffel, 2013). This systemic emphasis will likely continue because society can no longer ignore its members' psychosocial needs (Gutman and Raphael-Greenfield, 2014). As reported in this chapter, research strongly supports the relationships between occupational engagement, recovery, and life satisfaction and the distinct value and efficacy of occupational therapy in CMH programs. Substantial discipline-specific resources are available to support and promote best practice and research. Thus, it is an opportune time for occupational therapy practitioners to return to the profession's mental health roots and seize current and emerging CMH opportunities. The capacity for occupational therapy practitioners to make a transformative difference in the lives of people with SMI through the use of therapeutic occupations that enable and empower is limitless.

Summary

- Pervasive program gaps, funding inadequacies, and society's marginalization of people with mental illness have historically limited, and continue to constrain, the availability of CMH services.
- Key federal legislative initiatives and major paradigm shifts in mental health care have contributed to the development of community-based, person-directed, and recovery-oriented programs for persons with SMI.
- Best practice in CMH incorporates established mental health and occupational therapy practice models and evidence-based intervention approaches that promote empowerment, wellness, and recovery.
- Occupational therapy practitioners are well qualified to fulfill diverse roles in CMH programs to provide occupation-based evaluations and interventions that enable occupational performance and participation in desired roles.
- Multiple resources are available to develop practitioner competencies to meet the challenges and seize the opportunities afforded in CMH for the provision of effective recovery-oriented, person-directed, and evidence-based occupational therapy.

CASE STUDIES

CASE STUDY 18-1 Matt

Matt is 24 years old and has lived with schizophrenia for 4 years. Upon the onset of his illness, Matt received treatment in an IOP. He resumed college but struggled to meet the requirements of his environmental science major and part-time job. Matt dropped out and moved back home. He worked sporadically for his family's landscaping business but did not seek competitive employment. His parents supported Matt's unemployment and never asked him to do tasks (e.g., grocery shopping, preparing meals) that they believed would overstress him. Matt spent his days sleeping, smoking, and playing video games. When invited to engage in social activities, Matt declined because he had "nothing in common" with his high school friends, and noise made him "unfocused." Matt's sedentary lifestyle and antipsychotic medications contributed to him gaining over 35 pounds. His weight gain and isolated existence led to Matt discontinuing his medications and questioning if life with SMI was worth living. His concerned parents took him to the psychiatric emergency room for crisis intervention services, resulting in a 3-day hospitalization.

CASE STUDY 18-1 Matt

Upon discharge, Matt began a PHP that provides multidisciplinary recovery-oriented interventions to develop illness management, independent living, and participation skills. During the occupational therapy evaluation, Matt identified the past roles of student, worker, home maintainer, and friend as very valuable on the Role Checklist but did not see them in his future. When discussing his goals, Matt stated that he was "nervous about going it alone" but did not want to live with his parents "because they baby me." He expressed a desire to "be more productive" but reported "feeling tense around people because they judge me." The occupational therapist and Matt collaborated to formulate an intervention plan focused on enabling role engagement.

Discussion Questions

1. Which assessments can be used to obtain additional relevant information about Matt's capabilities and needs to guide the development of a person-directed intervention plan?
2. Referring to Tables 18-1 and 18-2, where does Matt seem to be in his recovery? Describe occupational therapy interventions that can help Matt move to the next stage of recovery along each scale and develop his competencies for desired role engagement.
3. The occupational therapist provides consumer psychoeducation. Applying the stress-vulnerability/coping-competence and recovery models, describe specific strategies for Matt to develop his stress management and coping skills and acquire competencies for a productive, satisfying, and healthy life.
4. As Matt approaches discharge from the PHP, which program(s) and service(s) would be relevant for the occupational therapist to explore with Matt to support his continued recovery?

CASE STUDY 18-2 Professional Rehabilitation Consultants

Professional Rehabilitation Consultants (PRC) is a Medicare-certified outpatient rehabilitation agency that specializes in providing mental health occupational therapy. PRC was founded in 1989 by an occupational therapist and certified occupational therapy assistant who collaborated with the owners of a board-and-care home to provide occupational therapy services to adults diagnosed with SMI. Located in Saint Paul, Minnesota, this freestanding, community-based psychiatric clinic is administered by an occupational therapist; all service providers are occupational therapy practitioners. People are referred to PRC after crisis intervention services or inpatient hospitalization, after symptom exacerbation, or upon receiving a new diagnosis.

Typical reasons for seeking services include decreased ADL and IADL functioning, increased need for caregiver support, limited structure, housing changes, poor interpersonal skills, a desire for more independence, and/or a change in overall health. Individualized person-directed services include the evaluation of independent living, social, cognitive, and sensory-processing skills to develop intervention plans tailored to each person's needs. Interventions include skills training, relapse prevention, illness management, and crisis intervention education. A variety of occupation-based modalities (e.g., crafts, ADLs and IADLs, psychoeducation) are provided in a structured setting to improve cognitive, social, emotional, and physical capabilities; develop and/or restore independent living, leisure, and community participation skills; create and engage in healthy lifestyle habits and routines; establish job readiness capabilities; and explore community supports and opportunities (e.g., volunteering). Most services are provided within the occupational therapy clinic; however, home visits and consultations with external agencies are also provided as needed to meet individual goals (Haertl et al., 2009; Professional Rehabilitation Consultants, n.d.).

CASE STUDY 18-2 Professional Rehabilitation Consultants

Discussion Questions

1. What needs assessment and program development strategies can be used to replicate this program exemplar?
2. What resources and partnerships are necessary to successfully establish an outpatient mental health rehabilitation agency?
3. How would you market a freestanding occupational therapy mental health clinic to the other CMH service providers?

Learning Activities

1. Read a first-person account of a person living with SMI. What gives meaning and purpose to this person's life? What are the individual's strengths and limitations? How could an occupational therapy practitioner engage with this person to support occupational engagement, health, and wellness?
2. Identify community resources people with SMI can use to attain their goals. Visit the location of one of these and engage in an activity typically performed there (e.g., requesting information at the Social Security office, shopping in a thrift store). Complete an analysis of the sensory, cognitive, perceptual, physical, and psychosocial demands of your activity performance. How might SMI affect a person's ability to meet these demands? What recommendations would you make to the person and facility to ensure full access to this resource and its activities?
3. Review your state's department of mental health website and the NAMI website to obtain more information about CMH services in your state. What are the similarities and differences between your state's stated aspirations and its service delivery realities? How do these compare to SAMHSA's recommended evidence-based services?
4. Visit one of the following websites to obtain the perspectives of people living with SMI. Review the site's resources that enable recovery. Describe how these perspectives and resources can be integrated into occupational therapy practice.
   a. Mental Health America (2018): www.mentalhealthamerica.net/
   b. National Coalition for Mental Health Recovery (2016): www.ncmhr.org/
   c. National Empowerment Center (2018): www.power2u.org

REFERENCES

Accreditation Council for Occupational Therapy Education. (2017). *Draft III revisions—December 2017.* Retrieved from www.aota.org/~/media/Corporate/Files/Education Careers/Accredit/StandardsReview/Draft-III-ACOTE-Standards-12-2017.pdf

Ahern, L., and Fisher, D. (2001). An alternative to PACT: Recovery at your own PACE. *Mental Health Special Interest Section Quarterly, 24*(4), 3–4.

American Occupational Therapy Association. (2011). *Definition of occupational therapy practice for the AOTA Model Practice Act.* Retrieved from www.aota.org/~/media/Corporate/Files/Advocacy/State/Resources/PracticeAct/MODEL%20PRACTICE %20ACT%20FINAL%202007.pdf

American Occupational Therapy Association. (2014). Occupational therapy practice framework: Domain and process (3rd ed.). *American Journal of Occupational Therapy, 68*(Suppl. 1), S1–S48.

American Occupational Therapy Association. (2015). Occupational therapy code of ethics. *American Journal of Occupational Therapy, 69*(Suppl. 3), 6913410030. doi:10.5014/ajot.2015.696S03

American Occupational Therapy Association. (2016a). *Occupational therapy's role in mental health recovery.* Rockville, MD: American Occupational Therapy Association.

American Occupational Therapy Association. (2016b). *Occupational therapy service outcome measures for certified community behavioral health centers (CCBHCs): Framework for occupational therapy service with rationale for outcome measures selection and listing of occupational therapy outcome measure tools.* Rockville, MD: American Occupational Therapy Association.

American Occupational Therapy Association. (2017). *Occupational therapy recognized in federal behavioral health programs.* Retrieved from www.aota.org/~/media/Corporate/Files/Advocacy /Federal/Federal-Actions.pdf

American Occupational Therapy Association. (2018). *Occupational therapy's role in case management position paper.* Rockville, MD: American Occupational Therapy Association.

Arbesman, M., and Logsdon, D. (2011). Occupational therapy interventions for employment and education for adults with serious mental illness: A systematic review. *American Journal of Occupational Therapy, 65,* 238–246.

Asher, I. E. (2007). *An annotated index of occupational therapy evaluation tools* (3rd ed.). Bethesda, MD: AOTA Press.

Association for Ambulatory Behavioral Healthcare. (2010). *Fast facts about partial hospitalization.* Retrieved from www.aabh.org/content/fast-facts-php

Azok, S. D., and Tomlinson, J. (1994). Occupational therapy in a multidisciplinary psychiatric home health care service. *Mental Health Special Interest Newsletter, 17*(2), 1–3.

Bassett, H., Lampe, J., and Lloyd, C. (2001). Living with underfives: A programme for parents with a mental illness. *British Journal of Occupational Therapy, 64,* 23–28.

Bjørkedal, S. T. B., Torsting, A. M. B., and Møller, T. (2016). Rewarding yet demanding: Client perspectives on enabling occupations during early stages of recovery from schizophrenia. *Scandinavian Journal of Occupational Therapy, 23,* 97–106.

Bourke, C., Sanders, B., Allchin, B., Lentin, P., and Lang, S. (2015). Occupational therapy influence on a carer peer support model in a clinical mental health service. *Australian Occupational Therapy Journal, 62,* 299–305.

Brown, C., Gelszer, L., Lewis, K., and Arbesman, M. (2018). Effectiveness of interventions for weight loss for people with serious mental illness: A systemic review and meta-analysis. *American Journal of Occupational Therapy, 72,* 7205190030p1–7205190030p9.

Case Management Society of America. (2016). *Standards of practice for case management.* Little Rock, AR: Case Management Society of America.

Centers for Medicare and Medicaid Services. (n.d.). *Medicare and home health care.* Retrieved from www.medicare.gov/Pubs/pdf/10969-Medicare-and-Home-Health-Care.pdf

Centers for Medicare and Medicaid Services. (2012). *Medicare and your mental health benefits.* Retrieved from www.medicare.gov/pubs/pdf/10184.pdf

Chandler, D. (2008). *Supported education for persons with psychiatric disabilities.* Retrieved from www.cimh.org

Chapleau, A., Seroczynski, A. D., Meyers, S., Lamb, K., and Buchino, S. (2012). The effectiveness of a consultation model in community mental health. *Occupational Therapy in Mental Health, 28*(4), 379–395.

Chapleau, A., and Tessel, R. (2010). Meeting the needs of the client with a co-occurring psychiatric condition: The role of the occupational therapist. *Home and Community Health Special Interest Section Quarterly, 17*(3), 1–4.

Chinman, M., George, P., Dougherty, R. H., Daniels, A. S., Ghose, S. S., Swift, A., and Delphin-Rittmon, M. E. (2014). Peer support services for individuals with serious mental illnesses: Assessing the evidence. *Psychiatric Services, 65,* 429–441.

Clay, P. (2013, December). Shared principles: The recovery model and occupational therapy. *Mental Health Special Interest Section Quarterly, 36*(4), 1–3.

Clubhouse International. (2016). *International standards for clubhouse programs.* Retrieved from www.clubhouse-intl.org/documents/standards_2016_eng.pdf

Commission for Case Management Certification. (2018). *Certification guide to the CCM® examination.* Retrieved https://ccmcertification.org/sites/default/files/docs/2018/ccmc-17-guide-certification-web.pdf

Copeland, M. (2001). Wellness recovery action plan: A system for monitoring, reducing, and eliminating uncomfortable or dangerous physical symptoms and emotional feelings. *Occupational Therapy in Mental Health, 17*(3/4), 127–150.

Cottrell, R. P. (2005). The issue is the Olmstead decision: Landmark opportunity or platform for rhetoric—our collective responsibility for community participation. *American Journal of Occupational Therapy, 59,* 561–568.

Cottrell, R. P. (2007). The New Freedom Initiative—transforming mental health care—will OT be at the table? *Occupational Therapy in Mental Health, 23*(2), 1–24.

Craig, D. G. (2012). Current occupational therapy publications in home health: A scoping review. *American Journal of Occupational Therapy, 66,* 338–347.

Crist, P., and Stoffel, V. (1992). The Americans With Disabilities Act of 1990 and employees with mental impairments: Personal efficacy and the environment. *American Journal of Occupational Therapy,46,* 435–443.

Dallas, J. (2011). Community-based case management. In C. Brown and V. Stoffel (Eds.), *Occupational therapy in mental health: A vision for participation* (pp. 571–581). Philadelphia, PA: F. A. Davis.

D'Amico, M. L., Jaffe, L. E., and Gardner, J. A. (2018). Evidence for interventions to improve and maintain occupational performance and participation for people with serious mental illness: A systematic review. *American Journal of Occupational Therapy, 72,* 7205190020.

Dasler, P. (1984). Deinstitutionalizing the occupational therapist. *Occupational Therapy in Mental Health, 1*(1), 31–40.

Deegan, P. (1988). Recovery: The lived experience of rehabilitation. *Psychosocial Rehabilitation Journal, 11,* 11–19.

Doroud, N., Fossey, E., and Fortune, T. (2015). Recovery as an occupational journey: A scoping review exploring the links between occupational engagement and recovery for people with enduring mental health issues. *Australian Occupational Therapy Journal, 62,* 378–392.

Dulay, J. L., and Steichen, M. (1982). Transitional employment for the chronically mentally ill. *Occupational Therapy in Mental Health, 2*(3), 65–77.

Dunton, W. (1919). N.S.P.O.T. *Maryland Psychiatric Quarterly, 13*(3), 68–73.

Earle, G. (1999, November). OT's role in mental health home care. *OT Practice,* 16–19.

Edward, K., Welch, A., and Chater, K. (2009). The phenomenon of resilience as described by adults who have experienced mental illness. *Journal of Advanced Nursing, 65*(3), 587–595.

Fleming-Castaldy, R. P. (2015). A macro perspective for client-centred practice in curricula: Critique and teaching methods. *Scandinavian Journal of Occupational Therapy, 22,* 267–276.

Foster, K., O'Brien, L., and Korhonen, T. (2012). Developing resilient children and families when parents have mental illness: A family-focused approach. *International Journal of Mental Health Nursing, 21,* 3–11.

Fox, V. (2013). Professional roles in community mental health practice: Generalist versus specialist. *Occupational Therapy in Mental Health, 29*(1), 3–9.

Gibson, R., D'Amico, M., Jaffe, L., and Arbesman, M. (2011). Occupational therapy interventions for recovery in community integration and normative life roles for adults with serious mental illness: A systematic review. *American Journal of Occupational Therapy, 65*(3), 247–256.

Goldman, H. H. (1988). Mental illness and family burden: A public health perspective. *Hospital and Community Psychiatry, 33,* 557–560.

Goodyear, M., Hill, T. L., Allchin, B., McCormick, F., Hine, R., Cuff, R., and O'Hanlon, B. (2015). Standards of practice for the adult mental health workforce: Meeting the needs of families where a parent has a mental illness. *International Journal of Mental Health Nursing, 24,* 1–12.

Gray, K., Haertl, K., Bowman, M. T., Leonard, L., and Leslie, C. A. (2018). Using interprofessional collaboration in occupational therapy mental health private practice. *SIS Quarterly Practice Connections, 3*(1), 15–17.

Gutman, S. (2011). Special issue: Effectiveness of occupational therapy services in mental health practice. *American Journal of Occupational Therapy, 65,* 235–237.

Gutman, S., Kerner, R., Zombek, I., Dulek, J., and Ramsey, C. A. (2009). Supported education for adults with psychiatric disabilities: Effectiveness of an occupational therapy program. *American Journal of Occupational Therapy, 63,* 245–254.

Gutman, S. A., and Raphael-Greenfield, E. I. (2014). Centennial vision—five years of mental health research in the *American Journal of Occupational Therapy. American Journal of Occupational Therapy, 68,* e21–e36.

Haertl, K., Behrens, K., Houtujec, J., Rue, A., and Ten Haken, R. (2009). Factors influencing satisfaction and efficacy of services at a free-standing psychiatric occupational therapy clinic. *American Journal of Occupational Therapy, 63,* 691–700.

Herron, J., Gioia, D., and Dohrn, B. (2009). A social enterprise model for employment. *Psychiatric Services, 60*(8), 1140.

Hinojosa. J., and Kramer, P. (2014). *Evaluation in occupational therapy: Obtaining and interpreting data* (4th ed.). Bethesda, MD: AOTA Press.

Hohl, W., Moll, S., and Pfeiffer, A. (2017). Occupational therapy in the treatment of people with severe mental illness. *Current Opinions in Psychiatry, 30,* 300–305.

Holmes, W., and Scaffa, M. E. (2009). The nature of emerging practice in occupational therapy: A pilot study. *Occupational Therapy in Health Care, 23*(3), 189–206.

Horvitz-Lennon, M., Normand, S., Gaccione, P., and Frank, R. (2001). Partial versus full hospitalization for adults in psychiatric distress: A systematic review of the published literature. *American Journal of Psychiatry, 158,* 676–685.

Iannelli, S., and Wilding, C. (2007). Health-enhancing effects of engaging in productive occupation: Experiences of young people with mental illness. *Australian Occupational Therapy Journal, 54,* 285–293.

Ikiugu, M. N., Nissen, R. M., Bellar, C., Maassen, A., and Van Peursem, K. (2017). Centennial topics—clinical effectiveness of occupational therapy in mental health: A meta-analysis. *American Journal of Occupational Therapy, 71,* 7105100020.

Kanter, J. (1989). Clinical case management: Definition, principles, components. *Hospital and Community Psychiatry, 40,* 361–368.

Kielhofner, G. (2009). *Conceptual foundations of occupational therapy practice.* Philadelphia, PA: F. A. Davis.

Krupa, T., Fossey, E., Anthony, W. A., Brown, C., and Pitts, D. B. (2009). Doing daily life: How occupational therapy can inform psychiatric rehabilitation practice. *Psychiatric Rehabilitation Journal, 32*(3), 155–161.

Krupa, T., McLean, H., Eastabrook, S., Bonham, A., and Baksh, L. (2003). Daily time use as a measure of community adjustment for persons served by Assertive Community Treatment teams. *American Journal of Occupational Therapy, 57,* 558–565.

Krupa, T., Radloff-Gabriel, D., Whippey, E., and Kirsh, B. (2002). Occupational therapy and assertive community treatment. *Canadian Journal of Occupational Therapy, 69,* 153–157.

Lancto, N., Durand, M. J., and Corbiere, C. (2012). The quality of work life of people with severe mental disorders working in social enterprises: A qualitative study. *Quality of Life Research, 21*(8), 1415–1423.

Leufstadius, C., and Eklund, M. (2008). Time use among people with persistent mental illness: Identifying risk factors for imbalance in daily activities. *Scandinavian Journal of Occupational Therapy, 15,* 23–33.

Liberman, R. P. (1988). *Psychiatric rehabilitation of chronic mental patients.* Washington, DC: American Psychiatric Press.

Lindström, M., Sjöström, S., and Lindberg, M. (2012). Stories of rediscovering agency: Home based occupational therapy interventions among people with severe psychiatric disability. *Occupation, Participation and Health, 32*(2), 5–12.

Lloyd, C., King R., and Ryan, L. (2007). The challenge of working in mental health settings: Perceptions of newly graduated occupational therapists. *British Journal of Occupational Therapy, 70*(11), 460–470.

Luciano, A., and Meara, E. (2014). The employment status of people with mental illness: National survey data from 2009 and 2010. *Psychiatric Services, 65,* 1201–1209.

Mahaffey, L., and Holmquist, B. (2011). Hospital-based mental health care. In C. Brown and V. Stoffel (Eds.), *Occupational therapy in mental health: A vision for participation* (p. 582–594). Philadelphia: F. A. Davis.

McKay, C., Nugent, K. L., Johnsen, M., Eaton, W. W., and Lidz, C. W. (2018). A systematic review of evidence for the clubhouse model of psychosocial rehabilitation. *Administration and Policy in Mental Health and Mental Health Services Research, 45,* 28–47.

Mental Health America. (2018). *About us.* Retrieved from www.mentalhealthamerica.net/

Merryman, M. B., and Riegel, S. K. (2007). Recovery process and people with serious mental illness living in the community: An occupational therapy perspective. *Occupational Therapy in Mental Health, 23*(2), 51–73.

Michetti, J., and Dieleman, C. (2014). Enabling occupational therapy: Moving beyond the generalist vs specialist debate in community mental health. *British Journal of Occupational Therapy, 77*(5), 230–233.

Myrick, K., and del Vecchi, P. (2016). Peer support services in the behavioral healthcare workforce: State of the field. *Psychiatric Rehabilitation Journal, 39,* 197–203.

National Alliance on Mental Illness. (2014). *Mental illness: NAMI report deplores 80 percent unemployment rate.* Retrieved from www.nami.org/Press-Media/Press-Releases/2014/Mental-Illness-NAMI-Report-Deplores-80-Percent-Une

National Alliance on Mental Illness. (2015). *State mental health legislation. 2015: Trends, themes and effective practices.* Arlington, VA: National Alliance on Mental Illness.

National Alliance on Mental Illness. (2018a). *Mental health by the numbers.* Retrieved from www.nami.org/Learn-More/Mental-Health-By-the-Numbers

National Alliance on Mental Illness. (2018b). *Find support.* Retrieved from www.nami.org/Find-Support/NAMI-Programs

National Coalition for Mental Health Recovery. (2016). *Home.* Retrieved from www.ncmhr.org

National Empowerment Center. (2018). *Home.* Retrieved from www.power2u.org

National Institute of Mental Health. (2017). *Mental illness.* Retrieved from www.nimh.nih.gov/health/statistics/mental-illness.shtml

Nelson, G. (2010). Housing for people with serious mental illness: Approaches, evidence, and transformative change. *Journal of Sociology and Social Welfare, 37*(4), 123–146.

Noyes, S., Sokolov, H., and Arbesman, M. (2018). Evidence for occupational therapy intervention with employment and education for adults with serious mental illness: A systematic review. *American Journal of Occupational Therapy, 72,* 7205190010.

O'Connell, J., and McKay, E. A. (2010). Profile, practice and perspectives of occupational therapists in community mental health teams in Ireland. *British Journal of Occupational Therapy, 73*(5), 219–228.

Palanker, D., Volk, J. A., Lucia, K., and Thomas, K. (2018). *Deregulating the individual market and the impact on mental health coverage: Mental health parity at risk.* Arlington, VA: National Alliance on Mental Illness.

Pettican, A., and Bryant, W. (2007). Sustaining a focus on occupation in community mental health practice. *British Journal of Occupational Therapy, 70*(4), 141–145.

Pitts, D. (2001). Assertive community treatment: A brief introduction. *Mental Health Special Interest Section Quarterly, 24*(4), 1–2.

Pitts, D. (2004). Understanding the experience of recovery for persons labeled with psychiatric disabilities. *OT Practice, 9*(5), CE-1–CE-8.

Professional Rehabilitation Consultants. (n.d.). *Occupational therapy specializing in your mental health.* Retrieved from www.prcstpaul.com/

Ragins, M. (2011). *Recovery with severe mental illness: Changing from a medical model to a psychosocial rehabilitation model.* Retrieved www.village-isa.org/Ragin's %20 Papers/recov.%20with%20 severe%20MI.htm

Ramsey, R. (2011). Voices of community practicing occupational therapists: An exploratory study. *Occupational Therapy in Health Care, 25*(2–3), 140–149.

Reed, K., and Anderson, L. (2017). *The history of occupational therapy: The first century.* Thorofare, NJ: SLACK.

Reeves, S., and Mann, L. S. (2004). Overcoming problems with generic working for occupational therapists based in community mental health settings. *British Journal of Occupational Therapy, 67*(6), 265–268.

Ringeisen, H., Langer Ellison M., Ryder-Burge, A., Biebel, K., Alikhan, S., and Jones, E. (2017). Supported education for individuals with psychiatric disabilities: State of the practice and policy implications. *Psychiatric Rehabilitation Journal, 40,* 197–206.

Roby, R., Goldstein, R., Rose, E., and Kerman, N. (2018). Post-discharge experiences of people with psychosis following partial hospital program completion. *Occupational Therapy in Mental Health, 34*(3), 272–284.

Rog, D., Marshall, T., Dougherty, R., George, P., Daniels, A., Ghose, S., and Dephin-Rittmon, M. (2014). Permanent supportive housing: Assessing the evidence. *Psychiatric Services, 65,* 287–294.

Rogers, S. E., and Swarbrick, M. (2016). Peer-delivered services: Current trends and innovations. *Psychiatric Rehabilitation Journal, 39,* 193–196.

Rossen, A., Mueser, K., and Teesson, M. (2007). Assertive community treatment: Issues from scientific and clinical literature with implications for practice. *Journal of Rehabilitation Research and Development, 44,* 813–826.

Russo, S. J., Murrough, J. W., Han, M. W., Charney, D. S., and Nestler, E. J. (2012). Neurobiology of resilience. *Nature Neuroscience, 15,* 1475–1484.

Salzer, M. S. (2012). A comparative study of campus experiences of college students with mental illness vs. a general college sample. *Journal of American College Health, 60*(1), 1–7.

Schene, A. (2004). The effectiveness of psychiatric partial hospitalization and day care. *Current Opinion in Psychiatry, 17,* 303–309.

Schindler, V. P. (2010). A client-centred, occupation-based occupational therapy programme for adults with psychiatric diagnoses. *Occupational Therapy International, 17,* 105–112.

Schindler, V. P. (2018). Service user perception of and satisfaction with programs having higher education and employment goals for people diagnosed with mental illness. *Occupational Therapy in Mental Health.* Retrieved from https://doi.org/10.1080/0164212X.2017. 1419900

Schindler, V., and Sauerwald, C. (2013). Outcomes of a 4-year program with higher education and employment goals for individuals diagnosed with mental illness. *Work: A Journal of Prevention, Assessment and Rehabilitation, 46*(3), 325–336.

Smith, D. L., Atmatzidis, K., Capogreco, M., Lloyd-Randolfi, D., and Seman, V. (2017). Increasing work participation for persons with various disabilities: A systematic review. *OTJR: Occupation, Participation and Health, 37*(2S), 3S–13S.

Social Security Administration. (2018). *The red book—a guide to work incentives.* Retrieved from www.ssa.gov/redbook/documents/TheRedBook2018.pdf

Spencer, B., Sherman, L., Nielsen, S., and Thormodson, K. (2018). Effectiveness of occupational therapy interventions for students with mental illness transitioning to higher education: A systematic review. *Occupational Therapy in Mental Health, 34*(2), 151–164.

Stoffel, V. C. (2013). Health policy perspectives—opportunities for occupational therapy behavioral health: A call to action. *American Journal of Occupational Therapy, 67,* 140–145.

Substance Abuse and Mental Health Services Administration. (2008). *Assertive community treatment: Building your program.* Washington, DC: Substance Abuse and Mental Health Services Administration.

Substance Abuse and Mental Health Services Administration. (2009). *Getting started with evidence-based practices: Supported employment.* Washington, DC: Substance Abuse and Mental Health Services Administration.

Substance Abuse and Mental Health Services Administration. (2010a). *Getting started with evidence-based practices: Illness management and recovery.* Washington, DC: Substance Abuse and Mental Health Services Administration.

Substance Abuse and Mental Health Services Administration. (2010b). *Getting started with evidence-based practices: Permanent supportive housing.* Washington, DC: Substance Abuse and Mental Health Services Administration.

Substance Abuse and Mental Health Services Administration. (2010c). *Getting started with evidence-based practices: Family psychoeducation.* Washington, DC: Substance Abuse and Mental Health Services Administration.

Substance Abuse and Mental Health Services Administration. (2011). *Getting started with evidence-based practices: Supported education.* Washington, DC: Substance Abuse and Mental Health Services Administration.

Substance Abuse and Mental Health Services Administration. (2012). *SAMHSA's working definition of recovery updated.* Retrieved from https://blog samhsa.gov/2012/03/23/defintion-of-recovery -updated/#.W67km_ZFzIU

Substance Abuse and Mental Health Services Administration. (2016). *Better outcomes through outreach and case management.* Retrieved from www.samhsa.gov/homelessness-programs-resources/hpr -resources/better-outcomes-through-outreach

Substance Abuse and Mental Health Services Administration. (2017). *Community mental health services block grant.* Retrieved from www.samhsa.gov/grants/block-grants/mhbg

Substance Abuse and Mental Health Services Administration. (2018). *Peer support and social inclusion.* Retrieved from www.samhsa.gov/recovery/peer-support-social-inclusion

Swarbrick, M. (2009). Historical perspective: from institution to community. *Occupational Therapy in Mental Health, 25*(3–4), 201–223.

Swarbrick, M. (2013). Wellness-oriented peer approaches: A key ingredient for integrated care. *Psychiatric Services, 64,* 723–726.
Swarbrick, M. (2016). Support models to enhance community transitions. *SIS Quarterly Practice Connections, 1*(2), 11–13.
Swarbrick, M., and Noyes, S. (2018). Guest editorial—effectiveness of occupational therapy services in mental health practice. *American Journal of Occupational Therapy, 72,* 7205170010.
Swarbrick, M., Tunner, T. P., Miller, D. W., Werner, P., and Tiegreen, W. W. (2016). Promoting health and wellness through peer-delivered services: Three innovative state examples. *Psychiatric Rehabilitation Journal, 39*(3), 204–210.
Swarbrick, P., and Pratt, C. (2006). Consumer-operated self-help services: Roles and opportunities for occupational therapists and occupational therapy assistants. *OT Practice, 11*(5), CE-1–CE-8.
Throckmorton, T., and Windle, P. E. (2009a). Evidenced-based case management practice, part I: The systematic review. *Professional Case Management, 14*(2), 76–81.
Throckmorton, T., and Windle, P. E. (2009b). Evidenced-based case management practice, part II: Meta-analysis a primer for case managers. *Professional Case Management, 14*(5), 226–232.
Torrey, E. F. (2013, February 3). Fifty years of failing America's mentally ill. *Wall Street Journal,* A15.
Treiger, T. M., and Fink-Samnick, E. (2014). COLLABORATE©: A universal competency-based paradigm for professional case management, part I: Introduction, historical validation, and competency presentation. *Professional Case Management, 18*(3), 122–135.
Turner, J. K., and TenHoo, W. J. (1978). The NIMH community support program: Pilot approach to a needed social reform. *Schizophrenia Bulletin, 4*(3), 319–349.
Urish, C., and Jacobs, B. (2011). Families living with mental illness. In C. Brown and V. Stoffel, (Eds.), *Occupational therapy in mental health: A vision for participation* (pp. 415–432). Philadelphia, PA: F. A. Davis.
Van Camp, D., Stubbs, B., Mitchell, A. J., De Hert, M., Wampers. M., Ward, P. B., . . . Correll, C. U. (2015). Risk of metabolic syndrome and its components in people with schizophrenia and related psychotic disorders, bipolar disorder and major depressive disorder: A systematic review and meta-analysis. *World Psychiatry, 14,* 339–347.
Ventura, J., Nuechterlein, K., Subotnik. K. L., Green, M., and Gitlin, M. J. (2004). Self-efficacy and neurocognition may be related to coping responses in recent-onset schizophrenia. *Schizophrenia Research, 69,* 343–352.
Wollenberg, J. (2002). Recovery and occupational therapy in the community mental health setting. *Occupational Therapy in Mental Health, 17*(3/4), 97–114.
World Health Organization. (2002). *Towards a common language for functioning, disability and health: ICF.* Geneva, Switzerland: World Health Organization.

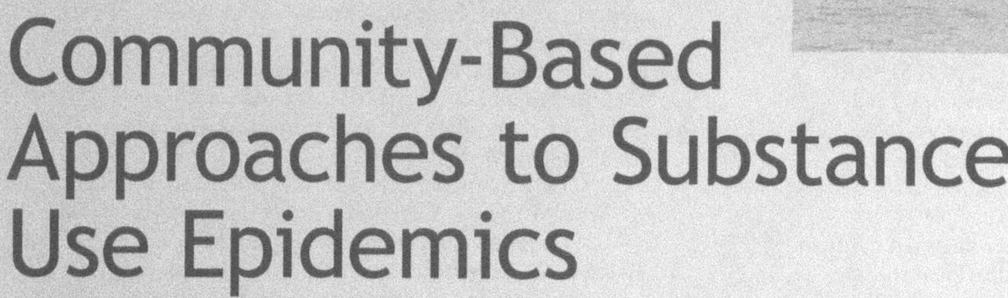

Chapter 19

Community-Based Approaches to Substance Use Epidemics

Sally Wasmuth, PhD, OTR

Bringing addiction under control depends on the success of a great variety of social and environmental movements that seek to reduce societal fragmentation in diverse ways. None of these movements can offer a short-term solution. However, they can offer both the possibility of success and the opportunity for enhancing our own belonging, identity, meaning, and purpose.

—Bruce Alexander (2015)

Learning Outcomes

This chapter is designed to enable the reader to:

19-1 Discuss the social history of drug use and its influence(s) on conceptualizations of addiction and resulting policies and practices.

19-2 Describe the current opioid epidemic that plagues the United States and other nations.

19-3 Identify several evidence-based practices for substance use disorders and their limitations.

19-4 Describe the meaning of a population health approach to address substance abuse.

19-5 List some population health and community-based practices that occupational therapy practitioners have used to address the opioid epidemic and their outcomes.

Key Terms

Addiction
Dislocation theory of addiction
Epidemic
Focused flexibility
Health inequities
Medical model
Medication-assisted therapies
Occupational justice
Opioids
Population health
Social determinants of health
Substance use disorders

Introduction

The **medical model** typically describes methods and classifications used by doctors and other health professionals such as psychologists and psychiatrists. The American Society of Addiction Medicine (ASAM, 2011) definition of addiction illuminates how addiction is understood from a medical model perspective:

> ***Addiction*** *is a primary, chronic disease of brain reward, motivation, memory and related circuitry.*

Dysfunction in these circuits leads to characteristic biological, psychological, social and spiritual manifestations. This is reflected in an individual pathologically pursuing reward and/or relief by substance use and other behaviors. Addiction is characterized by inability to consistently abstain, impairment in behavioral control, craving, diminished recognition of significant problems with one's behaviors and interpersonal relationships, and a dysfunctional emotional response. Like other chronic diseases, addiction often involves cycles of relapse and remission. Without treatment or engagement in recovery activities, addiction is progressive and can result in disability or premature death. (p. 1)

The medical model has been widely accepted by the general public and the research and science communities. However, ascription to this model has produced only moderate results with regard to decreasing the prevalence of substance use epidemics and related harms (Alexander, 2010; Shumway et al., 2013). Some suggest these unsatisfactory results are related to treating drug addiction as an individual rather than a population health problem, arguing that widespread systemic changes may be needed to improve addiction recovery outcomes and that interventions may need to target populations or societal structures rather than focusing on individual pathology (Alexander, 2010; Costanza et al., 2017). For instance, numerous studies have shown that individual recovery efforts are often not sustained because the contexts in which substances were introduced and abused remain (Fatseas et al., 2015; Panebianco, Gallupe, Carrington, and Colozzi, 2016; Wasmuth, Brandon-Friedman, and Olesek, 2016). According to the American Occupational Therapy Association (AOTA) *Occupational Therapy Practice Framework*, occupational therapy practitioners serve individuals, groups, and populations and emphasize that a "focus on the whole [including environmental context] is considered stronger than a focus on isolated aspects of human function" (AOTA, 2014, p. S4). As such, occupational therapy theory and practice may bolster addiction treatment services.

Kindig and Stoddart (2003) define **population health** as "the health outcomes of a group of individuals, including the distribution of such outcomes within the group" (p. 380). To conceive of the potential impact of a population health approach to addiction, it is important to understand how a population health perspective differs from the more typical individualistic view of addiction. Hawe and Potvin (2009) emphasized that population health intervention approaches should decrease **health inequities,** which are "systematic disparities in health . . . between groups with different levels of underlying social advantage/disadvantage" (Association of State and Territorial Health Officials [ASTHO], 2011, p. 1). In doing so, providers and policy-makers could "shift the distribution of health risk by addressing the underlying social, economic and environmental conditions" (p. 8). Likewise, as noted by Braveman and Gottlieb (2014), a large body of literature suggests that, in addition to medical care, **social determinants of health** such as income, wealth, education, neighborhood, access to healthy foods, and other factors have a significant impact on a wide range of health outcomes in numerous settings and populations. This differential access to resources has an impact on a person's ability to engage in meaningful occupations that support wellness and thus becomes an issue of **occupational justice**—the "the right to inclusive participation in everyday occupations . . . regardless of age, ability, gender, social class, or other differences" (Nilsson and Townsend, 2010, p. 57).

Social determinants of health, health inequities, and occupational injustice are particularly visible in addiction etiology and outcomes, suggesting the necessity of a population health approach. A population health approach to occupational therapy in addiction recovery moves beyond individual addiction treatments and addresses the social, cultural, and environmental factors responsible for health disparities and occupational injustices among and within populations. Shifting to a population health approach to treating addiction does not simply mean including family members in addiction recovery or utilizing group-based therapies, although both of these are evidence-based practices with a significant amount of supporting literature (Substance Abuse and Mental Health Services Administration [SAMHSA], 2018). A true population health approach to the problem of addiction alters not only the level at which intervention needs to occur but also the fact that addiction's causes, symptoms, and recovery outcomes are understood as societal, rather than individual.

Alexander (2010, 2015) and others have emphasized that addiction is a societal, rather than an individual, problem. Through the lens of Alexander's **dislocation theory of addiction,** people adopt addictive behaviors when they feel deeply isolated, detached, fragmented, or dislocated from meaningful participation in life. Abuse, trauma, natural disasters, cultural assimilation, globalization met with disruption of local economies, and numerous other factors may contribute to the onset and pains of dislocation. Of note is his claim that modernization and postmodernization expand worldwide dislocation by undercutting local economies via free market trade and celebrating immediate and limitless gratification. The growing prevalence of addictive behavior despite modest improvements in addiction medicine and individual treatment approaches are, for Alexander, indicators of larger social problems (Alexander, 2010). Dislocation theory provides a framework within which innovative population health approaches to addiction recovery focused on reducing dislocation and creating supportive, inclusive societal contexts can be conceptualized. The need for such innovation is evident in the growing number of drug-related deaths despite the billions of dollars invested in reducing addiction-related problems (Centers for Disease Control and Prevention [CDC], 2018b).

An understanding of addiction from a population health perspective can translate into interventions at multiple levels, including interventions designed for individual clients (microlevel), community-based interventions (mesolevel), and population-based interventions (macrolevel). For the occupational therapy practitioner, the ecological model of human performance (EHP; Dunn, Brown, McGuigan, 1994) may be a useful framework for adopting a population health approach to addiction prevention and intervention. The EHP encourages practitioners to consider how temporal, social, societal, historical, political, and other contexts influence task performance and thus participation in life. In addition, the model suggests skills, perceived roles, and abilities (all influenced by contextual factors) shape the occupations (tasks) available to a person and/or the way in which a person perceives and engages (or not) in those tasks. At the microlevel, an occupational therapist may assist a client in identifying contextual factors that have an impact on skill development, role identification, abilities, and availability of resources. Thus, even when treating at the individual level, addiction is viewed as a larger contextual problem. To apply a population health approach at the mesolevel, occupational therapists may develop community-based interventions designed to address the needs of a specific group within their local community context(s). A macrolevel population health approach using the EHP might aim to reduce health disparities and/or health-care inequities by examining, exposing, and correcting the social and occupational injustices that are contributing to the global substance use epidemic.

In small numbers, occupational therapy practitioners are currently developing and implementing multilevel interventions for problematic drug use that are rooted in their knowledge of how occupational justice and meaningful participation enhance community engagement and wellness (Boisvert, Martin, Grosek, and Clarie, 2008; Braveman and Suarez-Balcazar, 2009; Keightley et al., 2018; Wasmuth and Pritchard, 2016). Likewise, occupational therapy practitioners are uniquely positioned to intervene at the group and population level through their "consideration of co-occupations [that] supports an integrated view of the client's engagement in context in relationship to significant others" (AOTA, 2014, p. S6). An aim of this chapter is to support and expand the innovative efforts of occupational therapy practitioners by discussing current approaches and delineating ways in which occupational therapy practitioners may continue to contribute to population health approaches to addiction recovery in the future.

Substance Use: A Brief Social History

Addiction has many definitions. The definition of addiction offered by the *Diagnostic and Statistical Manual for Mental Disorders, Fifth Edition* (*DSM-5*) falls under the heading "substance-related and addictive disorders" (American Psychiatric Association [APA], 2013). Beneath this overarching heading, the *DSM-5* lists 10 **substance use disorders** (SUDs; see Box 19-1).

The *DSM-5* does not distinguish between substance use, misuse, abuse, and dependence. Instead,

Box 19-1 *DSM-5* Substance Use Disorders

- Alcohol use disorder
- Cannabis use disorder
- Phencyclidine use disorder
- Other hallucinogen use disorder
- Inhalant use disorder
- Opioid use disorder
- Sedative, hypnotic, or anxiolytic use disorder
- Stimulant use disorder
- Tobacco use disorder
- Other/unknown substance use disorder

From *Diagnostic and Statistical Manual of Mental Disorders (DSM-5),* by American Psychiatric Association, 2013, Washington, DC: American Psychiatric Association.

Box 19-2 Substance Use Disorder Diagnostic Criteria

Must meet at least *two* of the following 11 criteria in the same 12-month period:

Impaired Control

1. Substance used in larger amounts or for longer periods of time than was intended
2. Persistent desire to regulate use with multiple unsuccessful efforts to cut down or control use
3. Great deal of time spent in substance-related activities
4. Intense desire or urge to use/craving for the drug

Social Impairment

5. Recurrent use resulting in failure to fulfill major role obligations at work, school, or home
6. Continued use despite having persistent or recurrent social or interpersonal problems caused or exacerbated by the effects of the substance
7. Important social, occupational, or recreational activities are given up or reduced because of substance use

Risky Use

8. Recurrent use in situations in which it is physically hazardous
9. Continued use despite knowledge of having a persistent or recurrent physical or psychological problem that is likely to have been caused or exacerbated by substance use

Pharmacological Criteria

10. Tolerance (increased dose/frequency needed to achieve desired effect)
11. Withdrawal syndrome upon discontinuation of use

From *Diagnostic and Statistical Manual of Mental Disorders (DSM-5),* by American Psychiatric Association, 2013, Washington, DC: American Psychiatric Association.

based on the number of diagnostic criteria a person exhibits, a person is classified as having a mild, moderate, or severe SUD.

To be diagnosed with a mild substance-related or addictive behavior, a person must demonstrate at least two diagnostic criteria in any of the following groups: impaired control, social impairment, risky use, and pharmacological criteria such as neurobiological changes related to tolerance (see Box 19-2). Four to five criteria indicate a moderate SUD, and six or more suggest a severe SUD. In addition to the 10 substance-specific disorders, the *DSM-5* also includes a heading for addictive behaviors, although the only addictive behavior listed is gambling disorder. Both substance use and gambling disorder are thought to change neurobiological structure and function in maladaptive ways, producing the behavioral phenomena seen in addiction (APA, 2013).

This chapter uses SUD and addiction synonymously but also critically analyzes the evolving definitions of addiction as they emerged in sociohistorical contexts. A review of the history surrounding definitions of drugs, substances, and addiction illuminates how sociocultural influences have shaped the evolution of these constructs as well as the policies that direct how they are dealt with by society. For instance, Kushner (2006, 2010a, 2010b) argues:

> *The classification of certain substances as illicit or licit tells us more about social norms and power relationships than about the psychopharmacological properties of the substances themselves. (2010b, p. 8)*

In other words, as many anthropologists, historians, sociologists, and philosophers of science have pointed out, the path by which certain chemicals come to be defined as "substances" or "drugs" relies not necessarily on the physiological effects of using that chemical but rather on the social stigmas attached to the people who use those chemicals. As an example, Acker (2010) points out that many substances now considered to be psychoactive drugs first became the subject of concern because their use was linked to marginal racial groups. "Images of opium-smoking Chinese in the late nineteenth century, cocaine-maddened African Americans in the early twentieth century and marijuana-puffing Mexicans in the 1930s" (p. 73) contributed to perceptions that these substances threatened U.S. society, giving rise to modern-day drug policies. From this perspective, drug addiction cannot be understood outside the contexts in which drugs are conceptualized. Further emphasizing the influence of cultural contexts, Kushner (2010b) points out:

> *Social studies of addiction have examined past and current definitions of addiction and concluded that alcohol prohibition and the criminalization of narcotics and stimulants reflected dominant cultural values rather than robust scientific findings. (p. 8)*

In other words, definitions were based more on social stigmas attached to substances than scientific studies of how those substances affected health and well-being.

Why Race Matters

According to *DSM-5* criteria, for someone to be diagnosed with an SUD or addictive behavior the person must experience "harm" (which can be relatively subjective) as a result of the activity in question. Conventional models of addiction underscore the physiological harms that can result from chronic substance use, such as liver and kidney problems from excessive alcohol intake (Askgaard, Grønbæk, Kjær, Tjønneland, and Tolstru, 2015; Baffy, Brunt, and Caldwell, 2012) or cardiovascular problems and cancers related to smoking (Fabbri, 2016). However, depending on social, cultural, and political contexts, other factors may significantly contribute to whether a person experiences harm from substance use. Consider a person who regularly engages in marijuana use in a state where it is illegal. This person may experience recurring legal ramifications, posing potential financial and social burdens. The same person in a different context, such as a state where recreational marijuana use is legal, would not experience these harms. Thus, the first person would be classified as having an SUD, whereas the second person would not. This example illustrates how geographical and political contexts can play a role in diagnostic definitions (and experiences of harm) related to certain activities.

The ambiguity inherent in the term *harm* has been similarly discussed in occupational therapy literature. While the profession is rooted in the value of meaningful participation, it has recently begun to more deeply consider the impact of participation in occupations that provide identity and structure but are considered antisocial, harmful, illegal, unproductive, or deviant (Twinley, 2013). The importance of context in how occupational participation is experienced is evident in the above example of the daily marijuana user. The EHP's emphasis on context and how it influences the benefits and harms of occupational participation makes it a particularly relevant and applicable model for grappling with the complexities of understanding drug use, addiction, and recovery.

Engage Your Brain 19-1

Referring to the AOTA *Occupational Therapy Code of Ethics (2015)*, what ethical challenges might you face as an occupational therapy practitioner working with someone who has an SUD who is not ready to quit using?

One way in which race is related to experiences of harm has to do with biases of health-care professionals. Health-care professionals and consumers alike are situated within legal, political, and societal contexts that have a long-standing history of racial discrimination. Some of this history has affected the degree to which minorities experience harms related to drug use. For example, an overwhelming body of literature has suggested that implicit provider bias has an impact on health outcomes for black women in many areas, including but not limited to cardiac health, pre- and postnatal outcomes, mental health services, and pain management (Krieger, 2014). This has been especially true for black women with a history of substance misuse, particularly in the areas of pain management and prenatal care (e.g., Sacks, 2018; Wallace, Green, Richardson, Theall, and Crear-Perry, 2017). A recent study indicated peripartum cardiac mortality rates to be the highest for African American women (Sliwa et al., 2018), and some have suggested this is the result of social structures/institutional racism. Such findings again illustrate the impact of context described in the EHP framework (Dunn et al., 1994). In this case, social and historical contexts evoke harm in the occupational lives of black women as they engage in healthcare systems.

When literature first began to examine the impact of illicit substances on newborns, the women arrested in delivery rooms and charged with endangering their infants were almost exclusively poor and black crack users, despite the prevalence of white, pregnant powder cocaine users at the time (Acker, 2010, p. 84). Likewise,

> *longer sentences for crack possession compared to equivalent weights of powder cocaine contributed to disproportionate levels of African Americans incarcerated for drug convictions (Currie, 1993). These periods of incarceration, in turn, further reduced young black men's engagement in education or legitimate employment and deepened their criminal involvement. (p. 84)*

Such policies not only increased the direct harms associated with drug use (e.g., incarceration, financial impacts) but also further increased risk factors by imposing barriers to meaningful and efficacious participation in life.

Highlighting the relevance of race in discussions of addiction and health, Krieger (2014) emphasizes:

> *An important gap in current research . . . concerns the racialized health consequences of contemporary legal discrimination . . . [such as] the legally colorblind, albeit racially motivated, U.S. War on Drugs and its role in producing or exacerbating health-debilitating racial/ethnic inequalities. (p. 688)*

Krieger (2014) illuminates the importance of a population health approach to addiction; recognition of the ways in which race has contributed to policy decisions that have influenced health outcomes for minority populations is critical in understanding and addressing addiction. Therefore, a population health approach to addiction requires in-depth knowledge of the prevalence of addiction among different populations and the factors that differentially influence those populations. For example, experiences of crack addiction in impoverished black communities will likely differ greatly from experiences of alcohol addiction among middle-class white males in terms of legal policies related to each behavior, social norms and constructs, self-image, and contributing factors such as social history, environmental context, socioeconomic status, and access to recovery-related resources.

Guided by an EHP approach, occupational therapists can use the occupational profile and other holistic assessment tools to identify social, historical, and political contextual factors unique to an individual's experience of drug use and recovery in order to bring population-relevant insights into treatment planning. In addition, occupational therapy practitioners may learn about health disparities and relevant population-specific factors by engaging with community action groups, many of which have emerged in the past decade in response to the opioid epidemic. The activities of community action groups can help illuminate the specific needs within communities by illustrating the problems faced by their members. Occupational therapy practitioners can use this invaluable information in combination with information gleaned from occupation-based assessments in order to contribute to the efforts of community action groups, promoting occupational justice through targeted interventions. Some such approaches are described later in this chapter.

Understanding Evolving Definitions of Addiction and Substance Use

Perhaps the most significant change in the *DSM-5* pertaining to addiction is that the category under which it falls was retitled, eliminating the term *substance dependence* and replacing it with *substance use disorder*. This change was made because addiction connoted not only dependence but also harm. Additionally, a growing body of literature suggested that many forms of substance dependence actually supported rather than interfered with health. A classic example of this phenomenon was when dependence on opioid pain medication among people with severe chronic pain *facilitated* meaningful participation in life by allowing people to cope with their pain (Keane and Hamill, 2010).

The 10th revision of the World Health Organization (WHO) *International Classification of Diseases and Health Problems* (*ICD-10*) still uses the word *dependence* in its definition of addiction (dependence syndrome) but specifies it is "a cluster of physiological, behavioural, and cognitive phenomena in which the use of a substance or class of substances takes on a much higher priority for a given individual than other behaviors that once had greater value" (WHO, 2017, para. 1). This definition underscores that for something to be classified under dependence syndrome it must inhibit, not facilitate, participation in meaningful occupations, thus ruling out the above example of useful dependence on pain medication in those with chronic, debilitating pain.

In addition to removing the term *dependence,* the *DSM-5* definition of addiction also underscores neurobiological research that illuminates how certain substances and behaviors affect neurochemistry and, ultimately, behavior and lived experiences. It emphasizes that substance-related and addictive disorders are alike in the ways they intensely activate the midbrain reward system. Gambling disorder is listed as an addictive behavior on the basis that patterns of reward center activation observed in disordered gambling are similar to those seen in problematic drug use (Ross, Sharp, Vuchinich, and Spurrett, 2008). Other behaviors, including hypersexuality and compulsive Internet use, are receiving more scientific attention (e.g., Sussman, Lisha, and Griffiths, 2011).

Engage Your Brain 19-2

What occupations are currently being taken to extreme levels that could meet diagnostic criteria for addictive behaviors?

Opioid Epidemic

A 2015 report suggests that SUD prevalence among the general population is 8.4% in the United States (Center for Behavioral Health Statistics and Quality, 2016). However, prevalence varies between different types of SUD. For example, the above report proposes a prevalence of 8.5% for alcohol use disorder, 1.5% for cannabis use disorder, and only 0.37% for opioid use disorder. **Opioids** are "a class of drugs that include the illegal drug heroin, synthetic opioids such as fentanyl, and pain relievers available legally by prescription, such as oxycodone (OxyContin®), hydrocodone (Vicodin®), codeine, morphine, and many others" (National Institute on Drug Abuse [NIDA], 2018b, para. 1).

Despite this seemingly small percentage of people with problematic opioid use, the *Surgeon General's Report on Alcohol, Drugs, and Health* indicates "12.5 million Americans reported misusing prescription pain relievers in the past year [and that] seventy-eight people die every day in the United States from an opioid overdose. . . . Those numbers have nearly quadrupled since 1999" (U.S. Department of Health and Human Services [USDHHS], 2016, p. iii). Only 20% of those requiring opioid use disorder treatment actually receive help despite the existence of evidence-based treatment options. A more recent study suggests the prevalence of opioid use disorder to be 5% of the adult U.S. population (Srivastava and Gold, 2018).

According to the CDC (2018a), an **epidemic** "refers to an increase, often sudden, in the number of cases of a disease above what is normally expected in that population in that area" (para. 3). The opioid epidemic began in the 1990s and has continued for decades. It is marked by an exorbitant number of new addiction diagnoses and overdose-related deaths and is an unintended consequence, literature suggests, of "an enormous increase in the availability of prescription opiates" (Unick, Rosenblum, Mars, and Ciccarone, 2013, p. e54496) and the illegal manufacture and distribution of potent synthetic opioids (CDC, 2018b).

The prevalence of opioid use disorder among the U.S. population (primarily among middle-age whites in the United States) has skyrocketed. Many have suggested the cause to be related to "overinterpretation of a now infamous *New England Journal of Medicine* letter describing addiction as a rare occurrence in hospitalized patients treated with opioids" (Srivastava and Gold, 2018, p. 270). Others have attributed the epidemic to health-care initiatives to increase patient satisfaction by adequately medicating pain or, more generally, practices of overprescribing for pain instead of introducing alternative therapies (Kolodny et al., 2015; Manchikanti et al., 2012). Still others blame the introduction of extremely potent opioid derivatives such as fentanyl, which have also purportedly contributed to the critical rates of opioid overdoses (CDC, 2018b). According to CDC data from 2015 to 2016 (gathered from 31 states and Washington, DC):

> *Overall drug overdose death rates increased by 21.5 percent. The overdose death rate from synthetic opioids (other than methadone) more than doubled, likely driven by illicitly manufactured fentanyl (IMF). The prescription opioid-related overdose death rate increased by 10.6 percent [and] the heroin-related overdose death rate increased by 19.5 percent. (CDC, 2018b, para. 5)*

Thus, opioids are considered harmful substances that if ingested over time cause neurobiological alterations and, ultimately, addiction.

While it is clear that various drug and behavioral addictions demonstrate shared neurobiological characteristics (Ross et al., 2008), some potential problems arise when the neurobiology of addiction is emphasized outside the social contexts in which addictions manifest as lived experiences. This is particularly pertinent to understanding the opioid epidemic. For example, Keane and Hamill (2010) suggest:

> *In the context of pain treatment, opioids are not dangerous illicit substances but effective analgesics appropriate for long-term use. . . . Thus, pain medicine carefully separates the physiological and neural changes of long-term drug use from the psychological condition of "true addiction." (p. 58)*

From their perspective, opioids may produce neurochemical alterations seen in addiction, but these are not viewed as synonymous with addiction. Quite the contrary, proper opioid use in persons with chronic pain can support meaningful occupational participation. Their point is that brain states alone cannot be used to explain or predict human experiences. However, considering the concurrent rise in the availability of opioids and the increased prevalence of opioid addiction, this controversy deserves further exploration.

Opioid Crisis: A New Demographic

Opioid use among black Americans in the form of heroin was high in the 1970s and was treated as a criminal, rather than medical, issue (Arnold, 1990). The present-day opioid epidemic receiving widespread media attention and billions of research dollars to create innovative health-care solutions targets a new population of opioid users.

Who is most affected by the opioid epidemic in the United States? According to recent literature, postsurgical patients, adolescent athletes, and people with chronic pain who have been prescribed opioids are among those most affected (Brummett et al., 2017; NIDA, 2018a). According to NIDA (2018a), 21% to 29% of people with chronic pain with opioid prescriptions misuse them, and 8% to 12% develop an opioid use disorder. Approximately 4% to 6% of those who misuse their prescribed opioids transition to heroin use; conversely, 80% of heroin users first misused prescribed opioids. Brummett et al. (2017) reported that 5.9% to 6.5% of people who were prescribed opioids following a major or minor surgery demonstrated new, persistent opioid use—defined as those new to opioid use filling opioid prescriptions 90 to 180 days after surgery, long after postsurgery pharmacological pain relief would typically be needed. Incidences of persistent opioid use did not correlate with whether the participants of the study had a major or minor surgery. Instead, persistent opioid use was significantly linked to the presence of another SUD, anxiety, depression, or preoperative pain disorders, such as chronic neck or back pain or arthritis. Literature suggests that the duration of use (22.1 months or more) positively affects the likelihood of developing an addiction (Fishbain, Cole, Lewis, Rosomoff, and Rosomoff, 2007).

According to Srivastava and Gold (2018), opioid misuse and addiction is predominantly occurring in middle-aged white men and women. Interestingly, Case and Deaton (2015) recently reported a significant increase in midlife mortality and morbidity between 1999 and 2013 among middle-aged white non-Hispanics that, surprisingly, differed from other race groups in the United States, who were demonstrating decreased midlife mortality and morbidity. In this study, increased reports of pain paralleled increasingly poor health among middle-aged white people, suggesting that an increase in opioid prescriptions in the mid-1990s may have contributed to these poor midlife health trends. However, the authors note that their data cannot clarify which came first, the increase in pain or the increase in opioids. They point out that increases in pain may have been even higher without the influx of opioid prescriptions, or on the contrary, long-term opioid use may have exacerbated pain in some people. In either scenario, understanding the opioid epidemic calls for further examination of why pain levels are increasing among those living in the United States. Furthermore, as many others have suggested, finding alternative solutions to pain that address its root causes will be critical in making real progress toward eliminating the opioid epidemic (NIDA, 2018a; Srivastava and Gold, 2018).

Responses to the Opioid Epidemic

The majority of opioid epidemic initiatives target opioid use, adopting the perspective that if opioid use and availability are eliminated or replaced with other controlled substances such as methadone, the problem of addiction will decrease. Interventions aim to change provider practices (i.e., decrease opioid prescriptions), increase the number of available detoxification beds (the President's Commission on Combating Drug Addiction), or increase access to **medication-assisted therapies** (MATs)—pharmacological interventions that can reduce cravings and withdrawal—such as methadone (opioid agonist) and buprenorphine (partial agonist (NIDA, 2018a; Tetrault and Fiellin, 2018).

By contrast, in line with Keane and Hamill's (2010) perspective, others argue addiction has more to do with environmental contexts and client factors (Acker, 2010; Alexander, 2010; Wasmuth, Crabtree, and Scott, 2014). For example, studies suggest illicit drug use is higher among unemployed people (17.5%) than those employed full-time (8.4%) or part-time (11.2%) (Manchikanti et al., 2012). Likewise, the *Surgeon General's Report on Alcohol, Drugs, and Health* suggests several community and individual-level factors can be protective, such as access to opportunities for leisure, education, and social participation and good coping skills (Murthy, 2017).

From this perspective, detoxification or MAT only addresses a small portion of the experience of addiction—the physiological cravings. As Acker (2010) points out, "The push for pharmacotherapies contrasts with an earlier history in which addiction treatment addressed the whole person" (p. 72). Others have emphasized that tighter regulations on opioid prescriptions, along with rising heroin quality and lower prices (Case and Deaton, 2015), have led to the increased availability of heroin in areas where it has previously been virtually absent, suggesting that even if the opioid epidemic was brought about by excessive prescribing, reversing this trend has had limited impact on ameliorating the problem. In contrast to MAT and regulation-based approaches to substance use epidemics, occupational therapists help people identify "priorities and desired targeted outcomes that will lead to . . . engagement in occupations that support participation in life" (AOTA, 2014, p. S13). This approach is based on the perspective that those in recovery should be the ones to decide what activities bring them meaning, and goals and priorities of recovery must be identified by clients (p. S13).

Evidence-Based Practices for Substance Use Disorders

According to CDC Principal Deputy Director Anne Schuchat, MD, "all branches of the federal government are working together to reduce the availability of illicit drugs, prevent deaths from overdoses, treat people with substance-use disorders, and prevent people from starting using drugs in the first place" (CDC, 2018b, para. 4). Reducing the availability of opioids, as mentioned above, has largely been accomplished by educating providers to modify prescribing practices. Preventing deaths from opioid overdose has been addressed via widespread generic naloxone distribution. Naloxone (brand name *Narcan*®) is an opioid antagonist that can prevent death from overdose by counteracting the central nervous system and respiratory system depression resulting from excessive opioid use (CDC, 2018b).

Preventing people from starting to use drugs in the first place has been a challenge primarily addressed through educational and community-based programs for adolescents that provide positive opportunities for leisure and social participation (Murthy, 2017). Regarding opioids in particular, the literature suggests that education about the potential harms and risks of addiction for persons who are opioid-naïve, as well as the provision of pain relief alternatives such as nonopioid medications and other therapeutic modalities, is effective (AOTA, 2018).

For people who have developed an SUD, the literature supports several evidence-based approaches

Box 19-3 Goals of Recovery

- Enabling independent living and social participation within the community
- Increasing a person's ability to respond to and manage problems such as drug cravings and distress resulting from physiological and/or psychosocial factors
- Instilling a sense of hope, meaning, self-efficacy, personal responsibility, and engagement in one's own health

From "Recovery From Severe Mental Illness: An Intrapersonal and Functional Outcome Definition," by D. Noordsy, W. Torrey, K. Mueser, S. Mead, C. O'Keefe, and L. Fox, 2002, *International Review of Psychiatry, 14*(4), 318–326.

Box 19-4 Evidence Based Practices for Addiction Recovery

- MAT for opioid and alcohol use disorders
- Motivational interviewing
- Cognitive behavioral therapy
- Peer support
- Drug and alcohol counseling
- Education about drug use risks
- Family-based therapies
- Integrated therapies that include care for physical or other mental health issues

From *Finding Quality Treatment for Substance Use Disorders*, by Substance Abuse and Mental Health Services Administration, 2018.

and emphasizes the importance of a recovery-oriented approach to care, which addresses overall well-being rather than the mere removal of disease (Noordsy et al., 2002; Box 19-3).

SAMHSA (2018) suggests using a recovery-oriented approach that includes evidence-based practices for addiction (Box 19-4). Additionally, SAMHSA emphasizes that addiction treatment programs should provide options for long-term treatment, such as "ongoing counseling or recovery coaching and support [that] helps in meeting other basic needs like sober housing, employment supports, and continued family involvement" (SAMHSA, 2018, p. 1). Other evidence-based practices include contingency management (Prendergast, Podus, Finney, Greenwell, and Roll, 2006), housing first (Padgett, Stanhope, Henwood, and Stefancic, 2011), and mindfulness training (Garland, Roberts-Lewis, Tronnier, Graves, and Kelley, 2016).

Addiction rarely occurs in the absence of comorbid conditions. Dual diagnosis refers to a person with an addiction and severe mental illness (SMI). The literature suggests that dually diagnosed clients have had difficulties accessing care because some addiction treatment facilities are ill-equipped to treat persons with SMI, and conversely, SMI facilities are ill-equipped to address problems inherent in addiction recovery. Often SMI treatment centers require drug abstinence, which may not be realistic for someone with an SUD. Integrated dual disorder treatment (IDDT) is an evidence-based practice developed to concurrently address addiction and SMI (Kubek, Kruszynski, and Boyle, 2003). Providers are trained to address all aspects of addiction and SMI and understand the ways in which SMI may influence addictive behaviors while also recognizing how substance use may affect SMI symptoms and recovery. IDDT uses a stage-based approach to care and facilitates stable housing (despite drug use), harm reduction, employment, family involvement, continuity of care, and perhaps most importantly, true integration of services (Drake et al., 2001). IDDT treatment stages are described in Table 19-1. All providers are trained to treat both addiction and SMI. In addition to IDDT, widespread federal funding supports the development of integrated community behavioral health clinics that, recognizing the frequency with which physical and mental health conditions co-occur, bring together physical and mental health evaluation and treatment (Barnett et al., 2012).

Limitations of Current Practice

Despite many evidence-based practices for addiction recovery, SUD and associated harms remain a significant concern. This may be due to challenges in translating emerging research into practice. According to Becker et al. (2016), "the gap between research and clinical practice is vast across all fields of healthcare, but few areas are characterized by gaps as large and complex as addiction treatment in general and opioid addiction treatment in particular" (p. 135). In other words, scientific studies examining the effectiveness of new and existing addiction interventions are slow to translate into applicable,

Table 19-1 Integrated Dual Disorders Treatment (IDDT) Stages

Treatment Stage (Associated Transtheoretical Stage)	Intervention Description
Engagement (precontemplation)	Form client-therapist alliance, reduce harm, offer/identify support mechanisms
Persuasion (contemplation and preparation)	Motivate interested/engaged clients to abstain from or reduce addictive behaviors; enhance/facilitate participation in occupations and implement other recovery-oriented interventions
Active treatment (action)	Focus on skill building, pursuit of client goals, and SUD/SMI symptom management
Relapse prevention (maintenance)	Assist clients in developing strategies to sustain recovery and in integrating strategies into personal contexts

Adapted from *Integrated Dual Disorder Treatment (IDDT): An Overview of the Evidence-Based Practice,* by P. M. Kubek, R. Kruszynski, and P. E. Boyle, 2003, Cleveland, OH: Center for Evidence-Based Practices, Case Western Reserve University; E. A. McConnaughy, C. C. DiClemente, J. O. Prochaska, and W. F. Velicer, 1989, "Stages of Change in Psychotherapy: A Follow-Up Report," *Psychotherapy, 26*(4), 494–503; and J. C. Norcross, P. M. Krebs, and J. O. Prochaska, 2011, "Stages of Change," *Journal of Clinical Psychology, 67*(2), 143–154.

evidence-based treatment protocols with training manuals for preparing providers to deliver them. Becker and colleagues (2016) also suggest that "simply offering counselors didactic training is not sufficient to close the research to practice gap, and that the level and quality of training support affects implementation adoption" (p. 135). Thus, it is difficult to move beyond the status quo for addiction treatment to implement innovative and/or potentially more effective methods.

Moreover, despite the many existing evidence-based treatment approaches for addiction, treatment satisfaction and compliance remain relatively low. Approximately 60% of people in recovery are dissatisfied with their care and discontinue treatment (Shumway, Bradshaw, Harris, and Baker, 2013), and recovery outcomes are modest at best, with many studies indicating an 80% to 90% relapse rate (Bart, 2012). Others have pointed out that the SUD population is characterized as having poor metacognitive mastery—that is, the ability to put metacognitive knowledge to use (to support occupational participation, for example; Wasmuth et al., 2015). As a result, some people recovering from SUD may not experience significant and ongoing benefits from didactic methods without opportunities for real-time occupational performance through occupation-based intervention (Gutman and Schindler, 2007; Wasmuth et al., 2014; Wasmuth and Pritchard, 2016). Ultimately, despite ongoing efforts to solve the substance use epidemics in the United States and globally, drug overdoses, SUD diagnoses, and new substance use outbreaks continue to increase in alarming numbers.

Population Health Approach

Can a population health approach to addiction treatment address some of the limitations of current practice? As noted above, the literature suggests that psychosocial influences have a significant role in determining the influence that drug-induced neurological alterations will have on a person. In other words, brain changes that result from compulsive or chronic illicit drug use do not, in themselves, constitute addiction. It is only when those neurological changes negatively affect the experiences of the person (i.e., evoke harm) that they are defined as an SUD. Adopting a population health approach to substance use epidemics, psychosocial influences become central in defining differences. For instance, high rates of drug addiction in a particular region may indicate similarly high rates of occupational deprivation and dislocation; variable rates of drug addiction may warrant exploration of differential access to resources within a population; and increasing rates of drug use could indicate structural or societal factors influencing a population as a whole.

Social Determinants of Addiction

Many scholars have suggested that a number of modern or postmodern social institutions (and their incentive structures) parallel (or capitalize on) the characteristics of addiction observed in individuals (Costanza et al., 2017; Alexander, 2010; Ross et al., 2008). For example, it is well established that small, transient but immediate rewards can appear more attractive (and thus drive behavior) than smaller but more sustained long-term rewards (Ross et al., 2008). This is true for people with and without addictions. Bickel and colleagues have repeatedly shown that the tendency to devalue long-term rewards and continually choose immediate gratification centrally characterizes substance and behavioral addictions (Bickel, Jarmolowicz, Mueller, Koffarnus, and Gatchalian, 2012).

Social norms and structures in the United States have capitalized on the human desire for immediate reward through marketing, traditions such as Black Friday shopping, nearly immediate access to high-interest loans and credit cards with minimum payoff requirements, and, until the recent housing market crash, home mortgages with ultimately unachievable payoffs, considering a person's financial circumstances.

In Costanza et al.'s (2017, p. 48) words, many 21st-century social institutions and incentive structures offer "short-term rewards [that] are sometimes so powerful that other, more adaptive actions are diminished and damaging activities continue despite evidence of longer-term negative consequences" such that "entire societies might also be thought of as addicted to specific modes of behavior." Recalling that addictions are characterized by continued participation in an activity despite persistent harms, Costanza et al. (2017) and others (e.g., Alexander, 2010) offer several potential examples of societal addictions, such as fossil fuel consumption, leading to climate change; overfishing, leading to exploitation of resources to the point of collapse; overconsumption; and fetishization of gross domestic product (GDP) growth (Costanza et al., 2017). They suggest:

> *Social traps [societal addictions] occur when local or individual incentives that guide behavior are inconsistent with the overall goals of the individual, society, or system [and explore how] societies can go about changing entrapping rules and incentives, rather than changing individual behaviors in spite of the entrapping rules and incentives. (p. 48)*

In other words, they suggest it may be necessary to address the addictive aspects of societal structure in order for widespread individual addiction recovery efforts to truly be sustainable within populations.

A closer examination of the emerging literature on behavioral addictions illustrates the vastness of the problem of addiction and may illuminate factors that innovative intervention approaches could address.

Behavioral Addictions

Over the past decade, the literature has noted an increasing prevalence of behavioral addictions, also referred to as process addictions (Sussman et al., 2011). As mentioned above, the *DSM-5* lists gambling disorder as the only non-substance-related addictive behavior on the basis that research has illustrated neurobiological alterations in both SUD and problematic gambling that are similar (Ross et al., 2008). Behavioral phenomena resembling SUD have also been observed, such as a preoccupation with gambling, the development of tolerance (a need to gamble with larger amounts of money to evoke excitement), symptoms of withdrawal when abstaining from gambling (restlessness, irritability), and repeated unsuccessful attempts to abstain (APA, 2013).

A systematic literature review by Sussman et al. (2011) suggested that several other behaviors meet diagnostic criteria for addictive behaviors among a significant portion of the population. In addition to SUD and gambling, these include eating, Internet use, love, sex, exercise, work, and shopping. In the same way substance use can alter neurochemistry and, in certain contexts, contribute to addictive behaviors and harm, so, too, can other occupations that are popular in modern society.

The term *process addictions* highlights behavioral addictions that arise and are accompanied by neurobiological process changes without the introduction of a substance. In other words, it is the nature of the behavior—the way in which the person engages in the activity—that contributes to the neurobiology of addiction. These neurobiological processes are not unique to addiction. The midbrain reward system involved in addiction is the same system involved in learning, memory, and experiences of activities as rewarding, aversive, or uninteresting (Ross et al., 2008). In other words, alterations (both adaptive and maladaptive) in the midbrain reward system are central to all kinds of occupational participation, including drug use and addictive behaviors such as gambling.

Studies suggest frequent Internet use by adolescents and young adults may alter neurobiological structures in ways that contribute to chronic dysfunction (Yuan et al., 2011). Likewise, frequent Internet use can negatively affect analytical thinking (Rahwan, Krasnoshtan, Shariff, and Bonnefon, 2014) and result in decreased understanding of interpersonal cues and decreased feelings of bonding and affiliation (Sherman, Michikyan, and Greenfeld, 2013). Studies also suggest increased reactivity to feelings of rejection and increased frustration intolerance (Ko et al., 2014; Ko, Yen, Yen, Chen, and Wang, 2008; Silk et al., 2012).

Sussman et al. (2011) found that when behavioral addictions are included, "47% of the U.S. adult population suffers from maladaptive signs of an addictive disorder over a 12-month period" and that "it may be useful to think of addictions as due to problems of lifestyle as well as to person-level factors" (p. 3). However, Billieux, Schimmenti, Khazaal, Maurage, and Heeren (2015) suggest such studies "overpathologize everyday life" (p. 119). One longitudinal study suggests that most behavioral addictions in adults resolve over time and are "rather transient" (Thege, Woodin, Hodgins, and Williams, 2015, p. 4). Nonetheless, it is worth exploring why nearly half of the U.S. adult population is experiencing harms—transient or not—as a result of engaging addictively in a behavior. What does this reflect about modern society?

These claims raise several questions pertinent to a population health approach to addiction recovery. First, to what extent are societal structures/incentives responsible for ongoing addiction epidemics and challenges that individuals experience in sustaining recovery efforts? A second, related question arises: Who is addiction treatment for? Who (and what level) should addiction interventions target?

Occupational Therapy Research and Practice

Considering the previously mentioned concerns about the widespread nature of addiction and its relationship with societal and population-level factors, the remainder of this chapter considers ways in which occupational therapy may have a larger influence on addiction in society at the population level.

Over a decade ago, Stoffel and Moyers (2004) suggested that occupational therapy practitioners adopt the evidence-based practices of brief interventions, cognitive behavioral therapy, motivational strategies, and 12-step facilitation, with a focus on returning recovering individuals to meaningful occupational participation. Occupational therapy practitioners are ideal for implementing addiction recovery methods based on the holistic nature of the profession and its focus on addressing social, emotional, psychological, physical, and cognitive aspects of mental illness while supporting independent participation in daily life in given contexts (AOTA, 2017). Recently, the AOTA published a press release on the role of occupational therapy in addressing the opioid epidemic, emphasizing how "occupational therapy uses education, functional goal setting, and training to reduce the need for opioids or other potentially harmful approaches to managing chronic or severe pain" (AOTA, 2018, para. 5).

Likewise, Wasmuth et al. (2014) suggested that addiction is an occupation that requires new, meaningful opportunities for participation in early recovery to sustain recovery efforts. In the framework, "the term *occupation* denotes life engagements that are constructed of multiple activities. Both occupations and activities are used as interventions by practitioners" (AOTA, 2014, p. S6). Wasmuth, Pritchard, and Kaneshiro (2016) examined the effectiveness of occupation- and activity-based interventions for SUD implemented by a wide range of practitioners and found that all social participation interventions elicited superior outcomes compared to non-occupation-based treatment-as-usual methods. A narrative review of psychosocial occupational therapy interventions for SUD found that occupational therapy life skills interventions could "enhance functional independence and occupational performance for individuals recovering from SUD" (Amorelli, 2016, p. 167).

Screening and Evaluation

The AOTA has highlighted several occupational therapy screening and assessment tools that can be uniquely helpful in uncovering functional limitations accompanying an SUD and in developing an intervention plan. During the administration of an occupational profile, "the client, with the assistance of the occupational therapy practitioner, identifies priorities and desired targeted outcomes that will lead to the client's engagement in occupations that support participation in life" (AOTA, 2014, p. S13). Occupational therapy practitioners can examine current and future roles via the role checklist (Oakley, Kielhofner, Barris, and Reichler, 1986) to help people in recovery restructure their identity and participation as they embark on their recovery journeys. Assessing factors such as sensory processing, volition, and cognition (e.g., the capacity for planning, organizing and performing daily routines, and sequencing tasks to engage in community events) can provide helpful information about challenges a person might face in recovery efforts. Occupational therapy practitioners can also uncover valuable information via functional assessments that break the performance of occupations down into discrete steps that can be practiced and observed to determine the potential need for assistance or intervention (AOTA, 2017).

Some literature has also suggested that assessing readiness to change can be useful in determining what type of interventions would be most helpful to a person with an SUD at a given time. The University of Rhode Island Change Assessment (URICA) is a 32-item questionnaire (McConnaughy, DiClemente, Prochaska, and Velicer, 1989) that helps categorize a person into one of four change-readiness stages (precontemplation, contemplation, action, or maintenance) and is, according to Norcross, Krebs, and Prochaska (2011), the most commonly used readiness-to-change assessment. The Stages of Change and Treatment Eagerness Scale (SOCRATES) is also frequently used for this purpose (Miller and Tonigan, 1996). Additionally, one item on the Occupational Circumstances Assessment Interview and Rating Scale (OCAIRS) examines readiness to change based on feedback from others about the effectiveness or ineffectiveness of one's thoughts and actions (Forsyth et al., 2005).

Addiction as Occupation

Conceptualizing addiction as an occupation can help frame the substance use epidemic as a population health problem related to societal structure and human experiences among entire populations. This is in contrast to a view of addiction as an individual problem primarily resulting from the neurochemical alterations brought about by drug use.

Wasmuth, Crabtree, and Scott (2014) proposed the notion of addiction-as-occupation to underscore that when a person engages in an addiction, it becomes a central activity that shapes a person's identity; structures that person's time by creating habits, roles, and routines related to engaging in the addiction; serves as a source of volition; and has meaning for the person. Considering addiction as an occupation does not preclude it is harmful; rather, it contextualizes addiction on a scale with other occupations with varying degrees of gains and harms. The concept of addiction as an occupation is not new. Sackman, Sackman, and DeAngelis (1978) conceptualized addiction in this way decades ago, and Kiepek and Magalhães (2011) examined whether activities classified as addictions and impulse control disorders were occupations, finding that they "meet the criteria of occupation, in that they give meaning to life; are important determinants of health, well-being and justice; organize behaviour; develop and change over a lifetime; shape and are shaped by environments and have therapeutic potential" (p. 254).

The impetus for conceptualizing addiction-as-occupation from Wasmuth et al.'s (2014) perspective is to underscore early addiction recovery as a period of marked occupational deficit. As people endeavor to abstain from what were previously central occupations (addictions), they experience the loss of meaning, structure, and identity anyone experiences upon losing the ability to perform a meaningful occupation. Thus, "even when provided with effective, evidence-based interventions (for example, cognitive behavioral therapy for changing problematic thinking, medications to remove biologically-based cravings, and social skills training), attempts at abstinence may still be profoundly distressing" (Wasmuth et al., 2014, p. 607) due to the profound need for new occupations to replace the addictive behaviors. The person has a dire need for occupations to provide new meaning, structure, and a means for establishing, essentially, an entirely new identity rooted in new habits, roles, and routines. Qualitative explorations of addiction recovery experiences support that such a profound change is necessary (Wasmuth, Brandon-Friedman, and Olesek, 2016).

Occupation-Based Population Health Approaches

The model of addiction-as-occupation contextualizes addiction on a scale that delineates the degree to which occupations facilitate or deter wellness within environmental contexts. It is important to keep in mind that wellness is a fluid concept that can mean different things for different people in different settings. However, the construct of flexibility has been linked to health and wellness in many areas of psychological health (Bond and Flaxman, 2006; Fledderus, Bohlmeijer, Smit, and Westerhof, 2010) and overall adaptiveness of humans and other organisms (Moss, 2006) and therefore serves as a placeholder for wellness on the addiction-as-occupation scale depicted in Figure 19-1.

Figure 19-1 suggests that an absence of occupational participation (*top far left*) and rigid participation in one or few all-encompassing occupations (*top far right*) compromises overall wellness. While flexibility (considering its relationship to wellness) is desired, total flexibility or lack of structure (*far left*) has detrimental consequences such as contributing to lack of structure or routines, poor volition, symptoms of depression, social isolation, and related mental health concerns (Kielhofner, 2008). Likewise, participation in one or few stringent, rigid, or all-encompassing occupations (Fig. 19-1, *far right*) may result in a sense of belonging or mastery over one or a few occupations but provides little flexibility to adapt if these occupations are interfered with and may limit opportunities for reflection and the development of a person's most authentic beliefs, interests, values, and occupational paths (Kielhofner, 2008; Wasmuth, 2015). It is worth noting that people whose lives are characterized by the far left of the scale are at risk of compensating by adopting rigid or addictive occupations, shifting their experience to the far right of the scale.

Wasmuth (2015), building on the concept of occupational balance (Matuska and Christiansen, 2008), introduced the concept of **focused flexibility** to describe the middle of the scale, in which a person participates in a variety of meaningful occupations that can provide some structure and focus while still maintaining a degree of flexibility and adaptiveness. The person is not rigidly tied to any one all-encompassing occupation, such as an addiction. In a space of focused flexibility, if an injury or contextual factor prevents participation in one occupation, the person is afforded a degree of flexibility to continue participation in other meaningful occupations in order to maintain a consistent but fluid sense of meaning and personal identity matched with activities that can structure time and contribute to established routines and roles.

While this figure suggests the center of the scale to be indicative of wellness, it is essential to recognize that many individuals may operate successfully at different points on this scale, given supporting environmental circumstances. It is also important to note that the degree to which an occupation or set of occupations constrains an individual (or promotes

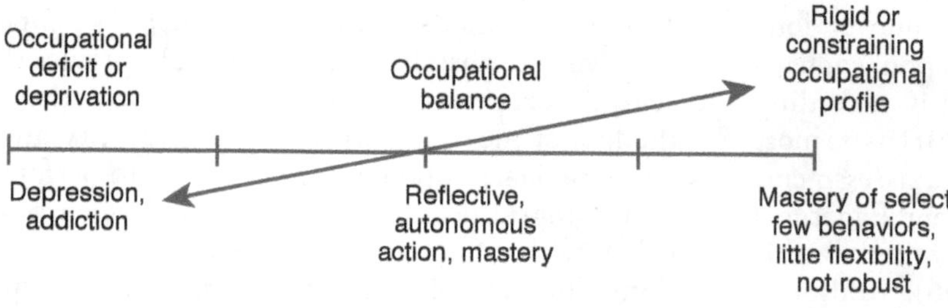

Figure 19-1 Normative scale of occupations.

flexibility and wellness) may be a result of the demands/dictates of the occupation, the impact it has on the individual's psyche, the temporal constraints it imposes, the associated environments, or some combination of these and other factors, such as the person's stage of recovery.

One benefit of this normative scale in the context of population health and addiction is that it conceptualizes addiction in the context of everyday occupations that vary in the degree to which they foster focused flexibility and therefore wellness. Such a scale can be used to remove stigma from conversations about addictive behaviors and their potential harms and benefits by placing addiction on a spectrum with other nonstigmatized activities as they relate to flexibility. The scale can be used to guide discussions about wellness goals and can help occupational therapy practitioners and clients identify alternative occupations that have the potential to promote wellness by focusing on the construct of focused flexibility. Likewise, the scale can assist individuals and societies in reflecting about the degree to which their current occupational lives or societal structures facilitate the desired degree of flexibility and freedom while avoiding overemphasis on the direct health-related harms of addictive substances that research literature suggests can actually impede recovery efforts (Costanza et al., 2017).

Along these lines, Costanza et al. (2017) emphasize that the evidence-based tenets of motivational interviewing, such as positive discussion of goals, motives, and futures, that have been highly effective with facilitating individual addiction recovery may be helpful at the societal level. They argue that efforts to promote societal change regarding issues like overconsumption, structures fostering ongoing social inequality, practices related to problematic climate change, and "misplaced use of GDP growth as a societal goal" (p. 47) by scientists and activists have been more confrontational and judgmental. Drawing an analogy between individual and societal addiction recovery, they emphasize that just as such stigmatizing and domineering approaches toward eliciting change in addicted individuals have often produced resistance to change, so, too, might these approaches impede societal-level change. They suggest community-engaged scenario planning as a potential solution for "engaging entire communities in building consensus about preferred alternative future via public opinion surveys and forums," noting:

> *Effective therapies for societal addictions are possible but require re-balancing effort away from only pointing out the dire consequences of current behavior and toward also building a truly shared vision of a positive future and ways to get there. (Costanza et al., 2017, p. 47)*

Kronenberg, Pollard, and Sakellariou (2011) have outlined several ways in which occupational therapy practitioners can contribute to engaging communities and societies in healing practices. They encourage using participation in occupations of daily life to enable people to overcome the limits imposed by marginalization and decrease feelings of dependency. Many of the interventions they outline focus on allowing voices of marginalized populations to be heard through theater and other expressive arts.

Engage Your Brain 19-3

What additional competencies would help occupational therapists be more prepared to work with a person recovering from an SUD?

Likewise, Wasmuth and Pritchard (2016) developed a theater protocol that specifically targets aspects of substance and process addictions, such as decreased volition, social isolation, a need for new habits and routines (and temporal structure), self-efficacy, and the tendency to devalue future rewards. The intervention builds on memory-training interventions shown to counteract the pathological consequences of drug use at the neurological level (Bickel et al., 2012) by having participants memorize scripts. It enhances volition by giving people a specific role to play, increasing their sense of relevance and thus promoting attendance. Participants gain habits and routines, as they are expected to adhere to a rigorous rehearsal schedule, and experience a decrease in isolation as they regularly engage with others. Finally, it enhances community engagement via public performances in the community, during which participants and audience members discuss the impacts of addiction on society and society's roles in promoting and sustaining innovative solutions.

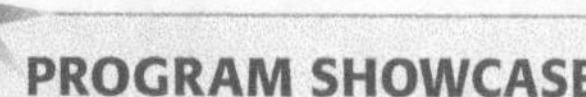

PROGRAM SHOWCASE

Integrating Occupational Therapy Into Adolescent SUD Recovery

Literature suggests that occupational therapists can be invaluable in facilitating SUD recovery (Costa, 2017). However, few addiction rehabilitation facilities employ occupational therapy services. A team of three occupational therapists addressed this discrepancy in an ongoing community partnership project from 2015 to 2018, described below.

In 2015, an occupational therapist and researcher collaborated with Fairbanks Alcohol and Drug Addiction Treatment Center in Indianapolis, Indiana, to provide an occupation-based theater intervention to facilitate recovery (Wasmuth and Pritchard, 2016). Fairbanks houses one of the only addiction recovery high schools in the country—Hope Academy. A second occupational therapist and researcher, Victoria Wilburn, began regularly meeting with Hope Academy personnel to provide education on the potential role of occupational therapy with adolescents in recovery. A level-one occupational therapy doctoral student was integrated into this process and assisted in conducting a needs assessment at the site that revealed a dire need among adolescents at Hope Academy to have their stories heard, told, empathized with, and learned from. For 6 months, an occupation-based approach bolstered by principles of narrative medicine (Charon and Marcus, 2016) was offered on a weekly basis, and after 6 months, occupational therapy services were written into Hope's summer budget. Additional grant funding was obtained to continue building occupational therapy's role at the site, with the goal of increasing client engagement and retention by attuning to the nuanced, intricate details of clients' unique individual stories. Clients valued occupational therapy services, especially their role in improving social participation. One stated, "Occupational therapy helped me grow my confidence—I am no longer afraid of public speaking," and another noted, "Occupational therapy helped me make friends."

Summary

- Many substances are considered illicit drugs based not on their physiological effects but rather on their historical prevalence within and among marginalized racial groups. Institutional racism has contributed to drug policy development, which, in addition to various social determinants of health, has affected the degree to which different social groups experience harm from drug use.
- The current opioid epidemic—marked by exponential increases in opioid use disorders and opioid-related deaths—emerged alongside increased rates of opioid prescriptions for acute and chronic pain and increased illicit production and distribution of high-potency opiates.
- In some cases, opioids can alleviate pain and promote meaningful occupational participation, even though their neurobiological consequences resemble the neurobiology of addiction. However, when matched with psychosocial and environmental risk factors, opioid use can negatively affect individuals, families, communities, and societies.
- Several evidence-based practices for SUD have elicited modest positive outcomes and include recovery-oriented care, education regarding risk for providers and potential substance users, MAT, motivational interviewing, CBT, peer support, family-based therapies, integrated therapies, long-term counseling or recovery coaching, contingency management, supportive housing, 12-step programs, and mindfulness training. Treatment satisfaction, engagement, and long-term recovery outcomes remain relatively poor.
- A population health approach to addiction treatment recognizes that populations' risk and experiences of addiction differ based on structural, social, environmental, and political forces; many aspects of modern society mirror addictive tendencies and may contribute to ongoing substance use epidemics.
- Conceptualizing addiction as an occupation suggests that recognizing the occupational deficit in early recovery and providing new occupations can bolster recovery outcomes.
- Scholars have used community engagement modalities such as theater productions and scenario planning to involve populations in critical conversations about substance use epidemics, societal addiction, and desired society-level changes.

- Occupational therapists have suggested conceptualizing substance use and other addictions on a continuum with other occupational engagements, distinguished based on the degree to which they promote focused flexibility and thus health, in order to address the widespread societal effects of different forms of addiction.

CASE STUDIES

CASE STUDY 19-1 Michael

Michael is a 39-year-old male admitted to inpatient rehab from acute care 6 weeks after sustaining a traumatic brain injury. Michael was a passenger in a car that reportedly crashed into a tree. He has a history of type 2 diabetes, cocaine use disorder, alcohol use disorder, and bipolar II disorder. After reviewing his chart, you learn Michael declined his physical therapy evaluation and has been refusing services from a speech language pathologist (SLP). You consult with the SLP to obtain more information, and she informs you that he has no diet restrictions but that SLP services were ordered by the physician because the client has not been eating, stating he has no appetite. She notes that sugar should be limited due to his diabetes diagnosis. You are able to motivate Michael to participate in an initial occupational therapy evaluation by having him make pancakes in the kitchen. Michael requires moderate assistance in the task during your initial evaluation due to deficits in sitting and standing balance and sequencing deficits.

You gather occupational profile information while Michael is eating his pancakes. You learn that he hopes to return home to the one-story house he shares with his 40-year-old cousin and 42-year-old sister. You ask Michael to tell you about the events leading up to his injury. He ignores you while quietly eating his pancakes, but after a few minutes have passed, you ask if the car accident was scary. "Not really," he says. "To be honest, we were all so high I don't really remember anything except the car moving real fast, and I had the door open and the wind was hitting my face and it felt amazing!" You engage him in a conversation about the experience, asking him questions about his drug use and what he enjoys about it. Through this discussion he reveals that he is really looking forward to getting out of the hospital so that he can get high.

Discussion Questions

1. What might you focus on during Michael's next therapy session? Hint: consider the transtheoretical (stages of change) model.
2. What client factors will you target during intervention sessions to support Michael's desire for home discharge?
3. What obstacles exist to Michael's desired discharge?

CASE STUDY 19-2 Recidivism Reduction Community Center

A new facility has just opened with a mission to decrease recidivism and improve recovery-related outcomes among offenders with SUD. If a person is stopped by law enforcement and determined to be intoxicated, that person can be brought to the facility (as an alternative to jail or the public hospital emergency department) for a 72-hour stay for substance detoxification (detox) and then moved to a recovery-supportive discharge site. The site has commissioned you to provide

CASE STUDY 19-2 Recidivism Reduction Community Center

occupational therapy consultant services. Upon visiting the site and conducting a needs assessment, you learn that staff consists of an administrative team, emergency medical services (EMS) personnel, and a nurse practitioner. The administrators are responsible for discharge decisions; clients are discharged when beds become available within the community. The nurse practitioner is responsible for MAT and monitoring vital signs during detoxification, and EMS staff provide medical and safety oversight within the facility. Administrative staff members collect basic medical history and demographic information upon intake. No mental health staff members are employed at the site, and no therapeutic or recreational activities are offered. From a literature review and interviews with residents, you learn that many residents are homeless or live in unsafe conditions, have a history of trauma and abuse, and are chronic drug users with numerous comorbid physical and mental health conditions such as depression, psychosis, COPD, asthma, chronic pain, and personality disorders. Many residents smoke cigarettes and report multiple unsuccessful attempts at SUD recovery. Residents report boredom and increased symptoms of anxiety and depression while staying in the facility. The site director expresses that she does not want therapists to conduct activities or assessments that could "open up old wounds or delve into psychiatric issues" because the facility lacks a permanent, on-site mental health practitioner to support people who may become triggered from such instances after therapists have left the facility.

Discussion Questions

1. As an occupational therapy consultant, what recommendations would you make to improve the site's ability to address clients' needs while also accommodating the director's requests?
2. What types of therapeutic groups might benefit residents while accommodating the director's requests?
3. In what ways might discharge processes at the site be improved?

Learning Activities

1. Use current literature, your occupational therapy education, and your clinical reasoning skills to create an occupation-based group intervention aimed at addressing the needs of one of the following specific populations:
   1) Women who are pregnant and abuse substances
   2) Middle-aged adults with chronic pain and newly prescribed opioids
   3) Adolescents in a correctional facility for illegal drug use or possession

   Using tenets of the model of human occupation (Kielhofner, 2008), consider how you might design the group to address volition, target the performance capacity needs of the population, and promote the healthy establishment of roles, routines, and habits among group members.

   Questions to consider:
   a. What characteristics of this population are important to consider according to recent literature?
   b. What will motivate participants to attend?
   c. How will the group design affect participants' habits, roles, and routines?
   d. In what ways does the group intervention specifically address performance capacity issues of the population in question?
2. Using Figure 19-1 and the list of occupations that follows, first consider where these occupations may fall on the scale. Discuss factors that may influence where they fall and why and the potential occupational gains and harms of each as they relate to focused flexibility and health. The occupations include Olympic athlete, graduate student, freelance writer, evangelist, Buddhist monk, self-employed actor working

intermittently, heroin addict, others? Next, reflect on how you might use this visual diagram to guide a community conversation about social responsibility for health disparities or climate change.

REFERENCES

Acker, C. J. (2010). How crack found a niche in the American ghetto: The historical epidemiology of drug-related harm. *BioSocieties, 5*(1), 70–88.

Alexander, B. K. (2010). *The globalization of addiction: A study in poverty of the spirit.* Oxford, United Kingdom: Oxford University Press.

Alexander, B. K. (2015). *Healing addiction through community: A much longer road than it seems?* Retrieved from www.brucekalexander.com/articles-speeches/healing-addiction-through-community-a-much-longer-road-than-it-seems2

American Occupational Therapy Association. (2014). Occupational therapy practice framework: Domain and process (3rd ed.). *American Journal of Occupational Therapy, 68*(Suppl. 1), S1–S48. https://doi.org/10.5014/ajot.2014.682006

American Occupational Therapy Association. (2015). Occupational therapy code of ethics (2015). *American Journal of Occupational Therapy, 69*(Suppl. 3), 6913410030. http://dx.doi.org/10.5014/ajot.2015.696S03

American Occupational Therapy Association. (2017). *The occupational therapy advantage for certified community behavioral health clinics.* [PowerPoint Slides]. Bethesda, MD: American Occupational Therapy Association.

American Occupational Therapy Association. (2018). *Opioids legislation including occupational therapy services, advances in House Committee.* Retrieved from www.aota.org/Advocacy-Policy/Congressional-Affairs/Legislative-Issues-Update/2018/opioids-legislation-includes-occupational-therapy-OT-services.aspx18&utm_medium=email&utm_campaign=Congress%20Sees%20OT%20as%20a%20Part%20of%20Opioids%20Solution

American Psychiatric Association. (2013). *Diagnostic and statistical manual of mental disorders (DSM-5).* Washington, DC: American Psychiatric Association.

American Society of Addiction Medicine. (2011). *Definition of addiction.* Retrieved from www.asam.org/quality-practice/definition-of-addiction

Amorelli, C. R. (2016). Psychosocial occupational therapy interventions for substance-use disorders: A narrative review. *Occupational Therapy in Mental Health, 32*(2), 167–184.

Arnold, R. A. (1990). Processes of victimization and criminalization of black women. *Social Justice, 17*(3), 153–166.

Askgaard, G., Grønbæk, M., Kjær, M. S., Tjønneland, A., and Tolstrup, J. S. (2015). Alcohol drinking pattern and risk of alcoholic liver cirrhosis: A prospective cohort study. *Journal of Hepatology, 62*(5), 1061–1067.

Association of State and Territorial Health Officials. (2011). *Health Equity Position Statement.* Retrieved from http://astho.org/Programs/Health-Equity/Affiliate-Health-Equity-Position-Statement/

Baffy, G., Brunt, E. M., and Caldwell, S. H. (2012). Hepatocellular carcinoma in non-alcoholic fatty liver disease: An emerging menace. *Journal of Hepatology, 56*(6), 1384–1391.

Barnett, K., Mercer, S. W., Norbury, M., Watt, G., Wyke, S., and Guthrie, B. (2012). Epidemiology of multimorbidity and implications for health care, research, and medical education: A cross-sectional study. *Lancet, 380*(9836), 37–43.

Bart, G. (2012). Maintenance medication for opiate addiction: The foundation of recovery. *Journal of Addictive Diseases, 31*(3), 207–225.

Becker, S. J., Squires, D. D., Strong, D. R., Barnett, N. P., Monti, P. M., and Petry, N. M. (2016). Training opioid addiction treatment providers to adopt contingency management: A prospective pilot trial of a comprehensive implementation science approach. *Substance Abuse, 37*(1), 134–140.

Bickel, W. K., Jarmolowicz, D. P., Mueller, E. T., Koffarnus, M. N., and Gatchalian, K. M. (2012). Excessive discounting of delayed reinforcers as a trans-disease process contributing to addiction and other disease-related vulnerabilities: Emerging evidence. *Pharmacology and Therapeutics, 134,* 287–297. Retrieved from http://dx.doi.org/10.1016/j.pharmthera.2012.02.004

Billieux, J., Schimmenti, A., Khazaal, Y., Maurage, P., and Heeren, A. (2015). Are we overpathologizing everyday life? A tenable blueprint for behavioral addiction research. *Journal of Behavioral Addictions, 4*(3), 119–123.

Boisvert, R. A., Martin, L. M., Grosek, M., and Clarie, A. J. (2008). Effectiveness of a peer support community in addiction recovery: Participation as intervention. *Occupational Therapy International, 15*(4), 205–220.

Bond, F. W., and Flaxman, P. E. (2006). The ability of psychological flexibility and job control to predict learning, job performance, and mental health. *Journal of Organizational Behavior Management, 26*(1–2), 113–130.

Braveman, B., and Suarez-Balcazar, Y. (2009). Social justice and resource utilization in a community-based organization: A case illustration of the role of the occupational therapist. *American Journal of Occupational Therapy, 63*(1), 13–23.

Braveman, P., and Gottlieb, L. (2014). The social determinants of health: It's time to consider the causes of the causes. *Public Health Reports, 129*(Suppl. 1), 19–31.

Brummett, C. M., Waljee, J. F., Goesling, J., Moser, S., Lin, P., Englesbe, M. J., . . . and Nallamothu, B. K. (2017). New persistent opioid use after minor and major surgical procedures in US adults. *JAMA Surgery, 152*(6), e170504.

Case, A., and Deaton, A. (2015). Rising morbidity and mortality in midlife among white non-Hispanic Americans in the 21st century. *Proceedings of the National Academy of Sciences, 112*(49), 15078–15083.

Center for Behavioral Health Statistics and Quality. (2016). *2015 National survey on drug use and health: Detailed tables.* Rockville, MD: Substance Abuse and Mental Health Services Administration.

Centers for Disease Control and Prevention. (2018a). *Principles of epidemiology in public health practice, third edition: An introduction to applied epidemiology and biostatistics.* Retrieved from www.cdc.gov/ophss/csels/dsepd/ss1978/lesson1/section11.html

Centers for Disease Control and Prevention. (2018b). *U.S. drug overdose deaths continue to rise; increase fueled by synthetic opioids.* Retrieved from www.cdc.gov/media/releases/2018/p0329-drug-overdose-deaths.html

Charon, R., and Marcus, E. R. (2016). *The principles and practice of narrative medicine.* Oxford: United Kingdom: Oxford University Press.

Costa, D. (2017). Occupational therapy's role in countering opioid addiction. *OT Practice, 22*(1), 12–16.

Costanza, R., Atkins, P. W., Bolton, M., Cork, S., Grigg, N. J., Kasser, T., and Kubiszewski, I. (2017). Societal addiction therapy: From motivational interviewing to community engaged scenario planning. *Current Opinion in Environmental Sustainability, 26,* 47–53.

Currie, E. (1993). *Reckoning: Drugs, the cities, and the American future.* New York, NY: Hill and Wang.

Drake, R. E., Essock, S. M., Shaner, A., Carey, K. B., Minkoff, K., Kola, L., . . . and Rickards, L. (2001). Implementing dual diagnosis services for clients with severe mental illness. *Psychiatric Services, 52*(4), 469–476.

Dunn, W., Brown, C., and McGuigan, A. (1994). The ecology of human performance: A framework for considering the effect of context. *American Journal of Occupational Therapy, 48*(7), 595–607.

Fabbri, L. M. (2016). Smoking, not COPD, as the disease. *New England Journal of Medicine, 374*(19), 1885–1886.

Fatseas, M., Serre, F., Alexandre, J. M., Debrabant, R., Auriacombe, M., and Swendsen, J. (2015). Craving and substance use among patients with alcohol, tobacco, cannabis or heroin addiction: A comparison of substance-and person-specific cues. *Addiction, 110*(6), 1035–1042.

Fishbain, D. A., Cole, B., Lewis, J., Rosomoff, H. L., and Rosomoff, R. S. (2007). What percentage of chronic nonmalignant pain patients exposed to chronic opioid analgesic therapy develop abuse/addiction and/or aberrant drug-related behaviors? A structured evidence-based review. *Pain Medicine, 9*(4), 444–459.

Fledderus, M., Bohlmeijer, E. T., Smit, F., and Westerhof, G. J. (2010). Mental health promotion as a new goal in public mental health care: A randomized controlled trial of an intervention enhancing psychological flexibility. *American Journal of Public Health, 100*(12), 2372–2378.

Forsyth, K., Deshpande, S., Kielhofner, G., Henriksson, C., Haglund, L., Olson, L., . . . Kulkarni, S. (2005). *The Occupational Circumstances Assessment Interview and Rating Scale Vol. 4.0.* Chicago: University of Illinois at Chicago.

Garland, E. L., Roberts-Lewis, A., Tronnier, C. D., Graves, R., and Kelley, K. (2016). Mindfulness-oriented recovery enhancement versus CBT for co-occurring substance dependence, traumatic stress, and psychiatric disorders: Proximal outcomes from a pragmatic randomized trial. *Behaviour Research and Therapy, 77,* 7–16.

Gutman, S. A., and Schindler, V. P. (2007). The neurological basis of occupation. *Occupational Therapy International, 14*(2), 71–85.

Hawe, P., and Potvin, L. (2009). What is population health intervention research? *Canadian Journal of Public Health, 100*(1), 8–14.

Keane, H., and Hamill, K. (2010). Variations in addiction: The molecular and the molar in neuroscience and pain medicine. *BioSocieties, 5*(1), 52–69.

Keightley, M., Agnihotri, S., Subramaniapillai, S., Gray, J., Keresztesi, J., Colantonio, A., . . . and Wiseman-Hakes, C. (2018). Investigating a theatre-based intervention for Indigenous youth with fetal alcohol spectrum disorder: Exploration d'une intervention basée sur le théâtre auprès de jeunes Autochtones atteints du syndrome d'alcoolisme fœtal. *Canadian Journal of Occupational Therapy, 85*(2), 128–136.

Kielhofner, G. (2008). *Model of human occupation: Theory and application.* Baltimore, MD: Lippincott Williams and Wilkins.

Kiepek, N., and Magalhães, L. (2011). Addictions and impulse-control disorders as occupation: A selected literature review and synthesis. *Journal of Occupational Science, 18*(3), 254–276. doi:10.1080/14427591.2011.581628

Kindig, D., and Stoddart, G. (2003). What is population health? *American Journal of Public Health, 93*(3), 380–383.

Ko, C. H., Liu, T. L., Wang, P. W., Chen, C. S., Yen, C. F., and Yen, J. Y. (2014). The exacerbation of depression, hostility, and social anxiety in the course of Internet addiction among adolescents: A prospective study. *Comprehensive Psychiatry, 55*(6), 1377–1384.

Ko, C. H., Yen, J. Y., Yen, C. F., Chen, C. S., and Wang, S. Y. (2008). The association between Internet addiction and belief of frustration intolerance: The gender difference. *Cyberpsychology and Behavior, 11*(3), 273–278.

Kolodny, A., Courtwright, D. T., Hwang, C. S., Kreiner, P., Eadie, J. L., Clark, T. W., and Alexander, G. C. (2015). The prescription opioid and heroin crisis: A public health approach to an epidemic of addiction. *Annual Review of Public Health, 36,* 559–574.

Krieger, N. (2014). Discrimination and health inequities. *International Journal of Health Services, 44*(4), 643–710.

Kronenberg, F., Pollard, N., and Sakellariou, D. (Eds.). (2011). *Occupational therapies without borders—volume 2 e-book: Towards an ecology of occupation-based practices.* Edinburgh, Scotland: Elsevier Health Sciences.

Kubek, P. M., Kruszynski, R., and Boyle, P. E. (2003). *Integrated dual disorder treatment (IDDT): An overview of the evidence-based practice.* Cleveland, OH: Center for Evidence-Based Practices, Case Western Reserve University.

Kushner, H. (2006). Taking biology seriously: The next task for historians of addiction? *Bulletin of the History of Medicine, 80*(Spring), 114–143.

Kushner, H. I. (2010a). Historical perspectives of addiction. In B. A. Johnson (Ed.), *Addiction medicine: Science and practice.* New York, NY: Springer.

Kushner, H. I. (2010b). Toward a cultural biology of addiction. *BioSocieties, 5*(1), 8–24.

Manchikanti, L., Helm, S., Fellows, B., Janata, J. W., Pampati, V., Grider, J. S., and Boswell, M. V. (2012). Opioid epidemic in the United States. *Pain Physician, 15,* ES9–ES38.

Matuska, K. M., and Christiansen, C. H. (2008). A proposed model of lifestyle balance. *Journal of Occupational Science, 15*(1), 9–19.

McConnaughy, E. A., DiClemente, C. C., Prochaska, J. O., and Velicer, W. F. (1989). Stages of change in psychotherapy: A follow-up report. *Psychotherapy, 26*(4), 494–503.

Miller, W. R., and Tonigan, J. S. (1996). Assessing drinkers' motivation for change: The Stages of Change Readiness and Treatment Eagerness Scale (SOCRATES). *Psychology of Addictive Behaviors, 10*(2), 81.

Moss, L. (2006). Redundancy, plasticity, and detachment: The implications of comparative genomics for evolutionary thinking. *Philosophy of Science, 73*(5), 930–946.

Murthy, V. H. (2017). Surgeon general's report on alcohol, drugs, and health. *Journal of the American Medical Association, 317*(2), 133–134.

National Institute on Drug Abuse. (2018a). *Opioid overdose crisis.* Retrieved from www.drugabuse.gov/drugs-abuse/opioids/opioid-overdose-crisis

National Institute on Drug Abuse. (2018b). *Opioids.* Retrieved from www.drugabuse.gov/drugs-abuse/opioids

Nilsson, I., and Townsend, E. (2010). Occupational justice—bridging theory and practice. *Scandinavian Journal of Occupational Therapy, 17*(1), 57–63.

Noordsy, D., Torrey, W., Mueser, K., Mead, S., O'Keefe, C., and Fox, L. (2002). Recovery from severe mental illness: An intrapersonal and functional outcome definition. *International Review of Psychiatry, 14*(4), 318–326.

Norcross, J. C., Krebs, P. M., and Prochaska, J. O. (2011). Stages of change. *Journal of Clinical Psychology, 67*(2), 143–154.

Oakley, F., Kielhofner, G., Barris, R., and Reichler, R. K. (1986). The Role Checklist: Development and empirical assessment of reliability. *Occupational Therapy Journal of Research, 6*(3), 157–170.

Padgett, D. K., Stanhope, V., Henwood, B. F., and Stefancic, A. (2011). Substance use outcomes among homeless clients with serious mental illness: Comparing housing first with treatment first programs. *Community Mental Health Journal, 47*(2), 227–232.

Panebianco, D., Gallupe, O., Carrington, P. J., and Colozzi, I. (2016). Personal support networks, social capital, and risk of relapse among individuals treated for substance use issues. *International Journal of Drug Policy, 27,* 146–153.

Prendergast, M., Podus, D., Finney, J., Greenwell, L., and Roll, J. (2006). Contingency management for treatment of substance use disorders: A meta-analysis. *Addiction, 101*(11), 1546–1560.

Rahwan, I., Krasnoshtan, D., Shariff, A., and Bonnefon, J. F. (2014). Analytical reasoning task reveals limits of social learning in networks. *Journal of the Royal Society Interface, 11*(93), 20131211.

Ross, D., Sharp, C., Vuchinich, R. E., and Spurrett, D. (2008). *Midbrain mutiny: The picoeconomics and neuroeconomics of disordered gambling: Economic theory and cognitive science.* Cambridge, MA: MIT Press.

Sackman, B. S., Sackman, M. M., and DeAngelis, G. G. (1978). Heroin addiction as an occupation: Traditional addicts and heroin-addicted polydrug users. *International Journal of the Addictions, 13*(3), 427–441.

Sacks, T. K. (2018). Performing black womanhood: A qualitative study of stereotypes and the healthcare encounter. *Critical Public Health, 28*(1), 59–69.

Sherman, L. E., Michikyan, M., and Greenfeld, P. M. (2013). The effects of text, audio, video, and in-person communication on bonding between friends. *Cyberpsychology: Journal of Psychosocial Research on Cyberspace, 7*(2). Retrieved from www.cyberpsychology.eu/view.php?cisloclanku=2013071101&article=1

Shumway, S. T., Bradshaw, S. D., Harris, K. S., and Baker, A. K. (2013). Important factors of early addiction recovery and inpatient treatment. *Alcoholism Treatment Quarterly, 31*(1), 3–24.

Silk, J. S., Stroud, L. R., Siegle, G. J., Dahl, R. E., Lee, K. H., and Nelson, E. E. (2012). Peer acceptance and rejection through the eyes of youth: Pupillary, eyetracking and ecological data from the Chatroom Interact task. *Social Cognitive and Affective Neuroscience, 7*(1), 93–105. doi:10.1093/scan/nsr044

Sliwa, K., Azibani, F., Baard, J., Osman, A., Zühlke, L., Lachmann, A., . . . and Johnson, M. R. (2018). Reducing late maternal death due to cardiovascular disease—a pragmatic pilot study. *International Journal of Cardiology, 272,* 70–76.

Srivastava, A. B., and Gold, M. S. (2018, March). Beyond supply: How we must tackle the opioid epidemic. *Mayo Clinic Proceedings, 93*(3), 269–272.

Stoffel, V. C., and Moyers, P. A. (2004). An evidence-based and occupational perspective of interventions for persons with substance-use disorders. *American Journal of Occupational Therapy, 58*(5), 570–586.

Substance Abuse and Mental Health Services Administration. (2018). *Finding quality treatment for substance use disorders.* Retrieved from https://store.samhsa.gov/system/files/pep18-treatment-loc.pdf

Sussman, S., Lisha, N., and Griffiths, M. (2011). Prevalence of the addictions: A problem of the majority or the minority? *Evaluation and the Health Professions, 34*(1), 3–56.

Tetrault, J. M., and Fiellin, D. A. (2018). More beds or more chairs? Using a science-based approach to address the opioid epidemic. *Annals of Internal Medicine, 168*(1), 73–74.

Thege, B. K., Woodin, E. M., Hodgins, D. C., and Williams, R. J. (2015). Natural course of behavioral addictions: A 5-year longitudinal study. *BMC Psychiatry, 15*(1), 4–18.

Twinley, R. (2013). The dark side of occupation: A concept for consideration. *Australian Occupational Therapy Journal, 60*(4), 301–303.

Unick, G. J., Rosenblum, D., Mars, S., and Ciccarone, D. (2013). Intertwined epidemics: National demographic trends in hospitalizations for heroin- and opioid-related overdoses, 1993–2009. *PloS One, 8*(2), e54496.

U.S. Department of Health and Human Services Office of the Surgeon General. (2016). *Facing addiction in America: The surgeon general's report on alcohol, drugs, and health.* Washington, DC: U.S. Department of Health and Human Services.

Wallace, M. E., Green, C., Richardson, L., Theall, K., and Crear-Perry, J. (2017). "Look at the whole me": A mixed-methods examination of black infant mortality in the US through women's lived experiences and community context. *International Journal of Environmental Research and Public Health, 14*(7), 727.

Wasmuth, S. (2015). Gehlen's philosophical anthropology: Contemporary applications in addiction research. In P. Honenberger (Ed.), *Naturalism and philosophical anthropology* (pp. 147–170). London, United Kingdom: Palgrave Macmillan.

Wasmuth, S., Brandon-Friedman, R. A., and Olesek, K. (2016). A grounded theory of veterans' experiences of addiction-as-occupation. *Journal of Occupational Science, 23*(1), 128–141.

Wasmuth, S., Crabtree, J. L., and Scott, P. J. (2014). Exploring addiction-as-occupation. *British Journal of Occupational Therapy, 77*(12), 605–613.

Wasmuth, S., and Pritchard, K. (2016). Theater-based community engagement project for veterans recovering from substance use disorders. *American Journal of Occupational Therapy, 70*(4), 7004250020p1–7004250020p11.

Wasmuth, S., Pritchard, K., and Kaneshiro, K. (2016). Occupation-based intervention for addictive disorders: A systematic review. *Journal of Substance Abuse Treatment, 62,* 1–9.

Wasmuth, S. L., Outcalt, J., Buck, K., Leonhardt, B. L., Vohs, J., and Lysaker, P. H. (2015). Metacognition in persons with substance abuse: Findings and implications for occupational therapists: La métacognition chez les personnes toxicomances: Résultats et conséquences pour les ergothérapeutes. *Canadian Journal of Occupational Therapy, 82*(3), 150–159.

World Health Organization. (2017). Management of substance abuse. *Dependence Syndrome.* Retrieved from www.who.int/substance_abuse/terminology/definition1/en/

Yuan, K., Qin, W., Wang, G., Zeng, F., Zhao, L., Yang, X., . . . and Gong, Q. (2011). Microstructure abnormalities in adolescents with Internet addiction disorder. *PloS One, 6*(6), e20708.

Chapter 20

Addressing the Needs of the Homeless

Thaddeus Parker, MS, OTR/L, and Marjorie E. Scaffa, PhD, OTR/L, FAOTA

Give me your tired, your poor,
Your huddled masses yearning to breathe free,
The wretched refuse of your teeming shore.
Send these, the homeless, tempest-tossed to me,
I lift my lamp beside the golden door!

—Emma Lazarus, "The New Colossus," Statue of Liberty, New York City Harbor

Learning Outcomes

This chapter is designed to enable the reader to:

20-1 Analyze structural, personal, and cultural factors that influence homelessness.
20-2 Describe populations at risk for experiencing homelessness.
20-3 Discuss effective responses to homelessness.
20-4 Describe the roles of occupational therapy in addressing the needs of the homeless population.
20-5 Analyze barriers to occupational engagement for persons who are homeless.
20-6 Apply theoretical and conceptual models to the development of occupational therapy services for the homeless.
20-7 Demonstrate the ability to develop client-centered, occupation-based interventions for persons and families who are homeless.

Key Terms

Adverse childhood experiences
Ecological model of homelessness
Empowerment
Fair market rent
Homeless
Housing First
Model of occupational empowerment
Poverty
Trauma-informed care

Introduction

Although the issue of homelessness affects nearly every community in the United States, it often goes unacknowledged, with members of the homeless population living out their daily lives in the margins of society. The U.S. Department of Housing and Urban Development (USDHUD, 2017) conducted a point-in-time count and estimated that nearly 550,000 people were experiencing homelessness on a single night in January in the United States. Approximately 68% of the homeless were sheltered for the night, with the remaining 32% sleeping in unsheltered locations. The majority of the homeless are individuals; however, families with children account for approximately 33% of the homeless population.

Box 20-1 Demographic Characteristics of the Homeless in the United States

Gender
60% male
40% female

Age
22% under age 18
9% ages 18–24
69% over age 24

Race
48% white
39% African American
22% Hispanic
7% multiracial
3% Native American
2% Pacific Islander
1% Asian

Data from *The 2017 Annual Homeless Assessment Report to Congress,* by U.S. Department of Housing and Urban Development, 2017.

Approximately 1 in 30 children are homeless annually, and 10% of homeless individuals are unaccompanied youth under the age of 25. Additional demographics are presented in Box 20-1. Five states (i.e., California, New York, Florida, Texas, and Washington) account for more than half of the homeless population in the United States (USDHUD, 2017).

According to federal legislation, a person or family is **homeless** if they lack a fixed, regular, and adequate nighttime residence. For example, individuals are considered homeless if their primary nighttime residence is:

- "A public or private place not designed for or ordinarily used as a regular sleeping accommodation for human beings, including a car, park, abandoned building, bus or train station, airport, or camping ground"
- "A publicly or privately-operated shelter designated to provide temporary living arrangements" (USDHUD, 2013, pp. 2–3)

Homelessness has a temporal dimension. The three basic temporal categories of homelessness are chronic, transitional, and episodic. The causes and stressors are different for each type of homelessness, as are the intervention needs. People who are chronically homeless tend to be older, unemployed, and often mentally ill and/or physically disabled. Although a small percentage of the homeless (10%), these are people who have been homeless for a year or more. Those who are transitionally homeless tend to be younger and become homeless because of some catastrophic event, such as a house fire or job loss. They use the shelter system temporarily before transitioning into more stable housing and represent the largest percentage (80%) of the homeless population. The episodically homeless (10%) are typically persons who are chronically unemployed, often due to medical, mental health, and substance use disorders. They may stay with family and friends intermittently and frequently move in and out of homelessness. The episodically homeless are at risk for becoming chronically homeless if the issues that caused their homelessness are not resolved (National Coalition for the Homeless [NCH], 2018).

Each community that receives federal funds is required to have a continuum of care for the homeless population. Although each continuum of care is tailored to specific community needs, most have the following components:

- Homeless prevention services
- Street outreach and assessment
- Emergency shelter programs
- Transitional housing programs
- Permanent supportive housing

These services are typically provided by government agencies (i.e., federal, state, and local) and nonprofit organizations. There are potential roles for occupational therapy in addressing all five components. The U.S. Interagency Council on Homelessness (USICH) works at the national level to coordinate the federal response to homelessness across 19 federal agencies and to create partnerships at every level of government and with the private sector to end homelessness (Livingston and Miller, 2006; USICH, 2018).

Factors and Perspectives Influencing Homelessness

Homelessness is the result of a complex interaction of structural factors, personal characteristics and vulnerabilities, and cultural influences (Petrenchik,

Box 20-2 Person-Environment Factors That Impact Homelessness

Structural/Socioenvironmental Factors

- Poverty
- Social and racial inequality and discrimination
- Lack of affordable housing
- Fewer employment opportunities for persons with a high school education or less
- Low federal minimum wage
- Insufficient housing assistance programs
- Reductions in social welfare programs
- Lack of affordable health care

Personal Characteristics and Vulnerabilities

- Limited education
- Poor skills
- Physical disability
- Mental illness
- Substance abuse
- Domestic violence

2006). Structural factors emerge from the social and environmental conditions in which people live, such as a lack of affordable housing. Personal vulnerabilities, such as mental illness, place individuals at greater risk for homelessness. A holistic understanding requires consideration of the various structural factors and personal characteristics that precipitate homelessness and their interactions. Examples are provided in Box 20-2.

Structural Factors

Structural factors that influence the rate of homelessness are the product of various governmental institutions, the laws they enact, and the policies that result from these laws. Poverty, the reduction of entitlement programs, a lack of affordable housing, and social and racial inequality are commonly accepted as structural factors associated with an increased risk for experiencing homelessness (Chard, Faulkner, and Chugg, 2009; Cronley, 2010; Johnson, Scutella, Tseng, and Wood, 2015; Nooe and Patterson, 2010).

Poverty, a primary factor contributing to homelessness, is a condition in which a person's basic needs for food, shelter, and clothing are not met due to a lack of income. The U.S. Census Bureau (2018a) uses "a set of money income thresholds that vary by family size and composition to determine who is in poverty. If a family's total income is less than the family's threshold, then that family and every individual in it is considered in poverty" (para. 1). Although unemployment often results in poverty, not all who fall below the poverty threshold are without a job. Rather, there are jobs that provide insufficient wages with little or no benefits (Nooe and Patterson, 2010). The effects of poverty are further compounded by cuts to social welfare programs, an extremely low federal minimum wage, and the presence of high unemployment rates (Ji, 2006).

The World Federation of Occupational Therapists' (2006) position statement on human rights views poverty as a barrier to participation in occupations, making its eradication particularly relevant to ensuring occupational justice for those who experience homelessness. It is well established that areas with higher poverty rates have a higher rate of homelessness (Carter, 2011; Ji, 2006). According to the U.S. Census Bureau (2018b), 12.3% of people in the United States (approximately 40,000,000 people) live in poverty. The federal government establishes poverty thresholds by analyzing several key indicators, including how many people reside in a given household, the number of children under their care, and the annual income of the household. Although the correlation between poverty and homelessness is well established, not everyone who experiences poverty will eventually experience homelessness. However, poverty greatly increases the risk that someone will experience homelessness for the first time (Thompson, Wall, Greenstein, Grant, and Hasin, 2013).

An important structural factor that increases the rate of homelessness is cuts to social welfare programs. According to Petrenchik (2006), as state governments in the United States seek to conserve limited resources, funding for welfare programs is often the first to be reduced, resulting in less spending on programs intended to benefit the poor. In particular, funding for Medicaid, low-income housing, food stamps, and child welfare programs is often targeted by these efforts, further weakening the protections they provide. Petrenchik (2006) notes that education spending is also a frequent target, with cuts to elementary, secondary, and higher education directly affecting homeless children, who are already at a disadvantage. Some of the school-related programs that are targeted by budget reductions and affect low-income and homeless children include meals, transportation, and other special services. According to Blank (2010), the reduction of entitlement programs—for example, Medicaid and the Supplemental Nutrition Assistance Program (food stamps)—is particularly detrimental to families in the United States, where eligibility for social support may be contingent on employment. This makes it increasingly difficult for low-income families struggling to find employment to benefit from these support systems. Without these benefits, families that are already facing uncertainty are made even more vulnerable, with even a slight decrease in aid increasing the odds that they will experience homelessness.

After the first instance of homelessness, it becomes more difficult for families to recover, making recurrent bouts of homelessness more likely (Petrenchik, 2006). This is less often observed in the United Kingdom and other European countries, where spending on welfare programs for families is significantly higher than in the United States (Shinn, 2010). However, higher spending on Social Security and Medicare in the United States has served to reduce poverty rates among older adults who qualify for these services. Higher spending on welfare programs for the elderly coupled with spending cuts to programs benefiting low-income families is one explanation for why families represent the fastest-growing subset of the homeless population (Blank, 2010).

In addition to fewer social benefits, poverty is inextricably linked to lower wages, with the ability to afford housing determined directly by income (Shinn, 2007). The federal minimum wage is currently $7.25 per hour. In the event that a state, city, or county minimum wage rate is higher than the federal rate, the employer must pay the higher rate (U.S. Department of Labor [USDOL], n.d.). Beginning January 1, 2018, Executive Order 13658 increased the minimum wage to $10.35 per hour for those performing work covered by federal contracts. In addition, tipped employees performing work covered by federal contracts must be paid $7.25 per hour (USDOL, 2018).

A sharp decline in affordable housing in the United States also means fewer individuals working for minimum wage can afford rent (Burt, 2001). The impact this has on securing affordable housing is made increasingly clear when comparing the federal minimum wage to the **fair market rent** (FMR; Petrenchick, 2006). The FMR is determined by the USDHUD and is the amount needed to rent privately owned, modest housing that is safe and sanitary. FMR varies by geographic location and type of housing and is adjusted annually (RentData.org, 2018). According to the National Low-Income Housing Coalition (NLIHC, 2018), the housing wage needed for a modest two-bedroom apartment is $22.10, $14.85 higher than the federal minimum wage. As of 2018, there was no state in which a full-time employee making $7.25 per hour could afford a modest two-bedroom apartment at the current FMR (NLIHC, 2018).

Belonging to a racial minority is a structural factor for homelessness due to the fact that minorities are more likely to experience poverty (Nooe and Patterson, 2010). In 2017, the poverty rate for blacks was 21.2%, for Hispanics,18.3%, and for Asians, 10%. During the same period, the poverty rate among non-Hispanic whites was 8.7% (U.S. Census Bureau, 2018b). The poverty rate for males in 2017 was 11%, while the poverty rate for females was 13.6%. While homelessness is primarily associated with poverty, housing policies that discriminate on the basis of race, ethnicity, and socioeconomic status have also contributed to the homeless rate (da Costa Nunez, 2012).

Personal Characteristics and Vulnerabilities

Homeless people experience health disparities. Mental illness, substance abuse, physical disabilities (Shinn, 2007), and chronic conditions (Burt, 2001) are all more common among the homeless population. Low education levels also increase the risk of experiencing homelessness (Nooe and Patterson, 2010).

The number of individuals with a mental illness who are homeless is significantly high compared to the population at large (Lee et al., 2010). In the United States, approximately one-third of homeless individuals have a severe chronic mental illness (Gutman and Raphael-Greenfield, 2017). Similar numbers have been reported in other industrialized nations (Teesson, Hodder, and Buhrich, 2004). Determining the prevalence of mental disorders among the homeless population has been the subject of several studies intended to inform policy solutions. A systematic review conducted by Fazel, Khosla, Doll, and Geddes (2008) revealed that 12.7% of homeless individuals had a psychotic illness, 11.4% reported major depression, 23.1% had a personality disorder, 24.4% suffered from drug dependence, and 37.9% suffered from alcohol dependence. In another study, persons with schizophrenia and bipolar disorder were 2.4 and 1.6 times more likely to have reported experiencing homelessness, respectively, than those with depression (Folsom et al., 2005), indicating that some mental illnesses, more than others, may increase a person's susceptibility to experiencing homelessness.

Substance use disorders have been found to predict risk for first-time homelessness (Thompson et al., 2013). Substance abuse can also result from having experienced homelessness. Among the homeless population of Melbourne, Australia, Johnson and Chamberlain (2008) found that 34% of people reported having developed an alcohol use or other drug use disorder before becoming homeless, whereas 66% of those surveyed had developed a substance use disorder during or after a period of homelessness. The authors attributed this difference to substance use as a form of coping, as well as a homeless subculture that promotes drug use. They also noted that people who first became homeless as teenagers were more than three times as likely to develop a substance use disorder compared with those who first became homeless as adults (Johnson and Chamberlain, 2008).

In addition to the negative health effects associated with substance use disorders, other physical problems are also known to increase one's risk of experiencing homelessness. In a systematic review and meta-analysis of 43 studies on the prevalence of infectious diseases and homelessness, Beijer, Wolf, and Fazel (2012) observed that tuberculosis, hepatitis C, and HIV were among the most common. The homeless are also more likely to experience respiratory infections such as tuberculosis, pneumonia, and influenza, and rates of chronic obstructive pulmonary disease (COPD) are higher in this population (Landon, 2017). Although the prevalence of high cholesterol, diabetes, and hypertension among the homeless is similar to that of the general population, homeless individuals are less likely to properly manage these conditions. Cardiovascular disease is also more prevalent among this population, and insufficient treatment is associated with higher mortality rates among the homeless than the general population (Lee et al., 2005).

Low levels of educational attainment increase a person's chances of experiencing homelessness (Nooe and Patterson, 2010). In a study of 65 participants of an occupational therapy employment program for persons who were homeless, Muñoz, Garcia, Lisak, and Reichenbach (2006) reported that 34% of participants had never finished high school. Of those who had completed high school, only 5% had completed some college. Educational attainment can also serve as a protective factor. However, after analyzing data from 10,340 patients with serious mental illness, Folsom et al. (2005) found that the average number of years of education achieved among homeless persons and those who were not homeless was nearly the same (12.1 and 12.3 years, respectively). Overall, these findings highlight the role education plays in protecting against homelessness while also challenging the misconception that individuals experiencing homelessness are not educated.

Cultural Influences

Structural factors affecting the homeless population are the result of social policies, which are themselves a product of sociocultural beliefs and attitudes. Perspectives on the causes of homelessness are important because they ultimately determine how societies address the problem (Petrenchick, 2006). According to Cronley (2010), the extent to which structural and personal factors cause homelessness has been heavily debated among policy-makers, the media, social scientists, and the general public. As a result of this ongoing debate, Cronley notes that two competing interpretations have emerged. The structural interpretation places a greater emphasis on external factors, such as a lack of affordable housing, as the primary cause of homelessness. According to this interpretation, inaction on the part of national, state, and local governments and policymakers places individuals at a greater risk for homelessness.

In contrast, the personal interpretation places greater emphasis on factors unique to each individual, viewing homelessness as a result of deviant behavior and poor lifestyle choices (Cronley, 2010). Both interpretations are shaped by political trends. During periods of social reform, societies are more likely to attribute homelessness to structural factors while advocating for the creation and expansion of social welfare programs to address the issue. The USDHUD, with its mission to reduce the rate of homelessness by increasing the availability of affordable housing, is an example of one such program. During politically conservative periods, societies are more likely to emphasize intrapersonal factors while advocating for privatization and cuts to social welfare programs in an effort to reduce government spending (Shinn, 2007).

These competing structural and personal interpretations of homelessness have been observed in other countries as well. In an effort to understand how cultural perspectives of homelessness differed among various industrialized nations, Toro et al. (2007) analyzed interview responses of adults from Belgium, Germany, Italy, the United Kingdom, and the United States. In doing so, they found that public opinion among U.S. and UK respondents differed significantly on certain issues when compared with the other countries represented. In particular, U.S. and UK respondents were more likely to view homelessness as a result of personal failings. They were also more likely to view the average homeless person as having a criminal record and issues with substance abuse. On the other hand, respondents from Germany, with its well-established and well-funded system of social welfare programs, were more likely to view homelessness as a result of structural factors. German respondents also displayed the highest levels of compassion among those surveyed from all five countries. The authors attributed these differences to whether the culture of each country valued individualism and personal freedoms versus social welfare and the well-being of the group (Toro et al., 2007).

The emergent consensus among researchers is that homelessness is the result of a complex interplay of structural factors, personal characteristics, and cultural influences. According to Petrenchik (2006),

> *the primary goal of occupational therapy programs and services for persons who are homeless, whether at the systems level or the individual, is assisting fellow citizens to return to and participate in the economy, their community, and in society as a whole. (p. 27)*

Populations at Risk of Experiencing Homelessness

The homeless population consists of culturally and ethnically diverse groups of men, women, and children. Each group has distinct needs and confronts unique challenges. Because the homeless population is not homogeneous, a "one size fits all" solution is likely to be unsuccessful at best and harmful at worst. Several subpopulations among the homeless are at higher risk for negative outcomes. Five groups will be discussed here: homeless families and youth, sexual minority youth, persons with mental illness, older adults, and Veterans.

Homeless Families and Youth

On average, a homeless family consists of three people, most frequently a single mother with two children, often under the age of 6. The mothers often have low levels of education, are unemployed, and are without adequate transportation. Many of these women are survivors of intimate partner violence (IPV) who fled a dangerous home situation. Women who have been subjected to IPV are four times more likely to experience housing instability than those who have not. Not surprisingly, they have disproportionately high rates of anxiety, depression, and posttraumatic stress disorder, and many self-medicate their distress with alcohol and other drugs (Bassuk, DeCandia, Beach, and Berman, 2014). Homeless women and adolescents may also be victims of the sex trade, exchanging sex for money to obtain food, shelter, and other basic needs (Nooe and Patterson, 2010).

In a study of homeless youths 25 years old or younger, Walls and Bell (2011) found that race, a history of personal or family drug use, and previous suicide attempts were associated with survival sex behavior. In particular, the researchers found that African American youth were significantly more likely to have engaged in survival sex than their white peers. Participants with a history of using methamphetamines and/or inhalants were also more likely to have engaged in survival sex (Walls and Bell, 2011). Refer to Chapter 22 for more information on the impact of human trafficking on occupational engagement.

Children in homeless families are often hungry, sick, and worried about where and when they will eat and sleep again. Many of these children are frequently absent from school and need to repeat grades, if they do not drop out of school entirely. In addition, children experiencing homelessness experience high levels of stress and recurrent exposure to violence, which have significant mental health consequences. **Adverse childhood experiences** (ACEs) are correlated with social, emotional, and cognitive impairments in children and adolescent risk-taking behaviors. ACEs are defined as "stressful or traumatic events, including abuse and neglect" (Substance Abuse and Mental Health Services Administration [SAMHSA], 2018a, para. 2). Many runaway and homeless youth (60% to 80%) are victims of emotional, physical, and/or sexual abuse in the home environment. Additionally, the loss of safety, privacy, possessions, friends, pets, and routines creates a life-altering experience, inflicting deep and enduring emotional scars on these individuals and families (Bassuk et al., 2014).

Adolescents who are homeless often lack the basic life skills necessary for school and work. While homeless, they have difficulty building and maintaining routines and habits that are healthy, adaptive, and functional. The lack of normative developmental experiences and the loss of traditional roles, such as student, family, and friend, often preclude homeless youth from maturing into healthy adults (Aviles and Helfrich, 2006).

Unaccompanied homeless youth are at high risk for injuries, sexually transmitted infections, pregnancy, malnutrition, suicide, and homicide. However, they are highly unlikely to seek out medical care due to mistrust of adults. Because they are minors, treatment may require parental consent, which further interferes with their ability to obtain health care. Rather than seeking mental health services, homeless youth often self-medicate with alcohol and street drugs (Aviles and Helfrich, 2006).

Sexual Minority Youth

According to the USDHUD (2016), youth who are lesbian, gay, bisexual, or transgender, or who are questioning their sexual orientation or gender (LGBTQ), are disproportionately represented in the homeless population. Composing 7% of the general youth population, they represent nearly 40% of the youth experiencing homelessness. Rosario, Schrimshaw, and Hunter (2012) suggest there are two pathways to homelessness among LGBTQ youth, the first being sexual abuse and the second being an earlier age of sexual development. LGBTQ youth often leave home after being rejected by family members (Cochran, Stewart, Ginzler, and Cauce, 2002; Kipke, Weiss, and Wong, 2007), and they are more likely to have been sexually abused prior to becoming homeless (Nolan, 2006; Rosario et al., 2012).

As with their heterosexual counterparts, there are several known risk factors associated with being LGBTQ and homeless. LGBTQ youth are at an increased risk for suicide (Nolan, 2006; Van Leeuwen, Boyle, Salomonsen-Sautel, and Baker, 2006), having multiple sex partners (Cochran et al., 2002; Kipke et al., 2007), engaging in unsafe sex, being victimized, and experiencing health and psychological problems (Cochran et al., 2002; Noell and Ochs, 2001). LGBT youth are also more likely to engage in survival sex in exchange for money, food, or shelter (Nolan, 2006; Van Leeuwen et al., 2006). As a result of having multiple sex partners, LGBTQ youth are also at an increased risk of contracting HIV/AIDS and other sexually transmitted infections (Kipke et al., 2007; Nolan, 2006). They are also more likely to use drugs (Kipke et al., 2007; Rosario et al., 2012) and to have left homes where drugs are frequently used (Van Leeuwen et al., 2006). LGBTQ youth experiencing homelessness must deal with issues arising from their sexual orientation and/or gender identity while simultaneously coping with the hardships of life on the street. As a result of leaving home and dropping out of school, these individuals also lack a stable support system and adult role models (Cochran et al., 2002; Nolan, 2006).

Persons With Mental Illness

The diagnosis of a mental illness often increases a person's chances of experiencing homelessness for several reasons. Self-care and home-management skills are often learned during the transition from adolescence to adulthood. This is also the period of human development during which the onset of a mental illness normally occurs. As a result, these individuals often display performance deficits in the instrumental activities of daily living (IADLs), including financial management, home establishment and maintenance, and health management and maintenance (Gutman and Raphael-Greenfield, 2017).

In addition to skill deficits, behaviors common to acute psychosis, such as a disregard for hygiene, paranoid delusions, hallucinations, and agitation can make it difficult to interact with neighbors and tenants. Individuals with schizophrenia may also find it difficult to engage in home-management tasks, such as paying rent and resolving disputes (Lee et al., 2010). However, when asked why they are experiencing homelessness, these individuals are more likely to cite financial and interpersonal problems, a lack of adequate housing, and unemployment as reasons for their housing status, rather than having a mental illness (Mojtabai, 2005).

Older Adults

As the median age of the U.S. population is shifting upward, the number of older adults living in poverty and experiencing homelessness is also increasing. The demand for housing for low-income older adults exceeds the supply. The mortality rate of older adults who are homeless is three to four times higher than for those living in safe housing (Nooe and Patterson, 2010). A cross-sectional study by Brown, Kiely, Bharel, and Mitchell (2012) found that common geriatric conditions were more prevalent among older homeless adults than others in the general population who were in their same age group. Of 247 homeless adults between the ages of 50 and 69, 30% reported experiencing difficulty performing one or more activities of daily living (ADLs). Participants were more likely to have experienced urinary incontinence (49.8%), major depression (39.8%), and vision loss (30.0%) compared to their population-based cohorts. Other common conditions among homeless adults were hearing loss (29.7%) and cognitive impairment (24.3%). Of the older adults studied, 53% had experienced a fall in the prior year (Brown et al., 2012).

The high prevalence of alcohol and drug use among this population is one explanation for the early occurrence of these functional deficits (Fazel, Geddes, and Kushel, 2014). In addition to other chronic conditions observed among the homeless population, it is important for occupational therapy practitioners to consider the unique ways in which this population experiences age-related cognitive and functional declines.

Veterans

Veterans account for nearly 10% of the homeless population. Of the Veterans who are homeless, 90% are men, 60% are white, 33% are African American, and the remainder are multiracial. The number of homeless Veterans increased by 18% between 2016 and 2017 (USDHUD, 2017). About half of Veterans who are homeless served during the Vietnam era; two-thirds of homeless Veterans served for at least 3 years, and one-third were stationed in a war zone. Approximately half of first episodes of homelessness occur within 3 years post-discharge from active duty (National Coalition for Homeless Veterans ([NCHV], n.d.).

All of the structural factors previously described—poverty, lack of affordable housing, and an unlivable federal minimum wage—have an impact on Veterans. In addition, Veterans contend with the lingering effects of posttraumatic stress disorder (PTSD) and substance use disorders and often have limited family and social support networks; 50% of Veterans who are homeless have serious mental illness, 70% have substance abuse problems, and 51% have service-connected disabilities (predominantly traumatic brain injury). A history of military sexual trauma is a predisposing factor for homelessness, particularly among female Veterans. Furthermore, military training and job classifications do not always transfer to the civilian workforce, making finding and securing positions that pay a living wage difficult (NCHV, n.d.). More information regarding community-based services for Veterans can be found in Chapter 21.

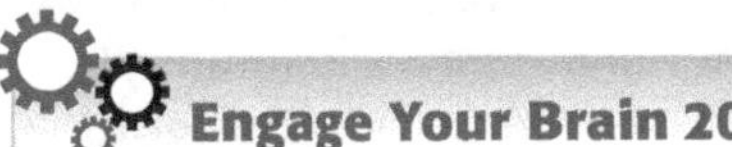
Engage Your Brain 20-1

What are the cultural competencies needed when working with homeless populations?

Effective Responses to Homelessness

Safe and affordable housing is a necessary, but insufficient, first step to ending individual and family homelessness. In order to ensure ongoing residential stability, individuals and families must also be provided with supports, resources, and trauma-informed services tailored to their specific needs.

Housing First

The **Housing First** model is an evidence-based approach that "offers people experiencing homelessness permanent housing as quickly as possible. It also provides people with the supportive services and connections to community-based resources they need to keep their housing and avoid returning to homelessness" (USICH, 2018a, para. 2). Other goals of Housing First are to remove barriers to housing entry and promote consumer choice, recovery from mental and substance use disorders, and community integration. Typically, Housing First programs do not require employment, sobriety, or treatment compliance as prerequisites for housing eligibility (Nooe and Patterson, 2010).

Providing educational and employment opportunities enhances the likelihood that individuals and families will be able to maintain housing stability. Job skills training, job placement assistance, childcare, and transportation are required for parents, particularly mothers, to obtain and maintain employment. Stable housing and related supports are prerequisites for social and community participation (Petrenchik, 2006).

Trauma-Informed Care

Prior to becoming homeless, many individuals have childhood histories of trauma, particularly physical and sexual abuse. Other traumas happen after becoming homeless—for example, physical assault, robbery, and rape. Due to the high prevalence of exposure to trauma and high rates of trauma symptoms, services provided to persons who are homeless should be based on the principles of **trauma-informed care.** A trauma-informed approach acknowledges the widespread prevalence and impact of trauma in society, recognizes the signs and symptoms of trauma in all individuals involved with the program, including its own workforce, integrates knowledge of trauma into policies and practices, and actively prevents retraumatization (SAMHSA, 2018b).

Trauma-informed care is a strengths-based and client-centered service delivery approach that is responsive to the impact of trauma, emphasizes the psychological and emotional safety of participants, and creates opportunities for trauma survivors to gain a sense of control and empowerment. Evidence-based practices for trauma-specific therapy can be present-focused, past-focused, or a combination. Present-focused therapies facilitate the development of coping skills and the management of symptoms to improve the client's ability to function. Past-focused therapies emphasize how understanding the trauma influences present-day thoughts, feelings, and behaviors. Depending on the client's needs and the nature of the trauma, one approach may be more appropriate than the other (SAMHSA, 2014).

Community Practice Settings and Occupational Therapy Roles

Occupational therapy practitioners must tailor their roles and interventions to address the needs of a specific community of persons who are homeless and the client(s) to be served. When working with a homeless population, clients may be "identified as individual direct service recipients, intervention groups, and service provider agencies and public/private organizations" (Herzberg and Petrenchik, 2010, p. 438).

Grandisson, Mitchell-Carvalho, Tang, and Korner-Bitensky (2009) conducted a study of occupational therapists to determine their perceptions of the role of occupational therapy with people who are homeless. The qualitative focus group and questionnaire responses fell into two broad categories—traditional roles and emerging roles. Traditional roles included direct services—for example, evaluation of and intervention for occupational performance deficits through group and individual sessions. Emerging roles included indirect services such as advocacy, education, outreach, and case management (Van Oss, Condoluci, and Annino, 2018).

Direct services are provided to homeless individuals and families in a variety of settings, including emergency shelters, transitional housing, health-care clinics, food pantries, meal distribution centers, mental health and alcohol/drug programs, and community drop-in centers. However, the homeless shelter is the most common location for occupational therapy service provision (Petrenchik, 2006). Shelter services are variable but may range from basic beds and meals to more comprehensive programs that include case management, housing assistance, substance abuse treatment, and job placement (Nooe and Patterson, 2010).

The organization's culture, mission, staffing patterns, and resources influence the types of direct occupational therapy services provided. Occupational therapy services are designed to capitalize on client strengths, minimize performance limitations, and promote community integration. Direct services for individual clients may include individual and group intervention, life skills training, and prevocational and vocational evaluation and training (Herzberg and Petrenchik, 2010).

Direct services can also be provided to organizations and agencies that provide assistance to the homeless population. These systems-level interventions may take the form of consultation, staff training, and program development services. Consultation may be provided to address system-level problems, such as:

- Meeting the needs of persons with disabilities or chronic diseases who are homeless
- Identifying needs assessment strategies, analyzing data, and interpreting results
- Designing, establishing, and evaluating a volunteer program

Staff and volunteer education and training might include responding therapeutically to a variety of mental health issues, engaging clients in goal-directed activities, and identifying needs and developing strategies to address these needs. Program development assistance would be appropriate for a shelter wanting to expand the types of services provided.

Meaningful Occupations of the Homeless

An occupational perspective of homelessness is important because it enhances the development of more comprehensive policy solutions while also enhancing efforts to understand the issue of homelessness (Marshall, Lysaght, and Krupa, 2017). In developing and providing client-centered interventions for those experiencing homelessness, it is helpful to understand how this population perceives barriers to occupational engagement and the occupations to which they ascribe meaning. It is also necessary to consider the opportunities that arise from increased engagement in meaningful occupations, as well as the consequences of being deprived of the right to do so.

Occupation within the context of homelessness is defined by M. Whiteford (2010) as "any form of social or cultural activity that purposefully aims to empower people experiencing homelessness to build self-esteem, develop skills and reconnect with mainstream social networks" (p. 195). The meaningful occupations of the homeless have been researched very little (Zufferey and Kerr, 2004), and current policies aimed at reducing the rate of homelessness focus very little on meaningful occupations other than those required for basic survival (Thomas, Gray, and McGinty, 2017). However, persons who are homeless often perceive engagement in meaningful occupations as being more important than the need to secure housing (Marshall et al., 2017).

Due to a lack of housing and the resources needed to satisfy basic needs, occupations that ensure survival are particularly meaningful to the homeless population (Marshall et al., 2017; Thomas et al., 2017). Occupations of survival are intended to satisfy immediate needs, and they rely on routines that are both consistent and reliable. They include securing food, finding a place to stay, completing personal hygiene and grooming tasks, staying out of trouble with law enforcement (Thomas et al., 2017), and seeking safety. Participation in these occupations often represents an undue burden for persons who are homeless, with the time and energy spent securing shelter, food, clothing, and relief from extreme temperatures leaving very little energy for securing housing. Participants of a recent study assessing meaningful occupations of the homeless noted that a great deal of time was spent waiting to receive services at various shelters, meal programs, and other resource centers. They also noted that interacting with other homeless individuals, especially those with a mental illness or criminal backgrounds, made securing safety a particularly important occupation. This was due, in part, to the conflict that often results from limited access to basic resources (Marshall et al., 2017).

Chard et al. (2009) note that occupational participation is particularly meaningful to persons who are homeless because it reduces feelings of boredom. These occupations include contributing to shelter life in various ways, socializing with others, and searching for work. Similarly, Marshall et al. (2017) note that productive occupations such as collecting bottles and aluminum cans, participating in research studies, donating plasma, checking parking meters for loose change, and participating as a volunteer represent ways not only to avoid feelings of boredom but also to fulfill the desire to be productive.

Marshall et al. (2017) note "non-traditional forms of employment such as bottle collecting are a part of the occupational repertoire of homeless persons, and represent a legitimate form of contributing work, albeit outside of the mainstream social economic system" (p. 178). Chard et al. (2009) observed that volunteer participation fulfilled the desire to be productive among their research participants. Although most participants were not gainfully employed, they often engaged in volunteer participation as a means of satisfying their desire to work. One participant stated: "Work means, to me, it's just like going to church. You feel good when you come out. Yeah. It gives you that feeling, good feeling. I've done something today" (p. 121). Studies of substance abuse among the homeless suggest that feelings of boredom, which often lead to alcohol and drug use, can be decreased by providing opportunities to engage in meaningful occupations (Marshall and Rosenberg, 2014).

Social participation is also a meaningful occupation for the homeless. Thomas et al. (2017) note that occupations of social connectedness provide a way for homeless individuals to overcome being marginalized and excluded by society. They also provide a sense of family and belonging. In particular, the occupation of maintaining social relationships with others who are homeless contributes to a sense of well-being. This is particularly true regarding participation in family routines among single mothers and their children (Thomas et al., 2017). Similarly, time spent sharing resources, caring for others who are homeless (Chard et al., 2009; Marshall et al., 2017), and caring for pets are also meaningful occupations. Meeting others' needs is viewed by persons who are homeless as a way to ensure that one's own needs will be met in the future.

Substance use occurs frequently among the homeless and often results from the close contact residents have with one another in a shelter setting (Chard et al., 2009). Drinking is often used as a preparatory method for engaging in sleep (Thomas et al., 2017) and is often considered by the homeless as necessary for survival (Marshall et al., 2017). Despite the negative health consequences of substance abuse, Kiepek and Magalhaes (2011) note that alcohol and drug use may qualify as a meaningful occupation among those experiencing homelessness. Substance use as an occupation is not a new concept. Moyers (1992, 1997) described the many tasks and activities that make up the occupation of substance use, including raising money to purchase alcohol or other drugs, protecting the supply from others, seeking persons with whom to use, and recovering from the effects of using substances.

The occupation of persevering through difficult circumstances is also meaningful among those experiencing homelessness. A single mother who participated in a recent study by Thomas et al. (2017) noted that her role as a mother and her desire to provide stable routines for her children empowered her to persevere. Other participants of the study noted that remaining positive about their circumstances, as opposed to succumbing to feelings of fear and hopelessness, helped them persevere. Similarly, the occupations of spending time alone, connecting with one's surroundings, and reading were cited as resulting in a sense of peace and contentment among participants. Occupations that help develop a positive self-identity are also meaningful to those experiencing homelessness. These occupations, which conform to social and cultural values, often challenge stereotypes of the homeless and include staying clean, visiting the library, reading, remaining physically fit, and painting (Thomas et al., 2017). The occupation of listening to music is also used as a way to cope with feelings of anger and stress (Marshall et al., 2017).

Perceived Barriers to Occupational Engagement

According to Marshall et al. (2017), feelings of being marginalized and alienated often result from an inability to engage in meaningful occupations, particularly occupations of productivity and self-care. The authors note that a lack of access to showers represents a barrier to performing bathing, showering, personal hygiene, and grooming activities, often resulting in feelings of shame and the use of drugs as a form of coping.

Muñoz et al. (2006) performed a descriptive study of retrospective data collected by occupational therapists using the Canadian Occupational Performance Measure (COPM). The data were collected as part of an occupational therapy intervention program serving the homeless population of Pittsburgh, Pennsylvania. The authors reported that just over half of all occupational performance problems identified by participants were in the domain of self-care. The domains of productivity (26.3%) and leisure (23.4%) accounted for the remaining self-perceived problems among participants. When participants were asked to select problem areas most important to them, a similar pattern emerged, with 57% choosing problems in the domain of self-care, 32% choosing problems in the area of productivity, and 11% choosing problems related to leisure. The authors noted that the most commonly cited self-care goals were related to achieving sobriety, securing housing, and improving one's physical and mental health. The most commonly cited productivity goals were related to securing a job, obtaining a GED (or similar educational goal), and becoming a volunteer. Goals related to leisure mostly centered on improving interpersonal relationships.

Environments unique to the experience of homelessness also have an impact on the repertoire of occupations available to this population. The shelter environment is governed by strict rules regarding mealtimes, curfews, and check-in times, resulting in very little freedom to engage in meaningful occupations. These rules also limit the residents' ability to make choices for themselves, often resulting in occupational deprivation (Chard et al., 2009; Marshall et al., 2017). G. Whiteford (2000) defines occupational deprivation as

> *a state in which a person or group of people are unable to do what is necessary and meaningful in their lives due to external restrictions. It is a state in which the opportunity to perform those occupations that have social, cultural and personal relevance is rendered difficult if not impossible. (p. 200)*

Marshall et al. (2017) note that occupational deprivation often results in feelings of boredom, with drug use serving as a source of stimulation that might otherwise be found through engagement in occupations. A lack of privacy in shelters affects participation in occupations, resulting in some homeless individuals choosing to engage in sleep in unsheltered locations. A lack of privacy also affects routines associated with maintaining self-care needs.

Those experiencing homelessness often desire to participate in the occupations of mainstream society. The inability to do so has been noted as a source of depression and feelings of increased isolation, with prolonged periods of homelessness being associated with a loss of occupational skills. Public misperceptions of the homeless also lead to feelings of increased isolation and difficulty securing employment (Marshall et al., 2017). As a result of these misperceptions, local governments often enact policies that contribute to the marginalization of the homeless, such as programming sprinkler systems to activate at night and locking public bathrooms at night. These and similar policies decrease the number of public spaces available to the homeless (Thomas et al., 2017).

According to Chard et al. (2009), participation in meaningful occupations is also limited by the stresses associated with being homeless. These stresses are often the result of missed opportunities and a loss of personal freedoms and relationships. Regarding a loss that had shaped his life, one homeless man recalled:

> *So my Mom drowned in her bathtub when I was 18 . . . I was trying to get [her] off [drugs and alcohol] and having a bath causes seizures and she had a seizure in her tub and drowned the day before her 40th birthday. (p. 122)*

This narrative underscores the importance of considering the lived experiences of the homeless and how loss has contributed to their individual circumstances.

Theoretical and Conceptual Models

A variety of theories and models can be used by occupational therapy practitioners when working with people who are homeless. A few of these will be described briefly, including the ecological model of homelessness, the empowerment model, and four occupation-based models.

Ecological Model of Homelessness

Nooe and Patterson (2010) propose an **ecological model of homelessness** (EMH) for interpreting how various personal and structural factors result in homelessness. Their proposed model consists of four components, with individual and structural factors grouped into a single component: biopsychosocial risk factors (see Fig. 20-1). Regarding this component, the authors state:

> *Biopsychosocial risk factors encompass a range of factors including individual biology and development and circumstances such as poverty and its many facets to housing availability and stability. . . . It recognizes the interaction of multiple factors on different levels, including individual factors (e.g., personality, developmental experiences, health-mental health, race, and ethnicity) and social factors, such as resource availability, policies, culture, discrimination, and social situations. (p. 106)*

The other three components of the model include the individual and social outcomes of homelessness, the temporal nature of homelessness (i.e., first time, episodic, and chronic), and the various levels of housing status experienced (e.g., shared dwelling, emergency shelter, permanent housing). These four components account for the complex interactions and relationships of numerous factors related to homelessness and provide a more accurate and holistic interpretation of the phenomenon. The EMH attempts to represent the "complexity of homelessness; its multiple, interacting causes; diverse manifestations; variable duration; and costly financial and social consequences" (Nooe and Patterson, 2010, p. 138). Petrenchik (2006) advocates that occupational therapy practitioners use an ecological approach in working with persons who are homeless because this approach emphasizes person-environment-occupation fit.

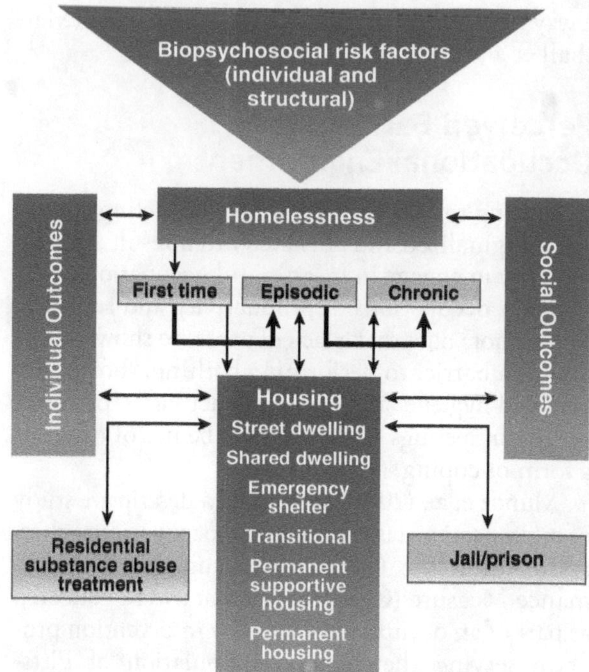

Figure 20-1 Ecological model of homelessness. *(Adapted from "The Ecology of Homelessness," by R. M. Nooe and D. A. Patterson, 2010,* Journal of Human Behavior in the Social Environment, *20[2], 105–152. Used with permission.)*

Empowerment Model

The model most often used for programs directed to the homeless population is the empowerment model. In public health, **empowerment** refers to "a social action process by which individuals, communities, and organizations gain mastery over their lives in the context of changing their social and political environment to improve equity and quality of life" (Minkler, 1997, p. 7). The characteristics of an ecological-empowerment approach include but are not limited to:

- Full participation
- Collaborative nonhierarchical roles

- Development of mutual and reciprocal alliances
- Focus on capacity building
- Ecological competence—having the skills needed for effective action in one's environment
- Development of personal and collective resources for action
- Linkages with larger systems to increase social equity and access (Herzberg and Petrenchik, 2010)

The National Coalition for the Homeless (2007) offers opportunities for people who have experienced homelessness to become part of the solution to end homelessness. These opportunities, called empowerment projects, are designed to change systems to make them more responsive to the needs of the homeless. Examples of empowerment projects include community organizing, homeless voter registration, homeless civil rights, policy advocacy and lobbying, and public education.

Model of Occupational Empowerment

The **model of occupational empowerment** (MOE) is the newest occupation-based model to be used with the homeless population. Based on the basic principles of an empowerment approach, Fisher and Hotchkiss (2008) developed a grounded-theory model of occupational empowerment for marginalized populations living in communities. The components of the MOE (see Fig. 20-2) include disempowering environments, occupational deprivation, learned helplessness, occupational empowerment, and occupational change. The authors suggest that persons living in disempowering environments

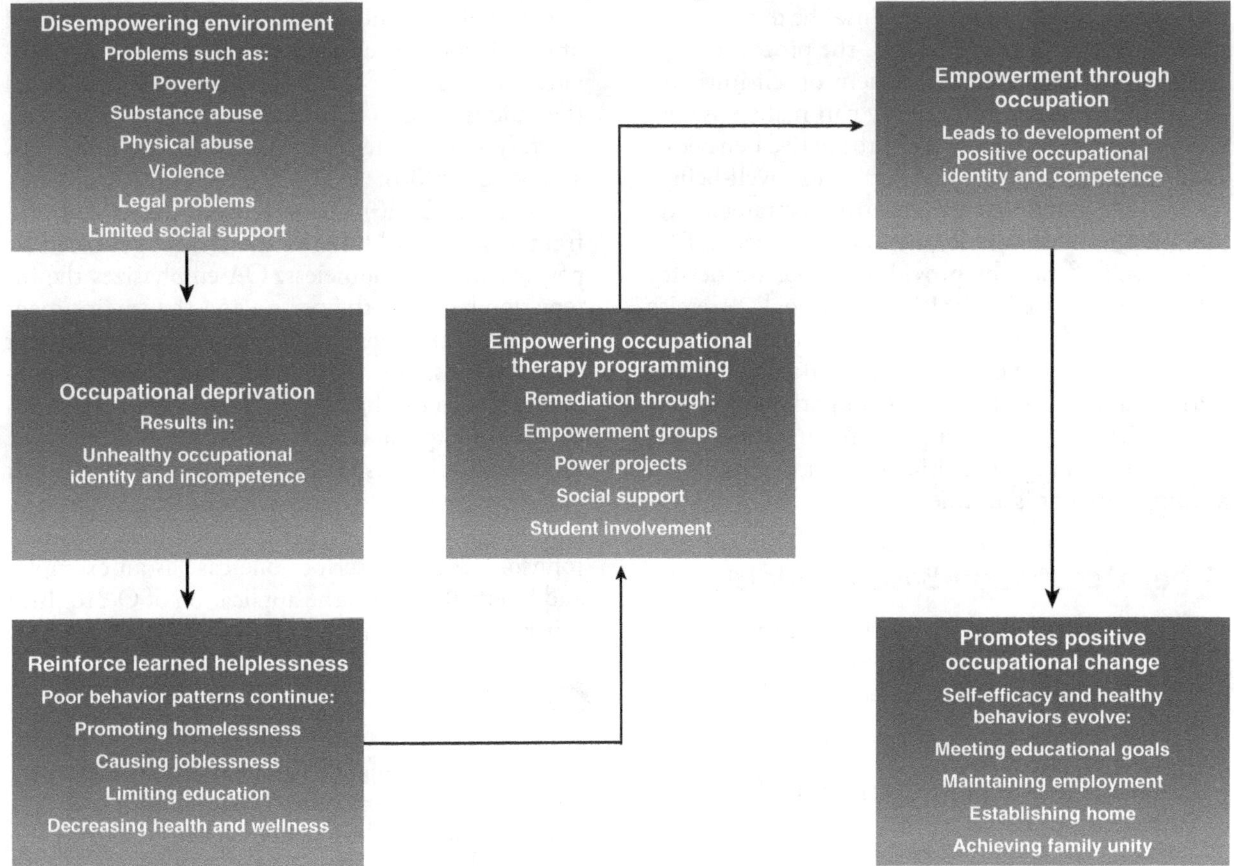

Figure 20-2 Model of occupational empowerment.

experience occupational deprivation and develop learned helplessness. Occupational empowerment strategies can be utilized to create healthy occupational change.

Disempowering environments are characterized by negative environmental influences that contribute to social marginalization—for example, poverty, unsafe living situations, crime, violence, and a lack of access to education and employment. These conditions place harmful limitations on a person's access and ability to engage in meaningful and purposeful occupations and create occupational deprivation. As a result of maladaptive occupational routines and poor occupational performance, individuals may develop learned helplessness (Fisher and Hotchkiss, 2008). Learned helplessness occurs when humans are conditioned to think, feel, and act as if they have no control over environmental circumstances or what happens to them. Long-term, chronic feelings of helplessness are highly correlated with symptoms of depression (Ackerman, 2018).

Fisher and Hotchkiss (2008) use the term *occupational empowerment* to describe "the process of supporting others in the development of self-initiative and independence, so that they can make wise decisions, manifest healthy and productive behaviors, and increase self-fulfillment and well-being" (p. 65). Occupational empowerment strategies are designed to overcome learned helplessness and facilitate self-efficacy by providing opportunities for individuals to make decisions, set goals, exercise control while engaging in self-chosen healthy occupations, and experience successful occupational performance and enjoyable occupational participation. Through this empowerment process, occupational change is initiated, and occupational accomplishment is attained.

Other Occupation-Based Models

Other occupation-based theories and models frequently used by occupational therapy practitioners working with homeless persons include the following:

- Canadian model of occupational performance (CMOP)
- Model of human occupation (MOHO)
- Occupational adaptation (OA) model

The client-centered CMOP is particularly useful with the homeless population. The application of this model promotes empowerment by ensuring that clients identify problems and their importance, as well as goals and the means to achieve them. In addition, the CMOP emphasizes the dynamic interaction of person-occupation-environment and places spirituality at the core of the physical, cognitive, and affective components of occupational performance (Herzberg and Petrenchik, 2010). Others who have advocated the use of the CMOP with homeless populations include Chan, Garland, Ratansi, and Batsheva (2007) and Tryssenaar, Jones, and Deanne (1999).

The MOHO has been used with a variety of homeless populations and found to be effective. Life skills interventions such as money management, food and nutrition, and employment were developed based on the MOHO and provided to three homeless populations—adults with mental illness, women exposed to domestic violence, and youth living in shelters. The 4-week intervention consisted of four 1-hour group sessions and four 1-hour individual sessions. Of the participants who completed the modules, 62% demonstrated increases in their mastery scores (Helfrich, Aviles, Badiani, Walens, and Sobol, 2006).

Johnson (2006) suggests that OA is a useful framework for addressing the challenges faced by persons who are homeless. OA emphasizes the interaction between the person and the environment (i.e., physical, social, cultural). The environment creates a press for mastery that produces an occupational goal or challenge. Through the use of adaptation energy and adaptive response modes, the individual achieves relative mastery. The end result of the process is OA. The goal of intervention is to enhance a client's internal adaptation capabilities. Johnson (2006) describes one case as an exemplar and briefly illustrates the application of OA to three other cases. In all cases, clients had dysfunctional

Engage Your Brain 20-2

What are the similarities and differences between an occupational empowerment approach and other occupation-based approaches (such as CMOP, MOHO, OA, etc.) to intervention?

role performance during their homeless episodes and difficulties with interpersonal relationships. Fostering adaptation "allows individuals to meet the demands of the environment, cope with the problems of everyday living, and fulfill age-specific roles" (Johnson, 2006, p. 75).

Client-Centered Evaluation and Evidence-Based Intervention Approaches

Occupational therapists have an educational background encompassing the medical, psychological, psychosocial, social behavioral, and occupational sciences that uniquely prepares them to evaluate the needs of individuals who are experiencing homelessness and develop interventions designed to maintain and improve their health (World Federation of Occupational Therapists, 2010).

Evaluation

Meeting the needs of persons and families who are homeless begins with a comprehensive evaluation process. This process should include the development of an occupational profile (American Occupational Therapy Association [AOTA], 2014) and the use of assessments to measure mental health functioning, developmental levels in children, occupational performance, occupational participation, and independent living skills. Mental health assessments should include screening for depression, anxiety, posttraumatic stress disorder, and substance abuse. Developmental assessments are important when evaluating the needs and abilities of children who are homeless. It is well documented that children living in impoverished environments often experience developmental delays (Black, Hess, and Berenson-Howard, 2000; Murnane, 2007; National Institute of Child Health and Human Development, 2005). A list of potentially useful mental health and developmental assessment tools can be found in Table 20-1.

Measures of occupational performance, occupational participation, and independent living skills that have been used with this population include the COPM, the Ansell-Casey Life Skills Assessment (ACLSA), and the Occupational Self-Assessment (OSA).

Muñoz et al. (2006) conducted a study using the COPM to identify the self-perceived occupational performance problems of adults who were homeless. Using the COPM, the occupational therapy practitioners engaged participants in discussions of their perceived problems in activities they wanted to or were expected to perform. On average, they identified 9.3 problems. Clients rated their problems in terms of importance, their perception of how well they perform the activity, and satisfaction with their performance for each problem area. Over half (57%) of the identified problems were in the self-care domain, 32% were related to productivity, and 11% were associated with leisure. The mean importance rating on the identified problems was 8.84 (on a

Table 20-1 Mental Health and Developmental Assessment Tools

Mental Health Assessments	Developmental Assessments
Patient Health Questionnaire-9 (for depression)	Ages and Stages Questionnaire (ASQ)
Generalized Anxiety Disorder-7 (GAD-7)	Pediatric Symptom Checklist
Alcohol Use Disorders Identification Test (AUDIT)	Developmental Assessment of Young Children, 2nd Ed. (DAYC-2)
Drug Abuse Screen Test (DAST)	Early Coping Inventory
PC-PTSD	Whole Child Assessment
SAFE-T (suicide assessment)	Miller Assessment of Preschoolers

Data from *Asher's Occupational Therapy Assessment Tools: An Annotated Index* (4th ed.), by I. E. Asher, 2014, Bethesda, MD: AOTA Press.

10-point scale). Muñoz et al. (2006) suggest that "practitioners must recognize and may need to prioritize the person's basic self-care needs before addressing limitations in productive roles such as student, worker, or volunteer" (p. 147).

The most frequent self-care goals identified by participants were maintaining sobriety, obtaining housing, maintaining physical and mental health, and managing legal problems. Productivity goals were related to household management, education, and employment. Leisure goals were primarily improving the quality of interpersonal relationships, particularly with family members, and engaging in more quiet-time recreation. Although minor modifications to the subcategories of the domains of occupational performance were necessary to improve the relevance of the assessment to the homeless population, Muñoz et al. (2006) assert that "the COPM can facilitate person-centered, culturally responsive assessment with individuals who are homeless" (p. 136).

The ACLSA was used by Aviles and Helfrich (2006) to evaluate the independent living skills of homeless adolescents. The ACLSA assesses self-care, money management, work and study habits, food and nutrition management, social development, housing, and community resources. There are four age-specific versions to account for normative developmental changes. The ACLSA is normed, allowing for comparison of individual performance scores to others of a similar age.

Aviles and Helfrich (2006) also used the OSA, an assessment based on the MOHO. The OSA is designed to obtain clients' perceptions of their occupational competence and OA. Clients assess their level of ability to perform a variety of everyday occupations and the value they place on those activities. This instrument enables the occupational therapy practitioner to identify not only areas of deficit but also client strengths. The OSA was also used by Schultz-Krohn, Drnek, and Powell (2006) to facilitate the development of goal-setting skills for mothers who were homeless. Other assessments based on MOHO might be useful. These include the Role Checklist (Oakley, Kielhofner, Barris, and Reichler, 1986) and the Interest Checklist–UK (Heasman and Brewer, 2008).

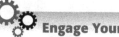

Engage Your Brain 20-3

What are some ethical considerations when designing occupational therapy programs for individuals and families who are homeless? Refer to the AOTA (2015) *Occupational Therapy Code of Ethics (2015)* to formulate your response.

Occupation-Based Interventions

According to Petrenchik (2006), "the overarching goal of occupational therapy interventions with persons living in homeless shelters is to maximize person-environment-occupation fit to enable participation in the immediate shelter environment and to reconfigure person-environment-occupation fit to enable greater participation in the community" (p. 25). Herzberg and Petrenchik (2010) provide examples of group interventions that facilitate community reintegration (see Box 20-3). Research

Box 20-3 Themes of Group Interventions With Adults

- Stress management (leisure skills, time management, coping skills)
- Self-care training (nutrition/cooking, health and safety, medication management, hygiene, grooming, dressing)
- Community-living skills training (clothing care, money management, shopping, public transportation, landlord and roommate issues)
- Prevocational services (task skills, aptitude testing, job structuring, interviewing and application activities, job coaching)
- Social and interpersonal skills (assertiveness, self-expression, conflict resolution, basic conversational skills, friendships)
- Home and neighborhood familiarization for those individuals transitioning into permanent housing to increase knowledge of local resources and transportation
- Individualized assistance to secure needed home items (furniture, bedding, kitchen items, etc.) and create a pleasant, livable, and personalized environment

Data from "Health Promotion for Individuals and Families Who Are Homeless," by G. Herzberg and T. Petrenchik, 2010, in M. E. Scaffa, S. M. Reitz, and M. A. Pizzi (Eds.), *Occupational Therapy in the Promotion of Health and Wellness*. Philadelphia, PA: F. A. Davis.

confirming the effectiveness of occupational therapy interventions used with the homeless population remains limited (Roy et al., 2017), and there is a great need for higher-level research into effective occupational therapy interventions (Thomas, Gray, and McGinty, 2011).

Roy et al. (2017) performed a scoping review of occupation-based interventions being used in community-based settings and found that current and potential interventions include:

- Life skills training
- Enrichment of occupational repertoire
- Education and employment services
- Child and family services
- Transition to stable housing

Life Skills Training

Individuals experiencing homelessness often have deficits in independent living skills. Life skills interventions provide the knowledge needed to perform living skills independently, teach clients how to use this knowledge, and provide opportunities for clients to practice newly learned skills during therapy sessions. Helfrich and Fogg (2007) implemented a program, based on empowerment and situated learning principles, teaching "skills in room and self-care management, food management, money management, and safe community participation" (p. 318). Teaching clients these skills not only increases participation in meaningful and necessary occupations but also serves a preventative function by reducing the recurrence of homelessness (Davis and Kutter, 1998). For clients experiencing homelessness, there are numerous areas where a deficit in life skills may be interfering with occupational performance. Based on the unique needs of those experiencing homelessness, meaningful and necessary life skills include safety planning, drug and alcohol awareness, self-advocacy, coping skills, money management, health management, medication management, safer sex practices, personal hygiene, and leisure exploration (Davis and Kutter, 1998; Gutman et al., 2004).

Gutman et al. (2004) provided a range of life skill interventions to homeless women who had experienced domestic violence. Interventions were identified through the literature and selected based on an initial needs assessment completed by each participant. Among the intervention topics selected, the authors found that stress management, anger management, and personal boundary setting were effective. All modules implemented during the study were found to improve life skills among participants, and data collected at 6 months post-study indicated that skills continued to improve after the intervention. Other intervention topics included safety planning, safety in the community, safer sex practices, assertiveness and personal advocacy, vocational and educational training, money management, housing applications, and leisure exploration (Gutman et al., 2004).

In another study, Helfrich et al. (2006) assessed the effectiveness of life skills interventions in improving housing independence among homeless persons with mental illness. The authors also wanted to examine whether participants would retain and implement the skills they had learned. Intervention topics included self-care, food management, money management, and safety in the community. The self-care module included public hygiene, personal health, clothing management, and home-management skills. The food-management module consisted of meal planning and preparation, food budgeting, food safety, nutrition, and cooking using a microwave. The money-management module addressed advertising gimmicks, budgeting, shopping, banking, credit scores, and tools to manage money. The safe community participation module included personal protection, safety in the home, safety in the community, and self-advocacy. Participants were reassessed 3 and 6 months postintervention. Based on their findings, the authors concluded that participants had maintained and applied the skills they had learned 6 months postintervention. Participants also reported the continued use of session materials to guide them through challenging situations (Helfrich et al., 2006).

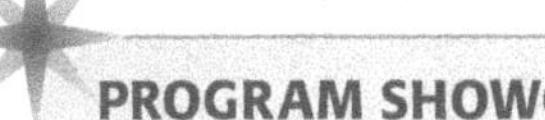

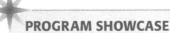

PROGRAM SHOWCASE

Providing Occupational Therapy to the Homeless in a Community-Based Setting

In response to a lack of access to affordable health care in the United States, student-run free medical clinics represent a sustainable model of collaborative local programs designed to provide care to the uninsured (Beck, 2005). Studies indicate that clients who visit student-run free clinics are satisfied with the care they receive (Ellett, Campbell, and Gonsalves, 2010).

The Student-Run Free Clinic (SRFC) of the University of South Alabama provides free health-care services to the homeless population of Mobile, Alabama. The clinic is located in the Salvation Army of Coastal Alabama, which also provides emergency shelter, job training and placement, social services, seasonal assistance for families in need, and group and individual therapy for men recovering from addictions. The need for these services was identified from data collected for the Point-in-Time (PIT) Count (Housing First Inc., n.d.), an annual survey of the homeless population of Mobile and Baldwin Counties. The most recent data indicated that there are 606 homeless persons in Mobile and Baldwin Counties, with 486 of those individuals residing in the city of Mobile. The SRFC receives support from the University of South Alabama and routinely solicits medical supplies and financial donations from various groups and organizations in the community.

The SRFC provides services on Fridays from 12:00 p.m. to 4:30 p.m., and the clinic utilizes an interprofessional team of students from the colleges of medicine, nursing, and allied health professions at the University of South Alabama. Students from the Harrison School of Pharmacy at Auburn University also volunteer to provide services. A total of nine disciplines are represented: pharmacy, medicine, nursing, physician assistant, physical therapy, occupational therapy, audiology, recreational therapy, and clinical mental health counseling. Clinic operations are overseen by a faculty member from Nursing and the Student Board, with each discipline electing at least one liaison to serve. All members of the Student Board receive Mental Health First Aid training to prepare them to respond effectively to mental health emergencies.

Students volunteer in examination rooms, provide educational sessions, conduct research, collect and sort donations, and inform clinic policies and procedures. In the examination room, students take vital signs, obtain medical and occupational histories, and perform physical exams (see Fig. 20-3). Information is then presented to the attending health-care professional, who is usually a physician, physician assistant, or nurse. Afterward, the student team returns to the client and provides information about the person's health status and relevant services. Occupational therapy students have been providing educational sessions on a variety of topics, including sleep hygiene, chronic disease self-management, and nutrition. Information about community resources, including public transportation, support groups for substance abuse, and mental health services, is also provided. Clients have access to a library of books and games maintained by occupational therapy students, allowing them to participate in leisure occupations while waiting to be seen for a medical appointment.

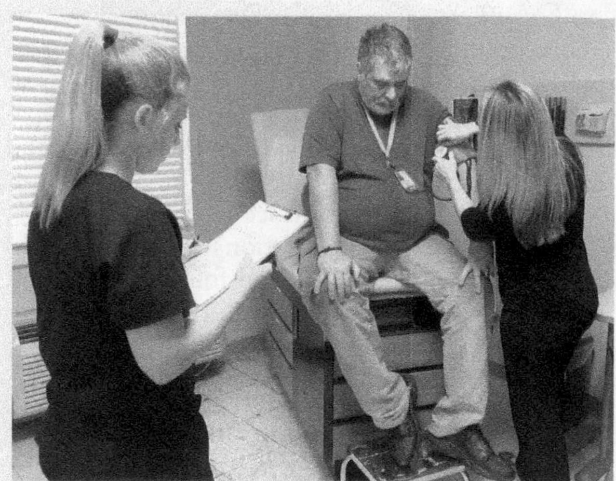

Figure 20-3 University of South Alabama occupational therapy students volunteering at the student-run free clinic for the homeless. *(Photo courtesy of Thaddeus Parker.)*

In the future, occupational therapy students and faculty hope to provide additional individual and group interventions at the SRFC. Interventions will focus on community living skills, prevention and health promotion, interpersonal skills, and health literacy.

Enrichment of Occupational Repertoire

Occupational imbalance among the homeless is often related to a narrowing repertoire of occupations. This often occurs due to substance abuse and the routines developed to support addiction (Heuchemer and Josephsson, 2006). Enriching the occupational repertoire of those experiencing homelessness is an effective intervention approach used by practitioners (Illman, Spence, O'Campo, and Kirsh, 2013; Roy et al., 2017).

Thomas, Gray, McGinty, and Ebringer (2011) conducted a study to assess how art interventions can lead to increased interpersonal functioning and social participation of people experiencing homelessness. Participants were given access to various media for sketching and painting on paper or canvas. The authors observed that participating in the art program allowed participants to establish routine behaviors that were purposeful and goal directed, resulting in a sense of accomplishment. In addition, participants were willing to forgo substance use in order to participate in the art program, and the creative process allowed them to develop the skills needed to envision a future in which they are no longer homeless or using drugs. Participants were also recognized for their creativity and abilities, leading to the development of a new and positive self-image. This new identity counteracts the marginalization that homeless individuals often experience (Thomas et al., 2011).

For persons who are homeless, involvement in sporting activities provides opportunities for social bonding that have been shown to reduce both substance abuse and symptoms of mental illness. This has been observed at the international level with the Homeless World Cup (HWC), which, utilizing a network of 73 organizations from 73 nation-states, including the United States, hosts an annual international soccer tournament. The HWC is made possible by numerous grassroots efforts to recruit 500 players to compete in the tournament. Teams consist of players who have either experienced homelessness in the past 2 years or are receiving rehabilitation for substance abuse (Magee, 2011). Sherry (2010) studied the Street Socceroos, Australia's HWC team, to determine the benefits of participating in sports. The author found that the friendships among participants served as a support system during times of hardship. Participants cited a sense of obligation to their teammates, which served as a source of positive peer pressure. Participants also reported an increased sense of well-being after participating in the games. Involvement in the HWC later resulted in increased access to stable housing, education, and employment resources (Sherry, 2010).

Education and Employment Services

The literature confirms that individuals around the world who experience homelessness greatly desire to find meaningful work but often lack the skills and support needed to do so (Boland and O'Mahony, 2002; Malekpour, 2008; Muñoz et al., 2006). Malekpour (2008) conducted a descriptive study to assess the occupational performance needs of homeless women residing in state-run shelters in Mashhad, Iran. Among the 44 participants, 81.8% indicated a desire to secure meaningful work. Studies show that supportive employment programs that provide life skills and professional skills training in conjunction with adequate support services are both viable and effective (Burt, 2012; Marrone, 2005; Muñoz, Reichenbach, and Hansen, 2005).

Project Employ is a grant-funded supportive employment program that is the result of a collaboration between Duquesne University's Department of Occupational Therapy and Bethlehem Haven, a shelter providing services to the homeless population of Pittsburgh, Pennsylvania (Muñoz et al., 2005). The program is staffed by a full-time occupational therapist serving as program coordinator, a part-time occupational therapy assistant, and a full-time employment specialist. The program offers both individualized and group training sessions that focus on the development of life skills and professional development. Participants are allowed to remain in the program for up to 18 months, and the program has enrolled up to 50 participants at one time.

The program consists of four phases. During the pre-enrollment phase, participants are referred to Project Employ by area service providers and other homeless shelters. Bethlehem Haven also requires some of its residents to participate. Participants are provided with information about the program and a copy of the program's curriculum. Once a participant decides to commit to the program, the second phase begins, which consists of professional development and skills training. The training sessions are offered over the course of 12 weeks and include games, role-playing to practice new skills, writing assignments, and life skills. Job-searching skills, resume and cover letter writing, and interview skills are also addressed. Staff also ensure that participants acquire any necessary documents needed to secure employment (e.g., photo ID/Social Security card). The 12-week curriculum used by Project Employ can be found in Box 20-4.

During the third phase of the program, participants begin searching for employment opportunities that incorporate their personal strengths. Once an employer is identified, participants begin a paid

Box 20-4 Project Employ Life Skills Curriculum

- Where Do I Begin?
- Setting Goals/Creating Action Plans
- Developing Your Resume
- Writing Effective Cover Letters and Thank You Notes
- Time Management and Prioritizing
- Developing Professional Responsibility
- Selling Yourself at an Interview
- Dress for Success
- Employment With a Criminal Record
- Strategies for Staying Motivated
- Promotion and Career Advancement
- Preventing Relapse
- Conversation/Listening Skills
- Stress Management
- Relationship Building
- Health and Wellness
- Community Resources
- Decision-making
- Coping With Change
- Successful Budgeting
- Being Assertive
- Anger Management
- Conflict Resolution
- Having Fun

Data from "Project Employ: Engineering Hope and Breaking Down Barriers to Homelessness," by J. Muñoz, D. Reichenbach, and A. M. Hansen, 2005, *Work, 25*(3), 241–252.

work experience (PWE). At the end of 6 months, participants may be hired by the company where they are completing their PWE. Throughout this entire process, the occupational therapist and employment specialist provide support and monitor each participant's performance to ensure success. Support continues during the fourth phase to aid participants in integrating the role of being a worker within their existing roles. This involves one-on-one meetings to problem-solve issues affecting success, as well as conducting performance evaluations.

Even after the fourth phase, participants continue meeting with staff twice a month to maintain progress. Outcome data suggest the program is viable and effective, with 96% of clients having assumed a productive role at the time of publication (Muñoz et al., 2005). A similar program focusing on homeless individuals with significant disabilities has also proven effective. Marrone (2005) reports the *Hope, Vocations, Progress* (HVP) program of Columbia River Mental Health Services in Vancouver, Washington, helped 129 participants secure employment over a 5-year period. Of those, 93 (72%) had retained their jobs after 90 days (Marrone, 2005).

Child and Family Services

The stress that homeless families experience often negatively affects family routines. Sources of stress include, among others, a lack of housing and the strict rules governing life in a homeless shelter. Such policies often result in a lack of privacy and choice among residents. Interventions for families experiencing homelessness involve aiding parents in constructing and maintaining family roles and routines. Interventions should also facilitate connection with the community (Mayberry, Shinn, Benton, and Wise, 2014). In a study seeking to better understand parenting roles within the context of a homeless shelter, Schultz-Krohn (2004) notes that occupational therapy interventions at a homeless shelter provided support to parents as they preserved existing routines while establishing new routines. The strategies and resources needed to maintain stability in daily family routines were also offered. These routines included promoting intimacy among parents and children, developing a family legacy, and engaging with the community. An example of an individual intervention involved providing parents with basic massage techniques to be used with their children and information about the importance of gentle touch in order to improve bonding and soothing. Interventions were also provided in small groups, covering topics such as appropriate child discipline strategies.

Another effective intervention approach included involving parents in the promotion of literacy development among their children. Providing parents with strategies to increase literacy, along with any necessary materials and books, can aid parents in assuming the role of literacy mentor (Di Santo, 2012).

Transition to Stable Housing

Securing stable housing is essential for individuals and families to be able to fully participate in their communities. One of the primary roles of occupational therapy practitioners working with homeless populations is utilizing and developing occupation-based interventions that ensure a successful transition to stable housing. This can be achieved by utilizing intervention strategies that develop the skills needed to adopt and maintain a new identity as a housed person through engagement in occupations (Petrenchik, 2006). Although research focusing on the transition to becoming housed is limited, programs that provide permanent supportive housing for the homeless represent an opportunity for practitioners to implement such interventions.

Activities that result in increased socialization and engagement with the community can support the development of new social roles, thereby reducing the chances of becoming homeless again. Another role for occupational therapy practitioners is to inform support workers of the importance of occupations and occupational engagement to clients making the transition to stable housing. This can be achieved through consultation with support workers and developing training initiatives that inform support staff of the role occupational engagement plays in the establishment of a housed identity (Marshall and Rosenberg, 2014).

Raphael-Greenfield and Gutman (2015) conducted in-depth interviews with four formerly homeless adults who had secured stable housing to better understand supports and barriers to transitioning, as well as occupations that establish and maintain a housed identity. Based on their findings, the authors identified factors that either promote or inhibit a successful transition. Factors valued by participants that promoted a successful transition included the occupation of maintaining abstinence from drugs/alcohol and housing that provided opportunities to socialize and reengage with the community. Participants also valued support staff who were nonjudgmental and kind. Factors identified by participants as inhibiting their transition included high levels of anxiety from having endured life on the street and age-related disease and changes in functioning.

Using this information to inform intervention strategies, Raphael-Greenfield and Gutman (2015) recommend interventions that create opportunities for clients to volunteer, socialize, and reengage with their communities. Interventions that help clients identify coping strategies to manage their anxiety, as well as promote leisure exploration and participation, are also recommended. Helping clients manage age-related changes in function through environmental modifications, energy conservation strategies, compensatory strategies, and access to health care can make it easier to remain housed (Raphael-Greenfield and Gutman, 2015).

Summary

- Homelessness is the result of a complex interaction of structural factors, individual characteristics and vulnerabilities, and cultural influences.
- Populations at high risk for homelessness include women and children who have experienced domestic violence, individuals with mental illness, sexual minority youth, low-income older adults with chronic health conditions, and Veterans.
- Research has demonstrated that the Housing-First approach combined with trauma-informed care is the most effective strategy for reducing homelessness.
- When working with the homeless population, occupational therapy practitioners may provide direct services—for example, the evaluation and treatment of occupational performance deficits through group and individual sessions. In addition, emerging roles include providing indirect services such as advocacy, education, outreach, and case management.
- Barriers to occupational engagement include skill deficits, environmental limitations, lack of access, and poor mental and physical health. These barriers result in occupational deprivation.
- Ecological and empowerment models are highly recommended for use with marginalized populations like the homeless. Occupation-based theories and models are appropriate adjuncts in the development of occupational therapy services for this population.
- A scoping review of occupation-based interventions being used in community-based settings found that current and potential interventions include life skills training, enrichment of the occupational repertoire, education and employment services, child and family services, and transitions to stable housing (Roy et al., 2017).

CASE STUDIES

CASE STUDY 20-1 Rachel

Rachel is a 35-year-old single mother of three whose family has been homeless for three weeks. Rachel's late husband, David, recently succumbed to a rare form of lung cancer, leaving the family saddled with debt from the accumulated medical bills. David and Rachel, both from Detroit, Michigan, graduated from high school but chose not to pursue college after they were able to secure good-paying jobs in the automotive manufacturing industry. After saving enough money, the couple bought a house and started a family. Rachel was the first to lose her job after the company she worked for moved its operations overseas. The company David worked for was next to move, leaving both jobless and struggling to find work. David started driving a delivery truck for a major shipping company, while Rachel was able to find a job at a fast-food restaurant chain. David's job paid roughly $20 an hour with benefits, just barely supporting the family's needs. After David became sick and had to quit his job, the family was forced to survive on Rachel's salary of $9.15 an hour. With David's passing, Rachel suddenly found herself lost and alone amid a mountain of bills and three children for whom she was responsible. After the family was evicted from their home due to missed payments, a friend told Rachel about Shelter Michigan, a homeless shelter for families. Despite worrying about what her friends and family would think, Rachel took her children to the shelter.

During the day, she works her job at the fast-food restaurant, researching additional sources of income during her lunch break while the children attend school. In the afternoon, Rachel has the opportunity to participate in group occupational therapy sessions. During a session on gardening, Rachel learns how to tend to the community garden at the shelter. Produce grown in the garden is purchased and used at a local farm-to-table restaurant, making Rachel feel she is one step closer to realizing her childhood dream of owning her own restaurant.

The occupational therapist also offers courses on coping strategies to manage stress as well as courses on child literacy. Based on what she learns from the course on literacy, Rachel is able to start a new routine of reading a book to her two youngest children each night before bed. Although the shelter offers protection for her family, Rachel finds some of the policies to be invasive. Rachel's oldest child, Devon, has just turned 14. Based on shelter policy, Rachel is required to accompany Devon to the restroom since he is under the age of 18. This humiliates Devon while making Rachel feel like she is violating her son's right to privacy. She expresses this concern to the staff at the shelter.

Discussion Questions

1. What structural factors, personal characteristics, and cultural influences have contributed to Rachel's experience with homelessness? In particular, how has an unlivable minimum wage affected Rachel's ability to provide for her family?
2. As a community-based occupational therapy practitioner, you are working with Rachel and her children as your clients. Describe potential interventions to help them engage with their community. What other types of interventions would help Rachel preserve existing family routines while establishing new ones?
3. How would you as an occupational therapy practitioner advocate for Rachel and her family in this setting? In particular, how would you advocate for Devon's request for privacy while using the restroom?

CASE STUDY 20-2 Family Village

The Family Village is a transitional living program for women and children who are homeless and have been living in shelters. The majority of women who reside in Family Village apartments have experienced intimate partner violence and have symptoms of posttraumatic stress disorder. In addition, approximately 20% of the women have substance use disorders. Program participants can stay in the Family Village for up to 18 months provided they are making progress toward educational and/or employment goals. Each apartment has two bedrooms, a full kitchen, one bathroom, and a small living room. All furniture and basic kitchen items are provided. The facility has a laundry room, a multipurpose room with a large-screen TV, computers, and a kitchen. There is a small library of books, DVDs, and table games. The program is funded through the United Way, grants, and donations.

A needs assessment was conducted, and the women indicated they could benefit from training in the following: parenting, coping skills, money management, meal planning and preparation, nutrition, job searching, job application and interviewing, self-advocacy skills, health and safety, public transportation, and community engagement. In addition, staff at the facility have identified developmental delays and psychosocial problems with many of the children.

The vast majority of the staff are nonprofessional. Occupational therapy students have been volunteering in the program for the past 2 years, and the director has noticed significant improvements in the women's goal attainment. As a result, the director decides to write a grant proposal to hire a full-time occupational therapist. You are asked to be a consultant.

Discussion Questions

1. What qualifications and responsibilities would you include in a job description for an occupational therapist at this facility?
2. What theoretical approach would you use and why?
3. What services would the occupational therapist provide?

Learning Activities

1. Volunteer at a homeless shelter or soup kitchen in your area. Identify what services an occupational therapy practitioner might provide in this setting.
2. Interview occupational therapists who work in urban school settings to find out how they address the needs of children who are homeless.
3. Contact your local housing board and explore the availability of low-income housing in your area.

REFERENCES

Ackerman, C. (2018). *Learned helplessness: Seligman's theory of depression.* Retrieved from https://positivepsychologyprogram.com/learned-helplessness-seligman-theory-depression-cure/#definition-learned-helplessness

American Occupational Therapy Association. (2014). Occupational therapy practice framework: Domain and process. *American Journal of Occupational Therapy, 68*(Suppl. 1), S1–S51.

American Occupational Therapy Association. (2015). Occupational therapy code of ethics (2015). *American Journal of Occupational Therapy, 69*(Suppl. 3), 6913410030. http://dx.doi.org/10.5014/ajot.2015.696S03

Asher, I. E. (2014). *Asher's occupational therapy assessment tools: An annotated index* (4th ed.). Bethesda, MD: AOTA Press.

Aviles, A. M., and Helfrich, C. A. (2006). Homeless youth: Causes, consequences and the role of occupational therapy. *Occupational Therapy in Health Care, 20*(3–4), 99–114.

Bassuk, E. L., DeCandia, C. J., Beach, C. A., and Berman, F. (2014). *America's youngest outcasts: A report card on child homelessness.* Waltham, MA: National Center on Family Homelessness at American Institutes for Research.

Beck, E. (2005). The UCSD student-run free clinic project: Transdisciplinary health professional education. *Journal of Health Care for the Poor and Underserved, 16*(2), 207–219.

Beijer, U., Wolf, A., and Fazel, S. (2012). Prevalence of tuberculosis, hepatitis C virus, and HIV in homeless people: A systematic review and meta-analysis. *Lancet Infectious Diseases, 12*(11), 859–870.

Black, M. M., Hess, C., and Berenson-Howard, J. (2000). Toddlers from low income families have below normal mental, motor, and behavior scores on the revised Bayley Scales. *Journal of Applied Developmental Psychology, 21,* 655–666.

Blank, R. M. (2010). The New American model of work-conditioned public support. In J. Alber and N. Gilbert (Eds.), *United in diversity: Comparing social models in Europe and America* (pp. 176–198). New York, NY: Oxford University Press.

Boland, L., and O'Mahony, P. (2002). A study of experiences and expectations of homeless men with schizophrenia. *Irish Journal of Occupational Therapy, 32,* 2–9.

Brown, R. T., Kiely, D. K., Bharel, M., and Mitchell, S. L. (2012). Geriatric syndromes in older homeless adults. *Journal of General Internal Medicine, 27*(1), 16–22.

Burt, M. (2001). *What will it take to end homelessness?* Washington, DC: Urban Institute. Retrieved from www.urban.org/research/publication/what-will-it-take-end-homelessness/view/full_report.

Burt, M. R. (2012). Impact of housing and work supports on outcomes for chronically homeless adults with mental illness: LA's HOPE. *Psychiatric Services, 63*(3), 209–215.

Carter, G. R. (2011). From exclusion to destitution: Race, affordable housing, and homelessness. *Cityscape, 13*(1), 33–70.

Chan, K., Garland, K., Ratansi, K., and Batsheva, Y. (2007). Viewing youth homelessness through an occupational lens. *Occupational Therapy Now, 9*(4), 14–15.

Chard, G., Faulkner, T., and Chugg, A. (2009). Exploring occupation and its meaning among homeless men. *British Journal of Occupational Therapy, 72*(3), 116–124.

Cochran, B. N., Stewart, A. J., Ginzler, J. A., and Cauce, A. M. (2002). Challenges faced by homeless sexual minorities: Comparison of gay, lesbian, bisexual, and transgender homeless adolescents with their heterosexual counterparts. *American Journal of Public Health, 92*(5), 773–777.

Cronley, C. (2010). Unraveling the social construction of homelessness. *Journal of Human Behavior in the Social Environment, 20*(2), 319–333.

da Costa Nunez, R. (2012). *Homelessness: It's about race, not just poverty.* Retrieved from https://citylimits.org/2012/03/05/homelessness-its-about-race-not-just-poverty/

Davis, J., and Kutter, C. J. (1998). Independent living skills and posttraumatic stress disorder in women who are homeless: Implications for future practice. *American Journal of Occupational Therapy, 52*(1), 39–44.

Di Santo, A. (2012). Promoting preschool literacy: A family literacy program for homeless mothers and their children. *Childhood Education, 88*(4), 232–240.

Ellett, J. D., Campbell, J. A., and Gonsalves, W. C. (2010). Patient satisfaction in a student-run free medical clinic. *Family Medicine, 42*(1), 16–18.

Fazel, S., Geddes, J. R., and Kushel, M. (2014). The health of homeless people in high-income countries: Descriptive epidemiology, health consequences, and clinical and policy recommendations. *Lancet, 384*(9953), 1529–1540.

Fazel, S., Khosla, V., Doll, H., and Geddes, J. (2008). The prevalence of mental disorders among the homeless in western countries: Systematic review and meta-regression analysis. *PLoS Medicine, 5*(12), e225.

Fisher, G. S., and Hotchkiss, A. (2008). A model of occupational empowerment for marginalized populations in community environments. *Occupational Therapy in Health Care, 22*(1), 55–71.

Folsom, D. P., Hawthorne, W., Lindamer, L., Gilmer, T., Bailey, A., Golshan, S., . . . Jeste, D. V. (2005). Prevalence and risk factors for homelessness and utilization of mental health services among 10,340 patients with serious mental illness in a large public mental health system. *American Journal of Psychiatry, 162*(2), 370–376.

Grandisson, M., Mitchell-Carvalho, M., Tang, V., and Korner-Bitensky, N. (2009). Occupational therapists' perceptions of their role with people who are homeless. *British Journal of Occupational Therapy, 72*(11), 491–498.

Gutman, S. A., Diamond, H., Holness-Parchment, S. E., Brandofino, D. N., Pacheco, D. G., Jolly-Edouard, M., and Jean-Charles, S. (2004). Enhancing independence in women experiencing domestic violence and possible brain injury: An assessment of an occupational therapy intervention. *Occupational Therapy in Mental Health, 20*(1), 49–79.

Gutman, S. A., and Raphael-Greenfield, E. I. (2017). Effectiveness of a supportive housing program for homeless adults with mental illness and substance use: A two-group controlled trial. *British Journal of Occupational Therapy, 80*(5), 286–293.

Heasman, D., and Brewer, P. (2008). *Interest Checklist (UK).* Retrieved from www.moho.uic.edu/productDetails.aspx?aid=39

Helfrich, C. A., Aviles, A. M., Badiani, C., Walens, D., and Sabol, P. (2006). Life skill interventions with homeless youth, domestic violence victims and adults with mental illness. *Occupational Therapy in Health Care, 20*(3–4), 189–207.

Helfrich, C. A., and Fogg, L. F. (2007). Outcomes of a life skills intervention for homeless adults with mental illness. *Journal of Primary Prevention, 28*(3–4), 313–326.

Herzberg, G., and Petrenchik, T. M. (2010). Health promotion for individuals and families who are homeless. In M. E. Scaffa, S. M. Reitz, and M. A. Pizzi (Eds.), *Occupational therapy in the promotion of health and wellness.* Philadelphia, PA: F. A. Davis.

Heuchemer, B., and Josephsson, S. (2006). Leaving homelessness and addiction: Narratives of an occupational transition. *Scandinavian Journal of Occupational Therapy, 13*(3), 160–169.

Housing First Inc. (n.d.). *Point-in-time count.* Retrieved from www.hfal.org/point-in-time-count/

Illman, S. C., Spence, S., O'Campo, P. J., and Kirsh, B. H. (2013). Exploring the occupations of homeless adults living with mental illnesses in Toronto: Explorer les occupations d'adultes sans-abri atteints de maladies mentales vivant à Toronto. *Canadian Journal of Occupational Therapy, 80*(4), 215–223.

Ji, E. G. (2006). A study of the structural risk factors of homelessness in 52 metropolitan areas in the United States. *International Social Work, 49*(1), 107–117.

Johnson, G., and Chamberlain, C. (2008). Homelessness and substance abuse: Which comes first? *Australian Social Work, 61*(4), 342–346.

Johnson, G., Scutella, R., Tseng, Y., and Wood, G. (2015). *Entries and exits from homelessness: A dynamic analysis of the relationship between structural conditions and individual characteristics, AHURI Final Report No. 248.* Melbourne: Australian Housing and Urban Research Institute. Retrieved from www.ahuri.edu.au/research/final-reports/248.

Johnson, J. A. (2006). Describing the phenomenon of homelessness through the theory of occupational adaptation. *Occupational Therapy in Health Care, 20*(3–4), 63–80.

Kiepek, N., and Magalhaes, L. (2011). Addictions and impulse-control disorders as occupation: A selected literature review and synthesis. *Journal of Occupational Science, 18*(3), 254–276.

Kipke, M. D., Weiss, G., and Wong, C. F. (2007). Residential status as a risk factor for drug use and HIV risk among young men who have sex with men. *AIDS and Behavior, 11*(2), 56–69.

Landon, C. (2017). Homelessness as a positive influence on pulmonary health in COPD. *Chest, 152*(4), A981.

Lee, S., Castella, A. D., Freidin, J., Kennedy, A., Kroschel, J., Humphrey, C., . . . Kulkarni, J. (2010). Mental health care on the streets: An integrated approach. *Australian and New Zealand Journal of Psychiatry, 44*(6), 505–512.

Lee, T. C., Hanlon, J. G., Ben-David, J., Booth, G. L., Cantor, W. J., Connelly, P. W., and Hwang, S. W. (2005). Risk factors for cardiovascular disease in homeless adults. *Circulation, 111*(20), 2629–2635.

Livingston, B. W., and Miller, K. S. (2006). Systems of care for persons who are homeless in the United States. *Occupational Therapy in Health Care, 20*(3–4), 31–46.

Magee, J. (2011). Disengagement, de-motivation, vulnerable groups and sporting inclusion: A case study of the Homeless World Cup. *Soccer and Society, 12*(2), 159–173.

Malekpour, M. (2008). Needs assessment of runaway females in Iran from an occupational therapy perspective. *Occupational Therapy International, 15*(4), 232–252.

Marrone, J. (2005). Creating hope through employment for people who are homeless or in transitional housing. *American Journal of Psychiatric Rehabilitation, 8*(1), 13–35.

Marshall, C. A., Lysaght, R., and Krupa, T. (2017). The experience of occupational engagement of chronically homeless persons in a mid-sized urban context. *Journal of Occupational Science, 24*(2), 165–180.

Marshall, C. A., and Rosenberg, M. W. (2014). Occupation and the process of transition from homelessness: L'occupation et le processus de transition de l'itinérance au logement. *Canadian Journal of Occupational Therapy, 81*(5), 330–338.

Mayberry, L. S., Shinn, M., Benton, J. G., and Wise, J. (2014). Families experiencing housing instability: The effects of housing programs on family routines and rituals. *American Journal of Orthopsychiatry, 84*(1), 95.

Minkler, M. (1997). *Community organizing and community building for health.* New Brunswick, NJ: Rutgers University Press.

Mojtabai, R. (2005). Perceived reasons for loss of housing and continued homelessness among homeless persons with mental illness. *Psychiatric Services, 56*(2), 172–178.

Moyers, P. A. (1992). *Substance abuse: A multidimensional assessment and treatment approach.* Thorofare, NJ: SLACK.

Moyers, P. A. (1997). Occupational meanings and spirituality: The quest for sobriety. *American Journal of Occupational Therapy, 51*(3), 2070214.

Muñoz, J. P., Garcia, T., Lisak, J., and Reichenbach, D. (2006). Assessing the occupational performance priorities of people who are homeless. *Occupational Therapy in Health Care, 20*(3–4), 135–148.

Muñoz, J. P., Reichenbach, D., and Hansen, A. M. W. (2005). Project Employ: Engineering hope and breaking down barriers to homelessness. *Work, 25*(3), 241–252.

Murnane, R. J. (2007). Improving the education of children living in poverty. *Future Child, 17,* 161–182.

National Coalition for Homeless Veterans. (n.d.). *Background and Statistics.* Retrieved from http://nchv.org/index.php/news/media/background_and_statistics/

National Coalition for the Homeless. (2007). *Homeless self-help and empowerment projects, NCH fact sheet # 17.* Retrieved from www.nationalhomeless.org/publications/facts/Self_Help.pdf

National Coalition for the Homeless. (2018). *Homelessness in America.* Retrieved from https://nationalhomeless.org/about-homelessness/

National Institute of Child Health and Human Development. (2005). Duration and developmental timing of poverty and children's cognitive and social development from birth through third grade. *Child Development, 76,* 795–810.

National Low-Income Housing Coalition. (2018). *Out of reach: 2018.* Retrieved from http://nlihc.org/sites/default/files/oor/OOR_2018.pdf

Noell, J. W., and Ochs, L. M. (2001). Relationship of sexual orientation to substance use, suicidal ideation, suicide attempts, and other factors in a population of homeless adolescents. *Journal of Adolescent Health, 29*(1), 31–36.

Nolan, T. C. (2006). Outcomes for a transitional living program serving LGBTQ youth in New York City. *Child Welfare, 85*(2), 385.

Nooe, R. M., and Patterson, D. A. (2010). The ecology of homelessness. *Journal of Human Behavior in the Social Environment, 20*(2), 105–152.

Oakley, F., Kielhofner, G., Barris, R., and Reichler, R. (1986). The Role Checklist: Development and empirical assessment of reliability. *Occupational Therapy Journal of Research, 6,* 157–170.

Petrenchik, T. (2006). Homelessness: Perspectives, misconceptions, and considerations for occupational therapy. *Occupational Therapy in Health Care, 20*(3–4), 9–30.

Raphael-Greenfield, E. I., and Gutman, S. A. (2015). Understanding the lived experience of formerly homeless adults as they transition to supportive housing. *Occupational Therapy in Mental Health, 31*(1), 35–49.

RentData.org. (2018). *2018 rent data by state.* Retrieved from www.rentdata.org/states/2018

Rosario, M., Schrimshaw, E. W., and Hunter, J. (2012). Risk factors for homelessness among lesbian, gay, and bisexual youths: A developmental milestone approach. *Children and Youth Services Review, 34*(1), 186–193.

Roy, L., Vallée, C., Kirsh, B. H., Marshall, C. A., Marval, R., and Low, A. (2017). Occupation-based practices and homelessness: A scoping review: Pratiques fondées sur l'occupation et itinérance: Un examen de la portée. *Canadian Journal of Occupational Therapy, 84*(2), 98–110.

Schultz-Krohn, W. (2004). The meaning of family routines in a homeless shelter. *American Journal of Occupational Therapy, 58*(5), 531–542.

Schultz-Krohn, W., Drnek, S., and Powell, K. (2006). Occupational therapy intervention to foster goal setting skills for homeless mothers. *Occupational Therapy in Health Care, 20*(3–4), 149–166.

Sherry, E. (2010). (Re)engaging marginalized groups through sport: The Homeless World Cup. *International Review for the Sociology of Sport, 45*(1), 59–71.

Shinn, M. (2007). International homelessness: Policy, socio-cultural, and individual perspectives. *Journal of Social Issues, 63*(3), 657–677.

Shinn, M. (2010). Homelessness, poverty and social exclusion in the United States and Europe. *European Journal of Homelessness, 4,* 19–44.

Substance Abuse and Mental Health Services Administration. (2014). *Trauma-informed care in behavioral health services: Treatment improvement protocol (TIP) series 57.* HHS Publication No. (SMA) 13–4801. Rockville, MD: Substance Abuse and Mental Health Services Administration.

Substance Abuse and Mental Health Services Administration. (2018a). *Adverse childhood experiences.* Retrieved from www.samhsa.gov/capt/practicing-effective-prevention/prevention-behavioral-health/adverse-childhood-experiences

Substance Abuse and Mental Health Services Administration. (2018b). *Trauma-informed approach and trauma-specific interventions.* Retrieved from www.samhsa.gov/nctic/trauma-interventions

Teesson, M., Hodder, T., and Buhrich, N. (2004). Psychiatric disorders in homeless men and women in inner Sydney. *Australian and New Zealand Journal of Psychiatry, 38*(3), 162–168.

Thomas, Y., Gray, M. A., and McGinty, S. (2011). A systematic review of occupational therapy interventions with homeless people. *Occupational Therapy in Health Care, 25*(1), 38–53.

Thomas, Y., Gray, M. A., and McGinty, S. (2017). The occupational wellbeing of people experiencing homelessness. *Journal of Occupational Science, 24*(2), 181–192.

Thomas, Y., Gray, M. A., McGinty, S., and Ebringer, S. (2011). Homeless adults engagement in art: First steps towards identity, recovery and social inclusion. *Australian Occupational Therapy Journal, 58*(6), 429–436.

Thompson, R. G., Jr., Wall, M. M., Greenstein, E., Grant, B. F., and Hasin, D. S. (2013). Substance-use disorders and poverty as prospective predictors of first-time homelessness in the United States. *American Journal of Public Health, 103*(S2), S282–S288.

Toro, P. A., Tompsett, C. J., Lombardo, S., Philippot, P., Nachtergael, H., Galand, B., . . . Harvey, K. (2007). Homelessness in Europe and the United States: A comparison of prevalence and public opinion. *Journal of Social Issues, 63,* 505–524. doi:10.1111/j.1540–4560.2007.00521.x

Tryssenaar, J., Jones, E., and Deanne, L. (1999). Occupational performance needs of a shelter population. *Canadian Journal of Occupational Therapy, 66*(4), 188–196.

U.S. Census Bureau. (2018a). *How the Census Bureau measures poverty.* Retrieved from www.census.gov/topics/income-poverty/poverty/guidance/poverty-measures.html

U.S. Census Bureau. (2018b). *Income and poverty in the United States.* Retrieved from www.census.gov/content/dam/Census/library/publications/2018/demo/p60–263.pdf

U.S. Department of Housing and Urban Development. (2013). *Guidance on housing individuals and families experiencing homelessness through the public housing and housing choice voucher programs.* Retrieved from www.hud.gov/sites/documents/PIH2013–15.PDF

U.S. Department of Housing and Urban Development. (2016). *Review of the LGBTQ youth homelessness prevention initiative planning phase: Summary of findings.* Retrieved from www.hudexchange.info/resources/documents/Review-of-LGBTQ-Youth-Homelessness-Prevention-Initiative.pdf

U.S. Department of Housing and Urban Development. (2017). *The 2017 annual homeless assessment report to Congress.* Retrieved from www.hudexchange.info/resources/documents/2017-AHAR-Part-1.pdf

U.S. Department of Labor. (n.d.). *Minimum wage.* Retrieved from www.dol.gov/general/topic/wages/minimumwage

U.S. Department of Labor. (2018). *Minimum wage for contractors; updating regulations to reflect Executive Order 13838.* Retrieved from www.federalregister.gov/documents/2018/09/26/2018–20757/minimum-wage-for-contractors-updating-regulations-to-reflect-executive-order-13838

U.S. Interagency Council on Homelessness. (2018). *Deploy housing first systemwide.* Retrieved from www.usich.gov/solutions/housing/

Van Leeuwen, J. M., Boyle, S., Salomonsen-Sautel, S., and Baker, D. N. (2006). Lesbian, gay, and bisexual homeless youth: An eight-city public health perspective. *Child Welfare, 85*(2), 151.

Van Oss, T., Condoluci, S., and Annino, R. (2018). Homelessness and the role of occupational therapy. *SIS Quarterly Practice Connections, 3*(2), 11–13.

Walls, N. E., and Bell, S. (2011). Correlates of engaging in survival sex among homeless youth and young adults. *Journal of Sex Research, 48*(5), 423–436.

Whiteford, G. (2000). Occupational deprivation: Global challenge in the new millennium. *British Journal of Occupational Therapy, 63*(5), 200–204.

Whiteford, M. (2010). Hot tea, dry toast, and the responsibilization of homeless people. *Social Policy and Society, 19,* 193–205.

World Federation of Occupational Therapists. (2006). *Position statement human rights.* Retrieved from www.wfot.org/AboutUs/PositionStatements.aspx

World Federation of Occupational Therapists. (2010). *Statement on Occupational Therapy.* Retrieved from www.wfot.org/Portals/0/PDF/STATEMENT%20ON%20OCCUPATIONAL%20THERAPY%20300811.pdf

Zufferey, C., and Kerr, L. (2004). Identity and everyday experiences of homelessness: Some implications for social work. *Australian Social Work, 57*(4), 343–353.

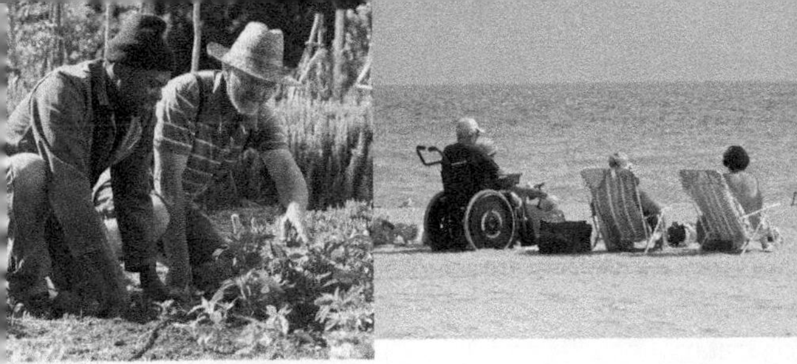

SECTION VII

Rehabilitation and Participation

Chapter 21

Community Reintegration Services for Military Veterans

Marjorie E. Scaffa, PhD, OTR/L, FAOTA, Jeremy Fletcher, PT, DPT, OCS, Major, U.S. Army Reserve, and John F. Kilpatrick, MSW, Lieutenant Colonel, U.S. Army Reserve

With malice toward none; with charity for all; with firmness in the right, as God gives us to see the right, let us strive on to finish the work we are in; to bind up the nation's wounds; to care for him who shall have borne the battle, and for his widow, and his orphan—to do all which may achieve and cherish a just, and a lasting peace, among ourselves, and with all nations.

–Abraham Lincoln, Second Inaugural Address, 1865

Learning Outcomes

This chapter is designed to enable the reader to:

21-1 Appreciate the impact of military culture and the context of military service on reintegration into civilian life.
21-2 Describe common mental and physical health conditions with which Veterans return home.
21-3 Illustrate how various aspects of the transition model apply to Veteran reintegration.
21-4 Compare the transitions experienced by the Veteran to those experienced by the family upon the service member's return home.
21-5 Discuss the impact of reintegration on occupational performance and participation.
21-6 Describe evidence-based evaluation and intervention strategies appropriate for this population.
21-7 Appreciate the importance of a population-based approach to community reintegration for Veterans.

Key Terms

Anticipated transitions
Chronic pain
Community (re)integration
Complicated grief
Deployment
Moral injury
Nonevent transitions
Occupational deprivation
Occupational disruption
Occupational imbalance
Peer support specialist
Polytrauma
Polytrauma triad
Transitions
Unanticipated transitions
Veteran identity

Introduction

Returning from extended deployments or transitioning to live outside military installations requires Veterans and their families to adapt and reintegrate into their new communities. Reintegration into the civilian community post-deployment can be a complex, lengthy, and nonlinear adjustment process involving changes in life relationships and responsibilities. In the rehabilitation literature, community integration refers to "being part of the mainstream of family and community life, discharging normal roles and responsibilities, and being an active and contributing member of one's social groups and of society as a whole" (Dijkers, 1998, p. 1). **Community (re)integration** (CR) as it relates to Veterans refers to "returning to participation in home, social and community living after deployment and, in many cases, after injury" (Hawkins, McGuire, Linder, and Britt, 2015, p. 527) and being "happily situated, productively occupied, and effectively supported in the community" (McColl, Davies, Carlson, Johnston, and Minnes, 2001, p. 429). **Deployment** refers to the movement of military personnel and equipment into places where they can be used when needed. The focus of this chapter is on military service members who were deployed and are returning from war zones in the Middle East. However, many of the topics covered in the chapter could easily be applied to Veterans who served in other conflicts.

Over 2,700,000 service members have served on 5,400,000 individual deployments in support of overseas military operations since September 11, 2001, with nearly half of these being from the U.S. Army (including the Reserve and National Guard). The majority of soldiers were deployed at least two to three times, with Special Forces deploying even more frequently (McCarthy, 2018). Of those who have served, approximately 200,000 persons will transition annually from military life to new civilian roles and responsibilities.

Although many military service members adjust seamlessly into civilian life, others struggle to transition back into family life, work, and community. It is not uncommon for those returning home after long deployments to experience disruption in daily life occupations, habits, roles, and routines. When working with Veterans who are transitioning to civilian life, occupational therapy practitioners have the knowledge and skills to:

- Foster Veterans' engagement in health-enhancing occupations, habits, roles, and routines
- Promote mental health
- Enable occupational participation
- Encourage community reintegration
- Facilitate the recovery process (American Occupational Therapy Association [AOTA], 2018)

The military has its own culture, with a distinct set of values and norms, which is significantly different from mainstream society. Therefore, the CR process could be considered a cross-cultural transition, making it multidimensional and highly complex (Zarecky, 2014). Although initial military training is designed to facilitate the transition into military culture, there is no corresponding mechanism to assist Veterans in successfully reintegrating into civilian life. To work effectively with Veterans, it is important to understand military culture, the context of their overseas military deployment, the physical and mental health conditions with which they return home, and the psychosocial stressors they experience.

Military Culture

Military culture has been described as more delineated than most cultures, having an overt set of values and normative behaviors and a code of ethics supported by its own judicial system. Individuals seek military service for a variety of reasons, such as a desire to serve their country and improve their employment prospects. Some feel compelled to serve to fulfill a sense of legacy established by previous familial service, while others seek to escape from adverse childhood experiences. While reasons for service may vary, each service member enters into an indoctrination process that often challenges an individual's worldview.

Military cultural competence is essential to caring for the biopsychosocial needs of military and Veteran populations (Meyer, Writer, and Brim, 2016). Veterans continue to be seen in many sectors of the health-care system, including both Veterans Health Administration (VHA) and non-VHA facilities. According to the U.S. Census Bureau (n.d.), Veterans experience a disparity in health-care coverage based on age and employment status. For example, in 2016 about one-half of Veterans received medical coverage through Medicare because they were 65 years or older. The other half of Veterans of working age (19 to 64) were covered by employer sponsored, TRICARE, direct purchase, or Medicaid insurance, with 5.5% of Veterans remaining uninsured.

Health care for Veterans is not guaranteed by military service alone. Eligibility and health-care benefits requirements vary by whether or not the Veteran's disability is related to military service (service connection), period of service, employment status, and income.

Since a large portion of Veterans will seek care outside of the VHA system, civilian health-care providers will benefit from additional training on military culture. To address the need for culturally competent care for Veterans, the Uniformed Services University has developed the Center for Deployment Psychology (CDP, n.d.). The mission of the CDP is to lead the development of a community of culturally mindful and clinically competent providers through the delivery of high-quality training and education, the convening of experts, and the dissemination of research-based treatment and the latest topics in military behavioral health. Resources, including self-assessments and health-care provider training, can be found at its website.

In addition to the need for culturally competent care, it is important to understand that health status and health behaviors differ among U.S. military, Veteran, and civilian men. Population data collected in conjunction with the VHA and the Centers for Disease Control and Prevention (CDC) Behavior Risk Factor Surveillance System found that male Veterans reported poorer overall health, health-related functional limitations, and lifetime health conditions (e.g., cardiovascular disease, arthritis, cancer, depression, and anxiety) more frequently than civilian men. Given these findings, efforts to address health disparities among Veteran populations are critical to improve Veteran well-being (Hoerster et al., 2012). Very little information specific to female Veterans is available.

Recent Military Combat Deployments

Military operations in Afghanistan began on October 7, 2001, designating the beginning of Operation Enduring Freedom (OEF), also known as the War in Afghanistan. In mid-2002, Congress signed into law authorization for the use of military force against the Saddam Hussein regime in Iraq, resulting in Operation Iraqi Freedom (OIF), also known as the War in Iraq.

Military deployment experiences vary widely by military branch of service, as well as other demographic variables. From 2001 to 2015, the U.S. Army provided approximately 58% of the total deployments. Across all services, there are 528,000 active component service members who have deployed more than three times. Over 80% of those who have deployed are enlisted personnel and 10% are female. On average, deployed persons are under 30 years old, more than half are married, and about half have children at the time of deployment (Wenger, O'Connell, and Cottrell, 2018).

Gulf War–era (1990 through the present) Veterans now comprise the largest demographic of the Veteran population, accounting for nearly 7,200,000 of the 20,000,000 Veterans. According to the U.S.

Department of Veterans Affairs (VA, 2018a), the total Veteran population is predicted to decrease from 20,000,000 in 2017 to 13,600,000 in 2037. As these trends emerge, Veteran culture may be affected by generational differences and race and ethnicity, as well as geographical location from where a service member currently resides. For example, Veterans from underrepresented groups are predicted to increase from 23.3% of the total Veteran population in 2017 to 32.8% in 2037, as the proportion of white Veterans declines. Additionally, 50% of Veterans live within 10 states, with the largest concentration residing in the West and South (VA, 2018a). Understanding the nuances of Veteran culture should better inform community health promotion programming, resulting in improved health outcomes.

Polytrauma

Compared to other conflicts, recent advances in battlefield medicine and protective armor have improved the ability of OIF/OEF Veterans to survive common mechanisms of injury, including small arms fire and explosive munitions (e.g., blasts from improvised explosive devices [IEDs]). Although lives have been saved, **polytrauma,** defined as "two or more injuries to physical regions or organ systems one of which may be life threatening, resulting in physical, cognitive, psychological, or psychosocial impairments and functional disability," has become the signature injury of the Wars in Iraq and Afghanistan (VA, n.d., para. 2). The **polytrauma triad** of mild traumatic brain injury (mTBI), chronic pain, and posttraumatic stress disorder (PTSD) have proven to be a difficult diagnostic and therapeutic challenge for the current medical system (Cifu et al., 2014). To address these challenges, the VHA Polytrauma System of Care has been established to provide an integrated network of specialized rehabilitation programs dedicated to serving Veterans and service members with both combat- and civilian-related traumatic brain injury (TBI) and polytrauma.

mTBI is experienced by 12% to 23% of Veterans who served in Afghanistan and Iraq. The VA definition of traumatic brain injury is "a traumatically induced structural injury and/or physiological disruption of brain function as a result of an external force" (O'Neil et al., 2013a, para. 1). External forces may include forces generated by a blast or explosion, the head being hit by an object or the head striking an object, or a foreign object penetrating the brain. mTBI is characterized by loss of consciousness for 0 to 30 minutes, altered mental state of a moment up to 24 hours, posttraumatic amnesia of 0 to 1 day, and a Glasgow Coma Scale score of 13 to 15 in the first 24 hours (O'Neil et al., 2013a).

Many Veterans recover spontaneously from mTBI within 3 months; however, 10% to 20% continue to experience long-term symptoms. Cognitive symptoms may include difficulties with attention, concentration, and visuospatial abilities. Physical symptoms may include headaches, pain, vestibular (balance) problems, and hearing and vision impairments. Other problems experienced by Veterans with mTBI include higher unemployment than their counterparts without TBI and moderate to severe sleep disturbance (O'Neil et al., 2013b).

According to the Institute of Medicine (2011), 25% of the U.S. population experiences chronic pain; however, 50% of Veterans are affected by chronic pain. The prevalence of moderate to severe chronic pain in the Veteran population is approximately 27%. **Chronic pain** is defined as "ongoing or recurrent pain, lasting beyond the usual course of acute illness or injury or more than 3 to 6 months, and which adversely affects the individual's wellbeing" (American Chronic Pain Association, n.d., para. 1). Chronic pain is pain without biological value that has persisted past the expected time for tissue healing. Of the types of chronic pain, musculoskeletal (61%) and back pain (24%) have the highest prevalence in VA primary care settings. Factors associated with chronic pain in both Veteran and civilian populations are lower levels of education, smoking, and emotional distress (Van Den Kerkhof, Carley, Hopman, Ross-White, and Harrison, 2014).

Chronic pain can affect many aspects of function (physical, emotional, and social) and has an impact on a variety of facets of a person's life. A person's perception of and response to pain are influenced by the dynamic and reciprocal interactions of biological, psychological, and sociological variables. Chronic pain is considered a complex biopsychosocial condition and therefore must be addressed holistically. Unremitting chronic pain increases the risk of substance abuse, depression, and suicide among Veterans (Blakey et al., 2018).

In addition to the polytrauma triad, extremity injuries are also very common; 54% of evacuated wounded service members have extremity injuries, and 26% of all extremity war injuries involve fractures. The majority of combat casualties are the result of a blast injury. After sustaining a fracture from a blast injury, casualties are evacuated from the theater of operations (i.e., the region in which military actions are in progress), medically stabilized, and returned to a definitive care facility, where management may include amputation or limb salvage. In a 4-year retrospective cohort study of 324 service members deployed to Afghanistan and Iraq who sustained a lower-limb injury requiring either amputation or limb salvage, patients were found to score significantly lower than population norms on the Short Musculoskeletal Function Assessment (SMFA). Compared to civilian populations with similar injury types, patients who received amputations reported higher functional outcomes than those with limb salvage. Additionally, several other factors had significant influence on functional outcomes. Higher military rank was positively correlated with a lower probability of depression and PTSD and with a higher probability of working/on active duty or in school and being engaged in vigorous activities. More intense combat experiences were associated with worse functional scores and a higher likelihood of PTSD. Strength of social support was a strong and consistent correlate of both physical and psychosocial functioning (Finley et al., 2015).

These findings highlight the need for a comprehensive, biopsychosocial approach to the rehabilitation of Veterans and military service members. While these wounds of war may take time to heal, the health-care system has learned valuable lessons surrounding the necessity to function within an interdisciplinary team to help Veterans achieve optimal mental, physical, and emotional recovery. Occupational therapy practitioners are particularly adept at integrating all of these aspects in recovery to improve or restore the functional performance of persons who have sustained polytrauma and enable them to participate in valued roles and activities at home, at school, in the workplace, and in the community (AOTA, 2014a).

Mental Health Conditions

According to the Defense Health Agency, the prevalence of active duty service members (ADSM) diagnosed with any mental health condition varies by military force (i.e., Army, Navy, Air Force, Marines) and has increased from 2005 to 2012, with a reported decline from 2013 to 2016. For example, the peak point prevalence for ADSM was 30% in 2013. The most common diagnoses across all services include anxiety disorders (5%), depressive disorders (7%), insomnia (5%), and PTSD (2.5%). Other diagnoses related to alcohol and substance abuse ranged from 0% to 1.5% (Crum-Cianflone, Powell, LeardMann, Russell, and Boyko, 2016).

The prevalence of mental health conditions among Veterans is much higher than in active-duty military service members and civilian populations. The 12-month prevalence of mental health disorders in a population of 4,400,000 Veterans seeking care through the VHA was found to be 25.7% for one of five mental health conditions: major depressive disorder (13.5%), PTSD (9.3%), substance use disorder (8.3%), anxiety disorders (4.8%), and serious mental illness, such as schizophrenia and bipolar disorder (3.7%). Mental health conditions often present with medical comorbidities, including pain (43%), hypertension (33%), and diabetes (32%; Trivedi et al., 2015).

PTSD and depression are major risk factors for suicide among Veterans. Other risk factors include "feelings of being a burden or lack of belonging during the transition to Veteran status, social isolation, and relationship problems" (Kashiwa, Sweetman, and Helgeson, 2017, p. 1). According to the VA (2018b), 20 Veterans die each day by suicide. Male Veterans ages 18 to 34 have the highest rates, and 69% of all Veteran suicide deaths are by firearms. The suicide rate among female Veterans is 1.8 times higher than non-Veteran adult women and 1.4 times higher among male Veterans compared to their non-Veteran counterparts (VA, 2018b). The Veteran suicide rate is increasing at a faster pace than civilian suicide (VA, 2016). In a sample of over 1,700 Veterans, 51% reported the loss of a friend to suicide. Veterans who know someone who has committed suicide are at higher risk for suicide, and the closer the suicide decedent, the higher the risk (Hom, Stanley, Gutierrez, and Joiner, 2017). There is a high likelihood that occupational therapy practitioners will encounter Veterans in a variety of practice settings. Therefore, Kashiwa et al. (2017) advocate entry-level programs to prepare graduates for the real possibility of encountering clients, both Veterans and non-Veterans, at risk for suicide.

Psychosocial Stressors

Even if service members return home without any physical injuries or diagnosable mental health disorders, they are likely to be coping with a variety of psychosocial stressors that produce confusion, frustration, and distress. These include but are not limited to grief and bereavement, loss of military self-identity, and moral injury. If these concerns are not addressed, significant mental health problems can result.

Grief and Bereavement

Reports indicate that nearly 90% of bereaved Veterans knew someone seriously injured or killed during their most recent deployment. Among soldiers returning home from combat, over 20% reported difficulty coping with grief 6 months later. The death of a team member in combat can be as emotionally significant as losing a close family member. Grief has been linked to negative health outcomes and functional impairment (Mobbs and Bonanno, 2018; Toblin et al., 2012).

In a study by Toblin et al. (2012), infantry brigade soldiers experiencing combat-related grief were at least 2.4 times more likely to experience negative health outcomes as those who reported no difficulty with grief. The top five physical health symptoms reported by those having difficulty coping with grief were fatigue (58.1%), sleep problems (55.4%), musculoskeletal pain (49.7%), back pain (41.3%), and headaches (32.7%). Other symptoms associated with grief included feeling easily annoyed or irritated (62.3%), concentration problems (37.3%), and memory problems (24.0%). Toblin et al. (2012) indicated it was the emotional reaction of grief, rather than the actual experience of loss, that was associated with diminished physical health.

Not everyone who experiences a loss has trouble coping with grief; therefore, interventions should be specifically directed at persons distressed by grief and loss. The majority of bereaved individuals return to previous levels of functioning without intervention. However, for those with **complicated grief** (CG), individual and group intervention may prove beneficial. CG is a persistent and impairing condition, often in response to a traumatic death, that is characterized by intense emotional pain and sorrow, avoidance of reminders of the deceased, role and identity confusion, and a wish not to live without the deceased. Although some of the symptoms of CG overlap with depression and PTSD and these conditions often co-occur, CG can arise independently from these mental disorders (Simon et al., 2018).

A study by Simon et al. (2018) found that 31% of Veterans with PTSD in a sample of 204 met the criteria for CG. The prevalence of CG was higher among those who had lost a fellow service member (FSM; nearly half of the study participants) than those who had not. CG in this Veteran population was associated with elevated levels of trauma-related guilt and distress, higher PTSD severity scores, and greater impairment in psychosocial functioning. In addition, Veterans with CG were not more likely to report current suicidal ideation; however, they were more likely to report one or more lifetime suicide attempts compared to those without CG. Exposure to the death of an FSM was associated with double the rate of CG when compared to other losses. Many Veterans may not initiate discussion about the death of an FSM with a health-care professional; therefore, it is important to specifically ask this question during evaluation interviews and screen for associated grief reactions (Simon et al., 2018).

Loss of Military Self/Identity

The process of training for the armed services strips away a person's civilian identity and requires rapid adjustment to a regimented lifestyle. Recruits are not only trained in the tasks and skills needed for service but also indoctrinated into the military culture. Military culture emphasizes duty, honor, loyalty, discipline, readiness, accountability, dedication, commitment to comrades, and unit cohesiveness. These values and experiences become a central component of a service member's military identity, which does not easily translate into civilian life (Demers, 2011). Veterans often reflect on their military service as a time that fostered personal maturation (93%), teamwork and collaboration (90%), and self-confidence (90%; Pew Research Center [PRC], 2011).

Veteran identity has been defined as a "Veteran's self-concept that derives from his or her military experience within a sociohistorical context" (Harada et al., 2002, p. 118). Combat experiences have lifelong influences on Veterans. Veteran identity is affected by sociocultural factors, such as race, ethnicity, gender, education, military status (i.e., rank, branch of service), combat exposure, and the time period (war era) in which the service occurred. While in the military, Veterans were highly trained, respected in their roles, and believed they had a purpose. Upon returning home, Veterans often feel misunderstood and disrespected by civilians who have difficulty comprehending and appreciating the Veterans' combat experiences. These changes in status can precipitate a loss of self-esteem and self-worth. There can be significant disparity between their military identity and who they are expected to be in the civilian world. Even though they were civilians before entering the military, due to their training and experiences, Veterans are no longer the same individuals who went off to war. Veterans often hold themselves to higher standards than the typical civilian. Creating an effective hybrid or integrated identity requires incorporating both "military and civilian cultural knowledge, values and practices" (Demers, 2011, p. 174).

The "warrior" persona and the attitudes and behaviors associated with this identity can translate into a positive or negative reentry into civilian life. For example, the "can-do" attitude may make adjustment more successful if used to learn a new skill but can be detrimental if it prevents needed help-seeking behavior. Newly returning Veterans often need to renegotiate their identities and roles at home as providers, spouses, and parents (Atherton, 2009).

According to Mobbs and Bonnano (2018), "Veterans may experience grief-like symptoms in response to the perceived loss of their military self . . . and the roles, values, and sense of purpose this lifestyle may have held for them" (p. 139). Grief symptoms may be triggered by any loss that affects a person's sense of stability and continuity of life. Grief can result from any event that produces a significant disruption in self-image, self-worth, and/or worldview. Separation from the military, even if done voluntarily, is one such event.

Moral Injury

According to Litz and colleagues (2009), **moral injury** is a consequence of "perpetrating, failing to prevent, bearing witness to acts that transgress deeply held moral beliefs and expectations" (p. 695). Acts that may precipitate moral injury include incidents causing harm to civilians during war, friendly fire deaths, military sexual assaults, and betrayals by leadership. Moral injury is a "broad clinical concept that exists in the intersection of multiple emotional, cognitive and social pathways" (Farnsworth, Drescher, Nieuwsma, Walser, and Currier, 2014, p. 258). It is a state of inner conflict and turmoil that often precipitates feelings of shame, guilt, grief, anxiety, anger, and remorse. Other reactions include purposelessness and alienation from self and others. Behavioral manifestations of moral injury may include self-harm, social withdrawal, substance abuse, and social instability. Although moral injury and PTSD have some common characteristics, "each has unique components that make them separable consequences of war" (Maguen and Litz, 2012, para. 6). PTSD is emotionally characterized by fear, while moral injury is emotionally characterized by shame. Moral injury can co-occur with depression and substance use disorder, as well as in the absence of active PTSD symptoms (Farnsworth et al., 2014).

Other manifestations of moral injury identified by Drescher et al. (2011) include social and relationship problems, difficulty trusting others, self-deprecation, a sense of betrayal, and spiritual and/or existential issues, such as a loss of faith and a sense of meaninglessness. Currier, Holland, and Malott (2015) postulate that experiences of moral injury may disrupt the coherence and stability of a Veteran's sense of global meaning. Global meaning refers to "a person's fundamental beliefs/values, goals, and subjective sense of purpose—all of which function together to infuse life with security and significance" (p. 231). As a result of the damage to this sense of global meaning, a Veteran may have difficulty maintaining "predeployment values and goals and regaining a sense of purpose and hope about the future," which can complicate adjustment to civilian life (Currier et al., 2015, p. 237).

In order to repair moral injury and experience spiritual renewal, the following three aspects of intervention appear to be useful:

- Emotional and psychological processing of the morally injurious event and its impact
- Exposure to and participation in positive moral experiences, such as giving and receiving love and engaging in altruistic behaviors
- Fostering reparation and the practice of forgiveness of self and others (Litz et al., 2009)

In addition, interventions that promote mindfulness and elicit positive moral emotions may enhance psychological, social, and spiritual functioning. Mindfulness practices may include sitting and walking meditations and yoga, among others (see Fig. 21-1). Mindfulness helps to focus attention, increase body awareness, and enhance emotion regulation. Nonjudgmental awareness of self can reduce emotional distress, including self-blame, and thereby make psychological change possible (Kopacz et al., 2016).

The experience of positive emotions, particularly compassion (including self-compassion), elevation, and pride, may assist in moral injury repair, increase cognitive flexibility, and promote social cohesion. Compassion is the desire to ameliorate the suffering of another; elevation is the feeling of warmth one gets from witnessing human goodness or moral beauty; and pride is the sense of the self as being good, competent, and virtuous. Providing opportunities and contexts to practice mindfulness and experience these emotions can be an important aspect of intervention (Farnsworth et al., 2014).

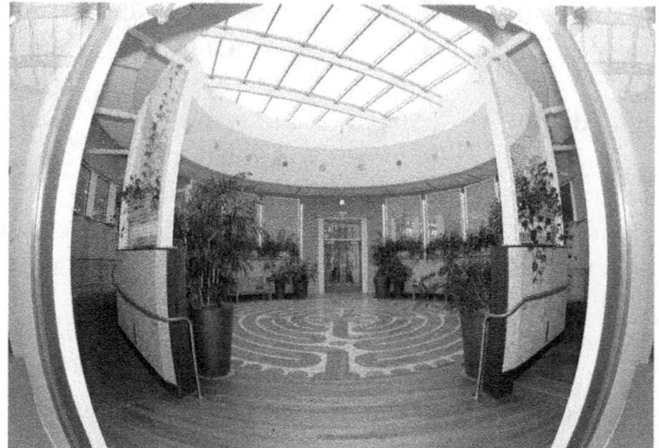

Figure 21-1 A labyrinth for mindful walking at the Walter Reed National Military Medical Center. *(Photo courtesy of the National Intrepid Center of Excellence, Walter Reed National Military Medical Center.)*

Reintegration Into Civilian Life

The majority of people who serve in the military do not make it a career. Military service often occurs during the developmental stage between high school and adult life. Even those who leave the military after a career of 20 years or more are likely to transition into civilian work roles, as they are typically underage for retirement or have too small a pension to live comfortably (Kelty, Kleykamp, and Segal, 2010).

Approximately 44% of Veterans who have served since the 2001 terrorist attacks report that reentry into civilian life has been difficult for them. According to a study by the PRC (2011), four factors were associated with a more difficult readjustment experience. These included:

- Being seriously injured in the line of duty
- Serving in the military while married
- Knowing someone who was killed or seriously injured in military service
- Experiencing a traumatic event during military service

Of the Veterans who have served since September 11, 2001, 43% report having had a military-related experience that was emotionally traumatic, and nearly half of these Veterans say they have suffered from posttraumatic stress as a result. Veterans who reported a relatively easy transition were more likely to be commissioned officers, have a college degree, and attend religious services a least once a week. Variables that appear to have no effect on ease of transition were race/ethnicity, length of service, age at discharge, and number of deployments (Morin, 2011).

Moving out of a military culture, with its hierarchical structure that has clear rules and expectations, into a civilian culture that appears to be lacking order and predictability can be very challenging. Knobloch and Theiss (2012) suggest that many of "the very behaviors that may be functional during deployment may be dysfunctional during reintegration" (p. 445). In order to understand the challenges Veterans face and facilitate their reentry into society, an understanding of the transition process is helpful.

Transitions Model

Transitions are turning points between two periods of relative stability. **Transitions** are life events or nonevents that require change, changes in relationships, assumptions, roles, and/or routines. Transitions provide unique challenges and opportunities for growth, adaptation, and transformation. They are frequently stressful even when freely chosen and deemed desirable. Moving through a transition requires relinquishing aspects of the self and former roles and learning new skills and developing a new identity. Multiple transitions can occur simultaneously, and often do. Transitions can be normative, anticipated, and expected or unpredictable, unanticipated, and unexpected (Anderson, Goodman, and Schlossberg, 2012).

Anticipated transitions are typically normative, meaning they predictably occur during the life course, and the vast majority of people experience them. Anticipated transitions are often self-initiated and planned; there is usually time to prepare. Examples of anticipated transitions are graduation, marriage, starting a job, the birth of a child, and retirement. **Unanticipated transitions** are nonnormative, have a low probability of occurrence, and often involve crises. Unanticipated transitions are outside of one's control and offer little or no opportunity to prepare. Unanticipated transitions may occur at the individual, family, community, or societal level. Examples of unanticipated transitions are divorce, the premature death of a spouse, the death of a child, natural and technological disasters, being laid off or fired from a job, war, and terrorism.

Nonevent transitions are expected or hoped for events that did not occur. These nonevent transitions also alter a person's life and require change and adaptation. The four types of nonevents are personal, ripple, resultant, and delayed. Personal nonevents are those individual aspirations that are not realized—for example, never marrying or having a baby or not being promoted. Ripple nonevents are personal nonevents of people close to us that require us to change or adapt—for example, a spouse not receiving a promotion at work. Resultant nonevents are the result of some event that occurs that causes an aspiration or expectation to remain unfulfilled. The event itself has a beginning and an end, but the nonevent lasts a lifetime—for example, not graduating from college because of an acquired brain injury due to an automobile crash. Delayed nonevents are those events that do not happen at the expected or desired time but are still hoped for and aspired to. The demarcation of when a dream delayed becomes a nonevent is idiosyncratic (Anderson et al., 2012).

In addition to the type of transition, additional factors determine the influence a transition has on a person's life. These factors are perspective, context, and impact. The person's appraisal and perception of the event or transition is critical. Does the person perceive the event/transition or nonevent as positive, negative, or benign? The same transition might be perceived as an opportunity by one person and as a crisis and disaster to another person. Context refers to the setting in which the transition takes place. Contextual factors can influence a person's appraisal of an event or transition and the person's response to it. Differences in access to resources, for example, can have an impact on one's ability to successfully navigate transitions. Impact can be positive or negative and refers to the degree to which the transition alters one's daily life. The greater the impact, the more coping resources are needed and the longer it will take for adaptation and assimilation. Understanding the meaning of a transition for a particular individual requires an assessment of the type of transition being experienced, the perspective the person holds regarding the transition, the context in which the transition is occurring, and the impact of the transition on the person's life (Anderson et al., 2012).

Reintegration Transitions for Veterans

A recent survey of active duty service members and Veterans identified the most significant challenges of the transition from military to civilian life as navigating VA programs, benefits, and services (60%); finding a job (55%); adjusting to civilian culture (41%); addressing financial challenges (40%); and applying military-learned skills to civilian life (39%; Zoli, Maury, and Fay, 2015).

Transitions require adapting to unanticipated gains and inescapable losses across many areas of life. In the highly structured military setting, in contrast to civilian life, all of the basic necessities, such as food, clothing, housing, work, health care, and social life, are provided (Zarecky, 2014). In a research study by Ahern et al. (2015), nearly half of the Veterans reported that the military structure "provided clarity and simplicity to decisions and procedures" (p. 5). Civilian life may seem chaotic to the Veteran, and attempting to impose structure and organization may feel overwhelming. The majority of service members entered the military during the developmental period of emerging adulthood (ages 18 to 25). Approximately half of active duty service members are 25 years of age or younger. When leaving the service, they may not have developed the life skills necessary to assume societal roles in the civilian sector (Resnick et al., 2012). In addition, they may lack confidence and clarity regarding what to do next (Zarecky, 2014). However, they often have strengths, of which they may be unaware, developed in the military to draw upon during the transition.

Even for those who have highly evolved life skills, the expectations and demands of reintegration can be daunting. Challenging transitions for Veterans during reintegration include leaving behind a built-in social support system, a steady income, and accessible resources. In the military, each person is part of a team, and each team member is important. Team members become as close as, if not more so than, family members. Leaving active duty means leaving a support system, which may feel much like abandonment and isolation and can have a profoundly negative effect on mental health (Anderson and Goodman, 2014).

Veterans may experience a return to civilian life and culture as alien, as many aspects of civilian life no longer feel normal to them. This is due to the reality that the Veteran, the family, and the home environment have changed while the service member was deployed. Veterans may feel disconnected from family and friends who have not shared the deployment experience. This is one reason they may gravitate toward and spend more time with military "buddies" than with family members (Sayer et al., 2011). Feelings of alienation increase the likelihood of engaging in risky behaviors that hinder reintegration and diminish well-being. Frequently, Veterans and their family members experience a mismatch between their expectations and reality when the person returns home. Adjustment requires time, patience, and the establishment of a "new normal" that satisfies the needs of the Veteran and the family (Ahern et al., 2015).

Some Veterans report feeling that they no longer matter. Mattering means "having attention paid to you, having a sense of importance, being appreciated, having people who depend on you, and having pride in what you do" (Anderson and Goodman, 2014, p. 42). Family members may have learned to manage without them, and employers may not value their military experience. Approximately half of the Veterans interviewed by Ahern et al. (2015) experienced civilian life as meaningless in comparison to combat missions. These feelings are intensified when Veterans cannot find meaningful work that utilizes their skills and values their contribution to the team.

Female Veterans may face some unique challenges. Among female Veterans, the rate of military sexual trauma is estimated to be in the 20% to 30% range (Kelty et al., 2010). The experience of sexual trauma can negatively affect female Veterans' physical and emotional health, relationships with family and friends, and ability to work, making successful readjustment to civilian life less likely (Katz, Bloor, Cojucar, and Draper, 2007).

The transition to civilian life is further compounded by the disconnect between service members and the general public; 84% of Gulf War–era Veterans believe the civilian population does not understand the challenges and problems faced by service members, Veterans, and their families. This belief is shared by 71% of the general public (PRC, 2011). However, "soldiers and Veterans are undeniably resilient, both by selection and by training" (Mobbs and Bonanno, 2018, p. 142).

Reintegration Transitions for Families

The U.S. Department of Defense (2016) estimates that nearly 35% of military personnel are married with children, 16% are married without children, and more than 6% are single parents. Every member of the family can be significantly affected by the prolonged separations associated with combat deployments, creating strain when the service member

Box 21-1 10 Categories of Relationship Change (% of thematic units in qualitative data)

Relationship is stronger (18%)
Value the relationship more (14.7%)
Problems reconnecting (11.8%)
Difficulty communicating (10.9%)
Increased autonomy (10.4%)
Changes in finances and employment (9.5%)
Changes in sexual behavior (7.6%)
Problems reintegrating the service member into daily life (5.7%)
Heightened conflict (5.7%)
Separation or divorce (5.7%)

Data from "Experiences of U.S. Military Couples During the Post-Deployment Transition: Applying the Relational Turbulence Model," by L. K. Knobloch and J. A. Theiss, 2012, *Journal of Social and Personal Relationships, 29*(4), 430–434.

returns home (Cogan, 2014). Although many military couples and families eagerly await a joyful reunion upon return from deployment, the transition and reintegration into family life is challenging for the family as well as the Veteran. Relationship distress and emotional turmoil are not uncommon during the 6 months following a return from a tour of duty (Knobloch and Theiss, 2012). In a study of 250 individuals, half of whom were in the military and half of whom were partners of service members (not necessarily matched couples), participants identified several ways their relationships had changed after deployment. These changes are listed in Box 21-1 (Knobloch and Theiss, 2012). Role changes affect both male and female Veterans. However, upon returning home, women Veterans face the civilian expectation of "traditional" caregiver female gender roles. In the military, women often work in job positions that would typically be considered male domains in the civilian world, thus making reintegration more challenging.

Upon return from deployment, service members and spouses expressed relationship uncertainty. Research participants expressed concerns about commitment, reintegration, household stressors, personality changes in partners, sexual behavior and infidelity, communication problems, and the service member's mental health. They also identified ways in which their partners made it more difficult to complete everyday activities. Interference from partners took a variety of forms, including differences in parenting, control issues, spending time with family and friends, and household chores. It is notable that participants' descriptions of the reentry transition were consistent across age, marital status, relationship length, length of deployment, and military branch (Knobloch and Theiss, 2012). The primary underlying theme regarding the transition was the need for changes in family members' occupational performance patterns (i.e., habits, routines, rituals, roles) upon the service member's return, a distinct opportunity for occupational therapy intervention (AOTA, 2014b).

Importance of Veteran Peer Support

Veterans experiencing anguish related to the mental, physical, emotional, and spiritual wounds of war tend to isolate themselves from society. The existing research indicates that successful recovery occurs when facilitated by social support within the context of a community. Peer support services provide a flexible and adaptable solution to address the current needs of Veterans and guide them along their path to recovery. However, peer support services are a complement to, not a substitute for, professional care. In this context peers are individuals who are stable in their recovery from mental illness and/or addiction and use their lived experience to promote mind-body recovery and resilience. A peer has the ability to extend care beyond the walls of the clinic, entering into the everyday life of the Veteran. Peers can participate in recovery centers, religious institutions, child welfare organizations, recovery homes, drug courts, behavioral health agencies, and other community organizations (see Fig. 21-2). Peers serve in

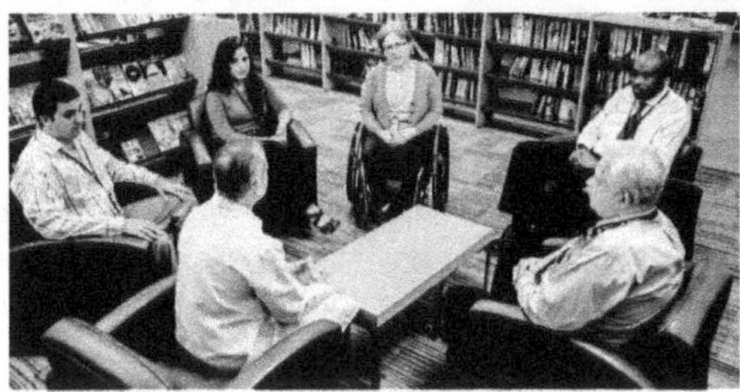

Figure 21-2 Peer support. *(Courtesy of the U.S. Department of Veterans Affairs.)*

the roles of allies and advocates on the road to recovery. Both parties in a peer relationship reap the benefits of their interactions, and the recovery of each is strengthened (Substance Abuse and Mental Health Services Administration [SAMHSA], 2009).

A **peer support specialist** "is a person who uses his or her lived experience of recovery from mental illness and/or addiction, plus skills learned in formal training, to deliver services in behavioral health settings to promote mind-body recovery and resiliency" (SAMHSA, n.d., para. 1). Peer specialists receive training in peer support competencies and must pass an exam to become certified. Peer support services have been designated by the Centers for Medicare and Medicaid Services (CMS) as an evidence-based practice. Services delivered by certified peer specialists have been shown to increase active engagement in treatment, reduce recurrent hospitalizations, improve relationships with health-care providers, enhance self-management skills, and reduce health-care costs. In some states, the services provided by a certified peer specialist are reimbursable (Daniels, Ashenden, Goodale, and Stevens, 2016).

SAMHSA, the leading national authority on mental health recovery, has identified four types of social support (emotional, informational, instrumental, affiliational) peers can provide within the context of community (see Table 21-1). Combining these types of peer support is more powerful than using any one type alone. For example, for a Veteran who is considering going to college, a peer specialist might:

- Offer a list of websites for colleges in the area (informational support)
- Provide transportation to a college for the Veteran to talk to a person in the Admissions Office (instrumental support)
- Connect the Veteran with a peer who is already enrolled at that university (affiliational support)
- Encourage and support the Veteran in applying to a college (emotional support)

Peer support programs can offer a variety of services, including providing supportive peer mentoring or coaching, facilitating connections with recovery resources in the community, leading recovery education and support groups, and building a

Table 21-1 Type of Social Support and Associated Peer Recovery Support Services

Type of Support	Description	Peer Support Service Example
Emotional	Demonstrate empathy, caring, or concern to bolster person's self-esteem and confidence	Peer mentoring Peer-led support groups
Informational	Share knowledge and information and/or provide life or vocational skills training	Parenting class Job readiness class Wellness seminar
Instrumental	Provide concrete assistance to help others accomplish tasks	Childcare Transportation Help accessing community health and social services
Affiliation	Facilitate contacts with other people to promote learning of social and recreational skills, create community, and acquire a sense of belonging	Recovery centers Sports league participation Alcohol and drug-free socialization opportunities

From *What Are Peer Recovery Support Services?* (p. 2), by Substance Abuse and Mental Health Services Administration, HHS Publication No. (SMA) 09-4454, 2009.

social network and community of recovery. Peer support services can be adapted to meet the needs of people at different stages of the recovery process: prior to formal treatment to increase motivation for change, as an adjunct to treatment to provide a connection to the community, following treatment for relapse prevention, and apart from treatment for those who cannot or choose not to enter the formal treatment system.

Regardless of the services provided, effective peer support programs share certain values, including:

- Maintaining a focus on recovery rather than on pathology or diagnoses
- Embracing diversity and inclusion, recognizing there are many routes to recovery
- Involving the recovery community in the design, implementation, and evaluation of the program
- Recognizing the power of mutuality in peer relationships to engender hope and motivation for recovery
- Building leadership capacity among members of the recovery community and empowering them to guide and direct the program

Peer recovery support services incorporate a strengths-based approach to build resiliency and capacity rather than focus on correcting deficits, disabilities, or problems. The process begins with a conversation about the peer's values, interests, goals, and abilities. Once a person's goals are clear, the peer specialist can help the peer identify the resources and skills necessary to achieve those objectives. In addition, peer support programs share a philosophy of self-direction, choice, and empowerment. Individuals seeking recovery are believed to be fully capable of making informed decisions, and their preferences and choices are respected (SAMHSA, 2009).

Recognizing the importance of peer support and its potential impact on occupational engagement and community reintegration, an occupational therapist who is an Olympic athlete and a Veteran herself established the Veterans Adaptive Sports and Training Program (VAST). She designed the program to help Veterans find friendship and healing and reintegrate into the community as full participants by eliminating as many barriers as possible (Yamkovenko, 2013).

Impact on Occupational Performance and Participation

During deployment, a service member's daily occupations are dictated by the exigencies of military operations. Long work hours, with little discretionary time, are typical of most military deployments. Furthermore, the range of leisure pursuits and the opportunities to engage in them are also typically limited during deployment. Upon returning home, service members have a greater opportunity to select occupations that are meaningful to them and to create their own daily routines. With the absence of structured time, which had been driven by military operation, returning Veterans are now expected to choose, schedule, and engage in self-care, work, and leisure occupations that are personally meaningful. Both during and following deployment, unmet occupational needs can lead to occupational deprivation, imbalance, and/or disruption. **Occupational disruption** "occurs when a person's normal pattern of occupational engagement is disrupted due to significant life events" (Whiteford, 2000, p. 201). Occupational disruptions are typically temporary and can occur due to a variety of situations—for example, moving to a new military base, changing job positions, losing a comrade, or transitioning to civilian life.

Occupational imbalance happens "when a person is unoccupied, underoccupied, or overoccupied" (Brown and Hollis, 2013, p. 1247). A lack of access to leisure or work opportunities can cause occupational imbalance. Occupational imbalance has a detrimental effect on health and well-being. The military is cognizant of the impact of occupational imbalance and goes to great effort to provide opportunities for service members to engage in meaningful leisure and social interaction. **Occupational deprivation** is a "state in which a person or group of people are unable to do what is necessary and meaningful in their lives due to external restrictions" (Whiteford, 2000, p. 200). This is a problem faced by most deployed service members. Physical disability and mental health challenges encountered by Veterans with polytrauma can also preclude active engagement in meaningful occupations, thereby producing occupational deprivation. If unresolved, occupational disruption, imbalance, and deprivation can result in depression, maladaptive coping such as excessive alcohol consumption, and increased potential for suicide (Brown and Hollis, 2013).

Client-Centered Evaluation and Evidenced-Based Intervention Approaches

The occupational therapy literature lacks research evidence regarding effective treatment for Veterans with combat-related mental health issues. As a result, practitioners working with this population are forced "to make treatment decisions without the benefit of supporting evidence of treatment efficacy" (Gerardi, 2017, p. 24). Evidence is included where it exists, but most of the information provided here is based on the authors' combined experience working with this population. The authors are members of a clinical team for a nonprofit, community-based organization called Veterans Recovery Resources (see the Program Showcase).

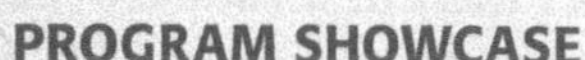

PROGRAM SHOWCASE

Veterans Recovery Resources

Beginning in 2014, several key events sparked action that led to the creation of Veterans Recovery Resources (VRR). The Veterans Access, Choice and Accountability Act of 2014 (Choice Act) became law and created a mechanism to compensate community organizations to treat Veterans. In 2018, two important reports regarding Veterans' health were released. The VA published a report that year stating that an average of 20 Veterans died from suicide each day and only six of these were users of VA services (VA, 2018b). In addition, a research study by the RAND Corporation concluded that only 13% of surveyed civilian providers met all the readiness criteria necessary to deliver culturally competent, quality mental health care to Veterans and their families. This limited cultural competency causes many Veterans to feel their providers do not understand or cannot relate (Tanielian et al., 2018).

Overall, while the VHA will continue to shoulder the primary responsibility in caring for persons who served in the U.S. military, no single organization can be expected to unilaterally address all of the mental health needs of Veterans and their families. Moreover, beyond increasing the quantity of treatment options, there is a need for innovative models of providing culturally sensitive and effective mental health care for Veterans. Looking ahead, community-based mental health services are needed to both complement and augment existing care options from the VHA. Combining the physical, mental, emotional, and moral injuries resulting from sustained combat operations, it is easy to see how the needs of our Veteran population have overwhelmed the current system of care.

The Gulf Coast region has one of the highest concentrations of Veterans in the country (5,000,000), yet there is no Veteran-specific residential substance abuse program in the region. Veterans are being lost to suicide, posttraumatic stress, and substance abuse at an alarming rate. These individuals are not outliers but mainstream professionals who have honorably served our country and deserve our help. VRR aims to address some of these very important gaps in services to Veterans by increasing the local community's capacity to address their needs.

VRR is a nonprofit organization, based in Mobile, Alabama, offering a unique, community-based, integrated model of primary care and mental wellness and substance abuse services developed for Veterans by Veterans. The concept for VRR grew out of the founder's personal, lived experience spanning over 32 years of mental health issues, addiction, military service, multiple deployments, physical injuries, and, most importantly, recovery. Having served first as an enlisted marine during Operations Desert Shield and Desert Storm and then as a Medical Service Corps officer in the U.S. Army, he developed a unique perspective of the military service member and Veteran.

The mission of VRR is "to accelerate Veteran wellbeing by removing barriers to care for Veterans, their families and caregivers suffering from substance abuse, post-traumatic stress and other mental wellness issues" (VRR, 2018, para. 1). VRR is designed to deliver the highest quality, evidence-based, compassionate services to all Veterans who need help regardless of their ability to pay. The goal of VRR is to create a vibrant network of Veterans and their families who support each other over a lifetime and work together to strengthen and contribute to their local communities and economy. VRR provides individual and group counseling, primary medical care, occupational and physical therapy, peer support, care for families, and opportunities for community engagement.

VRR purchased a 3-acre campus with two buildings in midtown Mobile, located in one of the most underserved areas of town, on a major thoroughfare, with a bus stop and easy access. The buildings were dilapidated and historic and qualified for several funding programs. VRR successfully opened an outpatient clinic in November 2018 and served over 50 Veterans and their families in the first 2 months of operation.

First and foremost, VRR was created by Veterans, for Veterans. Veterans make up less than 10% of the total U.S. adult population (Bialik, 2017), which causes many Veterans to believe others will never understand how it feels or what it is like. Military service members are trained in self-sacrifice and teamwork and to focus on accomplishing the mission. They are also taught to care for other members of the team. Transitioning from military service often leaves many service members feeling lost and alone, separated from their team and its support. VRR immediately removes this barrier because the majority of program staff and all of the peer support specialists are Veterans who understand the issues and challenges. This approach accelerates Veterans' recovery.

Second, VRR services are comprehensive and holistic. Experience and research show that Veterans who suffer with addiction, posttraumatic stress, or chronic pain almost always have co-occurring conditions, many of which are medical in nature (Stecher, Fortney, Owen, McGovern, and Williams, 2010). To treat one condition and not the others is counterproductive to the VRR way. The VRR team strives to treat the whole person in a coordinated and client-centered approach, driven by the Veteran. As such, VRR has developed an interprofessional team with expertise in primary care, clinical psychology, physical therapy, occupational therapy, counseling, and social work—all with one goal, to "return to duty," whatever that may be for the individual. VRR's unique, comprehensive three-stage treatment approach starts with a 360° (holistic) assessment of the Veteran's physical, mental, emotional, spiritual, and social well-being. An individual plan is developed that prioritizes the Veteran's goals in all aspects of life. Concurrently, services are offered to family members and caregivers to ensure their recovery as well.

Third, VRR is a community-based program. Many Veterans who have transitioned back to civilian life struggle to find the sense of community they once experienced in the military. Recovery in isolation is difficult; most mental illnesses get worse in isolation—never better. By establishing VRR directly in the community served, barriers separating Veterans from their communities are reduced. Several studies indicate Veterans serve their communities at a much higher rate than nonmilitary citizens. Veterans coach Little League sports, serve in churches, teach, are active in community service, and seek elected positions—it is in the military service member/Veteran DNA to serve. Therefore, community engagement is a significant component of the recovery process.

To ensure a sustainable model for VRR, it is important to provide services that payers are willing to fund. Initially, the goal was to extend and complement the VA and Veterans' service providers with evidence-based, culturally competent treatment by an interprofessional team of health professionals. This proved to be more challenging than expected.

Experience in military medicine frames the philosophy and expectations for how VRR will deliver this unique approach to care. In military medicine (especially in a deployed environment), there is little concern about payment for services. The goal is to treat the service member as effectively as possible so the individual can return to duty. To facilitate this return-to-duty mentality, almost all of the services necessary are located in one place. A team of multidisciplinary providers work together to ensure each service member gets all necessary treatment as quickly as possible in order to return to the fight. Typically, the service members' commanders or first sergeants interact with the treatment team to make sure the treatment plan meets the needs of the member, the unit, and the mission. Those leaders also ensure the service members' compliance, which greatly increases the efficacy of the treatment. At VRR, peer support specialists perform this role.

Despite troubling rates of mental health problems among Veterans, research has consistently revealed that struggling with such issues can lead to posttraumatic growth in the form of improved relationships, hopeful views of the future, enhanced self-confidence, greater appreciation of life, and stronger religious and/or spiritual commitments (Tsai, El-Gabalawy, Sledge, Southwick, and Pietrzak, 2015). While VRR services initially aim to reduce unhealthy coping strategies for managing problems and revisiting painful traumas/losses that might maintain substance use disorders, VRR seeks to cultivate a *recovery ethos* that honors the seeds of growth and character development in each person's pain and suffering. Hence, from the start of seeking care with VRR, Veterans' struggles are honored as sources of both pain and transformative potential. Rather than feeling shame about being "disordered," Veterans will instead be encouraged and challenged to seek a new diagnosis of *posttraumatic growth* in their recovery that can only be gained through healing from deep struggle. In committing to this new mission in life, the VRR way will rely on physical, mental, emotional, and spiritual therapeutic and community-based strategies for Veterans to embark on a recovery journey that will lead to a renewal of pride, belonging, and purpose in life.

VRR rests on the foundational belief that the country needs the strengths, skills, and abilities of military service members and Veterans to make communities stronger. In these ways, the VRR way aims to reclaim healthy aspects of the *warrior ethos* by inviting Veterans into a new mission and a shared sense of identity as sources of integrity, service, and wholeness.

"I am so grateful for everything you guys have done for me and how much I learned. Things are going very well. Back at work and have a good personal routine. Life is definitely easier and I have much more peace. I am thankful for Veterans Recovery Resources and what it has done for me."—Veteran who completed VRR program, December 2018.

In a Delphi study conducted by Gerardi (2017), Canadian occupational therapists ranked theories that could be used for intervention with Veterans with PTSD. The theoretical framework that was most highly supported for this purpose was the Canadian model of occupational performance and engagement (CMOP-E). Other theories identified included the recovery model and the model of human occupation (MOHO). In an earlier study conducted with occupational therapists in the United States, the MOHO was the most highly ranked theoretical framework for potential use as part of a manualized occupational therapy intervention for clients with PTSD (Gerardi, 2016).

Evaluation

Meeting the needs of Veterans and their families begins with a comprehensive evaluation process. This process should include the development of an occupational profile (AOTA, 2014b) and the use of assessments to measure mental health, cognitive function, occupational performance and participation, and community integration. Mental health assessments should include screening for depression, anxiety, PTSD, and substance abuse. Cognitive assessments should be considered for Veterans with mTBI. A list of potentially useful mental health and cognitive assessment tools can be found in Table 21-2.

Regarding occupation-based assessments, Gerardi (2017) found that the majority of occupational therapists endorsed the use of the following assessments for Veterans with PTSD: the Canadian Occupational Performance Measure (COPM), Modified Interest Checklist, Occupational Questionnaire, Self-Efficacy Scale, and Role Checklist. In addition, a significant percentage of occupational therapists recommended a "functional assessment of the impact of stress triggers and avoidance behaviors on occupational functioning" (Gerardi, 2016, p. 41). The COPM identifies occupational performance

Table 21-2 Mental Health and Cognitive Assessment Tools

Mental Health Assessments	Cognitive Assessments
Patient Health Questionnaire-9 (PHQ-9 for depression)	Allen Cognitive Level Screen (ACLS)
Generalized Anxiety Disorder-7 (GAD-7)	Montreal Cognitive Assessment (MOCA)
Alcohol Use Disorders Identification Test (AUDIT)	Bay Area Functional Performance Evaluation (BaFPE)
Drug Abuse Screen Test (DAST)	Toglia Category Assessment (TCA)
PTSD Checklist—Military Version (PCL-M)	Comprehensive Trailmaking Test
SAFE-T (suicide assessment)	Lowenstein OT Cognitive Assessment (LOTCA)
	Brief Traumatic Brain Injury Screen (BTBIS)

From *Asher's Occupational Therapy Assessment Tools: An Annotated Index* (4th ed.), by I. E. Asher, 2014, Bethesda, MD: AOTA Press; *VA/DoD Clinical Practice Guideline for Management of Post-Traumatic Stress*, by U.S. Department of Veterans Affairs, 2010.

problems and measures changes in clients' perception of their performance and satisfaction over time. The COPM is the only occupation-based assessment demonstrated through research to be useful with Veterans who are in the process of reintegrating into civilian life.

In one study, the COPM was used with young Veterans 20 to 29 years old to determine occupational performance challenges they encountered during their first year back in civilian life after service in a combat zone. The majority of difficulties they identified were in the area of self-care, particularly driving, sleeping, and health maintenance. Related to productivity, over 90% of the respondents indicated that transitioning to a student role was a significant obstacle—specifically, having the necessary academic skills to succeed and relating to younger classmates. In the area of leisure, social participation and relationships were often challenging, especially relating to people outside of the Veteran peer network (Plach and Sells, 2013).

The COPM was also used in an interdisciplinary residential treatment program for Veterans with PTSD and TBI and found to be effective in identifying each individual's unique set of goals and as an outcome measure of the efficacy of treatment (Speicher, Walter, and Chard, 2014). Residential program participants identified an average of 3.85 occupational performance areas to address during intervention (Speicher et al., 2014). The most frequently cited problem areas are listed in Box 21-2. Sleep disturbance is highly correlated with suicide among Veterans, which makes it a priority for intervention (Pigeon, Britton, Ilgen, Chapman, and Conner, 2012).

In addition to mental health, cognitive, and occupation-based assessments, evaluation of community integration is an important component of overall well-being and quality of life. From an occupational therapy perspective, community reintegration is a dynamic adaptation process that facilitates participation in culturally appropriate and personally meaningful roles and full engagement in community life. An assessment that may be useful in working with Veterans is the Community Integration Questionnaire (CIQ). The CIQ consists of 15 questions and three subscales (i.e., home integration, social integration, and productivity outside of the home). The questions are designed to ascertain whether the person performs a certain activity alone or with another person. The higher the score, the greater the integration into the community. Although the assessment was originally developed for use with clients with head injuries, it can be adapted for other populations (Dijkers, 2000).

Box 21-2 Occupational Performance Problem Areas Identified by Veterans (in order of frequency)

Rest and sleep
Leisure and social participation
Health management and maintenance
Education participation
Work participation
Household management tasks
Community mobility
Meal planning
Financial management
Volunteer exploration

Data from "Interdisciplinary Residential Treatment of Posttraumatic Stress Disorder and Traumatic Brain Injury: Effects on Symptom Severity and Occupational Performance and Satisfaction," by S. M. Speicher, K. H. Walter, and K. M. Chard, 2014, *American Journal of Occupational Therapy, 68*(4), 412–421.

An instrument specifically designed for Veterans is the Community Reintegration for Service Members (CRIS) assessment. The CRIS was developed based on the International Classification of Functioning, Disability and Health (ICF) and measures both objective and subjective aspects of participation. The assessment has three scales: extent of participation, perceived limitations in participation, and participation satisfaction. Preliminary research has demonstrated good reliability and validity of the instrument (Resnick, Plow, and Jette, 2009). Another tool under development is the Military to Civilian Questionnaire that measures self-perceived difficulties with reintegration into civilian life. The scale consists of 16 items rated on a 5-point scale of no difficulty to extreme difficulty. Sample items include doing what you need to do for work or school, enjoying or making good use of free time, and finding meaning and purpose in life (Sayer et al., 2011).

It is important to recognize that barriers to community reintegration may vary across subgroups. Differences in barriers and needs may exist between male and female Veterans, and service members from underrepresented groups may face additional challenges. Another factor that appears to influence community reintegration is family composition. Needs are likely to vary across service members depending on whether they are single, married, or divorced and members of traditional or nontraditional families (Crocker, Powell-Cope, Brown, and Besterman-Dahan, 2014).

Intervention

In a study of combat Veterans, Sayer et al. (2010) identified common experienced community reintegration problems. Many of the problems were interpersonal in nature—for example, difficulty sharing personal thoughts and feelings; making new friends; and getting along with a spouse, children, and other relatives. Other problem areas included managing anger, finding or keeping a job, taking care of domestic chores, getting involved in community activities, taking care of personal health, enjoying or making good use of leisure time, and finding meaning or purpose in life. Many of these concerns are appropriate for occupational therapy intervention.

Participants in Gerardi's (2017) study were asked to rank order occupational therapy interventions that should definitely be included in an outpatient intervention for Veterans with PTSD. The three top-ranked interventions endorsed by occupational therapists were:

- Engaging in goal-directed meaningful occupations and activities
- Developing occupational roles, habits, and routines
- Meditating or using other mindfulness techniques

No published models of occupational therapy intervention specifically designed to facilitate the reintegration of Veterans into civilian life have been located. For the purposes of the occupational therapy component of the program at Veterans Recovery Resources (2018), it was decided to integrate the concepts and principles of the CMOP-E, the MOHO (described in Chapter 3), and the Lifestyle Redesign® approach (LR; described in Chapter 24). The CMOP-E, MOHO, and LR have extensive research evidence supporting the efficacy of these approaches with a variety of populations. Aspects of the unpublished treatment template described by Gerardi (2017) have also been included. The program is in the early stages of implementation, and therefore, only anecdotal evidence regarding effectiveness is available at this time.

The CMOP-E is an expanded version of the CMOP. Engagement was added to the original model as a conceptual advancement, emphasizing the importance of occupational engagement as well as performance. Occupational performance is what a person is able to do; occupational engagement refers to the activities a person participates in on a regular basis. Occupational engagement, like performance, is an outcome of the dynamic interaction of person, occupation, and environment (Polatajko, Townsend, and Craik, 2007).

The primary contribution of the MOHO to the program is the concept of performance patterns and habituation. Veterans are often highly skilled individuals who are accustomed to functioning within a military structure. When they return home, they may find the need to adapt to new roles and develop new habits and routines in the absence of their former military structure. In order to develop new performance patterns, it is important to recognize the important impact of volition. Motivation, in the form of values, interests, goals, and self-efficacy, is a critical factor that drives roles and routines and should be considered critical to the development of an intervention plan.

The LR format for group and individual sessions is incorporated in the program. Each 90-minute group session consists of a didactic presentation, peer exchange, personal exploration, and direct experience (Mandel, Jackson, Zemke, Nelson, and Clark, 1999). The didactic presentations are on topics identified by the literature as relevant to Veterans reintegrating into civilian life, as well as on topics requested by participants. Peer exchange is a very important aspect of the program at Veterans Recovery Resources. In group sessions, Veterans are encouraged to share stories about their lives, the challenges they experience, and the ways in which they are trying to meet those challenges. Telling their stories provides continuity of identity and a sense of moving forward in life.

Personal exploration opportunities are provided during group sessions and through homework assignments. Veterans reflect on the relevance, importance, and meaningfulness of the topic discussed to their own lives. This is often accomplished through written exercises. Direct experience takes multiple forms—for example, participation in community outings, meditation, yoga, Internet searches, physical activities, volunteer work, and group games.

Individual sessions are designed to enable the client "to discover, plan, and implement a personalized program of lifestyle redesign" (Mandel et al., 1999, Appendix 1, para. 2). It provides an opportunity for the client to share information and ask questions they might not be comfortable addressing in a group setting. These sessions are tailored to the client's specific self-identified goals. The basic design of the occupational therapy component of the program at Veterans Recovery Resources is outlined in Box 21-3.

Box 21-3 Occupational Therapy Component of the Veterans Recovery Resources Program

The purpose of occupational therapy is to promote:

- Posttraumatic growth and resilience
- Healthy lifestyle choices
- Increased self-efficacy
- Occupational participation
- Community reintegration

Assessments used:

- Canadian Occupational Performance Measure
- Role Checklist
- Modified Interest Checklist
- Self-Efficacy Scale
- Occupational Questionnaire (activity log)
- Occupational Self-Assessment
- Community Integration Checklist
- Mental health and cognitive assessments as needed

Group topics:

- Psychoeducation regarding mental health conditions
- Goal setting
- Life skills training (stress management, anger management, communication and interaction skills, etc.)
- Mindfulness techniques
- Cognitive and sensory-grounding techniques
- Engagement in meaningful occupations and activities to support occupational roles, habits, and routines
- Nutrition and meal planning
- Emotion regulation and distress tolerance
- Relapse prevention
- Sleep hygiene
- Job search and acquisition

Occupational Challenges to Community Reintegration

Based on the literature, two specific occupational challenges to community reintegration have been chosen for more detailed explanation. These are civilian employment and return to school.

Civilian Employment

Work and volunteer occupations are of critical importance to Veterans as they reintegrate into their families and civilian communities. However, translating military strengths and skills to civilian life can be challenging. Many military specialties (e.g., field artillery operations chief, antitank missile gunner, fire control technician, combat control specialist) are not easily transferable to jobs in the civilian sector. In the military, a chain of command is in place, and the service member's rank in the hierarchy is observable. In civilian employment, the chain of command is not as outwardly obvious. As a member of the civilian workforce, a Veteran (regardless of military rank) will likely start lower on the hierarchy than previously and will need to work her or his way up to higher levels and more lucrative positions (Gaither, 2014).

Zarecky (2014) conducted a qualitative study evaluating the effectiveness of a coaching model using a strengths-based intervention to enhance Veterans' awareness of their personal strengths and help them gain clarity on future career aspirations. Working in careers chosen based on personal values, interests, and strengths enhanced worker well-being and increased the likelihood of performance excellence.

If a Veteran is not able to or does not want to seek paid employment, volunteer work is a health-promoting alternative. In one large study, over 300 participants provided 20 hours per week of volunteer service through The Mission Continues, a national nonprofit organization that deploys Veteran volunteers on specific projects for up to 6 months. Veterans were trained and provided a stipend to participate in the Fellowship Program, which is designed to promote career and educational development.

Overall, 86% of the participants indicated that volunteer service was a positive, life-changing experience; specifically, they reported that the program helped them become leaders in their communities. Veterans who participated demonstrated improvements in overall health, mental health, and social functioning. After completing their service, 71% furthered their education, 86% obtained civilian employment, and 91% intended to continue to engage in volunteer activities (Matthieu, Lawrence, and Robertson-Blackmore, 2017).

Return to School

The VA administers the Post-9/11 GI Bill to financially assist Veterans transitioning to student status. The Post-9/11 GI Bill provides significant financial educational benefits, including full tuition and fees, a monthly housing allowance, and up to $1,000 a year to use for books and supplies. While these financial resources are a valuable asset to student Veterans transitioning from "boots to books," transitioning requires additional personal and social capital to adapt to the academic environment (see Fig. 21-3). For example, Shiavone and Gentry (2014) performed a qualitative case study with six transitioning military members through the lens of Schlossberg's transitions theory, also referred to as the 4S system, to better understand the struggles of student Veterans. Situation, self, support, and strategies are concepts used to describe the transition process. Successful transitions require a balance of assets and liabilities in each of these categories.

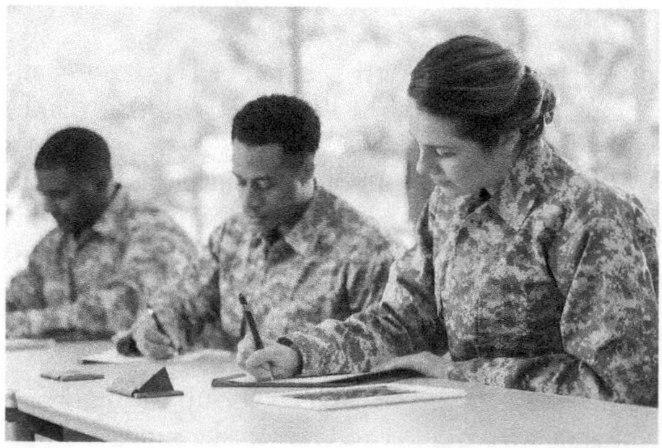

Figure 21-3 Boots to books. (*asiseeit/E+/Getty Images.*)

Situations, the first *S* in the model, consists of seven variables: trigger, timing, control, role change, duration, previous experience, and concurrent stress. Some military members may find purpose in their roles in the military, thus "triggering" a desire to transition those skills to a civilian occupation. Others may have benefited from the self-discipline instilled through military service and want to grow in new areas. Student Veterans are nontraditional students, and the timing of their transition produces challenges to managing jobs and relationships with a spouse and/or children. Additionally, student Veterans possess a variety of life experiences that shape their worldview, which may alienate them from their college peer group, creating role changes, relational conflict, and difficult social interaction (Shiavone and Gentry, 2014).

Self, the second *S* in the model, can be described in terms of resources, or personal assets necessary for successful transition, and deficits, or liabilities serving as roadblocks to transition. Psychological status varies among student Veterans and may hinder the transition process (Shiavone and Gentry, 2014). In a study of two university campuses in the southeastern United States, 56.9% of a sample of 538 student Veterans identified as having at least one mental health problem. Deficits in help-seeking behavior may also negatively affect the transitioning process. Of the one-third of student Veterans having a mental health problem requiring treatment, only one-third participated in an adequate number of treatment sessions to receive any benefit (Currier, McDermott, and McCormick, 2017). An additional liability is the emotional and psychological trauma experienced in combat, often leading to insomnia and difficulty managing relationships. Despite these challenges, student Veterans possess many assets to assist the transitioning process. Global awareness, maturity, and self-discipline can serve to open new opportunities with other student groups across campus while modeling behaviors necessary for academic success (Shiavone and Gentry, 2014).

Support, the third *S* in the model, refers to the encouragement, assistance, and options that are available in the environment. For example, campus administration and staff have an opportunity to create Military Friendly® schools. Using public data, Military Friendly schools assist student Veterans in locating schools that meet criteria across six categories: academic policy and compliance, admissions and orientation, culture and commitment, financial aid and loan repayment, graduation and career outcomes, and military student support and retention. Institutions may apply for designation as Military Friendly by meeting benchmarks related to student retention, graduation, job placement, loan repayment, and persistence (Blyth, n.d.). Strategies, the fourth *S* in the model, are the coping resources available to the person as he or she moves through the transition. These coping strategies can be health enhancing, such as humor and physical activity, or detrimental, such as excessive alcohol consumption and isolation (Shiavone and Gentry, 2014).

While this innovative approach to advocacy may guide student Veterans during their transition process, Van Dusen (2011) has created a Veteran-friendly environment model to address the policy-, institutional-, departmental-, and individual-level actions necessary to create an environment supportive of student Veterans that will lead to degree completion (see Box 21-4).

In summary, periods of transition often challenge existing individual resources while providing opportunity for growth. When student Veterans are faced with these challenges to adapt to a new environment, understanding their current assets and liabilities may serve as a catalyst to thrive in a new environment through increased self-awareness. Using individual strengths of global awareness, maturity, and self-discipline to engage in social organization may improve academic success.

Box 21-4 Veteran-Friendly Environment Model

At each level, interventions are proposed and summarized below:

Policy Level

- Create flexibility in general education requirements, allowing for the transfer of military credits and residency requirements

Institutional

- Educate and acclimate student Veterans on campus
- Establish a mentor program
- Create "Green Zones"—faculty trained on military culture competency and transitions

Departmental

- Develop a system to track academic success
- Develop a formal referral protocol

Individual Level

- Summer reading program
- Commemorate Veteran's holidays
- Establish institutional traditions

From *A Quantitative Study of Student Veterans' Intent to Persist,* by R. L. Van Dusen, 2011, unpublished doctoral dissertation, Texas Tech University, Lubbock, TX.

A Population-Based Approach to Community Reintegration

The Veterans Administration Office of Rehabilitation Research and Development (VA-RR&D) convened a working group to study the state of the art in community reintegration and make recommendations for future research and policy. The working group chose to use the ICF, developed by the World Health Organization (Resnick et al., 2012), as the theoretical basis of its investigation. In the process, it identified key dimensions of participation applicable to service members attempting to reintegrate into civilian society (see Box 21-5). The term *participation* in this context refers to the quantity and quality of a person's involvement in society (Resnick et al., 2012).

Successful community reintegration is not simply a matter of individual function but also the readiness of a community to embrace Veterans and their needs. Contextual factors—physical, social, and attitudinal—can have a profound effect on degree and ease of community reintegration for Veterans. It is therefore necessary to conduct a community assessment to identify the resources and barriers the environment presents to the Veteran who is trying to adjust to civilian life. Environmental barriers may include, but are not limited to, negative attitudes of civilians, a lack of available services and assistance, physical and structural obstructions, and policy limitations (Resnick et al., 2012).

Hawkins et al. (2015) conducted qualitative interviews of Veterans who had single or multiple physical or psychological injuries due to military service and were living in the community. The data analysis

Box 21-5 Dimensions of Participation

- Social: engaging with friends and family members
- Work: engaging in paid and unpaid employment
- Education: engaging in formal and informal learning activities
- Parental: caring for and supervising the raising of children
- Spouse/significant other: engaging in a long-term relationship
- Spiritual/religious: engaging in activities that address spiritual needs
- Leisure: engaging in preferred avocational activities
- Domestic life: engaging in activities to maintain the home and live in the community
- Civic: engaging in activities focused on the betterment of society and the responsibilities of citizens
- Self-care: engaging in activities to maintain societal standards of hygiene and maintain health
- Economic: engaging in simple and complex economic transactions and having command over economic resources

Participation in some of these role functions occurs in interaction with other people, while other roles may be performed without social interaction.

Data from "Issues in Defining and Measuring Veteran Community Reintegration: Proceedings of the Working Group on Community Reintegration," by L. Resnick, D. W. Bradford, S. M. Glynn, A. M. Jette, C. J. Hernandez, and S. Wills, 2012, *Journal of Rehabilitation Research and Development, 49*(1), p. 89.

yielded six themes that influenced community reintegration:

- personal factors;
- social support;
- adaptive sport, recreation, and other social programs;
- rehabilitation programs and therapists;
- school, work, and volunteering; and
- organizations and policies.

The structure of these contextual factors is illustrated in Figure 21-4.

It was determined that two elements directly influenced CR—personal factors (i.e., self-efficacy, motivation) and social support (i.e., family, friends, and peers). Personal factors that acted as facilitators of CR included participants' sense of self-efficacy, motivation to be productive, and ability to self-regulate and set goals. Social support and connections with others acted as both barriers and facilitators of CR. Spouses and children often facilitated the Veterans' participation in community activities. Connecting with Veteran peers provided an opportunity to regain a sense of personal identity as part of the military family. However, social support, or lack thereof, could also be an inhibiting factor or barrier to CR. Negative attitudes, misconceptions, and stigma related to military service and/or the physical and psychological injuries sustained by the

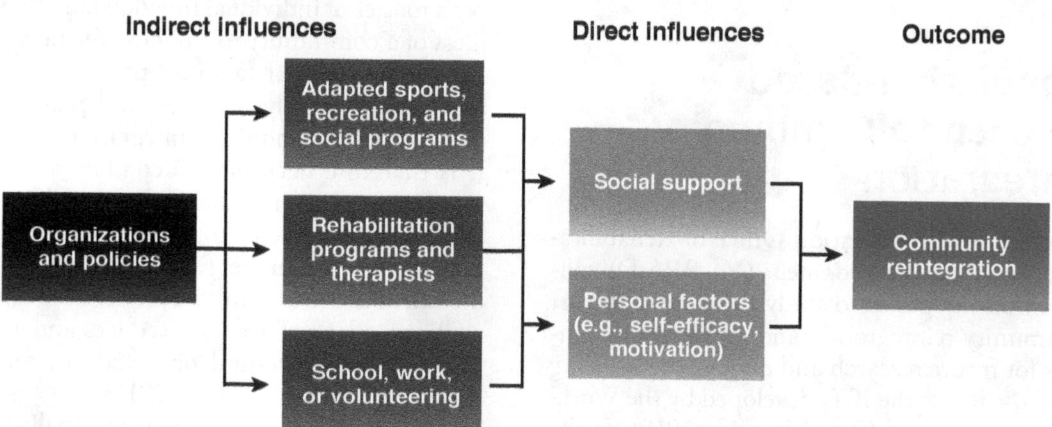

Figure 21-4 Thematic structure of contextual factors related to community reintegration. *(From "Understanding Contextual Influences of Community Integration Among Injured Service Members," by B. L. Hawkins, F. A. McGuire, S. M. Linder, and T. W. Britt, 2015,* Journal of Rehabilitation Research and Development, 52*[5], p. 532. Used with permission.)*

Veterans made CR more difficult (Hawkins et al., 2015).

The availability of adapted sports and recreation, access to rehabilitation (physical and psychological), and opportunities to participate in school, work, and volunteer activities indirectly affected CR. Sports and recreation served a larger purpose than mere participation; these activities provided opportunities to gain self-efficacy and develop social connections for support. Effective rehabilitation is more than simply treating medical conditions. It requires an understanding of how to treat mental health issues in addition to physical injuries and an emphasis on CR as a lifestyle change process. Participation in school, work, and volunteer experiences creates opportunities to give and receive social support, develop self-efficacy, and become part of the daily life of a community. However, many Veterans are exposed to barriers at work, such as mental health stigma on the part of employers and coworkers that affect job performance and make it difficult to maintain employment.

Organizations and policies had indirect effects on CR and direct effects on other factors. For example, one of the most commonly reported organizational barriers to CR was the difficulty encountered when trying to access federal programs and services (Hawkins et al., 2015). Community-based organizations and programs that contributed to CR included, but were not limited to, primary care services, mental health services, sport and recreation programs, tuition assistance programs, job placement services, and case management. Organizations and programs specifically designed for Veterans (e.g., Wounded Warriors; Team Red, White and Blue) also helped to facilitate CR.

One goal of occupational therapy intervention is to maximize the person-environment fit to enhance quality of life. This may mean intervening on a community or population level. One strategy for assessing the community is through the use of the PRECEDE-PROCEED planning model (described in Chapter 3).

Summary

- Military culture has been described as more delineated than most cultures, having an overt set of values, normative behaviors, and a code of ethics supported by its own judicial system. Therefore, the community reintegration process could be considered a cross-cultural transition. Although initial military training is designed to facilitate the transition into military culture, there is no corresponding mechanism to assist Veterans to successfully reintegrate into civilian life.
- As compared to the civilian population, Veterans experience poorer overall health and greater health-related functional limitations. Common war-related injuries include mTBI, extremity fractures, limb amputation, and chronic pain. Prevalent mental health conditions related to service include depression, anxiety, PTSD, and substance abuse.
- Transitions provide unique challenges, as well as opportunities for growth, adaptation, and transformation. Transitions are frequently stressful even when they are freely chosen and deemed desirable. Moving through a transition requires relinquishing aspects of the self and former roles and learning new skills and developing a new identity. All of these apply to a Veteran's community reintegration transition.
- Although many military couples and families eagerly await a joyful reunion upon the end of deployment, the transition and reintegration into family life is challenging for the family as well as the Veteran. Relationship distress and emotional turmoil are not uncommon during the 6 months following return from a tour of duty. Family relationships change in a variety of ways after deployment.
- During deployment, daily occupations are dictated and scheduled by the military. Upon returning home, service members are expected to choose, schedule, and engage in self-care, work, and leisure occupations that are personally meaningful. Unmet occupational needs can lead to occupational deprivation, imbalance, and/or disruption.
- The occupational therapy literature lacks research evidence regarding effective interventions for Veterans with combat-related mental health issues. As a result, practitioners working with this population are forced "to

make treatment decisions without the benefit of supporting evidence of treatment efficacy" (Gerardi, 2017, p. 24).

- Successful community reintegration is not simply a matter of individual function but also the readiness of a community to embrace Veterans and their needs. Contextual factors—physical, social, and attitudinal—can have a profound effect on degree and ease of community reintegration for Veterans. Thus, a population-based approach is warranted.

CASE STUDIES

CASE STUDY 21-1 Michael

Michael is a 48-year-old male with chronic pain, hypertension, PTSD, and depression who presents to his primary care provider with complaints of decreased mood, difficulty concentrating, marital stress, and life stressors, including a fear of homelessness, graduate school, and relationships with his children. He reports sleeping for 4 to 5 hours per night, awakening because of pain, and never feeling fully refreshed. Michael is a Veteran of the War in Afghanistan and served for 22 years as an information systems analyst in the military. During his service, he was airborne qualified and deployed twice to Afghanistan. He is married with three children, one from his current marriage and two from a previous marriage. Michael is currently in graduate school pursuing a master's degree in information systems. Michael has been referred for occupational therapy by the primary care provider to assist in the management of his life stressors.

The occupational therapist conducts an interview, administers several assessments, including the COPM, and develops an occupational profile. Michael lives with his wife and children in a second-story apartment. During his transition from military to civilian life, Michael experienced significant challenges. He was unable to find full-time employment, so he worked multiple low-paying jobs. He currently has very little leisure time. Michael describes himself as a "get it done" person and very rarely seeks assistance from others. He has a military pension and good insurance and receives supplemental disability payments from Veterans Health Affairs.

In collaboration with Michael, the occupational therapist develops an intervention plan that includes the following:

- Self-regulation skill training to include deep-breathing relaxation and mindfulness-based stress reduction
- Psychoeducation to improve sleep quality and explore additional stress management options
- Consultation, cotreatment, and/or referral to the physical therapist on the team regarding chronic pain
- Peer support services to decrease barriers to seeking mental health services and increase social connection and community engagement

Discussion Questions

1. What options may be available in the community to help Michael positively reengage in leisure and social participation?
2. What specific assessments, in addition to the COPM, would you use with this client and why did you choose these?
3. What other problems might occupational therapy address that are not accounted for in the current treatment plan? How would you address these?
4. When would you consider referring Michael to a psychologist for additional treatment for PTSD and depression?

CASE STUDY 21-2 Veterans Initiative in Southwest Alabama

The Community Foundation of South Alabama initiated a 4-year project to identify and address the unmet needs of the over 60,000 Veterans and their families in an eight-county region of South Alabama. Over half of the Veterans surveyed in Southwest Alabama reported a previous mental health diagnosis (e.g., PTSD) and/or recent thoughts of suicide and problem drinking. Over one-third of student Veterans surveyed at two Gulf Coast universities reported problem drinking and clinical levels of PTSD, major depressive disorder (MDD), and/or risk of suicidal behavior that indicated a probable need for treatment.

In a comprehensive community-based needs assessment, Veterans reported the following:

- Difficult adjustment to civilian life (40.7%)
- Extra time needed to figure out "what to do with my life" (45%)
- Employment instability (8.7% of Veterans as compared to the 3.9% state of Alabama unemployment rate)
- Food insecurity ("ran out of food") sometimes or often in the past 12 months (28.8%)
- Housing insecurity in the past 2 months (12.8%)
- Mental disorder diagnoses of PTSD (35.4%), TBI (13.8%), anxiety (42.4%), and/or bipolar disorder (7.7%)
- Suicidal ideation (36.4%)
- Alcohol consumption four or more times per week (16.3%)

Based on the findings of the needs assessment, the Community Foundation of South Alabama established the following primary objectives:

- Improve awareness of available services
- Address the underlying causes of substance abuse
- Provide therapy for mental health issues
- Offer treatment for substance abuse

The Community Foundation of South Alabama (2018) awarded over $450,000 in grants from the endowed Veterans Fund to local nonprofit organizations to support the development, implementation, and evaluation of innovative programs designed to meet the needs of Veterans and their families in the Gulf Coast region of Alabama.

Discussion Questions

You are planning on submitting a grant proposal to the Community Foundation of South Alabama.

1. In the development of an occupational therapy program for this Veteran population, what occupation-based goals would you write to be consistent with the Community Foundation's objectives?
2. Based on the needs assessment results, what innovative health promotion and restorative interventions might occupational therapy offer this Veteran population?
3. How will you evaluate the effectiveness of the occupational therapy program?

Learning Activities

1. Create a list of agencies and organizations in your community that serve Veterans. Interview someone who works with Veterans at one of these locations to identify any unmet needs.
2. Contact your university's community involvement office or search the dav.org website to identify volunteer opportunities to work with Veterans.
3. Interview a Veteran to determine the factors that impede or facilitate their adjustment into civilian life. Based on this information, consider how occupational therapy might assist with the community reintegration process.

REFERENCES

Ahern, J., Worthen, M., Masters, J., Lippman, S. A., Ozer, E. J., and Moos, R. (2015). The challenges of Afghanistan and Iraq

Veterans' transition from military to civilian life and approaches to reconnection. *PLoS ONE 10*(7), e0128599. doi:10.1371/journal.pone.0128599

American Chronic Pain Association. (n.d.). *Chronic pain.* Retrieved from www.theacpa.org/conditions-treatments/conditions-a-z/chronic-pain/

American Occupational Therapy Association. (2014a). *Occupational therapy in polytrauma.* Retrieved from www.aota.org/~/media/Corporate/Files/AboutOT/Professionals/WhatIsOT/RDP/Facts/Polytrauma%20fact%20sheet.pdf

American Occupational Therapy Association. (2014b). Occupational therapy practice framework: Domain and process. *American Journal of Occupational Therapy, 68*(Suppl. 1), S1–S51.

American Occupational Therapy Association. (2018). AOTA's societal statement on stress, trauma, and posttraumatic stress disorder. *American Journal of Occupational Therapy, 72*(Suppl. 2), 7212410080.

Anderson, M. L., and Goodman, J. (2014). From military to civilian life: Applications of Schlossberg's model for Veterans in transition. *Career Planning and Adult Development Journal, 30*(3), 40–51.

Anderson, M. L., Goodman, J., and Schlossberg, N. K. (2012). *Counseling adults in transition: Linking Schlossberg's theory with practice in a diverse world* (4th ed.). New York, NY: Springer.

Asher, I. E. (2014). *Asher's occupational therapy assessment tools: An annotated index* (4th ed.). Bethesda, MD: AOTA Press.

Atherton, S. (2009). Domesticating military masculinities: Home, performance and the negotiation of identity. *Social and Cultural Geography, 10*(8), 821–836.

Bialik, K. (2017). *The changing face of America's Veteran population.* Retrieved from www.pewresearch.org/fact-tank/2017/11/10/the-changing-face-of-americas-Veteran-population/

Blakey, S. M., Wagner, H. R., Naylor, J., Brancu, M., Lane, I., Sallee, M., . . . Elbogen, E. B. (2018). Chronic pain, TBI, and PTSD in military Veterans: A link to suicidal ideation and violent impulses? *Journal of Pain, 19*(7), 797–806.

Blyth, I. (n.d.). *Homepage.* Retrieved from http://militaryfriendly.com/

Brown, H. V., and Hollis, V. (2013). The meaning of occupation, occupational need, and occupational therapy in a military context. *Physical Therapy, 93,* 1244–1253.

Center for Deployment Psychology. (n.d.). *About CDP.* Retrieved from https://deploymentpsych.org/

Cifu, D., Taylor, B., Carne, W., Bidelspach, D., Sayer, N., Scholten, J., and Hagel-Campbell, E. (2014). TBI, PTSD, and pain diagnoses in OEF/OIF/OND Veterans. *Journal of Rehabilitation Research and Development, 50*(9), 1169–1176.

Cogan, A. M. (2014). Supporting our military families: A case for a larger role for occupational therapy in prevention and mental health care. *American Journal of Occupational Therapy, 68*(4), 478–483.

Community Foundation of South Alabama. (2018). *Veterans initiative.* Retrieved from https://communityfoundationsa.org/Veterans-initiative/

Crocker, T., Powell-Cope, G., Brown, L. M., and Besterman-Dahan, K. (2014). Toward a Veteran-centric view on community (re) integration. *Journal of Rehabilitation Research and Development, 51*(3), xi–xviii.

Crum-Cianflone, N. F., Powell, T. M., LeardMann, C. A., Russell, D. W., and Boyko, E. J. (2016). Mental health and comorbidities in U.S. military members. *Military Medicine, 181*(6), 537–545. Retrieved from https://doi.org/10.7205/MILMED-D-15-00187

Currier, J. M., Holland, J. M., and Malott, J. (2015). Moral injury, meaning making, and mental health in returning Veterans. *Journal of Clinical Psychology, 71*(3), 229–240. doi:10.1002/jclp.22134

Currier, J. M., McDermott, R. C., and McCormick, W. H. (2017). Mental health treatment-related stigma and professional help seeking among student Veterans. *Psychological Services, 14* (4), 531–542.

Daniels, A. S., Ashenden, P., Goodale, L., and Stevens, T. (2016). *National survey of compensation among peer support specialists.* Retrieved from www.leaders4health.org/images/uploads/files/PSS_Compensation_Report.pdf

Demers, A. (2011). When Veterans return: The role of community in reintegration. *Journal of Loss and Trauma, 16,* 160–179.

Dijkers, M. (1998). Community integration: Conceptual issues and measurement approaches in rehabilitation research. *Topics in Spinal Cord Injury Rehabilitation, 4,* 1–15.

Dijkers, M. (2000). *The Community Integration Questionnaire.* New York, NY: The Center for Outcome Measurement in Brain Injury. Retrieved from www.tbims.org/combi/ciq

Drescher, K. D., Foy, D. W., Kelly, C., Leshner, A., Schutz, K., and Litz, B. (2011). An exploration of the viability and usefulness of the construct of moral injury in war Veterans. *Traumatology, 17,* 8–13.

Farnsworth, J. K., Drescher, K. D., Nieuwsma, J. A., Walser, R. B., and Currier, J. M. (2014). The role of moral emotions in military trauma: Implications for the study and treatment of moral injury. *Review of General Psychology, 18*(4), 249–262.

Finley, E. P., Bollinger, M., Noël, P. H., Amuan, M. E., Copeland, L. A., Pugh, J. A., . . . Pugh, M. J. V. (2015). A national cohort study of the association between the polytrauma clinical triad and suicide-related behavior among us Veterans who served in Iraq and Afghanistan. *American Journal of Public Health, 105*(2), 380–387. https://doi.org/10.2105/AJPH.2014.301957

Gaither, D. (2014). Military transition management. *Career Planning and Adult Development Journal,* 215–239.

Gerardi, S. M. (2016). *Development of a manualized occupational therapy intervention for posttraumatic stress disorder.* (Unpublished doctoral capstone project). South University, West Palm Beach, FL.

Gerardi, S. M. (2017). *Development of a consensus based occupational therapy treatment template for Veterans with combat-related posttraumatic stress disorder: A Delphi study.* (Doctoral dissertation). Retrieved from https://twu-ir.tdl.org/handle/11274/9382

Harada, N. D., Damron-Rodriguez, J., Villa, V. M., Washington, D. L., . . . Anderson, R. (2002). Veteran identity and race/ethnicity: Influences on VA outpatient care utilization. *Medical Care, 40*(Suppl. 1), 117–128.

Hawkins, B. L., McGuire, F. A., Linder, S. M., and Britt, T. W. (2015). Understanding contextual influences of community integration among injured service members. *Journal of Rehabilitation Research and Development, 52*(5), 527–542.

Hoerster, K. D., Lehavot, K., Simpson, T., McFall, M., Reiber, G., and Nelson, K. M. (2012). Health and health behavior differences: U.S. military, Veteran, and civilian men. *American Journal of Preventive Medicine, 43*(5), 483–489. Retrieved from https://doi.org/10.1016/j.amepre.2012.07.029

Hom, M. A., Stanley, I. H., Gutierrez, P. M., and Joiner, T. E. (2017). Exploring the association between exposure to suicide and suicide risk among military service members and Veterans. *Journal of Affective Disorders, 207,* 327–335.

Institute of Medicine. (2011). *Relieving pain in America: A blueprint for transforming prevention, care, education, and research.*

Washington, DC: National Academies Press. Retrieved from https://doi.org/10.17226/13172

Kashiwa, A., Sweetman, M. M., and Helgeson, L. (2017). Centennial topics—occupational therapy and Veteran suicide: A call to action. *American Journal of Occupational Therapy, 71,* 7105100010. Retrieved from https://doi.org/10.5014/ajot.2017.023358

Katz, L. S., Bloor, L. E., Cojucar, G., and Draper, T. (2007). Women who served in Iraq seeking mental health services: Relationships between military sexual trauma, symptoms and readjustment. *Psychological Services, 4,* 239–249.

Kelty, R., Kleykamp, M., and Segal, D. R. (2010). The military and the transition to adulthood. *Future of Children, 20*(1), 181–207.

Knobloch, L. K., and Theiss, J. A. (2012). Experiences of U.S. military couples during the post-deployment transition: Applying the relational turbulence model. *Journal of Social and Personal Relationships, 29*(4), 423–450.

Kopacz, M. S., Connery, A. L., Bishop, T. M., Bryan, C. J., Drescher, K. D., Currier, J. M., and Pigeon, W.R. (2016). Moral injury: A new challenge for complementary and alternative medicine. *Complementary Therapies in Medicine, 24,* 29–33.

Lincoln, A. (1865). *Second inaugural address.* Retrieved from www.ourdocuments.gov/doc.php?flash=false&doc=38&page=transcript

Litz, B. T., Stein, N., Delaney, E., Lebowitz, L., Nash, W. P., Silva, C., and Maguen, S. (2009). Moral injury and moral repair in war Veterans: A preliminary model and intervention strategy. *Clinical Psychology Review, 29*(8), 695–706.

Maguen, S., and Litz, B. (2012). *Moral injury in the context of war.* Washington, DC: U.S. Department of Veterans Affairs. Retrieved from www.ptsd.va.gov/professional/treat/cooccurring/moral_injury.asp

Mandel, D. R., Jackson, J. M., Zemke, R., Nelson, L., and Clark, F. A. (1999). *Lifestyle Redesign: Implementing the well elderly program.* Bethesda, MD: American Occupational Therapy Association.

Matthieu, M. M., Lawrence, K. A., and Robertson-Blackmore, E. (2017). The impact of a civic service program on biopsychosocial outcomes of post 9/11 U.S. military Veterans. *Psychiatry Research, 248,* 111–116.

McCarthy, N. (2018). *2.77 million service members have served on 5.4 million deployments since 9/11.* Retrieved from www.forbes.com/sites/niallmccarthy/2018/03/20/2-77-million-service-members-have-served-on-5-4-million-deployments-since-911-infographic/#2a14c57350db

McColl, M. A., Davies, D., Carlson, P., Johnston, J., and Minnes, P. (2001). The Community Integration Measure: Development and preliminary validation. *Archives of Physical Medicine and Rehabilitation, 82,* 429–434.

Meyer, E. G., Writer, B. W., and Brim, W. (2016). The importance of military cultural competence. *Current Psychiatry Reports, 18*(26), 1–8. https://doi.org/10.1007/s11920-016-0662-9

Mobbs, M. C., and Bonanno, G. A. (2018). Beyond war and PTSD: The crucial role of transition stress in the lives of military Veterans. *Clinical Psychology Review, 59,* 137–144.

Morin, R. (2011). *The difficult transition from military to civilian life.* Retrieved from www.pewresearch.org/wp-content/uploads/sites/3/2011/12/The-Difficult-Transition-from-Military-to-Civilian-Life.pdf

O'Neil, M. E., Carlson, K., Storzbach, D., Brenner, L., Freeman, M., Quiñones, A., . . . Kansagara, D. (2013a). *Complications of mild traumatic brain injury in Veterans and military personnel: A systematic review.* Washington, DC: U.S. Department of Veterans Affairs, Appendix C. Retrieved from https://europepmc.org/books/NBK189784

O'Neil, M. E., Carlson, K., Storzbach, D., Brenner, L., Freeman, M., Quiñones, A., . . . Kansagara, D. (2013b). *Complications of mild traumatic brain injury in Veterans and military personnel: A systematic review.* Washington DC: Department of Veterans Affairs; Executive Summary. Retrieved from https://europepmc.org/books/NBK189789

Pew Research Center. (2011). *Social and demographic trends, the military-civilian gap: War and sacrifice in the post-9/11 era.* Retrieved from www.pewsocialtrends.org/2011/10/05/war-and-sacrifice-in-the-post-911-era/

Pigeon, W. R., Britton, P. C., Ilgen, M. A., Chapman, B., and Conner, K. R. (2012). Sleep disturbance preceding suicide among Veterans. *American Journal of Public Health, 102*(Suppl. 1), S93–S97.

Plach, H. L., and Sells, C. H. (2013). Occupational performance needs of young Veterans. *American Journal of Occupational Therapy, 67,* 73–81.

Polatajko, H. J., Davis, J., Stewart, D., Cantin, N., Amoroso, B., Purdie, L., and Zimmerman, D. (2007). Specifying the domain of concern: Occupation as core—specification of an occupational perspective. In E. A. Townsend and H. J. Polatajko (Eds.), *Enabling occupation II: Advancing an occupational therapy vision of health, well-being, and justice through occupation* (pp. 13–21). Ottawa, ON: CAOT Publications ACE.

Polatajko, H. J., Townsend, E. A., and Craik, J. (2007), Canadian model of occupational performance and engagement. In E. A. Townsend and H. J. Polatajko (Eds.), *Enabling occupation II: Advancing an occupational therapy vision of health, well-being, and justice through occupation* (pp. 22–36). Ottawa, ON: CAOT Publications ACE.

Resnick, L., Bradford, D. W., Glynn, S. M., Jette, A. M., Hernandez, C. J., and Wills, S. (2012). Issues in defining and measuring Veteran community reintegration: Proceedings of the working group on community reintegration, VA Rehabilitation Outcomes Conference, Miami, Florida. *Journal of Rehabilitation Research and Development, 49*(1), 87–100.

Resnick, L., Plow, M., and Jette, A. (2009). Development of the CRIS: Measure of community reintegration of injured service members. *Journal of Rehabilitation Research and Development, 46*(4), 469–480.

Sayer, N. A., Frazier, P., Orazem, R. J., Murdoch, M., Gravely, A., Carlson, K. F., . . . Noorbaloochi, S. (2011). Military to civilian questionnaire: A measure of post-deployment community reintegration difficulty among Veterans using Department of Veterans Affairs medical care. *Journal of Traumatic Stress, 24*(6), 660–670.

Sayer, N. A., Noorbaloochi, S., Frazier, P., Carlson, K., Gravely, A., and Murdoch, M. (2010). Reintegration problems and treatment interests among Iraq and Afghanistan combat Veterans receiving VA medical care. *Psychiatric Services, 61*(6), 589–597.

Schiavone, V., and Gentry, D. (2014). Veteran-students in transition at a midwestern university. *Journal of Continuing Higher Education, 62*(1), 29–38.

Simon, N. M., O'Day, E. B., Helberg, S. N., Hoeppner, S. S., Charney, M. E., Robinaugh, D. J., . . . Rauch, S. A. M. (2018). The loss of a fellow service member: Complicated grief in post-9/11 service members and Veterans with combat-related posttraumatic stress disorder. *Journal of Neuroscience Research, 96*(1), 5–15.

Speicher, S. M., Walter, K. H., and Chard, K. M. (2014). Interdisciplinary residential treatment of posttraumatic stress disorder and traumatic brain injury: Effects on symptom severity and occupational performance and satisfaction. *American Journal of Occupational Therapy, 68*(4), 412–421.

Stecher, T., Fortney, J., Owen, R., McGovern, M. P., and Williams, S. (2010). Co-occurring medical, psychiatric, and alcohol-related disorders among Veterans returning from Iraq and Afghanistan. *Psychosomatics, 51,* 503–507.

Substance Abuse and Mental Health Services Administration. (n.d.). *Peer providers*. Retrieved from www.integration,samhsa.gov/workforce/team-members/peer-providers

Substance Abuse and Mental Health Services Administration. (2009). *What are peer recovery support services?* HHS Publication No. (SMA) 09-4454. Retrieved from https://store.samhsa.gov/system/files/sma09-4454.pdf

Tanielian, T., Farmer, C. M., Burns, R. M., Duffy, E. L., and Setodji, C. M. (2018). Ready or not? Assessing the capacity of New York State health care providers to meet the needs of Veterans. Santa Monica, CA: RAND. Retrieved from www.rand.org/pubs/research_reports/RR2298.html

Toblin, R. L., Riviere, L. A., Thomas, J. L., Adler, A. B., Kok, B. C., and Hoge, C. W. (2012). Grief and physical health outcomes in U.S. soldiers returning from combat. *Journal of Affective Disorders, 136*(3), 469–475.

Trivedi, R. B., Post, E. P., Sun, H., Pomerantz, A., Saxon, A. J., Piette, J. D., . . . Nelson, K. (2015). Prevalence, comorbidity, and prognosis of mental health among U.S. Veterans. *American Journal of Public Health, 105*(12), 2564–2569.

Tsai, J., El-Gabalawy, R., Sledge, W. H., Southwick, S. M., and Pietrzak, R. H. (2015). Post-traumatic growth among Veterans in the USA: Results from the National Health and Resilience in Veterans Study. *Psychological Medicine, 45*(1), 165–179.

U.S. Census Bureau. (n.d.). *Health insurance coverage of Veterans.* Retrieved from www.census.gov/newsroom/blogs/random-samplings/2017/09/health_insurancecov0.html

U.S. Department of Defense. (2016). *2016 demographics: Profile of the military community.* Retrieved from http://download.militaryonesource.mil/12038/MOS/Reports/2016-Demographics-Report.pdf

U.S. Department of Veterans Affairs. (n.d.). *Enhancing care for Veterans with polytrauma and blast-related injuries.* Retrieved from www.hsrd.research.va.gov/news/feature/pt-bri.cfm?_ga=2.192742319.480293028.1545507117-954101287.1536435951

U.S. Department of Veterans Affairs. (2010). *VA/DoD clinical practice guideline for management of post-traumatic stress.* Retrieved from www.rehab.research.va.gov/jour/2012/495/pdf/VADODclinicalguidlines495.pdf

U.S. Department of Veterans Affairs. (2016). *VA conducts nation's largest analysis of Veteran suicide.* Retrieved from www.va.gov/opa/pressrel/includes/viewPDF.cfm?id=2801

U.S. Department of Veterans Affairs. (2018a). *Veteran population—National Center for Veterans Analysis and Statistics [General information].* Retrieved from www.va.gov/vetdata/Veteran_population.asp

U.S. Department of Veterans Affairs. (2018b). *VA national suicide data report 2005–2018.* Retrieved from www.mentalhealth.va.gov/docs/data-sheets/OMHSP_National_Suicide_Data_Report_2005-2016_508.pdf

Van Den Kerkhof, E. G., Carley, M. E., Hopman, W. M., Ross-White, A., and Harrison, M. B. (2014). Prevalence of chronic pain and related risk factors in military Veterans: A systematic review. *JBI Database of Systematic Reviews and Implementation Reports, 12*(10), 152–186.

Van Dusen, R. L. (2011). *A quantitative study of student Veterans' intent to persist.* (Unpublished doctoral dissertation). Texas Tech University, Lubbock, TX. Retrieved from http://citeseerx.ist.psu.edu/viewdoc/download?doi=10.1.1.918.7468&rep=rep1&type=pdf

Veterans Recovery Resources. (2018). *Outpatient services.* Retrieved from https://Veteransrecoveryresources.org/wp-content/uploads/2018/11/VRR_Level-One-Outpatient_Program-Description-Marketing_October-2018.pdf

Wenger, J. W., O'Connell, C., and Cottrell, L. (2018). *Examination of recent deployment experience across the services and components.* Retrieved from www.rand.org/pubs/research_reports/RR1928.html

Whiteford, G. (2000). Occupational deprivation: Global challenge in the new millennium. *British Journal of Occupational Therapy, 63,* 200–204.

Yamkovenko, S. (2013). *Veterans helping Veterans: Adaptive sports program shows power of occupation.* Retrieved from www.aota.org/Publications-News/AOTANews/2013/Adaptive-Sports-for-Veterans-Power-of-Occupation.aspx

Zarecky, A. (2014). How strengths-focused coaching can help military personnel in their transition to "civvy street." [Special issue]. *International Journal of Evidence-Based Coaching and Mentoring, 8,* 54–66.

Zoli, C., Maury, R., and Fay, D. (2015). *Missing perspectives: Service members' transition from service to civilian life.* Retrieved from https://surface.syr.edu/cgi/viewcontent.cgi?referer=&httpsredir=1&article=1006&context=ivmf

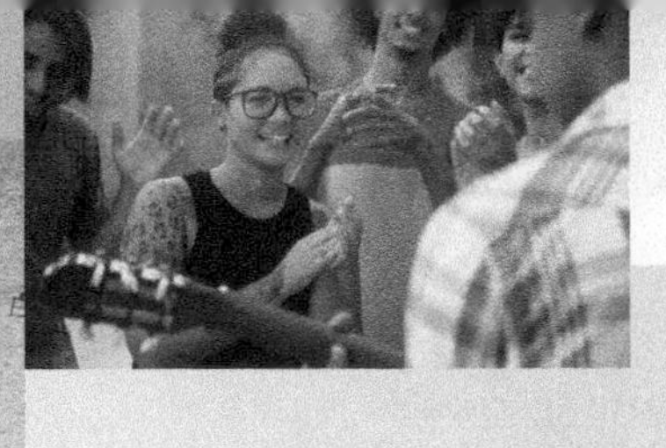

Chapter 22

Promoting Occupational Participation in Marginalized Populations

Stephen B. Kern, PhD, OTR/L, FAOTA, S. Maggie Reitz, PhD, OTR/L, FAOTA, Francine M. Seruya, PhD, OTR/L, Jillian Silveira, OTR/L, Betsey C. Smith, PhD, OTR/L, Toni Thompson, DrOT, OTR/L, C/NDT, Kevin Kilkuskie, BA, MAT, Gabriella Santos, BS, and Anton Nguye, BA

Compromise is often necessary [in politics], but entire marginalized identities are not expendable chess pieces.

—Sarah McBride

Learning Outcomes

This chapter is designed to enable the reader to:

22-1 Identify the role of occupational therapy in advocating for policy that addresses the occupational freedom of marginalized communities and populations.

22-2 Appreciate the lived experiences of marginalized groups and populations.

22-3 Understand the occupational risk factors such as occupational deprivation, alienation, and imbalance in the lives of marginalized groups and populations.

22-4 Describe innovative strategies to address harassment and health inequities among marginalized groups and populations.

22-5 Design occupation-based, theory-driven community- and population-based interventions for marginalized groups and populations.

Key Terms

Asexual
Asylum seekers/refugees
Bisexual
Cisgender
Cisnormative
Community assets
Community organization
Correctional system
Drag queens
Gender nonconforming
Gender queer
Heteronormativity
Human trafficking
Intersex
Marginalized population
Migration
Minority stress
Occupational apartheid
Occupational justice
Pansexual
Protracted refugee situations
Recidivism
Same-gender-loving couples
Structural violence
Transgender
Transsexual
Violence of uncertainty

Introduction

Marginalized populations are ignored in terms of health equity and occupational justice. The principles (see Box 22-1) of the World Health Organization (WHO, 1948/2018) clearly articulate the right for access to health. While the WHO focuses on health equity for all—including marginalized groups and populations—it is occupational therapy's role and responsibility to address access to health, health care, and occupational injustice. This is supported by the core values and ethical standards for the profession (AOTA, 2015).

Descriptions of the terms *marginalized population, occupational apartheid,* and *occupational justice* set the stage for the discussions in this chapter. A **marginalized population** is a group of people with similar characteristics who are less accepted by the dominant population(s) and are pushed and confined to the periphery of a society. As such, the marginalized community is restricted from equal opportunities to engage in the society's mainstream economic, political, cultural, and social activities (Reference, 2018). The definition of **occupational apartheid,** while similar, focuses specifically on the lack of access to meaningful occupational participation. According to Kronenberg and Pollard (2005),

> *occupational apartheid refers to the segregation of groups of people through the restriction and denial of access to dignified and meaningful participation in occupations of daily life on the basis of race, color, disability, national origin, age, gender, sexual preferences, religion, political beliefs, status in society, or other characteristics. (p. 67)*

Another related construct is that of **occupational justice,** a term that has evolved over time and is based on the work of Wilcock and Townsend (2014) beginning in the 1990s. Within the occupational therapy practice framework (American Occupational Therapy Association [AOTA], 2014b), occupational justice is defined as "a justice that recognizes occupational rights to inclusive participation in everyday occupations for all persons in society, regardless of age, ability, gender, social class, or other differences" (Nilsson and Townsend, 2010, p. 58, as cited in AOTA, 2014b, p. S43). It includes the availability of resources to support full participation in culturally relevant occupations that an individual, community, or population chooses that affords the entity social and physical health and well-being within a political economic context as an equal (Wilcock and Townsend, 2014).

Occupational therapy as a profession has historically advocated for certain marginalized

Engage Your Brain 22-1

Which AOTA core values and ethical principles support the profession's work with marginalized populations?

Box 22-1 Constitution of the World Health Organization: Principles

- Health is a state of complete physical, mental, and social well-being and not merely the absence of disease or infirmity.
- The enjoyment of the highest attainable standard of health is one of the fundamental rights of every human being without distinction of race, religion, political belief, or economic or social condition.
- The health of all peoples is fundamental to the attainment of peace and security and is dependent on the fullest cooperation of individuals and states.
- The achievement of any state in the promotion and protection of health is of value to all.
- Unequal development in different countries in the promotion of health and control of diseases, especially communicable disease, is a common danger.
- Healthy development of the child is of basic importance; the ability to live harmoniously in a changing total environment is essential to such development.
- The extension to all peoples of the benefits of medical, psychological, and related knowledge is essential to the fullest attainment of health.
- Informed opinion and active cooperation on the part of the public are of the utmost importance in the improvement of the health of the people.
- Governments have a responsibility for the health of their peoples that can be fulfilled only by the provision of adequate health and social measures.

From *Constitution of the World Health Organization,* by the World Health Organization, 1948/2018. Reprinted with permission.

populations—most often people and groups with disabilities or in specific age groups (e.g., vulnerable youth and older adults). Internationally, the profession's concerns have broadened beyond these groups to include displaced people (World Federation of Occupational Therapists [WFOT], 2014). The ability of the profession "to respond to the occupational needs of displaced people demands that the profession engage the socio-political context of displacement. The profession's approach must be critical as well as constructive" (WFOT, 2014, p. 2). The profession cannot be apolitical in addressing the occupational rights of displaced persons and other marginalized communities and populations. The WFOT (2018) *Position Statement on Human Rights* further supports this belief and upholds the United Nations (UN, 1948) *Universal Declaration of Human Rights.*

Position papers, statements, and societal statements by professional organizations can draw attention to discriminatory practices that negatively affect health and inclusion in a society with both external and internal audiences. For example, the AOTA's *Societal Statement on Health Disparities* clearly communicates the responsibility of occupational therapy practitioners "to intervene with individuals and communities to limit the effect of inequalities that result in health disparities" (2013, p. S7). In an AOTA (2014a) position paper, *Occupational Therapy's Commitment to Nondiscrimination and Inclusion,* occupational therapy practitioners are reminded that nondiscrimination and inclusion practices are an expectation not only for the provision of professional services but also for interactions between professional colleagues. This includes colleagues with disabilities, an area where work needs to be done, as marginalization has been reported (Heffron, The, and Harrison, 2018).

Position and policy statements are an important step in addressing the needs of marginalized groups, communities, and populations. However, documents are only one small step; they need to be followed by consistent, unapologetic acts by individual practitioners as well as occupational therapy and occupational science professional organizations. Actions should include addressing concerns as they are brought to the forefront through accreditation standards, annual conferences, scholarship, and business meetings.

While the peoples marginalized vary by geography (e.g., continents and countries), socioeconomic and political climate, and historical time frames, this chapter will focus on the following populations that have been marginalized consistently over time and space: asylum seekers and refugees; immigrants; the lesbian, gay, bisexual, transgendered, and queer or questioning (LGBTQ+) communities; incarcerated people; and people who have been trafficked. While occupational therapy practitioners could work with, or expand their work with, other forgotten or ignored marginalized populations, such as individuals and groups with disfigurements (Changing Faces, n.d.), indigenous people, and survivors of infectious diseases (e.g., severe acute respiratory syndrome [SARS], Ebola), they will not be addressed in this chapter. This chapter begins with a discussion of the theoretical frameworks that can be used in collaboration with other social justice advocacy groups and professions, as well as oppressed people.

Theoretical Frameworks

The occupational therapy theoretical frameworks discussed in Chapter 3 of this text can be used to support work by occupational therapy practitioners to address occupational injustice. In addition, the non–occupational therapy frameworks discussed in that chapter can also be used to understand social health disparities and needs; to develop services and advocacy efforts in partnership with a client group, community, or population; to assess the impact of the services and advocacy; and to publicize effective, innovative solutions. Community organization approaches and the participatory occupational justice framework (POJF) will be discussed next.

Community Organization Approaches[1]

Community organization approaches are essential in assisting with the advancement of oppressed marginalized groups, communities, and organizations.

1. Portions of this section first appeared in Reitz, S. M., Scaffa, M. E., Campbell, R. M., and Rhynders, P. A. (2010). Health behavior frameworks for health promotion practice. In M. E. Scaffa, S. M. Reitz, and M. A. Pizzi (Eds.), *Occupational therapy in community-based practice settings* (pp. 46–69). Philadelphia, PA: F. A. Davis.

The principles of these approaches work well with occupational therapy theoretical perspectives due to shared values such as empowerment, client centeredness, and the long-term goal of sustainability. **Community organization** has been defined as "the process by which community groups are helped to identify common problems or goals, mobilize resources, and in other ways develop and implement strategies for reaching goals they have set" (Minkler and Wallerstein, 2005, p. 26). It is "a participatory decision-making process that empowers communities to improve health" (Rural Health Information Hub, 2019, para. 1). The goals of community organization include solving current community problems, building permanent organizational and community capacity for ongoing problem-solving, and empowering individuals and neighborhoods to act collectively in their own best interest (Rubin and Rubin, 2005). Before initiating a community organization effort, familiarity with the community, as well as the language of community development and the values and assumptions of community organization, is important.

The majority of theoretical approaches to community organization are need- or problem-based and involve identification and remediation of deficits in a community. However, Kretzmann and McKnight (2005) propose a strengths-based approach that involves identifying and mobilizing all of the existing and potential, but often unrecognized, assets in a community. This approach is very much in alignment with the profession's values. **Community assets** include personal attributes and skills, relationships among people, local associations, and informal networks. Connecting community assets and strengths creates a synergy and multiplies their power and efficacy.

Community organizing strategies take many forms but typically involve consensus, collaboration, and advocacy. Examples of effective strategies include developing critical awareness, creating community identity, building relationships, mapping community assets, organizing coalitions, identifying community successes, and leveraging resources and investments from outside the community, as well as leadership development and political and legislative action (Mathie and Cunningham, 2003; Minkler and Wallerstein, 2005).

Participatory Occupational Justice Framework

While the POJF was developed by occupational therapists as a "conceptual tool for doing justice" (Whiteford and Townsend, 2011, p. 65), it is intended for use by a variety of people in partnership who are interested in promoting action to address meaningful change to eradicate occupational injustice (Whiteford and Townsend, 2011). This theoretical approach is also discussed in Chapters 3 and 4. The POJF promotes the value of an occupational lens to adequately identify, describe, and address specific impacts of occupational injustice. Similar to community organization approaches, recognizing and raising consciousness about an injustice is the first meaningful step toward action and, ultimately, transformational change. The next steps include:

- Engaging collaboratively with partners
- Mediating agreement on a plan
- Strategizing resource-finding actions
- Supporting implementation and continuous evaluation of the plan
- Inspiring advocacy for sustainability or closure (Whiteford and Townsend, 2011, pp. 73–74)

Populations

The following populations will be described in this next section: asylum seekers and refugees; immigrants; LGBTQ+ communities; incarcerated people; and people who have been trafficked. Their lived experiences, together with the occupational performance and participation challenges they face, are detailed.

Asylum Seekers, Refugees, and Other Migratory Populations

Migration is the movement of people from one place to another. Throughout history, there have always been migratory populations—some who immigrate by personal choice and others who are displaced or forced to leave their countries of origin. The majority of this migratory population are displaced people (i.e., refugees, asylum seekers, and stateless people) who remain close to home, with only a small proportion seeking resettlement to another country. According to the United Nations High Commission for Refugees (UNHCR, 2018), the global population of forcibly displaced people reached 68,500,000 people in 2017. "While the Syrian conflict contributed significantly to this increase, there have been other major displacements throughout the world over the last five years, notably in and from Burundi, Central African Republic, the Democratic Republic of the Congo, Iraq, Myanmar, South Sudan, Sudan, Ukraine, and Yemen" (UNHCR, 2018, p. 4). As a result of armed and unarmed internal conflicts and shifting political environments, the trend in human migration does not seem to be slowing down. The majority of displaced people (i.e., refugees, asylum seekers, and stateless people) remain close to home, with only a small proportion seeking resettlement to another country. The UNHCR reported that at the end of 2017 the global refugee population was 20,000,000 people. This figure represents the highest known total to date (UNHCR, 2018). Table 22-1 provides examples of the definitions that have been developed to differentiate the different types of displaced persons.

Lived Experience

Globally, there are high rates of human migration. With this migration, which frequently is abrupt and unplanned, comes a disruption in established occupations (Huot, Kelly, and Park, 2016). Huot et al. (2016) assert that this disruption also "challenges one's identity, sense of competence, health, and

Table 22-1 Migration Terms and Definitions

Term	Definition
Asylum seeker[1]	"A person who seeks safety from persecution or serious harm in a country other than his or her own and awaits a decision on the application for refugee status under relevant international and national instruments. In case of a negative decision, the person must leave the country and may be expelled, as may any non-national in an irregular or unlawful situation, unless permission to stay is provided on humanitarian or other related grounds." (para. 3)
Internally displaced persons[1]	"Persons or groups of persons who have been forced or obliged to flee or to leave their homes or places of habitual residence, in particular as a result of or in order to avoid the effects of armed conflict, situations of generalized violence, violations of human rights or natural or human-made disasters, and who have not crossed an internationally recognized State border." (para. 15)
Migrant[1]	"Any person who is moving or has moved across an international border or within a State away from his/her habitual place of residence, regardless of (1) the person's legal status; (2) whether the movement is voluntary or involuntary; (3) what the causes for the movement are; or (4) what the length of the stay is. IOM concerns itself with migrants and migration-related issues and, in agreement with relevant States, with migrants who are in need of international migration services." (para. 19)
Refugee[1]	"A person who, 'owing to a well-founded fear of persecution for reasons of race, religion, nationality, membership of a particular social group or political opinions, is outside the country of his nationality and is unable or, owing to such fear, is unwilling to avail himself of the protection of that country.'" (para. 26)
Stateless individuals[2]	An individual who is not a citizen of any country

[1] From *Glossary on Migration*, International Migration Law Series No. 25, by International Organization on Migration, 2011.
[2] From *The 10-Point Plan in Action, 2016—Glossary*, by United Nations High Commissioner for Refugees, 2016.

well-being" (p. 186). Along with these rates of migration, there is an increase in **protracted refugee situations,** defined by the UNHCR (2018) as situations "in which 25,000 or more refugees from the same nationality have been in exile for five consecutive years or more in a given asylum country" (p. 22). Many of these individuals and families live in displaced persons camps, where participation in daily activities is heavily restricted. They experience limitations and barriers in access to schools and education, employment, health care, and social services. Play and leisure activities are also restricted or denied (Steindl, Winding, and Runge, 2008). An example of prolonged displacement can be seen in African nations where generations of people are born, raised, and grow to adulthood in camps. As a result of extended periods of occupational injustices, such as occupational deprivation, marginalization, imbalance, and impoverished environments, they experience deficits in client factors, performance skills, and patterns (McElroy, Muyinda, Atim, Spittal, and Blackman, 2012).

Trauma is a common experience for many refugees and asylum seekers. Unfortunately, it can occur multiple times during their migration experience: in their home countries, on their journey to resettlement, and during resettlement (Jani and Reisch, 2018). While many people focus on the trauma that occurred in their home countries, it has been found that stressors occurring after resettlement can have as much of an impact on the mental health of refugees (Copley, Turpin, Gordon, and McLaren, 2011; Heptinstall, Sethna, and Taylor, 2004).

Health Inequalities

By the time refugees arrive in countries of resettlement, they have experienced many prolonged physical and mental health concerns. Im (2018) reports that refugees' health issues, deteriorated by chronic poverty, malnutrition, and poor living conditions, are further exacerbated by acculturative challenges, such as cultural and language barriers, stigma, and a lack of resources and information. Additionally, unattended and untreated health needs tend to induce a high risk for poor social functioning and public health concerns (Vaage et al., 2010).

Posselt, Galletly, de Crespigny, and Procter (2014) describe the higher risk for mental health and substance use problems experienced by young people of refugee backgrounds. They found that as a result of having to navigate refugee background, cultural, and linguistic barriers in their daily lives, as well as barriers to health-care access and service, they may be at higher risk for developing these comorbidities. Others have found that as a result of forced migration and traumatic experiences preflight and during the flight from their home countries, many refugees from Asian and African nations fail to access mental health services due to stigma, a lack of knowledge of mental health, shame and fear, and a history of political repression (Shannon, Wieling, Simmelink-McCleary, and Becher, 2015).

Studies of the health disparities of people forced to migrate from their countries of origin have highlighted the vast number and types of barriers and violence faced throughout the phases of preflight to the resettlement phases of forced human migration.

Farmer (1996) introduced to the health disparities literature the concept of **structural violence,** which recognizes the harm and suffering inherent in health disparities that are both caused and obscured by inequality. Grace, Bais, and Roth (2018) reported on the **violence of uncertainty** inflicted on these groups through "systematic personal, social, and institutional instability that exacerbates inequality and injects fear into the most basic of daily interactions" (p. 904). Grace et al. (2018) report that these policies harm people's mental and physical health. They state that "taken together, the two crises create a vicious cycle that plays out partly in the health care system; policies of uncertainty enact the violence of uncertainty" (p. 379). They further state that violence of uncertainty is perpetuated by policies of uncertainty intended to create systematic insecurity by constantly changing the terms of daily life and targeting what matters most to people. Policies to separate immigrant children from their parents, for instance, or end the reunification of refugee families are recent examples of the process of systematic insecurity. This violence, along with the stress experienced by these populations as a result of posttraumatic stress, depression, and substance use, further exacerbates their health status and negatively affects participation in everyday, culturally sanctioned daily occupations.

Marginalized populations, such as people who are trafficked, refugees, and asylum seekers, experience a wide variety of physical and mental health conditions at much higher rates than the overall population. These include but are not limited to sexually transmitted diseases, eating disorders, headaches, backaches, abdominal pain, nausea, musculoskeletal and skin problems, respiratory disease, substance misuse, mental health and emotional issues, anxiety, panic attacks, insomnia, depression, and low self-esteem (George and Stanley, 2018; Turner-Moss, Zimmerman, Howard, and Oram, 2014). Additionally, these populations have little or no access to medical care and nutrition, further exacerbating health inequalities (Turner-Moss et al., 2014). These health issues are exacerbated among youth, as chronic stress can affect the development of the prefrontal cortex (Purvis, Cross, Dansereau, and Parris, 2013). This area of the brain is the last portion of the brain to develop and is responsible for many of the complex cognitive processes, such as memory and perception (Siddiqui, Chatterjee, Kumar, Siddiqui, and Goyal, 2008), that are linked to the success of future occupational performance.

Occupational Performance and Participation Challenges

The concept of occupational justice, which first emerged in professional discourse in the late 1990s, is still being developed and debated in occupational therapy and occupational science (Whalley Hammell, 2016). An early description of occupational justice was given by Wilcock and Townsend (2000) as "equitable opportunity and resources to enable people's engagement in meaningful occupations" (p. 85). Occupational justice recognizes that "individuals are different and have different needs" (Stadnyk, Townsend, and Wilcock, 2010, p. 334). Because all people have different needs, occupational justice requires the ability to access and engage in occupations that one finds personally meaningful. The ability to engage in individually meaningful occupations is inherently linked to both the health and quality of life of the individual (Stadnyk et al., 2010). Therefore, when individuals are prevented from engaging in occupations they find meaningful, their health and quality of life will be negatively affected. Forms of occupational injustice have been identified and categorized as occupational deprivation, occupational marginalization, occupational imbalance, and occupational apartheid (Kronenberg and Pollard, 2005; Townsend and Wilcock, 2004; Whiteford, 2005) and are frequently experienced by marginalized populations.

It is important to draw a distinction between being unable to engage in meaningful occupations and being unengaged from occupation. Occupational disruption can lead to a decrease in occupation via inefficient time use, causing a person to feel insufficient in valued life roles (Smith, Cornella, and Williams, 2014). Because of this decrease in occupation, the affected individual can also have less community involvement, serving to further isolate and marginalize the person, which perpetuates health inequalities and an overall loss of opportunity (Morville and Erlandsson, 2013; Smith et al., 2014). This is often common in asylum seeker and refugee populations, who may spend years in prolonged migration and waiting before resettlement to a host country.

However, "both doing and a lack of doing can negatively impact health and well-being" (George and Stanley, 2018, p. 10). Construction work, a common setting for labor trafficking, is highly demanding both physically and temporally. Overwork and improper safety procedures can lead to increased musculoskeletal injuries and chronic respiratory disease, as well as chronic stress caused by having pay withheld and travel documents seized while working (George and Stanley, 2018; Turner-Moss et al., 2014). Individuals who have occupations imposed on them also suffer from occupational injustice. Occupation without autonomy can be just as negatively impactful as a lack of occupation.

As Whiteford noted in a case study involving a refugee from Kosovo, "occupational deprivation is . . . a process as well as an outcome" (2005, p. 86). As an outcome, it is associated with physical and mental health conditions as well as harmful coping strategies that are ineffective in an individual's current life (Smith et al., 2014). Individuals who have gone through a difficult migration are likely to have undergone different traumas in addition to their occupational deprivation, resulting in coping strategies that are better suited to ensure survival than to enable participation in meaningful occupations for maximum health and quality of life (Cerny, 2016).

All of these factors combine to entrench occupational injustice as an outcome and a cycle, which must be broken by intervention in order to address its underlying health conditions.

Occupational Risk Factors

Marginalized populations have many risk factors that can increase their chances of experiencing occupational injustice and its attendant physical and mental health conditions. Chief among them are deprivation and isolation and the effects of these risk factors before, during, and after extended migration experiences. Refugee populations often experience isolation due to the language barriers and technology barriers caused by settling in a new country, as well as social isolation because of participating in an underrepresented group or population, and the effects of mental health issues (McAllister, Penn, Smith, Van Dort, and Wilson, 2010; Smith et al., 2014).

A difficult and/or prolonged migration itself is a risk factor for occupational injustice, with many asylum seekers saying their lives were "interrupted, on hold, or blown off course" (Morville and Erlandsson, 2013) as they resettled and attempted to have their legal and immigration status decided. While in the process of migrating or seeking asylum, however, they were still dealing with trauma experienced premigration, enduring new traumas, and continuing to experience trauma postmigration (Copley et al., 2011). Additionally, the experience of migration in itself requires a change in environment, which will always affect participation in daily occupations (Gupta, 2012; Morville and Erlandsson, 2013). Thorton and Spalding (2018) identified that once in the host country—whether in detention centers, refugee camps, or in the community—both asylum seekers and refugees have limited or no (human) rights, few opportunities for living a normal life, nothing to do, little financial support to facilitate activities, a lack of choices, and limited overall control over their lives.

Once approved for resettlement to the United States, the individual goes through additional security checks and clearances, which can take an additional 12 to 24 months. The U.S. Department of State (USDOS, n.d.a) reports that the total time from displacement from home to resettlement is on average 26 years. These marginalized individuals or populations experience prolonged environmental barriers to health promotion, education, employment, and occupational justice. When seeking asylum or migrating as a refugee, individuals' lack of citizenship in their current environment often leads to segregation, isolation, and a reduction in the number of occupations available to them (Crawford, Turpin, Nayar, Steel, and Durand, 2016).

After resettlement, refugees and asylees continue to experience isolation and its related occupational injustice, often restricting the occupation in which a refugee or asylee participates (Smith et al., 2014). The process of being immersed in a new culture and expected to learn its language, food, traditions, and norms is a large stressor in itself (Brymer, Steinberg, Sonoborger, Layne, and Pynoos, 2008; Copley et al., 2011). Because of this isolation and local stigmas, refugees and asylees are frequently isolated by the community they have resettled in and are unable to participate in its functioning and betterment (Morville and Erlandsson, 2013).

Youth who are refugees or asylees have additional needs, as their development, physical health, and mental health are affected by trauma (Brymer et al., 2008; Copley et al., 2011). Compounding these needs is the fact that trauma is not explicitly addressed in many current policies, which are admittedly more person centered than in the past yet still not as proactive and culturally relevant as is necessary to meet the multidimensional needs of asylum seekers and refugees of different backgrounds (Jani and Reisch, 2018). Refugees and asylum seekers often have limited access to occupation in general, as well as to paid work and education (Morville, 2014). Long term, creating an environment that supports asylees and refugees holistically as they attempt to integrate into a new culture and community is necessary in order for them to discover or resume meaningful occupations and roles in their new environments (Huot and Laliberte Rudman, 2010; Morville and Erlandsson, 2013). As 20 people are newly displaced every minute (UNHCR, 2016), occupational therapy practitioners must rise to the challenge to build, study, and reform the systems in place to ensure that all individuals have access to occupational justice, its meaningful occupation, and the human rights and freedom, positive health, and quality of life it inherently brings.

Human Trafficking

"**Human trafficking** is the acquisition of people by improper means such as force, fraud or deception, with the aim of exploiting them" (United Nations Office on Drugs and Crime [UNDOC], 2018, para. 1). A heinous human rights violation that results in pervasive occupational injustice, human trafficking affects persons in every country within and across all borders in the world (Bryant et al., 2015; Gorman and Hatkevich, 2016; Thompson, 2017). "Today, in too many places around the world—including right here in the United States—the injustice of modern slavery and human trafficking still tears at our social fabric" (The White House, 2016, para. 1).

In order to meet the UN definition for human trafficking, there must be movement, coercion, and exploitation of the person (George and Stanley, 2018; UN, 2000). Using this definition, multiple subtypes of trafficking exist, including labor trafficking, sex trafficking, domestic servitude, forced marriage, organ trafficking, and child soldiers (Cockbain and Bowers, 2015; Cockbain, Bowers, and Dimitrova, 2018; International Labor Organization [ILO], 2012). Sex trafficking involves coerced sexual activity up to 40 times per day (Alvarez and Alessi, 2012; Bryant et al., 2015; ILO, 2012; Meshkovska, Siegel, Stutterheim, and Bos, 2015; WHO, 2012). Due to the recent increase in labor trafficking, international governments have been increasing both their attention and resources toward this issue (Cockbain et al., 2018).

Description of the Problem

The UN defines human trafficking as

> *trafficking in persons, as the recruitment, transportation, transfer, harbouring or receipt of persons, by means of the threat or use of force or other forms of coercion, of abduction, of fraud, of deception, of the abuse of power or of a position of vulnerability or of the giving or receiving of payments or benefits to achieve the consent of a person having control over another person, for the purpose of exploitation. Exploitation shall include, at a minimum, the exploitation of the prostitution of others or other forms of sexual exploitation, forced labour or services, slavery or practices similar to slavery, servitude or the removal of organs. (UNODC, 2018)*

The mix of physical and mental health issues of marginalized populations is often complex and not easily resolved. Because of this complexity and the severity of trauma suffered by individuals in recovery from being trafficked, these individuals' health conditions are frequently long-term (George and Stanley, 2018). Oram et al. (2012) found that 88% of women in a sample of individuals in recovery from human trafficking "met ICD-10 criteria for a mental disorder" (p. 4). Women who had received 6 months of posttrafficking support services still reported high levels of symptoms such as headache, memory problems, stomach and back pain, loss of appetite, tooth pain, weight loss, chest pain, and breathing difficulties (Oram et al., 2012). Posttraumatic stress disorder (PTSD) is also a large concern with this population, with high levels of hyperarousal, feelings of hopelessness, and the re-experiencing of traumatic events (Turner-Moss et al., 2014).

Lived Experiences

Just as with other marginalized migration groups, human trafficking involves trauma occurring to individuals over multiple stages. George and Stanley (2018) report the incidence of a "chain of traumatizing events" that occur to an individual during the three main stages of trafficking: recruitment, travel, and transit. Furthermore, once people find themselves "victims" of trafficking, they are more likely to experience *repeat victimization* and *polyvictimization*, with men more likely to experience this than women (deVries and Farrell, 2018).

It follows, then, that the longer that one is actively being trafficked, the more likely one is to suffer from trauma (George and Stanley, 2018). Victims and survivors of trafficking endure severe restrictions for opportunities to participate in activities of daily living (ADLs), educational pursuits, social participation, and other occupations, often for years (Bryant et al., 2015; Macy and Johns, 2011; Muraya and Fry, 2016; Thompson, 2017). This pervasive occupational deprivation can cause extensive biopsychosocial impairments, including but not limited to depression, dissociation, PTSD, cognitive deficits, educational lags, developmental delays, sensory impairments, dental problems, gastrointestinal difficulties, gynecological disorders, and extensive medical ailments (Abas et al., 2013; Gorman and Hatkevich, 2016; Meshkovska et al., 2015; Trickett, Noll, and Putnam, 2011). "Service providers assert that the needs of trafficking survivors are far greater than those of other marginalized groups . . . because they have lived under the abusive control of others and have been traumatized" (Shigekane, 2007, p. 122).

While being actively trafficked, individuals often face isolation through physical imprisonment and debt bondage, insecure legal status, and no knowledge of how or when their debt will be paid (Cerny, 2016; George and Stanley, 2018). Forced occupation and isolation create occupational injustice, such as when individuals are not able to choose occupations in which they participate, leading to decreased satisfaction with roles and an inability to establish and maintain health-promoting routines and habits (George and Stanley, 2018). Occupational marginalization occurs during the cycle of active trafficking and recovery, as discrimination can prevent participation in meaningful occupations and paid labor at home, putting one at risk for recruitment into trafficking. Occupational deprivation occurs primarily during active trafficking, as individuals can no longer choose their own occupations that allow doing, being, becoming, and belonging in a chosen environment. Forced work often occurs over long hours with few breaks, leading to occupational imbalance.

These conditions produce long-term negative effects on body functions, daily activities, participation, and environmental factors as defined by the WHO (2014) in the *International Classification of Functioning, Disability and Health.* The repercussions of trafficking on each person contribute to significant personal, familial, community, national, regional, and international disorganization and dysfunction. Furthermore, resolution of one's active status as an asylum seeker or refugee, or a person who has been trafficked, does not mean an end to physical or mental health difficulties. Additionally, individuals in recovery from human trafficking often self-isolate, preferring to "keep their 'victim-status' a secret . . . to avoid blame, stigma, rejection, or even violence and abuse" (Brunovskis and Surtees, 2013, as cited in George and Stanley, 2018, p. 8). In a 2013 study of individuals who were receiving services while in recovery from labor trafficking, four-fifths of participants reported having experienced at least one symptom of poor physical health in the previous two weeks, and nearly one-third reported having experienced five or more symptoms (Turner-Moss et al., 2014).

Bryant et al. (2015) developed a formative societal statement directed to the AOTA that encouraged the association to pursue formal action to address intervention, research, and education focused on sex trafficking. Sex-trafficked persons live for years incurring the "loss of the roles and occupations associated with their ages and typical developmental stages" (Bryant et al., 2015, p. 18). The authors contended that occupational therapy practitioners could provide evidence-based interventions and opportunities to enhance meaningful occupations for survivors of trafficking.

Engage Your Brain 22-2

Has the AOTA issued a societal statement or official document on human trafficking? What other mechanisms can an AOTA member use to advocate for the AOTA's action with this or other marginalized populations?

Occupational Performance and Participation Challenges

To address the international scope of trafficking, the UN developed the guiding definition, directives, and international legal precedents embodied in the 3P Protocol. The purpose of the protocol is to promote cooperation among nations and professions in antitrafficking efforts, focusing on the areas of prevention, punishment, and protection of survivors (United Nations Office of High Commission on Human Rights [UNOHCHR], 2000). The United States built upon the UN 3P Protocol and added a fourth *P* to the paradigm of prosecution, protection, and prevention—partnership—"to achieve progress across the 3Ps and enlist all segments of society in the fight against modern slavery" (USDOS, n.d.b, para. 1). The occupational therapy literature shows minimal involvement in programs to address trafficking in the three areas delineated in the protocol (Bryant et al., 2015; Gorman and Hatkevich, 2016; Thompson, 2017). To address the pervasive biopsychosocial deficits that result from trafficking, occupational therapy practitioners have the skills, knowledge, and experience to develop extensive practice, research, and education methods that encompass cultural components, gender differences, and individual differences. Potential options for developing a distinct occupational approach within multidisciplinary efforts can encompass intervention, education, and research in the following areas.

Prevention

Current prevention programs specifically focus on young girls. An occupation-based approach to develop prevention programs can be extended to other at-risk populations, including boys, men, women, and the LGBTQ+ communities. Martinez and Kelle (2013) and Shigekane (2007) have identified the need for dedicated services to address the distinct needs of girls, women, boys, men, and the LGBTQ+ communities. Prevention includes both organized and informal efforts directed at vulnerable persons to decrease their recruitment into trafficking activities (USDOS, n.d.b). Informal prevention efforts can include information sessions about trafficking, technical training, educational programs, and microlending services (Kaufman and Crawford, 2011). Prevention program components include awareness of traffickers' recruitment techniques, trafficker identification, techniques to avoid entry into trafficking, and methods to enhance self-esteem. Gorman and Hatkevich (2016) described the potential value of occupational therapy in developing evidence-based programs and conducting and publishing research on prevention programs and education efforts. Occupational therapy practitioners have opportunities to play pivotal roles in developing awareness campaigns, educating medical and law enforcement personnel, and evaluating novel prevention efforts.

Protection

The umbrella of victim protection encompasses rescue that transforms victims into survivors, legal process management, recovery services, and community integration (USDOS, n.d.b). Rescue opportunities include law enforcement raids, organized victim rescues, informal street outreach services, strip club outreach initiatives, and other dedicated outreach programs (USDOS, n.d.b).

Occupational therapy practitioners can develop culturally sensitive programs for all populations to promote recovery and community integration for survivors. Prison alternative options, residential programs, outreach services, postrecovery support groups, alternative recovery programs, and advocacy efforts will benefit from an occupation-based approach. Occupational therapists can develop services to improve survivors' skills in self-care, education, vocational stability, financial management, cognition, stress management, community integration, and advocacy.

"Active participation in meaningful occupations offers a distraction from negative patterns of thinking and promotes feelings of confidence and control while learning new skills" (Gorman and Hatkevich, 2016, p. 3). Using a variety of sensory, musculoskeletal, and other occupation-based approaches, occupational therapy practitioners can provide immediate life skills training in basic self-care, emotional regulation, sleep, and physical stability. Intervention can focus on improving skills in education, employment, social participation, budgeting, home management, and executive function to assist survivors in achieving constructive personal roles, functional performance patterns, and a positive quality of life on a long-term basis. A growing need exists for programs to empower and educate survivors in maneuvering complex national and international legal processes.

Prosecution

Occupational therapy practitioners can serve as expert witnesses in legal proceedings for individual cases. Developing educational programs for persons working in various aspects of the legal system is an area that would benefit from occupational therapy expertise. A vastly underserved area includes the development of rehabilitation services for offenders, solicitors, and traffickers.

Human trafficking encompasses a reprehensible violation of human rights that result in comprehensive occupational deprivation. The literature currently shows minimal, but growing, occupational therapy involvement in the vast field of human trafficking. Using the guiding UN's protocol (UNOHCHR, 2000), occupational therapy practitioners can develop strategies, programs, and methods to enhance prevention, protection, and prosecution efforts. These approaches should consider the needs of each unique individual in light of trafficking within countries, across all international borders, with unique gender needs, and in various cultural settings.

Resources

A variety of resources are available for occupational therapy practitioners to prepare for engagement in this type of community-based and population-based service delivery. For example, an AOTA-approved online continuing education provider offers a course on human trafficking that focuses on the ability to identify, assess, and work with humans who have been trafficked (Sheridan, 2016). Through participation in international and national professional organizations such as those identified earlier in this chapter, practitioners can locate others who have interest and expertise in this population. Social media is another tool that can facilitate this type of communication. For example, four occupational therapists organized the Facebook™ site Occupational Therapy Human Trafficking Network (2018) as an international base to educate, network, and advocate for human trafficking efforts.

LGBTQ+ Communities

In order to understand the lived experience of the LGBTQ+ communities, a discussion of language and meaning is first needed, as well as a review of long-standing societal norms and beliefs. **Heteronormativity** is the belief in a binary system of gender; it assumes heterosexuality is the only sexual norm and that marriage is only acceptable for two persons of opposite sexes. Heteronormativity is linked to heterosexism, homophobia, and transphobia (Leap, 2007). **Cisgender** persons are those whose assigned sex (i.e., genitalia) and gender identity correlate; for example, a person assigned male at birth (i.e., the presence of a penis) and who identifies as of the male gender would be referred to as a cisgender male. Therefore, a cisgender woman who is attracted to men would be referred to as a heterosexual, cisgender woman, and conversely, a cisgender man who is attracted to other men would be a cisgender, gay man. **Cisnormative** is the assumption that all human beings are cisgender (Crethar and Vargas, 2007). Lesbian women and gay men are those individuals who have romantic and sexual attraction to others of the same gender; gay, lesbian, or **same-gender-loving couples** is a term coined by activist Cleo Manago (Black Men's Xchange National, 2012). **Bisexual** persons are attracted to both men and women. **Transgender** is an umbrella term for people whose gender identity and/or gender expression differs from what is typically associated with the sex they were assigned at birth. **Pansexual** persons are those who are open to romantic attachments with cisgender men and women as well as transgender men and transgender women.

Some individuals within the LGBTQ+ communities may identify as gender nonconforming, gender queer, and/or drag queens. **Drag queens,** typically, are gay men who wear clothing, makeup, and wigs to simulate a female or fantasy appearance, most often in the context of being a celebrity or performance artist within the LGBTQ+ community. In recent years, the drag community has come to be more accepted by the general population with the rise of weekly reality competition television shows and the popularity of restaurants that offer weekend brunches with drag performances as entertainment in most major cities across the country, including Los Angeles, Chicago, Philadelphia, Washington, DC, Baltimore, and more. Drag stars are making appearances at major awards events, including the 2019 Academy Awards, in movies such as *Hairspray* and the Academy-Award-nominated *A Star is Born,* and in television shows with drag queen stars such as Netflix's *Dancing Queen.* Other persons within the LGBTQ+ communities may identify as **gender queer** or **gender nonconforming.** These individuals may present variously in attire that is a mix of masculine and feminine; this may be an aspect of personal expression, a reflection of undetermined gender—as is the case with some intersex individuals—or an act of social rebellion and consciousness raising. **Intersex** is a general term used for a variety of conditions in which a person is born with a reproductive or sexual anatomy that does not seem to fit the typical definition of female or male. **Asexual** persons are those individuals who do not experience or act on sexual attraction to others but desire and likely seek intimate relationships that are of a nonsexual nature (Lesbian, Gay, Bisexual, Transgender, Queer, Intersex, Asexual [LGBTQIA] Resource Center, n.d.).

There are multiple forms of intersex, including:

- Klinefelter syndrome (a person with 47 XXY chromosomes)
- Androgen insensitivity syndrome (AIS; a person with 46 XY chromosomes, born with female external genitalia due to the inability of the developing fetus to process androgens or male hormones)
- Turner syndrome (a person with 46 XO chromosomes), hypospadias (where the urethral opening is located along the underside of the penis rather than the tip), aphallia (a person with 46 XY chromosomes, born without a penis)
- clitoromegaly (a person with 46 XX chromosomes, born with a large clitoris that may appear to be a penis)

Other conditions of intersex exist with variable differences in genitalia and the ability to procreate. Some conditions are readily visible, with the genitalia being ambiguous (not appearing male or female) at birth. (Intersex Society of North America, 2008)

Transgender persons may choose to socially, medically (via hormonal therapies), and physically (through surgical procedures) transition to becoming whole with their gender identities. Gender-confirming surgeries have been available in the United States since the early 1960s. In the past, such persons were referred to as transsexuals; this term came from the work of Dr. Harry Benjamin in the 1960s (GLAAD, 2017). The term **transsexual** referred to those persons that fully transitioned legally, socially, medically, and surgically. This term is not used much today, as it is too narrow a definition of the transgender experience. However, some people identify as transgender and live in their gender identity without hormonal therapies and/or surgeries for multiple reasons. These persons may feel that while they identify as a specific gender, their birth genitalia are not a source of dysphoria, or medical conditions may prohibit medical transition due to contraindications such as high blood pressure, a history of blood clotting, or heart disease (Futterweit, 1998). Cost might be another reason or barrier to surgery. Historically, health insurance companies have used language such as "experimental or cosmetic" to delegitimize gender-affirming surgeries in order to deny health insurance coverage for these procedures—a form of discrimination, as these procedures are well researched and are considered the medical standard (Lambda Legal, n.d.).

Lived Experience

Historically, the LGBTQ+ communities have been marginalized in most Judeo-Christian and Islamic cultures (Human Rights Campaign, n.d.). Sodomy laws were used to criminalize the actions of same-gender-loving individuals and those who wore clothing of the opposite sex (drag queens and transgender persons), leading to attempts at conversion therapies, public humiliation (e.g., names published in newspapers), loss of employment, limited access to housing, institutionalization, and even death. Discrimination, public condemnation, and outdated social norms would also often lead to the loss of family connections for individuals who identified as LGBTQ+. Shame, guilt, and rejection, historically, have been significant factors within the LGBTQ+ communities, leading to higher rates of depression and suicide (Centers for Disease Control and Prevention, 2017). The 1960s and early 1970s saw a debate within the American Psychological Association over the classification of homosexuality as a mental disorder; the debate ended in 1973 when homosexuality was removed from the *Diagnostic and Statistical Manual of Mental Disorders (DSM) II* (Drescher, 2015).

However, stigma and discrimination continue to linger. Recent examples include marriage licensees, gender definitions, bathroom access, and the ability to serve in the U.S. military. In 2015 in Rowan County, Kentucky, clerk Kim Davis refused to issue marriage licenses to same-sex couples, defying the Supreme Court; this event was well publicized in major media outlets (e.g., Blinder and Pérez-Peña, 2015). If reported draft policy changes to narrow the definition of gender are enacted, they would remove federal recognition of an estimated 1.4 people in the United States who choose to identify in terms other than male or female (Green, Benner, and Pear, 2018), leaving transgender persons in legal limbo related to passports, driver's licenses, and other legal documents. Transgendered individuals are being affected by a federal administration regulation. The

American Medical Association president criticized the transgender military ban, saying that "the only thing deficient is any medical science behind this decision" (Associated Press and Lyster, 2019).

> ***Minority stress*** *is the concept that stigma-related prejudice and discrimination experienced by LGBTQ people constitute chronically stressful events that can lead to negative health outcomes. Minority stress has been linked to psychological distress among gay men and lesbians and may contribute to elevated rates of distress frequently observed among LGBTQ. (Kelleher, 2009, p. 3)*

The LGBTQ+ communities are very diverse, and discrimination has existed between the various component groups. Today the communities are more cooperative in working together toward legal and civil rights. While same-gender-loving couples now have the right to legal marriage, discrimination in other forms remains. As of March 6, 2018, Idaho became the 47th state to allow transgender persons to legally change their gender on birth certificates; Ohio, Kansas, and Tennessee continue to prevent any changes to the birth records (Lambda Legal, 2018). Eighteen states do not protect LGBTQ+ from employment discrimination in any form, and 27 do not protect LGBTQ+ from discrimination in public accommodations (e.g., restaurants, hotels, entertainment), with two additional states only protecting lesbians, gays, and bisexuals but not transgender individuals. Ten states only offer protection in public sector employment, and only 17 states protect LGBT from employment discrimination in both public and private sectors (Lambda Legal, 2018).

Occupational Performance and Participation Challenges

Minority stress, discussed earlier, negatively affects the occupational engagement of members of the LGBTQ+ communities. For example, gay married men reported being "hyper-vigilant, uncomfortable, or unwelcome in public spaces" where they went to engage in instrumental activities of daily living (IADLs), such as grocery shopping and leisure occupations (Wrightsman, 2018, p. 105). This chronic impact on occupation choice and experience was buffered by positive feelings regarding time in the home and the role of spouse.

Multiple studies have shown that the LGBTQ+ communities have experienced, continue to experience, and fear experiencing discriminatory practices from health-care providers. This can lead to hiding their identities due to fear; this is especially of concern to LGBTQ+ seniors (Swiatek and Jewell, 2018). Suggested approaches to support ethical practice include the following (Swiatek and Jewel, 2018, pp. 17–18):

- Eliminating "heterosexist assumptions," or the assumption that heterosexuality is the only sexual norm and that marriage is only acceptable for two persons of opposite sexes
- "Encouraging sensitivity trainings for health care and social service providers to promote safe environments"
- Selecting updated assessment tools that avoid the use of binary exclusionary language
- Using inclusive language
- Developing "outreach programs and services that cater to" seniors in LGBTQ+ communities
- Creating an open and welcoming environment (e.g., post a rainbow or other LGBTQ+ symbol, acknowledge LGBTQ+ Awareness Day)

Additionally, individuals in marginalized communities often lack adequate health-care insurance coverage. Issues related to quality of care include a lack of provider knowledge of the medical and psychological needs of LGBTQ+ communities and violations of Health Insurance Portability and Accountability Act (HIPAA) standards for patient confidentiality, as well as outright hostility from caregiver and support staff (Grant, Mottet, Tanis, Herman, and Keisling, 2011; Gurmankin, Caplan, and Braverman, 2005; Harrison-Quintana and Herman, 2013; Kovacs, Stefaneau, Smyth, and Ezzat, 1994).

In recent years, transgender communities have become more vocal in terms of advocacy for acceptance and civil rights. This has led to a backlash from conservative groups and legislators, leading to multiple issues related to bathroom access in schools and the community at large. This debate is ongoing and emotion charged. For example, concerns about women and children being assaulted in restrooms have been cited as the impetus of efforts to legalize discrimination despite a lack of evidence to support these claims. Bathroom separation is historically not specific to the LGBTQ+ communities, as African Americans experienced these types of restrictions well into the 1960s.

Enhancing health-care providers' understanding of LGBTQ+-related language and their self-awareness of personal biases are key to offering improved standards of health care for the LGBTQ+ communities. Personal information related to an individual's sexuality, sexual habits, and genitalia can be titillating, and therefore there is an urge to share confidential information with coworkers. To improve quality of care, health-care providers will need to be mindful of and adhere to HIPAA standards, including those associated with need-to-know personal information and protected health information.

Health-care providers also need to be aware of the importance of asking clinically driven questions and mindful of what information is purely for curiosity. Questions unrelated to care should be minimal and mimic those asked in care scenarios with nontransgendered persons to avoid creating a negative encounter with the patient. For example, asking a trans person about plans for surgeries may be relevant to certain medical conditions if knowing what surgeries have or have not taken place would assist in reducing discomfort for the patient and the clinician prior to any procedure that involves disrobing (e.g., medical examinations, medical procedures, assisting with toileting). However, if an occupational therapy practitioner is not addressing activities that require disrobing, questions about surgeries are not relevant to care and are intrusive. Additionally, seemingly benign questions such as "What did your name use to be?" (referred to as dead naming) or "Do you have a picture of you before?" are also intrusive, as the person is being asked to identify with an earlier part of life that was likely painful and does not represent who they believe themselves to be or who the person presents as in all aspects of daily life. Some trans persons may choose to share this information freely, but these types of questions should be avoided.

Following gender-affirming surgeries, transgender persons may require ongoing personal care to maintain positive surgical outcomes. Postoperatively, trans women need to insert vaginal stents or dilators into the neovagina for several minutes several times a month to maintain depth and diameter to allow for penetration during sexual intercourse during times when medical needs prevent the individual from having an active sexual relationship. This maintenance becomes part of weekly ADL needs and may need to be addressed with a patient after an incapacitating medical procedure or medical event, such as a stroke, leading to the need for rehabilitation. In contrast, preoperative and nonoperative trans women may need assistance and training with donning and doffing a gaff (i.e., compression undergarment) and tucking to hide any genital bulge in clothing. Additionally, some transgender women who have not completed electrolysis or laser hair removal may place a high value on facial and body hair removal and the application of makeup to cover beard shadow, and some may wear wigs or hair pieces as part of their need to present at their best. Such accommodations may not be simply a desire to look their best but can also address social anxiety and personal safety and assist in presenting as their true selves. Trans men may need assistance and training in how to don and doff chest binders worn underneath clothing to present with a male-appearing chest. Additionally, some trans men may place a high value on the use of adaptive equipment (e.g., stand-to-urinate devices), again to address areas of self-concept and the ability to more fully function in the community as men. Many transgender persons have posted tutorial videos on YouTube as resources that can be used by occupational therapy practitioners to familiarize themselves with these processes. They may also be useful as teaching aids in a peer-to-peer manner. As with any online resource, the videos need to be screened for quality. Videos may be graphic—appropriately so—and some videos may be of limited usefulness.

In summary, while all persons have the right to their personal spiritual, religious, or moral beliefs, the occupational therapy practitioner is also responsible for being mindful of the needs, rights, and dignity of those who seek such expertise. Discrimination in any form, be it misgendering (i.e., referring to a transgender woman as he or a transgender man as she), disrespectfulness, or intentional or benign neglect, is discrimination. Health-care providers and all helping professionals need to seek appropriate education and training to assist the client to maximize independence and dignity in the community. The LGBTQ+ person is not there as a teacher, and therefore the occupational therapy practitioner must have sufficient familiarity to improve personal comfort to best serve their clients. Sensitivity and respect are key in all aspects of modern ethical health care. Additionally, each occupational therapy practitioner is also responsible for challenging any other colleague to be mindful of interactions and language both verbal and in documentation (AOTA, 2015). Discrimination is discrimination.

Incarcerated Communities and Post-Released Populations

Another marginalized population facing occupational injustices includes persons imprisoned in the correctional system. The **correctional system** is responsible for "apprehending, prosecuting, defending, sentencing, and punishing those who are suspected or convicted of criminal offences" (Oxford Dictionaries, 2018, para. 1). The United States currently has the highest level of incarceration compared to other countries, with an average of 2,300,000 individuals in jail or prison (Wagner and Sawyer, 2018).

Currently, there are 1,316,000 people held in state prisons, while 225,000 individuals are being held in federal jails and prisons. In addition, of those, 53,000 youth are being detained within the system (Courtney et al., 2017. Demographically, a disproportionate representation of people of color are incarcerated. In 2016, people who identified as African American represented 12% of the U.S. adult population but 33% of the sentenced prison population. People of Hispanic ethnicity represented 16% of the adult population but accounted for 23% of inmates. In contrast, people who identified as Caucasian accounted for 64% of the adult population but only 30% of the prison population (Gramlich, 2018). Women make up approximately 7% of the total prison population (Carson, 2018). Globally, the number of prisoners tracked by the Institute for Criminal Policy Research in 2015 was 10,350,000, but due to a variety of political realities, the actual number could be over 11,000,000 people (Walmsley, 2015).

Individuals convicted in the United States are serving long terms. However, the length of actual time served is closely linked to individual state policies. Of those serving the longest prison terms, 40% were incarcerated before the age of 25. Data indicate that the average time served across the country has increased, with many states reporting an average of 10 years served in prison for every 1 in 10 people incarcerated. Additionally, 33% of the people serving the longest terms are 55 and older, thereby indicating people are aging in prison (Courtney et al., 2017). The prison population in the United States is aging; people are incarcerated when they are young and are serving longer sentences.

Once an individual has served time in a penitentiary and been released, there is a high probability the person will be rearrested or returned to prison. **Recidivism,** the reengagement in criminal behavior after serving a sentence, is measured by criminal acts resulting in rearrests, reconviction, or a return to prison, with or without a new sentence, during a 3-year period following a prisoner's release (Durose, Cooper, and Snyder, 2014). Studies indicate that 44% of individuals who were released between 2005 and 2014 recommitted crimes within the first year of release. This number increases to 82% when examining the 3-year period after release (Alper, Durose, and Markman, 2018).

Lived Experiences

One of the primary purposes of prisons is punishment (Zoukis, 2014). Some justice systems include rehabilitation as a mission of their institutions although there are minimal opportunities provided to those incarcerated, and those provided are often not client or occupation centered. Decisions regarding time allocation and the way in which time is spent are dictated by prison resources. Programs offered to individuals are those that have been mandated or designed based on state or federally funded programs and offer little opportunity for choice regarding topic or content. This leads to occupational deprivation, which has been linked to prison violence, suicides, and psychosis (Molineux and Whiteford, 1999).

Prison life is extremely regimented. The typical freedoms and occupational choices many take for granted are not afforded to people living within a prison. The choice of when and how to perform basic self-care tasks is removed, and many decisions are made based on systemic issues such as staffing. For example, depending on the ratio of inmates to correctional officers, times allotted to basic self-care tasks, such as eating, may be significantly altered. The occupation of sleep is significantly affected within the prison setting as well. Inmates are typically awoken throughout the night by correctional officers conducting cell checks as well as by ongoing noises within the facility (Seruya et al., 2019).

Access to basic services such as health care, while available, is not easily obtained (Wilper et al., 2009) and often requires a co-pay from inmates (Zoukis, 2018). Those who require health care often must wait for extended periods of time prior to gaining access to a health provider. Due to the restrictive nature and lack of resources available in the prison setting, there are limited treatment options offered, other than pharmacological interventions, for those with chronic conditions such as diabetes, asthma, or cardiovascular disease. Individuals with physical needs are often not provided with the necessary adaptive or durable medical equipment.

In addition, minimal services are available to address psychosocial issues such as depression and anxiety or other more serious mental illnesses. Based on growing pressure to enhance the care of prisoners with mental health concerns, the Federal Bureau of Prisons instituted a new policy in 2014. This appears to have resulted in a decreased number of prisoners classified as needing regular mental health services; thus, fewer federal prisoners have access to treatment for serious mental health conditions on a regular basis (Thompson and Eldridge, 2018). After the start of the new policy, the number of federal prisoners needing regular mental health services was reported as 3%, while the rates for states with large penal populations in California (30%), Texas (20%), and New York (21%) reported much higher rates. While only 3% of federal prisoners are "deemed ill enough to merit regular therapy, officials acknowledge that 23 percent have been diagnosed with some type of mental illness" (Thompson and Eldridge, 2018, p. A4).

Prisons are intended to create social isolation, as the individual is removed from society. Inmates have minimal contact with the outside world and often must earn privileges, such as visitation from family and loved ones. Even in circumstances in which visitation may occur, interactions are monitored and frequently do not allow for intimacy or human physical contact. There are no means for those who are incarcerated to have regular access to independently controlled connections typical to daily life in the outside world, such as television, use of the Internet, or social media, further adding to social isolation and deprivation. Sensory deprivation is a significant concern in prolonged solitary confinement (Cloud, Drucker, Browne, and Parsons, 2015). Additionally, the physical environment of a prison lacks typical sensory exposure. The amount of time inmates are allowed outdoors and access to natural light, depending on the prison, may also be highly limited. In addition, with a large number of people confined to a closed, confined space, the environment creates continual auditory and visual stimulation.

Occupational Performance/Participation Challenges

While people who have been incarcerated demonstrate significant needs, the majority of prisoners in the United States are released without receiving services that help prepare them for life after prison. In addition, due to the restrictive nature of the prison setting, many individuals who are released do not recognize their occupational deficits until they are released and attempt to reintegrate (Williams, 2015). Adding to the lack of preparation and skill, people who are released from prison after serving a full term are often released without a plan to reenter the community. Further, individuals may be incarcerated in different geographic locations than where they had originally lived, making reentry all the more challenging (Seruya et al., 2019; Smith et al., 2018).

Once released, individuals who have been incarcerated experience numerous challenges in their everyday lives. After living in prison, many people experience anxiety when faced with having to make personal choices and decisions (Seruya et al., 2019). When individuals attempt to reintegrate into the community, they typically have both diminished skill sets and self-esteem. People who have been incarcerated may also demonstrate executive function disorders that have an impact on self-regulation, impulse control, and working memory (Meijers, Hsrte, Jonker, and Meynen, 2015). Therefore, in addition to environmental challenges, there may also be changes in the individual's internal capacity, affecting occupational function and successful reentry. The occupational deprivation that inmates endure while incarcerated can lower the ability of the individual to adapt. In a qualitative study, individuals incarcerated and eligible for parole indicated a preference to remain in prison due to fear of the challenges they would face upon release (Best, Wodahl, and Holmes, 2014).

After release, many individuals often find themselves without the skills to obtain the basic necessities of everyday life, including the ability to apply for housing or access health care. Those individuals with mental health needs, such as substance abuse or anxiety and depression that were not addressed while incarcerated, frequently continue to experience these issues, also leading to a negative impact on successful reintegration (Kim and Peterson, 2014). While there may be opportunities for public assistance in the community, the cognitive, physical, and environmental resources required to access these services often create barriers (Seruya et al., 2019; Smith et al., 2018). For example, travel to Social Service offices may require knowledge of the bus schedule and money for a bus pass. In addition, various community agencies may be located far away from each other. Furthermore, the ability to complete forms for housing or employment may require the ability to utilize online or computerized systems, to which these individuals would not have access while in prison.

By the time many people are released from prison, they are often of an age when most others would have established careers and social connections. Research has shown that individuals who have formerly been incarcerated are at a high risk of economic insecurity due to the challenges that exist while attempting to obtain gainful employment (Harding, Wyse, Dobson, and Morenoff, 2014). Although great strides have been made to provide equal employment opportunities for those who have been incarcerated through initiatives such as Ban the Box (see Box 22-2) on employment applications (Avery and Hernandez, 2018), those who have been incarcerated have lacked the opportunities to develop the skills, education, and experience needed to be competitive applicants for employment.

In 2008, legislation was passed to authorize the Second Chance Act (2008; U.S. Department of Justice [USDJ], 2018). This important legislation (see Box 22-3) authorized the provision of grant monies to develop services for individuals who

Box 22-2 Ban the Box

Have you ever been convicted?

In 2008, All of Us or None, a civil and human rights organization, began a campaign for fair and nondiscriminatory hiring policies for people previously incarcerated. Ban the Box advocated for removal of the question of whether a job applicant has ever been convicted. Given the high number of individuals in the United States who have been incarcerated, the addition of this question to job applications made it difficult for individuals to gain employment after incarceration.

This movement has largely been geared toward either governmental or public employment; however, more private employment agencies are voluntarily adopting this practice. In addition, the movement has begun to broaden to other areas of assistance, such as public housing. As of this writing, 33 states and over 150 cities have adopted Ban the Box as part of their fair hiring practices. It should be noted that although individuals may not need to indicate whether they have been incarcerated, employers still retain the right to complete criminal background checks, and some areas of employment require criminal background checks to be completed.

From *Ban the Box: U.S. Cities, Counties, and States Adopt Fair Hiring Policies to Advance Employment Opportunities for People With Past Convictions*, by B. Avery and P. Hernandez, 2018, National Employment Law Project.

Box 22-3 H.R. 1593—Second Chance Act of 2007

110th Congress (2007–2008)

Sponsor: Representative Danny K. Davis (D-IL)

The Second Chance Act of 2007 (H.R. 1593) was submitted to the House of Representatives in 2007 to amend the Omnibus Crime Control and Safe Streets Act of 1968. The purpose of the Second Chance Act was to address the increased rates of recidivism and public safety as well as the growing numbers of inmates reentering communities across the United States. The act included the ability to reauthorize, rewrite, and expand provisions for adult and juvenile offender reentry demonstration projects and to provide expanded services to offenders and their families for community reentry, including jobs, housing, and substance abuse and mental health treatment.

From Second Chance Act of 2007, Pub. L. 110–199, 122, Stat. 657 (2008).

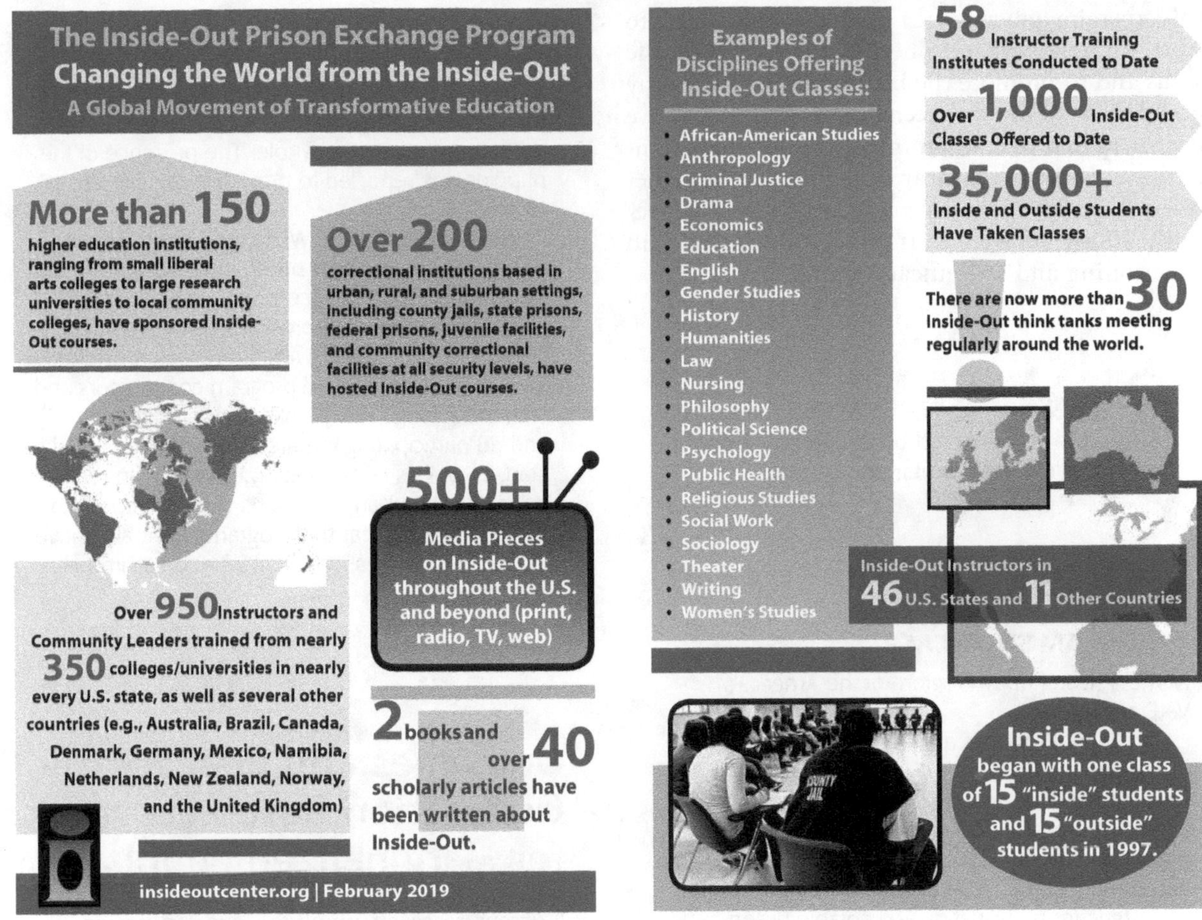

Figure 22-1 Inside-out prisoner exchange program data. *(From* About Us, *The Inside-Out Prison Exchange Program, 2018. Used with permission.)*

have been released from prison and appropriate programming to address their needs for housing, employment, and health care (USDJ, 2018). The *Inside-Out Prison Exchange Program®*, which brings "incarcerated (inside) and non-incarcerated (outside) people together for engaged and informed dialogue [and] allows for transformative learning experiences" (Inside-Out, 2018, para. 2), and other programs that provide educational opportunities, allowing prisoners to obtain college degrees while in prison, have demonstrated positive outcomes. The reach of the Inside-Out Prison Exchange Program® is shown in Figure 22-1. Those involved in educational programs have lower levels of recidivism and higher employment rates than those who do not participate in these programs (Mastrorilli, 2016).

Molineux and Whiteford (1999) promoted the use of occupational enrichment strategies to combat the negative impacts of occupational deprivation from prolonged incarceration. However, to date, there are scant data indicating how many occupational therapy practitioners currently work in the U.S. criminal justice system (Muñoz, Moreton, and Sitterly, 2015). There is increased interest and scholarship among educators and practitioners regarding occupational therapy's role within the correctional system, often within occupational therapy academic programs. Occupational therapy practitioners are able to address skills such as parenting, stress management, social skills, problem-solving, and wellness (Dailey, 2002; Dailey and Reitz, 2003; Rosenbaum et al., 2018), and life skills (Hetache-Pretzer and Jacob, 2018). Practitioners working within this emerging practice area have the opportunity to work directly with prisoners to develop basic life skills and to promote the incorporation of healthy occupations to improve reentry efforts. Studies have demonstrated that when inmates engage in meaningful activities while incarcerated they show higher levels of positive identity and adaptability (Whiteford, 2000), as well as improved executive skill functioning and self-efficacy (Bradbury, 2015).

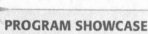

Engage Your Brain 22-3

How are the issues faced by the various populations in this chapter similar and different?

PROGRAM SHOWCASE

Name: Prison Puppy Program of the America's VetDogs (n.d.)

Location: Programs are located in correctional institutions from Maine to Florida.

Goal: To raise and train future service dogs for wounded veterans while providing inmates with the opportunity to participate in an altruistic occupation and develop job and life skills

Criteria for participation: Acceptable prison behavioral records

Application process: Inmates are required to write a letter of intent, which they submit to a liaison. A selection committee of health-related and custody professionals and program staff reviews the letter and records. Inmates who are veterans with an honorable discharge are given preference.

Inmate handler training: Inmate handlers learn to teach the puppies through a series of weekly 2-hour classes. The inmate handlers learn how to teach basic obedience skills and service dog tasks (e.g., opening doors, providing physical support for standing and stair use, picking up dropped items). The curriculum also contains material on puppy development, behavior theory, socialization, and basic first aid.

Puppy training: A group of three to four puppies begin the program at age 8 to 9 weeks. Puppies live in the inmate handler's cell on weekdays, where crate training and other housebreaking and puppy skills start immediately. On weekends, puppies visit "weekend puppy raiser" families to extend their training into the broader world, so the puppies can acclimate to traffic, car rides, and community settings.

Outcomes: Prison officials remarked on the benefit of the program to the inmate handlers and for the institution as a whole. The presence of the puppies was reported to provide a calming effect to all.

Research evidence: While there is anecdotal, positive evidence from other correctional officials involved in similar service-dog-training programs and from dog-training-program administrators (Hogle, 2009), there is limited research evidence. Studies that interviewed program coordinators and staff in 13 programs (Cooke and Farrington, 2014) and 38 participating inmates, administrators, and staff, as well as community members who received dogs from two Kansas prisons (Britton and Button, 2005), indicate that the programs have a positive impact on inmates, prison staff, and community participants.

Outcomes and Challenges of Occupation-Based Programs for Marginalized Populations

Current research involving the evaluation of programs for marginalized populations remains extremely limited for all fields, especially occupational therapy. For example, a systematic review examining the European evidence base regarding human trafficking and labor exploitation found that "publications typically described trafficking's problem profile and/or discussed interventions; they rarely assessed trafficking's impacts or evaluated interventions . . . The quality of evidence was variable and often low" (Cockbain et al., 2018, p. 319).

Previous research has found that by working with refugees, practitioners' cultural awareness and confidence can increase (Jani and Reisch, 2018). However, there are also many challenges that can accompany working with marginalized populations. For example, difficulty establishing a clear history, ongoing risky behavior, increased social needs, a lack of trained practitioners, a lack of engagement, and a lack of interagency collaboration have been found to be challenges when working with individuals in recovery from human trafficking (Abas et al., 2013; Domoney, Howard, Abas, Broadbent, and Oram, 2015; Thompson and Haley, 2018). When examining access to mental health care for individuals in recovery from human trafficking, difficulty in navigating the system of services has led to inconsistent and sometimes unsafe care. Difficulty scheduling intake, coordinating care, making referrals, and a lack of organizational support with regard to working with this population can add unnecessary complexity to treating already complex individuals and is an issue ripe for advocacy (Cheshire, 2017; Domoney et al., 2015; Thompson and Haley, 2018).

Further challenging working with marginalized populations is the paucity of standardized occupational therapy assessments to measure baseline client factors, performance skills and patterns, and participation that do not rely on the client's ability to communicate in written or spoken English. Inmates have lower literacy rates, higher rates of learning disabilities (11% compared to 3% for the general population), and fewer opportunities to read the type of documents needed upon release for the IADLs (National Center for Education, 1994)

Evidence is lacking that addresses the best interventions to use with clients during the resettlement period. In addition to absent or severely limited English literacy, many clients seen are preliterate in their native language as well. Assessment tools and methods that have been adapted are utilized in practice; however, the degree of diagnostic accuracy following subsequent administration may not be as high as one would typically observe in the absence of those adaptations. Occupational profiles, along with skilled observation of the individual performing the activities/occupations, are utilized to obtain the best assessment data.

The needs of marginalized populations are as broad as they are deep. One of the great challenges of the current time will be how governments, nongovernmental organizations, and health-care systems respond to the proven physical and mental health inequalities experienced by populations such as inmates, LGBTQ+ communities, asylum seekers, and refugees, as well as individuals who have experienced human trafficking.

Development of Occupation-Based Programs for Marginalized Populations

Most policies and programs designed to assist marginalized populations have focused solely on physical health needs and have not addressed all the issues that are influencing the health and quality of life of marginalized populations (Cerny, 2016; Hom and Woods, 2013; Konstantopoulos et al., 2013). However, as has been described, their needs are complex and may require an interprofessional team involving physical medical care, psychosocial support, and counseling in order to enable holistic services that can facilitate full participation in meaningful occupation (Oram et al., 2012).

As with all aspects of occupational therapy, practitioners must consider all of the contexts in which an individual participates. Recognizing the role that power plays in occupational injustice and understanding that injustice is socially constructed, one must consider the socioeconomic context, political context, and social determinants of health in addition to the more obvious physical and social contexts (George and Stanley, 2018). In order to address this, occupational therapy practitioners must collaborate with local organizations (through training and outreach), serve in positions in which they can make and affect policy, obtain funding to complete research, and contact legislators to address issues affecting marginalized populations (Cerny, 2016). Once exposed to the population, learning about and understanding the experiences of their migration, their personal strengths and challenges, the environmental (including political and policy) affordances and barriers to resettlement, and the successful integration into the local culture and customs required for self-sufficiency, the occupational needs of these groups and individuals become clear.

Summary

- Occupational therapy practitioners are ethically bound to support the eradication of occupational apartheid and the promotion of occupational freedom for marginalized persons, communities, and populations.

- Marginalized persons, communities, and populations live lives challenged by bias and restricted access to resources.
- Occupational injustice impedes the ability of marginalized persons, communities, and populations to participate and benefit from occupational engagement.
- Occupational therapy practitioners have the expertise to develop innovative strategies to address harassment, health inequities, and occupational apartheid among marginalized persons, communities, and populations. They also have the skills to replicate, adapt, and evolve programs described in this chapter.
- Occupational therapy theories combined with those from other disciplines provide support for the development of innovative strategies to address the needs of marginalized persons, communities, and populations.

CASE STUDIES

CASE STUDY 22-1 History and Recovery of a Survivor of Sexual Trafficking

Family history: Chris is one of four children in a well-established family, living with one biological parent and one stepparent who joined the family when Chris was an infant. Chris's stepparent began fondling Chris during the preschool years, which advanced to sexual penetration by the age of 8. By age 11, the stepparent trafficked Chris several times per week within a 50-mile radius of the home and during family vacations. During this time, Chris attended school, played soccer and lacrosse, joined in social activities with friends, and participated in family celebrations.

The trafficking journey: At age 14, Chris told the biological parent about the sexual abuse. The biological parent accused Chris of making up stories and seeking attention. The trafficking continued. Within 1 year, Chris ran away from home by taking a bus to a larger city. Upon arrival at the bus station, a kind stranger offered Chris a meal, which progressed to a bed for the night. Within 1 week, the stranger bought Chris new clothes and professed "special feelings." A few weeks later, the stranger asked Chris to entertain a friend with sexual favors "just one time." Within 2 weeks, the stranger was trafficking Chris to upscale clients on a daily basis, up to 30 times per day, moving Chris from city to city under the direction of managers, often called bottom bitches. The upscale settings included elegant parties, chic hotel rooms, yachts, and elaborate homes. When Chris showed reluctance to perform the sexual activities, the bottom bitch beat Chris and laced Chris's food with drugs.

Chris became friends with several others who were trafficked by this group, even though the bottom bitches shifted the victims around often to prevent bonding. Chris tried to run away and use the cell phone for purposes other than business, which resulted in beatings and demands for more nontraditional sexual activities.

After 2 years of being trafficked, Chris showed decreases in physical attractiveness, performance skills, and cognitive function due to repeated sexual trauma and coerced drug addiction. Chris was then moved to the street level of trafficking in cheap hotels, backstreets, and shoddy brothels. After 5 more years of being trafficked, Chris showed poor ability to continue performing sexual and daily activities due to untreated anal problems. The traffickers discarded Chris to the street one night, after having made well over $750,000 from Chris's unpaid, coerced work.

Detox phase of recovery: Chris had the advantage of being discarded, while most trafficked victims cannot escape "the life." Chris showed cognitive disintegration, signs of substance withdrawal, sensory-processing difficulties, flashbacks, PTSD symptoms, memory impairment, and decreased self-esteem. After three nights on the street, Chris met another kind stranger who guided Chris to a shelter. Shelter staff arranged for Chris to attend a detox facility and to receive treatment for severe gastrointestinal problems, including anal difficulties.

CASE STUDY 22-1 History and Recovery of a Survivor of Sexual Trafficking

Assessment phase of recovery: After completing detox, Chris entered a residential assessment program for survivors of trafficking. In the assessment program, Chris performed basic household tasks, such as cleaning the room shared with a peer, as well as group meal preparation and cleanup. Daily activities included reflection time, group and individual therapies, exercise activities, nutrition, and life planning. A volunteer occupational therapy practitioner worked with each resident to develop a personal life plan.

Chris became aware that certain activities, perfumes, and phrases served as "triggers" that caused immediate reactionary increases in anxiety, rapid heart rate, flashbacks, and an inability to cope with current environmental demands. Through daily occupations, Chris worked to be more aware of methods to manage anxiety attacks, depression, mood changes, flashbacks, cognitive lapses, triggers, and weight gain despite a healthy nutritional regimen. The volunteer occupational therapy practitioner developed a comprehensive, multidisciplinary program with an occupational base, a sensory-processing element, and a trauma-informed approach to assist survivors in the assessment phase. The management staff accepted the program proposal but were unable to implement it due to a lack of financial resources.

Residential recovery phase: After three weeks, Chris qualified for a 12- to 24-month residential recovery program. In the program, Chris completed household tasks decided by the group, including shopping, meal planning, meal preparation, and home management. Chris chose to care for all the houseplants for the mandatory in-house volunteer project. To comply with program requirements, Chris worked on getting a general education diploma GED™ with a tutor, found health-care resources with the help of a technology volunteer, and participated in group and individual therapies. With the assistance of a volunteer attorney, Chris had legal charges dismissed, pressed charges against the traffickers, and filed a lawsuit to seek restitution, including coverage of occupational therapy services, a right secured by the passage of the Trafficking Victims Protection Reactivation Act. A volunteer occupational therapy practitioner worked with Chris to develop advocacy strategies and coping skills to manage this strenuous legal process.

Chris secured a part-time job in a veterinary clinic affiliated with the recovery program, for which he volunteered to walk dogs at a shelter once a week and participated in the therapeutic equine program. An occupational therapy practitioner completed a needs assessment and proposed an occupational approach to recovery, but funding allocations were not available to implement the services.

Transitional living phase: After 15 months, Chris graduated from the residential program and earned a place in the transitional program. Upon completion of the GED, Chris began a 1-year veterinary technician program at the community college while continuing work at the vet clinic and animal shelter, as well as continuing therapies and participation in a substance abuse support group. Within 1 month, Chris entered into a dating relationship that resulted in emotional turmoil and a relapse of substance abuse. Chris spent 1 week in the recovery program, then progressed back to transitional living. In the community integration group led by an occupational therapy practitioner, Chris identified sources of healthy relationships and developed a plan to select a safe independent living setting.

Independent living: After 1 year in the transitional living program, Chris moved into an apartment, completed a veterinary tech program, secured full-time employment at the veterinary clinic, began volunteering at a therapeutic equine center, and joined a community activity center with a gym and leisure activity offerings. Other ongoing activities included individual psychotherapy, participation in a substance abuse support group, and periodic speeches at events about trafficking recovery. After an arduous legal battle, Chris won a judgment to receive financial restitution but has been unable to collect because the traffickers are imprisoned.

CASE STUDY 22-1 History and Recovery of a Survivor of Sexual Trafficking

Discussion Questions

1. What occupation-based theoretical frameworks would guide the occupational therapy volunteer's work with Chris? What occupation-based theoretical frameworks could be used to support practice for the marginalized population of people who have been sexually trafficked?
2. What research methodology would be most appropriate in investigating the efficacy of occupational therapy services focused on the complex biopsychosocial needs of this marginalized population?
3. Which methods are the most effective at ensuring the reliable measurement of and efficacy of these outcomes?
4. What ethical principles support and guide work by occupational therapy practitioners with people who have been sexually trafficked?
5. What support services exist in your community for people who have been sexually trafficked?

CASE STUDY 22-2 Malik and Safiya

Malik, a friendly, outgoing 20-year-old male with Down syndrome, was in his fifth month of recovery from open-heart surgery. He and his family were refugees from Syria by way of Jordan. The family had been placed in a duplex home in the far northeast section of Philadelphia 5 months earlier (Philadelphia is the U.S. resettlement destination of many refugees who have more complex medical conditions as a result of the breadth of medical services available in the city). This section of the city was isolated from Center City Philadelphia, which affected the accessibility of community services. Malik's father was working. His mother, Safiya, who was a teacher in Syria, stayed home with Malik. His younger brother was enrolled in and attending a Philadelphia public school.

Upon first meeting Malik and his mother in their home, Sam, the occupational therapy supervisor, and Liz, the fieldwork student assigned to the family, were met with a spread of coffee, fruit, cookies, and nuts, typical of Syrian culture. Liz conducted an occupational profile and learned more about the family, Malik, and the family's expectations for care. This was facilitated through the use of a telephonic Arabic interpreter via the student's cell phone. Meanwhile, Malik was excitedly smiling and using his iPad to show pictures of his life in Syria to Sam. The pictures he had stored on his iPad depicted a life in Syria full of social, educational, and leisure occupations with his extended family, as well as his intellectually disabled and nondisabled peers.

When asking Safiya to talk about her expectations for Malik in the future, she became tearful and said, "What will happen to him when his father and I are no longer here?" The student asked her, "When you think about Malik in a year or two, what do you see him to be doing?" Her response provided a strong indication of a good way to work with the family. Safiya indicated she wanted him to be finished with school, working, taking care of himself, and living on his own (but nearby!).

The initial assessment revealed that Malik had many skills from his life prior to resettlement. He received physical and cognitive assistance from his family to perform self-care activities. His family was protective of him and his personal health and safety, especially because he was not able to communicate in English, was unfamiliar with U.S. cultural customs and norms, and did not leave the home. Additionally, the home was limited in objects and access to occupations in which Malik had previously participated, and he was still recovering from his heart surgery 5 months earlier. The family had a car, which Malik's father used to drive himself to work each

CASE STUDY 22-2 Malik and Safiya

day. Safiya was afraid to leave the immediate physical environment due to her lack of familiarity; inability to communicate in English; little to no knowledge of public services such as transportation, the library, the markets, and other stores; and a general fear of the new, unfamiliar human and nonhuman environment.

Based on the assessment results and the family's preferences, the team identified activities of daily living (ADLs) and limited IADLs goals for Malik. His mother was adamant that he not participate in activities that would put him at risk for injury (e.g., preparing food with a knife, cooking food on the stove or in the oven, or shaving). It was agreed to develop strategies for him to facilitate ADLs and IADLs with his mother's supervision and cuing. One of the first new roles Malik was given was to fold the laundry and deliver it to each family member's room. He mastered this activity immediately. He was eager to do more, so activities of upgraded complexity were initiated. He began showering and dressing with Safiya's distant supervision and the use of visual aids to cue him to activity sequences. Slowly, Safiya believed he could do these activities without supervision, and Malik demonstrated to her that he could perform them independently. The same strategy was applied to moving Malik from dependent shaving to independence. His father viewed shaving his son as his role. However, both parents supported Malik's independent performance by allowing him to perform more and more of each activity independently.

In the 5 months since resettlement, Malik had undergone successful heart surgery and recovery. He had not been enrolled in public school. Liz went with Safiya and Malik to the public school to enroll him in class. Since an interpreter was needed to facilitate enrolling Malik in class, Liz acted as a role model and demonstrated assertive communication and advocacy. After two sessions, Safiya was able to complete the written forms, with assistance from an Arabic-speaking interpreter, and enroll Malik in school. Safiya successfully advocated and applied for Malik to attend an extended school year and arranged for the school bus to pick up Malik outside of their home, at the end of the driveway. Malik's younger brother also rode this bus to school. Safiya would walk both boys to the end of the driveway and wait with them until they safely boarded the bus. Eventually, with Liz's encouragement, Safiya developed a sufficient level of comfort with watching from a window inside the home as the boys boarded the bus independently like their peers.

Malik flourished at school. His English-speaking and reading skills steadily progressed. He made friends easily in his classroom and added a rich array of educational and leisure occupations to his repertoire. However, back at home, Malik remained physically isolated. Liz worked with Malik's mother to locate and access the local gym, where they could both participate in health-promoting occupations. Together, using the iPad and a smartphone supported through the Low Income Program of the Universal Service Fund (Universal Service Administration, 2008), Liz and Safiya learned of a nearby gym and how to use public transportation to get there. Due to their limited family income, they also found that the membership fees could be greatly reduced. Safiya made an appointment for her, Malik, and Liz to tour the facility. They rehearsed how to use public transportation to get to and from the gym, identified bus stops, and located the bus route on a map application on the phone. Upon arriving for the first time at the gym, Safiya met another mother who also spoke Arabic and was from Syria. She showed them around the gym and facilitated their signing up for membership.

Eventually, Malik was assisting Safiya with meal preparation—preparing cold foods, setting the table for meals, and cleaning up after meals. It was then time for Malik to begin moving into those activities that posed a potential risk of injury. Liz suggested Safiya create visual instructions (with English and Arabic words) for Malik to prepare simple hot foods. Using the visual cue strategies that were successful for ADLs, Safiya

CASE STUDY 22-2 Malik and Safiya

created instructions for Malik to cook rice for the family dinner. Due to his unfamiliarity with cooking hot items, he required close supervision when interacting around the stovetop, oven, and knives. The final activity for meal preparation was Malik successfully cooking pizza "from scratch" for himself, his mother, and the occupational therapy team to eat together. Malik continues to regularly prepare hot meals for his family. He is independent in all self-care activities. His mother has not achieved complete comfort with him using public transportation independently, but he continues to ride city buses safely under her supervision.

In order for all family members to improve their English communication, they created a game using flash cards and labels with English and Arabic words printed on them. Liz had an (in-person) interpreter phonetically write the English word in Arabic too. Malik and his mother are now more confident in their use of English both in and outside the home.

Due to system bureaucracy, Malik, now 21 years old, was unable to be placed in a work-training program after he completed the extended school year (and simultaneously aged out of attending school). A year later, he works 3 days a week at the Refugee Resettlement Organization as an office volunteer. With an assigned "coach," Malik is developing and practicing work skills that he can apply to future paid employment and using his English communication skills. The family moved to a less isolated neighborhood in Philadelphia. There are other Arabic-speaking residents in this neighborhood who are now friends with the family. Safiya has more time to devote to her role as home manager. She and her husband drive to the market weekly, as well as other stores, for her to shop for the family's needs. The family located and applied for membership at a new local gym. Malik now resembles the outgoing, social, participatory person in his pictures from life in Syria. He continues to expand his knowledge and English communication in his daily round of occupations.

Discussion Questions

1. Liz, the fieldwork student, asks Safiya to talk about her expectations for Malik in the future. Reflecting on this, what might Liz's intent be for asking this question?
2. What are the benefits to the day-to-day occupations and overall health of the family as a result of Liz's therapeutic activities of upgraded complexity and safety risk?
3. What additional goals around community mobility might the occupational therapist work on with Malik in order for him to secure paid employment and move closer to Safiya's vision of him in the future?

Learning Activities

1. What areas of occupational therapy can practitioners draw upon to develop services in the area of human trafficking? How can practitioners conserve the unique value and contribution of occupational therapy in working with a team of multiple professional and medical services in this area?
2. Do student groups or student affairs staff at your college or university promote Valentine's Day events? Do any of the events have the potential to marginalize individuals from the LGBTQ+ communities or members of other underrepresented groups? If so, what actions would be supported and encouraged by the AOTA *Occupational Therapy Code of Ethics (2015)*?
3. As future occupational therapy practitioners, how can you balance the use of holiday celebrations as an important occupation-based strategy with avoiding the marginalization of populations?

REFERENCES

Abas, M., Ostrovschi, N. V., Prince, M., Gorceag, V. I., Trigub, C., and Oram, S. (2013). Risk factors for mental disorders in women survivors of human trafficking: A historical cohort study. *BMC Psychiatry, 13,* 1–11. doi:10.1186/1471-244X-13-204

Alper, M., Durose, M., and Markman, J. (2018, May). *2018 update of prisoner recidivism: A nine-year follow-up period (2005–2014).* Washington, DC: U.S. Department of Justice. Retrieved from www.bjs.gov/content/pub/pdf/18upr9yfup0514.pdf

Alvarez, M. B., and Alessi, E. J. (2012). Human trafficking is more than sex trafficking and prostitution: Implications for social work. *Affilia: Journal of Women and Social Work, 27*(2), 142–152. doi:10.1177/0886109912443763

American Occupational Therapy Association. (2013). AOTA's societal statement on health disparities. *American Journal of Occupational Therapy, 67*(Suppl. 6), S7–S8. doi:10.5014/ajot.2013.67S7

American Occupational Therapy Association. (2014a). Occupational therapy's commitment to nondiscrimination and inclusion. *American Journal of Occupational Therapy, 68*(Suppl. 3), S23–S24. doi:10.5014/ajot.2014.686S05

American Occupational Therapy Association. (2014b). Occupational therapy practice framework: Domain and process (3rd ed.). *American Journal of Occupational Therapy, 68*(Suppl. 1), S1–S48. http://dx.doi.org/10.5014/ajot.2014.682.006

American Occupational Therapy Association. (2015). Occupational therapy code of ethics (2015). *American Journal of Occupational Therapy, 69*(Suppl. 3), 6913410030. http://dx.doi.org/10.5014/ajot.2015.696S03

America's VetDogs. (n.d.). *Learn more about our prison puppy program.* Retrieved from www.vetdogs.org/AV/DogPrograms/PrisonPuppyProgram.aspx

Associated Press, and Lyster, L. (2019, April 12). *American Medical Association blasts transgender military ban.* Retrieved from https://ktla.com/2019/04/12/american-medical-association-blasts-transgender-military-ban/

Avery, B., and Hernandez, P. (2018, September). *Ban the box: U.S. cities, counties, and states adopt fair hiring policies to advance employment opportunities for people with past convictions.* National Employment Law Project. Retrieved from www.nelp.org/publication/ban-the-box-fair-chance-hiring-state-and-local-guide/

Best, B. L., Wodahl, E. J., and Holmes, M. D. (2014). Waiving away the chance of freedom: Exploring why prisoners decide against applying for parole. *International Journal of Offender Therapy and Comparative Criminology, 58*(3), 320–347.

Black Men's Xchange National. (2012). *What is same gender loving?* Retrieved https://web.archive.org/web/20131015005535/http://bmxnational.org/faqs/what-is-same-gender-loving/

Blinder, A., and Pérez-Peña, R. (2015, September 1). Kentucky clerk denies same-sex marriage licenses, defying court. *New York Times.* Retrieved from www.nytimes.com/2015/09/02/us/same-sex-marriage-kentucky-kim-davis.html

Bradbury, R. (2015). *The role of occupational therapy in corrections settings* (Master's thesis.) Retrieved from https://digitalcommons.ithaca.edu/ic_theses/3/

Britton, D. M., and Button, A. (2005). Prison pups: Assessing the effects of dog training programs in correctional facilities. *Journal of Family Social Work, 9*(4), 79–95.

Bryant, C., Freeman, L., Granata, M., He, A., Hough, H., Patel, S., . . . Tran, M.-L. (2015). Societal statement on the role of occupational therapy with survivors of human sex trafficking in the United States. *OCCUPATION: A Medium of Inquiry for Students, Faculty and Other Practitioners Advocating for Health Through Occupational Studies, 1*(1), 18–19.

Brymer, M., Steinberg, A., Sonoborger, J., Layne, C., and Pynoos, R. (2008). Acute interventions for refugee children and families. *Child and Adolescent Psychiatry Clinics of North America, 17,* 625–640.

Carson, A. E. (2018, August 7). *Prisoners in 2016.* Washington, DC: U.S. Department of Justice. Retrieved from www.bjs.gov/content/pub/pdf/p16.pdf

Centers for Disease Control and Prevention. (2017, March 09). *Gay and bisexual men's health: Suicide and violence prevention.* Retrieved from www.cdc.gov/msmhealth/suicide-violence-prevention.htm

Cerny, S. (2016). The role of occupational therapy within the Federal Strategic Action Plan on Services for Victims of Human Trafficking in the United States. *Occupational Therapy in Mental Health, 32*(4), 317–328. doi:10.1080/0164212X.2016.1172998

Changing Faces. (n.d.). *About us.* Retrieved from www.changingfaces.org.uk/about-us

Cheshire, W. P. (2017). Group think: How should clinicians respond to human trafficking? *Medicine and Society, 19*(1), 91–97.

Cloud, D. H., Drucker, E., Browne, A., and Parsons, J. (2015). Public health and solitary confinement in the United States. *American Journal of Public, 105*(1), 18–26.

Cockbain, E., and Bowers, K. (2015). *The faces and places of trafficking for labour exploitation: A large-scale analysis.* Paper presented at the meeting of the European Society of Criminology, Porto, Portugal.

Cockbain, E., Bowers, K., and Dimitrova, G. (2018). Human trafficking for labour exploitation: The results of a two-phase systematic review mapping the European evidence base and synthesising key scientific research evidence. *Journal of Experimental Criminology, 14*(3), 1–42. doi:10.1007/s11292-017-9321-3

Cooke, B. J., and Farrington, D. P. (2014). Perceived effects of dog-training programmes in correctional settings. *Journal of Forensic Practice, 16*(3), 171.

Copley, J., Turpin, M., Gordon, S., and McLaren, C. (2011). Development and evaluation of an occupational therapy program for refugee high school students. *Australian Occupational Therapy Journal, 58*(4), 310–316. doi:10.1111/j.1440-1630.2011.00933.x

Courtney, L., Eppler-Epstein, S., Pelletier, E., King, R., and Lei, S. (2017). *A matter of time: The causes and consequences of rising time served in America's prisons.* Washington, DC: Urban Institute. Retrieved from http://apps.urban.org/features/long-prison-terms/a_matter_of_time.pdf

Crawford, E., Turpin, M., Nayar, S., Steel, E., and Durand, J.-L. (2016). The structural-personal interaction: Occupational deprivation and asylum seekers in Australia. *Journal of Occupational Science, 23*(3), 321–338. doi:10.1080/14427591.2016.1153510

Crethar, H. C., and Vargas, L. A. (2007). Multicultural intricacies in professional counseling. In J. Gregoire and C. Jungers (Eds.), *The counselor's companion: What every beginning counselor needs to know* (pp. 52–71). Mahwah, NJ: Erlbaum.

Dailey, B. (2002). *Occupational therapy services within the criminal justice system: Healthy life skills beyond the walls* (Unpublished graduate project paper). Towson University, Towson, MD.

Dailey, B., and Reitz, S. M. (2003, June). *Occupational therapy services in the criminal justice system: Healthy life skills beyond the walls.* Poster presented at the 83rd AOTA Annual Conference and Exposition, Washington, DC.

de Vries, I., and Farrell, A. (2018). Labor trafficking victimizations: Repeat victimization and polyvictimization. *Psychology of Violence, 8*(5), 630–638. doi:10.1037/vio0000149

Domoney, J., Howard, L. M., Abas, M., Broadbent, M., and Oram, S. (2015). Mental health service responses to human trafficking: A qualitative study of professionals' experiences of providing care. *BMC Psychiatry, 15,* 289.

Drescher, J. (2015). Out of DSM: Depathologizing homosexuality. *Behavioral Sciences (Basel, Switzerland), 5*(4), 565–575. doi:10.3390/bs5040565

Durose, M. R., Cooper, A. D., and Snyder, H. N. (2014, April). *Recidivism of prisoners released in 30 states in 2005: Patterns from 2005 to 2010.* Washington, DC: U.S. Department of Justice. Retrieved from www.bjs.gov/content/pub/pdf/rprts05p0510.pdf

Farmer, P. (1996). On suffering and structural violence: A view from below. *Daedalus, 125*(1), 261–283.

Futterweit, W. (1998). Endocrine therapy of transsexualism and potential complications of long-term treatment. *Archives of Sexual Behavior, 2,* 209–226.

George, E., and Stanley, M. (2018). Exploring the occupational injustices of human trafficking. *Journal of Occupational Science,* 1–14. doi:10.1080/14427591.2018.1515104

GLAAD. (2017, April 19). *GLAAD media reference guide—transgender.* Retrieved from www.glaad.org/reference/transgender

Goodreads. (2018). *Marginalization quotes.* Retrieved from www.goodreads.com/quotes/tag/marginalization

Gorman, K. W., and Hatkevich, B. A. (2016). Role of occupational therapy in combating human trafficking. *American Journal of Occupational Therapy, 70*(6), 7006360010p1–7006360010p6. doi: 10.5014/ajot.2016.016782.

Grace, B. L., Bais, R., and Roth, B. J. (2018). The violence of uncertainty—undermining immigrant and refugee health. *New England Journal of Medicine, 379*(10), 904–905

Gramlich, J. (2018, January 12). *The gap between the number of blacks and whites in prison is shrinking.* Retrieved from www.pewresearch.org/fact-tank/2018/01/12/shrinking-gap-between-number-of-blacks-and-whites-in-prison/

Grant, J. M., Mottet, L. A., Tanis, J., Harrison, J., Herman, J. L., and Keisling. (2011). *Injustice at every turn: A report of the national transgender discrimination study.* Washington, DC: National Center for Transgender Equity and National Gay Task Force. Retrieved from https://rhyclearinghouse.acf.hhs.gov/library/2011/injustice-every-turn-report-national-transgender-discrimination-survey

Green, E. L., Benner, K., and Pear, R. (2018). "Transgender" could be defined out of existence under Trump administration. *New York Times.* Retrieved from www.nytimes.com/2018/10/21/us/politics/transgender-trump-administration-sex-definition.html

Gupta, J. (2012). Human displacement, occupational disruptionsm and reintegration: A case study. *WFOT Bulletin, 66,* 27–29.

Gurmankin, A., Caplan, A., and Braverman, A. (2005). Screening practices and beliefs of assisted reproductive technology programs. *Fertility and Sterility, 83*(1), 61–67. doi:10.1016/j.fertnstert.2004.06.048

Harding, D. J., Wyse, J., Dobson, C., and Morenoff, J. (2014). Making ends meet after prison. *Journal of Policy Analysis and Management, 33*(2), 440–470.

Harrison-Quintana, J., and Herman, J. L. (2013). Still serving in silence: Transgender service members and veterans in the national transgender discrimination survey. In *LGBTQ Policy Journal at the Harvard Kennedy School* (Vol. 3, pp. 1–13). Retrieved from https://williamsinstitute.law.ucla.edu/wp-content/uploads/Harrison-Quintana-Herman-LGBTQ-Policy-Journal-2013.pdf

Heffron, J., The, K., and Harrison, E. (2018, April). *Room for change? Experiences of occupational therapy practitioners with disabilities.* Research poster presented at 2018 AOTA Annual Conference and Expo, Salt Lake City, UT.

Heptinstall, E., Sethna, V., and Taylor, E. (2004). PTSD and depression in refugee children: Association with pre-migration trauma and post-migration stress. *European Child and Adolescent Psychiatry, 13,* 373–380.

Hetache-Pretzer, E., and Jacob, J. (2018). From prison to the community: Programs for developing life skills. *OT Practice, 23*(7), 8–11.

Hogle, P. S. (2009, August). Going to the dogs: Prison-based training programs are win-win. *Corrections Today,* 69–72.

Hom, K. A., and Woods, S. J. (2013). Trauma and its aftermath for commercially sexually exploited women as told by front-line service providers. *Issues in Mental Health Nursing, 34*(2), 75–81. doi:10.3109/01612840.2012.723300

Human Rights Campaign. (n.d.). Retrieved from www.hrc.org/

Huot, S., Kelly, E., and Park, S. J. (2016). Occupational experiences of forced migrants: A scoping review. *Australian Occupational Therapy Journal, 63*(3), 186–205.

Huot, S., and Laliberte Rudman, D. (2010) The performances and places of identity: Conceptualizing intersections of occupation, identity and place in the process of migration, *Journal of Occupational Science, 17*(2), 68–77. doi: 10.1080/14427591.2010.9686677

Im, H. (2018). Constructing health capital in ecological systems: A qualitative evaluation of community-based health workshops in the refugee community. *Health and Social Care in the Community, 26,* e541–e551.

Inside-Out Prison Exchange Program®. (2018). *About.* Retrieved from www.insideoutcenter.org/index.html

International Labor Organization. (2012). *ILO global estimate of forced labour 2012: Results and methodology.* Geneva, Switzerland: International Labour Organization. Retrieved from www.ilo.org/wcmsp5/groups/public/---ed_norm/---declaration/documents/publication/wcms_182004.pdf

International Organization on Migration. (2011). *Glossary on migration.* International Migration Law Series No. 25. Geneva, Switzerland: International Organization on Migration.

Intersex Society of North America. (2008, June). *What is intersex?* Retrieved from www.isna.org/faq/what_is_intersex

Jani, J. S., and Reisch, M. (2018). Assisting the least among us: Social work's historical response to unaccompanied immigrant and refugee youth. *Children and Youth Services Review, 92*(C), 4–14.

Kaufman, M. R., and Crawford, M. (2011). Sex trafficking in Nepal: A review of intervention and prevention programs. *Violence Against Women, 17*(5), 651–665. doi:10.1177/1077801211407431

Kelleher, C. (2009). Minority stress and health: Implications for lesbian, gay, bisexual, transgender, and questioning (LGBTQ) young people. *Counselling Psychology Quarterly, 22*(4), 373–379. doi:10.1080/09515070903334995

Kim, K. D., and Peterson, B. (2014, September 5). *Aging behind bars: Trends and implications of graying prisoners in the federal prison system.* Washington, DC: U.S. Department of Justice. Retrieved from www.urban.org/research/publication/aging-behind-bars-trends-and-implications-graying-prisoners-federal-prison-system

Konstantopoulos, W., Ahn, R., Alpert, E. J., Cafferty, E., McGahan, A., Williams, T. P., . . . Burke, T. F. (2013). An international comparative public health analysis of sex trafficking of women and girls in eight cities: Achieving a more effective health sector response. *Journal of Urban Health, 90*(6), 1194–1204. doi:10.1007/s11524-013-9837-4

Kovacs, K., Stefaneanu, L., Smyth, H., and Ezzat, H. (1994). Prolactin-producing pituitary adenoma in a male-to-female transsexual patient with protracted estrogen administration: A morphologic study. *Archives of Pathology and Laboratory Medicine, 118*(5), 562–565.

Kretzmann, J. P., and McKnight, J. L. (2005). *Discovering community power: A guide to mobilizing local assets and your organization's capacity.* Evanston, IL: Asset-Based Community Development Institute in cooperation with the Kellogg Foundation.

Kronenberg, F., and Pollard, N. (2005). Overcoming occupational apartheid: A preliminary exploration of the political nature of occupational therapy. In F. Kronenberg, S. S. Algado, and N. Pollard (Eds.). *Occupational therapy without borders: Learning from the spirit of survivors* (pp. 58–86). New York, NY: Elsevier.

Lambda Legal. (n.d.). *Accessing coverage for transition-related health care.* Retrieved from www.lambdalegal.org/know-your-rights/article/trans-health-care

Lambda Legal. (2018, September 17). *Changing birth certificate sex designations: State-by-state guidelines.* Retrieved from www.lambdalegal.org/know-your-rights/article/trans-changing-birth-certificate-sex-designations

Leap, W. (2007). Language, socialization, and silence in gay adolescence: Charting a path through the "desert of nothing." In K. E. Lovaas and M. M. Jenkins (Eds.), *Sexualities and communication in everyday life: A reader* (pp. 98–103). Thousand Oaks, CA: Sage.

LGBTQIA Resource Center. (n.d.). *LGBTQIA Resource Center glossary.* Retrieved from https://lgbtqia.ucdavis.edu/educated/glossary.html

Macy, R. J., and Johns, N. (2011). Aftercare services for international sex trafficking survivors: Informing U.S. service and program development in an emerging practice area. *Trauma, Violence, and Abuse, 12*(2), 87–98.

Martinez, O., and Kelle, G. (2013). Sex trafficking of LGBT individuals: A call for service provision, research, and action. *International Law News, 42*(4), 1–6.

Mastrorilli, M. E. (2016). With Pell Grants rising: A review of the contemporary empirical literature on prison postsecondary education. *Journal of Correctional Education, 67*(2), 44–60.

Mathie, A., and Cunningham, G. (2003). From clients to citizens: Asset-based community development as a strategy for community-driven development. *Development in Practice, 13*(5), 474–486.

McAllister, L., Penn, C., Smith, Y., Van Dort, S., and Wilson, L. (2010). Fieldwork education in non-traditional settings or with non-traditional caseloads. In L. McAllister, M. Paterson, J. Higgs, and C. Bithell (Eds.), *Innovations in allied health fieldwork education: A critical appraisal* (pp. 39–47). Rotterdam, Netherlands: Sense.

McElroy, T., Muyinda, H., Atim, S. Spittal, P., and Blackman, C. (2012). War, displacement, and productive occupations in Northern Uganda. *Journal of Occupational Science, 19*(3), 198–212. doi:10.1080/14427591.2011.614681

Meijers, J., Harte, J. M., Jonker, F. A., and Meynen, G. (2015). Prison brain? Executive dysfunction in prisoners. *Frontiers in Psychology, 6,* 43.

Meshkovska, B., Siegel, M., Stutterheim, S. E., and Bos, A. E. (2015). Female sex trafficking: Conceptual issues, current debates, and future directions. *Journal of Sex Research, 52*(4), 380–395. doi:10.1080/00224499.2014.1002126

Minkler, M., and Wallerstein, N. (2005). Improving health through community organization and community building: A health education perspective. In M. Minkler (Ed.), *Community organizing and community building for health* (2nd ed., pp. 26–50). Rutgers, NJ: State University of New Jersey.

Molineux, M. L., and Whiteford, G. E. (1999). Prisons: From occupational deprivation to occupational enrichment. *Journal of Occupational Science, 6*(3), 214–130.

Morville, A-L. (2014). *Daily occupations among asylum seekers—experience, performance and perception.* Lund, Sweden: Department of Health Sciences, Lund University.

Morville, A.-L., and Erlandsson, L.-K. (2013). The experience of occupational deprivation in an asylum centre: The narratives of three men. *Journal of Occupational Science, 20*(3), 212–223. doi: 10.1080/14427591.2013.808976

Muñoz, J., Moreton, E., and Sitterly, A. (2015, March). *A survey of occupational therapy in the U.S. criminal justice system.* Poster presented at the meeting of the American Occupational Therapy Association, Nashville, TN.

Muraya, D. N., and Fry, D. (2016). Aftercare services for child victims of sex trafficking: A systematic review of policy and practice. *Trauma, Violence, and Abuse 17*(2), 204–220.

National Center for Education. (1994). *Literacy behind prison walls: Profiles of the prison population from the National Adult Literacy Survey.* Retrieved from https://nces.ed.gov/pubs94/94102.pdf

Occupational Therapy Human Trafficking Network. (2018). Retrieved from www.facebook.com/search/top/?q=occupational%20therapy%20human%20trafficking%20network

Oram, S., Ostrovschi, N. V., Gorceag, V. I., Hotineanu, M. A., Gorceag, L., Trigub, C., and Abas, M. (2012). Physical health symptoms reported by trafficked women receiving post-trafficking support in Moldova: Prevalence, severity and associated factors. *BMC Women's Health, 12,* 20. doi:10.1186/1472-6874-12-20

Oxford Dictionaries. (2018). *Correctional system.* Retrieved from https://en.oxforddictionaries.com/definition/us/criminal_justice_system

Posselt, M., Galletly, C., deCrespigny, C., and Procter, N. (2014). Mental health and drug and alcohol comorbidity in young people of refugee background: A review of the literature. *Journal of Mental Health and Substance Use, 7*(1), 19–30. doi.org/10.1080/17523281.2013.772914

Purvis, K., Cross, D., Dansereau, D. F., and Parris, S. R. (2013). Trust based relational intervention (TBRI): A systemic approach to complex developmental trauma. *Child and Youth Services, 34,* 360–386. doi:10.1080/0145935x.2013.859906

Reference. (2018). *What is a marginalized community?* Retrieved from www.reference.com/world-view/marginalized-community-517401cfa76aa4eb#

Rosenbaum, E., Robnett, R., Eades, J., Ellis, A., Emond, C., Chevalier, E., and Kramer, L. (2018, April). *Unlocking convictions: Opening minds through a weekly wellness program at a correctional facility.* Poster presented at the 2018 AOTA Annual Conference and Expo, Salt Lake City, Utah.

Rubin, H. J., and Rubin, I. S. (2005). The practice of community organizing. In M. Weil (Ed.), *The handbook of community practice* (pp. 189–203). Thousand Oaks, CA: Sage.

Rural Health Information Hub. (2019). *Community organization model.* Retrieved from www.ruralhealthinfo.org/toolkits/health-promotion/2/program-models/community-organization

Second Chance Act of 2007, Pub. L. 110–199, 122, Stat. 657 (2008).

Seruya, F. M., Smith, B., Caryon, A., Bailey, P., DiGiacomo, A., and Pyne, N. (2019, April). *Preparation for occupation upon community re-entry for individuals who have been previously incarcerated.* Poster presented at the meeting of the American Occupational Therapy Association, New Orleans, LA.

Shannon, P. J., Wieling, E., Simmelink-McCleary, J., and Becher, E. (2015). Beyond stigma: Barriers to discussing mental health in refugee populations. *Journal of Loss and Trauma, 20*(3), 281–296. doi.org/10.1080/15325024.2014.934629

Sheridan, T. (2016). *Human trafficking: Identification and assessment of victims essential.* Retrieved from www.continuingeducation.com/course/ot759/human-trafficking/

Shigekane, R. (2007). Rehabilitation and community integration of trafficking survivors in the United States. *Human Rights Quarterly, 29*(1), 112–126.

Siddiqui, S. V., Chatterjee, U., Kumar, D., Siddiqui, A., and Goyal, N. (2008). Neuropsychology of prefrontal cortex. *Indian Journal of Psychiatry, 50*(3), 202–208.

Smith, B., Seruya, F. M., Albee, H., Laprade, E., Mulry, E., and Zoulafy, S. (2018, April 19). *Inmate preparation for occupation upon community reentry.* Poster presented at the Annual Conference of American Occupational Therapy Association, Salt Lake City, UT.

Smith, Y. J., Cornella, E., and Williams, N. (2014). Working with populations from a refugee background: An opportunity to enhance the occupational therapy educational experience. *Australian Occupational Therapy Journal, 61*(1), 20–27. doi:10.1111/1440-1630.12037

Stadnyk, R. L., Townsend, E. A., and Wilcock, A. A. (2010). Occupational justice. In C. H. Christiansen and E. A. Townsend (Eds.), *Introduction to occupation: The art and science of living* (pp. 329–358). Upper Saddle River, NJ: Pearson.

Steindl, C., Winding, K., and Runge, U. (2008). Occupation and participation in everyday life: Women's experiences of an Austrian refugee camp. *Journal of Occupational Science, 15*(1), 36–42. doi:10.1080/ 14427591.2008.9686605

Swiatek, D., and Jewell, V. (2018, April). LGBT seniors: Including the invisible population. *OT Practice, 23*(6), 16–19.

Thompson, C., and Eldridge, T. E. (2018, November 22). New data link denial of care to inmate assault, self-harm. *Washington Post,* A4.

Thompson, J., and Haley, M. (2018). Human trafficking: Preparing counselors to work with survivors. *International Journal for the Advancement of Counselling, 40*(3), 1–12. doi:10.1007/ s10447-018-9327-1

Thompson, T. (2017). *Community living integration club for women in recovery from sex trafficking.* Fort Lauderdale, FL: Nova Southeastern University. Retrieved from http://nsuworks.nova.edu/hpd_ot_student_dissertations/47/

Thorton, M., and Spalding, N. (2018). An exploration of asylum seeker and refugee experiences of activity. *World Federation of Occupational Therapists Bulletin, 74*(2), 114–122. doi.org/10 .1080/14473828.2018.1539282

Townsend E., and Wilcock, A. A. (2004). Occupational justice and client-centred practice: A dialogue in progress. *Canadian Journal of Occupational Therapy, 71*(2), 75–87.

Trickett, P. K., Noll, J. G., and Putnam, F. W. (2011). The impact of sexual abuse on female development: Lessons from a multigenerational, longitudinal research study. *Developmental Psychopathology, 23*(2), 453–476. doi:10.1017/s0954579411000174

Turner-Moss, E., Zimmerman, C., Howard, L. M., and Oram, S. (2014). Labour exploitation and health: A case series of men and women seeking post-trafficking services. *Journal of Immigrant and Minority Health/Center for Minority Public Health, 16*(3), 473–480. doi:10.1007/s10903-013-9832-6

United Nations. (1948). *Universal declaration of human rights.* Retrieved from www.un.org/en/universal-declaration-human -rights/index.html

United Nations. (2000). *Protocol to prevent, suppress and punish trafficking in persons especially women and children, supplementing the United Nations Convention Against Transnational Organized Crime.* Retrieved from www.ohchr.org/EN/Professional Interest/Pages/ProtocolTraffickingInPersons.aspx

United Nations High Commissioner for Refugees. (2016). *The 10-point plan in action, 2016—glossary.* Retrieved from www.refworld.org/docid/59e99eb94.html

United Nations High Commissioner for Refugees. (2018). *Global trends: Forced displacement in 2017.* Retrieved from www.unhcr.org/en-us/statistics/unhcrstats/5b27be547/unhcr -global-trends-2017.html?query=global%20trends%202018

United Nations Office of High Commission on Human Rights. (2000). *Protocol to prevent, suppress and punish trafficking in persons, especially women and children.* Retrieved from www.ohchr.org/EN/ProfessionalInterest/Pages/ProtocolTraffickingInPersons.aspx

United Nations Office on Drugs and Crime. (2016). *United Nations convention against transnational organized crime and the protocols thereto.* Retrieved from www.unodc.org/unodc/en/treaties/CTOC/index.html

United Nations Office on Drugs and Crime. (2018). *UNODC on human trafficking and migrant smuggling.* Retrieved from www.unodc.org/unodc/human-trafficking/

Universal Service Administration. (2008). *Understand the benefits.* Retrieved from http://web.archive.org/web/20080315054050/http://www .lifelinesupport.org/li/low-income/benefits/default.aspx

U.S. Department of Justice. (2018, June). *Lessons learned from the second chance act: Moving forward to strengthen offender reentry.* Retrieved from www.ncjrs.gov/pdffiles1/nij/251704.pdf

U. S. Department of State. (n.d.a). *Protracted refugee situations.* Retrieved from www.state.gov/j/prm/policyissues/issues/protracted/

U.S. Department of State. (n.d.b). *3Ps: Prevention, protection, and prosecution.* Retrieved from www.state.gov/j/tip/3p/index.htm

Vaage, A. B., Thomsen, P. H., Silove, D., Wentzel-Larsen, T., Van Ta, T., and Hauff, E. (2010). Long-term mental health of Vietnamese refugees in the aftermath of trauma. *British Journal of Psychiatry, 196*(2), 122–125.

Wagner, P., and Sawyer, W. (2018, March 14). *Mass incarceration: The whole pie 2018.* Retrieved from www.prisonpolicy.org/reports/pie2018.html

Walmsley, R. (2015). *World prison population list* (11th ed.). Institute for Criminal Policy and Research. Retrieved from www.prisonstudies.org/sites/default/files/resources/downloads /world_prison_population_list_11th_edition_0.pdf

Whalley Hammell, K. R. (2016). Critical reflections on occupational justice: Toward a rights-based approach to occupational opportunities. *Canadian Journal of Occupational Therapy, 84*(1), 47–57. doi: 10.1177/0008417416654501.

Whiteford, G. E. (2000). Occupational deprivation: Global challenge in the new millennium. *British Journal of Occupational Therapy, 63*(5), 200–204.

Whiteford, G. E. (2005). Understanding the occupational deprivation of refugees: A case study from Kosovo. *Canadian Journal of Occupational Therapy, 72*(2), 78–88. doi:10.1177/000841740507200202

Whiteford, G. E., and Townsend, E. (2011). Participatory occupational justice framework (POJF): Enabling occupational participation and inclusion. In F. Kronenburg, N. Pollard, and D. Sakellariou (Eds.), *Occupational therapies without borders: Volume 2—toward an ecology of occupation-based practices* (pp. 65–84). New York, NY: Elsevier.

The White House. (2016, December. 28). *Presidential proclamation—National Slavery and Human Trafficking Prevention Month, 2017.* Retrieved from https://obamawhitehouse.archives.gov/the-press-office/2016/12/28/presidential-proclamation-national-slavery-and-human-trafficking

Wilcock, A. A., and Townsend, E. A. (2000). Occupational justice: Occupational terminology interactive dialogue. *Journal of Occupational Science, 7,* 84–86. doi:10.1080/144275591.2000.9686470

Wilcock, A. A., and Townsend, E. A. (2014). *Occupational justice.* In B. A. Boyt Schell, G. Gillen, and M. Scaffa (Eds.), *Willard and Spackman's occupational therapy* (12th ed., pp. 541–552). Philadelphia, PA: Lippincott, Williams and Wilkins.

Williams, R. (2015). Offenders given another chance in life through occupational therapy. *Guardian.* Retrieved from www.theguardian.com/social-care-network/2015/jan/28/prisoners-young-offenders-occupational-therapy

Wilper, A. P., Woolhandler, S., Boyd, J. W., Lasser, K. E., McCormick, D., Bor, D. H., and Himmelstein, D. U. (2009). The health and health care of U.S. prisoners: Results of a nationwide survey. *American Journal of Public Health, 99*(4), 666–672.

World Federation of Occupational Therapists. (2014). *Position statement: Human displacement* (Rev.). Retrieved from www.wfot.org/ResourceCentre.aspx

World Federation of Occupational Therapists. (2018). *World Federation of Occupational Therapists position statement on human rights.* Retrieved from www.wfot.org/ResourceCentre.aspx

World Health Organization. (1948/2018). *Constitution of the World Health Organization: Principles.* Retrieved from: www.who.int/about/mission/en/

World Health Organization. (2012). *Understanding and addressing violence against women: Human trafficking.* Geneva, Switzerland: International Labour Organization.

World Health Organization. (2014). *International classification of functioning, disability and health.* Retrieved from www.who.int/classifications/icf/en/

Wrightsman, W. B. (2018, October). *Home as a restorative place: Illuminating how stigmatization influences the occupational experience and well-being of gay married men.* Paper presented at the Society for the Study of the Occupation, Lexington, KY.

Zoukis, C. (2014). The purpose of prison and the measuring stick of recidivism. *Zoukis Prisoner Resources.* Retrieved from www.prisonerresource.com/prison-reform/the-purpose-of-prison-and-the-measuring-stick-of-recidivism/

Zoukis, C. (2018). Co-pays deter prisoners from accessing medical care. *Prison Legal News.* Retrieved from www.prisonlegalnews.org/news/2018/jan/31/co-pays-deter-prisoners-accessing-medical-care/

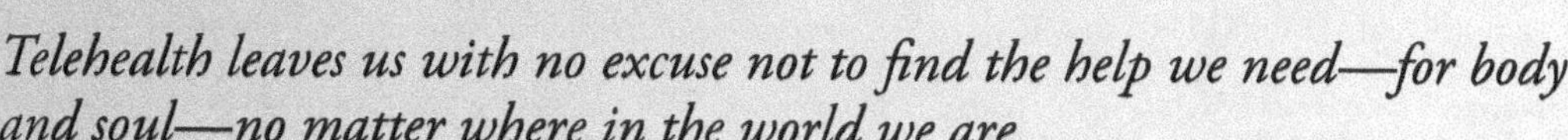

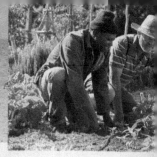

Chapter 23

Telehealth

Ranelle Nissen, PhD, OTR/L

Telehealth leaves us with no excuse not to find the help we need—for body and soul—no matter where in the world we are.

—Eric J. Hall, President and CEO of HealthCare Chaplaincy Network, Chairman of Alzheimer's Global Initiative

Learning Outcomes

This chapter is designed to enable the reader to:

23-1 Define the scope of telehealth services in occupational therapy.
23-2 Describe the benefits and limitations of telehealth.
23-3 Identify the legal and ethical issues of using telehealth to deliver occupational therapy services.
23-4 Identify current evidence to support the use of telehealth as an effective delivery model.
23-5 Describe the opportunities and challenges of using telehealth in population health.

Key Terms

Asynchronous
Information and communication technologies
Justice
Remote patient monitoring
Synchronous
Telehealth
Telemedicine
Telerehabilitation

Introduction

Information and communication technologies (ICTs) include technology that allows for the "transfer of information and various types of electronically mediated communication" (Zuppo, 2012, p. 19). This may include technology such as online video conferencing, telephone, e-mail, text messages, or remote monitoring systems (Center for Connected Health Policy, 2014; LeadingAge Center for Aging Services Technologies [LACAST], 2015). Professions such as education, business, and economics utilize ICTs to enhance workflow. Health care utilizes ICTs as a means to deliver services under the umbrella of telehealth. The American Occupational Therapy Association (AOTA, 2013) defines **telehealth** as "an emerging model of health care delivery . . . which involves health care services, health information, and health education" and "a mechanism to provide services at a location that is physically distant from the client, thereby allowing for services to occur where the client lives, works, and plays" (p. S69). Within the context of telehealth, **telerehabilitation** is a term used to identify the use of ICTs for the delivery of rehabilitative and habilitative services (American Telemedicine Association [ATA], 2010). In addition, various professional organizations use the term **telemedicine.** Some organizations differentiate the two terms of telehealth and telemedicine, but for the purpose of this chapter, telehealth and telemedicine are used interchangeably. The term telehealth is preferred because of the broader scope across all health-care disciplines and the scope of services provided implied by the term. It is important to note that telehealth only refers to the format of service delivery; the practice principles remain the same as practice using other formats.

Technology

The expanding field of technology allows for increasing flexibility in telehealth. Telehealth technology can vary from a low to high level of complexity. Higher levels of technology include equipment that has the capability of measuring a client's vital signs, a dynamometer for grip strength measurements, or goniometry to assess joint range of motion from a distance. This type of technology may not be appropriate or feasible for use with all clients in a community-based setting.

Technology that is more accessible may be a better fit because the client may already have access and be familiar with its use. This may lead to higher acceptance by the client of the use of telehealth to receive services (Demiris et al., 2010). More familiar types of technology include a telephone, videophone, or personal computer or tablet with video and audio capability. Through collaboration with the client, the occupational therapy practitioner can identify the type of technology the client is comfortable using. The client may also accept additional education on the use of less-familiar technology.

Other technology can track health information through remote patient monitoring. **Remote patient monitoring** (RPM) is the use of technology to collect and monitor a client's health data (Center for Connected Health Policy, 2014). RPM systems include devices the client can use to record health data, such as blood pressure, heart rate, and weight, to transmit to an off-site monitoring location for interpretation by a health-care professional. Other types of RPM systems can track safety indicators of the person and environment, such as falls, or carbon monoxide levels, or behavioral indicators of daily performance patterns (LACAST, 2015). Use of these systems is beneficial for older adults who are living alone but need additional supervision to track their safety and health. Systems can be set up in the client's home to provide continuous monitoring through the use of motion detection equipment or devices worn by the client to activate during an emergency. These systems can track the client's normal pattern of movement in the home, use of appliances, bathing patterns, and sleep. This information can identify when a normal pattern of behavior is disrupted by illness, declining health, or other concerns. Use of these monitoring systems can prevent hospitalization and allow the client to age in place (see Chapter 12).

Formats and Delivery Methods

Multiple formats of telehealth are available to individualize the services to a client in community-based practice. Telehealth can allow for a tailored approach to deliver services that best meet the client's needs. The practitioner can vary the timing of the services, utilize different technology formats, augment telehealth with in-person visits, and provide individual or group intervention.

Community-based services focus on clients in their natural environments. Telehealth allows for service delivery that is consistent with this focus by allowing for both synchronous and asynchronous timing of delivery. In **synchronous** telehealth delivery, the client and practitioner are both present, interacting at a designated time. Real-time videoconference or audio conference sessions are examples of synchronous telehealth sessions.

In certain contexts of service, **asynchronous** delivery of services may be a better fit to meet the client's needs. Asynchronous delivery does not require both parties to be present at the same time. For example, a client's caregiver may make a video recording of a walkthrough of the client's home and upload the recording for the therapist. The therapist then views the recording and makes recommendations for safety and home modification that support aging in place. The practitioner may send documents and resources electronically to the client and caregiver to review at their convenience. A hybrid approach using synchronous video may be used for additional discussion, clarifications, and observation of the client in the home following implementation of the recommendations. Furthermore, the team may collaborate asynchronously through the client's electronic medical record.

Telehealth as a Service Delivery Model

Telehealth has been gaining acceptance as an evidence-based, client-centered model of service delivery in occupational therapy. The AOTA (2013) and the World Federation of Occupational Therapists (WFOT, 2014) support the use of telehealth as a means to expand client access to occupational therapy services and promote a higher quality of care. Occupational therapy practitioners can improve the quality of care provided to clients by decreasing access barriers, increasing their reach to clients in rural and underserved communities, and consulting with practitioners with specialized expertise across the country. Telehealth can be used for evaluation, intervention, consultation, monitoring, and supervision. The flexibility of the options for services delivered through telehealth aligns with community-based practice and allows for modification to fit the client's needs. This can include timing the service delivery, varying the technology used, augmenting telehealth with in-person services (i.e., hybrid approach), and providing services to an individual or a group.

Telehealth is a delivery method and not a distinct service; the service is still occupational therapy. The practitioner collaborates with the client to determine the desired goals and uses clinical judgment to determine the best means to meet those goals. Telehealth may be the best alternative when in-person services are not feasible. The client and practitioner can determine if this means 100% telehealth delivery or a mix of telehealth and in-person services. Telehealth may be feasible for some types of services, while in-person services might be the best means to provide other types of services.

Telehealth can benefit clients when it is not feasible to have a health-care professional travel to their homes. It can also provide an alternative to travel for a client or occupational therapist in inclement weather or when the distance may be prohibitive. In addition, telehealth can provide a means to increase contact with the client by providing flexibility in timing and frequency of therapy or by adding extra sessions between in-person visits when using a hybrid therapy approach.

In community-based practice, a client can be a single person, a family, or a population of persons that may or may not be in the same physical location. Telehealth can be tailored to deliver services to any of these client types. One distinct advantage that telehealth offers is the ability of the practitioner to bring together a population of persons who are not able to come together otherwise in one physical location. This creates possibilities for a broader scope of services to meet the needs of the clients in the community when the population spans across locations. Likewise, it can bring together persons who are homebound; telehealth can bring a community of peers to the client.

Engage Your Brain 23-1

What additional competencies should an occupational therapy practitioner have to provide occupational therapy services by telehealth?

Service Delivery

It is important to identify the type of service for delivery through telehealth to determine the optimal approach. Providing an evidence-driven method of service delivery is still best practice in the telehealth model, as it is in the traditional in-person model. The growing evidence supporting the use of telehealth in the delivery of occupational therapy services provides more options of validated assessments, service approaches, and interventions for use in a virtual context (Kairy, Lehoux, Vincent, and Visintin, 2009; Little, Pope, Wallisch, and Dunn, 2018; Ng, Polatajko, Marziali, Hunt, and Dawson, 2013; Serwe, Hersch, Pickens, and Pancheri, 2017; Sundsli, Söderhamm, Espnes, and Söderhamm, 2014).

Evaluation

Evaluation of clients in a community-based setting focuses largely on the clients in their natural contexts. The occupational therapy practitioner will complete an occupational profile and evaluate the client's occupational performance. The focus of evaluation in the community-based setting may be more conducive to telehealth delivery than assessments completed in a traditional medical model context. The practitioner must first identify a means to build rapport with the client in this virtual context. With readily available technology, the gathering of information for an occupational profile is easily conducted through telehealth (Fig. 23-1). Furthermore, video-conferencing capabilities that include wide-angle views of the activity allow for observation of performance in occupations within

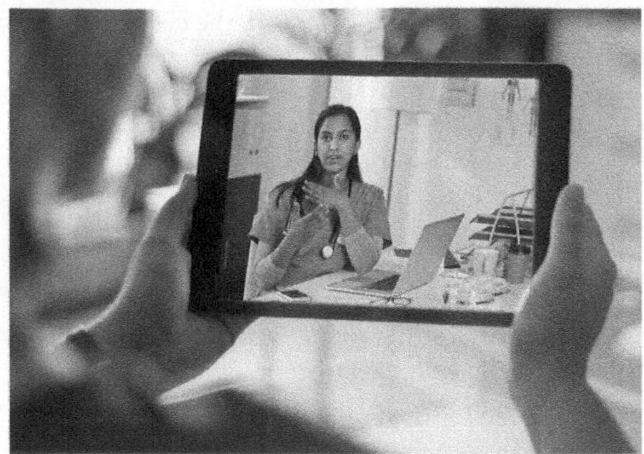

Figure 23-1 Delivery of occupational therapy services by telehealth allow the client and practitioner to connect from a distance. *(AAJ Watt/E+/Getty Images.)*

the client's natural environment. Additional physical supports provided by an aide, caretaker, or other health professional may be necessary to ensure the client's safety during the evaluation.

Evaluation of a group of individuals that may include the family or a population of individuals is also possible through telehealth. For example, if a client has a family member who is a caregiver to the client but that caregiver is not available to be physically present during the time of the evaluation, the use of telehealth provides an opportunity for the caregiver to connect through videoconferencing and participate in the session. If the client group is together in a space, then it is important to ensure that all individuals are in the view of the camera or able to access a microphone when speaking. If the client group is separated by physical distance, telehealth can bring them all together for the evaluation process through the use of a conference system with video and/or audio. In this situation, telehealth may hold an advantage over the traditional in-person evaluation process because of the ability to bring together the entire client group for increased collaboration in the health-care process.

In a similar way, telehealth can provide an opportunity to bring together one client with a group of health-care professionals. The completion of a community-based evaluation process also includes identifying the resources and means to facilitate the client's goals. This includes collaborating with other professionals who make up the community-based team and providing services to facilitate the client's desired goals. Telehealth allows for the interaction of the client with every member of the health-care team. Each member can join a video or a phone conference to participate in the evaluation process, which allows all team members to be present when distance or scheduling may be a limiting factor.

The client's environment can also be evaluated using telehealth. The occupational therapist can complete an interview-style assessment to gather all the necessary information about the client's environment. This would be a process similar to how a therapist would gather information about the client's home when completing an in-person evaluation at a hospital, skilled nursing facility, or outpatient clinic. Videoconferencing using a portable device such as an electronic tablet or smartphone can allow for observation of the physical space or community in which the client performs and participates in occupations. The occupational therapist can direct the client or a caregiver to move around the environment with the video camera pointed at the areas to be evaluated. One study conducted through the Durham Department of Veterans Affairs Medical Center (VAMC) demonstrated the use of a telephone and video camera to provide an evaluation of mobility throughout the home. The video was transmitted in real time to the therapist at the Durham VAMC (Hoenig et al., 2006). A technician assisted with camera placement, so the occupational therapist could observe the client completing tasks such as transfers in different areas of the home. The technician assisted during tasks that required physical assistance for safe completion (Hoenig et al., 2006).

Intervention

Telehealth can be a valuable tool for direct occupational therapy intervention services to a single client, family, or group of individuals within a population. Similar to conducting an evaluation, telehealth can provide a means to improve access to occupational therapy for clients and allows practitioners to provide interventions within clients' natural contexts, including their home and community. The practitioner can establish connection to a client through telehealth in home, school, work, and other contexts in the community where the client performs daily life occupations. Various types of technology, such as a tablet or laptop computer, can be loaned to clients to increase access to devices. Internet is available in many areas, with options such as air cards and hot spots available to expand access further. The Internet speed must be sufficient to assure adequate bandwidth for videoconferencing if a visual interaction is desired for intervention. The amount of bandwidth required will vary with the device, software, and features being used. For example, a low-bandwidth platform such as VSee (n.d.) requires a minimum bandwidth connection of 200 kilobits per second (kbps), while other platforms such as Zoom (n.d.) require 600 kbps. Bandwidth requirements can be reduced by eliminating the video stream and the use of audio and the screen share-only feature (50–75 kbps).

Similar to the use in evaluation, telehealth can bring together a population of individuals for intervention who may be physically present in different locations. A group session can be coordinated to provide direct intervention services to individuals with the same condition or needs. The benefit of providing occupational therapy services in a group is the addition of the social support the group members provide to one another. Telehealth also provides an alternative to the practitioner and clients traveling to a common location for group sessions. This can save on travel cost and time that may outweigh the cost of the telehealth system used. In rural areas or life situations that make it difficult for a population of individuals to come together at a community center or other location, telehealth bridges this gap. The occupational therapist can provide services such as education, training for occupations, preparatory methods, prevention services, and advocacy. Telehealth does present a unique challenge to developing the rapport and social support that is a hallmark of group-based interventions. The occupational therapist must take special care to provide a virtual environment that is open for dialogue and discussion as well as accessible to all participants.

Consultation

Consultation is a part of community-based practice that can be provided through telehealth. Occupational therapy practitioners with expertise in a service specific to a client's needs (e.g., complex seating systems) may not be available in a client's community. This would normally require the client to travel to where the service is provided, such as a larger medical facility. Treating practitioners can consult with the specialist to broaden their understanding of a client's needs in order to provide high-quality therapy services. The client may also be present during these sessions to provide full collaboration and to keep the client as the central focus of the services. This approach allows clients to remain in their communities while still having access to specialists. This approach is more consistent with a community-based model of service.

Benefits

The use of telehealth in the delivery of services in a community-based context provides many benefits. The benefits include improved access to services, decreased cost, reduction in time investment, and improved client outcomes (see Box 23-1).

Access

According to the 2015 AOTA Salary and Workforce Survey, 23.8% of occupational therapists and 23.8% of occupational therapy assistants report working in a community-based setting (AOTA, 2015b). This includes the settings of community, home health, early intervention, and schools. The greatest number of those practitioners identify with working in a school-based setting (19.9% of occupational therapists and 15% of occupational therapy assistants). This leaves a significantly low number of practitioners who work with clients in other community-based

Box 23-1 Selected Benefits and Limitations of Telehealth as a Service Delivery Model

Benefits	Limitations
Increased access to services	Technical constraints
Decreased cost	Limited client knowledge in the use of technology
Reduced time investment	Negative perceptions of telehealth by client and/or practitioner
Improved client outcomes	

settings across the country. One area of significant need is for occupational therapy practitioners in rural areas. The U.S. Census Bureau defines rural as an area that does not meet the definition of an urban area based upon set criteria of population, density, land use, and distance. Approximately 97% of the land in the U.S. is designated as rural (Ratcliffe, Burd, Holder, and Fields, 2016). However, according to the 2010 census, only approximately 19.3% (59,500,000) of the U.S. population live in rural areas. Though this is a relatively small number of people, it is a large area of need due to limited access to health-care services in rural areas (Health Resources and Services Administration, 2017). Telehealth can provide access in rural areas by connecting a practitioner in another rural area or larger urban location to clients in their home, work, or school setting.

Decreased Cost: Time and Financial

Access to clients in rural settings may include extensive amounts of travel for the practitioner. The clients may also need to travel to access services in a community center or other site. Telehealth can reduce the cost and time of travel for the clients and practitioner. The clients may get back to their meaningful daily activities if they do not need to spend excessive time traveling. Practitioners may be able to provide services to more clients during the time they would normally be traveling between locations. The cost of the equipment to utilize telehealth does not significantly increase the overall costs of the services. Depending on the type of technology and the distance needed to travel, the cost can be offset or reduced by using telehealth (Kairy et al., 2009; Pramuka and van Roosmalen, 2009).

Client Outcomes

In community-based care, it is important to meet the needs of clients in the context of their natural environments. Telehealth provides not only the access to achieve this goal when it may not be otherwise feasible but also a service that can be as effective as in-person care (Chumbler et al., 2012; Ng et al., 2013). When the client and practitioner collaborate to determine the best methods for using telehealth to deliver the services needed, telehealth can be just as effective and provide benefits that result in better outcomes than in-person services, in some situations.

Limitations

Telehealth may not be the best delivery method for all services provided to clients in the community-based setting. The practitioner and client need to weigh the limitations of telehealth against the benefits. Limitations include technical constraints, lack of client knowledge to manage the technology, and negative perceptions by the practitioner or client regarding the use of telehealth.

Technical Constraints

The use of technology has inherent limitations. Equipment failure, reduced or failed Internet service, and audio problems are a few technical issues that may arise. These issues will need to be resolved in order for the telehealth session to be successful. The ability of the practitioner or client to troubleshoot many of these issues is necessary in a community-based setting. There may not be an information technology (IT) specialist available to support the client or practitioner during the therapy session. Providing the client with a troubleshooting guide for common technology issues and developing a backup plan (e.g., use of telephone audio in the event of computer audio failure) are essential components of using telehealth in practice. If the occupational therapist is part of a larger health-care organization, he or she may have access to IT support to assist with troubleshooting technical issues. The support services available should be identified ahead of time to allow for timely assistance when needed. In addition, some companies provide telehealth equipment packages that come with different levels of support options.

Client Knowledge

Clients will have varying levels of knowledge about the use of technology. Many clients will have experience with using a phone, but not all may be comfortable using higher-level technology, such as a computer, smartphone, or tablet, for videoconference sessions. Tailoring the type and amount of technology used for client sessions to the client will make the experience more successful. If a client is not comfortable with technology, the practitioner may need to spend more time preparing the client to perform the basic functions needed to interact with the technology. This may include providing an additional session or extra time in the first session to educate the client on using the technology. For clients who are not knowledgeable at all or feel discomfort with the initial launch to enter the telehealth session, an in-person session to educate the client on the use of the technology may be necessary. An aide may also provide this service by being present during the initial sessions until clients feel comfortable operating the system on their own. This additional time and resource will need to be factored into the therapy process. Clients who are more comfortable with technology may not need as much initial education to participate in telehealth sessions.

Perceptions of Telehealth

Perceptions of technology and the use of telehealth to receive health-care services can vary based on each person's prior experience. If clients or practitioners had a negative experience with technology in the past, they may be less open to using technology for health-care services. In addition, limited experience with technology or the use of telehealth may make people more skeptical about its effectiveness when they compare it to their experience of receiving services in the traditional in-person model. Furthermore, clients and practitioners may be hesitant to use telehealth because of the perceived lack of a personal connection to build positive rapport or the risk to one's privacy (Cimperman, Brencic, Trkman, and Stanonik, 2013; Levy and Strachan, 2013). Building a telehealth program that incorporates user-centered design (e.g., the use of technology familiar to the client, intuitive software, etc.) with procedures in place to provide training and ongoing assessment can increase the overall success of the telehealth program by improving user perception (Demiris et al., 2010).

One population often thought to be most resistant to learning new technology is older adults. This may be because they often have more limited experience with technology use compared to younger generations, who grew up using technology in their everyday lives. However, there is evidence that older adults are willing to learn to use technology and that their perceptions are generally positive after receiving services through a telehealth service delivery model (Crotty et al., 2014). One study by Cimperman et al. (2013) found that older adults were likely to preevaluate the use of telehealth based upon perceived usefulness, effort expectancy, social influence, perceived security, computer anxiety, facilitating conditions, and physician opinion but not on their self-identified computer skill set.

Client and/or practitioner perceptions of telehealth can be identified through the technology acceptance model (TAM; Davis, 1985; Holden and Karsh, 2010). TAM posits that a person's attitude toward technology is influenced by the perceived ease of use and usefulness of the system for the intended purpose. This in turn directly affects the user's intent to use the system. A negative perception will lead to low intention to use the system. If the practitioner does not see telehealth as a useful tool to deliver health-care services, then telehealth will most likely not be used. Likewise, if clients do not see the value in telehealth as an effective means to receive health-care services, they are most likely not going to agree to use it. The practitioner should consider these perceptions when determining if telehealth is an appropriate delivery method and what additional actions are needed to increase the client's comfort with telehealth.

Engage Your Brain 23-2

What occupational therapy and other theories are conducive to guide services provided through telehealth and why?

Ethical and Legal Issues

The AOTA (2013) and the WFOT (2014) both emphasize that the use of telehealth must maintain the same practice standards as in-person services. This includes following ethical standards, protecting the client's health information, and abiding by licensure statutes and regulations.

Ethics

The AOTA (2015a) *Occupational Therapy Code of Ethics (2015)* calls for practitioners to practice in alignment with the principles of beneficence, nonmaleficence, autonomy, justice, veracity, and fidelity.

These ethical principles hold true regardless of the delivery method chosen—in-person or telehealth. One principle of ethical practice is beneficence. A standard of conduct pertaining to beneficence is the need for practitioners to "take steps (e.g., continuing education, research, supervision, training) to ensure proficiency, use careful judgment, and weigh potential for harm when generally recognized standards do not exist in emerging technology or areas of practice" (AOTA, 2015a, p. 3).

A second principle is autonomy. The practitioner is ethically bound to maintain the confidentiality of all aspects of the encounter (AOTA, 2015a; Estes, 2017). In the virtual environment of telehealth, this includes upholding all laws pertaining to protection of health information, providing the client full disclosure of the possibility of a technology breach, and informing the client of anyone else who may be present (i.e., in person or virtual) during the time of the encounter.

A third principle relevant to the use of telehealth is justice. **Justice** is "the fair, equitable, and appropriate treatment of persons" (AOTA, 2015a, p. 5). The practitioner must advocate for equal access to services for clients who may experience barriers to access. Telehealth may be the best option for healthcare access for clients who would otherwise not have access to services. The *Code of Ethics* also calls upon the practitioner to utilize standards of practice (AOTA, 2010). The practitioner must uphold the same standards of practice in the virtual context as in the in-person context.

Health Insurance Portability and Accountability Act

The Health Insurance Portability and Accountability Act (HIPAA) of 1996 includes protection of a client's health information from unauthorized disclosure and standards of security for all electronic documents. In 2009, HIPAA was expanded to include the Health Information Technology for Economic and Clinical Health (HITECH) Act. This act expanded HIPAA to include all business associates as covered entities that must adhere to the protection of client health information (U.S. Department of Health and Human Services, 2017). In the context of telehealth, this means the practitioner must utilize technology sources that are HIPAA compliant for all client information record-keeping and service delivery (Estes, 2017). The system must be secure against possible data breaches that would allow an unauthorized individual or entity to view the client session or documents. It is the practitioner's ethical obligation to let the client know that breaches are possible and that in the event of this occurring the practitioner will abide by the applicable laws regarding breaches of protected health information (Estes, 2017).

Engage Your Brain 23-3

What impact does each AOTA ethical principle have on the use of telehealth in occupational therapy practice?

Licensure

State licensure regulations have not caught up with the expanding use of telehealth in each state. Currently, state licensure regarding the use of telehealth to provide occupational therapy services varies greatly. Most state licensure boards either take no position, deem it out of their authority, or directly regulate the use of telehealth by occupational therapy practitioners. Direct regulation may include items of parity between traditional in-person services and those provided by telehealth, the physical location of the practitioner, and the requirement of state licensure in the state where the client is located (AOTA State Affairs, 2018). Before implementing the use of telehealth in any state, occupational therapy practitioners should review the current state licensure laws related to their own state as well as the state where the client is located. If the licensure laws are unclear, the practitioner should consult the professional licensing board(s).

Role of Telehealth in Community-Based Practice and Population Health

The AOTA (2018) *Vision 2025* states that "occupational therapy maximizes health, well-being, and quality of life for all people, populations, and communities through effective solutions that facilitate participation in everyday living" (p. 18). Telehealth can be used as a means to achieve the *AOTA Vision 2025* by focusing attention on four areas: effectiveness, leadership, collaboration, and accessibility (AOTA, 2018).

Current available evidence supports the use of telehealth as an effective means to provide services to community-based clients. Multiple studies demonstrate how services provided through telehealth are as effective or more effective than services provided in person (Bendixen, Horn, and Levy, 2007; Chumbler et al., 2012; Crotty et al., 2014; Dallolio et al., 2008; Hoenig et al., 2006; Kairy et al., 2009; Little et al., 2018; Ng et al., 2013; Sundsli et al., 2014). Telehealth offers a means to be client-centered by allowing clients to remain in their homes to receive services. Maintaining a client-centered approach to services in the client's natural context is also the focus of community-based service. In addition, telehealth can be a cost-effective approach, especially in rural areas where access to health-care services may be limited or unavailable.

Occupational therapy can be a leader in the area of developing telehealth for use in community-based practice to increase access to services to clients. Policies are continually changing in the area of telehealth utilization, and occupational therapy practitioners can continue to develop evidence and advocate for its expanded use.

Collaboration between the client and the health-care team is a key component in community-based practice. Telehealth can bring all team members together for more effective and collaborative care to meet the client's goals. Telehealth can be an option for the community-based practitioner to align the frequency and duration of services provided to best meet the client's needs and to access specialists who may not otherwise be available to the client.

Through collaboration with the client, telehealth can provide services that bring together team members who are not physically present in the same location. This flexibility and opportunity to facilitate interprofessional practice results in telehealth being an excellent option for the delivery of occupational therapy services to meet the AOTA's *Vision 2025*.

Applications Across Populations: Opportunities

Telehealth has applications in community-based practice across multiple populations. Telehealth is useful in a variety of practice areas, including early intervention, school-based services, mental health, adult rehabilitation, ergonomics, community reintegration, productive aging, and hospice care. Research in the area of telehealth provides evidence for its efficacy for use with clients in a community-based setting (Bendixen et al., 2007; Cason and Jacobs, 2014; Chumbler et al., 2012; Dallolio et al., 2008; Jenkins-Guarnieri, Pruitt, Luxton, and Johnson, 2015; Little et al., 2018; Ng et al., 2013).

Research supports the use of telehealth in the provision of occupation-based coaching to families with children who have autism spectrum disorder (ASD). An example is a program for families in rural and underserved areas. The occupation-based coaching model, which supports caregivers in identifying goals and strategies to support the child in his or her natural environments and family routines, was implemented through telehealth (Little et al., 2018). This program was delivered by an online teleconferencing system with 17 families. The 12-week program provided individualized sessions between the occupational therapist and each family, with a focus on authentic contexts; family interests and routines; caregiver interactions and responsiveness, reflection and feedback; and joint plans. The program delivered through telehealth was successful in improving parenting efficacy and children's participation in activity (Little et al., 2018).

A systematic review of psychotherapeutic interventions for adults demonstrates potential for the use of telehealth to provide services for clients with mental health diagnoses (Jenkins-Guarnieri et al., 2015). Completed in both urban and rural settings, the studies in this systematic review utilized both videoconference and phone-based interventions. The interventions were delivered by psychologists; however, the use of telehealth would also be applicable in the delivery of community-based occupational therapy mental health services (Cason and Jacobs, 2014).

Another area of community-based occupational therapy practice that is currently using telehealth as a delivery method is adult rehabilitation (Fig. 23-2).

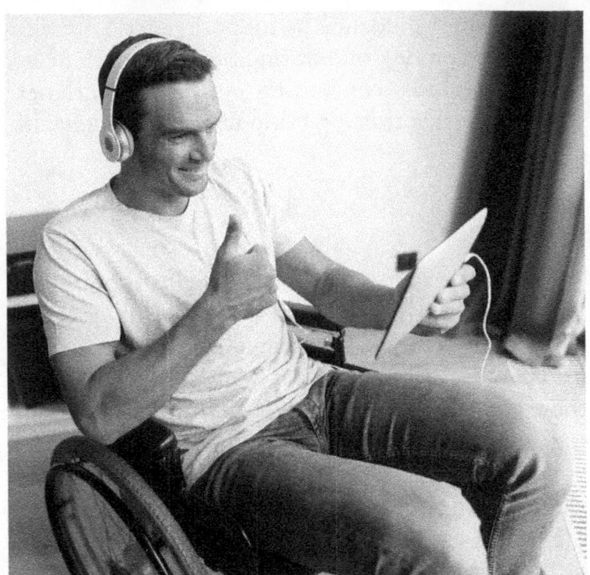

Figure 23-2 Clients can receive rehabilitative services at home. *(vadimguzhva/iStock/Getty Images Plus/ Getty Images.)*

Several researchers have demonstrated the efficacy of using telehealth to deliver rehabilitation services to clients in their home, with a focus on increasing participation in daily occupations at home, at work, and in the community (Chumbler et al., 2012; Dallolio et al., 2008; Ng et al., 2013). One program, the Stroke Telerehabilitation (STeleR) intervention, focused on improving functional mobility for stroke survivors who were living at home (Chumbler et al., 2012). The results of this program demonstrated the effectiveness of a telehealth program to improve self-care performance and social role tasks.

A program that worked with clients with spinal cord injuries also demonstrated good outcomes in the areas of functional mobility and activities of daily living (ADLs). Participants at one site of this multisite program, the Telerehabilitation Through Interactive Video Endorsement (THRIVE) Project, demonstrated significantly higher gains in Functional Independence Measure (FIM) scores and greater satisfaction with their provider interactions than the standard-care control group (Dallolio et al., 2008). A third example program is the use of the Cognitive Orientation to Daily Occupational Performance (CO-OP) approach with adults who had suffered a traumatic brain injury (TBI). The three participants in the study had improved executive function, better integration into their community, and some level of improvement in satisfaction with and performance of their occupation-based goals (Ng et al., 2013). These studies provide support for the use of telehealth as an effective intervention to improve occupational performance and client satisfaction.

Research also supports the use of telehealth in the area of productive aging. Telehealth can be useful in productive aging as a means to provide remote safety monitoring of older adult clients to allow them to remain in their homes and to provide recommendations for home modifications. One study by Bendixen et al. (2007) examined the Low ADL Monitoring Project (LAMP), a program that provided services to veterans who had at least two areas of ADL deficits. Results of the LAMP indicated that the application of remote monitoring improved care for veterans through care coordination and the provision of appropriate assistive technology and/or adaptive equipment. Bendixen, Levy, Olive, Kobb, and Mann (2009) also reported on a cost-analysis study of the LAMP. The analysis of 115 participants found that the cost of the LAMP was not significantly different than the cost of the same number of veterans receiving standard care. This demonstrates telehealth as a fiscally viable option for care in the client's home.

PROGRAM SHOWCASE

Powerful Tools for Caregivers

Contributed by Katrina Serwe, PhD, OTR/L

Caregivers are at greater risk for health problems, stress related to caregiving, and limited time to meet their own health-care, leisure, and social needs. **Powerful Tools for Caregivers** is a 6-week program that addresses the issue of caregiver health by promoting self-care behaviors. Collaborating community organizations offer the program at little to no cost. The in-person Powerful Tools for Caregivers program started in 1998 and now benefits caregivers across 40 states. Benefits of participation include improved self-care behaviors, increased self-efficacy, increased use of community resources, reduced caregiver burden, and improved psychological well-being (Boise,

Congleton, and Shannon, 2005; Savundranayagam, Montgomery, Kosloski, and Little, 2011; Won Won, Fitts, Favaro, Olsen, and Phelan, 2007). However, not all caregivers have equal access to this program. Class leaders are requesting a delivery format with the ability to reach caregivers who face barriers to attending a class, such as lack of respite care, limited time, mobility issues, limited transportation options, or a home in a rural area. Telehealth offers a delivery format capable of overcoming these barriers.

A telehealth delivery method for Powerful Tools for Caregivers was developed in response to this need, with a format as close to the in-person program as possible (Serwe, Hersch, and Pancheri, 2017). Participants use the free version of VSee (n.d.) software to participate in six weekly classes via synchronous videoconferencing. Class leaders share information via PowerPoint slides and model concepts and facilitate discussion. High class attendance (an average of 5.5 out of 6 classes) and high ratings on the Telehealth Usability Questionnaire demonstrated the telehealth method was feasible (Serwe, Hersch, and Pancheri, 2017). Furthermore, participants indicated in a focus group interview that the telehealth-delivered program was a positive experience and provided an opportunity they would not otherwise have had (Serwe, Hersch, Pickens, and Pancheri, 2017). Participants appreciated the social aspects:

"This is the first time I have been using it [VSee®] and I think it's very interesting because you can feel like you're in a group and you can talk about your problems and listen to what other people have gone through, so I thought it was quite a learning experience. . . . I felt very close to all our group and it was nearly like being face-to-face [in person]."

A pilot study was conducted in four states, and the results are being used to develop the next step of comparing outcomes from the telehealth and in-person delivery formats. If outcomes are comparable, the goal is to offer the program nationwide through community organizations at little to no cost to caregivers.

The evidence to support telehealth as a viable option to deliver services to community-based clients continues to expand. The studies highlighted in this section are only a small portion of the evidence available to support occupational therapy using telehealth in community-based practice. The occupational therapy practitioner must stay current with knowledge of emerging technologies for telehealth and the latest evidence to support practice in this area. This can be done through reading current literature, seeking continuing education, and networking with other practitioners using telehealth in practice.

Challenges

Though research provides evidence to support the use of telehealth in community-based practice, its use does not come without challenges. The occupational therapy practitioner will need to identify these challenges and work to minimize or avoid issues that may lead to a breakdown in the services provided to the client. Some of the challenges include the limitations noted earlier of technical issues, lack of client knowledge to manage the technology, and negative perceptions of the practitioner or client. Additional challenges may include concerns with legal and ethical adherence to client rights. The occupational therapy practitioner should also identify the funding or payer source prior to the implementation of services because funding varies by payer and by state. Medicare does not pay for occupational therapy services provided through telehealth unless services provided by an occupational therapy practitioner through telehealth are part of a bundled payment model (Cason and Richmond, 2016). Medicaid payment of services is limited or not available in many states (ATA, 2016; Centers for Medicare and Medicaid Services, 2016a, 2016b). Private health insurance coverage varies by state, company, and plan.

Outside of the traditional payer sources of Medicare, Medicaid, and private insurance exist other viable options for reimbursement of services provided through telehealth. The most direct option is to bill the client for services. A set fee can be established for direct pay; however, the practitioner must be aware of applicable laws that may require notification to the client. For example, the Centers for Medicare and Medicaid Services (2017) requires an Advance Beneficiary Notice (ABN) to notify Medicare recipients that the services provided are not reimbursable. Another alternative may be to identify funding sources, such as nonprofit organizations or grants, that will assist in supporting start-up costs; ongoing technology fees, such as those for Internet service; or equipment to provide for client use.

Table 23-1 Telehealth Resources

Organization	URL Address
American Occupational Therapy Association	www.aota.org/
American Telemedicine Association	www.americantelemed.org/home
Center for Connected Health Policy: The National Telehealth Policy Resource Center	www.cchpca.org/
Telehealth Resource Centers	www.telehealthresourcecenter.org/
World Federation of Occupational Therapists	www.wfot.org/

To minimize or avoid some challenges that may arise, the practitioner should collaborate with the client and other members of the health-care team to identify and address such challenges before implementing telehealth. Following recommendations for the implementation of services, such as those provided by the AOTA or the ATA, is key to providing effective service delivery through telehealth. Table 23-1 provides a list of organizations with resources to assist in the implementation of telehealth in practice.

Summary

- The information provided in this chapter demonstrates the scope of the use of telehealth as a viable delivery method to provide occupational therapy services to individual clients, families, and client populations in community-based environments.
- Benefits of telehealth include expanding the reach of occupational therapy to clients where they live, work, and play; decreasing costs; reducing time investment; and improving client outcomes. Limitations need to be addressed to provide successful implementation of services.
- The use of telehealth requires the practitioner to abide by the same standards of practice as in-person services and uphold the ethical and legal requirements of practice. Additional modifications may need to be made to ensure that privacy, security, and licensure laws are maintained in the virtual context.
- Evidence supports the use of telehealth to provide services to clients that are equivalent to or better than in-person services.
- Community-based practice is focused on clients in their natural environments, and telehealth can be a part of that service model to provide opportunities to improve services for better client outcomes.

CASE STUDIES

CASE STUDY 23-1 Vivian

Vivian is a 46-year-old woman with multiple sclerosis (MS). Her physician referred her to occupational therapy after an exacerbation of her symptoms left her with performance deficits in her daily occupations. Her largest barriers are in her home and work environments. Both environments are not conducive to her overall decline in strength, endurance, and coordination. Vivian lives in a single-story home with a four-step entry and no environmental modifications. She is an office assistant for a local certified public accountant. Vivian lives in a rural town that does not have access to outpatient occupational therapy services, and she does not qualify for home health services. The nearest clinic is 60 minutes away. Vivian's goals are to be independent at home and at work now and to prepare for future functional declines that may occur due to her MS.

CASE STUDY 23-1 Vivian

Discussion Questions

1. Why would telehealth be beneficial for Vivian?
2. How can you determine if Vivian's insurance company pays for occupational therapy services delivered by telehealth? What alternative options are available if services are not covered under her insurance but Vivian desires to receive services using telehealth?
3. What intervention strategies might be conducive to use with telehealth? Are there interventions that might need to be completed in person?

CASE STUDY 23-2 Alzheimer's Association

The staff of the local chapter of the Alzheimer's Association has identified a group of local caregivers who are in need of support and resources. The caregivers live in an urban area that provides in-person educational groups led by a team of health-care professionals, including an occupational therapist, social worker, and nurse. However, this particular group of caregivers does not attend these sessions on a consistent basis. Due to this inconsistent attendance, the caregivers often report feeling that they do not have the tools necessary to care for their loved ones.

Discussion Questions

1. Why might caregivers of persons with dementia find it difficult to access in-person services?
2. Why is telehealth beneficial to bring together a population of persons in urban settings who lack access to services due to their situations?
3. How would you design a group-based telehealth program to deliver occupational therapy services to a group of caregivers of persons with dementia?
4. What factors would you identify to select the appropriate technology system and protocol when designing such a program?

Learning Activities

1. Create a telehealth resource manual to guide the use of telehealth for clients in your community. Include items such as identifying the availability of technology, a systematic guide on using the technology, and education for the client.
2. Identify funding sources available to access and/or purchase the technology that is needed in your community to support the use of telehealth.
3. Participate in the opportunities for professional community networking available through different telehealth organizations.

REFERENCES

American Occupational Therapy Association. (2010). Standards of practice for occupational therapy. *American Journal of Occupational Therapy, 64*(Suppl. 6), S106–S111. doi:10.5014/ajot.2010.64S106-64S111

American Occupational Therapy Association. (2013). Telehealth. *American Journal of Occupational Therapy, 67*(Suppl. 6), S69–90.

American Occupational Therapy Association. (2015a). Occupational therapy code of ethics (2015). *American Journal of Occupational Therapy, 69*(Suppl. 3), 6913410030. doi:10.5014/ajot.2015.696S03

American Occupational Therapy Association. (2015b). *2015 American Occupational Therapy Association salary and workforce survey: Executive summary.* Retrieved from www.aota.org/Education-Careers/Advance-Career/Salary-Workforce-Survey.aspx

American Occupational Therapy Association. (2018). Vision 2025. *OT Practice, 23*(1), 18–19.

American Occupational Therapy Association State Affairs. (2018). *Occupational therapy and telehealth: State statutes, regulations and regulatory board statements.* Retrieved from www.aota.org/Advocacy-Policy/State-Policy/StateNews/2016/state-telehealth-law-chart-occupational-therapy.aspx

American Telemedicine Association. (2010). *A blueprint for telerehabilitation guidelines.* Retrieved from www.americantelemed.org/home

American Telemedicine Association. (2016). *State telemedicine gaps analysis: Coverage and reimbursement.* Retrieved from www.americantelemed.org

Bendixen, R. M., Horn, K., and Levy, C. (2007). Using telerehabilitation to support elders with chronic illness in their homes. *Topics in Geriatric Rehabilitation, 23*(1), 47–51.

Bendixen, R. M., Levy, C. E., Olive, E. S., Kobb, R. F., and Mann, W. C. (2009). Cost effectiveness of a telerehabilitation program to support chronically ill and disabled elders in their homes. *Telemedicine and e-Health, 15*(1), 31–38. doi:10.1089/tmj.2008.0046

Boise, L., Congleton, L., and Shannon, K. (2005). Empowering family caregivers: The powerful tools for caregiving program. *Educational Gerontology, 31,* 573–586. doi:10.1080/03601270590962523

Cason, J., and Jacobs, K. (2014). Snapshots of current telehealth applications in occupational therapy. *OT Practice, 19*(14), 7–12.

Cason, J., and Richmond, T. (2016, February). Innovative occupational therapy practice for patients with lower extremity joint replacement. *SIS Quarterly Practice Connections, 1*(1), 10–11.

Center for Connected Health Policy. (2014). *What is telehealth?* Retrieved from www.cchpca.org/what-is-telehealth

Centers for Medicare and Medicaid Services. (2016a). *Medicare benefit policy manual: Chapter 15—covered medical and other health services.*

Centers for Medicare and Medicaid Services. (2016b). *Medicare claims processing manual: Chapter 12—physicians/nonphysician practitioners.*

Centers for Medicare and Medicaid Services. (2017). *Medicare advance written notices of noncoverage.*

Chumbler, N. R., Quigley, P., Li, X., Morey, M., Rose, D., Sanford, J., . . . Hoenig, H. (2012). Effects of telerehabilitation on physical function and disability for stroke patients: A randomized, controlled trial. *Stroke, 43*(8), 2168–2174.

Cimperman, M., Brencic, M. M., Trkman, P., and Stanonik, M. D. L. (2013). Older adults' perceptions of home telehealth services. *Telemedicine and e-Health, 19*(10), 786–790. doi:10.1089/tmj.2012.0272

Crotty, M., Killington, M., van den Berg, M., Morris, C., Taylor, A., and Carati, C. (2014). Telerehabilitation for older people using off-the-shelf applications: Acceptability and feasibility. *Journal of Telemedicine and Telecare, 20*(7), 370–376. doi:10.1177/1357633X14552382

Dallolio, L., Menarini, M., China, S., Ventura, M., Stainthorpe, A., Soopramanien, A., . . . Fantini, M. P. (2008). Functional and clinical outcomes of telemedicine in patients with spinal cord injury. *Archives of Physical Medicine and Rehabilitation, 89,* 2332–2341. doi:10.1016/j.apmr.2008.06.012

Davis, F. D. (1985). *A technology acceptance model for empirically testing new end-user information systems: Theory and results.* Cambridge, MA: Massachusetts Institute of Technology. Research Gate Database.

Demiris, G., Charness, N., Krupinski, E., Ben-Arieh, D., Washington, K., Wu, J., and Farberow, B. (2010). The role of human factors in telehealth. *Telemedicine and e-Health, 16*(4), 446–453. doi:10.1089/tmj.2009.0114

Estes, J. (2017). *American Occupational Therapy Association advisory opinion for the Ethics Commission: Telehealth.* Retrieved from www.aota.org/Practice/Ethics/Advisory.aspx

Hall, E. J. (2015, May 19). Have you joined the telehealth revolution yet? *Huffington Post.* Retrieved from www.huffingtonpost.com/eric-j-hall/have-you-joined-the-teleh_b_6801226.html

Health Resources and Services Administration. (2017). *Defining rural population.* Retrieved from www.hrsa.gov/rural-health/about-us/definition/index.html

Hoenig, H., Sanford, J. A., Butterfield, T., Griffiths, P. C., Richardson, P., and Hargraves, K. (2006). Development of a teletechnology protocol for in-home rehabilitation. *Journal of Rehabilitation Research and Development, 43*(2), 287–298. doi:10.1682/JRRD.2004.07.0089

Holden, R. J., and Karsh, B. T. (2010). The technology acceptance model: Its past and its future in healthcare. *Journal of Biomedical Informatics, 43*(1), 159–172. doi:10.1016/j.jbi.2009.07.002

Jenkins-Guarnieri, M. A., Pruitt, L. D., Luxton, D. D., and Johnson, K. (2015). Patient perceptions of telemental health: Systematic review of direct comparisons to in-person psychotherapeutic treatments. *Telemedicine and e-Health, 21*(8), 652–660. doi:10.1089/tmj.2014.0165

Kairy, D., Lehoux, P., Vincent, C., and Visintin, M. (2009). A systematic review of clinical outcomes, clinical process, healthcare utilization, and costs associated with telerehabilitation. *Disability and Rehabilitation, 31*(6), 427–447. doi:10.1080/09638280802062553

LeadingAge Center for Aging Services Technologies. (2015). *Telehealth and remote patient monitoring for long-term and post-acute care: A primer and provider selection guide 2015.* Retrieved from www.leadingage.org

Levy, S., and Strachan, N. (2013). Child and adolescent mental health service providers' perceptions of using telehealth. *Mental Health Practice, 17*(1), 28–32.

Little, L. M., Pope, E., Wallisch, A., and Dunn, W. (2018). Occupation-based coaching by means of telehealth for families of young children with autism spectrum disorder. *American Journal of Occupational Therapy, 72,* 7202205020. doi:10.5014/ajot.2018.024786

Ng, E. M. W., Polatajko, H. J., Marziali, E., Hunt, A., and Dawson, D. R. (2013). Telerehabilitation for addressing executive dysfunction after traumatic brain injury. *Brain Injury, 27*(5), 548–564. doi:10.3109/02699052.2013.766927

Pramuka, M., and van Roosmalen, L. (2009). Telerehabilitation technologies: Accessibility and usability. *International Journal of Telerehabilitation, 1*(1), 85–98. doi:10.5195/ijt.2009.6016

Ratcliffe, M., Burd, C., Holder, K., and Fields, A. (2016). *Defining rural at the U.S. Census Bureau.* Retrieved from www.census.gov/geo/reference/urban-rural.html

Savundranayagam, M. Y., Montgomery, R. J. V., Kosloski, K., and Little, T. D. (2011). Impact of a psychoeducational program on three types of caregiver burden among spouses. *International Journal of Geriatric Psychiatry, 26,* 388–396. doi:10.1002/gps.2538

Serwe, K. M., Hersch, G. I., and Pancheri, K. (2017). Feasibility of using telehealth to deliver the "Powerful Tools for Caregivers" program. *International Journal of Telerehabilitation, 9*(1), 15–22. doi:10.5195/ijt.2017.6214

Serwe, K. M., Hersch, G. I., Pickens, N. D., and Pancheri, K. (2017). Brief report—caregiver perceptions of a telehealth wellness program. *American Journal of Occupational Therapy, 71,* 7104350010. doi:10.5014/ajot.2017.025619

Sundsli, K., Söderhamm, U., Espnes, G. A., and Söderhamm, O. (2014). Self-care telephone talks as a health-promotion intervention in urban home-living persons 75+ years of age: A randomized controlled study. *Clinical Interventions in Aging, 9,* 95–103. doi:10.2147/CIA.S55925

U.S. Department of Health and Human Services. (2017). *HIPAA for professionals.* Retrieved from www.hhs.gov/hipaa/for-professionals/index.html

VSee (n.d.). *Telehealth that works.* Retrieved from https://vsee.com/

Won Won, C., Fitts, S. S., Favaro, S., Olsen, P., and Phelan, E. A. (2007). Community-based "powerful tools" intervention enhances health of caregivers. *Archives Gerontology and Geriatrics, 46*(1), 89–100. doi:10.1016/j.archger.2007.02.009

World Federation of Occupational Therapists. (2014). World Federation of Occupational Therapists' position statement on telehealth. *International Journal of Telerehabilitation, 6*(1), 37–40. doi:10.5195/ijt.2014.6153

Zoom. (n.d.). *Flawless video. Clear audio. Instant sharing.* Retrieved from https://zoom.us

Zuppo, C. M. (2012). Defining ICT in a boundaryless world: The development of a working hierarchy. *International Journal of Managing Information Technology, 4*(3), 13–22. doi:10.5121/ijmit.2012.4302

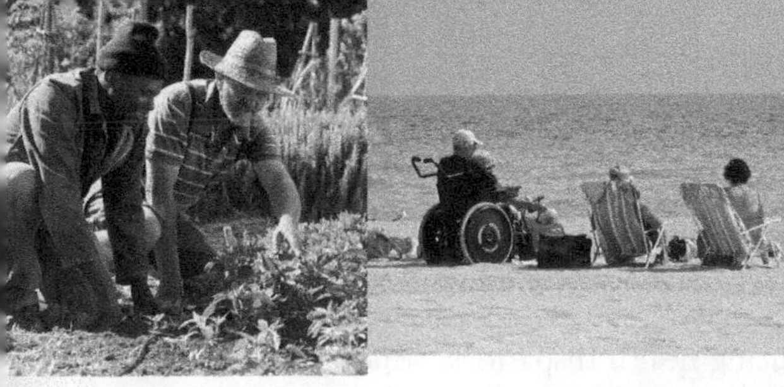

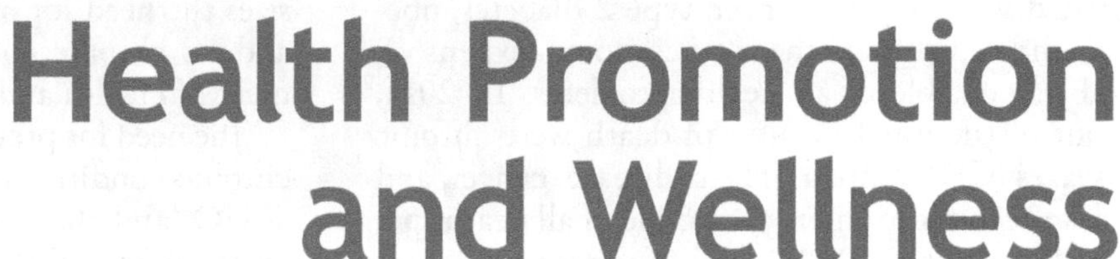

SECTION VIII

Health Promotion and Wellness

Chapter 24

Lifestyle Redesign® Programs

Camille Dieterle, OTD, OTR/L

Live a balanced life—learn some and think some and draw and paint and sing and dance and play and work every day some.

—Robert Fulghum, *All I Really Need to Know I Learned in Kindergarten*

Learning Outcomes

This chapter is designed to enable the reader to:

24-1 Explain the need for Lifestyle Redesign intervention.
24-2 Identify the key components that make up "lifestyle."
24-3 Describe the history and development of Lifestyle Redesign.
24-4 Describe different types of Lifestyle Redesign programs and how Lifestyle Redesign interventions can be applied to various populations and settings.
24-5 Identify reimbursement and education/marketing issues relevant to Lifestyle Redesign programming.

Key Terms

Accountability structures
Didactic presentation
Direct experience
Lifestyle
Lifestyle Redesign
Obesogenic
Occupational self-analysis
Occupational storytelling and story making
Peer exchange
Personal exploration
Wellness

Introduction

According to the Centers for Disease Control and Prevention (CDC, 2017a), chronic diseases such as heart disease, stroke, cancer, type 2 diabetes, obesity, and arthritis are the most common, expensive, and preventable of all health problems. In 2014, 7 out of the top 10 causes of death were chronic diseases (CDC, 2017a). Heart disease, cancer, and stroke account for more than 50% of all deaths per year (Kung et al., 2008), and of the top 30 causes of self-reported disability in adults, the following chronic conditions were ranked among the top 15: arthritis, spine and back pain, heart disease, lung and respiratory problems, mental health and emotional issues, diabetes, stroke, cancer, hypertension, and kidney problems (CDC, 2009). Additionally, the number of U.S. adults age 65 and older is projected to double by 2030, and experts are expecting to see an increase in the incidence of disability from chronic conditions (CDC, 2009). The top chronic conditions experienced by adults over the age of 65 are chronic obstructive pulmonary disease (COPD), Alzheimer's disease, depression, heart failure, chronic kidney disease, diabetes, ischemic heart disease, arthritis, high cholesterol, and hypertension (National Council on Aging, 2017).

Although the statistics within the United States alone are staggering, such health concerns appear internationally. The World Health Organization (WHO, 2019b) reports that noncommunicable diseases (NCDs), including heart disease, stroke, cancer, diabetes, and chronic lung disease, are collectively responsible for almost 71% of all deaths worldwide. Heart disease is the number one cause of death worldwide. In the United States, tobacco use, physical inactivity, unhealthy use of alcohol, and unhealthy diets, all of which are modifiable, are cited as the greatest risk factors for these diseases (WHO, 2019b). About 15% of the world's population has a disability. This rising number is due to aging populations and the increase in chronic disease (WHO, 2019a).

The CDC also describes the significant health disparities for chronic conditions. The following characteristics are associated with higher rates of disability related to chronic conditions: lower education levels; lower income; unemployment; living in southeastern states like Alabama, Mississippi, and Tennessee; and ethnic background (CDC, 2015). Non-Hispanic black and Hispanic adults are more likely to have a disability than non-Hispanic white adults (CDC, 2015). *Healthy People 2030* prioritizes reducing health disparities, which further emphasizes the need for occupational therapy services to address chronic conditions widely (U.S. Department of Health and Human Services, 2018).

The need for prevention and self-management of chronic conditions is paramount. The CDC, the WHO, and the occupational therapy profession, among others, are calling for additional health professionals to address these conditions with more vigor. According to the CDC (2009),

> *greater numbers of trained professionals will be needed to expand the reach of effective community-based programs to mitigate the effects of disability. Modifiable lifestyle characteristics (e.g., physical inactivity, obesity, and tobacco use) are major contributors to the most common causes of disability, and sometimes stem from a primary disabling condition. (editorial note, para. 4)*

Lifestyle Redesign is an occupational therapy approach to chronic condition self-management. Addressing common and expensive chronic diseases through Lifestyle Redesign programs is responsive, customized, collaborative, evidence-based, client centered, and cost-effective, which are priorities of the *Vision 2025* for occupational therapy (American Occupational Therapy Association [AOTA], 2018). With both the evidence to support their efficacy with certain populations and a practical format, Lifestyle Redesign programs are situated to directly address each of the goals in the AOTA's *Vision 2025* to "maximize health, well-being, and quality of life for all people, populations, and communities through effective solutions that facilitate participation in everyday living" (AOTA, 2018, p. 18).

With their emphasis on the impact of activity on health, occupational therapy practitioners are among the key health professionals to provide preventive interventions and management of chronic conditions. As a community-based occupational therapy approach and a set of techniques and tools specifically developed to address chronic conditions, Lifestyle Redesign intervention can both prevent chronic conditions and help to better manage them after onset.

Through clinical trial research, Lifestyle Redesign was demonstrated to be an effective preventive technique in community-based settings. It enhances health, improves quality of life, and reduces health-care costs (Clark et al., 1997; Mandel, Jackson, Zemke, Nelson, and Clark, 1999). Occupational therapy practitioners can use Lifestyle Redesign as an approach for widening the scope of occupational therapy practice to include facilitating the self-management of chronic conditions on a broader scale.

Presently, the University of Southern California (USC) Occupational Therapy Faculty Practice (OTFP) provides occupational therapy interventions for the prevention and management of chronic conditions. The OTFP is an outpatient clinic situated on the campus of USC, where occupational therapy practitioners utilize the Lifestyle Redesign approach to address chronic conditions.

Box 24-1 Lifestyle Components

- Attitude and mood
- Daily habits and routines
- Eating routines and nutrition
- Health status
- Meaningful activities
- Pacing and energy conservation
- Personal motivation and habit change
- Physical activity patterns
- Pleasure, play, and leisure
- Relaxation and sleep
- Roles and their impact on daily routines
- Social relationships, demands, support, and community
- Spirituality
- Stressors and stress management
- Time management

Additional client factors related to lifestyle:

- Abuse, trauma, violence, and discrimination
- Increased risk factors for chronic condition(s) and/or disability
- Occupational deprivation
- Occupational role overload
- Poverty
- Presence of chronic condition(s) and/or disability

Lifestyle Redesign Defined

Lifestyle Redesign is defined by Clark as "the process of developing and enacting a customized routine of health promoting and meaningful daily activities" (Mandel et al., 1999, Introduction page). The term **lifestyle** includes several occupational factors, such as activities of daily living (ADLs), instrumental activities of daily living (IADLs), habits, and routines, as well as other factors such as health status, environmental press, attitude, and mood. Lifestyle also refers to daily choices, great and small, and includes the tangible and intangible aspects of a person's occupational repertoire, such as nutritional choices, cultural preferences, physical activity patterns, and sources of pleasure and motivation. Lifestyle Redesign intervention uses the occupational therapy skill of activity analysis to address health-management occupations and often targets the performance patterns identified in the occupational therapy practice framework, including habits, routines, rituals, and roles (AOTA, 2014). The various components of lifestyle are listed in Box 24-1. Lifestyle is created by what individuals place their attention on throughout their daily and weekly occupations and routines. Lifestyle Redesign is the intentional process of analyzing occupations and lifestyle choices and then making changes based on articulated personal priorities, values, and health-related goals. Lifestyle Redesign places clients as the empowered directors over their own lives, health, and actions. It helps clients to become their own health advocate and to see how what they do affects their health and life satisfaction.

Often during the process of Lifestyle Redesign, a need to make considerable changes in lifestyle arises, such as a change in living environment, employment, relationship status, or a significant, meaningful occupation. Throughout this process of transformation, Lifestyle Redesign *always* targets the minutiae of life, such as monitoring daily water or caffeine consumption, reflecting on specific nutritional choices, taking the stairs to increase physical activity, taking deep breaths to relax while stuck in traffic, listening to a portable music device while engaged in an activity, or keeping a gratitude journal. Occupational therapy practitioners have an in-depth knowledge of the importance of detail and how it can completely change occupation or motivate one to stop an undesirable habit or begin to cherish a new one. It is these kinds of finely calibrated changes that can have powerful radiating effects on many aspects of lifestyle and lead to total lifestyle redesign.

The Lifestyle Redesign approach aims to facilitate gradual lifestyle changes over a prolonged period, which has a profound and extensive effect on occupation, health outcomes, and quality of life. The goal is to help clients determine lifestyle changes that *they want to make* and would like to maintain indefinitely since Lifestyle Redesign is an ongoing lifelong process. As clients undergo the process of Lifestyle Redesign, they acquire tools, including attitudes, beliefs, strategies, and actions, that will eventually allow them to continue this process for the rest of their lives.

Engage Your Brain 24-1

Think of a habit that you would like to start or stop. What are some accountability structures that you could set up to help you engage in or cease this habit?

The wellness construct is an important part of Lifestyle Redesign. The AOTA defines **wellness** as "more than a lack of disease symptoms. It is a state of mental and physical balance and fitness" (AOTA, 2014, p. S34). Clients can develop their own sense of what wellness means for them by taking into account individual factors, preferences, and situations. Occupational therapy practitioners can work with clients to analyze the activities, environments, and people that either energize and restore or drain and deplete. Then the client and therapist work to decrease any barriers to enacting a customized routine of health-promoting activities while utilizing supports. This analytic process becomes a practice or tool that the client can use perpetually.

Development of Lifestyle Redesign

In *Lifestyle Redesign: Implementing the Well Elderly Program,* Mandel and colleagues (1999) summarize four core ideas from the occupational therapy profession that shaped the development of Lifestyle Redesign:

- Occupation is life itself.
- Occupation can create new visions of possible lives.
- Occupation has a curative effect on physical and mental health and on a sense of life order and routine.
- Occupation has a place in preventive care (pp. 12–13).

Additionally, occupational science greatly influences Lifestyle Redesign (Carlson, Clark, and Young, 1998). Mandel et al. (1999) and Jackson, Carlson, Mandel, Zemke, and Clark (1998) describe four occupational science concepts that shape Lifestyle Redesign as:

- The "dynamic and generative quality of occupations," which have the power to create transformation
- The meaning evoked from occupation, including life narratives
- Dynamic systems theory
- The "view of the human as occupational being" (pp. 14–17)

Other theoretical and philosophical influences on Lifestyle Redesign are listed in Box 24-2.

With its many theoretical and philosophical influences, the Lifestyle Redesign approach was created to be the intervention for the USC Well Elderly Study, a randomized clinical trial conducted with community-dwelling seniors living in Los Angeles, California, from 1994 through 1997. The primary

Box 24-2 Lifestyle Redesign Theoretical and Philosophical Influences

- Grounded theory for qualitative research (Polkinghorne, 1988)
- Grounded theory for occupational narrative analysis (Clark, 1993; Clark, Ennevor, and Richardson, 1996)
- Narrative analysis and reasoning (Mattingly, 1991)
- Problematiques and technologies of the self (Foucault, 1984)
- Human condition—Heidegger (Calhoun and Solomon, 1984)
- Hermeneutics (Chessick, 1990)
- Positive psychology (Seligman, 2004)
- Self-determination theory (Deci, 2016)
- Stages of change (Prochaska and Norcross, 2001; Prochaska, Norcross, and DiClemente, 1995)
- Motivational interviewing—used more recently in treatment and in the Pressure Ulcer Prevention Study (PUPS) after the original development of Lifestyle Redesign (Miller and Rollnick, 2002)

Engage Your Brain 24-2

Review the theoretical and philosophical influences on the development of Lifestyle Redesign in Box 24-2. What other theoretical and philosophical influences could support this type of intervention? (Hint: see Chapter 3.)

objective of the study was to determine if occupational therapy was effective for preventing declines in function and well-being in a healthy aging population. Funded by the National Institutes of Health (NIH) and the American Occupational Therapy Foundation, the study had 361 men and women participants over the age of 60 (with a mean age of 74.4) who were African American, Asian, Caucasian, and Hispanic. The participants were randomly assigned to one of three groups: occupational therapy, social activities led by a nonprofessional, and no treatment. Treatment lasted 9 months, and groups of 8 to 10 participants met once per week for 2 hours and once per month individually with their occupational therapist.

The results demonstrated that the participants who received occupational therapy experienced greater gains or fewer declines in physical health, physical functioning, social functioning, vitality, mental health, and life satisfaction, with p values less than 0.05 (Clark et al., 1997). Not only were the results maintained after the 6-month follow-up period but additional findings also demonstrated that the Lifestyle Redesign intervention was cost-effective (Clark et al., 2001; Hay et al., 2002).

Several steps were taken to develop the Lifestyle Redesign intervention implemented in the study, including an extensive needs assessment, pilot study, qualitative studies, and literature review (Mandel et al., 1999). One of the qualitative studies examined the adaptive strategies that were being utilized by successful community-dwelling elderly persons *not living with disabilities.* Researchers interviewed 29 community-dwelling well older people and found that the following 11 life domains were most threatening to the participants: ADLs, adaptation to a multicultural environment, use of free time, grave illness and death, spirituality, health maintenance, mobility maintenance, personal finances, personal safety, psychological well-being and happiness, and relationships with others (Clark et al., 1996). This study was especially significant because it identified certain areas that occupational therapy had not traditionally addressed at the time with elders. These needs were specific to this particular group of elders and their environment, an urban, multicultural high-rise apartment building. This pilot study was important because it highlighted the need for occupational therapists to perform extensive needs assessments for the specific populations they work with to tailor interventions. Thorough needs assessments allow occupational therapists to identify significant factors affecting a unique population that may be different from those associated with the general population.

Another step was the development by Clark of **occupational self-analysis** in a course taught for several years at USC. The students were challenged to analyze their own occupational patterns and then make changes according to what they thought would make their lives more satisfying, productive, and meaningful. Specifically, they looked at how their childhood occupations shaped their current occupational choices, how their daily occupations and choices affected their health and well-being, and how their everyday routines were promoting or inhibiting the achievement of personal goals. Occupational therapy practitioners in the Well Elderly Study utilized this process throughout the sessions. Occupational self-analysis has become a central care process in the Lifestyle Redesign approach with all populations. Occupational therapy practitioners train their clients to examine their occupations, habits, and routines and how their daily choices are affecting their health and well-being. The clients then become more conscious of why and how they do the things they do and can bring more intention to their daily choices to create better health and quality of life.

Key Components of the Lifestyle Redesign Intervention Created for the USC Well Elderly Study

A summary of the work of Mandel et al. (1999) and Jackson et al. (1998) describing the Lifestyle Redesign intervention of the USC Well Elderly Study follows. As the process of Lifestyle Redesign unfolded, each client developed a personal action plan. The occupational therapist educated the client about how to harness the "power of ordinary occupations" in order to "optimize health and wellbeing" (Jackson et al., 1998, p. 329). For example, the occupational therapists educated the participants about how occupational engagement contributes to physical health, productivity, creativity, and satisfaction and, conversely, depression, loneliness, helplessness, and both physical and cognitive fatigue. The participants gained "occupational knowledge and reflective skills" and then could "imagine and enact healthy occupational lives as they age" (Jackson et al., 1998, p. 329).

Several components were crucial to the success of Lifestyle Redesign. The attitude of the therapist and the environment that she/he created for intervention was paramount. The therapist created an environment where the participant was the expert and where he or she felt safe and inspired to take risks and initiate change. For example, the occupational therapist would prepare a document of the participants' thoughts, feelings, and ideas from a previous session and then distribute them to the participants at the following session to create a notebook. Such physical representations validated their ideas and contributions (Mandel et al., 1999).

Service delivery incorporated four key methods, as outlined by Mandel et al. (1999): didactic presentation, peer exchange, direct experience, and personal exploration. **Didactic presentation** included new information about a topic relevant to the participant(s), as well as about occupation and how it affects each participant. Occupational therapists led the participants through a process of occupational self-analysis in regard to the topic (Mandel et al., 1999). The therapist facilitated **peer exchange,** where each participant had the opportunity to tell stories from his or her own life and how his or her experiences related to the topic at hand. Time was provided for group problem-solving, and group members were encouraged to offer solutions to each other. The Lifestyle Redesign intervention also provided **direct experience** through an activity or outing. Some examples from the Well Elderly Study include creating resource booklets with transportation information and inexpensive things to do in the community, performing the range-of-motion (ROM) dance, planning, shopping for and preparing a meal together, and creating and displaying personal history time lines. Direct experience, both inside and outside of sessions, provided participants with the opportunity to increase their self-efficacy and sense of control and to better self-regulate (Mandel et al., 1999).

Box 24-3 Outline of the Lifestyle Redesign® Intervention Process

1. Acquiring knowledge of the factors related to occupation that promote health and happiness
2. Performing a personal inventory and reflecting on one's fears and occupational choices, interests, life goals, and so forth (occupational self-analysis)
3. Overcoming one's fears by taking incremental risks in the real world of activity in small steps over time
4. Weaving together the outcomes of prior steps to develop a health-promoting daily routine

Data from "Practical Contributions of Occupational Science to the Art of Successful Aging: How to Sculpt a Meaningful Life in Older Adulthood," by M. Carlson, F. A. Clark, and B. Young, 1998, *Journal of Occupational Science, 5*, pp. 107–118; *Lifestyle Redesign®: Implementing the Well Elderly Program* (p. 29), by D. R. Mandel, J. M. Jackson, R. Zemke, L. Nelson, and F. A. Clark, 1999, Bethesda, MD: American Occupational Therapy Association.

Personal exploration and application happened throughout each of these processes and consisted of specific time for reflection on the content of each session. This reflection could take shape in a writing exercise, discussion, or another format. These activities allowed the participants to see how far they had come and increased their awareness of the graduated nature of the Lifestyle Redesign process (Mandel et al., 1999). The process of intervention is described in Box 24-3.

Four key ideas that participants learned that contributed to the success of the intervention were as follows:

1. Experience in occupation creates radiating, not linear change.
2. "Occupational self-analysis is possible," and through this process participants are encouraged to identify barriers to desired changes and the small next steps to get them there.

3. "When people understand the elements of occupation, they have the tool kit to redesign their lives." Selection of occupations becomes more intentional, and participants are guided through the process of recognizing and experiencing meaning in their selected occupations.
4. "Occupation is the impetus that propels people forward" (Mandel et al., 1999, pp. 30–31).

Both the therapist and the participant engage in **occupational storytelling and story making** to create the future lifestyle they will begin to enact. Through this approach, participants are able to see that their life, or story, is still moving forward and that they are experiencing transformation (Mandel et al., 1999, pp. 30–31).

Lifestyle Redesign interventions can be conducted in both group and individual formats, and often participants utilize both formats to maximize their experience. The benefits from group and individual formats share similarities and differences yet when done concurrently can enhance one another (Carlson, Fanchiang, Zemke, and Clark, 1996). Groups and individuals meet with their occupational therapist once per week for an extended period of time, usually 12 to 16 weeks or longer. In the group sessions, the same participants meet together for the duration and become sources of support for one another. This format intentionally allows for a feeling of both familiarity and novelty simultaneously. Meetings occur at the same location and time weekly; however, the occupational therapist presents a different topic each week, providing spontaneity and variation. Activities and outings also sprinkle the process with more variety, as does the continual social shifting as participants get to know one another better (Mandel et al., 1999).

Lifestyle Redesign Programs and Applications Since the USC Well Elderly Study

All of the Lifestyle Redesign programs created since the USC Well Elderly Study contain the same key components outlined previously. Differences include the content of the didactic material, which is based on each population's needs, and variations in format (e.g., individual, group, or a combination of both), frequency, duration, and location. The occupational therapy practitioners may see clients in an outpatient occupational therapy clinic, physician clinics, university offices and conference rooms, or clients' homes. A list of Lifestyle Redesign programs offered by the OTFP is provided in Box 24-4.

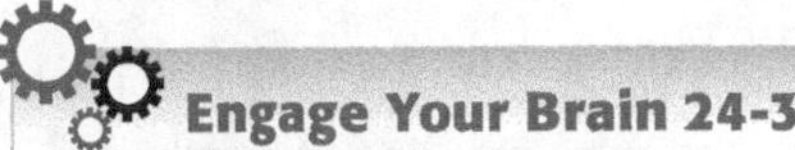

Engage Your Brain 24-3

Review the list of Lifestyle Redesign programs provided in Box 24-4. Identify two to three other populations that could benefit from this type of approach.

Lifestyle Redesign Weight Management Program

In 2015 and 2016, 39.8% of adults in the United States were categorized as obese (body mass index [BMI] greater than 30; Hales, Carroll, Fryar, and Ogden, 2017). Another 32.8% were categorized as overweight (BMI of 25 to 29.9; National Center for Health Statistics, 2017). The Lifestyle Redesign Weight Management Program was created to address the growing need to address overweight, obesity, and associated comorbid conditions. By far the largest program at the OTFP, its therapists have seen thousands of clients since its inception in 2000. Due to the chronic nature of overweight/obesity and common comorbidities, Lifestyle Redesign is an appropriate method and has yielded positive results. According to a 2006 analysis, after attending eight or more Lifestyle Redesign sessions, participants lost, on average, 4.2% of their original body weight and 7.5% of their original fat mass. The more sessions clients attended, the more weight they lost. Clients attend group or individual sessions for 16 consecutive weeks and often continue as needed. Because healthy weight loss (about 1 to 2 pounds per week) is critical (NIH, 1998), in a 16-week program clients lose a maximum of 32 pounds. As many clients have more weight to lose, they may choose to continue treatment and/or often continue to lose weight on their own following intervention.

Box 24-4 Lifestyle Redesign Programs Developed at the USC Occupational Therapy Faculty Practice

- *Weight Management, including bariatric surgery*—development and enactment of a customized routine of health-promoting and meaningful activities designed to result in weight loss and improved life satisfaction
- *Diabetes*—integration of health-promoting and meaningful activities into one's daily routine to prevent or manage diabetes, improve life satisfaction, and increase quality of life
- *Chronic Pain Management*—development and enactment of a customized routine of health-promoting and meaningful activities designed to decrease debilitating habits; reduce pain levels; increase ability to cope with pain; and utilize strategies including energy conservation, pacing, adaptive equipment, and time management
- *Chronic Headaches*—identification of triggers and other lifestyle factors associated with headaches and incorporation of strategies to prevent headaches throughout routines
- *College Student*—development and optimization of routines to improve overall well-being and academic performance through increasing time management, stress management, organization, lifestyle balance, motivation, and focus
- *Movement Disorders/Parkinson's Disease/Multiple Sclerosis*—integration of healthy routines and habits that focus on engagement in occupation, stress management, ergonomics, energy conservation, pacing techniques, healthy eating, relaxation, and fall safety
- *Mental Health*—integration of health-promoting and meaningful activities into one's daily routine to improve mental wellness, stress management, coping skills, lifestyle balance, time management, organization, and life satisfaction
- *Breast Cancer*—integration of healthy habits to support remission and life reintegration, increase functional and meaningful activity, and prevent chronic conditions through eating routines, physical activity, stress management, and more
- *Smoking Cessation and Relapse Prevention*—development of health-promoting daily habits and routines to replace smoking and manage triggers, including eating routines, physical activity, and stress management
- *Autism/Asperger's*—development of health-promoting daily habits and routines to support adolescents and adults to live independently and achieve education and/or career goals
- *Ergonomics*—assessment to address body mechanics, posture, safety, prevention of repetitive stress injuries, equipment recommendations, pacing, and energy conservation; follow-up to address stress management and pain
- *Green Lifestyle Redesign*—integration of environmentally sustainable activities into daily habits and routines to strengthen stewardship of the environment and improve physical and mental health and well-being.

The most common comorbid conditions associated with overweight/obesity include hypertension, hypercholesterolemia, heart disease, and type 2 diabetes. Other common diagnoses for weight management include prediabetes, glucose intolerance, metabolic syndrome, coronary heart disease (CHD), coronary artery disease (CAD), hypertriglyceridemia, fatty liver, morbid obesity, joint pain, sleep apnea, thyroid issues, depression, anxiety, and multiple sclerosis (MS), among others. A comorbid diagnosis is usually necessary for reimbursement by a third-party payer, since overweight/obesity is not currently considered a reimbursable diagnosis for occupational therapy in most cases. This requirement is especially challenging for pediatric clients who are overweight or obese but have not yet acquired a comorbid condition.

Weight management intervention is based on implementing gradual lifestyle changes that affect weight, comorbid conditions, overall physical and psychosocial health, self-efficacy, and life satisfaction. Emphasis is placed on goal setting and accountability during each session. First, clients learn to analyze their own habits and routines and relate their personal experience to the weekly topic. Topics include eating routines, meal/snack preparation, physical activity, time management, and addressing occupational role overload and deprivation. Throughout the intervention, clients consider how their routines and environments affect their weight management, sleep, relaxation, lifestyle balance, stress management, and emotional eating.

Through occupational self-analysis, clients can begin to enact change. They become savvy consumers regarding food labels, dining out, and fad diets. They address psychosocial and emotional issues related to healthy habit formation and find new healthy pleasures and meaningful activities to replace habits related to overeating. Weight Management Program occupational therapists ensure that clients have the experience and understanding to independently make the best choices for themselves to manage their weight effectively. Clients gain experience in reading food and menu labels and learn how to reach comfortable satiety while consuming fewer calories, balancing blood sugar, and choosing foods to decrease cholesterol and blood pressure. A registered dietitian provides consultation during the development of the program and approves an eating plan.

Next, the sessions focus on problem-solving with the occupational therapist and other participants (if applicable) on how to make the best choices within a client's current occupational repertoires and environments and how to overcome barriers to the changes the client has decided to make. The occupational therapist places emphasis on the relationship between stress, occupation, and eating and helps the client see and transform the reactionary eating patterns that contribute to weight gain. Clients establish **accountability structures** for their short-term, action-oriented goals each week.

The occupational therapist helps the client to create his or her own accountability structures in order to increase the likelihood of achieving short-term goals and to have accountability when occupational therapy intervention is complete. Examples of accountability structures include making an appointment to walk or exercise with a friend or family member; being responsible for walking the dog once or twice per day; or paying for a service, such as a class or massage, in advance. It is essential for clients to determine their own goals and accountability structures each week with the therapist and other group members (if applicable). Developing relationships with other group members and the occupational therapist, practicing the new habit, and performing the weekly check-in are each a crucial part of the habit change process (Clark, 2000).

Additionally, the weight management program places particular emphasis on the environments in which the clients are situated in their daily lives. The built environment includes the foods to which they are exposed and is a key contributor to weight gain or loss. The built environment also includes the sidewalks, transportation, local parks, neighborhood safety, and density of the surrounding area. Occupational therapists in Los Angeles frequently address the built environment because it has become so **obesogenic,** defined by the CDC as an environment that "offers access to high-calorie foods but limits opportunities for physical activity" (CDC, n.d., para. 1). Many clients find it impossible or inconvenient to walk or bike to their daily activities such as work, markets, restaurants, and other recreational areas. With longer commutes and more sedentary jobs, the physical activity embedded into daily routines can become very limited. The occupational therapist works with the client to increase physical activity in the home, work, and transportation environments when possible and advises how to navigate the deluge of calorie-dense food available at every turn (Clark, Saliman Reingold, and Salles-Jordan, 2007).

Bariatric Surgery

Many insurance companies now require lifestyle intervention/modification programs before authorizing bariatric surgery. Occupational therapy programs like the Lifestyle Redesign Weight Management Program can meet these requirements. Because bariatric surgery is only one of the tools clients may use to maintain a healthy weight, it is crucial for clients to learn and incorporate the skills and habits necessary to continue to lose and maintain their desired weight for life after surgery. The surgery is essentially a jump start and can enable clients to engage in physical activity more comfortably, as well as decrease or eliminate symptoms and comorbidities associated with type 2 diabetes and obesity. Lifestyle Redesign intervention for bariatric clients emphasizes preparation for engagement in increased meaningful activity that is not associated with food.

Because clients must drastically decrease their caloric intake and food options after surgery, many clients lose some of their cherished, meaningful occupations that revolve around mealtimes and pleasure from food. As a result, they must begin to identify other healthy pleasures, reward systems, and emotional outlets to replace eating. Similarly, eating routines change drastically. Prior to surgery, as part of the Lifestyle Redesign program, bariatric clients prepare to change their eating routines to eat more frequently, decrease portion sizes, and incorporate new nutritional needs such as supplements and protein. Clients who undergo bariatric surgery must also increase their physical activity in order to prevent muscle loss. The OTFP has partnered with the bariatric surgeons at USC to provide this service.

Lifestyle Redesign for Diabetes

The Lifestyle Redesign for Diabetes program naturally evolved from the weight management program to address the growing population with diabetes. In 2015, 9.4% of people in the United States, or 30,300,000, had diabetes (CDC, 2017b). This program utilizes similar didactic content but adds information about both preventing and managing diabetes and its associated comorbid conditions, sustaining healthy eating routines and blood sugar levels, and engaging in physical activity and stress management to help decrease blood sugar levels and symptoms of diabetes. The REAL Diabetes study demonstrated that a Lifestyle Redesign approach was effective in improving HbA1c levels and diabetes-related quality of life in ethnically diverse young adults who have diabetes (Pyatak et al., 2018).

Lifestyle Redesign for Chronic Pain

According to Nahin (2015), 11.2% of Americans suffer from chronic pain. Typically, physicians, often primary care providers, offer prescription pain medications as the only treatment (NIH, 2016). Both clients and providers are now seeking alternatives to opioid pain medications, whose use and overdose rates have reached epidemic proportions (CDC, 2016). Interdisciplinary pain programs have demonstrated better outcomes in reducing pain severity, improving mood, and restoring function than prescription medications alone (Gatchel and Okifuji, 2006; Morley, Eccleston, and Williams, 1999; Oslund et al., 2009). The OTFP partners with the USC Pain Center, whose staff consists of physicians who specialize in pain medicine, pain psychologists, physical therapists, and occupational therapists. Common diagnoses include fibromyalgia, complex regional pain syndrome, neuralgias, and other traumatic injuries. The Lifestyle Redesign for chronic pain program emphasizes quality of life, self-efficacy, and functional abilities (Uyeshiro Simon and Collins, 2017). Program topics include the following, as outlined by Uyeshiro Simon and Collins in their retrospective study: self-care and health management (eating, sleeping, physical activity routines, stress and mood management, medication management, energy and fatigue management, and time management), functional rehabilitation topics (ADLs, IADLs, home management, body mechanics, and posture), community integration (transportation, socialization, and paid or unpaid work), and general pain management topics (establishing a baseline, pain flare-up planning, assertive communication, and pain communication). This study, completed at the OTFP, demonstrated that clients significantly increased performance and satisfaction in the occupational areas of the Canadian Occupational Performance Measure (COPM), increased in the quality of life measure on the SF-36, and significantly increased their pain self-efficacy as measured by the Pain Self-Efficacy Questionnaire (PSEQ).

PROGRAM SHOWCASE

Program Name: Lifestyle Redesign® for Chronic Pain

City/State: Los Angeles, CA

Needs Assessment: Patients with chronic pain experience significant disruption to engagement in occupation, roles, and daily routines. These clients experience needs in multiple areas of life including self-care and health management, community participation and knowledge, and the execution of pain management techniques.

Goal: Address the lifestyle needs of people with chronic pain in order to increase participation, function, self-efficacy, and quality of life.

Population: Adults who have a chronic pain diagnosis and who are seeking care at the USC Pain Center. The most common diagnoses include lumbago, myalgia (including fibromyalgia), and complex regional pain syndrome. Typically, these clients have had their diagnosis for several years and have seen multiple doctors before finding the multidisciplinary pain center.

Participant's perspective (real quote): "Thank you for taking the time to get to know what my life is really like. You [the occupational therapist] are the one on the care team that really understands how it is for me."—Woman, age 62, with a diagnosis of fibromyalgia

Evaluation results: Data collected retrospectively from routine chronic pain treatment at the USC Occupational Therapy Faculty Practice indicate significant improvements in client functioning, self-efficacy, and quality of life (Uyeshiro Simon and Collins, 2017).

Funding: Occupational therapy treatment is covered by clients' Medicare and PPO insurance. Clients are referred by a pain physician specialist. Some clients have limitations on number of sessions, which, when shared with other disciplines (usually physical therapy), can be limiting.

Lifestyle Redesign for Chronic Headaches

The Lifestyle Redesign program for clients with headaches and migraines grew out of the pain management program. The prevalence of migraines in the United States is 19% of adult American women and 9% of men (Burch, Loder, Loder, and Smitherman, 2015). Inspired by the Lifestyle Redesign programs, a neurologist at USC requested occupational therapy for patients with headaches, where lifestyle factors play such an important part in pain and pain management. The chronic headache population lends itself well to a group format because of commonly shared traits and demographics. Depending on their needs, many clients with chronic headaches often choose individual or both group and individual sessions simultaneously. The program lasts for 8 weeks, though many clients continue for additional sessions. Topics covered are similar to the pain management program and also emphasize identifying and reducing headache/migraine triggers, which can significantly decrease headache incidence (Buse, Rupnow, and Lipton, 2009; Sahai-Srivastava, Sigman, Uyeshiro Simon, Cleary, and Ginoza, 2017; Sun-Edelstein and Maskop, 2009).

Lifestyle Redesign for the College Student

Out of 529 university and college counseling centers surveyed in 2016, 57% reported an increase in the severity of student mental health concerns (Association for University and College Counseling Center Directors Annual Survey, 2016). In 2015 college students reported that their greatest mental health concern was anxiety, and almost 9% had taken prescription medications prior to coming to college (American Psychiatric Association, 2015). College students experience frequent habit and routine changes every year and often every semester. Many students, away from home for the first time, have to learn how to engage in new occupations, create their own occupational routines, and structure their time independently. Lifestyle Redesign helps students acquire the skills to successfully meet academic, social, and other developmentally appropriate demands. The program helps students manage time, become more self-motivated, improve focus, problem-solve, better organize their activities, decrease procrastination, optimize study/work environments, reduce stress, engage in healthy dating and other social occupations, and promote lifestyle balance (see Fig. 24-1). Other topics include leisure, money management, community transportation, effective communication, eating routines/cooking, exercise, substance abuse, psychosocial issues, learning styles, and goal setting. Common diagnoses include

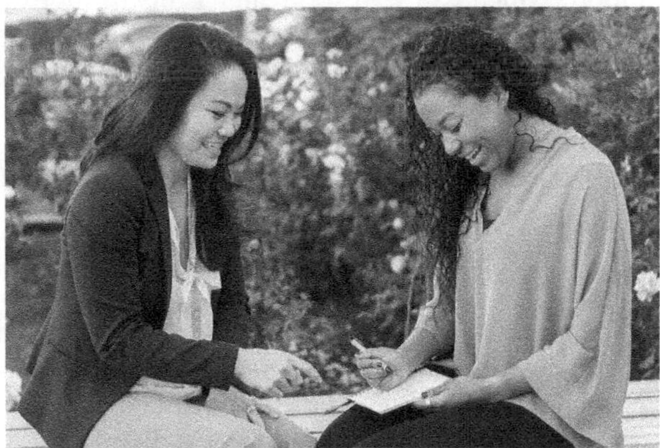

Figure 24-1 Lifestyle Redesign® for the college student. (*Photo courtesy of the University of Southern California, Janis Yue.*)

difficulty adjusting to college roles, learning disabilities, attention deficit disorder (ADD), attention deficit hyperactivity disorder (ADHD), mental health diagnoses, and acute reactions to stress, as well as diagnoses related to weight management and chronic pain.

The intervention is usually delivered individually because most students prefer this format. In addition, the OTFP offers six to eight open enrollment occupational therapy groups, in conjunction with counseling, per semester on topics such as lifestyle balance, time management, stress management, communication/conflict resolution, self-awareness, embracing diversity, and relationship success. In the community setting of a large university campus, intervention can conveniently occur in work, home, and leisure environments, including dorm rooms, eating places, grocery stores, and the student fitness center.

Lifestyle Redesign for Mental Health

Lifestyle Redesign for any population addresses the psychosocial realm of clients and their lifestyles, health status, and situations. This can be an appropriate intervention method for people who have moderate to mild symptoms from psychosocial disease. Intervention emphasizes using lifestyle factors and lifestyle changes as a way to improve self-regulation, coping skills, mood, attention, concentration, and motivation. For example, maintaining proper blood sugar and getting consistent physical activity can greatly improve concentration and mood, which can lead to greater gains in motivation and productivity. Addressing lifestyle factors also gives clients a sense of control over themselves and their daily lives. This population receives weekly individual sessions, usually over several months.

Lifestyle Redesign Interventions Outside of USC Settings

The name *Lifestyle Redesign* has been registered and trademarked by USC in order to maintain the precision and consistency of its successful clinical trial interventions. In addition to the Well Elderly Study, USC has created other Lifestyle Redesign research trials, such as the Pressure Ulcer Prevention Study (PUPS) and the REAL Diabetes study (Clark et al., 2014; Pyatak et al., 2018). Occupational therapy practitioners are encouraged to draw from the Lifestyle Redesign format and methods in their settings; however, they must use a different name.

The following are examples of interventions in other settings using a Lifestyle Redesign approach. At Rancho Los Amigos National Rehabilitation Center, there are eight programs informed by Lifestyle Redesign for groups and individuals, including stroke, chronic pain, diabetes, spinal cord injury, arthritis, epilepsy, cardiac rehab, and weight management. *Employee Wellness* is an 8-week program for employees at USC designed to encourage the acquisition of health-promoting habits in the workplace by Daley. *Lifestyle Matters* is an adapted version of the USC Well Elderly Study in Great Britain (Mountain, Craig, Mozley, and Ball, 2006). The California Institute for Technology now provides occupational therapy services for students in a program modeled after the USC college student program, and Dwelle Collective in Los Angeles provides a grant-funded program for women who were previously victims of sex trafficking and are transitioning to new careers. City of Hope Medical Center near Los Angeles also provides lifestyle programs delivered by occupational therapists for cancer survivors to prevent relapse.

Reimbursement for Lifestyle Redesign

Reimbursement for the Lifestyle Redesign programs offered at the OTFP primarily comes from the clients' preferred provider organization (PPO) health insurance. Common occupational therapy codes are used, such as evaluation, therapeutic group, functional therapeutic activity, ADLs, and therapeutic exercise. Even though the diagnoses treated using Lifestyle Redesign may be different than those of more traditional occupational therapy practice, many insurance companies pay for occupational therapy services for these diagnoses. For example, students who have the USC student health insurance are entitled to 26 visits per academic year for occupational therapy shared with physical therapy and chiropractic services and pay a small co-payment. Often students have not used any of these visits for other services, so they are able to come once per week for almost two full semesters per year.

Self-pay, grants, and special contracts have also been demonstrated to be viable methods of reimbursement. Grants may also be secured because there are many specific populations that need lifestyle interventions and are often prioritized by funding agencies.

Many potential referring providers do not know occupational therapy's efficacy in working with individuals and groups with chronic conditions. Significant education to referring providers is usually necessary in order to reach clients in need of Lifestyle Redesign occupational therapy intervention. This outreach may take many forms, including departmental in-services, one-on-one relationship building, and the creation of flyers or other written/electronic materials. The OTFP does ongoing outreach to both clients and referring providers in order to build programs that include a website, print brochures, ongoing relationship building with individual providers, in-services in various departments at the USC Keck Medical Center, a presence at health fairs and other community events, and participation in USC committees, symposiums, and other leadership opportunities to increase visibility.

Summary

- As the health and occupational needs of society shift, occupational therapy intervention must shift as well. With the sheer numbers of people living with chronic conditions and diseases and predicted to acquire chronic conditions in the coming years, the profession must more fully utilize its unique and effective Lifestyle Redesign approach to increase the role of occupational therapy practice in prevention and health promotion.
- Lifestyle includes performance patterns such as habits, routines, roles, and rituals; client factors such as values, beliefs, and spirituality; and the occupations one chooses to engage in. Lifestyle includes both controllable and uncontrollable life circumstances, health realities and goals, and the ways in which a person chooses to address these aspects of life and find meaning.
- Lifestyle Redesign draws from the roots of occupational therapy but also looks to the future by widening the scope of practice to include a much broader client base.
- Lifestyle Redesign was originally designed as an intervention for community-dwelling older adults to prevent and better manage chronic conditions and has since been applied to many diverse populations and problems.
- Lifestyle Redesign can benefit anyone who wants to live a healthier and happier life and prevent or better manage chronic conditions.
- Lifestyle Redesign interventions are occupational therapy treatment and can be paid for in the same way occupational therapy is paid for, including reimbursement by private and public health insurance. Limitations can include the presence of a diagnosis, the type of diagnosis, and the specific constraints of an individual's insurance policy.
- Other methods of reimbursement, such as grants, self-pay, and contracts designed to incentivize self-care/health behaviors, are also viable.
- Administrators, referring providers, and the general public are commonly not aware of Lifestyle Redesign or occupational therapy's ability to treat lifestyle-related diseases. Significant education and marketing may be necessary for program development and sustainability.

CASE STUDIES

CASE STUDY 24-1 Linda

Linda is a 58-year-old female with a diagnosis of obesity and diabetes. After being referred by her physician, Linda started the Lifestyle Redesign program for diabetes. Biomeasures on her first session were as follows: weight: 227.4 pounds, BMI: 37.8, fat mass: 102.8 pounds, and blood pressure: 142/72 (with medication). Her concerns included diabetes and escalating blood sugar, continued weight gain from the increased amounts of insulin required to manage her blood sugar, fatigue, and increased stress at work. Linda is a registered nurse and the manager of a large nursing unit in a hospital. Her work demands high energy, constant communication with others, and attention to detail. She attended a Lifestyle Redesign for Diabetes group for 24 sessions. During these sessions, Linda realized that she focused most of her attention throughout her long workday and at home on other people. She is a caregiver in some capacity for most of her time. Additionally, while completing a "balance wheel" activity in which she colored a circular picture of a wheel divided into 24 hours according to how she spends her typical day, Linda realized that she spends very little time engaging in leisure activities. In another session, she learned that her caffeine consumption of six to eight diet sodas per day was excessive and could be contributing to her weight gain.

Linda was guided in prioritizing her own health and well-being, planning ahead for healthy eating, engaging in consistent physical activity, improving self-esteem, managing stress and relaxation techniques, cultivating happiness in daily routines, and substituting new healthy pleasures for caloric rewards. After 24 weeks, Linda lowered and maintained her blood sugar to a level where she was able to stop using insulin completely. She also stopped her weight gain. She lost 2 pounds overall and 5 pounds of fat mass. She developed and maintained consistent exercise for 3 days per week. She started a routine at the YMCA, where she worked with a trainer who guided her through both cardiovascular and resistance exercises that were appropriate for her and made her feel good. Linda was able to reduce her caffeine consumption by 75%, and she reported that she felt happier at work and less stressed most of the time. When reflecting on her accomplishments, she wrote, "I feel great! I have so much more energy now."

Discussion Questions

1. Identify the lifestyle factors that contribute to Linda's concerns.
2. Identify the additional lifestyle factors that Linda discovered were contributing to her presenting concerns through occupational self-analysis.
3. Identify and discuss the lifestyle changes that Linda made and how they had radiating effects in other aspects of her lifestyle and health outcomes.
4. What do you think motivated Linda to stay consistent with her lifestyle changes over 24 weeks?

CASE STUDY 24-2 Lifestyle Redesign® for the College Student

The Lifestyle Redesign for the College Student program at USC serves several hundred undergraduate and graduate students per year on the university's two largest campuses. Developed and implemented by occupational therapy faculty and doctoral residents, the program helps students to establish health-promoting habits and to meet their personal, academic, and health goals. The service typically occurs in individual sessions about once per week throughout a semester. Some students find relief from one to two sessions, and others continue to utilize services for one, two, or more semesters.

CASE STUDY 24-2 Lifestyle Redesign® for the College Student

The most common topics include stress and anxiety management, time management and organization, focus and concentration, sleep hygiene, and overall lifestyle balance, including physical activity and healthy eating. Many students focus on managing a chronic mental or physical health condition, dealing with social or dating anxiety, or adjusting to the many transitions required in college life.

Students are referred by physicians and counselors from the student health center and also learn about occupational therapy services from word of mouth, faculty, residential advisors, and the student health center website. Most occupational therapy services happen in a clinic environment on campus, though sessions can occur in other settings on or near campus in order to engage in a particular activity related to the client's goals.

Common outcomes include improved academic performance; increased engagement in health-promoting activities such as sleep, healthy eating, and physical and social activities; and increased self-esteem. Since its inception over 15 years ago, faculty and occupational therapy doctorate graduates who provided services in this program have gone on to replicate this model on college campuses in other cities, states, and countries.

Discussion Questions

1. Does your university or college offer any program related to those offered by USC? If so, are occupational therapy faculty or practitioners involved in the program delivery?
2. Thinking back to the past when you were a student, or if you are a student now—How could you benefit from this type of occupational therapy service on your campus?
3. Describe a therapeutic activity you could do with a student who is struggling with time management.

Learning Activities

1. Find articles from popular media (e.g., newspapers, magazines, websites, etc.) about a situation, issue, or population that could benefit from Lifestyle Redesign both in the United States and in another country.
2. Create a list of 8 to 10 interview questions to use as part of a needs assessment for a particular community-based population that you think may have a need for a lifestyle intervention. Craft the questions in order to obtain specific, detailed information about this population's threats to health, well-being, and engagement in occupation as well as their current occupational patterns and lifestyle factors.
3. Plan a group activity for a specific population in a community-based setting that engages the participants in the process of occupational self-analysis. Determine the population and setting and take into consideration the clients' occupational and lifestyle factors.

REFERENCES

American Occupational Therapy Association. (2014). *Occupational therapy practice framework: Domain and process.* Retrieved from http://ajot.aota.org/ on 06/22/2016 Terms of Use: http://AOTA.org/terms

American Occupational Therapy Association. (2018). Vision 2025. *OT Practice, 23*(1), 18–19.

American Psychiatric Association. (2015). *College students: Coping with stress and anxiety on campus.* Washington, DC: American Psychiatric Association.

Association for University and College Counseling Center Directors. (2016). *The Association for University and College Counseling Center Directors Annual Survey, September 2016–June 1026.* Retrieved from www.aucccd.org/

Burch, R. C., Loder, S., Loder, E., and Smitherman, T. A. (2015). The prevalence and burden of migraine and severe headache in the United States: Updated statistics from government health surveillance studies. *Headache, 55*(2), 356. doi:10.1111/head.12482

Buse, D. C., Rupnow, M. F. T., and Lipton, R. B. (2009). Assessing and managing all aspects of migraine: Migraine attacks, migraine-related functional impairment, common comorbidities, and quality of life. *Mayo Clinic Proceedings, 84*(5), 422–435.

Calhoun, C., and Solomon, R. C. (1984). Martin Heidegger. In C. Calhoun and R. C. Solomon (Eds.), *What is an emotion? Classic readings in philosophical psychology* (pp. 229–243). New York, NY: Oxford University Press.

Carlson, M., Clark, F., and Young, B. (1998). Practical contributions of occupational science to the art of successful aging: How to sculpt a meaningful life in older adulthood. *Journal of Occupational Science, 5,* 107–118.

Carlson, M., Fanchiang, S., Zemke, R., and Clark, F. (1996). A meta-analysis of the effectiveness of occupational therapy for older persons. *American Journal of Occupational Therapy, 50*(2), 89–98.

Centers for Disease Control and Prevention. (n.d.). *Genomics and health: Genes and obesity.* Retrieved from http://cdc.gov/genomics/resources/diseases/obesity/obesedit.htm

Centers for Disease Control and Prevention. (2009). *The power of prevention: Chronic disease . . . the public health challenge of the 21st century.* Retrieved from www.cdc.gov/chronicdisease/pdf/2009-Power-of-Prevention.pdf

Centers for Disease Control and Prevention. (2015). *CDC: 53 million adults in the US live with a disability.* Retrieved from www.cdc.gov/media/releases/2015/p0730-US-disability.html

Centers for Disease Control and Prevention. (2016, January). Increases in drug and opioid overdose deaths—United States, 2000–2014. *Morbidity and Mortality Weekly Report, 64*(50), 1378–1382.

Centers for Disease Control and Prevention. (2017a). *Chronic disease overview.* Retrieved from www.cdc.gov/chronicdisease/overview/index.htm

Centers for Disease Control and Prevention. (2017b). *New CDC report: More than 100 million Americans have diabetes or prediabetes.* Retrieved from www.cdc.gov/media/releases/2017/p0718-diabetes-report.html

Chessick, R. D. (1990). Hermeneutics for psychotherapists. *American Journal of Psychotherapy, 44*(2), 256–273.

Clark, F. A. (1993). Occupation embedded in a real life: Interweaving occupational science and occupational therapy. *American Journal of Occupational Therapy, 47*(12), 1067–1078.

Clark, F. A. (2000). The concepts of habits and routine: A preliminary theoretical synthesis. *Occupational Therapy Journal of Research, 20*(Suppl. 1), 123S–137S.

Clark, F. A., Azen, S. P., Carlson, M., Mandel, D., LaBree, L., Hay, J., . . . Lipson, L. (2001). Embedding health-promoting changes into the daily lives of independent-living older adults: Long-term follow-up of occupational therapy intervention. *Journal of Gerontology: Psychological Sciences, 56,* 60–63.

Clark, F. A., Azen, S. P., Zemke, R., Jackson, J., Carlson, M., Mandel, D., . . . Lipson, L. (1997). Occupational therapy for independent-living older adults: A randomized control trial. *JAMA 278*(16), 1321–1326.

Clark, F. A., Carlson, M., Zemke, R., Frank, G., Patterson, K., Ennevor, L., . . . Lipson, L. (1996). Life domains and adaptive strategies of the low income well elderly. *American Journal of Occupational Therapy, 50,* 99–108.

Clark, F. A., Ennevor, L. E., and Richardson, P. (1996). A grounded theory of techniques or occupational storytelling and occupational story making. In R. Zemke and F. A. Clark (Eds.), *Occupational science: The evolving discipline* (pp. 373–392). Philadelphia, PA: F. A. Davis.

Clark, F. A., Pyatak, E. A., Carlson, M., Blanche, E. I., Vigen, C., Hay, J., Mallinson, T., . . . Azen, S. P. (2014). Implementing trials of complex interventions in community settings: The USC-Rancho Los Amigos Pressure Ulcer Prevention Study (PUPS). *Clinical Trials, 11*(2), 218–229.

Clark, F. A., Saliman Reingold, F., and Salles-Jordan, K. (2007). American Occupational Therapy Association obesity position paper. *American Journal of Occupational Therapy, 61*(6), 701–703. doi:10.5014/ajot.61.6.701

Deci, E. (2016). *A self-determination view of behavior change for health and work.* 25th USC Occupational Science Symposium, September 23, 2016, Los Angeles, CA.

Foucault, M. (1984). On the genealogy of ethics: An overview of work in progress. In P. Rabinow (Ed.), *The Foucault reader* (pp. 340–372). New York, NY: Pantheon Books.

Fulghum, R. (2004). *All I really need to know I learned in kindergarten* (15th anniversary ed.). New York, NY: Ballantine Books.

Gatchel, R. J., and Okifuji, A. (2006). Evidence-based scientific data documenting the treatment and cost-effectiveness of comprehensive pain programs for chronic nonmalignant pain. *Journal of Pain, 7*(11), 779–793.

Hales, C., Carroll, M., Fryar, C., and Ogden, C. (2017). Prevalence of obesity among adults and youth: United States, 2015–2016. *NCHS Data Brief.* No. 288. Hyattsville, MD: U.S. Department of Health and Human Services.

Hay, J., LaBree, L., Luo, R., Clark, F. A., Carlson, M., Mandel, D., . . . Azen, S. P. (2002). Cost-effectiveness of preventative occupational therapy for independent-living older adults. *JAGS, 50,* 1381–1388.

Jackson, J., Carlson, M., Mandel, D., Zemke, R., and Clark, F. A. (1998). Occupation in lifestyle redesign: The well elderly study occupational therapy program. *American Journal of Occupational Therapy, 52*(5), 326–336.

Kung H., Hoyert D., Xu, J., and Murphy, S. (2008). Deaths: Final data for 2005. *National Vital Statistics Reports: From the Centers for Disease Control and Prevention, National Center for Health Statistics, National Vital Statistics System, 56,* 1–120.

Mandel, D. R., Jackson, J. M., Zemke, R., Nelson, L., and Clark, F. A. (1999). *Lifestyle Redesign®: Implementing the Well Elderly program.* Bethesda, MD: American Occupational Therapy Association.

Mattingly, C. (1991). *Healing dramas and clinical plots: The narrative structure of experience.* Cambridge, UK: Cambridge University Press.

Miller, W. R., and Rollnick, S. (2002). *Motivational interviewing: Preparing people to change.* New York, NY: Guilford Press.

Morley, S., Eccleston, C., and Williams, A. (1999). Systematic review and meta-analysis of randomized controlled trials of cognitive behaviour therapy and behaviour therapy for chronic pain in adults, excluding headache. *Pain, 80,* 1–13.

Mountain, G., Craig, C., Mozley, C., and Ball, L. (2006). *Lifestyle matters: An occupational approach towards health and wellbeing in later life.* Sheffield, England: Sheffield Hallam University.

Nahin, R. L. (2015). Estimates of pain prevalence and severity in adults: United States, 2012. *Journal of Pain, 16*(8), 769–780.

National Center for Health Statistics. (2017). *Health, United States, 2016: With chartbook on long-term trends in health.* Hyattsville, MD: National Center for Health Statistics.

National Council on Aging. (2017). *Top 10 chronic conditions in adults 65+ and what you can do to prevent or manage them.* Retrieved from www.ncoa.org/blog/10-common-chronic-diseases-prevention-tips/

National Institutes of Health. (1998). *Clinical guidelines on the identification, evaluation and treatment of overweight and obesity in adults: The evidence report.* Publication No. 98-4083. Bethesda, MD: National Institutes of Health.

National Institutes of Health. (2016). *National pain strategy: A comprehensive population health-level strategy for pain.*

Retrieved from https://iprcc.nih.gov/sites/default/files/HHSNational_Pain_Strategy_508C.pdf

Oslund, S., Robinson, R. C., Clark, T. C., Garofalo, J. P., Behnk, P., Walker, B., . . . Noe, C. E. (2009). Long-term effectiveness of a comprehensive pain management program: Strengthening the case for interdisciplinary care. *Baylor University Medical Center Proceedings, 22,* 211–214.

Polkinghorne, D. (1988). *Narrative knowing and the human sciences.* Albany, NY: State University of New York Press.

Prochaska, J. O., and Norcross, J. C. (2001). Stages of change. *Psychotherapy, 38*(4), 443–448.

Prochaska, J. O., Norcross, J. C., and DiClemente, C. C. (1995). *Changing for good: A revolutionary six-stage program for overcoming bad habits and moving your life positively forward.* New York, NY: Avon Books.

Pyatak, E., Carandang, K., Vigen, C., Blanchard, J., Diaz, J., Concha-Chavez, A., . . . Peters, A. (2018, April). Occupational therapy intervention improves glycemic control and quality of life among young adults with diabetes: The Resilient, Empowered, Active Living With Diabetes (REAL Diabetes) Randomized Controlled Trial. *Diabetes Care, 41*(4), 696–704.

Sahai-Srivastava, S., Sigman, E., Uyeshiro Simon, A., Cleary, L., and Ginoza, L. (2017). Multidisciplinary team treatment approaches to chronic daily headaches. *Headache, 57*(9), 1482–1491.

Seligman, M. E. P. (2004). Can happiness be taught? *Daedalus, 133*(2), 80–87.

Sun-Edelstein, C., and Maskop, A. (2009). Foods and supplements in the management of migraine headaches. *Clinical Journal of Pain, 25,* 446–452. Retrieved from http://clinicalpain.com.

U.S. Department of Health and Human Services. (2018). *Healthy people 2030 framework.* Retrieved from www.healthypeople.gov/2020/About-Healthy-People/Development-Healthy-People-2030/Proposed-Framework

Uyeshiro Simon, A., and Collins, C. E. R. (2017). Lifestyle Redesign® for chronic pain management: A retrospective clinical efficacy study. *American Journal of Occupational Therapy, 71,* 1–7.

World Health Organization. (2019a). *Disability and health. WHO fact sheet.* Retrieved from www.who.int/news-room/fact-sheets/detail/disability-and-health

World Health Organization. (2019b). *Noncommunicable diseases and their risk factors.* Retrieved from www.who.int/en/news-room/fact-sheets/detail/noncommunicable-diseases

Chapter 25

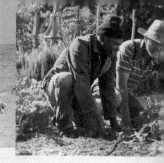

Occupational Therapy in Primary Health-Care Settings

Marjorie E. Scaffa, PhD, OTR/L, FAOTA, and S. Blaise Chromiak, MD

Primary health care is essential health care based on practical, scientifically sound and socially acceptable methods and technology made universally accessible to individuals and families in the community through their full participation and at a cost that the community and country can afford to maintain at every stage of their development in the spirit of self-reliance and self-determination.

—World Health Organization (1978, section VI)

Learning Outcomes

This chapter is designed to enable the reader to:

25-1 Describe primary health care, including the types of providers, settings, and populations served.
25-2 Discuss the most commonly addressed prevention and health-promotion issues in primary health-care practice.
25-3 Discuss potential roles for occupational therapy in primary care settings.
25-4 Explain the impact of health literacy on individual health and strategies for addressing the problem of health illiteracy.
25-5 Describe evidence-based practices that can be integrated into primary care.

Key Terms

Brief office interventions
Chronic disease self-management
Health literacy
Health risk appraisals
Integrated care
Medical home
Primary care physician
Primary health care
Teachable moments

Introduction

Advances in preventive medicine have significantly reduced or delayed the morbidity and mortality associated with several chronic conditions, including cardiovascular disease, hypertension, stroke, diabetes, and some types of cancer (Ganiats and King, 2003). Improved medications and technological breakthroughs have contributed to these health benefits. However, the stress of today's complex lifestyles is resulting in new epidemics of chronic illness that seriously endanger the health of individuals and families. Deleterious societal influences and unhealthy living conditions are accelerating the prevalence of risk factors for illness.

The incidence of obesity, poor nutrition, sedentary lifestyles, and diabetes is increasing and has negative implications for the cardiovascular system and other body structures. As a result, life expectancy at birth has declined for 3 years in a row, with increases in death rates at younger ages (Centers for Disease Control and Prevention [CDC], 2018b). In addition, other contributors to the decrease in life expectancy are the increasing numbers of deaths related to mental health conditions, such as opioid overdose and suicide (CDC, 2018a; CDC, 2018c). These physical and mental illnesses may present acutely, but their risk of morbidity may become chronic and persist throughout the life span.

Although the challenges of modern life may be a barrier to achieving sustained positive changes in health and quality of life, primary care physicians are ideally situated to address many types of medical problems and disabilities, both physical and/or mental and emotional. The focus of this chapter is on the most common lifestyle-related health problems seen in the primary health-care setting and the potential roles for occupational therapists as service extenders for individuals and families throughout the life span (see Box 25-1).

Primary Health-Care Services and Providers

Primary health care is the "provision of integrated, accessible health care services by clinicians who are accountable for addressing a large majority of personal health care needs, developing a sustained partnership with patients, and practicing in the context of family and community" (Institute of Medicine [IOM], 1994, p. 1). According to the American Academy of Family Physicians (AAFP, 2011),

> *primary care includes health promotion, disease prevention, health maintenance, counseling, patient education, diagnosis and treatment of acute and chronic illnesses in a variety of health care settings (e.g., office, inpatient, critical care, long-term care, home care, day care, etc.). Primary care is performed and managed by a personal physician often collaborating with other health professionals and utilizing consultation or referral as appropriate. (para. 3–4)*

This broader conceptualization provides opportunities for the infusion of occupational therapy services in primary health care. However, to be effective in this setting, "an occupational therapist must be a true generalist who is competent across all age spans and the entire domain of occupational therapy practice" (Muir, 2012, p. 509).

Primary health care is continuous, comprehensive care designed to maximize health and prevent disease that is provided near where people live, work, and play (Edelman and Mandle, 2002). The term **primary care physician** "is used to describe all physicians whose practice includes the provision of medical care for well individuals and who act as 'gatekeepers' to specialist services" (Goel and McIsaac, 2000, p. 230). The physicians who today provide the bulk of primary health care are family and general practitioners, medical internists, and pediatricians. In addition, there are obstetrician-gynecologists for women's primary health care and psychiatrists for primary mental health services. Physician extenders, such as nurse practitioners and physician assistants, are also involved in the delivery of primary care services.

A recent survey indicated that most physicians spend between 13 and 16 minutes with each patient during a primary care visit, and this feels inadequate to both participants (Peckham, 2016). There are many types of primary care settings. Usually, the physical setting is an office or hospital, but primary care physicians and physician extenders may provide services in the home and in assisted living, rehabilitation, long-term, and hospice care facilities. Patient populations span all age groups: infants, children, adolescents, pregnant women, adults, and older adults.

The long-term relationships that primary care physicians develop and share with those in their care make the primary physician the entry point in accessing the health-care system. Ideally, the primary physician's office is the patient's medical home. The primary care **medical home**

> *is accountable for meeting the large majority of each patient's physical and mental health care needs, including prevention and wellness, acute care, and chronic care. Providing comprehensive care requires*

Box 25-1 Selected Occupational Therapy Contributions to Health Promotion in Primary Care Settings Throughout the Life Span

Children

- Childhood developmental assessments, including infant reflexes
- Evaluation of and intervention for learning disabilities
- Identification of sensory integration deficits
- Assessment and intervention for infant and child feeding problems
- Safety and injury prevention education for parents, including the appropriate use of car safety seats, playground safety, stranger safety, etc.
- Childproofing strategies for the home and family childcare sites
- Provide parents with toilet-training strategies
- Facilitate parent-child attachment, bonding, and communication
- Parental education regarding developmental toys and facilitating age-appropriate play
- Identification of child neglect and abuse
- Guide families in their search for and evaluation of appropriate childcare services
- Assist families in identifying governmental and community resources
- Childhood mental health screenings
- Preschool readiness screening
- Educate parents regarding strategies for preventing childhood obesity
- Provide handwriting assessment and intervention for school-aged children
- Assist parents with problem behavior management

Adolescents

- Mental health screenings
- Sexuality education
- Prevention and intervention for tobacco, alcohol, and other drug use
- Identification of and intervention for eating disorders
- Encouraging the development of healthy habits
- Facilitating adaptive coping and use of healthy stress-management strategies
- Educating parents about signs of suicide and suicide prevention strategies
- Educating teens about injury prevention, including high-risk behaviors, sports injuries, etc.
- Development of conflict resolution skills and anger management
- Coping with peer pressure
- Promoting health literacy

Adults

- Work injury prevention, assessment, and treatment
- Chronic pain management
- Parenting training and support
- Ergonomics, body mechanics
- Facilitating adaptive coping and managing psychosocial stress
- Smoking cessation
- Prevention of and intervention for back pain
- Weight loss and healthy meal planning
- Mental health screening
- Promoting health literacy
- Identification of and intervention for alcohol and other drug abuse
- Identification of family violence
- Grief and bereavement support
- Identification of resources for elder care, evaluating assisted living and long-term care options
- Managing caregiver stress and preventing burnout
- Incorporating physical activity into the daily routine
- Reducing or managing disability associated with chronic conditions
- Promoting chronic disease self-management

Older Adults

- Medication management
- Energy conservation
- Joint protection
- Fall prevention
- Driving evaluations and identifying alternative transportation
- Low vision adaptations
- Retirement preparation and adjustment
- Adaptive equipment
- Dementia management
- Work simplification strategies
- Identification of elder neglect and abuse
- Mental health screening
- Identification of and intervention for alcohol and other drug abuse
- Grief and bereavement support
- Reducing or managing disability associated with chronic conditions
- Weight management
- Incorporating physical activity into the daily routine
- Managing health-care visits and insurance issues
- Home assessment and modification to increase safety and functional independence
- Incontinence management
- Assisting elders in identifying governmental and community resources
- Facilitating adaptive coping and managing psychosocial stress
- Facilitating aging in place
- Promoting health literacy
- Chronic disease self-management

a team of care providers. This team might include physicians, advanced practice nurses, physician assistants, nurses, pharmacists, nutritionists, social workers, counselors, educators, and care coordinators. Although some medical home practices may bring together large and diverse teams of care providers to meet the needs of their patients, many others, including smaller practices, will build virtual teams linking themselves and their patients to providers and services in their communities. (Agency for Healthcare Research and Quality [AHRQ], n.d., para. 2)

The CDC (2009) estimates that approximately 25% of persons with chronic diseases experience significant activity limitations that may make it difficult to effectively manage their conditions. The role of occupational therapy practitioners in primary care settings is not yet well defined. However, according to the American Occupational Therapy Association (AOTA, 2014), "occupational therapy practitioners are well prepared to contribute to interprofessional care teams addressing the primary care needs of individuals across the life span, particularly those with, or at risk for, one or more chronic conditions" (p. S25). In addition to providing services for persons with chronic diseases, occupational therapy can enhance health promotion efforts in primary care settings. Occupational therapists are in the unique position of being able to evaluate the impact of a patient's medical condition on their ability to complete daily activities and how participation in daily occupations influences the person's health (Dahl-Popolizio, Rogers, Muir, Carroll, and Manson, 2017).

Health Promotion in Primary Care Settings

Health promotion is an important component of helping patients reach their health goals. The purpose of health promotion is "to enable people to gain greater control over the determinants of their own health" (WHO, 1986, p. iii). According to the U.S. Preventive Services Task Force (USPSTF, 2007), modifying personal health behaviors is the most promising approach for health promotion within current medical practice. Health promotion and disease prevention activities in primary care settings are guided by *Healthy People 2030*, the national health agenda in the United States (U.S. Department of Health and Human Services [USDHHS], 2011). Many objectives in *Healthy People 2030* refer to primary care.

Primary care physicians' offices are ideal settings for disease prevention and health promotion. Physicians are generally viewed as authoritative and credible sources of information and advice on health and illness. A significant number of studies have demonstrated that physician advice is a strong determinant of adherence to preventive practices, such as mammograms. In addition, brief office interventions have demonstrated effectiveness for smoking cessation, reduced alcohol consumption, and other health-related behaviors. **Teachable moments,** when direct links can be made between symptoms, behavior, and outcome, occur routinely during office visits. For example, an office visit for angina is a teachable moment to address smoking cessation, nutrition, and weight loss with a patient. However, due to time constraints, physicians may not be able to utilize these opportunities effectively.

The role of occupational therapy in health promotion has been conceptualized as having three critical functions: promoting healthy lifestyles for all clients, emphasizing occupational participation as an essential component of health promotion efforts, and providing interventions for populations, particularly those experiencing health disparities (AOTA, 2013). Occupational therapists providing services in primary care settings need to recognize that health promotion and prevention interventions do not immediately resolve health problems and that individuals will progress in their own incremental and idiosyncratic ways. Appropriate health promotion theoretical approaches for use in primary care settings include the PRECEDE-PROCEED model (Green and Kreuter, 2004) and the transtheoretical (or stages of change) model (TTM) by Prochaska,

Engage Your Brain 25-1

Which occupational therapy theories would be appropriate for a primary care setting and why?

DiClemente, and Norcross (1992) described in Chapter 3.

Assessing the person's health-promotion needs includes identifying a readiness to change and the predisposing, reinforcing, and enabling factors that have an impact on the targeted health behavior. The TTM can be utilized to identify the individual's readiness to change. The health-promotion strategies used should correspond with the stage of readiness, whether precontemplation, contemplation, preparation, action, or maintenance. Acquiring the skills, habits, and lifestyle behaviors that promote health provides individuals with a sense of self-efficacy regarding their health that may lead to better and longer-lasting results and can be generalized to other health issues.

Applying the stages of change to prevention and health promotion involves:

- Bringing the risky behavior(s) to the person's attention
- Helping the person to determine the need to change these risky behaviors
- Facilitating the decision to change and selecting strategies for change
- Maintaining and reinforcing the new healthy behaviors
- Reinstituting the healthy behaviors when lapsing into old habit patterns and behaviors (Moyers and Stoffel, 2001, p. 329)

The health-promotion process in primary care consists of assessing the person's health-promotion needs; providing appropriate, culturally sensitive health education; setting realistic health goals collaboratively; facilitating the person's acquisition and development of the skills needed to implement health behaviors; assisting individuals and their families to integrate health-behavior change into their daily lives; facilitating access to and use of community resources; and evaluating outcomes through follow-up visits or contacts (Goel and McIsaac, 2000). This approach is consistent with occupational therapy's emphasis on client-centered care (AOTA, 2014). Occupational therapists can offer a wide variety of prevention, health-promotion, evaluation, and intervention services in primary care settings.

Some of the most common health concerns for lifestyle intervention in today's primary care medical practice include diabetes, weight management, chronic pain, and mental health problems, including substance abuse (Practice Fusion, 2011). These health problems and the role of occupational therapy in the primary care setting are discussed in the next section.

Diabetes

Diabetes affects approximately 9% of the population and is the seventh leading cause of death in the United States. Type 2 diabetes, or hyperglycemia, is a chronic metabolic disorder that results from a combination of resistance to the action of insulin on the body's cells and insufficient insulin production by the pancreas. Insulin is a hormone needed by cells in the body to absorb and convert glucose into energy. Signs and symptoms of diabetes include increased hunger and thirst, frequent urination, fatigue, irritability, dizziness, unexplained weight loss, frequent infections, slow wound healing, and visual and cognitive disturbances. The risk of developing diabetes increases with age, obesity, family history, high blood pressure, and inactivity. Persons of African American, Hispanic, Asian, and Native American descent are at higher risk for developing diabetes (National Institute of Diabetes and Digestive and Kidney Diseases [NIDDK], 2017).

The A1C, or glycated hemoglobin test, measures average blood glucose levels over a period of 2 to 3 months. It is considered the standard biomarker for adequate glycemic management and can be used to diagnose diabetes. An A1C level of 6.5% or higher is indicative of diabetes, between 5.7% and 6.4% is considered prediabetes, and below 5.7% is considered normal. Complications of diabetes due to poor blood sugar control develop gradually and may include neuropathy, cardiovascular conditions, retinopathy, kidney disease, and lower-extremity amputations due to nerve damage or poor blood flow. Treatment may include a combination of the following: blood glucose monitoring, oral medications, insulin injections, healthy eating, and physical activity (American Diabetes Association, 2010; Mayo Clinic, 2014).

Depression and/or anxiety are frequently comorbid with diabetes. Persons with diabetes have a 60% higher rate of major depressive disorder and a 123% higher rate of generalized anxiety disorder than the general population (Fisher et al., 2008).

The relationship between diabetes and depression is bidirectional. Individuals with depression are at higher risk for developing diabetes, and individuals with diabetes are at higher risk for developing depression, particularly if they are experiencing secondary complications. In addition, persons with diabetes and comorbid depression often have greater symptom severity and disease burden. This is likely due to the fact that depression often hinders a person's ability to initiate and maintain chronic disease self-management behaviors (Lin et al., 2010). This highlights the need for mental health services in addition to medical care for the management of diabetes.

Role of Occupational Therapy

Typically, occupational therapy practitioners do not treat diabetes as a primary diagnosis. More frequently, occupational therapy services are provided to persons who have experienced secondary complications from diabetes, such as amputation, low vision, stroke, myocardial infarction, and peripheral neuropathy. The AOTA (2011) affirms that occupational therapy practitioners "can effectively educate and train persons at risk for or who currently have diabetes to modify current habits and routines and develop new ones to promote a healthier lifestyle and minimize disease progression" (p. 1). There is some evidence of occupational therapists providing interventions focused on the self-management of diabetes, including blood glucose monitoring, nutrition, physical activity, and medication management (Pyatak, 2011).

Lifestyle changes are extremely difficult to make and maintain. Only when they are embedded into one's daily routine do they have a chance of success. Identifying the individual habits and routines needed to support diabetes self-management is critical (Thompson, 2014). Pyatak (2011) recommends that occupational therapy interventions focus attention on "both personal and contextual factors and provide opportunities for long-term support" (p. 94). Effective interventions are tailored to specific client needs and include educational and skill-building components. In a study by Hwand, Truax, Claire, and Caytap (2009), community-dwelling older adults with diabetes identified several areas in which they would like assistance, including managing blood sugar, foot care, fatigue management, pain management, and cholesterol control. Occupational therapy practitioners have the unique capacity to integrate the physical, psychosocial, and occupational aspects of diabetes management and to attend to both the primary diagnosis of diabetes and secondary complications.

Weight Management

Obesity has been a well-recognized concern since before the *Surgeon General's Call to Action on Obesity* (U.S. Public Health Service [USPHS], 2001) stated that reducing obesity was a national priority. Research has demonstrated that the risk of all causes of mortality increases significantly as weight and body mass index (BMI) increase. Specifically, for each five-unit increase in BMI over 25 kg/m^2 (considered healthy weight), the risk of death from cardiovascular disease increases by 49%, respiratory disorders increase by 38%, and cancer increases 19% (Global BMI Mortality Collaboration, 2016).

The National Heart, Lung, and Blood Institute (NHLBI) guidelines for the prevention of cardiovascular disease recommend a target BMI between 18.5 and 24.9 regardless of age (NHLBI, 2018). Of the approximately 70% of adults who are overweight (BMI greater than or equal to 25), 36% are obese (BMI greater than or equal to 30), 15% are very obese (BMI greater than or equal to 35), and 6% are extremely obese (BMI greater than or equal to 40; Flegal, Carroll, Kit, and Ogden, 2012). Several studies have indicated that abdominal obesity, regardless of overall weight, is a significant predictor of metabolic disturbances and disease risk. Even persons with a BMI in the normal range can be at higher risk if they have a large waist circumference. Therefore, waist circumference measurements are recommended as part of a routine physical examination (Dobbelsteyn, Joffres, MacLean, and Flowerdew, 2001). A waist circumference of more than 36 to 40 inches in men and more than 32 to 35 inches in women is highly correlated with obesity-related conditions such as hypertension, sleep apnea, diabetes, and heart disease (Dobbelsteyn et al., 2001; Mosley, Jedlicka, LeQuieu, and Taylor, 2008).

The medical approach to weight management combines healthy nutrition, appropriate physical activity, behavior modification, psychotherapy, hypnosis, and stress-reduction techniques. Medications that improve metabolic parameters, increase the sensation of fullness, and decrease cravings have been helpful for modest weight reduction prior to evaluation for bariatric surgery or procedures. Diet support groups, such as Weight Watchers, self-help, and 12-step groups (Overeaters Anonymous), may also be useful. Stimulant-based weight-loss medications may have severe risks or unpleasant side effects; thus, there is no safe, effective weight-loss drug for the general population.

Role of Occupational Therapy

Mosley et al. (2008) provide a succinct overview of the role of occupational therapy in prevention and intervention for obesity in children and adults. They address the importance of occupation in weight reduction and the prevention of obesity. In addition, they describe adaptations and modifications that can be made to facilitate bariatric clients' abilities to perform and participate in daily life activities. Occupational therapists can assess an individual's overall pattern of daily activity and make recommendations for occupational participation in instrumental activities of daily living (IADLs), work, and leisure that increase the level of physical activity in which the person engages. Increasing the frequency and duration of physical activity will enable a person to maintain or lose weight more easily.

Moderate intensity physical activity, such as a brisk walk for 150 minutes per week, is the level recommended by the American Heart Association (AHA) for raising the heart rate from 40% at baseline to 60% of its maximal capacity. Regular exercise, sports, yard work, and job activities may confer the benefits as well (AHA, 2018).

Occupational therapists can provide guidance to patients regarding incorporating physical activity into their daily routines. Integrating a variety of occupations into one's routine can provide needed physical activity—for example, washing and waxing a car, housework, gardening, pushing a stroller, raking leaves, and climbing stairs. Occupational therapists can introduce and encourage active leisure pursuits such as bicycling, volleyball, dancing, and swimming. Providing interventions that are developmentally and culturally appropriate while addressing safety issues are important considerations (Reitz, 2010).

Chronic Pain

According to the Interagency Pain Research Coordinating Committee (IPRCC, 2016) of the National Institutes of Health, chronic pain is a complex biopsychosocial condition that has reached an epidemic proportion in the United States. The overuse of opioid pain relievers has resulted in high levels of addiction and death. The CDC (2016) recommends the use of nonpharmacological interventions tailored to a person's specific type of pain. For example, interventions may include the use of low-impact aerobic activity for fibromyalgia, interdisciplinary rehabilitation and cognitive behavioral therapy for low back pain (LBP), biofeedback for migraine headaches, and weight loss for osteoarthritis.

LBP is the most common musculoskeletal complaint seen in primary care medical practice and is a major source of activity limitation and disability. LBP is experienced by one in five adults each year and affects 60% to 80% of adults at some time in their lives. It is often persistent or recurrent and is a significant cost to individuals, businesses, and society. It is the fifth most common reason to seek health care. LBP can be due to a single event resulting in acute injury or to a cumulative process of stress and strain (Gaunt, Herring, and O'Connor, 2008; Rosenwax, Semmens, and Holman, 2001).

The longer a person is out of work due to chronic pain, the more disabling the condition becomes and the less likely the person is to recover and return to work. A work absence of 1 to 3 months puts the worker at a 10% to 40% risk of remaining unemployed 1 year after injury. Returning to work after a 1- to 2-year absence is highly unlikely, even with further treatment (Waddell and Burton, 2001). Therefore, the primary goal of intervention is to return the worker to the job as soon as possible. Strong epidemiological evidence indicates that most workers with LBP can continue working or return to work within a few days or weeks of injury. There is no need for a person with LBP to wait for the complete resolution of pain prior to returning to work, as this does not increase the risk of reinjury and actually reduces recurrences and missed workdays during the next year. Due to the recurrent and persistent nature of LBP, a complete cure is an unrealistic expectation regardless of work status. Job reassessment, modified work, and employer support increase the likelihood of successful job reentry (Waddell and Burton, 2001).

Role of Occupational Therapy

Self-management programs for chronic pain can improve quality of life and reduce the need for pain medications (IPRCC, 2016). A study of client perceptions of chronic pain indicated that occupational therapy services should focus on improving quality of life by assisting clients to participate in occupations, particularly sleep and IADLs, that they were unable to perform without medication (Jehl et al., 2017). Simon and Collins (2017) evaluated the efficacy of a Lifestyle Redesign® program for chronic pain management that was integrated into the patients' medical plan of care. In this program, 45 clients with a variety of pain syndromes participated in individualized sessions on a variety of topics, such as sleep, physical activity, stress and mood management, medication management, energy conservation, body mechanics and posture, pain management, assertive communication, and community integration, depending on the needs identified during the initial occupational therapy evaluation. The mean number of sessions was nine, and the mode was eight. Outcome measures included the Canadian Occupational Performance Measure (COPM), the 36-item Short-Form Survey, the Brief Pain Inventory, and the Pain Self-Efficacy Questionnaire. Improvements were noted in occupational performance and satisfaction, energy and fatigue, general health, pain self-efficacy, and physical and social functioning.

According to Karjalainen et al. (2003, p. 4), "prolonged low back pain can lead to a combination of physical, psychological, occupational and social impairment." Therefore, a biopsychosocial approach, including psychological, behavioral, and educational interventions, is likely to produce the best results. Rosenwax et al. (2001) provide examples of how occupational therapists can adapt and apply clinical guidelines for LBP from evidence-based reviews to occupational therapy practice. For example, strong evidence exists that bed rest is counterproductive in the management of LBP. Occupational therapists can assess clients' functional limitations and lifestyles and modify activities to achieve a tolerable comfort level (not necessarily pain-free) that enables a person to maintain participation in a variety of occupations.

For persons with subacute LBP, the grading of activities as the client progresses can enable a return to work more quickly with less disability. In addition, there is moderate evidence to support workplace intervention involving the worker, medical team, and employer to facilitate a prompt return to work. Occupational therapists can make recommendations for workstation design and the modification of work tasks, provide instruction on appropriate body mechanics in job performance, and address psychosocial risk factors in the work environment (Rosenwax et al., 2001). For more information on the ergonomics and prevention of work-related injury, see Chapter 15.

Mental Health

Approximately 25% of patients seen by primary care providers present with physical and mental health comorbidities. According to the National Institute of Mental Health (NIMH, 2017), at least 50% of mental health care for common psychiatric disorders is provided in primary care settings. Mental health problems in primary health-care settings frequently manifest with physical symptoms such as chronic pain, insomnia, gastrointestinal disturbance, headaches, and difficulty breathing, among others. In addition, addressing the emotional and psychological issues related to chronic medical conditions has been shown to improve overall health and is cost-effective (Dahl-Popolizio, Doyle, and Wade, 2018).

The most common mental health problems encountered in primary care are depression, anxiety, substance abuse, eating disorders, and posttraumatic stress disorder (PTSD; Summergrad and Kathol, 2014). Excessive alcohol use is a concern because it is associated with a high rate of injuries and deaths, as well as liver disease, ischemic heart disease, cardiomyopathy, and hemorrhagic stroke (Jaen, 2003). The primary care office is an important setting for screening and brief interventions aimed at reducing alcohol and drug use (Jaen, 2003). When screening reveals at-risk drinking, the four-item CAGE questionnaire is very reliable in diagnosing problem drinking (National Institute on

Box 25-2 CAGE Substance Abuse Screening Tool

Ask your clients these four questions to determine if substance abuse exists and needs to be addressed:

1. Have you ever felt you ought to **cut down (C)** on your drinking or drug use?
2. Have people **annoyed (A)** you by criticizing your drinking or drug use?
3. Have you felt bad or **guilty (G)** about your drinking or drug use?
4. Have you ever had a drink or used drugs first thing when you wake up to steady your nerves or to get rid of a hangover (**eye opener**) (E)?

A total of two positive answers is considered clinically significant.

Reprinted with permission from Brown, R. L. and Rounds, L. A. (1995). Conjoint screening questionnaires for alcohol and drug abuse. *Wisconsin Medical Journal, 94*, 135–140.

Alcohol Abuse and Alcoholism, 2003). The CAGE-AID questionnaire is a modified version that includes drug use (see Box 25-2; Brown and Rounds, 1995).

Mental health problems, particularly major depressive disorder, impose a significant burden on society in terms of lost work productivity, increased use of health services, and increased morbidity and mortality from chronic illnesses and are a leading cause of disability. In addition, mental disorders have adverse effects on adherence to medical regimens and health habits, including poor diet, increased alcohol consumption and smoking, and sedentary lifestyle (NIMH, 2010). In order to meet the mental health needs of primary care patients, the collaborative care movement is developing and implementing models of integrated care. **Integrated care** "blends the expertise of mental health, substance use, and primary care clinicians, with feedback from patients and their caregivers. This creates a team-based approach where mental health care and general medical care are offered in the same setting" (NIMH, 2017, para. 3). Mental health professionals can address the psychosocial challenges that affect patient self-management and health behaviors, as well as address the needs of persons with psychiatric conditions. Integrated care has been shown to increase access to mental health services, improve patient outcomes, reduce hospital readmission rates, and lower health-care costs (Buche et al., 2017; Ward, Miller, Marconi, Kaslow, and Farber, 2015).

Role of Occupational Therapy

Although the United Kingdom has a different health-care system than the United States, occupational therapists in the United Kingdom have led the way in providing mental health services in primary care venues. Several models have been used, including:

- Providing services in primary care offices
- Direct referrals from physicians to a service provided at a community site
- Collaboration between a mental health service and primary care physicians (Creek, Beynon, Cook, and Tulloch, 2002)

In the first model, two occupational therapists working in an inpatient psychiatric unit of a hospital decided to pilot mental health services in a local general practice. They discussed the role of occupational therapy in mental health with the physicians and provided them with a written description of the services that could be provided, along with referral criteria. The potential benefits to the physician included "reduced time seeing patients with social and emotional problems, reduced prescriptions for anxiolytics and antidepressants, and status in offering an extra service to patients" (Creek et al., 2002, p. 457). The physicians agreed and the occupational therapists began providing evaluations and individual and group interventions. The patients (age 21 to 76) presented with a variety of problems, including anxiety, stress, obsessions, tranquilizer dependence, depression, postnatal depression, bereavement, marital disharmony, loneliness, child abuse, and lack of self-confidence. Some of the positive aspects of the service included:

- People needed fewer visits than in a hospital-based program because they were identified at an earlier stage
- People were more likely to accept the services provided in the primary care setting because the stigma of going to a mental health setting was eliminated (Creek et al., 2002).

The second model involved occupational therapists working for a home health-like agency that marketed their mental health services to physicians. They provided individual and group interventions in homes, physician offices, and other community settings. Several group interventions were run on a regular basis, including groups addressing anger management, anxiety management, and assertiveness skills. The types of client problems seen were similar to the first model, with the addition of some psychosocial issues, including women going through menopause, chronic fatigue syndrome, myocardial infarction (for stress management and lifestyle changes), PTSD, and employment/unemployment issues. The group used a biopsychosocial approach, with access to psychiatrists and primary care physicians readily available. Referring physicians noted that patients were requesting referral to the occupational therapy services because a friend, family member, or neighbor recommended it (Creek et al., 2002).

The third model utilized the services of a multidisciplinary Community Mental Health Team (CMHT) that provided services to eight primary care practices. The CMHT was composed of an occupational therapist, psychiatric nurse, and social worker. A pilot project was set up at one of the practice sites. The goals of the project were to increase access to mental health services, offer services within the familiar surroundings of a primary care office, provide timely and effective brief interventions, and develop stronger relationships with primary care providers. During the 6 months of the pilot program, referrals increased dramatically and necessitated the development of a waiting list. Patients expressed a need for evening hours due to work and school schedules and stated that attending mental health services provided in the primary care setting was convenient and less stressful than traveling to another location (Creek et al., 2002).

These models individually, or the development of a hybrid model, could be useful to occupational therapy practitioners in the United States as a starting point for establishing mental health services in primary care settings. The benefits of this type of program are impressive, including identifying clients with psychosocial problems early before the problems become severe and chronic, reducing the need for psychotropic medication prescriptions, and increasing quality of life.

Integration of Evidence-Based Health-Promotion Practices Into Routine Primary Care

Specific populations and the health-promotion services from which they could benefit were just described. In this next section, the following three evidence-based health-promotion approaches that can be used by occupational therapists are introduced: brief office interventions, health literacy interventions, and chronic disease self-management.

Brief Office Interventions

Brief office interventions are short, targeted interactions between patients and health-care professionals for the purpose of changing health behaviors. They are practical and cost-effective and can be implemented by a variety of health-care professionals, including occupational therapists (Moyers and Stoffel, 2001). The Counseling and Behavioral Interventions Work Group of the U.S. Preventative Services Task Force (USPSTF) evaluated the features of six models of behavior change and recommended an adaptation for brief office interventions in primary care settings. The model, briefly described in Table 25-1, is based on the five *A*s: assess, advise, agree, assist, and arrange (Jaen, 2003).

Medication adherence is a significant concern in primary care practice that can be addressed by occupational therapists through brief office interventions. Barriers to medication compliance, which are magnified with advancing age and increased medical, cognitive, and psychiatric problems, include multiple drugs, multiple doses per day, problematic side effects or interactions, and a lack of family/social support. Even a change from one medication to another, or from one dosing schedule to another of the same medication, may be confusing to some patients and provide a challenge to adherence. Effective motivational strategies to improve medication adherence include using daily reminder charts and daily pill holders, packaging medications in combination, training in self-determination, enlisting social/family support, and offering phone calls from nurses and phone-linked computer counseling (Domino, 2005).

Table 25-1 Brief Office Intervention Model: The Five *A*s

Step	Description
1. Assess	• Target a risky behavior identified by patient complaint and/or medical and social history
2. Advise	• Emphasize the importance of discontinuing the risky behavior, the improvements that can be gained in health status, and the willingness of the health-care provider to assist the patient in making the needed changes • Clear, simple, and personalized advice provided in a warm, empathic, nonjudgmental way
3. Agree	• Collaboratively design and agree upon a course of action to change the target risk behavior • Assess the patient's readiness to change and design interventions accordingly
4. Assist	• Provide specific behavioral interventions • Encourage and facilitate follow-up counseling and health education sessions • Assess the effectiveness of physician-provided medications in assisting behavior change
5. Arrange	• Reinforce positive changes • Revise intervention plans if necessary • Provide ongoing follow-up and support by telephone, electronic communication, or office visits

Data from "Integrating Health Behavior Counseling Into Routine Primary Care," by C. R. Jaen, 2003, *AAFP CME Bulletin, 2*(7), pp. 1–5, Leawood, KS: American Academy of Family Physicians.

Engage Your Brain 25-2

Based on the AOTA (2015) *Occupational Therapy Code of Ethics,* what are some ethical considerations in using brief office interventions in primary care settings?

Health Literacy Interventions

Health literacy refers to "the degree to which individuals have the capacity to obtain, process, and understand basic health information and services needed to make appropriate health decisions" (USDHHS, 2000, pp. 11–20). Osborne (2005) believes that health literacy goes beyond the individual and that it is the mutual responsibility of the health-care provider to communicate information in ways that can be understood and applied. The national emphasis on health literacy is based, in part, on research that demonstrates relationships among health literacy, health disparities, and health outcomes. According to the National Center for Education Statistics, "adults with low literacy levels are more likely than those with high literacy levels to be poor and to have health conditions which limit their activities" (National Network of Libraries of Medicine, 2006, p. 3). Low health literacy is also linked to higher hospitalization rates, more frequent use of emergency room services, less compliance with health recommendations, and more frequent errors with medication management. Studies on health literacy and health outcomes have elucidated the connections between low health literacy and cancer incidence, mortality and quality of life (Merriman, Ades, and Seffrin, 2002), glycemic control and rates of retinopathy in persons with type 2 diabetes (Schillinger et al., 2002), and other health conditions (Williams, Baker, Honig, Lee, and Nowlan, 1998; Williams, Baker, Parker, and Nurss, 1998).

Primary health-care settings provide an excellent opportunity for occupational therapists to promote health literacy, thereby enhancing health outcomes. Health literacy services may include:

- Informal assessment of health literacy
- Creation and provision of culturally relevant health communications
- Creation and provision of "plain-language" health communications for persons with limited health literacy
- Health information sessions on a variety of topics
- Office staff training in effective communication with patients

- Health counseling
- In-person and online self-help and support groups
- Patient education on how to prepare for and participate in health-care interactions with providers
- Assistance for patients with medication management
- Patient education on how to assess the relevance, quality, and credibility of health information, particularly on the Internet

Chronic Disease Self-Management

In the older adult population, approximately 80% have at least one of the following chronic diseases or conditions: arthritis, cancer, diabetes mellitus, heart disease, hypertension, respiratory disease, and cerebrovascular accident (CVA; National Council on Aging, 2016). In addition, chronic diseases are often accompanied by depression and other mental health problems. As a result of rising health-care costs, patient self-management of chronic disease is being increasingly emphasized. Varying definitions exist in the literature, but essentially, **chronic disease self-management** involves individuals and families actively participating in the health-care process, self-monitoring symptoms or physiological processes, making informed decisions about their health, and managing the impact of the disease on their daily lives. Chronic disease self-management programs are designed to enable individuals to prevent, control, and manage complications of their conditions, including the mental health sequelae (Chodosh et al., 2005).

Several reviews have been published regarding the nature and efficacy of chronic disease self-management programs, with mixed results. Program elements vary, but generally they feature:

- Tailoring the program and messages to specific individual needs and circumstances
- Grouping interventions in order to facilitate peer support
- Giving frequent feedback to the patient regarding progress in meeting self-management goals (including the use of technology applications for self-monitoring at home)
- Addressing psychosocial concerns
- Involving the health-care provider in program delivery (Chodosh et al., 2005)

It is important to note that the Lifestyle Redesign program includes all of these elements and incorporates occupational therapy principles and practices.

The School of Medicine at Stanford University (2006) has developed a model chronic disease self-management program (CDSMP). The program is provided in a workshop format for a total of 15 hours over several sessions and is facilitated by two trained leaders—one a health-care professional and the other a person with a chronic disease. The content of the program was derived from information provided by focus groups of people with chronic disease. The topics covered include:

- Techniques to deal with problems such as frustration, fatigue, pain, and isolation
- Appropriate exercise for maintaining and improving strength, flexibility, and endurance
- Appropriate use of medications
- Effectively communicating with family, friends, and health professionals
- Nutrition and meal planning
- Evaluating new treatments and making informed treatment decisions (Stanford University, 2006, para. 2)

More than 1,000 people participated in a randomized, controlled evaluation of the program. Participants were followed for up to 3 years. Those who participated in the program, as compared to those who did not, demonstrated significant improvements in a number of areas, as described in Box 25-3. Many of the improvements noted persisted for as long as 3 years. The study showed that for every dollar spent on the self-management program, 10 dollars were saved in health-care costs (Stanford University, 2006). Replications of the study yielded similar results (Lorig, 2015).

Occupational therapists have knowledge of chronic diseases and their effects on daily life functioning, which enables them to develop chronic disease self-management programs in primary care settings; train persons with chronic diseases to instruct and lead groups; and evaluate the outcomes. The research available supports the efficacy of generic

Box 25-3 Stanford University's Chronic Disease Self-Management Program

Participants in Stanford University's Chronic Disease Self-Management Program (2006) demonstrated improvements in the following:

Health status:

- Disability
- Social/role limitations
- Energy/fatigue
- Health distress
- Self-reported general health

Health-care utilization:

- Fewer hospitalizations
- Fewer days in the hospital
- Fewer outpatient visits

Self-management behaviors:

- Exercise
- Cognitive symptom management
- Communication with physician

Data from *Chronic Disease Self-Management Program,* 2006, Stanford University. Retrieved from http://www.selfmanagementresource.com/programs/small-group/chronic-disease-self-management/

chronic disease self-management programs and their cost-effectiveness. This is a service that occupational therapists could market to primary care providers.

Development of Evidence-Based Health-Promotion Programs for Primary Care

The nature of primary care is such that practitioners follow a panel of patients intermittently over an extended period, providing health-promotion, prevention, and treatment services at times of need. This is much different than typical occupational therapy services, which are often provided continuously and intensely over a short period. However, patients may need fewer visits for intervention because they are seen at an earlier stage of the health problem. Therefore, occupational therapists working in primary care settings must be flexible, adaptive, and readily available when the physician refers a person or family with a particular need.

Engage Your Brain 25-3

What additional competencies should an occupational therapy practitioner have in order to develop, implement, and evaluate health-promotion programs in a primary care setting?

Allowing the patient to leave the office and attempting to schedule a follow-up appointment for occupational therapy is likely to be unsuccessful. Patients fail to schedule, or miss follow-up appointments, for a variety of reasons, including time constraints, financial limitations, lack of transportation, confusion, and memory impairment.

A comprehensive health-promotion program in a primary care setting would include:

- Health risk appraisals, including mental health screenings
- Health education and counseling
- Caregiver education and training
- Phone call follow-up
- Home visits
- Brief office interventions

Health risk appraisals (HRAs) are assessments that profile an individual's risk factors and estimate the probabilities of certain diseases manifesting. HRAs ask the participant a number of questions related to health behaviors and thereby raise awareness about the impact of lifestyle on health. In addition, some HRAs provide suggestions for improving one's health status. These assessments are a useful tool for initiating dialogue about lifestyle concerns and may motivate the individual to action. Educating patients regarding their health status is the next logical step. Information tailored to the individual's needs can enable and empower the individual to assume more responsibility for his or her health.

Caregivers are also in need of health education and counseling regarding the needs of the care recipient and their own health needs as caregivers. Providing support, information about community resources, and training to prevent caregiver injury and stress can reduce caregiver burden and improve caregiver well-being. Follow-up phone calls to patients and caregivers can reinforce plans made

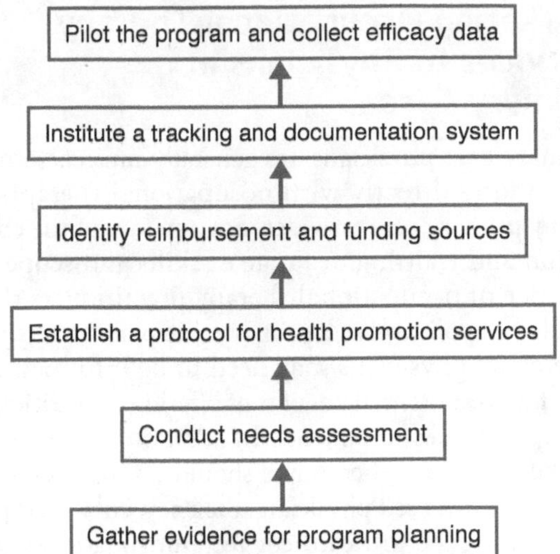

Figure 25-1 Developing a health-promotion program for the primary care setting.

during a health-promotion visit, encourage compliance with medical recommendations, and identify barriers to health behavior change. Home visits to assess safety, support systems, psychosocial issues, and home modification can also be helpful. Home visits are particularly beneficial for those who have a difficult time getting to health-care facilities and who might otherwise need to move to a long-term care facility (Devereaux and Walker, 1995). Brief office interventions, as described earlier, should be used routinely to address tobacco use, alcohol abuse, mental health, physical fitness, obesity, risky sexual behavior, and other health behaviors.

Developing a health-promotion program for a primary care setting is much like developing other community-based health initiatives, with a few additional considerations. The basic steps are outlined in Figure 25-1.

The first step is to be well informed and gather evidence for program planning. As is true in all areas of practice, preventive interventions should be based on the best research evidence available. Evidence on appropriate assessment strategies, early detection procedures, and effectiveness of known interventions is essential.

The second step is to conduct a needs assessment of the primary care physician's patient panel. This can be done in a variety of ways using surveys, focus groups, epidemiological data, and chart reviews (Scaffa and Reitz, 2014). The choice of targets for health-promotion interventions should be based on current morbidity and mortality profiles of the community in which the primary care practice is situated (Zapka, 2000). Health-promotion approaches are complex and must be flexible, adaptable, and tailored to the individual or group to be effective.

The third step is to establish a protocol that outlines how patients will be evaluated, potential interventions that may be used, and community resources that are available as support services. The protocol should include clear referral criteria and describe the services the occupational therapist can provide. Administering the COPM provides an excellent opportunity for the occupational therapist to gain an understanding of the patient's needs, desires, and priorities as a basis for individualized health-promotion planning (Law et al., 2005). Health behavior contracts that specify the number of sessions, goals, and strategies may enhance motivation and commitment to long-term change.

The fourth step is to identify reimbursement and funding sources for the program. In addition to private health insurance, Medicare, Medicaid, and other reimbursement mechanisms for billable services, sources of revenue may include grants, fee-for-service, and foundation funding. Next is establishing a tracking and documentation system. Tracking may involve creating flow sheets, checklists, and other strategies for monitoring the provision of screenings and other health-promotion services. Funding sources often dictate documentation style and content.

Finally, the health-promotion program is ready to be piloted and evaluated. Quarterly process assessments of services provided, patient satisfaction, and outcome measures are needed to document the efficacy and cost-effectiveness of the program. Data are collected and used to modify and enhance program components. An electronic health record that can track patients by age group, diagnosis, or other characteristics may be helpful for program evaluation purposes. Although program evaluation is the last step in this sequence, it must be systematically planned throughout the earlier stages of program development.

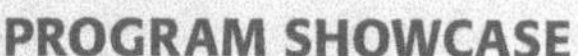

PROGRAM SHOWCASE

Submitted by Joy D. Doll, OTD, OTR/L

Infusing Occupational Therapy (OT) Into Primary Care

Meeting the needs of population health requires occupational therapy practitioners to think in a new way about care delivery. In this case, we will explore the impact of infusing OT into primary care at an ambulatory care clinic.

In 2013, a group of clinicians sat in a room with the task of designing a new ambulatory care clinic that would house an outpatient rehabilitation clinic with occupational and physical therapy (PT) services. In addition, the clinicians were challenged to consider how OT and PT services could be offered within a primary care model of delivery within a family medicine residency ambulatory care clinic. This is the story of how OT became part of a robust primary care rehabilitation approach to improving population health.

Many factors had to be considered, including clinical workflow, billing, documentation, and the availability of occupational therapists (OTs) to exit the outpatient clinic to go to the primary care floor. The team started with initial brainstorming of what would make an ideal clinical delivery model. This was followed by a literature review to explore best practices and identify leaders in OT primary care delivery. Phone interviews and e-mail surveys were sent to OTs with expertise in delivering primary care asking about lessons learned from their experiences.

The team also looked at current billing and documentation practices. Many of these would need to be altered to afford successful implementation. It was decided that the OT would participate in twice-daily clinic huddles, previsit planning, and once-a-week collaborative care planning for high patient utilizers. In addition, the OT would be available for 15 minutes on every hour to leave the outpatient clinic and provide care for patients in primary care.

Critical factors to success were related to roles and responsibilities. The providers and health-care team needed to understand the role of OT in order to refer appropriately. OT was highlighted in huddles, and patient stories of the impact OT had made on the patient's life were shared. Soon, referrals to outpatient OT surged. Another critical factor was ensuring legality and compliance for the OT to bill outside of the outpatient clinic. The OT was given the proper credentials and was able to bill for evaluations in the primary care and outpatient clinic settings. Currently, OT is provided in primary care in the ambulatory care clinic. Team members see the value of OT and its diverse roles in helping patients.

Marketing Occupational Therapy Services to Physicians in Primary Care

Primary care physicians are generally unaccustomed to working directly with occupational therapists. Many primary care providers are unaware of the education and training or range of skills and scope of practice of occupational therapy practitioners that would be applicable in a primary care practice setting. Therefore, physicians may need to be informed regarding the potential benefits of offering occupational therapy services to patients. In addition, the benefits to the physicians themselves should be stressed—for example, increased physician efficiency, enhanced patient adherence to treatment recommendations, and improved outcomes and patient satisfaction. Occupational therapy practitioners must be able to clearly articulate and support with evidence the unique value of occupational therapy in primary care. Muir (2012) encourages the profession to "make a coordinated and concerted effort to develop mechanisms to quantify not only the positive effects that we have on a specific client, but also the ripple effects that result when people and community populations change" (p. 510).

Attitudes, personal beliefs, and lifestyle habits of physicians have a major impact on the likelihood of implementing prevention and health-promotion strategies in their practices. Primary care physicians tend to be more prevention and health-promotion focused than physicians in other specialties. In addition, reimbursement issues and energy, time, and resource constraints also limit physicians' participation in patient-centered health promotion (Goel and McIsaac, 2000). Employing or collaborating with other professionals, such as occupational therapists, who have the expertise and time to address lifestyle modifications and health literacy can enhance the health outcomes in primary care settings. The physician can then focus on treating illness and preventing disease, identifying patients in need of specific prevention and health-promotion interventions, and referring these individuals for follow-up services.

The benefits to primary care physicians of utilizing occupational therapists (as an employee or a contractor) to provide health-promotion and prevention services in their practice settings potentially include:

- Availability of high-quality prevention and health-promotion services on-site, thus increasing the physician's time to focus on medical interventions

- Better patient health outcomes as a result of comprehensive health-promotion services
- Less need for medications and better compliance with self-management regimens
- Identification of patients who have mental health needs not readily recognizable in a short medical office visit, including alcohol and drug abuse problems, domestic violence, depression, anxiety, bereavement, etc.
- Detection of performance deficits that may affect safe participation in everyday activities
- Early identification of patient lack of adherence to medical treatment plans, thereby preventing secondary complications of medical conditions

In addition, it has been noted that providing occupational therapy and other services in-house can enhance a physician's earnings. Out of 11 factors that are associated with high-earning family physicians, the provision of adjunctive services ranks fourth, with occupational therapy specifically mentioned (Carter, 2005). The benefits to patients include more time with staff, immediate access to occupational therapy services without the need to leave the physician's office, opportunities to learn to manage their own health problems, and improved quality of life.

Funding Occupational Therapy Services in Primary Care

Funding for occupational therapy services in primary care can come from a number of sources. There are office visit and current procedural terminology (CPT) codes commonly billed in primary care, such as health counseling, that can be billed to insurance for either individual or group sessions. Dahl-Popolizio and colleagues (2017) estimated the net reimbursement for occupational therapy in a typical day in a primary care setting (see Table 25-2). Occupational therapy evaluation and treatment is a billable service under Medicare and many private health insurance plans. Many preventive interventions, such as energy conservation, work simplification, and safety awareness, are already being reimbursed through these mechanisms. However, before developing a health-promotion program, it is essential that occupational therapists are cognizant of, and adhere to, state licensure laws that define the scope of occupational therapy practice.

Other revenue sources may be foundation grants, fee-for-service plans, health maintenance organizations (HMOs), workers' compensation, and other government programs. In addition, many people may be able and willing to pay for occupational therapy services, as is evidenced by the amount spent

Table 25-2 A Typical Day With Occupational Therapy Available in Primary Care

CPT Code* (visit type)	Number of Patients	Minutes Spent With Patient	Per Unit Fee	Billed/Day/ Code	Hours/Day/ Code
97110 (ex)	2	30	$32.54/15 min	$130.16	1 hr
97535 (ADL)	4	30	$35.04/15 min	$280.32	2 hr
97530 (act)	5	30	$35.04/15 min	$350.40	2.5 hr
97150 (group)	10	60	$17.52 (untimed)	$175.20	1 hr
97003 (eval)	1	30	$85.45 (untimed)	$85.45	0.5 hr
97532 (cog tx	2	30	$26.82/15 min	$107.28	1 hr
Total net reimbursement for a typical 8 hr day				$1,128.81	
Total net reimbursement per year based on this typical day (50 weeks)					$282,202.50

Note: *CPT codes (all modifiers) retrieved from the Centers for Medicare and Medicaid Services, 2015. Salaries vary greatly and are dictated by setting and region.

Current salary range across the nation according to the U.S. Bureau of Labor Statistics (www.bls.gov) is approximately $50,000 to $98,000 per year, with 114,600 jobs in 2014, which is expected to increase by 27% by 2024. As primary care is an emerging practice setting, there are no current statistics regarding salaries in this setting.

From "Interprofessional Primary Care: The Value of Occupational Therapy," by S. Dahl-Popolizio, O. Rogers, S. L. Muir, J. Carroll, and L. Manson, 2017, *Open Journal of Occupational Therapy, 5*(3), article 11. Used with permission.

for complementary and alternative medical care, which typically is not reimbursed by insurance (National Center for Complementary and Alternative Medicine, 2006). More information about funding community-based occupational therapy services can be found in Chapter 8.

Summary

- Primary health care is continuous, comprehensive care designed to maximize health and prevent disease and disability.
- Traditionally, primary health care has been provided by physicians, nurse practitioners, and physician assistants in a variety of settings.
- Health promotion and the medical model can be effectively blended in primary care office practice.
- The most common health problems seen in primary care settings include diabetes, obesity, chronic pain conditions, and mental health disorders.
- Occupational therapists may be able to establish a niche on the primary health-care team by assisting primary care physicians by providing health education, prevention, health-promotion, and intervention services for patients in the physician office.
- Evidence-based practices such as brief office interventions, health literacy interventions, and chronic disease self-management strategies can be implemented by occupational therapists in primary care settings.
- Many of the objectives in *Healthy People 2030* that refer to primary health care can be addressed by occupational therapists.

Integrating occupational therapy and health-promotion services into primary care practice is an opportunity and challenge worth pursuing. According to Devereaux and Walker (1995), "occupational therapy can be a major force in the delivery of primary health care" (p. 393). Occupational therapy's focus on physical, cognitive, emotional, social, and spiritual well-being provides a useful, and increasingly necessary, adjunct to primary care medical services.

CASE STUDIES

CASE STUDY 25-1 Doris

Doris is a recently widowed 68-year-old woman with diabetes who presents to her family physician with complaints of fatigue, poor concentration, insomnia, and binge eating. She has gained 20 pounds in the 6 months since the death of her husband. The physician, a member of a multidisciplinary practice, diagnoses depression, prescribes an antidepressant medication, and refers the patient to an occupational therapist who works in the office. The occupational therapist conducts an interview, administers several assessments, including the COPM, and develops an occupational profile. Prior to her retirement, Doris worked as a middle school teacher. Doris lives alone and has two grown children and six grandchildren who live approximately 2 hours from her home. She enjoys movies, reading, gardening, and walking her dog. In the past, Doris was very active in her church, but over the past 2 years while caring for her ill husband, her participation diminished significantly. She has a limited income, but her home mortgage is paid off, and she has good health insurance coverage as a benefit of her teacher's retirement plan.

In collaboration with Doris, the occupational therapist develops an intervention plan that includes the following:

- Chronic disease self-management and health literacy to address the client's diabetes
- Lifestyle Redesign® for weight management to increase the client's level of physical activity, to encourage adherence to her food plan, and to improve the quality of her sleep
- Mental health services to facilitate the grief process and reestablish life goals
- Reengagement in meaningful occupations

CASE STUDY 25-1 Doris

Discussion Questions

1. What types of occupational therapy services could be provided to Doris in the primary care physician's office? How would the occupational therapy services be unique and different from services provided by other health-care professionals in this setting?
2. What intervention strategies would you use to improve Doris's health literacy and chronic disease self-management? To help Doris achieve her weight loss goals? To maximize her occupational performance?
3. What intervention strategies would you use to facilitate the grief process and improve her mental health?
4. How would the provision of occupational therapy services in this case benefit the primary care physician?

CASE STUDY 25-2 County Health Department

The County Health Department has had an influx of patients with chronic pain who are going through a planned, phased reduction (weaning) of narcotic pain medications. The director recently read an article on Lifestyle Redesign® and how it has been used effectively to manage chronic pain. He requests a meeting with you to discuss how occupational therapy might be incorporated into health department programs, particularly the chronic pain management program. The population served by the County Health Department is largely indigent and immigrant, with a small percentage being working adults who cannot afford health insurance for themselves and their families. There are five locations spread throughout the county. All patients with chronic pain are served at the downtown location, where there are three full-time physicians and five nurse practitioners.

Chronic pain can limit a person's occupational performance, disrupt sleep patterns, result in social isolation, and contribute to feelings of helplessness, anxiety, and depression. You describe to the director how occupational therapy might alleviate these problems through a variety of interventions addressing energy conservation, body posture and mechanics, stress management, emotion regulation, habits and routines, and the ergonomic assessment of home and work environments. The director is impressed and asks you to develop a proposal that includes a description of the services to be provided, the expected outcomes, and the costs associated with a Lifestyle Redesign–based chronic pain management program. Although you are familiar with the Lifestyle Redesign model, you do not feel competent to design and implement such a program.

Discussion Questions

1. What would be your next steps in this process?
2. How might you learn more about the design and implementation of a Lifestyle Redesign program?
3. What components of a Lifestyle Redesign program for the management of chronic pain would be appropriate in a primary care setting?
4. How would you market this service to the physicians and nurse practitioners?
5. What strategies would you use to evaluate the effectiveness of the program?
6. What are the costs and benefits of this program to the County Health Department?

Learning Activities

1. Write a brief article for *OT Practice* describing how the five *As* model of health behavior change could be applied to weight management in a primary care setting.
2. Interview a primary care physician to assess the potential services an occupational therapist could provide to patients in this setting.
3. Conduct a needs assessment and write a brief proposal for occupational therapy services in a primary care setting in your community.

REFERENCES

Agency for Healthcare Research and Quality. (n.d.). *Defining the patient centered medical home.* Retrieved from https://pcmh.ahrq.gov/page/defining-pcmh

American Academy of Family Physicians. (2011). *Primary care.* Retrieved from http://aafp.org/online/en/home/policy/policies/p/primarycare.html

American Diabetes Association. (2010). Diagnosis and classification of diabetes mellitus. *Diabetes Care, 33*(Suppl. 1), S62–S69. Retrieved from https://doi.org/10.2337/dc10-S062

American Heart Association. (2018). Getting active: It's easier than you think. Retrieved from www.heart.org/HEARTORG/HealthyLiving/PhysicalActivity/Physical-Activity_UCM_001080_SubHomePage.jsp

American Occupational Therapy Association. (2011). *Occupational therapy's role in diabetes self-management* [Fact sheet]. Retrieved from www.aota.org/~/media/Corporate/Files/AboutOT/Professionals/WhatIsOT/PA/Facts/Diabetes%20fact%20sheet.pdf

American Occupational Therapy Association. (2013). Occupational therapy in the promotion of health and well-being. *American Journal of Occupational Therapy, 67*(Suppl.), S47–S59.

American Occupational Therapy Association. (2014). The role of occupational therapy in primary care. *American Journal of Occupational Therapy, 68*(Suppl. 3), S25–S33.

American Occupational Therapy Association. (2015). Occupational therapy code of ethics (2015). *American Journal of Occupational Therapy, 69*(Suppl. 3), 6913410030p1-6913410030p8. doi:10.5014/ajot.2015.696S03

Brown, R. L., and Rounds, L. A. (1995). Conjoint screening questionnaires for alcohol and drug abuse. *Wisconsin Medical Journal, 94*, 135–140.

Buche, J., Singer, P. M., Grazier, K., King, E., Maniere, E., and Beck, A. J. (2017). *Primary care and behavioral health workforce integration: Barriers and best practices.* Retrieved from www.behavioralhealthworkforce.org/publications/

Carter, J. (2005). What makes a high-earning family physician? *Family Practice Management, 12*(7), 16–23.

Centers for Disease Control and Prevention. (2009). *Chronic diseases: The power to prevent, the call to control.* Atlanta, GA: Centers for Disease Control and Prevention.

Centers for Disease Control and Prevention. (2016). *Nonopioid treatments for chronic pain.* Retrieved from www.cdc.gov/drugoverdose/pdf/nonopioid_treatments-a.pdf

Centers for Disease Control and Prevention. (2018a). *Drug overdose deaths in the United States 1999–2017.* Retrieved from www.cdc.gov/nchs/products/databriefs/db329.htm

Centers for Disease Control and Prevention. (2018b). *Mortality in the United States, 2017.* Retrieved from www.cdc.gov/nchs/products/databriefs/db328.htm

Centers for Disease Control and Prevention. (2018c). *Suicide mortality in the United States 1999–2017.* Retrieved from www.cdc.gov/nchs/products/databriefs/db330.htm

Chodosh, J., Morton, S. C., Mojica, W., Maglione, M., Suttorp, M. J., Hilton, L., Rhodes, S., and Shekelle, P. (2005). Meta-analysis: Chronic disease self-management programs for older adults. *Annals of Internal Medicine, 143*, 427–438.

Creek, J., Beynon, S., Cook, S., and Tulloch, T. (2002). Occupational therapy in primary care. In J. Creek, *Occupational therapy and mental health.* Edinburgh, Scotland: Churchill Livingstone.

Dahl-Popolizio, S., Doyle, S., and Wade, S. (2018). The role of primary health care in achieving global healthcare goals: Highlighting the potential contribution of occupational therapy. *World Federation of Occupational Therapists Bulletin.* doi:10.1080/14473828.2018.1433770

Dahl-Popolizio, S., Rogers, O., Muir, S. L., Carroll, J., and Manson, L. (2017). Interprofessional primary care: The value of occupational therapy. *Open Journal of Occupational Therapy, 5*(3), article 11. Retrieved from https://doi.org/10.15453/2168-6408.1363

Devereaux, E. B., and Walker, R. B. (1995). The role of occupational therapy in primary health care. *American Journal of Occupational Therapy, 49*(5), 391–396.

Dobbelsteyn, C. J., Joffres, M. R., MacLean, D. R., and Flowerdew, G. (2001). A comparative evaluation of waist circumference, waist-to-hip ratio and body mass index as indicators of cardiovascular risk factors. *International Journal of Obesity, 25*(5), 652–661.

Domino, F. J. (2005). Improving adherence to treatment for hypertension. *American Family Physician, 71*(11), 2089–2090.

Edelman, C. L., and Mandle, C. L. (2002). *Health promotion throughout the lifespan.* St. Louis, MO: Mosby.

Fisher, L., Skaff, M. M., Mullan, J. T., Arean, P., Glasgow, R., and Masharani, U. (2008). A longitudinal study of affection and anxiety disorders, depressive affect and diabetes distress in adults with type 2 diabetes. *Diabetic Medicine, 25*(9), 1096–1101. https://doi.org/10.1111/j.1464-5491.2008.02533.x

Flegal, K. M., Carroll, M. D., Kit, B. K., and Ogden, C. L. (2012). Prevalence of obesity and trends in the distribution of body mass index among U.S. adults, 1999–2010. *Journal of the American Medical Association, 307*(5), 491–497.

Ganiats, T., and King, V. (2003, January). Prevention strategies in family practice. *AAFP Video CME Program.* Leawood, KS: American Academy of Family Physicians.

Gaunt, A. M., Herring, S. A., and O'Connor, F. G. (2008). Caring for patients who have acute and subacute low back pain. *AAFP CME Bulletin, 7*(2), 1–6.

Global BMI Mortality Collaboration. (2016). Body-mass index and all-cause mortality: Individual-participant meta-analysis of 239 prospective studies in four continents. *Lancet, 388*, 776–786.

Goel, V., and McIsaac, W. (2000). Health promotion in clinical practice. In B. D. Poland, L. W. Green, and I. Rootman (Eds.), *Settings for health promotion.* Thousand Oaks, CA: Sage.

Green, L., and Kreuter, M. (2004). *Health program planning: An educational and ecological approach* (4th ed.). New York, NY: McGraw-Hill.

Hwand, J. E., Truax, C., Claire, M., and Caytap, A. L. (2009). Occupational therapy in diabetic care—areas of need perceived by older adults with diabetes. *Occupational Therapy in Health Care, 23*(3), 173–188.

Institute of Medicine. (1994). *Defining primary care: An interim report.* Washington, DC: National Academy Press.

Interagency Pain Research Coordinating Committee. (2016). *National Pain Strategy: A comprehensive population health-level strategy for pain.* Retrieved from https://iprcc.nih.gov/sites/default/files/HHSNational_Pain_Strategy_508C.pdf

Jaen, C. R. (2003). Integrating health behavior counseling into routine primary care. *AAFP CME Bulletin, 2*(7), 1–5. Leawood, KS: American Academy of Family Physicians.

Jehl, E., Solger, E. Weaver, C., Oliveira, D., Kornblau, B., Mbiza, S., and Alexander, A. (2017). Chronic pain patients' perceptions of treatments that decrease pain and increase function. *American Journal of Occupational Therapy, 71,* 7111520297p.1. doi:10.5014/ajot.2017.7151-PO5160

Karjalainen, K., Malmivaara, A., van Tulder, M., Roine, R., Jauhiainen, M., Hurri, H., and Koes, B. (2003). Multidisciplinary biopsychosocial rehabilitation for subacute low-back pain among working age adults. *Cochrane Database of Systematic Reviews, 2,* Art. No.: CD002193. doi:10.1002/14651858.CD002193

Law, M., Baptiste, S., Carswell, A., McColl, M. A., Polatajko, H., and Pollock, N. (2005). *Canadian Occupational Performance Measure.* Ottawa: Canadian Association of Occupational Therapists.

Lin, E. H., Rutter, C. M., Katon, W., Heckbert, S. R., Ciechanowski, P., . . . Von Korff, M. (2010). Depression and advanced complications of diabetes: A prospective cohort study. *Diabetes Care, 33*(2), 264–269. https://doi.org/10.2337/dc09-1068

Lorig, K. R. (2015). Chronic disease self-management program: Insights from the eye of the storm. *Frontiers in Public Health.* Retrieved from https://doi.org/10.3389/fpubh.2014.00253

Mayo Clinic. (2014). *Diabetes.* Retrieved from www.mayoclinic.org/diseases-conditions/diabetes/symptoms-causes/syc-20371444

Merriman, B., Ades, T., and Seffrin, J. R. (2002). Health literacy in the information age: Communicating cancer information to patients and families. *CA: A Cancer Journal for Physicians, 52,* 130–133.

Mosley, L. J., Jedlicka, J. S., LeQuieu, E., and Taylor, F. D. (2008). Obesity and occupational therapy practice. *OT Practice, 13*(7), 8–15.

Moyers, P. A., and Stoffel, V. C. (2001). Community-based approaches for substance use disorders. In M. Scaffa (Ed.), *Occupational therapy in community-based practice settings.* Philadelphia, PA: F. A. Davis.

Muir, S. (2012). Occupational therapy in primary health care: We should be there. *American Journal of Occupational Therapy, 66*(5), 506–510.

National Center for Complementary and Alternative Medicine. (2006). *News and events: Use of complementary and alternative medicine in the United States.* Retrieved from http://nccam.nih.gov/news/camsurvey_fs1.htm#top

National Council on Aging. (2016). *Healthy aging facts.* Retrieved from www.ncoa.org/news/resources-for-reporters/get-the-facts/healthy-aging-facts/

National Heart, Lung, and Blood Institute. (2018). *Classification of overweight and obesity by BMI, waist circumference, and associated disease risks.* Retrieved from www.nhlbi.nih.gov/health/educational/lose_wt/BMI/bmi_dis.htm

National Institute of Diabetes and Digestive and Kidney Diseases. (2017). *Diabetes.* Retrieved from www.niddk.nih.gov/health-information/diabetes

National Institute of Mental Health. (2010). *Statistics.* Retrieved from http://nimh.nih.gov/statistics/index.shtml

National Institute of Mental Health. (2017). *Integrated care: Overview.* Retrieved from www.nimh.nih.gov/health/topics/integrated-care/index.shtml

National Institute on Alcohol Abuse and Alcoholism. (2003). *Helping patients with alcohol problems: A health practitioner's guide.* NIH Publication 03-3769. Bethesda, MD: National Institutes of Health.

National Network of Libraries of Medicine. (2006). *Health literacy.* Retrieved from http://nnlm.gov/outreach/consumer/hlthlit.html

Osborne, H. (2005). *Health literacy from A to Z: Practical ways to communicate your health message.* Boston, MA: Jones and Bartlett.

Peckham, C. (2016). *Medscape physician compensation report 2016.* Retrieved from www.medscape.com/features/slideshow/compensation/2016/public/overview

Practice Fusion. (2011). *The 25 most common medical diagnoses.* Retrieved from www.practicefusion.com/blog/25-most-common-diagnoses/

Prochaska, J. O., DiClemente, C. C., and Norcross, J. C. (1992). In search of how people change. *American Psychologist, 47,* 1102–1114.

Pyatak, E. A. (2011). The role of occupational therapy in diabetes self-management interventions. *OTJR: Occupation, Participation, and Health, 31*(2), 89–96.

Reitz, S. M. (2010). Promoting exercise and physical activity. In M. Scaffa, S. M. Reitz, and M. Pizzi (Eds.), *Occupational therapy in the promotion of health and wellness* (pp. 225–252). Philadelphia, PA: F. A. Davis.

Rosenwax, L. K., Semmens, J. B., and Holman, C. D. (2001). Is occupational therapy in danger of "ad-hocery"? An application of evidence-based guidelines to the treatment of acute low back pain. *Australian Occupational Therapy Journal, 48,* 181–186.

Scaffa, M. E., and Reitz, S. M. (2014). *Occupational therapy in community-based practice settings* (2nd ed.). Philadelphia, PA: F.A. Davis.

Schillinger, D., Grumbach, K., Piette, J., Wang, F., Osmond, D., Daher, C., Palacios, J., Sullivan, G. D., and Bindman, A. (2002). Association of health literacy with diabetes outcomes. *JAMA, 288*(4), 475–482.

Simon, A.U., and Collins, C. E. (2017). Lifestyle Redesign for chronic pain management: A retrospective clinical efficacy study. *American Journal of Occupational Therapy, 71,* 7104190040p1-7104190040p7. doi:10.5014/ajot.2017.025502

Stanford University. (2006). *Chronic disease self-management program.* Retrieved from http://patienteducation.stanford.edu/programs/cdsmp.html

Summergrad, P., and Kathol, R. G. (2014). *Integrated care in psychiatry: Redefining the role of mental health professionals in the medical setting.* New York, NY: Springer.

Thompson, M. (2014). Occupations, habits, and routines: Perspectives from persons with diabetes. *Scandinavian Journal of Occupational Therapy, 21*(2), 153–160. doi:10.3109/11038128.2013.851278

U.S. Department of Health and Human Services. (2000). *Healthy people 2010: Understanding and improving health.* Retrieved from http://healthdisparitiesks.org/download/Hllthy_People_2010_Improving_Health.pdf

U.S. Department of Health and Human Services. (2011). *Healthy people 2020.* Retrieved from http:// healthypeople.gov/2020/about/default.aspx

U.S. Preventive Services Task Force. (2007). *The guide to clinical preventive services—2007: Recommendations of the U.S. Preventive Services Task Force.* Rockville, MD: Agency for Healthcare Research and Quality.

U.S. Public Health Service. (2001). *Surgeon general's call to action on obesity.* Washington, DC: U.S. Public Health Service.

Waddell, G., and Burton, A. K. (2001). Occupational health guidelines for the management of low back pain at work: Evidence review. *Occupational Medicine, 51*(2), 124–135.

Ward, M. C., Miller, B. F., Marconi, V. C., Kaslow, N. J., and Farber, E. W. (2015). The role of behavioural health in optimizing care for complex patients in the primary care setting. *Journal of General Internal Medicine, 31*(3), 265–267. doi:10.1007/s11606-015-3499-8

Williams, M. V., Baker, D. W., Honig, E. G., Lee, T. M., and Nowlan, A. (1998). Inadequate literacy is a barrier to asthma knowledge and self-care. *Chest, 114,* 1008–1015.

Williams, M. V., Baker, D. W., Parker, R. M., and Nurss, J. R. (1998). Relationship of functional health literacy to patients' knowledge of their chronic disease: A study of patients with hypertension and diabetes. *Archives of Internal Medicine, 158,* 166–172.

World Health Organization. (1978). *Declaration of Alma-Ata.* Retrieved from www.who.int/hpr/NPH/docs/declaration_almaata.pdf

World Health Organization. (1986). Ottawa charter for health promotion. *Health Promotion, 1*(4), iii–v.

Zapka, J. G. (2000). Commentary: On finding common ground. In B. D. Poland, L. W. Green, and I. Rootman (Eds.), *Settings for health promotion.* Thousand Oaks, CA: Sage.

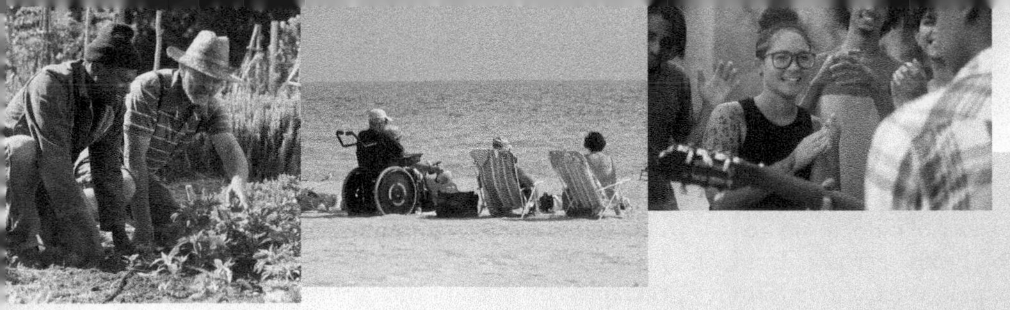

Chapter 26

Disaster Preparedness, Response, and Recovery

Theresa M. Smith, PhD, OTR, CLVT, and Marjorie E. Scaffa, PhD, OTR/L, FAOTA

When disaster comes, let it find us doing sensible and human things—praying, working, teaching, reading, listening to music, bathing the children, playing tennis, chatting to our friends over a pint and a game of darts. . . .

—C. S. Lewis

Learning Outcomes

This chapter is designed to enable the reader to:

26-1 Describe what is meant by an "all-hazards approach" to disaster management.
26-2 Identify the roles of governmental agencies and nonprofit organizations in disaster preparedness, response, and recovery.
26-3 Discuss the impact of disasters on occupational performance and occupational participation.
26-4 Describe evidence-based approaches to addressing acute stress reactions to disasters.
26-5 Describe potential roles for occupational therapy practitioners in addressing the needs of special populations affected by disasters.
26-6 Explain how the role of occupational therapy changes during disaster preparedness, response, and recovery.

Key Terms

All-hazards approach
Community emergency response teams
Disaster
Disaster medical assistance teams
Emergency Management Institute
Incident Command System
Mass shooting
National Disaster Medical System
National Incident Management System
National Response Framework
Posttraumatic growth
Psychological first aid
Resilience
Special needs populations
Trauma-informed care

Introduction

Communities across the world experience a wide range of threats and hazards with varying frequencies and complexities. According to the United Nations Centre for Research on the Epidemiology of Disasters (2018), "between 1998 and 2017 climate-related and geophysical disasters killed 1.3 million people and left a further 4.4 billion injured, homeless, displaced, or in need of emergency assistance" (p. 3). Although geophysical events, such as earthquakes and tsunamis, caused the majority of fatalities, climate-related disasters (e.g., floods and storms) accounted for 91% of all recorded events worldwide. The average number of climate-related disasters increased from 165 events per year from 1978 to 1997 to 329 events per year from 1998 to 2017. The knowledge of impending disasters and their resultant effects is now broadcast on a virtual 24/7 news cycle.

The term **disaster** refers to "dangerous accidental or uncontrollable situations or events that cause significant environmental destruction, loss of life, and disruption of social structure and daily life routines. Disasters overwhelm the local capacity to respond and necessitate requests for external assistance" (Smith and Scaffa, 2014, p. 964). Disasters affect the most vulnerable group—the poor—the hardest, particularly children, women, and the elderly. In New Orleans, the impact of Hurricane Katrina was felt most acutely by African Americans (both elderly and nonelderly) living in disadvantaged neighborhoods. The African American community experienced a disproportionately higher number of deaths than would be expected based on the demographics of the city (Sharkey, 2007). Disasters deplete financial and material assets quickly in the immediate aftermath of a crisis. Therefore, the effects of a disaster can last a long time, especially in areas with limited resources (World Health Organization [WHO], 2019).

Occupational therapy practitioners became particularly interested in disaster response and recovery following the terrorist attacks on September 11, 2001. In 2006, the American Occupational Therapy Association (AOTA) published its first official document on the role of occupational therapy in disaster preparedness, response, and recovery (DPRR). The document was revised (2011) and replaced with the *Societal Statement on Disaster Response and Risk Reduction* (2017). In the third edition of the *Occupational Therapy Practice Framework,* the definition of clients was modified to include persons, groups, and populations (AOTA, 2014). This concept of client better aligns with the role of occupational therapy practitioners in supporting communities, not just individuals, after traumatic events.

The World Federation of Occupational Therapists (WFOT, 2016b) also supports and promotes the involvement of occupational therapists in DPRR at local, district, and national levels. The WFOT published a document on "dos and don'ts" for rehabilitation professionals when responding to international disasters. In 2016, the WFOT (2016a) began offering online training for occupational therapists on disaster management.

Types and Stages of Disasters

Disasters occur in stages and are typically classified into three types: natural, technological, and intentional.

Natural

How much influence humankind has had on the number or severity of natural disasters is being debated, but there has been a gradual increase in natural disasters such as hurricanes, earthquakes, floods, and wildfires in the United States, from 60 recorded events in 1980 to 100 in 2016 (Insurance Information Institute [III], 2019b). Of the 10 most costly hurricanes on record, three occurred in 2017: Harvey, Irma, and Maria (Weather Channel, 2018). It is predicted that more of the worst type of wildfires with large, destructive blazes will spread secondary to rising temperatures (III, 2019a). Warmer temperatures improve the chances of wildfires by causing drier vegetation, more lightning strikes, a longer fire season, and intense winds. Over 90% of wildfires can be attributed to humans. In 2018, over 25,000,000 dollars in losses were estimated due to wildfires, heat waves, and drought (III, 2019a). Residents of the affected areas may be displaced temporarily or permanently.

Nearly 75% of the world's tornados occur in the United States. Tornados are unpredictable and can cause massive damage. The winds of a tornado can travel up to 250 miles per hour and can clear a path a mile wide and 50 miles long, destroying anything in its wake. In a typical year, tornados kill approximately 80 people and injure 1,500 more in the United States (National Geographic, n.d.b). A half-million earthquakes occur each year worldwide. Most are small, deep underground, and unnoticeable. However, 100,000 are closer to the earth's surface and strong enough to be felt, and about 100 are so strong they can level high-rise buildings and disrupt power, water, and communications. It is impossible to predict when and where an earthquake may happen (National Geographic, n.d.a).

Technological

Technological disasters are due to the "failure or breakdown of systems, equipment and engineering standards that harms people and the environment" (Emergency Management [EM], 2016, para. 2). A wide range of disasters are due to technology failures, such as structural collapses, hazardous materials (HAZMAT) spills, and nuclear explosions. It is sometimes difficult to determine who or what is ultimately responsible for the cause of a complex technological disaster and for assuming the personal, economic, and community costs of recovery (EM, 2016).

Technological disasters are human-made, usually not intentionally but often due to human error. Many are preventable and as a result, victims of technological disasters often feel angry toward the identified "perpetrators." Recovery from technological disasters tends to take longer, and conflict among community members is more common as compared to natural disasters (Lindsey, Donovan, Smith, Radunovich, and Gutter, 2017). It is not uncommon for a natural disaster to precipitate a technological disaster—for example, the 2011 earthquake and tsunami in Japan that caused nuclear accidents in three reactors at a power plant (see Fig. 26-1; CNN, 2018a).

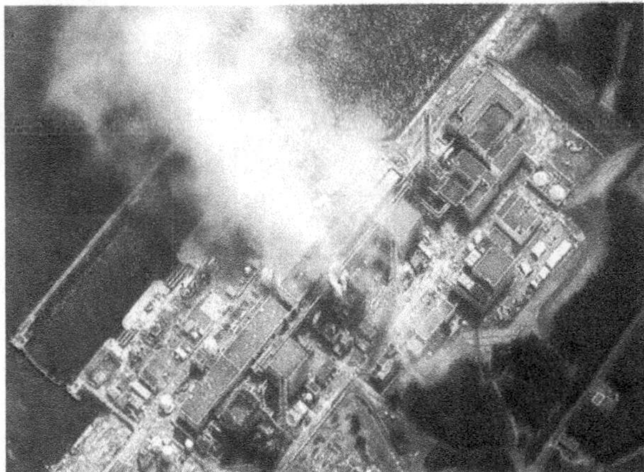

Figure 26-1 Explosions at a nuclear plant. *(From "Fukushima Explosions From Air, Taken by Global Hawk Drone," via https://www.flickr.com/photos/vizpix/5529038135. Used with permission.)*

Intentional

The United States has significantly more deaths by firearms (12 per 100,000) than any other developed country, and some of these deaths are the result of mass shootings (Vox, 2018). In 1999, the Columbine High School in Colorado was the site of a mass shooting that captured widespread attention and prompted a national debate on gun control; 13 people were killed, and 20 were injured by gunfire (History.com, 2018). A **mass shooting** is defined as an event in which four or more people, excluding the shooter, are shot but not necessarily killed at the same general time and location (Vox, 2018). Shootings have occurred in schools at every level of education. In 2007, a gunman killed 32 people at Virginia Tech University (History.com, 2018). More recently, in February 2018, 17 people were killed, and 17 were injured at the Parkland, Florida, school shooting (Westword, 2018). The Parkland school shooting was the 208th school shooting since Columbine in 1999. Not long afterward, in May 2018, 10 were killed and 10 injured in a school shooting in Santa Fe, Texas. Refer to Chapter 27 for more on violence prevention and mitigation.

Some mass shooting deaths in the United States are deemed to be "hate crimes"—for example, 50 deaths at a gay nightclub in Orlando, Florida (June 2016) and 11 deaths at a Jewish synagogue in Pittsburg, Pennsylvania (October 2018; CNN, 2018b; Johnston, 2018). The Federal Bureau of Investigation ([FBI], n.d.) defines a hate crime as a "criminal offense against a person or property motivated in whole or in part by an offender's bias against a race, religion, disability, sexual orientation, ethnicity, gender, or gender identity" (para. 4).

To date, the most destructive mass shooting occurred in October 2017 in Las Vegas, Nevada, with 59 deaths of concertgoers at a country music festival. Since 2012, there have been 1,929 mass shootings, with approximately 2,184 killed and 8,080 wounded (Vox, 2018). In the case of mass shootings, it is extremely difficult to effectively prepare, as it less a matter of who the person is than where the person is that makes a person a target.

Stages of Disaster

Disasters progress through three main stages, and different behavioral and organizational responses are needed for each stage. The first stage, disaster planning and preparedness, has two phases. The first phase, planning, occurs well in advance of a disaster and provides an opportunity for developing disaster response plans. The second phase, preparation, or the immediate preimpact period, occurs in the hours or days preceding the disaster and provides an opportunity for disaster preparation if time permits—for example, obtaining supplies in anticipation of a hurricane. In some cases, such as a school shooting or an earthquake, there may be no warning and therefore no ability to prepare.

The second stage, disaster response, includes the impact of the disaster and its immediate aftermath. This is the time when search and rescue operations and evacuation efforts are initiated, and emergency agencies and organizations are mobilized for response. The third stage, disaster recovery, has two phases. The first phase focuses on the short term and involves the clearing of debris and the restoration of basic necessities, such as shelter, water, food, and electricity. The second phase focuses on the long term and involves the reconstruction of physical structures and the rebuilding of individual lives, families, and community coherence.

Roles of Governmental Agencies and Nonprofit Organizations

A variety of governmental agencies and nonprofit organizations are involved in DPRR. The vast majority of these utilize the all-hazards approach to emergency preparedness advocated by the WHO (2018).

The **all-hazards approach** focuses on developing the generic capabilities that are critical to prepare for and respond to a full spectrum of emergencies and disasters: natural (e.g., hurricane), technological (e.g., oil spill), and intentional (e.g., terrorist bombing). This approach takes into consideration the population's vulnerability to specific hazards but does not specifically address every possible threat. Rather, an all-hazards approach seeks to ensure the community has the capacity to address a broad range of emergencies through maintaining certain core functions that will be needed in most disasters. These core functions include communication, evacuation, and shelter. Emergency plans need to be sufficiently flexible and scalable to adapt not only to the anticipated risks but also to the unexpected (Canton, 2013).

If occupational therapy practitioners want to become involved in DPRR, it is important to understand the roles of these governmental agencies and nonprofit organizations in emergency management, the ways in which occupational therapy might fit in with their missions, and the strategies to gain entry into these systems. Becoming affiliated with governmental agencies and nonprofit organizations involved in DPRR and participating in training increases the credibility of occupational therapy practitioners and facilitates participation when a disaster occurs.

Governmental Agencies

Although almost every federal agency has some role in DPRR, the governmental agencies with the majority of responsibility described here include the following:

- U.S. Department of Homeland Security (USDHS)
- Federal Emergency Management Agency (FEMA)
- U.S. Department of Health and Human Services (USDHHS) Office of Preparedness and Response (OPR)
- U.S. Public Health Service (USPHS)
- State- and local-level emergency management agencies (EMAs)

The overall mission of the USDHS (2017, para. 2) is stated as follows: "With honor and integrity, we will safeguard the American people, our homeland, and our values." The goals of the USDHS are to prevent terrorism, manage borders, administer immigration laws, secure cyberspace, and ensure disaster resilience.

President Jimmy Carter created FEMA in 1979 through executive order. In 2003, FEMA was subsumed administratively under the USDHS. FEMA

(2018a) leads and "coordinates the federal government's role in preparing for, preventing, mitigating the effects of, responding to, and recovering from all domestic disasters, whether natural or man-made, including acts of terror" (para. 3). FEMA operates under the all-inclusive concept of "whole community," meaning preparedness and response are shared responsibilities of government at all levels, businesses, faith-based organizations, nonprofit groups, schools, and the media.

The **National Response Framework** (NRF) developed by FEMA outlines principles, roles and responsibilities, and best practices for managing emergencies and disasters, ranging from serious, small-scale local incidents to large-scale catastrophes. The principles underlying the NRF include: "(1) engaged partnership, (2) tiered response, (3) scalable, flexible, and adaptable operational capabilities, (4) unity of effort through unified command, and (5) readiness to act" (USDHS, 2013, p. 5). The construct of Emergency Support Functions (ESFs) has proven to be an effective strategy for managing disaster-related resources. The ESFs group the coordinating agencies, resources, and capabilities into the functional areas frequently needed in disaster response. Federal ESF agencies and departments may be selectively activated depending on the nature and scope of the disaster. The NRF lists 15 ESFs (see Table 26-1; USDHS, 2013). ESFs #6 and 8 are of most interest to occupational therapy practitioners.

In 2004, the USDHS developed and released the **National Incident Management System** (NIMS), which established a standardized set of structures, processes, and procedures that enable emergency responders at all levels to collaboratively address incidents of all types and complexities more effectively and efficiently. Since then, FEMA has been responsible for its implementation. A recent update of NIMS policies and procedures outlined three major components of the system: resource management, command and coordination, and communication and information management (FEMA, 2017). Resource management guidelines standardize mechanisms to manage personnel, equipment, supplies, teams, and facilities during a disaster. Command and coordination principles describe leadership roles, processes, and organizational structures for managing all types of hazardous incidents. The **incident command system** (ICS) is a standardized approach to the on-site management of the disaster or hazardous situation. The ICS provides a common hierarchy through which multiple organizations can effectively participate. Communications and information management standards help to ensure that decision-makers have the data and means necessary to make and communicate their decisions during a disaster situation. Situation reports (SITREPs), or regular updates on incident details, are a function of communications and information management.

FEMA has two initiatives that are of particular interest to occupational therapy practitioners: **community emergency response teams (CERTs)** and the Emergency Management Institute. CERTs train volunteers to prepare for and respond safely and effectively to the specific types of disasters their communities are likely to experience. There are over 2,700 local CERT programs across the country. Occupational therapy personnel are eligible to participate in CERTs. CERT training includes the following topics:

- Disaster preparedness
- Fire suppression
- Medical operations
- Light search and rescue operations
- Psychology and team organization
- Course review and disaster simulation

CERT training materials are available online (USDHS., n.d.).

Engage Your Brain 26-1

After consulting the AOTA *Occupational Therapy Code of Ethics (2015)*, identify the ethical implications of arriving on the scene of a disaster to volunteer without the proper training.

The national **Emergency Management Institute** (EMI) is the lead agency providing all-hazards emergency management education and training. The EMI offers more than 600 courses (in person and web based) to government employees, first responders, and volunteer organizations throughout the United States, reaching nearly 2,000,000

Table 26-1 Emergency Response Functions (ESFs)

ESF	Federal Coordinating Agency	Basic Responsibility
#1 Transportation	Department of Transportation	Ensures safety, security, and restoration of the transportation infrastructure, including national airspace
#2 Communications	USDHS National Communications System	Coordinates disaster communications and reestablishment of communication infrastructure
#3 Public works and engineering	DoD/U.S. Army Corps of Engineers	Provides technical assistance, engineering expertise, and construction management postdisaster
#4 Firefighting	USDHS/FEMA/ U.S. Fire Administration	Coordinates support for the detection and suppression of fires
#5 Information and planning	USDHS/FEMA	Supports multiagency planning and coordination, including incident action planning and data collection, analysis, and dissemination
#6 Mass care, emergency assistance, temporary housing, and human services	USDHS/FEMA	Coordinates the delivery of public health and medical services, emergency transportation, human services, and disaster housing
#7 Logistics	USDHS/FEMA General Services Administration	Coordinates comprehensive incident resource planning, management, and capability to meet the needs of disaster survivors and responders
#8 Public health and medical services	USDHHS	Provides assistance in response to public health/ medical emergencies and disasters, including medical surge support and mass fatality management
#9 Search and rescue	USDHS/FEMA	Coordinates rapid deployment of search and rescue resources and provides specialized lifesaving assistance
#10 Oil and hazardous materials response	Environmental Protection Agency	Coordinates response to actual or potential release of oil or other hazardous materials and environmental decontamination and cleanup
#11 Agriculture and natural resources	Department of Agriculture	Protects the national food supply, protects natural and cultural resources, and responds to pest and disease outbreaks
#12 Energy	Department of Energy	Facilitates the reestablishment of damaged energy systems and provides technical assistance during incidents involving radiologic/nuclear materials
#13 Public safety and security	Department of Justice, Bureau of Alcohol, Tobacco, Firearms, and Explosives	Coordinates the safety and security of facilities, resources, and the public and manages traffic and crowd control
#14	No longer in effect—superseded by the National Disaster Recovery Framework	
#15 External affairs	USDHS	Coordinates the release of accurate, coordinated, timely, and accessible public information to affected audiences and works closely with state and local officials

From *National Response Framework* (2nd ed.), by U.S. Department of Homeland Security, 2013, pp. 31–35.

individuals each year. Training is offered at no cost. Courses are offered at three levels: awareness, performance, and management and planning. A few courses that may be of interest to occupational therapy practitioners include:

- Community Emergency Response Team Program Manager
- Community Emergency Response Team Train the Trainer
- Community Mass Care and Emergency Assistance
- Improving Preparedness and Resilience Through Public-Private Partnerships
- Management of Spontaneous Volunteers in Disasters
- Mass Care/Emergency Assistance Shelter Field Guide Training
- National Preparedness Goal and System Overview
- Religious and Cultural Literacy and Competency in Disaster (FEMA, 2018b)

Two entities within the USDHHS have DPRR as an element of their missions: the OPR and the USPHS. The OPR is responsible for coordinating the medical response to disaster, including integrating medical response capabilities, enhancing medical surge capabilities, engaging and training first responders, and building on regional health-care coalitions. The OPR manages the **National Disaster Medical System** (NDMS), which augments local health and medical systems during federally declared disasters when local resources are overwhelmed. NDMS professionals also provide health care/emergency services behind the scenes at national events, such as presidential inaugurations. Nationwide, nearly 6,000 health-care professionals and paraprofessionals serve with the NDMS and are organized into units called **disaster medical assistance teams** (DMATs). DMATs are deployed during disasters, disease outbreaks, and special events. These teams are typically activated for 2 weeks at a time.

The USPHS includes the following federal agencies: the National Institutes of Health, Centers for Disease Control and Prevention, Food and Drug Administration, Health Resources and Services Administration, and Substance Abuse and Mental Health Services Administration (SAMHSA), among others. The USPHS's mission is to protect and promote the nation's health through rapid and effective responses to public health emergencies, leadership and excellence in public health practices, and the advancement of public health science (USDHHS, n.d.).

The USPHS workforce, including occupational therapists, can be mobilized and deployed during disasters or other public health emergencies. USPHS occupational therapists have served on disaster mental health teams under the auspices of FEMA and the American Red Cross (ARC) during a number of natural disasters, including Hurricane Katrina in 2005 and other hurricanes in Florida. For example, occupational therapists were deployed to a very large emergency shelter for older adults with special needs in Florida and to a National Guard unit in Mississippi to assist "first responders, caregivers, and service providers, many of whom had witnessed trauma or were victims of loss themselves" (Oakley, Caswell, and Parks, 2008, p. 363).

In addition to federal agencies, state and local agencies are also involved in DPRR. Each state, and often local municipalities, have EMAs that coordinate their activities with FEMA. The state and local EMAs are responsible for comprehensive disaster planning, response, and recovery efforts in their jurisdictions. These agencies also serve as a communications and operations hub during disasters and provide information to their constituents on a variety of disaster-related topics.

Nonprofit Organizations

Although there are hundreds of community-based organizations that respond to disasters, the most active and visible in emergency situations are the ARC and the Salvation Army (SA). Other lesser-known nonprofit organizations described here include:

- National Voluntary Organizations Active in Disaster
- International Critical Incident Stress Foundation
- Humane Society of the United States (HSUS)

The ARC is probably the most well-known disaster relief organization in the United States. Its purpose is to "meet the immediate disaster-caused needs of individuals, families, and communities" (ARC, 2018, para. 3). Volunteers make up 95% of the ARC disaster workforce. During the disaster response phase, the ARC provides shelter, food, emergency supplies, emergency response vehicles, health care, and mental health services. During the recovery phase, the ARC provides financial aid for households that need extra assistance and grants to nonprofit organizations for community-based services (ARC, 2018).

The SA gathers donations, resources, and volunteers to be ready to assist in disasters. During the disaster response phase, the SA provides food, water, and shelter; assists with cleanup efforts; and helps victims make connections with family members. The SA collaborates with local, state, and federal governments to develop and execute a long-term disaster recovery plan. Recovery services provided include restoring and rebuilding structures, covering health-care expenses, reducing funeral costs, and distributing in-kind donations to needy families. In addition, the SA provides emotional support and spiritual comfort to disaster survivors and first responders (SA, 2018).

The National Voluntary Organizations Active in Disaster (NVOAD) is an association of organizations that are involved in DPRR. The coalition consists of 56 nationally reputable faith-based and community-based organizations and many state-level VOADs. The NVOAD (2014) "provides a forum, promoting cooperation, communication, coordination, and collaboration; and fosters more effective delivery of services to communities affected by disaster" (para. 2).

The International Critical Incident Stress Foundation (ICISF, n.d.a) provides "leadership, education, training, consultation, and support services in comprehensive crisis intervention and disaster behavioral health services to the emergency response profession, other organizations, and communities worldwide" (para. 2). The ICISF (n.d.b) provides training and support for Critical Incident Stress Management (CISM) teams around the world and every 2 years sponsors an international conference.

The HSUS is also responsive in emergencies where animals' lives are endangered, such as when hurricanes, tornados, wildfires, floods, and earthquakes strike. Frequently, families must leave cherished pets behind when they evacuate, as shelters and hotels often have policies prohibiting animals. The HSUS rescues and evacuates and shelters all types of animals during disasters, including farm animals. In addition, the HSUS supplies emergency funding to local animal shelters and provides food for displaced animals. The HSUS was instrumental in the enactment of the Pet Evacuation and Transportation Standards Act (PETS), which requires states seeking FEMA funds to accommodate pets and service animals in their disaster evacuation plans (HSUS, 2018).

Impact of Disasters on Occupational Performance and Participation

Some survivors may have physical injuries and/or suffer emotional distress that can last for years and impair their occupational performance. In addition, changes in the survivors' contexts may affect role participation. Therefore, it is important for occupational therapy practitioners to facilitate resumption in valued roles, help with the adoption of new roles to adapt to their changed contexts, and assist survivors in ensuring a healthy balance of future roles (Smith, Dreyfus, and Hersch, 2011).

Damage to home and property may make it difficult to perform normal daily activities, including basic self-care and instrumental activities of daily living (IADLs; see Fig. 26-2). Depending on the extent of the damage to one's home, some of the IADLs likely to be affected include caring for others,

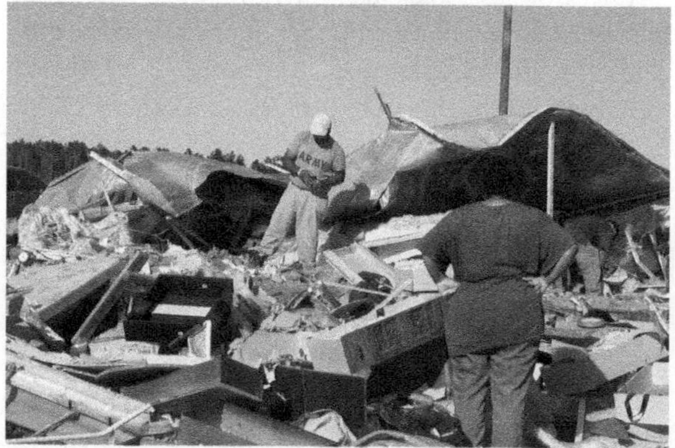

Figure 26-2 Searching for personal belongings after a tornado spawned by Hurricane Irene. *(Photo by FEMA.)*

PROGRAM SHOWCASE

Occupational Therapy Participation in Hurricane Recovery

Submitted by Lindsey H. D. Telg, MOT, OTR/L, Adjunct Faculty, University of Florida

On October 10, 2018, Hurricane Michael, a Category 4 storm, tore through the Florida Panhandle. In its wake, at least 60 individuals lost their lives; the state of Florida and portions of Central America incurred an estimated 15,000,000,000 dollars in damages. But it was not until nearly a month later that the occupational therapy program at the University of Florida had the opportunity to participate in recovery efforts.

On conference calls between numerous local, state, and federal entities, concern arose regarding the accessibility of the largest remaining shelter in Panama City Beach. Someone needed to complete an "Access and Functional Needs Assessment." This seemed to be a perfect role for occupational therapy. Within 48 hours a team was assembled that consisted of an adjunct occupational therapy faculty member, six occupational therapy students, and one nurse. Only the nurse had been directly involved in disaster relief efforts previously.

There was no set form for the "Access and Functional Needs Assessment," and different entities had different perspectives on its purpose. A month had passed and Hurricane Michael's effect on the Panhandle was no longer in the news, so the team was not sure of the status of the area at that point. Contacts in the Panhandle advised that housing was scarce. In fact, the team could not secure a hotel until the morning of its departure. Some restaurants in parts of the city were open, while other parts were destroyed. It was difficult to identify contacts at the shelter as the turnover in volunteer staffing was high, meaning staff may have only been on-site for a few days and knew little more than the team. Just planning for the trip was an exercise in adaptability and flexibility.

The "Access and Functional Needs Assessment" was modeled after the Canadian Occupational Performance Measure (COPM), analyzing both institutional and personal factors. It was not uncommon for shelter residents to mistrust the team's intentions, roles, affiliations, and the purpose of documentation. The primary goal for most residents was to find housing, which was an almost insurmountable goal given the environmental and societal factors. The shelter had no case managers on-site, and this proved a big challenge.

The team overheard an interaction between Shirley and a shelter volunteer in which Shirley adamantly stated she was not going to an assisted living facility. It was learned from volunteers that Shirley was struggling with her personal hygiene at the shelter, including changing her clothes routinely and bathing. The team befriended Shirley; members stopping by frequently throughout the day to chat with her allowed the team to assess her cognition. The shelter volunteers were concerned about Shirley and the team's interactions. Later, a shelter official asked the team to attend a meeting with Shirley and FEMA; she was to receive some benefits and had to make some important decisions about her living arrangements. The team helped ensure the information was presented at an appropriate cognitive level, advocated for the involvement of Elder Affairs, and recommended transportation be provided to her hotel as the team did not believe Shirley was fit to drive her own vehicle. Later, the team personally followed up with her at her hotel and provided some basic groceries to limit her need to drive. In addition, advocacy helped to ensure Shirley received some special funding to support her in her housing transition. This story highlights occupational therapy's contribution—cognitive and physical assessment, case management, safety recommendations, and advocacy.

At the shelter, the team was given a table in a long hallway full of other resource tables. The shelter residents were required to visit this hallway every 48 hours to self-identify resources that might help them move out of the shelter. Residents referred to this place as "the Hallway of Doom." They felt exhausted at having to recount their stories over and over to each resource table and reported feeling defeated at being denied some services. Some residents expressed that they did not understand the processes, in terms of applying to different state and federal entities. The team observed the process and also found it overwhelming; perhaps that was the inherent nature of trying to piece together services for housing, health care, and other needs postdisaster. The team wondered whether some environmental and procedural adaptations might help. For example, an occupational profile on each client placed in the client's personal folder might help limit the need to relay the client's story repeatedly, reducing the cumulative effect of reliving the trauma. An environmental adaptation, such as organizing the resource tables by type of resource (housing, healthcare, youth needs, clothing, etc.) would limit the cognitive and emotional burden of searching for the correct or most helpful resource.

meal preparation and cleanup, financial management, health management and maintenance, and home maintenance. Unfortunately, when an individual's occupational performance and participation are negatively affected, occupational identity often is impacted as well. During the disaster recovery stage, occupational performance and participation in a variety of occupations are essential to manage the chaos and disruption created by the disaster (Smith and Scaffa, 2014).

Disasters not only have an impact on individuals. They "impact whole communities, resulting in potential community-wide economic, environmental, governmental, social and cultural disruptions" (Smith and Scaffa, 2014, p. 965). In the same way that performance patterns of individuals are interrupted by disaster, the roles and routines in the community are also affected. The roles and routines of community agencies, worksites, and places of worship must also adapt to address the challenges presented by disasters. The destruction of schools and worksites due to a disaster may make it challenging or impossible to participate in education and work-related occupations. Social participation and co-occupations with family, friends, and neighbors may be affected by widespread evacuations.

Impact of Disasters on Mental Health

The emotional impact of disaster can sometimes be more devastating than the loss of home and personal property and often lasts longer than the physical manifestations (Carroll, Morbey, Balogh, and Araoz, 2008). Typical emotional reactions to acute stress include fear, anger, depression, anxiety, grief, confusion, helplessness, hopelessness, and emotional numbing. These "traumatic stress reactions are normal reactions to abnormal circumstances" (SAMHSA, 2014. p. 59). If the emotional reactions are severe, these feelings can interfere with occupational performance, especially sleep, and cognitive functions such as decision-making and concentration. Children, older adults, and persons with physical and mental health challenges are especially at risk. If symptoms persist for more than 1 month and cause distress and/or impair social or work functioning, then a person may be diagnosed with post-traumatic stress disorder (PTSD). The mental health impact of a disaster is a function of proximity, intensity, and duration. The greater the intensity, the longer the duration, and the closer the proximity of the disaster, the more likely a person is to experience mental health problems (Hobfoll and De Vries, 2013).

Nearly 80% of people are exposed to some type of traumatic event in their lifetime; however, not everyone will develop mental health problems as a result (Rollins, 2012). An internal protective factor against the development of mental illness is self-compassion (Maheux and Price, 2016). Neff (2004) describes three elements of self-compassion: being kind and understanding toward oneself during difficult times, being mindful of painful thoughts and feelings, and accepting one's emotions as a normal part of the universal human experience. Social support is positively related to self-compassion (Maheux and Price, 2016).

Considerable evidence identifies social support as a protective factor against the development of mental health problems postdisaster (Neria, Besser, Kiper, and Westphal, 2010; Ozer, Best, Lipsey, and Weiss, 2003). Social support can come from individuals and the community. The community provides a sense of belonging and can offer communal coping in the event of shared traumatic experiences (Houston, First, and Danforth, 2018) or a sense of shared responsibility in response to disasters. Communities can exist in many forms, such as neighborhoods, cities, schools, workplaces, churches, professional associations, and virtual support groups.

Only about 10% of trauma/disaster survivors develop PTSD (Meyers, 2017). Yet it is still important to provide **trauma-informed care** (TIC) following a disaster. TIC is a strengths-based approach

> *that is grounded in an understanding of and responsiveness to the impact of trauma, that emphasizes physical, psychological, and emotional safety for both providers and survivors, and that creates opportunities for survivors to rebuild a sense of control and empowerment. (Hopper, Bassuk, and Olivet, 2010, p. 82)*

TIC has become the standard of care in mental health services and represents a paradigm shift from a focus on dysfunction and diagnosis (i.e., what is wrong with the person) to a focus on what has happened to the person (Smith and Scaffa, 2014). TIC emphasizes the importance of avoiding processes and practices that may retraumatize persons who already have histories of trauma (SAMHSA, 2014). TIC adheres to six important principles, rather than a prescribed set of practices or procedures. The principles include:

- Safety
- Trustworthiness and transparency
- Peer support
- Collaboration and mutuality
- Empowerment, voice, and choice
- Sensitivity to cultural, historical, and gender issues (SAMHSA, 2018)

One example of a TIC approach is psychological first aid.

Engage Your Brain 26-2

What mental health competencies should an occupational therapy practitioner have to volunteer in disaster situations? How does one acquire these competencies?

Psychological first aid (PFA) is designed to reduce the initial distress experienced with trauma and to facilitate positive adaptive functioning in the short and long term. PFA is appropriate for all age groups and developmental levels. It is flexible and applicable in a variety of disaster situations. There are five essential elements to PFA: (a) providing a sense of safety, (b) promoting calming, (c) fostering a sense of self- and community efficacy, (d) encouraging connectedness, and (e) instilling hope (Hobfoll et al., 2007). Trained volunteers offer PFA immediately postdisaster (usually within 48 hours) after the basic needs for food, shelter, and safety are met, and people are working to reestablish their daily routines. It provides information, comfort, and practical support tailored to the needs of individual survivors (SAMHSA, 2014).

PFA intervention strategies "represent the approaches most consistently supported by research and practice" (Vernberg et al., 2008, p. 387) and are grouped into eight core actions or modules:

- Contact and engagement
- Safety and comfort
- Stabilization
- Information gathering (current needs and concerns)
- Practical assistance
- Connection with social supports
- Information on coping
- Linkage with collaborative services (Vernberg et al., 2008)

PFA attempts to foster resilience. **Resilience** refers to "the ability to bounce back or rise above adversity as an individual, family, community, or provider. Well beyond individual characteristics of hardiness, resilience includes the process of using available resources to negotiate hardship and/or the consequences of adverse events" (SAMHSA, 2014, p. xviii). More simply, resilience is the ability to return to baseline functioning after trauma. However, in addition to facilitating resilience, mental health intervention postdisaster can foster **posttraumatic growth** (PTG), improvement beyond pretrauma adaptation that can sometimes be deeply profound (Tedeschi and Calhoun, 2004).

PTG is a "positive psychological change experienced as the result of the struggle with highly challenging life circumstances" (Tedeschi and Calhoun, 2004, p. 1). It is the *cognitive* and *emotional* "*struggle* [emphasis added] with the new reality in the aftermath of trauma" (p. 5) that is crucial for PTG to occur. The five domains in which positive changes typically take place in the PTG process include:

- Greater appreciation of life and a changed sense of priorities
- Greater sense of personal strength and capabilities
- Deeper, more meaningful relationships with others
- Recognition of new possibilities or paths for one's life
- Richer spiritual life and/or renewal (Rollins, 2012).

Three factors appear to facilitate PTG:

1. The individual personality characteristics of extraversion, positive affect, optimism, ability to manage distressing emotions, and openness to experience
2. The degree to which a person discloses her or his feelings and perceptions of the

traumatic event (tells the story) and the social support the person receives in response to that disclosure

3. Cognitive processing of the event/trauma in which resolving discrepancy and developing new life schemas are the outcomes (Tedeschi and Calhoun, 2004).

An occupational therapy approach to addressing mental health needs postdisaster and facilitating PTG is the use of the recovery model outlined by SAMHSA (Pizzi, 2015). The recovery model consists of 10 components: self-directed, individualized and client centered, empowerment, holistic, nonlinear, strengths-based, peer support, respect, responsibility, and hope. The recovery model can be used as a frame of reference for community- and population-based occupational therapy intervention in disaster recovery. Based on research of survivors' reactions to Hurricane Sandy, Pizzi (2015) identified potential occupational therapy interventions for each of the 10 components.

Populations With Special Needs

FEMA (2016) defines **special needs populations** as

> *those whose members may have additional needs before, during, and after an incident in functional areas, including but not limited to: maintaining independence, communication, transportation, supervision, and medical care. Individuals in need of additional response assistance may include those who have disabilities, live in institutionalized settings, are elderly, are children, are from diverse cultures, have limited English proficiency or are non-English speaking, or are transportation disadvantaged. (para. 42)*

People with disabilities (PWD) are at particular risk during disaster situations. Evacuation is often challenging at best and unsafe at worst. In addition, PWD often find themselves in emergency locations or shelters not specifically designed to accommodate their needs (AOTA, 2011). The collapse of infrastructure common in disasters affects everyone, "but it disadvantages persons with disabilities disproportionately" (Smith and Scaffa, 2014, p. 968). Since there are an infinite number of activity limitations, no one solution is appropriate for all persons with disabilities in DPRR. Occupational therapy practitioners can modify and adapt shelter, home, and community environments to promote safety and more independent function.

Older adults, particularly those who are homebound, are at high risk. The number of older adults is increasing with the aging of the baby boomers, yet little attention is being given to disaster resilience for older adults (Shih et al., 2018). Occupational therapy practitioners can not only help individuals prepare for disasters in at-risk areas but also work in coordination with public health departments and age-friendly communities to add disaster preparation to aging-in-place plans (see Chapter 12 for more information on aging in place).

Children have been disproportionally affected by disasters, as they are affected by all types, including school shootings. Schools provide students a sense of community and are frequently part of a community emergency plan. Occupational therapy practitioners working in the school system need to help allay students' fears following a disaster. Students need to be able to express their emotions and ask questions; however, school staff have expressed a need for assistance with this type of communication. Researchers have also found that providing students an opportunity to help others affected by disaster helps students address feelings of helplessness and powerlessness (Houston et al., 2018).

Others who are vulnerable, but not included in the FEMA definition of special needs populations, are the disaster relief workers. Disaster relief workers, both volunteer and professional, are usually the first on the scene of a disaster and may witness a variety of traumatic events (Lanza, Roysircar, and Rodgers, 2018). They work long hours under difficult conditions and are frequently expected to engage in tasks that could potentially result in injury or even death. Even though the emergency management system has procedures in place for debriefing professional first responders following traumatic events, approximately 30% develop mental health problems such as depression and PTSD, compared with 20% in the general population (Abbott et al., 2015). First responders are at high risk for vicarious traumatization, compassion fatigue, and burnout.

Each disaster situation is different, and as a result the needs of disaster relief workers and volunteers will vary from disaster to disaster. For this reason, Lanza et al. (2018) recommend psychoeducation for responder self-care to maintain resilience prior to deployment to the area, immediately after the trauma exposure, and long-term, if necessary. Self-care areas upon which to focus are "self-reflection journaling, eating well, prioritizing sleep and rest, expressing emotions, attending to family relationships, connecting with friends and one's community, embracing religion or spirituality, engaging in cognitive activities, and attending to financial and physical security" (Lanza et al., 2018, p. 196).

Role of Theory in Disaster Preparedness, Response, and Recovery

Best practice in DPRR involves using theory-based interventions. Concepts inherent in occupation-based models include the interaction of person, occupation, and environment. Choosing the most appropriate occupation-based model is dependent upon how the person, occupation, and environment or their interactions have been affected by the disaster. The model of human occupation (Kielhofner, 2009) can be very helpful in focusing on the importance of establishing routines in temporary shelters or in regaining a balance of roles in the disaster recovery stage. In the case of forced relocation, the model of occupational adaptation (OA; Schkade and Schultz, 1992; Schultz and Schkade, 1992) is useful in understanding the press for mastery the new environment demands. Through OA, mature adaptive response behaviors can be facilitated.

It is common for disaster survivors to gain a new or renewed spiritual focus following a traumatic event. For this reason, the Canadian model of occupational performance and engagement having spirituality at its core (Polatajko et al., 2007) may be the most appropriate approach to use. Spirituality is often associated with improved mental health outcomes; it contributes to recovery by providing comfort and hope. The ecology of human performance model (Dunn, Brown, and McGuigan, 1994), with its levels of intervention such as restore and create, may fit well when occupational therapy practitioners are working with a community.

One means of coping with a disaster is by sense making or narrative making (Houston et al., 2018). According to Pizzi (2015), "personal narratives about living through a natural disaster can assist in the recovery" of the persons affected (p. 9). This type of communication can transpire interpersonally or in social systems in the community. The process of sense making or narrative reasoning can lead to benefit finding, or finding an upside to a traumatic event, but this occurs only over time (Nolen-Hoeksema and Davis, 2002).

Engage Your Brain 26-3

Considering the types of disasters that are likely to occur in your state, which theory or combination of theories would you choose to use with disaster survivors? Why?

Disaster Preparedness

Disaster preparedness involves planning at the household, organizational, and community levels before the disaster in order to enable an effective population-based response when an emergency occurs. This requires planned interventions designed to address system-level concerns. For example, organizations and businesses should develop emergency response plans, train employees how to manage emergency situations, acquire needed supplies and equipment, and conduct response drills and exercises (AOTA, 2011; Tierney, Lindell, and Perry, 2001).

Schools are often the most likely place that children will be when a disaster occurs. School disaster planning is essential and typically consists of identifying school crisis teams, delineating the roles of staff during an emergency, and establishing processes for reuniting children with their parents. Occupational therapy practitioners who work in academic settings (e.g., grades K through 12 schools, universities) can assist in school planning regarding the requirements of students with special needs (AOTA, 2011).

Carra, Hyett, Kenny, and Curtin (2018) recommend occupational therapists work with communities to support their recovery from collective trauma. Three strategies they suggest require planning and include working with communities to design programs aligned with community strengths and weaknesses, using therapeutic occupations in the recovery, and developing a strong community network system (Carra et al., 2018, p. 2).

It is also important for occupational therapy practitioners to have disaster plans in place for themselves and their families, as they may need to remain on duty at their workplaces for an extended period of time during a disaster (AOTA, 2011). For more examples of potential occupational therapy roles during disaster preparedness, see Table 26-2.

Disaster Response

Emergency response consists of actions taken just prior to, during, and shortly after disaster impact to address the immediate needs of victims and to reduce damage, destruction, and disruption. Disaster response activities include the detection of threats, dissemination of warnings, evacuation of vulnerable populations, search for and rescue of victims, provision of emergency medical care, and furnishing of food and shelter for displaced persons (AOTA, 2011; Tierney et al., 2001). It is important to prioritize interventions based on a hierarchy of needs. Most important are survival, safety, and security, followed by food, shelter, and

Table 26-2 Potential Occupational Therapy Roles During Disaster Preparedness, Response, and Recovery

Stage of Disaster	Occupational Therapy Roles
Preparedness	• Assist businesses and employers in developing plans for emergency evacuation of employees with disabilities • Design and adapt spaces in health-care facilities for emergency response and plan support services for patients, families, and caregivers • Participate in facility-level and community-wide disaster-planning efforts • Design special needs shelters to minimize environmental barriers and train staff and volunteers • Educate families/clients about creating a family disaster plan and strategies for sheltering in place
Response	• Assist in the evacuation of vulnerable populations and their service animals and medical equipment • Modify and adapt shelter environments to promote safety and more independent function • Provide supportive mental health services to victims and their families, first responders, and volunteers • Provide support and assistance to those sheltering in place • Provide occupation-based interventions in shelters • Facilitate support groups designed to reduce anxiety and stress • Supervise staff and volunteers at special needs shelters
Recovery	• Help people resume participation in occupations, reestablish meaningful routines, and redesign/adapt lifestyles to the new reality • Provide occupation-based, psychoeducational mental health services • Facilitate adaptation to temporary housing (e.g., FEMA trailers) or assist individuals and families to transition out of shelters into permanent housing • Encourage community leaders and others to reorganize community supports and routines to meet the needs of those affected by the disaster

Sources: "The Role of Occupational Therapy in Disaster Preparedness, Response, and Recovery," by American Occupational Therapy Association, 2011, *American Journal of Occupational Therapy, 65*(Suppl. 6), pp. S11–S25.
Disaster Preparedness and Response (DP&R), by World Federation of Occupational Therapists, 2016b. Retrieved from www.wfot.org/Practice/DisasterPreparednessandResponseDPR.aspx

health care (National Institute of Mental Health [NIMH], 2002).

Occupational therapy practitioners are especially qualified to provide disaster response services for people with special needs. These include persons with physical, mental, or medical-care needs who may require assistance before, during, or after a disaster when they have exhausted their usual resources and support systems. People with special needs may be evacuated to general public shelters or shelters for people with special needs, or they may shelter in place (i.e., remain in their personal homes, assisted living facilities, foster and group homes, or long-term care facilities). Occupational therapy expertise is useful in all of these settings and situations (AOTA, 2011).

After conducting a quick, basic needs assessment, occupational therapy practitioners can provide appropriate interventions wherever people are sheltering. These might include identifying and emphasizing people's strengths, encouraging the creative expression of feelings, providing structure in daily routines, coordinating age-appropriate play for children, and offering opportunities for stress management. Therapeutic play should be initiated with children, so they can express themselves (Smith and Picone, 2018). Engaging survivors in purposeful and meaningful occupations and routines as they adjust to the disaster-imposed changes in their lives can help them regain a sense of mastery and relieve stress. For more examples of potential occupational therapy roles during disaster response, see Table 26-2.

Disaster Recovery

Recovery is often a long-term process of addressing physical, psychological, emotional, social, and spiritual needs. It involves the repair and rebuilding of property, restoration of public utilities, and reestablishment of social and economic activities that were disrupted by the disaster. Occupational therapy practitioners can advocate for accessible environments postdisaster—for example, in displaced persons camps and in rebuilding homes and community facilities (WFOT, 2016b).

Children need to return to school and its routine even if classes are held in temporary quarters (Rao, 2006). Reopening schools as soon as possible provides age-appropriate occupational engagement for children (Hobfoll et al., 2007). According to the American Academy of Pediatrics Council on School Health (2008), "although returning to the classroom does not ensure that children are ready to address learning tasks, evidence points to the restorative power of the educational routine in guiding children through emotional crises" (p. 898).

Recovery efforts are designed to reduce acute stress, foster resilience, reestablish roles and routines, and enhance the psychosocial well-being and the quality of life of the community members affected (Tierney et al., 2001). Occupational engagement reduces the intensity of stressful events and helps reestablish a sense of mastery in a situation in which a child or adult feels a loss of control (AOTA, 2011).

Occupational therapy practitioners can also address the short-term and long-term mental health sequelae of disasters. Examples include assessing the mental health status of survivors and first responders, with subsequent referral for mental health services as needed or training volunteers to administer quick mental health screening tools in order to provide more immediate services for greater numbers of people (WFOT, 2016b). Developing and implementing occupation-focused mental health services in the community is another possibility. Unfortunately, occupational therapists are not considered certified mental health service providers in many states, which is a barrier to the profession's full participation in DPRR. The AOTA is working toward solving this problem (Smith and Scaffa, 2014).

Disasters often disrupt the habits and routines that sustain role enactment. Roles contribute to one's identity and sense of self and help identify the responsibilities associated with that identity (Deeny and McFetridge, 2005; Kielhofner, Forsyth, and Barrett, 2003). After a disaster, roles, such as student or worker, may be permanently or temporarily lost. If displaced from one's home and community, some roles, like those of family member or friend, may need to be adapted or maintained from a distance. Other roles may also need to be adapted or expanded. Changes in context may require the adoption of new roles, such as volunteer, renter, or home remodeler. Occupational therapy practitioners are skilled at helping clients successfully navigate periods of transition and can help clients adjust to the role changes necessitated by a disaster. Through engagement in occupation, survivors can restructure their habits and routines to participate in their valued life roles (AOTA, 2011). For more examples of potential occupational therapy roles during disaster recovery, see Table 26-2.

Summary

- The purpose of an all-hazards approach is to develop the capabilities and strategies to prepare for and respond to a variety of potential disasters (i.e., natural, technological, and intentional), rather than creating a specific plan for each different type of emergency.
- If occupational therapy practitioners want to become involved in DPRR, it is important to understand the roles of the governmental agencies and nonprofit organizations in emergency management, how occupational therapy might fit in with their missions, and strategies to gain entry into these systems.
- Disasters have "significant negative impact, both short- and long-term, on the health and occupational engagement of individuals, families, and communities," and therefore occupational therapy practitioners have a role in disaster planning, response, and recovery (AOTA, 2011, p. S11).
- TIC is an evidence-based practice that has become the standard of care in mental health services. TIC represents a paradigm shift from a focus on dysfunction and diagnosis (what is wrong with the person) to a focus on what has happened to the person.
- Occupational therapy practitioners are especially qualified to provide disaster response services for people with special needs. These include persons with physical, mental, or medical-care needs who may require assistance before, during, or after a disaster when they have exhausted their usual resources and support systems.
- Occupational therapy practitioners can use their professional expertise in all stages of DPRR—for example, assisting in planning for the evacuation of persons with disabilities in the disaster preparation stage, managing special needs shelters in the disaster response stage, and facilitating the normalization of habits, roles, and routines in the disaster recovery stage.

CASE STUDIES

CASE STUDY 26-1 Lydia

Lydia, age 55, lives in a suburb of Houston, Texas, in a neighborhood that incurred heavy flooding from Hurricane Harvey. Her neighborhood had never flooded before, so she did not evacuate ahead of the hurricane and required rescue, along with her two dogs, by the Cajun Navy in a privately owned speedboat. She and her dogs were taken to a shelter that allowed pets and then later housed in a hotel room with an apartment-sized refrigerator and microwave until her home could be repaired. She returned home after 6 months.

Lydia has changed her routine since returning home. She no longer stays after work to socialize with coworkers, stating she needs to leave and catch the bus home because she lost her car in the flood. She is having difficulty getting to sleep and on average has a nightmare every 3 weeks. Lydia has gained 15 pounds and is no longer coloring her hair. Although she used to stay in frequent contact with her family in Florida and close friends in Texas and California, she no longer does. Lydia is worried that she is no more prepared for the next hurricane season than she was in 2017.

Discussion Questions

1. How could an occupational therapy practitioner help Lydia improve her sleep?
2. What occupational therapy theory or model would you use in Lydia's treatment, and how would you apply it?
3. How could the occupational therapy practitioner help Lydia prepare for the next hurricane season?
4. What should Lydia do now to prepare for the next hurricane season?

CASE STUDY 26-2 Impact of Oil Spill Disaster on Occupational Engagement

On April 20, 2010, the Deepwater Horizon oil rig exploded in flames, spilling at least 20,000 barrels, or 840,000 gallons, of oil each day into the Gulf of Mexico. The oil spill is noted as one of the largest environmental disasters in history. A group of occupational therapy students and their instructor designed a research project to:

- Assess the impact of the 2010 Deepwater Horizon oil spill disaster on the daily lives, roles, habits, routines, and occupational participation of persons living and working on the Gulf Coast
- Identify the psychosocial impact of the disaster on Gulf Coast residents, identifying the stressors they experience and their emotional reactions to those stressors and the adaptation and coping strategies used
- Identify potential interventions to improve the health of individuals, families, and the community (Scaffa and Sasse, 2011)

For this needs assessment, the students employed a phenomenological approach using semistructured interviews of 31 persons (15 women, 16 men) aged 31 to 75 living and working on the Gulf Coast in Orange Beach, Alabama. Work occupations of the participants were diverse and included law enforcement, boat captain, reservationist, real estate broker, plant operator, cashier/sales clerk, college instructor, firefighter, insurance agent, information technology and web developer, mural painter, offshore oil field supplier, recreation center attendant, and restaurant cook.

During the interviews, many of the residents who initially stated they were not affected by the oil spill disaster realized that even though they had not experienced financial or employment losses, they were affected in other ways. For example, they described loss of leisure opportunities, decreased social interactions with family and friends, stress-related illnesses, and feelings of frustration and sadness over the "loss of a way of life." Many expressed gratitude and relief for the opportunity to talk about their concerns and experiences.

The research results indicated that the most frequent losses/stressors experienced by residents were financial losses, relationship stressors, lost leisure activities, health problems, and legal issues. Their most prevalent emotional reactions were anger, anxiety, depression, pessimism, fear, helplessness, and cynicism. Overwhelmingly, they responded with positive and healthy coping strategies—for example, cognitive reframing, optimism, behavioral adaptations, spirituality, altruism, and social support.

Some quotes from the interviewees include:

- "Right now I am basically working for a paycheck. Before, I had everything planned out, what I wanted to do, and uh, I just don't have any hopes of meeting those goals. I've had to readjust everything."
- "My main desire is to paint. And that is where it has affected me. With the oil spill, restaurants and businesses on the beach scene where I contract to paint murals, well, those businesses folded. The people just cannot use the paintings anymore."
- "I probably sleep more on my off days than I used to. All you want to do is rest and sleep. You know, you just don't want to do anything else."
- "It affected our summer because our routine during the summer is to spend our time at the beach and in the water. We are boating people, so it was pretty traumatic in the sense that we and our friends really didn't know what to do with ourselves because there's really not a lot to do down here unless you're involved in water activity."
- "My husband loves to fish, and he actually sold his boat because he didn't think he wanted to catch those fish."
- "I'm actually on two different medications for anxiety. I can't sleep at night, I'm grinding my teeth at night, or not sleeping at all."
- "I lost my job. Lost my income, about to lose my house, about to lose the only car that I have."

The majority of participants had intact skills following the disaster but had difficulty in the area of habituation. Disruption in roles, routines, and daily habits were experienced by a significant number of interviewees. In addition, some expressed a lack of motivation to participate in occupations and decreased self-efficacy and the need to adjust their goals for the future (Scaffa and Sasse, 2011).

CASE STUDY 26-2 Impact of Oil Spill Disaster on Occupational Engagement

Discussion Questions

1. What other strategies might the students have used to address their research questions?
2. What occupational therapy and/or population health theories or models might you use to understand and explain the results? Why did you choose these, and how do they apply?
3. Based on the research results, what occupational therapy interventions might be appropriate for this population?

Learning Activities

1. Contact a local governmental agency or nonprofit organization involved in disaster response (e.g., the ARC, your local EMA, the SA) and interview a relief worker about a disaster during which they provided services.
2. Take an online course from the Emergency Management Institute or review training materials for becoming a member of a CERT.
3. Create your own disaster readiness plan or disaster kit. There are templates and instructions for these on a number of websites, including FEMA, the American Red Cross, and Ready.gov.

REFERENCES

Abbott, C., Barber, E., Burke, B., Harvey, J., Newland, C., Rose, M., and Young, A. (2015). *What's killing our medics? Ambulance service manager program.* Conifer, CO: Reviving Responders. Retrieved from www.revivingresponders.com/originalpaper/pt5lehsknczsaofld89leijbmehz3c

American Academy of Pediatrics Council on School Health. (2008). Disaster planning for schools. *Pediatrics, 122*(4), 895–901.

American Occupational Therapy Association. (2006). The role of occupational therapy in disaster preparedness, response, and recovery. *American Journal of Occupational Therapy, 60*(6), 642–649.

American Occupational Therapy Association. (2011). The role of occupational therapy in disaster preparedness, response, and recovery. *American Journal of Occupational Therapy, 65*(Suppl. 6), S11–S25.

American Occupational Therapy Association. (2014). Occupational therapy practice framework: Domain and process (3rd ed.). *American Journal of Occupational Therapy, 68*(Suppl. 1), S1–S48.

American Occupational Therapy Association. (2015). Occupational therapy code of ethics (2015). *American Journal of Occupational Therapy, 69*(Suppl. 3), 6913410030.

American Occupational Therapy Association. (2017). AOTA's societal statement on disaster response and risk reduction. *American Journal of Occupational Therapy, 71*(Suppl. 2), 7112410060

American Red Cross. (2018). *Disaster relief.* Retrieved from www.redcross.org/about-us/our-work/disaster-relief.html

Canton, L. G. (2013). "All-hazards" doesn't mean "plan for everything." *Emergency Management.* Retrieved from www.govtech.com/em/emergency-blogs/managing-

Carra, K., Hyett, N., Kenny, A., and Curtin, M. (2018). Strengthening occupational therapy practice with communities after traumatic events. *British Journal of Occupational Therapy, 0*(0), 1–4. doi:10.1177/0308022618795594

Carroll, B., Morbey, H., Balogh, R., and Araoz, G. (2008). Flooded homes, broken bonds, the meaning of home, psychological processes and their impact on psychological health in disaster. *Health and Place, 15,* 540–547. doi:10.1016/j.healthplace.2008.08.009

CNN. (2018a). *2011 Japan earthquake—tsunami fast facts.* Retrieved from www.cnn.com/2013/07/17/world/asia/japan-earthquake—tsunami-fast-facts/index.html

CNN. (2018b). *U.S. terrorist attacks fast facts.* Retrieved from www.cnn.com/2013/04/18/us/u-s-terrorist-attacks-fast-facts/index.html

Deeny, P., and McFetridge, B. (2005). The impact of disaster on culture, self, and identity: Increased awareness by health care professionals is needed. *Nursing Clinics of North America, 40*(3), 431–440.

Dunn, W., Brown, C., and McGuigan, A. (1994). The ecology of human performance: A framework for considering the effect of context. *American Journal of Occupational Therapy, 48,* 595–607.

Emergency Management. (2016). *What is a technological disaster?* Retrieved from www.emergency-management-degree.org/faq/what-is-a-technological-disaster/

Federal Bureau of Investigation. (n.d.). *What we investigate: Hate crimes.* Retrieved from www.fbi.gov/investigate/civil-rights/hate-crimes

Federal Emergency Management Agency. (2016). *Glossary/acronyms of key terms for the national disaster housing strategy.* Retrieved from www.fema.gov/glossary/acronyms-key-terms-national-disaster-housing-strategy

Federal Emergency Management Agency. (2017). *National Incident Management* System (3rd ed.) Retrieved from www.fema.gov/media-library-data/1508151197225-ced8c60378c3936adb92c1a3ee6f6564/FINAL_NIMS_2017.pdf

Federal Emergency Management Agency. (2018a). *Agency: History.* Retrieved from www.fema.gov/about-agency

Federal Emergency Management Agency. (2018b). *Welcome to the Emergency Management Institute.* Retrieved from https://training.fema.gov/emi.aspx

History.com. (2018). *Columbine shooting.* Retrieved from www.history.com/topics/1990s/columbine-high-school-shootings

Hobfoll, S. E., and de Vries, M. W. (2013). *Extreme stress and communities: Impact and intervention.* New York, NY: Springer.

Hobfoll, S. E., Watson, P. E., Bell, C. C., Bryant, R. A., Brymer, M. J., Friedman, M. J., . . . Ursano, R. J. (2007). Five essential elements of immediate and mid-term mass trauma intervention: Empirical evidence. *Psychiatry: Interpersonal and Biological Processes, 70,* 283–315.

Hopper, E. K., Bassuk, E. L., and Olivet, J. (2010). Shelter from the storm: Trauma-informed care in homelessness services settings. *Open Health Services and Policy Journal, 3,* 80–100.

Houston, J. B., First, J., and Danforth, L. M. (2018). Students coping with the effects of disaster media coverage: A qualitative study of school staff perceptions. *School Mental Health.* Retrieved from https://doi.org/10.1007/s12310-018-9295-y

Humane Society of the United States. (2018). *Disaster relief.* Retrieved from www.humanesociety.org/disaster-relief

Insurance Information Institute. (2019a). *Background on: Wildfires.* Retrieved from www.iii.org/article/background-on-wildfires

Insurance Information Institute. (2019b). *Facts+statistics: U.S. catastrophes.* Retrieved from www.iii.org/fact-statistic/facts-statistics-us-catastrophes

International Critical Incident Stress Foundation. (n.d.a). *What is critical incident stress management?* Retrieved from https://icisf.org/about-us/

International Critical Incident Stress Foundation. (n.d.b). *What we offer.* Retrieved from https://icisf.org/

Johnston, W. J. (2018). Terrorist attacks and related incidents in the United States. Retrieved from www.johnstonsarchive.net/terrorism/wrjp255a.html

Kielhofner, G. (2009). *Conceptual foundations of occupational therapy practice* (4th ed.). Philadelphia, PA: F. A. Davis.

Kielhofner, G., Forsyth, K., and Barrett, L. (2003). The model of human occupation. In E. B. Crepeau, E. S. Cohn, and B. A. Boyt Schell (Eds.), *Willard and Spackman's occupational therapy* (pp. 212–219). Philadelphia, PA: Lippincott Williams and Wilkins.

Lanza, A., Roysircar, G., and Rodgers, S. (2018). First responder mental healthcare: Evidence-based prevention, postvention, and treatment. *Professional Psychology: Research and Practice, 49*(3), 193–204. https://doi.org/10.1037/pro0000192

Lewis, C. S. (1986). *Present concerns: A compelling collection of timely journalistic essays.* London, United Kingdom: C. S. Lewis PTE.

Lindsey, A. B., Donovan, M., Smith, S., Radunovich, H., and Gutter, M. (2017). *Impacts of technological disasters.* Retrieved from http://edis.ifas.ufl.edu/pdffiles/FY/FY123000.pdf

Maheux, A., and Price, M. (2016). The indirect effect of social support on post-trauma psychopathology via self-compassion. *Personality and Individual Differences, 88,* 102–107. http://dx.doi.org/10.1016/j.paid.2015.08.051

Meyers, L. (2017). Lending a helping hand in disaster's wake. *Counseling Today.* Retrieved from https://ct.counseling.org/2017/07/lending-helping-hand-disasters-wake/

National Geographic. (n.d.a). *Earthquakes can happen in more places than you think.* Retrieved from https://news.nationalgeographic.com/2017/08/earthquake-fault-quakeland-kathryn-miles

National Geographic. (n.d.b). *Tornadoes.* Retrieved from www.nationalgeographic.com/environment/natural-disasters/tornadoes/

National Institute of Mental Health. (2002). *Mental health and mass violence: Evidence-based early intervention for victims/survivors of mass violence.* Publication No. 02-5138. Washington, DC: U.S. Government Printing Office.

National Voluntary Organizations Active in Disaster. (2014). *Who we are.* Retrieved from www.nvoad.org/about-us/

Neff, K. D. (2004). Self-compassion and psychological well-being. *Constructivism in the Human Sciences, 9,* 27–37.

Neria, Y., Besser, A., Kiper, D., and Westphal, M. (2010). A longitudinal study of posttraumatic stress disorder, depression, and generalized anxiety disorder in Israel civilians exposed to war trauma. *Journal of Traumatic Stress, 23*(3), 322–330. http://doi.org/10.1002/jts.20522

Nolen-Hoeksema, S., and Davis, C. G. (2002). Positive responses to loss perceiving benefits and growth. In C. R. Snyder and S. J. Lopez (Eds.), *Handbook of positive psychology* (pp. 584–597). New York, NY: Oxford University Press.

Oakley, F., Caswell, S., and Parks, R. (2008). The issue is . . . occupational therapists' role on U.S. Army and U.S. Public Health Service Commissioned Corps disaster mental health response teams. *American Journal of Occupational Therapy, 62*(3), 361–364.

Ozer, E. J., Best, S. R., Lipsey, T. L., and Weiss, D. S. (2003). Predictors of posttraumatic stress disorder and symptoms in adults: A meta-analysis. *Psychological Bulletin, 129*(1), 52–73.

Pizzi, M. A. (2015). Hurricane Sandy, disaster preparedness, and the recovery model. *American Journal of Occupational Therapy, 69,* 6904250010. http://dx.doi.org/10.5014/ajot.2015.015990

Polatajko, H. J., Davis, J., Stewart, D., Cantin, N., Amoroso, B., Purdie, L., and Zimmerman, D. (2007). Specifying the domain of concern: Occupation as core. In E. A. Townsend and H. J. Polatajko (Eds.), *Enabling occupation II: Advancing an occupational therapy vision for health, well-being, and justice through occupation* (pp. 13–36). Ottawa, Canada: CAOT Publications ACE.

Rao, K. (2006). Psychosocial support in disaster-affected communities. *International Review of Psychiatry, 18,* 501–505. doi:10.1080/0954020601038472

Rollins, J. (2012). The transformative power of trauma. *Counseling Today.* Retrieved from https://ct.counseling.org/2012/02/the-transformative-power-of-trauma/

Salvation Army. (2018). *After the unspeakable, we speak hope.* Retrieved from www.salvationarmyusa.org/usn/help-disaster-survivors/

Scaffa, M. E., and Sasse, C. S. (2011, April). *Impact of the Gulf of Mexico oil spill on occupation.* Poster presentation at the American Occupational Therapy Association Annual Conference, Philadelphia, PA.

Schkade, J. K., and Schultz, S. (1992). Occupational adaptation: Toward a holistic approach for contemporary practice, part 1. *American Journal of Occupational Therapy, 46*(9), 829–837. https://doi.org/10.5014/ajot.46.9.829

Schultz, S., and Schkade, J. K. (1992). Occupational adaptation: Toward a holistic approach for contemporary practice, part 2. *American Journal of Occupational Therapy, 46*(10), 917–925. https://doi.org/10.5014/ajot.46.10.917

Sharkey, P. (2007). Survival and death in New Orleans: An empirical look at the human impact of Katrina. *Journal of Black Studies, 37*(4), 482–501.

Shih, R. A., Acosta, J. D., Chen, E. K., Carbone, E. G., Xenakis, L., Adamson, D. M., and Chandra, A. (2018). Improving disaster resilience among older adults: Insights from public health departments and aging-in-place efforts. *Rand Health Quarterly, 8*(1), 3.

Smith, T. M., Drefus, A., and Hersch, G. (2011). Effects of hurricane Ike on graduate students' habits, routines and roles. *Occupational Therapy in Health Care, 25*(4), 283–297.

Smith, T. M., and Picone, N. (2018). Providing occupational therapy for disaster survivors. In B. Schell and G. Gillen (Eds.), *Willard and Spackman's occupational therapy* (13th ed., pp. 1065–1077). Baltimore, MD: Wolters Kluwer.

Smith, T. M., and Scaffa, M. E. (2014). Providing occupational therapy for disaster survivors. In B. Schell, G. Gillen, and M. Scaffa (Eds.), *Willard and Spackman's occupational therapy* (12th ed., pp. 962–972). Baltimore, MD: Wolters Kluwer.

Substance Abuse and Mental Health Services Administration. (2014). *Trauma-informed care in behavioral health services: Treatment Improvement Protocol (TIP) Series 57.* HHS Publication No. (SMA) 13-4801. Rockville, MD: Substance Abuse and Mental Health Services Administration.

Substance Abuse and Mental Health Services Administration. (2018). *Trauma-informed approach and trauma-specific interventions.* Retrieved from www.samhsa.gov/nctic/trauma-interventions

Tedeschi, R. G., and Calhoun, L.G. (2004). Posttraumatic growth: Conceptual foundations and empirical evidence. *Psychological Inquiry, 15*(1), 1–18.

Tierney, K. J., Lindell, M. K., and Perry, R. W. (2001). *Facing the unexpected: Disaster preparedness and response in the United States.* Washington, DC: Joseph Henry Press.

United Nations Centre for Research on the Epidemiology of Disasters. (2018). *Economic losses, poverty and disasters, 1998–2017.* Retrieved from cred.be/unisdr-and-cred-report-economic-losses-poverty-disasters-1998-2017

U.S. Department of Health and Human Services. (n.d.). *Commissioned Corps of the U.S. Public Health Service: Mission and core values.* Retrieved from https://usphs.gov/aboutus/mission.aspx

U.S. Department of Homeland Security. (n.d.). *Community emergency response team.* Retrieved from www.ready.gov/community-emergency-response-team

U.S. Department of Homeland Security. (2013). *National response framework* (2nd ed.). Retrieved from www.fema.gov/media-library-data/20130726-1914-25045-8516/final_national_response_framework_20130501.pdf

U.S. Department of Homeland Security. (2017). *About DHS.* Retrieved from www.dhs.gov/about-dhs

Vernberg, E. M., Steinberg, A. M., Jacobs, A. K., Brymer, M. J., Watson, P. J., Osofsky, J. D., . . . Ruzek, J. I. (2008). Innovations in disaster mental health: Psychological first aid. *Professional Psychology: Research and Practice, 39*(4), 381–388.

Vox. (2018). *After Sandy Hook, we said never again.* Retrieved from www.vox.com/a/mass-shootings-america-sandy-hook-gun-violence

Weather Channel. (2018). *New list of the costliest U.S. hurricanes includes 2017's Harvey, Irma, Maria.* Retrieved from https://weather.com/storms/hurricane/news/2018-01-29-americas-costliest-hurricanes

Westword. (2018). *Parkland school shooting 208th since Columbine: The tragic list.* Retrieved from www.westword.com/news/parkland-to-columbine-school-shootings-list-9993641

World Federation of Occupational Therapists. (2016a). *Disaster management for occupational therapists.* Retrieved from https://dmot.wfot.org/

World Federation of Occupational Therapists. (2016b). *Disaster preparedness and response (DP&R).* Retrieved from www.wfot.org/Practice/DisasterPreparednessandResponseDPR.aspx

World Health Organization. (2018). *Disaster preparedness and response: Policy.* Retrieved from www.euro.who.int/en/health-topics/emergencies/disaster-preparedness-and-response/policy

World Health Organization. (2019). *Myths and realities in disaster situations.* Retrieved from www.who.int/hac/techguidance/ems/myths/en/

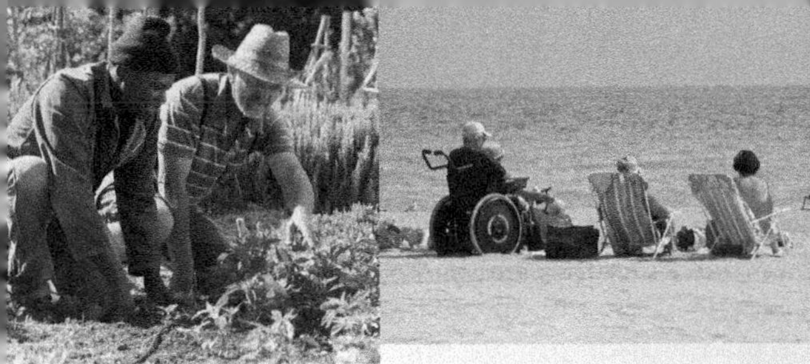
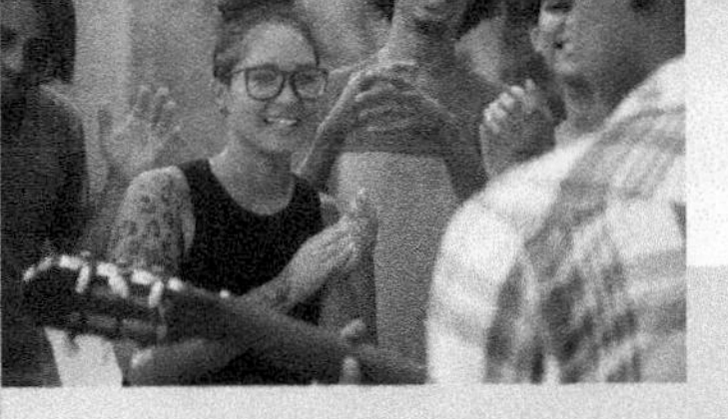

Chapter 27

Violence Prevention and Mitigation

Susan Cahill, PhD, OTR/L, FAOTA, Janie B. Scott, MA, OT/L, FAOTA, S. Maggie Reitz, PhD, OTR/L, FAOTA, and Leah K. Cox, PhD

But no one knows me no one ever will
If I don't say something, if I just lie still
Would I be that monster, scare them all away
If I let them hear what I have to say
I can't keep quiet, no oh oh oh oh oh oh
I can't keep quiet, no oh oh oh oh oh oh
A one woman riot, oh oh oh oh oh oh oh
I can't keep quiet
For anyone
Anymore

—From the song "Quiet," by MILCK (2017)

Learning Outcomes

This chapter is designed to enable the reader to:

27-1 Define and differentiate terms related to violence.
27-2 Discuss causal links to violence.
27-3 Identify the prevalence rates for harassment and violence among at-risk populations.
27-4 Describe evidence-based and evolving innovative strategies to address violence in families, schools, sports and leisure venues, online, and the workplace.
27-5 Develop occupation-focused and occupation-based community-based and population health strategies for violence prevention and mitigation.

Key Terms

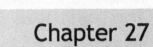

Ageism
Bullying
Child mistreatment
Cyberbullying
Direct bullying
Elder abuse
Family violence
Homicide
Indirect bullying
Intimate partner violence
Suicide
Violence
Workplace violence

Introduction[1]

Violence can be defined as "the intentional use of physical force or power, threatened or actual, against oneself, another person, or against a group or community, that either results in or has a high likelihood of resulting in injury, death, psychological harm, maldevelopment, or deprivation" (World Health Organization [WHO], 2002, p. 4). Although the media often portrays violence perpetrated by strangers, in reality the majority of violence occurs within families and among acquaintances (Christoffel and Gallagher, 2006). Elders, women, and children are most frequently the targets of violence, and the perpetrators are often people they know. LGBTQ+ youth face bias, which may place them at greater risk for a variety of physical and mental violence, including being threatened with a weapon and being bullied via electronic means, as well as dating violence (Centers for Disease Control and Prevention [CDC], 2017). In addition, people with disabilities are more often the targets of violence than their nondisabled counterparts. The social context of disability, including factors such as poverty, isolation, and dependence on support services, significantly increases a person's risk for abuse.

Violence is pervasive in U.S. society and globally and comes in a variety of forms and types, including homicide, suicide, domestic and family violence, sexual violence, youth and school violence, elder abuse, and workplace violence. According to the CDC (2019a), "in 2016, more than 19,000 people were victims of homicide," and approximately 45,000 committed suicide (para. 1). The leading causes of violence-related deaths by age group appear in Figure 27-1. The trend of suicides outnumbering homicides shown in this figure is also seen globally. Worldwide, 470,000 individuals die annually as a result of homicide (WHO, 2019a, para. 1), while it is estimated that about 800,000 people commit suicide (WHO, 2019b). A summary of the impact of violence globally, as well as ideas for mitigation, is presented in Figure 27-2.

A public health approach to violence includes the identification of risks and protective factors in order to design programs based on epidemiological data, the evaluation of program effectiveness, and the modification of prevention strategies based on evidence. Risk elements associated with violence include personal factors, such as male gender, alcohol abuse, and childhood trauma, as well as environmental and social factors, such as access to guns and poverty. A theoretical model that matches this approach and that has been used to develop programs to address complex health problems such as violence mitigation is the social ecological model (CDC, n.d.b; Reitz, Scaffa, Campbell, and Rhynders, 2010). This approach simultaneously examines individual, environmental, and broader societal aspects of health behavior and promotes the use of multiple intervention strategies to address community and population health needs. Health interventions that examine the interrelationships between these social and physical contextual factors tend to demonstrate higher-level success. The key concepts in this model are identified in Table 27-1. The social ecological model of violence prevention is recommended as an approach for community and population health-change advocates to examine the connections between individuals, relationships between individuals and groups, the community, and society in approaches to violence mitigation (CDC, n.d.b). An interactive tool that provides additional information on the model and its use in violence mitigation is available (CDC, n.d.a).

The chapter begins with a review of the prevalence of the two methods to intentionally kill individuals or groups. This discussion is followed by examining many types of violence, including violence in and around the home (i.e., child abuse and neglect, intimate partner violence, elder abuse), violence at school (i.e., bullying, shootings), and violence in the workplace.

Methods of Violence That Result in Death

People die from two methods of intentional violence—homicide and suicide. Both methods have been used to kill one or more people. While suicide most frequently results in the death of one

1. Portions of this chapter first appeared in Scaffa, M. E., Chromiak, S. B., Reitz, S. M., Blair-Newton, A., Murphy, L., and Wallis, C. B. (2010). Unintentional injury and violence. In M. E. Scaffa, S. M. Reitz, and M. A. Pizzi (Eds.), *Occupational therapy in community-based practice settings* (pp. 350–375). Philadelphia, PA: F. A. Davis.

10 Leading Causes of Injury Deaths by Age Group Highlighting Violence-Related Injury Deaths, United States–2017

Rank	<1	1–4	5–9	10–14	15–24	25–34	35–44	45–54	55–64	65+	Total
1	Unintentional suffocation 1,106	Unintentional drowning 424	Unintentional MV traffic 327	Unintentional MV traffic 428	Unintentional MV traffic 6,697	Unintentional poisoning 16,478	Unintentional poisoning 15,032	Unintentional poisoning 14,707	Unintentional poisoning 10,581	Unintentional fall 31,190	Unintentional poisoning 64,795
2	Homicide unspecified 139	Unintentional MV traffic 362	Unintentional drowning 125	Suicide suffocation 280	Unintentional poisoning 5,030	Unintentional MV traffic 6,871	Unintentional MV traffic 5,162	Unintentional MV traffic 5,471	Unintentional MV traffic 5,584	Unintentional MV traffic 7,667	Unintentional MV traffic 38,659
3	Unintentional MV traffic 90	Homicide unspecified 129	Unintentional fire/burn 94	Suicide firearm 185	Homicide firearm 4,391	Homicide firearm 4,594	Suicide firearm 3,098	Suicide firearm 3,937	Suicide firearm 4,219	Suicide firearm 5,996	Unintentional fall 36,338
4	Homicide other spec., classifiable 76	Unintentional suffocation 110	Homicide firearm 78	Homicide firearm 126	Suicide firearm 2,959	Suicide firearm 3,458	Suicide suffocation 2,562	Suicide suffocation 2,294	Unintentional fall 2,760	Unintentional unspecified 5,125	Suicide firearm 23,854
5	Undetermined suffocation 56	Unintentional fire/burn 95	Unintentional suffocation 36	Unintentional drowning 110	Suicide suffocation 2,321	Suicide suffocation 3,063	Homicide firearm 2,561	Suicide poisoning 1,604	Suicide suffocation 1,631	Unintentional suffocation 3,920	Homicide firearm 14,542
6	Unintentional drowning 43	Unintentional pedestrian, Other 88	Unintentional other land transport 25	Unintentional other land transport 66	Unintentional drowning 469	Undetermined poisoning 887	Suicide poisoning 1,089	Homicide firearm 1,447	Suicide poisoning 1,459	Adverse effects 2,902	Suicide suffocation 13,075
7	Undetermined unspecified 37	Homicide other spec., classifiable 49	Homicide suffocation 15	Unintentional fire/burn 56	Suicide poisoning 463	Suicide poisoning 788	Undetermined poisoning 792	Unintentional fall 1,248	Homicide firearm 824	Unintentional poisoning 2,871	Unintentional suffocation 6,946
8	Homicide suffocation 26	Homicide firearm 44	Homicide cut/pierce 14	Suicide poisoning 39	Undetermined poisoning 280	Unintentional drowning 479	Unintentional fall 522	Undetermined poisoning 887	Unintentional suffocation 811	Unintentional fire/burn 1,278	Unintentional unspecified 6,606
9	Unintentional natural/ environment 18	Unintentional natural/ environment 34	Unintentional firearm 14	Unintentional poisoning 39	Homicide cut/pierce 266	Homicide cut/pierce 404	Unintentional drowning 397	Unintentional drowning 451	Adverse effects 773	Suicide poisoning 1,111	Suicide poisoning 6,554
10	Three Tied 16	Unintentional firearm 31	Two Tied 13	Unintentional suffocation 35	Unintentional fall 212	Unintentional fall 351	Homicide cut/pierce 337	Unintentional suffocation 441	Undetermined poisoning 732	Suicide suffocation 919	Adverse effects 4,459

Data Source: National Center for Health Statistics (NCHS), National Vital Statistics System.
Produced by: National Center for Injury Prevention and Control, CDC using WISQARS™.

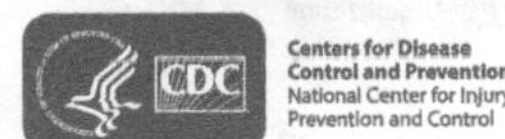

Figure 27-1 Leading causes of violence-related deaths highlighted by age. *(From the Centers for Disease Control and Prevention, 2017.)*

individual, it, as well as homicide, can result in multiple deaths. Mass suicides can be grouped into two broad categories by two very different catalysts—one, called hetero-induced, is a reaction to oppression, as happens under colonization or with the threat of an approaching hostile armed force. The second category has been labeled as self-induced, as it is the result of a "distorted evaluation of reality, without there being either an intolerable situation or real risk of death" (Mancinelli, Comparelli, Girardi, and Tatarelli, 2002, p. 91).

Homicide

Homicide is "death resulting from injuries inflicted by another person with the intent to injure or kill" (Christoffel and Gallagher, 2006, p. 106). It occurs when "a person knowingly, purposefully, recklessly or negligently causes the death of another human being" (Gellert, 2002, p. 240). In 2017 in the United States, 19,000 deaths, an average of 50 per day, were attributable to homicide. Firearms were used in approximately 80% of murders. Males account for 78% of the homicide victims and 62% of the perpetrators. Female perpetrators account for 20% of homicides, with the remaining 18% of unknown gender. In 2017, 52% percent of homicide victims were African American, 43% were white, and 5% were of unknown race (CDC, 2019c; Federal Bureau of Investigation [FBI], 2019). Overall, the rate of homicide in the United States, 5.4 per 100,000 people, is much higher than in Canada (1.7/100,000), the United Kingdom (1.2/100,000), and Australia (0.9/100,000; United Nations Development Programme, 2016).

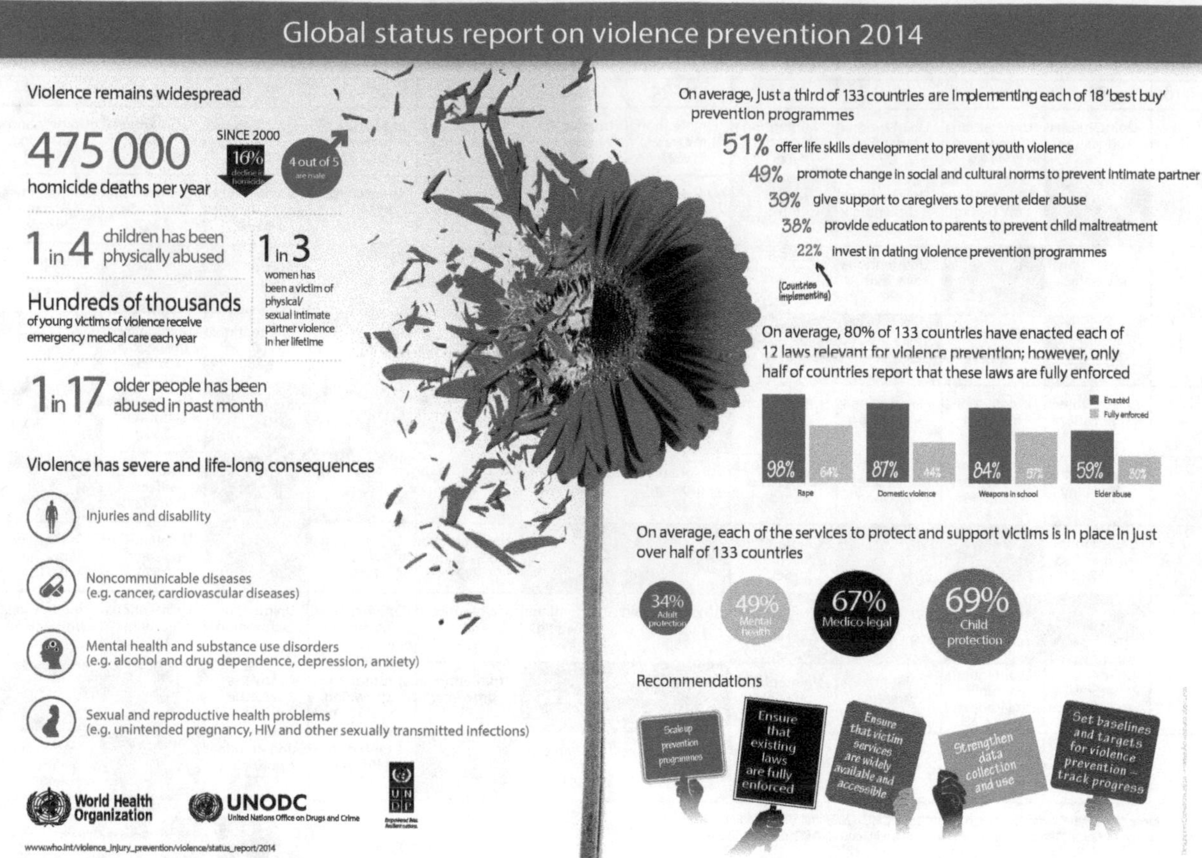

Figure 27-2 Global status report on violence prevention, 2014. *(Graphic from World Health Organization, 2014b. Reprinted with permission.)*

Table 27-1 An Ecological Perspective: Levels of Influence

Concept	Definition
Intrapersonal level	Individual characteristics that influence behavior, such as knowledge, attitudes, beliefs, and personality traits
Interpersonal level	Interpersonal processes and primary groups, including family, friends, and peers that provide social identity, support, and role definition
Community level	
Institutional factors	Rules, regulations, policies, and informal structures, which may constrain or promote recommended behaviors
Community factors	Social networks and norms, or standards, that exist as formal or informal among individuals, groups, and organizations
Public policy	Local, state, and federal policies and laws that regulate or support healthy actions and practices for disease prevention, early detection, control, and management

From *Theory at a Glance: A Guide for Health Promotion Practice* (2nd ed., p. 11), by National Cancer Institute, 2005, Bethesda, MD: National Institutes of Health.

Most homicides are not the result of organized criminal activity but rather of family dysfunction, alcohol and drug use, and poverty. In 2017, 28% of homicides were perpetrated by friends or acquaintances, 12% by family members, and 10% by strangers. In the remaining 50%, the relationship between the victim and perpetrator was unknown (FBI, 2019). Low-income neighborhoods are disproportionately affected by violent crimes, particularly homicide. Social organizations, job opportunities for youth, and residential stability are associated with lower crime rates (U.S. Department of Housing and Urban Development, 2016). Alcohol and drugs are frequently associated with homicide deaths. A meta-analysis of case files, self-reports, and toxicology data indicated that 37% of perpetrators were under the influence of alcohol at the time of the murder (Johns Hopkins University, 2015).

Suicide

Suicide is "death from intentional self-inflicted injury" (Christoffel and Gallagher, 2006, p. 103) and is the cause of over 47,000 deaths annually (American Foundation for Suicide Prevention [AFSP], 2019). Every 11 minutes in the United States, a person commits suicide. It is the second leading cause of death for persons ages 10 to 34 and the 10th leading cause of death overall. Suicide occurs almost three times as often as homicide (CDC, 2019c). Over 50% of suicides are committed with firearms. The next two most frequent means of suicide are suffocation (28%) and poisoning (14%). Globally, an estimated 800,000 people die as a result of suicide each year, and, as is the case in the United States, suicide is the second leading cause of death for youth and young adults between the ages of 15 and 29. The most frequent methods include purposefully ingesting pesticides; hanging, causing suffocation; and using a firearm (WHO, 2018).

Persons living in households that contain guns have a suicide risk that is five times greater than those living in households without firearms. Other risk factors include previous suicide attempts; psychiatric disorders, especially depression; alcohol and substance abuse; a family history of suicide or abuse; physical illness; feelings of hopelessness or isolation; and emotional or financial loss; among others (Christoffel and Gallagher, 2006). Males are three to four times more likely than females to die from suicide, yet females attempt suicide more often. White males account for 78% of all suicides (AFSP, 2019). Among teenagers, suicide is the third leading cause of death (11%); only unintentional injuries (48%) and homicides (13%) kill more adolescents (Miniño, 2010). Among youth, the most common correlates of suicide are depression, behavioral problems, impulsivity, neurocognitive difficulties, family adversity, substance abuse, and the availability of guns (Brent and Mann, 2006). Suicide rates also vary by geography (see Fig. 27-3).

Other at-risk groups include middle and older adults and veterans. Suicide rates in England and Wales were examined to determine if there was a link to the 2008 economic recession (Coope et al., 2014). While no such relationship was found for females, unemployment and economic burden on males between the ages of 35 and 44 were linked to an increase in suicide rates in that age group. A systematic review of literature on suicide among older adults 65 years of age and older indicates that changes in health (i.e., the onset of dementia, cognitive impairment, or physical illness) and social engagement, often due to a change in marital status or bereavement, may be linked to suicidal behavior (Conejero, Olié, Courtet, and Calati, 2018).

Veterans have higher rates of suicide than nonveterans, with "more than 6,000 Veteran suicides each year from 2008 to 2016" (U.S. Department of Veterans Affairs [USDVA] Office of Mental Health and Suicide Prevention, 2018, p. 6). From 2015 to 2016, the suicide rate for Veterans between the ages of 18 and 34 "increased substantially, from 40.4 suicide deaths per 100,000 in 2015 to 45 suicides per 100,000" the next year (USDVA, 2018, p. 7). Risk factors vary by age and ethnicity. Acute and general warning signs of suicide (American Association of Suicidology [AAS], 2019) are displayed in Box 27-1. The AAS also provides information on risk factors by groups as well as data to combat typical myths on its website.

The phenomena of taunting individuals who appear to be contemplating suicide was documented as early as the 1920s (Mann, 1981). This taunting usually occurred when people were contemplating jumping to their deaths in a public place with a crowd. Mann suggested that crowd size, leading to anonymity, and adverse temperatures may lead to taunting. Mann also suggested that a lengthy waiting time to observe the conclusion (i.e., the person

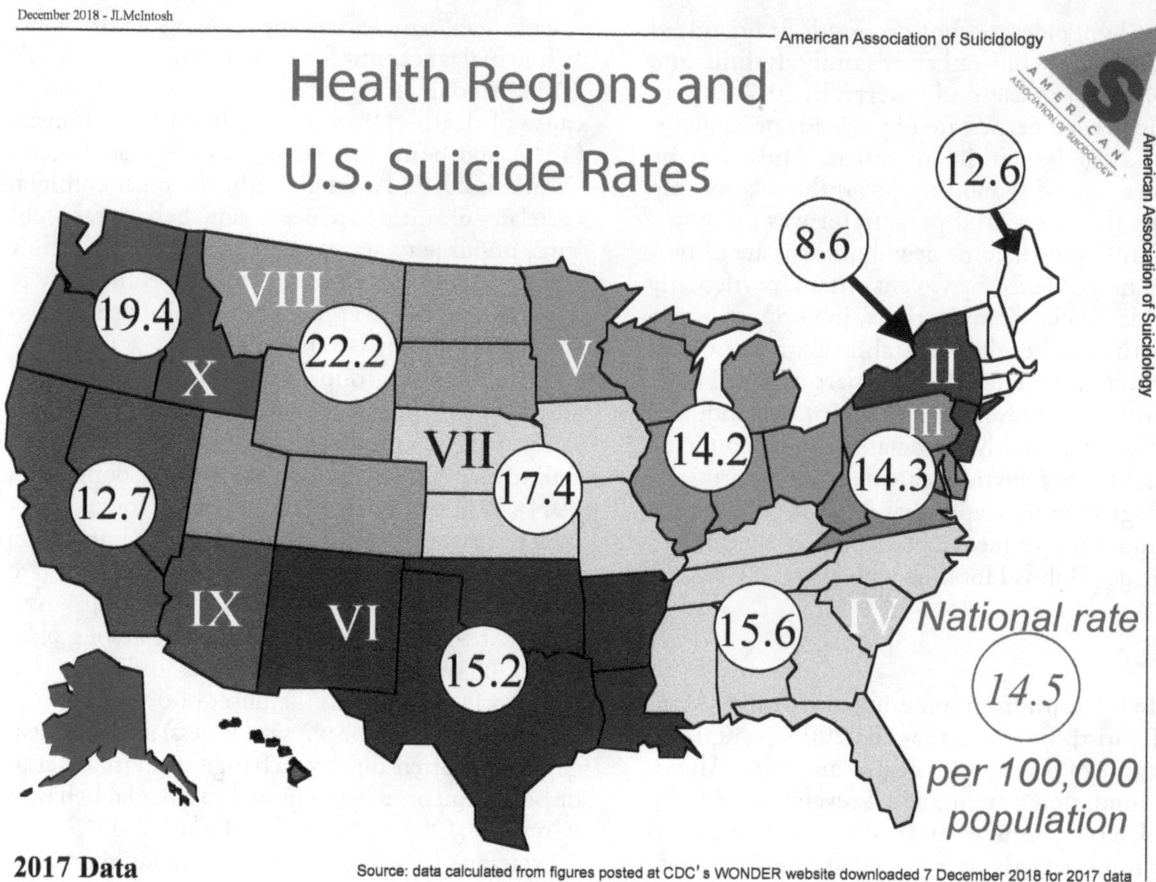

Figure 27-3 Health regions and U.S. suicide rates. *(From the American Association of Suicidology, 2018. Reprinted with permission.)*

threating to jump is indecisive over a prolonged period) also may lead to taunting, as the crowd becomes impatient while awaiting the event's conclusion. This phenomena seems to have evolved with the advent of social media. More recently, cyberbullying (Milosevic and Livingstone, 2018) and taunting by phone have been linked to suicides (Harvard Law Review, 2018). This new type of taunting will need to be monitored and prevention initiatives modified to address this suicide threat. Suicide is a public health problem that requires evolving community-based prevention strategies.

Populations and Settings

The next section of the chapter focuses on populations and settings where violence occurs. The populations include children and youth, sexual partners, and the elderly. The settings include homes, schools, and workplaces.

Families/Home/Domestic Violence

Family violence takes the form of child abuse and neglect, IPV, and elder abuse. According to the National Coalition Against Domestic Violence (NCADV), each year 10,000,000 people, or an average of 20 people every minute, experience physical abuse at the hands of an intimate partner. A perpetrator's access to a firearm increases the risk of homicide by 500% (NCADV, n.d.). Individuals with disabilities are at a higher risk of domestic violence, especially women (AOTA, 2017). These numbers may only approximate the true scope within the United States because domestic violence often remains hidden within the community, as it is difficult for many people to leave these unsafe

Box 27-1 Acute and Expanded Warning Signs of Suicide

Acute Warning Signs
- Threatening to do harm to self, including killing self
- Looking for ways to harm or kill self
- Writing or discussing death or suicide

Expanded Warning Signs
- "Increased **substance** (alcohol or drug) **use**"
- "No reason for living; no sense of **purpose** in life"
- "**Anxiety,** agitation, unable to sleep or sleeping all of the time"
- "Feeling **trapped**—like there's no way out"
- "**Hopelessness**"
- "**Withdrawal** from friends, family and society"
- "Rage, uncontrolled **anger,** seeking revenge"
- "Acting **reckless** or engaging in risky activities, seemingly without thinking"
- "Dramatic **mood changes**"

From *Knowing the Warning Signs of Suicide* (para. 3), by American Association of Suicidology, 2019.

situations. Thomas, Goodman, and Putnins (2015) explored the required "trade-offs" faced by survivors of domestic violence. While safety is the primary focus of domestic violence programs, it is also important to understand the impact of forfeiting housing and financial stability for safety. Thomas et al. (2015) found that for some survivors, safety "comes at a cost so high that it does not seem worth pursuing" (p. 170), which leads them to call for a break-down of the silos of social service provision.

The aftermath of domestic violence involves several negative consequences for those who have been victimized. The survivors typically exhibit limitations in daily occupations, particularly in work performance; instrumental activities of daily living (IADLs), such as health management and maintenance, home establishment and management, child rearing, care of others, community mobility, and financial management; social participation; rest and sleep; and leisure. These limitations are often due to difficulty with decision-making, problem-solving, direction following, task initiation, and judgment. Problems with self-confidence, interpersonal relationships, stress management, and coping skills are also prevalent (AOTA, 2017; Gorde, Helfrich, and Finlayson, 2004). Limitations may also exist in important prevocational skills, such as acquiring and maintaining a job to provide for the family.

Child Abuse and Neglect

Extent of the Problem

Child mistreatment "is the abuse and neglect that occurs to children under the age of 18" (WHO, 2016, para. 2). Worldwide, it is estimated that 22.6% of children under the age of 18 have experienced physical abuse, 36.3%, emotional abuse, and 16.3%, physical neglect (WHO, 2014a). In the United States in 2012, out of 1,000 children under age 18, 9.2 were reported victims of child maltreatment. This same year it is estimated that 2.2 children per 100,000 died of abuse. For these children, maltreatment was evident in several forms, including neglect (70%) and physical abuse (44%), with some children also experiencing another form of or a combination of maltreatment. Overall, girls are at slightly higher risk for child maltreatment than boys. The highest rate of child maltreatment is for children from birth to 3 years of age, and the rates decline as children get older. In most cases, the perpetrator of child abuse is a family member. In 80% of the cases, the parents were the abusers; in 10% of the cases, they were other relatives; and in 4%, they were unmarried partners of a parent (CDC, 2014). Child abuse can be found in all socioeconomic groups, and family stress, particularly economic stress, is a major determinant in abuse. Children who are abused often become abusive parents themselves and also have a higher likelihood of committing other violent acts (Christoffel and Gallagher, 2006).

Risk Factors

A variety of factors increase a child's risk for abuse or neglect. Children from unplanned pregnancies, children of single parents, children cared for by transient caregivers, and children who have disabilities are all at higher risk. Family risk factors that predispose children to abuse include social isolation, parent stress, poor parent-child relationships, family disruption, and poverty (CDC, 2019b). According to Gellert (2002), "in homes where child abuse occurs, violence among siblings is not uncommon" (p. 27). Children who are being abused can be identified by a wide range of signs and symptoms. Physical signs of broken bones, lacerations, and bruises may be infrequent. More subtle signs may include malnutrition, failure of the child to develop properly, bed-wetting, thumb-sucking, poor school performance, and difficulty forming meaningful relationships (Gellert, 2002).

Consequences

Children who have been mistreated experience disruptions in health, occupational performance, and roles, with the impact continuing into their adult years (AOTA, 2017). Impacts on long-term health include:

- Depression and anxiety
- Eating disorders
- Posttraumatic stress disorder (PTSD)
- Chronic pain and fibromyalgia
- Somatic symptoms
- Functional bowel disorders (Springer, Sheridan, Kuo, and Carnes, 2003)

Child abuse negatively affects childhood and adult occupations. A study of 219 dancers in California (Thomson and Jaque, 2018) found that dancers who had experienced multiple childhood adversities displayed greater internalized shame and anxiety. Through studies of children's play habits, it has been found that an abused child's play tends to be impulsive, disorganized, and lacking a theme (Cooper, 2000), in comparison to the play of a nonabused child. This is of great concern because for young children, play is the most important means of adapting and developing the skills needed to prepare for more advanced tasks. Unhealthy occupational engagements, which include smoking and alcohol and drug use, as well as unsafe sex behaviors, are also associated with childhood abuse (Springer et al., 2003). Since occupational therapy practitioners provide services to individuals with these health conditions, it is important for occupational therapy practitioners to be aware of these links to child abuse.

Evidence-Based Prevention/ Mitigation Strategies

Evidence-based programs and strategies are available to help reduce child abuse and child maltreatment (National Center for Injury Prevention and Control [NCIPC], 2019). In the NCIPC (n.d.) document *Essentials for Childhood: Creating Safe, Stable, Nurturing Relationships and Environments for All Children,* specific evidence-based examples are provided. Examples of such programs include Parent-Child Interaction Therapy (PCIT); Safe Environment for Every Kid (Seek), which uses a self-administered questionnaire during an office visit with a trained primary care provider supplemented by resources and follow-up; and the Nurse-Family Partnership (NFP), which utilizes home visits to first-time mothers and their infants. The programs and strategies are geared toward providing parents with information to better equip them to cope with the various challenges and stresses associated with parenting. They pertain to just two of the strategies (i.e., parent and caregiver support and education and life skills initiative) identified by the WHO (2016) in *INSPIRE: Seven Strategies for Ending Violence Against Children* (see Table 27-2). The WHO (2014a, 2016) and the NCIPC (n.d., 2016, 2019) offer a variety of resources to assist in the development of programs to mitigate and prevent child maltreatment.

While no evidence-based occupational therapy prevention strategies for child mistreatment or domestic violence could be found, one potential intervention for enhancing mother and child interaction following domestic violence was located (Waldman-Levi and Weintraub, 2015). The intervention, Family Intervention for Improving Occupational Performance (FIOP), was compared to participation of a control group in a play area program. Both programs were conducted in the same domestic shelter. Improvements in the interaction between mothers and children, as well as play skills in children, were noted in the groups receiving the FIOP intervention. However, playfulness did not improve in the FIOP group but did in the comparison group (Waldman-Levi and Weintraub, 2015). These findings warrant the further refinement and investigation of this promising approach to improving the relationship of children with their mothers following domestic violence.

Occupational Therapy's Role

The role of occupational therapy practitioners is to facilitate the continued development and optimal occupational participation of parents and children recovering from domestic violence. Facilitating co-occupations between parents and children in domestic violence shelters is one potential way to

Table 27-2 The Inspire Strategies

Strategy	Approach	Sector	Crosscutting Activities
Implementation and enforcement of laws	Laws banning violent punishment of children by parents, teachers, or other caregivers	Justice	Multisectoral actions and coordination
	Laws criminalizing sexual abuse and exploitation of children		
	Laws that prevent alcohol misuse		
	Laws limiting youth access to firearms and other weapons		
Norms and values	Changing adherence to restrictive and harmful gender and social norms	Health, education, social welfare	
	Community mobilization programs		
	Bystander interventions		
Safe environments	Reducing violence by addressing "hot spots"	Interior, planning	
	Interrupting the spread of violence		
	Improving the built environment		
Parent and caregiver support	Delivered through home visits	Social welfare, health	
	Delivered in groups in community settings		
	Delivered through comprehensive programs		
Income and economic strengthening	Cash transfers	Finance Labor	Monitoring and evaluation
	Group saving and loans combined with gender equity training		
	Microfinance combined with gender norm training		
Response and support services	Counseling and therapeutic approaches	Health, justice, social welfare	
	Screening combined with interventions		
	Treatment programs for juvenile offenders in the criminal justice system		
	Foster-care interventions involving social welfare services		
Education and life skills	Increase enrolment in preschool, primary schools, and secondary schools	Education	
	Establish a safe and enabling school environment		
	Improve children's knowledge about sexual abuse and how to protect themselves against it		
	Life and social skills training		
	Adolescent intimate partner violence prevention programs		

From *INSPIRE: Seven Strategies for Ending Violence Against Children* (p. 24), by World Health *Organization,* 2016. Reprinted with permission.

fulfill this role. De Brun (2017) identified internal characteristics and the past experience of domestic violence as major barriers for mothers in finding time for maternal-child co-occupational experiences. In addition, the high levels of rules and regulations in domestic violence shelters and a lack of needed resources also affected the pursuit of maternal-child co-occupations. Occupational therapy practitioners have the knowledge and expertise to address these challenges and to enhance parent-child co-occupations in families who have experienced domestic violence.

A primary role of occupational therapy practitioners is in fulfilling their role as mandated health-care providers to report suspected child abuse and neglect. This is a serious legal and ethical responsibility. Procedures for reporting may vary across health-care facilities and from state to state, so practitioners must familiarize themselves with state law and regulatory acts. Reports of child abuse and neglect should always be documented. Failure to do so would place the occupational therapy practitioners in violation of laws and the AOTA *Occupational Therapy Code of Ethics (2015)*. In addition, given the high representation of women in the occupational therapy profession, it is statistically likely that a peer is currently or has previously experienced domestic violence (AOTA, 2017). Occupational therapy practitioners also have a responsibility beyond the care of individual clients or families in the prevention of child maltreatment and domestic violence. Other actions highlighted in Table 27-2 (WHO, 2016) are within the expertise and responsibility of occupational therapy practitioners, such as advocating for policies and laws as well as participating in and providing bystander training. A technical package provided by the NCIPC (2016) is a useful tool for the development of policy, advocacy, and programming activities.

Engage Your Brain 27-1

What are the ethical implications of confronting a coworker with the fact that she repeatedly appears with bruises sustained by "accidents" after her husband returns from business trips? Refer to the AOTA *Occupational Therapy Code of Ethics (2015)* to formulate your response.

Intimate Partner Violence

Intimate partner violence (IPV) is "physical violence, sexual violence, stalking and psychological aggression by a current or former intimate partner" (CDC, 2018c, slide 1). IPV includes behaviors that occur when the individuals are physically in the same space as well as when they are apart. Aggression, coercion, and stalking can also occur from a distance over social media and through the use of mobile electronic devices (Niolon et al., 2017).

Extent of the Problem

IPV occurs more frequently in adolescence and young adulthood, with prevalence decreasing as people age. Among U.S. high school students who had dated in the previous year, 10% experienced physical dating violence, and 11% reported sexual dating violence. These reports vary by gender, with 21% of girls who had dated the previous year reporting physical and or sexual violence, compared to 10% of boys (Niolon et al., 2017). Worldwide, almost a third of women who have been in a relationship have experienced a form of IPV in their lifetimes. The prevalence rates of IPV vary globally by geographical and economic region (see Fig. 27-4). War, the period shortly afterward, and human displacement may increase and expand IPV and other violence (WHO, 2017).

Risk Factors

There are risk factors associated with being a victim and being a perpetrator of IPV. In the United States, the risk of IPV is higher among certain groups of people. Lifetime prevalence is highest among bisexual women (61%), multiracial women (57%), American Indian/Alaska Native women (48%), non-Hispanic black women (45%), multiracial men (42%), lesbian women (44%), and bisexual men (37%; Niolon et al., 2017). Risk factors of becoming a perpetrator include age (i.e., youth, young adult); low income and educational achievement; exposure to aggression and violence in the family; being a victim of violence, including IPV; belief in strict gender roles; substance abuse history; and demonstrating behaviors such as hostile communication patterns (Niolon et al., 2017).

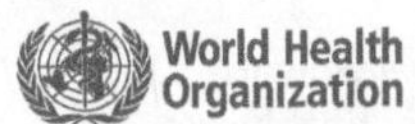

VIOLENCE AGAINST WOMEN: GLOBAL PICTURE HEALTH RESPONSE

PREVALENCE →

1 in 3 women throughout the world will experience physical and/or sexual violence by a partner or sexual violence by a non-partner

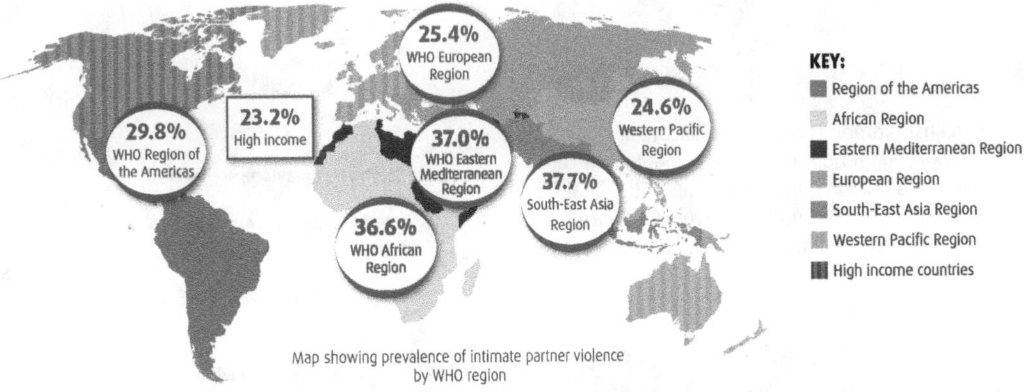

KEY:
- Region of the Americas
- African Region
- Eastern Mediterranean Region
- European Region
- South-East Asia Region
- Western Pacific Region
- High income countries

Map showing prevalence of intimate partner violence by WHO region

HEALTH IMPACT: Women exposed to intimate partner violence are →

Mental health

TWICE as likely to experience depression

ALMOST TWICE as likely to have alcohol use disorders

Sexual and reproductive health

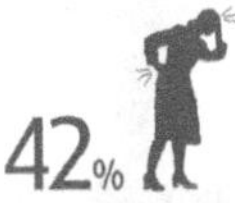

16% more likely to have a low birth-weight baby

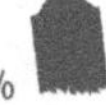

1.5 TIMES more likely to acquire HIV and 1.5 times more likely to contract syphilis infection, chlamydia, or gonorrhoea

Death and injury

42% of women who have experienced physical or sexual violence at the hands of a partner have experienced injuries as a result

38% of all murders of women globally were reported as being committed by their intimate partners

Figure 27-4 Violence against women: prevalence. *(Fact sheet from the World Health Organization, n.d. Reprinted with permission.)*

Continued

GUIDELINES FOR HEALTH SECTOR RESPONSE ➔

WHO's new clinical and policy guidelines on the health sector response to partner and sexual violence against women emphasize the urgent need to integrate these issues into clinical training for health care providers. WHO has identified the key elements of a health sector response to violence against women which have informed the following recommendations:

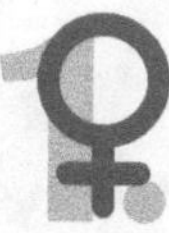

Women-centred care:

Health-care providers should, at a minimum, offer first-line support when women disclose violence (empathetic listening, non-judgmental attitude, privacy, confidentiality, link to other services).

Identification and care for survivors of intimate partner violence:

Health-care providers should ask about exposure to intimate partner violence when assessing conditions that may be caused or complicated by intimate partner violence, in order to improve diagnosis/identification and subsequent care.

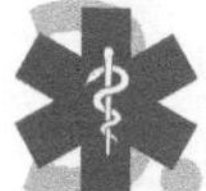

Clinical care for survivors of sexual violence:

Offer comprehensive care, including first-line support, emergency contraception, and STI and HIV prophylaxis by any perpetrator, and take a complete history, recording events to determine what interventions are appropriate.

Training of health-care providers on intimate partner violence and sexual violence:

Training at pre-qualification level in first-line support for women who have experienced intimate partner violence and sexual assault should be given to healthcare providers.

Health-care policy and provision:

Care for women experiencing intimate partner violence and sexual assault should, as much as possible, be integrated into existing health services rather than as a stand-alone service.

Mandatory reporting of intimate partner violence:

Mandatory reporting to the police by the health-care provider is not recommended. Health-care providers should offer to report the incident if the woman chooses.

HEALTH-CARE WORKER INTERVENTION ➔

Violence against women is a global public health problem of epidemic proportion requiring urgent action. Health-care providers are in a unique position to address the health and psychosocial needs of women who have experienced violence, provided certain minimum requirements are met:

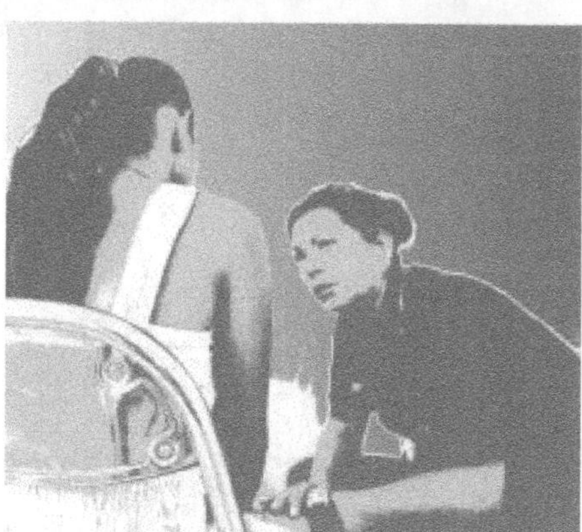

- ✓ Health-care providers are trained
- ✓ Standard operating procedures are in place
- ✓ Consultation takes place in a private setting
- ✓ Confidentiality is guaranteed
- ✓ A referral system is in place to ensure that women can access related services
- ✓ Health-care settings are equipped to provide a comprehensive response, addressing both physical and mental health consequences
- ✓ Health-care providers gather forensic evidence when needed

All statistics can be found in the report entitled Global and regional estimates of violence against women: Prevalence and health effects of intimate partner violence and non-partner sexual violence, by the World Health Organization, the London School of Hygiene & Tropical Medicine, and the South African Medical Research Council, found here: http://www.who.int/reproductivehealth/publications/violence/en/index.html

Figure 27-4 *cont'd*

Consequences

The consequences of IPV include adverse immediate and long-term health outcomes and health behaviors. Negative health outcomes include "cardiovascular, gastrointestinal, reproductive, musculoskeletal, and nervous system conditions" (Niolon et al., 2017, p. 10). Survivors of IPV are also more likely to engage in unhealthy behaviors such as smoking and binge drinking (Niolon et al., 2017, p. 10). These adverse health outcomes and habits can have negative impacts on occupational role performance. In addition to the impacts on survivors of IPV, children exposed to IPV frequently experience sleep and eating disturbances and have difficulty self-calming. They also may exhibit developmental delay, maladaptive behaviors, limited social skills, and poor academic performance (AOTA, 2017).

Evidence-Based Prevention/Mitigation Strategies

No evidence-based occupational therapy programs or strategies could be located in the literature at the time of publication. There are other resources available from the CDC, including a technical package of programs, policies, and practices (Niolon et al., 2017). Included in this package is a table of strategies to prevent IPV, which is replicated in Table 27-3.

Occupational Therapy's Role

Occupational therapists play an important role in their clients' lives and often assist with both private and personal areas of their occupational functioning. Because of this, many clients may feel more comfortable opening up to their occupational therapist

Table 27-3 ***Preventing Intimate Partner Violence Strategies and Approaches***

Strategy	Approaches
Teach safe and healthy relationship skills	Social-emotional learning programs for youth Healthy relationship programs for couples
Engage influential adults and peers	Men and boys as allies in prevention Bystander empowerment and education Family-based programs
Disrupt the developmental pathways toward partner violence	Early childhood home visitation Preschool enrichment with family engagement Parenting skill and family relationship programs Treatment for at-risk children, youth, and families
Create protective environments	Improve school climate and safety Improve organizational policies and workplace climate Modify the physical and social environments of neighborhoods
Strengthen economic supports for families	Strengthen household financial security Strengthen work-family supports
Support survivors to increase safety and lessen harm	Victim-centered services Housing programs First responder and civil legal protections Patient-centered approaches Treatment and support for survivors of IPV, including TDV

From *Preventing Intimate Partner Violence Across the Lifespan: A Technical Package of Programs, Policies, and Practices* (p. 12), by P. H. Niolon, M. Kearns, J. Dills, K. Rambo, S. Irving, T. L. Armstead, and L. Gilbert, 2017, Atlanta, GA: National Center for Injury Prevention and Control: Division of Violence Prevention.

concerning their experience with sexual abuse/violence. Reports of sexual violence should always be documented.

For primary prevention of violence, a focus on decreasing risk factors and increasing protective factors is also appropriate. Improving assertiveness and interpersonal skills, increasing safety awareness, and building self-defense skills are protective factors that offer appropriate prevention opportunities for occupational therapy. These decrease personal vulnerability and the likelihood of becoming a victim of violence. Life skills training, anger management, conflict resolution, and coping and relaxation skill development may decrease the probability of some forms of violence by providing the potential perpetrator with alternative strategies for dealing with stress. These approaches can also be used for victims and perpetrators of violence as secondary prevention to reduce the likelihood of reoccurrence.

As was mentioned earlier, serious injury and violence often have significant psychological and emotional health consequences. If left unaddressed, these emotional symptoms and responses can result in long-term psychological sequelae that have negative impacts on a person's occupational and social functioning. It is therefore important to address these issues and mediate these emotional responses in order to prevent occupational dysfunction and to rebuild a sense of empowerment and self-worth. Expressive therapy techniques such as music, dance, drawing, painting, journaling, and so on are particularly beneficial for this purpose. Songs such as "Quiet" by MILCK have been used worldwide in communities to promote the healing and empowerment of women who are survivors of sexual harassment and abuse (Blair, 2019).

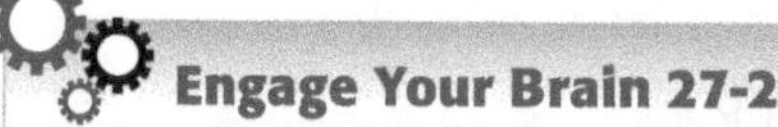

Engage Your Brain 27-2

Can you identify three songs other than "Quiet" that could be used in either a violence prevention program or violence mitigation program?

Elder Abuse

The number of older adults is growing worldwide, placing a strain on both family and national fiscal and human resources. This burden can result in untrained and stressed professional and family caregivers, as well as violence toward vulnerable older adults.

> *Globally, the number of persons aged 80 or over is projected to triple by 2050, from 137 million in 2017 to 425 million in 2050. By 2100 it is expected to increase to 909 million, nearly seven times its value in 2017. (United Nations Department of Economic and Social Affairs, 2017, para. 4)*

The responsibility to address the public health problem of elder abuse is the responsibility of all health professionals and communities.

Extent of the Problem

"Abuse can happen to anyone—no matter the person's age, sex, race, religion, or ethnic or cultural background. Each year, hundreds of thousands of adults over the age of 60 are abused, neglected, or financially exploited. This is called **elder abuse**" (National Institute on Aging [NIA], 2016, para. 3). Since 95% of older adults live outside of institutions such as nursing homes or assisted living facilities, it is not surprising that the majority of such abuse occurs in the home (American Psychological Association [APA], 2012). The perpetrator is most frequently a professional or family caregiver (National Institutes of Health [NIH], 2017). According to the NIA (2016), women are abused more frequently than men. It has been reported that

> *approximately 1 in 10 Americans aged 60+ have experienced some form of elder abuse. Some estimates range as high as 5 million elders who are abused each year. One study estimated that only 1 in 14 cases of abuse are reported to authorities. (National Council on Aging [NCOA], n.d.a, para. 2)*

Elder abuse can go unnoticed and, as mentioned, is thought to be grossly underreported (Hayslip, Reinberg, and Williams, 2015). Abusers can be family members (e.g., spouses, children); paid and unpaid caregivers; or staff at nursing, hospice, and assisted living facilities. It has been reported that "70 to 80 percent of community care for older adults is provided by informal caregivers as opposed to formal care providers" (Ploeg and Markle-Reid, 2018, p. 2). The causes of elder abuse range from societal, such as ageism, to personal (e.g., caregiver stress, resentment of the elder). Financial stress can be overwhelming for family caregivers, especially as half of caregivers are between 45 and 65 years of age, in the peak of their earning years" (Ploeg and Markle-Reid, 2018, p. 4).

Ageism, negative attitudes toward older adults and their place in society, as well as the stresses that caregivers often experience, may make the elderly more vulnerable to caregiver abuse. Even when the informal caregiver cares deeply about the person they care for, their own unmanaged or poorly regulated coping skills from emotional, financial, and other factors may result in abuse. The range of abuse can be broad and include one or more of the aspects defined in Box 27-2.

"Elders who have been abused have a 300% higher risk of death when compared to those who have not been mistreated" (NCOA, n.d.b, para. 5). In addition to the risk of shortened life spans, the elderly also face high rates of financial abuse and fraud that drain their resources. It has been reported that in the United States these costs range from $2,900,000,000 to $36,500,000,000 annually and may be higher, as this type of abuse is likely under-reported. "Yet, financial exploitation is self-reported at rates higher than emotional, physical, and sexual abuse or neglect" (NCOA, n.d.b, para. 1).

Risk Factors

A wide variety of risk factors exist for elder abuse. Some of these risk factors focus on the older adult, such as poor physical health, cognitive impairments, fragility, self-neglect, loneliness, and depression (APA, 2012). Caregivers' physical, emotional, and financial conditions and impaired ability to manage stress may make one more prone to become an abuser. "Family stressors that may contribute to elder abuse include discord created by a pattern or history of violent interactions with family, lifestyle adjustments and accommodations to living in a multigenerational household, and social isolation" (APA, 2012, p. 8).

When there is little engagement from family or friends with an older adult and when their ability to get out into the community is restricted, social isolation can occur. A lack of oversight regarding the care of an older adult may provide opportunities for unscrupulous people to take advantage and abuse the individual. Families need to be educated to the risk factors and signs of abuse, both of which are summarized in an infographic by the NIA (n.d.).

Background checks are imperative when hiring a caregiver. The backgrounds of perpetrators may reveal problems with substance abuse, lack of training, or mental illness (CDC, 2018b). Educating and cautioning the service recipient and/or family members against hiring people from newspaper ads or by word of mouth may prevent future problems.

Box 27-2 Types of Elder Abuse

- Physical: The use of physical force that might result in bodily injury, physical pain, or impairment. Physical punishments of any kind are examples of physical abuse.
- Emotional or psychological abuse: The infliction of anguish, pain, or distress.
- Neglect: The refusal or failure to fulfill any obligations or duties to an elder.
- Self-neglect: The behaviors of an elderly person that threaten his or her health or safety. The definition of self-neglect excludes a situation in which a mentally competent older person who understands the consequences of his or her decisions makes a conscious and voluntary decision to engage in acts that threaten his or her own health or safety.
- Abandonment: The desertion of an elderly person by an individual who had physical custody or otherwise had assumed responsibility for providing care for an elder or by a person with physical custody of an elder.
- Social isolation: The absence of contact with others, whether or not it is intentional (Nugent, 2013).
- Sexual abuse: Nonconsensual sexual contact of any kind with an elderly person.
- Financial or material exploitation: The illegal or improper use of an elder's funds, property, or assets.
- Health-care fraud: "An intentional deception or misrepresentation that the individual or entity makes knowing that the misrepresentation could result in some unauthorized benefit to the individual, or the entity or to some other party" (National Health Care Anti-Fraud Association, 2018, para. 1).

Content adapted from "Elder Abuse and Neglect: An Overview," by M. J. Gorbien and A. R. Einstein, 2005, *Clinics in Geriatric Medicine, 21,* pp. 279–292, unless otherwise indicated.

Hiring assistants through an agency or hospital who complete comprehensive background investigations may help reduce the likelihood of victimization. If problems occur, the family can turn to the agency to help or intervene. When abuse is suspected from an independent provider, the family recourse is more cumbersome.

Consequences

Little is written about the consequences of elder abuse. The CDC indicates that there are physical and psychological impacts on the individual who is abused. The physical consequences of abuse are broad and include bruises, fractures, increased susceptibility to illness, difficulty sleeping, and premature death. Psychological manifestations of abuse include PTSD, fear, anxiety, and increased dependence (CDC, 2018a). Elder abuse and neglect may also result in social isolation, greater propensity for falls, and financial vulnerability due to theft.

Evidence-Based Prevention/ Mitigation Strategies

Older adults can help prevent health-care fraud by not sharing their personal information (e.g., Social Security, Medicare, or bank account information) with others without confirming their need to know. Seniors are encouraged to write and regularly update their living wills, medical powers of attorney, and other documents that protect their finances and express their wishes when a time arrives when they may be unable to speak for themselves. The prevention of elder abuse includes education of the family and elder; respite care for caregivers to provide stress relief; social contact; support for both the elder and the caregiver; and individual, family, and/or group counseling (APA, 2012). Physical activities may keep the elder safe by increasing stability and reducing vulnerability to falls—for example, being less likely to fall if pushed.

Research into prevention and mitigation strategies is limited, and the outcomes are not overwhelmingly positive thus far. Some of the research is reviewed below. It is important to note that the researchers hope that studies will continue to explore methods to intervene before abuse occurs and to minimize the impact when it does.

In the Impact of Elder Abuse Education on Young Adults study (Hayslip et al., 2015), the authors examined the effectiveness of three different educational interventions (i.e., elder abuse education, aging education, family education) in changing the attitudes of traditionally aged college students toward elder abuse. While one of the three showed promise (i.e., the elder abuse education), its impact decreased over time, indicating the potential need for subsequent education. "Findings clearly suggest that gerontological interventions geared specifically toward elder abuse are needed for the minimization of elder abuse behaviors" (p. 246), with the primary education target being caregivers.

Cooper et al. (2015) acknowledged that many family caregivers become abusers when providing care for their loved ones with dementia. They "investigated whether START (STrAtegies for RelaTives), a psychological intervention which reduces depression and anxiety in family carers also reduces abusive behavior in carers of people living in their own homes" (p. 2). The authors focused on caregivers of persons with dementia, as they are frequent abusers of this population. They hoped that the use of START would reduce the occurrences of abuse. "This is the first study to consider outcomes for carers based on whether they reported behaving abusively at baseline. A quarter of carers still reported significant abuse after two years, but those not acting abusively at baseline did not become abusive. START decreased anxiety and depression and increased quality of life in family carers" (p. 7). There was no evidence that this intervention reduced abusive behaviors.

In long-term care living (e.g., nursing homes), "resident-to-resident elder mistreatment (R-REM), although not often studied, occurs with relatively high frequency" (Teresi et al., 2018, p. 15). The study acknowledged that R-REM acts of aggression like pushing often result in falls and other injuries. The study authors aimed to use the education of frontline staff (e.g., certified nursing assistants) focused on anticipating and intervening with R-REM to reduce falls and injuries. There was a reduction in falls in facilities where staff received the training. The authors hypothesized that this program might also be of use in assisted living and acute care settings.

Occupational Therapy's Role

Signs of elder abuse observable by the occupational therapy provider include bruises, fractures, social withdrawal or isolation, and fear of physical contact. When an occupational therapy practitioner determines that an elder is vulnerable to abuse due to caregiver stress, a referral to respite care, Adult Protective Services (APS), or social supports may be valuable. The occupational therapy practitioner can refer the caregiver to the local Area Agency on Aging, Eldercare Locator, APS, or community support groups for the elder and their caregiver. The practitioner should review personal as well as professional, legal, and ethical obligations and act accordingly.

The use of nonpharmaceutical interventions such as New Ways for Better Days: Tailoring Activities for Persons With Dementia and Their Caregivers (TAP), an evidence-based program to decrease caregiver stress while providing structured activities for people with dementia, is seen as beneficial in helping the caregiver and elder maintain a more satisfying quality of life. The protocol and clinical reasoning processes of TAP underlie the use of tailored activities as a therapeutic intervention designed to address dementia-related neuropsychiatric behaviors (Marx, Scott, Piersol, and Gitlin, 2019). The reduction of these behaviors makes management of the person with dementia easier, reducing the potential for caregiver stress and, by extension, abuse.

Occupational therapy practitioners, along with other health professionals, are mandatory reporters when abuse is suspected. Each state board of occupational therapy practice has specific reporting requirements. The American Occupational Therapy Association's *Occupational Therapy Code of Ethics (2015)* includes principles and related standards of conduct (RSC) to guide occupational therapy students and practitioners in ways to protect and advocate for clients and families. One of several principles and the corresponding RSC applicable to situations in which elder abuse is possible are identified in Box 27-2.

APS is an important resource for practitioners and families alike. The mission of APS is to protect older adults and people with disabilities from mistreatment. There are offices in every state, although programs vary from state to state. Clients' safety is promoted through APS's collaboration with professionals and clients. Information on programs, mandatory reporting and investigation processes, and other helpful information appears on the website of the National Adult Protective Services Association (n.d.). Its interdisciplinary focus is to prevent abuse, neglect, and exploitation through collaborative interventions (Ramsey-Klawsnik, Dayton, Gregorie, and Koontz, 2018a, 2018b).

If social isolation is a risk factor for elder abuse, occupational therapy practitioners should access the social participation of their older clients. Engaging these clients in occupation-based activities with their peers may reduce isolation and, ultimately, vulnerability to elder abuse. Furthermore, following the work of researchers like Landeiro, Barrows, Musson, Gray, and Leal (2017), who conducted Reducing Social Isolation and Loneliness in Older People: A Systematic Review, may provide the occupational therapy practitioner with a protocol for using their results to benefit occupational therapy practice and the people served.

Occupational therapy students and practitioners should also review the work of Gitlin (Johns Hopkins University, n.d.), which has included studying the use of tailored activities to reduce behaviors of people living with dementia and cared for in the community. The occupation-based assessment and intervention processes are geared to the needs of persons with dementia and their caregivers.

"Elder abuse will not stop on its own. Someone else needs to step in and help" (NIH, 2017, para. 4). If an occupational therapy practitioner determines that the older adult is in imminent danger, 9-1-1 should be contacted. If abuse is suspected, follow the guidelines established for mandatory reporters and the principles and RSC in the AOTA *Occupational Therapy Code of Ethics (2015)* for guidance.

Engage Your Brain 27-3

Has the AOTA issued a societal statement or official document on violence? What other mechanisms can an AOTA member use to advocate for the AOTA's action to protect individuals with disabilities and other marginalized populations from violence?

Bullying

Bullying is a term used to describe a collection of unwanted and aggressive behaviors that cause harm or distress to a targeted individual (Gladden, Vivolo-Kanor, Hamburger, and Lumpkin, 2014). These intentional and repeated acts of aggression can greatly affect both the victim's and the perpetrator's mental and physical health (Gladden et al., 2014; Volk, Veenstra, and Espelage, 2017), even into adulthood (Byjos, Dusing, Zartman, and Cahill, 2016). Acts of bullying can be classified into three distinct categories: direct, indirect, and cyberbullying (AOTA, 2013). **Direct bullying** includes physical acts of aggression and verbal taunting or name-calling. **Indirect bullying** is characterized by relational acts of aggression like spreading rumors. Finally, **cyberbullying** involves threatening or hurtful messages or images that are posted on social media or received through text or e-mail.

Extent of the Problem

Nearly 20% of all children and youth in the United States experience some form of bullying (CDC, 2018d), and around 40% of middle school students report being bullied or engaging in bullying on a weekly basis (Domino, 2013). The number of victims who experience cyberbullying may be as much as twice that of those bullied directly in a school setting (Chang et al., 2013).

Risk Factors

Children and youth who engage in bullying behaviors often do so in order to gain peer acceptance and obtain a higher social status than others (Thornberg, 2011). Once individuals are viewed as bullies by their peer group, it is often difficult to be viewed differently (Burns, Maycock, Cross, and Brown, 2008). Some literature suggests that children and youth who bully are more likely to have a lower socioeconomic status and come from homes where parents have less education (Verlinden et al., 2014). Parents who demonstrate too little supervision and control (Verlinden et al., 2014) and those who are overcontrolling and abusive are both associated with having children who bully (Gladstone, Parker, and Malhi, 2006).

Children and youth are bullied for many reasons, such as their appearance, the amount and types of friends they have, and their perceived social status (Lemstra, Nielsen, Rogers, Thompson, and Moraros, 2012). Females are generally thought to experience indirect bullying (i.e., gossip) and verbal bullying, while males are generally thought to experience physical aggression (Maynard, Vaughn, Salas-Wright, and Vaughn, 2016). Children and youth with some disabilities are particularly at risk for experiencing bullying due to experiencing peer rejection, possessing decreased social skills, and occupying lower social status (Zablotsky, Bradshaw, Anderson, and Law, 2014). For example, children with autism spectrum disorders, particularly those who are found to be high functioning and integrated into general education programs, are more at risk for bullying than lower-performing peers (Zablotsky et al., 2014). In addition, children and youth in the United States with immigrant status are often marginalized and more at risk for bullying than native-born children (Maynard et al., 2016). Children and youth with immigrant status who have poor health and are overweight report greater marginalization, dissatisfaction with peer relationships, and loneliness (Maynard et al., 2016). Other risk factors for bullying include being perceived as different by peers (Jansen et al., 2012). Examples of differences included lower socioeconomic status (Jansen et al., 2012) and differences in appearance (i.e., perceived attractiveness, height, and weight; Frisen, Johnsson, and Persson, 2007).

Consequences

The consequences children and youth experience as a result of bullying vary based on the type of bullying and a variety of personal factors (Byjos et al., 2016). For example, some children and youth may shy away from social situations, avoid peers, or be hesitant to advocate for themselves. Children and youth who have strong attachments, higher levels of intelligence, and better coping skills generally respond more adaptively to bullying (Byjos et al., 2016).

Bullying affects mental and physical health as well as occupational performance. Victims of bullying report depression, anxiety, poor relationships, and a higher risk for suicide (Lemstra et al., 2012). In addition, victims often experience sleep disturbances, abdominal pain, and headaches (Lemstra et al., 2012). School attendance and performance often suffer because of the consequences of being bullied, and some victims go on to have difficulty completing school and maintaining employment in adulthood (Lemstra et al., 2012). Victims of bullying may not always seek help from others due to fear of retaliation and feelings of insecurity (Lemstra et al., 2012). Victims often have difficulty with trust and forming relationships (Schafer et al., 2004). As a result of ongoing bullying, some victims narrow their social circles and tend to surround themselves with others who may share the same bullying experiences (Schafer et al., 2004).

Evidence-Based Prevention/ Mitigation Strategies

Both universal and focused interventions have been designed to address bullying. Universal interventions are those provided at the school-wide level. The focus of universal interventions is to establish social environments where bullying is not tolerated and generally include clear rules and consequences associated with bullying behaviors (Cantone et al., 2015). Curricula, such as the Positive Action program (Lewis et al., 2013), are often incorporated into universal strategies to provide a framework for formal instruction on topics such as self-concept, social responsibility, positive mental health, and getting along with others.

Focused interventions often center around the early identification of children and youth at risk for bullying (Jansen et al., 2012) and teaching social skills to potential victims (Cantone et al., 2015). However, the literature suggests that such bullying-prevention programs are only somewhat effective and that more effective programs target potential victims and perpetrators and focus on the development of empathy (Evans, Fraser, and Cotter, 2014). Effective programs teach children and youth to experience what others feel and include empathic skills training in a group setting (Van Noorden, Haselager, Cillessen, and Bukowski, 2015).

Occupational Therapy's Role

Occupational therapy practitioners can be instrumental in helping children and youth to develop empathy and other social skills (e.g., negotiation, cooperation, asking for help) to reduce the likelihood of engaging in bullying behavior and increasing the chances of early reporting. Occupational therapy practitioners address volitional development and identity formation through the use of intentionally selected occupations and occupational challenges (Byjos et al., 2016). In addition, occupational therapy practitioners can promote social relationships and foster friendships during opportunities to participate in enjoyable occupations, both of which are important mediators in the promotion of mental health and the prevention of bullying (AOTA, 2013).

Shootings

The CDC (2018d) views violence against children and youth as a leading cause of injury and death for this population. In 2017, 6% of high school students report being threatened or injured with a weapon on school property (CDC, 2018d). Gun violence, in particular, is viewed as a serious threat to children and youth, and there is a need for improved policies and strategies to reduce unintentional access to firearms by this population (National Association of School Psychologists, 2013).

Types of Shootings

The two types of gun violence perpetrated by youth are street shootings and school shootings (Bushman et al., 2016). Street shootings are often concentrated in urban environments and are typically performed by individuals who have previously been exposed to crime and violence and have access to illegally obtained firearms (Bushman et al., 2016; Butts, Roman, Bostwick, and Porter, 2015). Low socioeconomic status, low levels of education, and substance use are commonly associated with individuals who perform street shootings (Bushman et al., 2016).

In contrast, school shootings are often concentrated in suburban and rural environments and are typically performed by white, middle-class individuals whose family members obtained firearms through legal channels (Bushman et al., 2016). Access to multiple firearms, including semiautomatic weapons, high levels of academic achievement, and symptoms of mental illness are commonly associated with individuals who perform school shootings (Bushman et al., 2016; Ferguson, Coulson, and Barnett, 2011).

Risk Factors

Several risk factors are common to youth who commit gun violence, regardless of the type. Some common characteristics of street and school shooters include a lack of empathy, a drive to obtain power, and a sense of entitlement (Bushman et al., 2016). In addition to personality characteristics, family relationships play a large role. Family violence, inconsistent discipline, abuse, neglect, and regression are associated with youth who commit gun violence (Bushman et al., 2016; Stoddard et al., 2013).

Peer rejection, or the fear of peer rejection, devaluation, bullying, and disrespect have also been found to be risk factors for gun violence (Bushman et al., 2016). Youth involved in bullying, either as the victim or the perpetrator, are five times more likely to carry weapons than peers who have no experience with bullying (van Geel, Vedder, and Tanilon, 2014). Individuals who experienced bullying or distrust formal systems of justice are more likely to seek retaliation (Bushman et al., 2016).

Evidence-Based Prevention/ Mitigation Strategies

Several interventions have been found to reduce the likelihood of youth violence. Like interventions to address bullying, antiviolence interventions can be universal or focused. Universal interventions include limiting access to guns and substances and improving school climate (Bushman et al., 2016).

The majority of homicides that take place in the United States are committed with guns (FBI, 2013). Although youth engaging in violence may have more ready access to other weapons (e.g., knives), guns are considered the most lethal (Bushman et al., 2016). More stringent policies regarding the ownership and transfer of firearms could potentially reduce youths' access to guns (Bushman et al., 2016). However, stricter gun reform is just one factor associated with universal youth violence prevention.

Youth violence and aggression is associated with alcohol and substance use (Bushman et al., 2016). Alcohol and other substances can reduce judgment and heighten feelings like aggression and fear. Policies and interventions that deter youth from using alcohol and drugs may also have the potential for lowering the risk of violence in certain youth populations (Bushman et al., 2016).

Creating positive school environments that foster a sense of belonging for all students is an important universal intervention associated with reducing school violence (Bushman et al., 2016). The most effective interventions build a foundation of trust between youth and the adults who work in the school and include mechanisms to address peer conflict management (Bushman et al., 2016). Examples of ways conflict management is effectively addressed are through the use of peer juries, group conferencing, and peer mediation (Braithwaite, 1999).

Focused interventions to prevent school violence are often directed toward the development of empathy, perspective taking, anger management, and skills for coping with social rejection (Bushman et al., 2016). Such interventions should target children and youth who are at risk for violence early, and additional support for the use of the acquired skills should be provided throughout their educational experience (Conduct Problems Prevention Research Group, 2011).

Occupational Therapy's Role

Occupational therapy practitioners can work with children and youth to promote participation in meaningful occupations and develop habits and routines around conflict management and coping during stressful or unpleasant social situations (AOTA, 2018). Such interventions have the potential to increase occupational engagement at school, as well as provide a foundation for habits and routines that youth can use into adulthood. Occupational therapy practitioners may also work with schools and communities to screen children and youth for indicators of mental health (i.e., subjective well-being) and signs of mental illness (Cahill and Egan, 2017).

Workplace Violence

Workplace violence is a significant employee issue, with long-lasting and damaging effects on morale, time away from work, injury, and illness. As defined by the Occupational Safety and Health Administration (OSHA, 2015), **workplace violence** is any act or threat of physical violence, harassment, intimidation, or other threatening, disruptive behavior that occurs at the workplace (National Institute for Occupational Safety and Health, 2002). This includes both physically or psychologically damaging actions. Examples of workplace violence include direct physical assaults, written or verbal threats, physical or verbal harassment, and homicide (OSHA, 2015).

Extent of the Problem

The U.S. Bureau of Labor Statistics releases an annual report about injuries and illnesses resulting in time away from work in the United States due to workplace violence. It is estimated that approximately 2,000,000 people report some type of workplace violence each year, while 25% goes unreported (U.S. Bureau of Labor Statistics, 2014). Nearly half (48%) of military women who served in a war zone report being sexually harassed, and 22.8% report experiencing sexual assault while there (Spivak, 2017). Mullen (2019), in an article citing a poll of active duty and veteran members, found that 66% of women in the military say they have personally experienced sexual assault or sexual harassment, compared to just 6% of men.

In recent years, the frequency of workplace violence has increased, and the number of mass shooting events in the workplace has trended upward. The Gun Violence Archive (2019) reported 346 mass workplace shootings in 2017, compared to 270 in 2014. The U.S. Bureau of Labor Statistics (2014) also reports that 13% of the days away from work in 2013 were due to violence, and the rate is increasing. OSHA (2014) also reported an increased frequency of workplace violence for those in the health-care and social assistance sectors. These episodes are characterized by either verbal or physical assaults perpetrated by patients, coworkers, and visitors against providers.

The published data from the Bureau of Labor Statistics revealed that health-care workers were nearly four times more likely to require time away from work because of violence. Nearly 75% of the workplace assaults occurred in a health-care setting. For example, OSHA (2015) reports show that between 2011 and 2013, U.S. health-care workers suffered 15,000 to 20,000 serious workplace-violence-related injuries. The latest workplace violence statistics indicate that 80% of emergency medical services personnel are attacked by patients, while 78% of emergency department physicians have been attacked by patients (Lebron, 2017). Studies show that between 35% and 80% of hospital staff have been physically assaulted at least once during their careers (Clements, DeRanieri, Clark, Manno, and Kuhn, 2005).

The latest statistics on workplace violence also indicate that there is underreporting of nonfatal injuries and illnesses. This underreporting creates a misleading picture of violence in the workplace, which results in employers failing to adequately manage risk and protect employees. A study conducted by Peek-Asa et al. (2009) found that 80% of the nurses surveyed did not feel safe in their work environments. Many health-care workers underreport, believing that "violence is a part of the job" (McPhaul and Lipscomb, 2004).

Risk Factors

The violence experienced at workplaces is often overlooked and, as mentioned above, underreported. The use of different definitions and data collection and measurement methods and the differences in cultural contexts may often contribute to employers' lack of attention to workplace violence. In health care, reasons for underreporting workplace violence have included lack of injury or time lost and time-consuming incident-reporting procedures (Arnetz, 1998; Gates, 2004), as well as the belief that reporting will not lead to positive change (Arnetz et al., 2015). In addition, it is difficult to identify specific warning signs, so they are often misread or ignored. The presence of overly stressed work environments and unstable individuals creates an explosive combination. According to the National Safety Council (2019), approximately 2,000,000 workers per year report having been victims of workplace violence. Employees are faced with threats, harassment, bullying, verbal and physical intimidation, stalking, and other forms of unacceptable behavior that often have the potential to lead to significantly more violent behavior.

While violence can take place in any work setting, some occupations are more at risk than others. Occupations that involve face-to-face interaction with clients, customers, or others outside the work organization increase the risk of violent incidents (i.e., "third-party" violence). Risk sectors include education, health care and social work, transport and communication services, and hotels and restaurants, as well as shop workers and assistants. It is reported that younger workers appear to be more at risk than older ones (Estryn-Behar et al., 2008).

Research results are varied concerning the role of gender (Estryn-Behar et al., 2008). It is suggested that because women are overrepresented in high-risk jobs, they are at greater risk of exposure to violence than men. However, studies in the health-care sector reveal higher risk levels for male workers than for female workers (Di Martino, Hoel, and Cooper, 2003). Overall, women are more at risk of other types of violence and discrimination—in particular, sexual harassment and victimization (European Foundation for the Improvement of Living and Working Conditions, 2013).

Current research does not always focus on the longitudinal relationships that may explain the results. However, the available evidence highlights a number of individual, organizational, and societal-level factors that have been found to be associated with higher exposure to workplace violence. Some of these factors are presented below.

Individual Factors

Several individual factors are believed to increase the risk of exposure to workplace violence. For example, lower levels of education and training, as well as limited work experience, previous exposure to violence, inadequate conflict management skills, and low self-esteem can be associated with a higher risk of workplace violence (Hahn et al., 2008).

Organizational Factors

A wide range of factors related to specific tasks or situations and the organization of work have been identified as potential antecedents of workplace violence. Individuals working with people in need of physical or emotional care or with substance or drug addiction are at greater risk. Other specific high-risk tasks and situations include evening and night work, delivery of goods and services, shift work or working alone, on-location work, valuables handling, jobs that exercise physical control over others, and specific physical design features of the workplace (Chappell and Di Martino, 2006). Often, the potential for violence also arises when an employee needs to deny an individual's request or when a request is made to do something an individual does not want to do. Conditions that may lead to higher stress levels in the workplace may include interpersonal conflicts, constant contact with the public, role ambiguity, low job control, time pressure, low-quality teamwork, and high workloads; situations such as these increase the risk of both external and internal violence. Terminations, demotions, layoffs, disciplinary actions, and unresolved or unsatisfied resolution of employee complaints and grievances are also considered contributing factors to incidents of workplace violence (Calabro and Baraniuk, 2003). For health-care providers, the quality of health care received by patients, which may include long waiting times and satisfaction with treatment, has been linked to workplace violence. Fatigue or stress resulting from high-strain work may also undermine the conflict management skills of workers, decreasing their ability to defuse potentially violent situations. Finally, workers may actually be the instigators of violent interactions due to anger or frustration caused by working under strain.

Social and Economic Level Factors

Social- and economic-level factors have an impact on workplace violence. There are numerous cultural norms and values. Individualization, the violence that is embedded in societies, globalization, media attention, and governmental decisions that have an impact on society and population density are all noteworthy factors related to workplace violence. These issues can help to create a climate of violence. The increased concentrations of poverty, along with diminished economic opportunities, create an atmosphere for those working in emergency services or health care that can lead to potential violence. Hoobler and Swanberg (2006) suggest that public sector employees were only 16% of the workforce from 1992 to 1996; however, they were victims of 37% of the incidents of workplace violence. This increase in violence may be due to antigovernmental sentiments involving frustrated clients, terrorist groups, and those who may be angry with bureaucrats.

Consequences

Violence in the workplace may have serious consequences for individuals, families, friends, coworkers, witnesses, supervisors, organizations, and society. According to OSHA (2014), approximately 75% of nearly 25,000 workplace assaults reported annually occurred in health-care and social service settings. The effects of workplace violence can lead to physical and psychological health problems. In a study by De Puy et al. (2015), the consequences of psychological violence were deemed to be serious and often long lasting, which is consistent with studies by Hogh and Viitasara (2005). Physical consequences depend upon the severity of the incident and can range from bruising to death. Psychological consequences can include anxiety, fear, increased irritability, concentration difficulties, reduced self-confidence, fatigue, sleeping problems, stress reactions, depression, and PTSD. The exposure to violence may also lead to lowered motivation, increased absenteeism, and diminished performance. The psychological effects of violence will differ from person to person. However, the effects can be long lasting and often overwhelming for all the individuals involved in or witnessing the violence. In the study by De Puy et al. (2012), individuals cited financial constraints related to the loss of their job due to workplace violence, while other individuals in the study reported fears related to personal safety concerns and job insecurity, as well as fear and lasting psychological conditions.

There are multiple costs to organizations due to workplace violence. Organizations may experience higher sickness-related absence rates, higher turnover rates (replacement costs and skills loss), and reduced job satisfaction, as well as decreased motivation and productivity of victimized workers and their colleagues. Additionally, increased insurance premiums may result in economic loss for organizations. The consequences of workplace bullying, harassment, and incivility may lead to litigation costs, grievance/compensation costs, property damage or damaged equipment, training costs, rehabilitation costs, and loss of public goodwill and reputation.

Evidence-Based Prevention/ Mitigation Strategies

The imperative for management to understand and implement prevention strategies continues to grow in importance. Support from top leadership is necessary to ensure that adequate resources are provided to facilitate success in programs and prevention strategies so that programs have a top-down approach and the prevention strategies will potentially be accepted throughout the organization (OSHA, 2014). Research by Lipscomb et al. (2006) determined that interventions, such as improved management commitment to a violence prevention program and employee engagement, can lead to enhanced employee perceptions of safety. Buy-in and employee participation in the planning, development, and implementation of programs and strategies are critical to success. Creating an environment of commitment in the prevention of workplace violence is fundamental to establish a culture of awareness and prevention in the workplace.

A multidisciplinary approach with individuals who have diverse knowledge and experiences will provide the most beneficial approach to help people understand the complexity of the various types of workplace violence. The collaboration of multiple units and departments within an organization is key to planning and implementing education, practices, and programs to address intervention and response (Clements et al., 2005). A collaborative approach will also support the creation of a threat assessment team to review and respond to reports of physical or verbal threats of violence. Key offices that should be part of a multidisciplinary approach include management, labor representatives, human resources, safety and health, security, medical/psychology, legal, communications, and worker assistance. Memorandums of understanding may be arranged to help obtain outside expertise from local law enforcement and local service providers. Prearranged collaboration with local law enforcement will assist with incidents that require police response and intervention.

Organizations must commit to developing strong policies and procedures to address workplace violence. Such policies must include unambiguous definitions of the behaviors that are indicative of workplace violence and the consequences of those actions. Clear information must be provided that outlines the review and response system for all reported violent incidents. Additionally, well-defined guidelines to assist those tasked with the responsibility to review and respond are essential; such procedures are necessary for reviewing all reported incidents. Multiple response mechanisms should be available and in place to support and protect all affected persons.

Communication to all members of the organization is also key to assisting employees with reporting and responding to workplace violence. Effective communication, confidentiality, teamwork, and accountability must be exercised regularly.

Communication to employees should be provided in multiple ways, and organizations utilizing creative communication strategies may assist with employee comprehension of policies and procedures for response and reporting.

Training both supervisors and employees regularly is an important element in prevention (Gallant-Roman, 2008). Both supervisors and employees must participate in the training so that buy-in is created from the top down. Training must be provided annually, and the content should focus on hazards found in the workplace, as well as the organization's prevention policies and procedures, highlighting reporting, review, response, and evaluation procedures.

Employers must determine if there are cultural barriers (Neuman and Baron, 1998) to the awareness, prevention, and response to workplace violence. Changes in the workplace culture must occur to foster an atmosphere that provides support for victims and increased clarification of acceptable and unacceptable behaviors, reporting mechanisms, and help or sanctions for perpetrators.

Finally, every program must employ an evaluation system that is evidence based. Companies must make the effort to evaluate policies, procedures, and programs. Organizations may waste valuable resources on prevention mechanisms and training if evaluation procedures are not integrated into programs to measure impact. Effective programs and strategies need to be shared across industries, sectors, units, and within the organization. The evaluation and evidence of the success and failure of programs can become key to both prevention and the support of victims.

Occupational Therapy's Role

There is very limited discussion within the discipline's literature of the impact of workplace violence on occupational therapy practitioners and occupational therapy's role in addressing that violence. A survey of 283 occupational therapy practitioners within Canada and the United States (Brown and Rivard, 2017) indicated that bullying and mobbing were the most frequently experienced type of workplace violence, with the perpetrator being a coworker or manager 90% of the time. The vast majority did not report the incident because they either did not believe anything would change (64%) or they felt ashamed (21%). These results indicate a need for further study and the development of interventions to address the violence experienced by occupational therapy practitioners.

There also is limited literature on occupational therapy's broader role in workplace violence prevention and mitigation. Rai (2002) articulated the education and expertise (e.g., task analysis, reduction of workers' physical or psychological stress) of occupational therapy personnel that is beneficial to violence prevention in the workplace. There is logic in advocating for the extension of occupational therapy's role in workplace ergonomic consultation to include workplace violence prevention and mitigation.

Twinley and Addidle (2012) highlighted the need to discuss and study antisocial occupations such as violence. They pointed out that while occupational therapy researchers study the impact of violence on survivors, the profession has neglected to "acknowledge the individual or collective experience of violence as an occupation from the perspective of those who are violent" (2012, p. 203). Twinley and Addidle acknowledge that there will be legal and practical barriers, as well as ethical considerations, in conducting this work but stress the need for the profession to understand the impact of engaging in violence on perpetrators' health and well-being. The authors clearly stated that this call to action in no way condones violent behavior.

While there is limited literature on the role of occupational therapy in workplace violence prevention and mitigation, it is clear that there is a need. First, there is a need for an active expansion of occupational therapy's work in ergonomics and industrial consultation to include risk assessments for and the mitigation of violence. Second, there is a need for continued research on the impact of workplace violence on survivors and the factors that promote resiliency among survivors to inform future interventions and research. Third, occupational therapy practitioners should advocate for policies, such as the California Hospital Safety and Security Act, which may decrease assaults on staff (Casteel et al., 2009). In addition, an understanding of the catalysts for perpetrators engaging in workplace violence is needed both to inform policy and prevention strategies for others as well as to provide an opportunity for perpetrators to reassess choices related to occupational engagement.

PROGRAM SHOWCASE

The Family Village is a transitional living facility for women and children who are homeless, the majority of whom have experienced domestic violence.

The goals of the Family Village program are to:

- Meet families' immediate needs for stable housing so they are free to work on overcoming obstacles to self-sufficiency
- Help family members obtain job skills and educational skills so they can financially support their families
- Overcome obstacles, such as lack of affordable childcare, so parents may work outside the home
- Facilitate recovery from and avoid the trauma which homelessness and economic instability cause to their health, self-esteem, and emotional development and
- Help families secure and retain permanent housing when they complete the Family Village program.

Transitional housing and program participation are provided for up to 24 months. The site has 18 apartments, a playground/courtyard, laundry facilities, a community room with a kitchen, 2 small conference rooms, and staff offices.

When the program began, no occupational therapy services were offered. Seeing this as an opportunity to develop a community-based occupational therapy program, occupational therapy faculty and students at a local university offered to conduct a needs assessment and volunteered their services.

The needs assessment methodology included a review of existing literature, record reviews/data mining, key informant interviews with stakeholders and service providers, and focus groups consisting of family members living at the facility. In addition, mothers were asked to complete questionnaires designed to measure (a) the physical and mental health of the women and their children, and (b) their perceived needs for job-related and independent living skills.

Based on the results of the needs assessment, occupational therapy faculty and students proposed the development of an occupational therapy program to address the following goals:

- Improve the mental health, life skills, quality of life and overall health and well-being of the women and children residing in the Family Village.
- Facilitate independent living in the community, job acquisition and retention, and full participation in society.

A health fair was conducted at the facility as a means of collecting additional health data and to launch the occupational therapy program. The health fair was provided by an interprofessional group of faculty and students and included the following services:

- Hearing screening provided by the Audiology department
- Developmental screening
  - Gross motor screening provided by the Physical Therapy department
  - Fine motor and ADL screening provided by the Occupational Therapy department
- General health screening provided by the Physician Assistant Studies department
- Mental health screening provided by the Occupational Therapy department
- Dental hygiene screening by the Occupational Therapy department and local dentists

In addition, healthy snacks and balloons were donated by local vendors.

Occupational therapy students developed skill-based group interventions in the areas of money management, household management, parenting, and nutrition/meal planning. These sessions were provided during both daytime and evening hours to accommodate the mothers' school and work schedules. Clients were scheduled for individual sessions as needed. The site was established as a Level I fieldwork experience for students.

Future plans for occupational therapy services at the facility include creating programs for children based on developmental level, expanding opportunities for mothers to acquire job acquisition and retention skills, and providing supports to address trauma and substance abuse recovery and to promote positive mental health. Sources of funding are being sought to hire a full-time occupational therapist for the facility.

Summary

- Violence is pervasive worldwide. It is observed across all groups in the United States and comes in a variety of forms and types, including homicide, suicide, domestic and family violence, sexual violence, youth and school violence, elder abuse, and workplace violence.
- Causal links to committing violence include personal (e.g., childhood trauma, male gender, substance abuse and use) as well as social and environmental factors, including poverty and access to guns.
- While prevalence rates of violence vary by geography, economic level, and ethnicity, women are the group most affected by violence.
- The provision of occupational therapy interventions to survivors of violence can lessen the negative impact of these incidents on social, emotional, and occupational functioning. Additional theory-based strategies need to be developed and studied to serve the growing number of survivors of violence.
- In order to be maximally effective, occupational therapy violence prevention efforts should not focus solely on individuals. Due to the inextricable links between persons and their environments, prevention strategies should also address families, groups, organizations, communities, and policy-makers.

CASE STUDIES

CASE STUDY 27-1 Bully Mediation

Peter is a sixth-grade student who recently moved from a nearby town, which caused him to change schools in the middle of the academic year. Peter is tall for his age, has asthma, and is slightly overweight. Peter struggles to keep up with his classmates during physical education and is frequently chosen last for teams. Recently, another sixth-grade student, named James, has begun to tease Peter in the locker room while the students are changing for physical education class. James makes fun of Peter's appearance and asks the other boys in the locker room if they can help him "find Peter's bra." The taunting has caused Peter to change in a bathroom stall. The boys pound on the stall door while he changes and have sometimes held the door shut so he cannot get out.

Peter is extremely upset about the teasing. However, he does not feel like he can tell Mr. Jones, the physical education teacher, because the teacher has commented on his weight before, and Peter fears further embarrassment and retaliation from James and his group of friends. Peter begins to tell his mom that he is sick and asks to stay home. Peter's mom allows him to stay home for 2 days. On the third day, Peter's mom takes him to his pediatrician. Peter confides in his mother on the way home from the appointment, once it has been determined by the physician that he is not ill.

Upon learning about the bullying, Peter's mother calls the school principal. The principal puts her in touch with the school social worker. The social worker convinces Peter's mom to send him to school the next day. Once Peter returns to school, he meets with the school social worker for one-on-one sessions to discuss the bullying and his feelings about it. The social worker refers Peter to the occupational therapy practitioner for a friendship-promotion group.

The friendship-promotion group meets two times a week during an advisory period. The focus of the group is on fostering friendships in a safe and predictable environment. The occupational therapy practitioner works with the students to identify interests and then selects activities (e.g., games, crafts, and projects) for them to work on during the groups. The occupational therapy practitioner facilitates friendship skills during the group, and the group members have opportunities to practice entering a group, giving compliments, cooperating, and demonstrating empathy.

CASE STUDY 27-1 Bully Mediation

While attending the friendship group, Peter meets Henry. Henry and Peter share many common interests and enjoy each other's company. Henry is well liked by many of his classmates and is in the same physical education class as Peter. Henry invites Peter to play on the playground, and the two boys make plans to see each other outside of school. Despite Peter's friendship with Henry, and warnings provided by Mr. Jones, James continues to bully Peter.

With permission from the principal, the social worker and the occupational therapy practitioner work to set up a system for peer mediation. One student from each sixth-grade classroom is elected by classmates to serve on a panel. The panel acts like a jury to determine who is at fault in a given situation and provides recommendations to the principal regarding consequences. The occupational therapy practitioner works with the panel to establish ground rules and procedures for assuming the role of peer mediators. The social worker works with Peter and James on an individual basis to process the situation and prepare them for their presentations to the panel.

The peer mediation panel hears from Peter and James and finds James guilty of bullying Peter. The panel recommends that James serves a week of in-school detention and lose the opportunity to go on an upcoming field trip. The principal supports this recommendation, as do James's parents. The other sixth-grade students become aware of the panel's decision, and other students begin to come forward with problems for the panel to consider.

James is upset with the decision and tries to bully Peter in the locker room shortly after their peer mediation. However, this time the other boys in the locker room do not participate in the bullying, and two boys encourage James to stop and remind him of his consequences. Without the support of his friends, James stops bullying Peter in the locker room. Peter continues to feel better when he has the opportunity to change in a stall, and Mr. Jones permits him to do so. Mr. Jones is now careful with the comments he makes when Peter struggles to keep up with his peers and now understands he is accountable for creating a climate of inclusion during physical education class.

Discussion Questions

1. What unique knowledge and skills do the social worker and the occupational therapist bring to Peter's situation? How do these professional disciplines complement each other?
2. What are the pros and cons of peer mediation? Who in the school might be supportive of peer mediation? Who might be opposed to peer mediation?
3. What are some games or activities that are appropriate for Peter's age range that could be included in the friendship groups?
4. Changing for physical education is stressful for many children and youth. What are some strategies the physical education teacher could use to create a safe and supportive locker room climate?

CASE STUDY 27-2 Caregiver Stress

Sonny, an 81-year-old man, lives with his wife of 50 years. Sonny began showing signs of dementia more than 10 years ago. His wife, Margo, was initially able to cope with her husband's memory loss and occasional word-finding problems. As time went on, his symptoms increased, and he had difficulty concentrating for sustained periods of time. Nevertheless, Margo and Sonny continued to enjoy outings together, and Sonny could stay at home occupying himself for hours at a time.

CASE STUDY 27-2 Caregiver Stress

Margo came home one day from lunch with friends and discovered Sonny gone. He had never left the house before without letting her know. She drove around their neighborhood and found him wandering in the park. Sonny was quite confused and afraid, stating that he was trying to find her. Following this episode Sonny wanted to always be at Margo's side. This was such a change in their relationship that Margo had difficulty coping with this "closeness."

Sonny's symptoms were reported to his doctor, who prescribed medication to reduce his anxiety and help him calm down. One of the side effects was that the medication was somewhat sedating. Margo began giving Sonny his medication more frequently than prescribed, as it helped give her a break from his closeness. As time went on and his disease progressed, Margo increased the use of the antianxiety medication and supplemented this with over-the-counter sleep medications. Finally, Margo was getting a break from Sonny, who needed to be with her constantly, and the day-to-day stressful consequences of his disease. Although she recognized that the medication impaired his balance and made him more confused, the medication regime helped to decrease her own stress.

Penny, Margo and Sonny's daughter, came to visit her parents from another state. She had become concerned that her dad was less available when she called, and when they did talk, his speech was slurred, and he seemed drowsy and out of touch. Penny knew a little about dementia; however, these symptoms did not fit her expectations. She wanted to see her dad in person to find out what was going on.

Margo initially reduced Sonny's medication after Penny's arrival, as she was worried that their daughter might become concerned. Sonny resumed his habit of following Margo around the house due to his need for close and constant contact. Margo's tolerance for this behavior was low, and she began gradually increasing Sonny's medication again. Penny observed these changes, reviewed the signs and symptoms of dementia again, and began to wonder if something else was occurring. She began to suspect that her mother was overmedicating her dad. As painful as this suspicion was, Penny knew that it had to be investigated and stopped if it was true. She tried to discuss her concerns with her mother but felt that she was being stonewalled. Penny developed a plan to call her dad's doctor and Adult Protective Services for help. She was willing to do whatever was necessary to keep her father safe and support her mother.

Discussion Questions

1. Based on your reading of the studies presented in the elder abuse section, project whether elder abuse education might benefit Penny, Margo, or both? Please provide a brief explanation to support your projections.
2. If Penny sought consultation with an occupational therapist who has expertise in working with older adults with dementia, what legal and ethical standards must the occupational therapist observe?
3. Identify three resources or organizations that would benefit this family through education and intervention.

Learning Activities

1. Use the Connections Selector located at https://vetoviolence.cdc.gov/apps/connecting-the-dots/node/5 to explore the relationships between types of violence and various risk and protective factors. Based on this review and the content of this chapter and Chapter 22, identify a population and its corresponding risk and protective factors to consider in the development of a proposal for a violence mitigation program.
2. Contact your state APS office. Review the services available and the number and type of

staff and compare this to another state with similar state demographics. If there are differences, explore the possible reasons for the differences through an interview with a staff member of your state APS.

3. Review the process and directions to make a Title IX complaint at your school or workplace. Using the SMOG Readability Formula (National Cancer Institute, 2001) or another assessment tool for reading level, determine the reading level of the directions. Develop a memo to compliment or to provide feedback on the access (e.g., how many clicks to reach the directions), readability of the instructions, ease of comprehension of the directions, or any other features.

REFERENCES

American Association of Suicidology. (2018). *Health regions and USA suicide rates.* Retrieved from www.suicidology.org/Portals/14/docs/Resources/FactSheets/2017/2017HEALTHregions.pdf

American Association of Suicidology. (2019). *Know the warning signs of suicide.* Retrieved from www.suicidology.org/resources/warning-signs

American Foundation for Suicide Prevention. (2019). *Suicide statistics.* Retrieved from https://afsp.org/about-suicide/suicide-statistics/

American Occupational Therapy Association. (2013). *Bullying prevention and friendship promotion.* Retrieved from www.aota.org/~/media/Corporate/Files/Practice/Children/SchoolMHToolkit/BullyingPreventionInfoSheet.pdf

American Occupational Therapy Association. (2015). Occupational therapy code of ethics (2015). *American Journal of Occupational Therapy, 69*(Suppl. 3), 6913410030. http://dx.doi.org/10.5014/ajot.2015.696S03

American Occupational Therapy Association. (2017). Occupational therapy services for individuals who have experienced domestic violence. *American Journal of Occupational Therapy, 71*(Suppl. 2), 7112410037.

American Occupational Therapy Association. (2018). *AOTA's societal statement on youth violence.* Retrieved from www.aota.org/~/media/Corporate/Files/Secure/Practice/OfficialDocs/Soc%20Statements/Soc-Stmt-Youth-Violence-fin.pdf

American Psychological Association. (2012). *Elder abuse and neglect: In search of solutions.* Retrieved from www.apa.org/pi/aging/resources/guides/elder-abuse.aspx

Arnetz, J. E. (1998). The Violent Incident Form (VIF): A practical instrument for the registration of violent incidents in the health care workplace. *Work Stress, 12*(1), 17–28.

Arnetz, J. E., Hamblin, L., Ager, J., Luborsky, M., Upfal, M. J., Russell, J., and Essenmacher, L. (2015). Underreporting of workplace violence comparison of self-report and actual documentation of hospital incidents. *Workplace Health and Safety, 63*(5), 200–210.

Blair, E. (2019, March 8). *"Quiet": A global anthem for victims of sexual harassment and abuse* [Rebroadcast interview with MILCK]. Retrieved from www.npr.org/2019/03/08/701409825/quiet-a-global-anthem-for-victims-of-sexual-harassment-and-abuse

Braithwaite, J. (1999). Restorative justice: Assessing optimistic and pessimistic accounts. *Crime and Justice, 25,* 1–127. doi:10.1086/449287

Brent, D. A., and Mann, J. J. (2006). Familial pathways to suicidal behavior: Understanding and preventing suicide among adolescent. *New England Journal of Medicine, 355*(26), 2719–2721.

Brown, C. A., and Rivard, A. (2017). *Violence in the occupational therapy workplace: Background to the project and survey report 2016.* Alberta, Canada: University of Alberta Department of Occupational Therapy. Retrieved from https://cbotlabs.wixsite.com/ot-work-violence/module-sessions

Burns, S., Maycock, B., Cross, D., and Brown, G. (2008). The power of peers: Why some students bully others to conform. *Qualitative Health Research, 18*(12), 1704–1716. doi:10.1177/1049732308325865

Bushman, B. J., Newman, K., Calvert, S. L., Downey, G., Dredze, M., Gottfredson, M., and Romer, D. (2016). Youth violence: What we know and what we need to know. *American Psychologist, 71*(1), 17–39. doi:10.1037/a0039687

Butts, J. A., Roman, C. G., Bostwick, L., and Porter, J. R. (2015). Cure violence: A public health model to reduce gun violence. *Annual Review of Public Health, 36,* 39–53.

Byjos, O., Dusing, J., Zartman, C., and Cahill, S. (2016). Perspectives of individuals who experienced bullying during childhood. *Open Journal of Occupational Therapy, 4*(4), article 2. doi:10.15453/2168-6408.1249

Cahill, S., and Egan, B. (2017). Identifying youth with mental health concerns. *OT Practice, 22*(5), CE1–CE7.

Calabro, K., and Baraniuk, S. (2003). Organizational factors related to safety in a psychiatric hospital: Employee perceptions. *AAOHN Journal: Official Journal of the American Association of Occupational Health Nurses, 51,* 425–432.

Cantone, E., Piras, A. P., Vellante, M., Preti, A., Daníelsdóttir, S., D'Aloja, E., . . . Bhugra, D. (2015). Interventions on bullying and cyberbullying in schools: A systematic review. *Clinical Practice and Epidemiology in Mental Health, 11*(Suppl. 1 M4), 58–76. doi:10.2174/1745017901511010058

Casteel, C., Peek-Asa, C., Nocera, M., Smith, J. B., Blando, J., Goldmacher, S., . . . Harrison, R. (2009). Hospital employee assault rates before and after enactment of the California Hospital Safety and Security Act. *Annals of Epidemiology, 19*(2), 125–133.

Centers for Disease Control and Prevention. (n.d.a). *Injury prevention and control: Division of violence prevention—connecting the dots.* Retrieved from https://vetoviolence.cdc.gov/apps/connecting-the-dots/node/5

Centers for Disease Control and Prevention. (n.d.b). *Violence prevention: Social ecological model.* Retrieved from https://vetoviolence.cdc.gov/violence-prevention-basics-social-ecological-model

Centers for Disease Control and Prevention. (2014). *Child maltreatment: Facts at a glance.* Retrieved from www.cdc.gov/violenceprevention/pdf/childmaltreatment-facts-at-a-glance.pdf

Centers for Disease Control and Prevention. (2016). *10 leading causes of injury deaths by age group highlighting violence-related injury deaths, United States—2016.* Retrieved from www.cdc.gov/injury/images/lc-charts/leading_causes_of_death_highlighting_violence_2016_1030w800h.gif

Centers for Disease Control and Prevention. (2017). *Lesbian, gay, bisexual, and transgendered health: LGBT youth.* Retrieved from www.cdc.gov/lgbthealth/youth.htm

Centers for Disease Control and Prevention. (2018a). *Elder abuse: Consequences.* Retrieved from www.cdc.gov/violenceprevention/elderabuse/consequences.html

Centers for Disease Control and Prevention. (2018b). *Elder abuse: Risk and protective factors.* Retrieved from www.cdc.gov/violenceprevention/elderabuse/riskprotectivefactors.html

Centers for Disease Control and Prevention. (2018c). *Violence prevention: Intimate partner violence—what is intimate partner violence?* [PowerPoint slide show]. Retrieved from www.cdc.gov/violenceprevention/intimatepartnerviolence/index.html

Centers for Disease Control and Prevention. (2018d). *Youth risk behavior survey: Data summary and trends report 2007–2017.* Retrieved from www.cdc.gov/healthyyouth/data/yrbs/pdf/trendsreport.pdf

Centers for Disease Control and Prevention. (2019a). *Violence prevention at the CDC.* Retrieved from www.cdc.gov/violenceprevention/overview/index.html

Centers for Disease Control and Prevention. (2019b). *Violence prevention: Child abuse and neglect—risk and protective factors.* Retrieved from www.cdc.gov/violenceprevention/childabuseandneglect/riskprotectivefactors.html

Centers for Disease Control and Prevention. (2019c). *Violence prevention: Frequently asked questions.* Retrieved from www.cdc.gov/violenceprevention/datasources/nvdrs/faqs.html

Chang, F., Lee, C., Chiu, C., Hsi, W., Huang, T., and Pan, Y. (2013). Relationships among cyberbullying, school bullying, and mental health in Taiwanese adolescents. *Journal of School Health, 83*(6), 454–462. doi:10.1111/josh.12050

Chappell, D., and Di Martino, V. (2006). *Violence at work* (3rd ed.). Geneva, Switzerland: International Labour Organization.

Christoffel, T., and Gallagher, S. S. (2006). *Injury prevention and public health: Practical knowledge, skills and strategies* (2nd ed.). Gaithersburg, MD: Jones and Bartlett.

Clements, Paul T., DeRanieri, J. T., Clark, K., Manno, M. S., and Kuhn, D. W. (2005). Workplace violence and corporate policy for health care settings. *Nursing Economics, 3*(23), 1–10.

Conduct Problems Prevention Research Group. (2011). The effects of the fast track preventive intervention on the development of conduct disorder across childhood. *Child Development, 82,* 331–345. doi:10.1111/j.1467-8624.2010.01558.x

Conejero I., Olié, E., Courtet, P., and Calati, R. (2018). Suicide in older adults: Current perspectives. *Clinical Interventions in Aging, 13,* 691–699.

Coope, C., Gunnell, D., Hollingworth, W., Hawton, K., Kapur, N., Fearn, V., . . . Metcalfe, C. (2014). Suicide and the 2008 economic recession: Who is most at risk? Trends in suicide rates in England and Wales 2001–2011. *Social Science and Medicine, 117,* 76–85.

Cooper, C., Barber, J., Griffin, M., Rappaport, P., and Livingstone, G. (2015). Effectiveness of START psychological intervention in reducing abuse by dementia family carers: Randomized controlled trial. *International Psychogeriatrics, 11,* 1–7. Retrieved from www.ncbi.nim.nih.gov/pubed/26652193

Cooper, R. J. (2000). The impact of child abuse on children's play: A conceptual model. *Occupational Therapy International, 7*(4), 259–276.

De Brun, J. (2017). Maternal-child co-occupation within a domestic violence shelter. *American Journal of Occupational Therapy, 71,* 1.

De Puy, J., Romain-Glassey, N., Gut, M., Wild, P., Dell'Eva, A. S., and Asal, V. (2012). Clinically assessed consequences of workplace physical violence. *International Archives of International and Environmental Health, 88,* 213–224.

De Puy, J., Romain-Glassey, N., Gut, M., Wild, P., Mangin, P., and Danuser, B. (2015). Erratum to: Clinically assessed consequences of workplace physical violence. *International Archives of International and environmental Health, 88*(2), 225.

Di Martino, V., Hoel, H., and Cooper, C. L. (2003). *Preventing violence and harassment in the workplace (report).* Dublin: Ireland: European Foundation for the Improvement of Living and Working Conditions.

Domino, M. (2013). Measuring the impact of an alternative approach to school bullying. *Journal of School Health, 83*(6), 430–437. doi:10.1111/josh.12047

Estryn-Behar, M., van der Heijden, B., Camerino, D., Fryl, C., Le Nezet, O., Conway, P. M., and Hasselhorn, H-M. (2008). Violence risks in nursing—results from the European "NEXT" Study. *Occupational Medicine, 58,* 107–114.

European Foundation for the Improvement of Living and Working Conditions. (2013). *Physical and psychological violence at the workplace.* Dublin, Ireland: European Foundation for the Improvement of Living and Working Conditions.

Evans, C. B., Fraser, M. W., and Cotter, K. L. (2014). The effectiveness of school-based bullying prevention programs: A systematic review. *Aggression and Violent Behavior, 19*(5), 532–544. doi:10.1016/j.avb.2014.07.004

Federal Bureau of Investigation. (2013). *Uniform crime reports.* Washington, DC: Government Printing Office.

Federal Bureau of Investigation. (2019). *2017 crime in the United States: Murder.* Retrieved from https://ucr.fbi.gov/crime-in-the-u.s./2017/crime-in-the-u.s.-2017/topic-pages/murder

Ferguson, C. J., Coulson, M., and Barnett, J. (2011). Psychological profiles of school shooters: Positive directions and one big wrong turn. *Journal of Police Crisis Negotiations, 11*(2), 141–158. doi:10.1080/15332586.2011.581523

Frisén, A., Jonsson, A., and Persson, C. (2007). Adolescents' perception of bullying: Who is the victim? Who is the bully? What can be done to stop bullying? *Adolescence, 42*(168), 749–761.

Gallant-Roman, M. (2008). Strategies and tools to reduce workplace violence. *Workplace Health and Safety, 56*(11), 449–454.

Gates, D. M. (2004). The epidemic of violence against healthcare workers. *Occupational and Environmental Medicine, 61,* 649–650.

Gellert, G. A. (2002). *Confronting violence* (2nd ed.). Washington, DC: American Public Health Association.

Gladden, R., Vivolo-Kantor, A., Hamburger, M., and Lumpkin, C. (2014). *Bullying surveillance among youths: Uniform definitions for public health and recommended data elements, Version 1.0.* Atlanta, GA: National Center for Injury Prevention and Control, Centers for Disease Control and Prevention, and U.S. Department of Education.

Gladstone, G., Parker, G., and Malhi, G. (2006). Do bullied children become anxious and depressed adults? *Journal of Nervous and Mental Disease, 194*(3), 201–208.

Gorbien, M. J., and Einstein, A. R. (2005). Elder abuse and neglect: An overview. *Clinics in Geriatric Medicine, 21,* 279–292.

Gorde, M. W., Helfrich, C. A., and Finlayson, M. L. (2004). Trauma symptoms and life skills needed of domestic violence victims. *Journal of Interpersonal Violence, 19,* 691–708.

Gun Violence Archive. (2019). *Past summary ledgers.* Retrieved from www.gunviolencearchive.org/past-tolls.

Hahn, S., Zeller, A., Needham, I., Kok, G., Dassen, T., and Halfens, R. J. G. (2008). Patient and visitor violence in general hospitals: A systematic review of the literature. *Aggression and Violent Behavior, 13,* 431–441.

Harvard Law Review. (2018). *Criminal law—liability for physical harm—trial court convicts defendant of involuntary manslaughter based on encouragement of suicide, 131*(3), 918–925.

Hayslip, B., Reinberg, J., and Williams, J. (2015). The impact of elder abuse education on young adults. *Journal of Elder Abuse and Neglect, 27*(3), 233–253.

Hogh A., and Viitasara E. (2005). A systematic review of longitudinal studies of nonfatal workplace violence. *European Journal Work Organizational Psychology, 14*(3), 291–313.

Hoobler, J., and Swanberg, J. (2006). The enemy is not us: Unexpected workplace violence trends. *Public Personnel Management, 35*(3), 229–246.

Jansen, P., Verlinden, M., Dommisse-van Berkel, A., Mieloo, C., van der Ende, J., Veenstra, R., and Tiemeier, H. (2012). Prevalence of bullying and victimization among children in early elementary school: Do family and school neighbourhood socioeconomic status matter? *BMC Public Health, 12,* 494. doi:10.1186/1471-2458-12-494

Johns Hopkins University. (n.d.). *Laura N. Gitlin.* Retrieved from https://jhu.pure.elsevier.com/en/persons/laura-n-gitlin/publications/

Johns Hopkins University. (2015). *Alcohol and violence.* Retrieved from www.camy.org/resources/fact-sheets/alcohol-violence

Landeiro, F., Barrows, P., Musson, E. N., Gray, A. M., and Leal, J. (2017). Reducing social isolation and loneliness in older people: A systematic review. *BMJ Open, 2017,* e013778. doi:10.1136/bmjopen-2016-013778

Lebron, A. (2017). *The latest on workplace violence statistics.* Retrieved from www.ravemobilesafety.com/blog/latest-workplace-violence-statistics

Lemstra, M., Nielsen, G., Rogers, M., Thompson, A., and Moraros, J. (2012). Risk indicators and outcomes associated with bullying in youth aged 9–15 years. *Canadian Journal of Public Health, 103*(1), 9–13.

Lewis, K. M., Schure, M. B., Bavarian, N., DuBois, D. L., Day, J., Ji, P., and Flay, B. R. (2013). Problem behavior and urban, low-income youth: A randomized controlled trial of positive action in Chicago. *American Journal of Preventive Medicine, 44*(6), 622–630.

Lipscomb, J., McPhaul, K., Rosen, J., Brown, J. G., Choi, M., Soeken, K., . . . Porter, P. (2006). Violence prevention in the mental health setting: The New York State experience. *Canadian Journal of Nursing Research, 38*(4), 96–117.

Mancinelli, I., Comparelli, A., Girardi, P., and Tatarelli, R. (2002). Mass suicide: Historical and psychodynamic considerations. *Suicide and Life-Threatening Behavior, 32*(1), 91–100.

Mann, L. (1981). The baiting crowd in episodes of threatened suicide. *Journal of Personality and Social Psychology, 41*(4), 703–709.

Marx, K. A., Scott, J. B., Piersol, C. V., and Gitlin, L. N. (2019). Tailored activities to reduce neuropsychiatric behaviors in dementia: Case report. *American Journal of Occupational Therapy, 73*(2), 1–9.

Maynard, B. R., Vaughn, M. G., Salas-Wright, C. P., and Vaughn, S. (2016). Bullying victimization among school-aged immigrant youth in the United States. *Journal of Adolescent Health, 58*(3), 337–344. doi:10.1016/j.jadohealth.2015.11.013

McPhaul, K. M., and Lipscomb, J. A. (2004). Workplace violence in health care: Recognized but not regulated. *Online Journal of Issues in Nursing, 9*(3), 7.

MILCK. (2017). *#ICANTKEEPQUIET.* Retrieved from www.icantkeepquiet.org/song

Milosevic, T., and Livingstone, S. (2018). Cyberbullying, dignity, and children's rights. In *Protecting children online?* (pp. 1–20). Cambridge, MA: MIT Press.

Miniño, A. M. (2010). *Mortality among teenagers aged 12–19 years: United States, 1999–2006.* NCHS Data Brief No. 37. Hyattsville, MD: National Center for Health Statistics.

Mullen, C. (2019, January 7). Two-thirds of military women say they've been assaulted, harassed. *Bizwomen.* Retrieved from www.bizjournals.com/bizwomen/news/latest-news/2019/01/two-thirds-of-military-women-say-theyve-been.html?page=all

National Adult Protective Services Association. (n.d.). *About NAPSA.* Retrieved from www.napsa-now.org/about-napsa/

National Association of School Psychologists. (2013). *Youth gun violence fact sheet.* Retrieved from http://webcache.googleusercontent.com/search?q=cache:7WMgN16TB8wJ:www.nasponline.org/assets/documents/Resources%2520and%2520Publications/Handouts/Safety%2520and%2520Crisis/Youth_Gun_Violence_Fact_Sheet.pdf+&cd=1&hl=en&ct=clnk&gl=us

National Cancer Institute. (2001). *Making health communication programs work: A planner's guide* [Reprinted 2004]. Retrieved from www.cancer.gov/publications/health-communication/pink-book.pdf

National Cancer Institute. (2005). *Theory at a glance: A guide for health promotion practice.* (2nd ed.). Retrieved from https://cancercontrol.cancer.gov/brp/research/theories_project/theory.pdf

National Center for Injury Prevention and Control. (n.d.). *Essentials for childhood: Creating safe, stable, nurturing relationships and environments for all children.* Retrieved from www.cdc.gov/violenceprevention/pdf/essentials-for-childhood-framework508.pdf

National Center for Injury Prevention and Control. (2016). *Preventing child abuse and neglect: A technical package for policy, norm, and programmatic activities.* Retrieved from www.cdc.gov/violenceprevention/pdf/can-prevention-technical-package.pdf

National Center for Injury Prevention and Control. (2019). *Violence prevention: Child abuse and neglect prevention.* Retrieved from www.cdc.gov/violenceprevention/childabuseandneglect/index.html

National Coalition Against Domestic Violence. (n.d.). *National statistics domestic violence* [Fact sheet]. Retrieved from https://ncadv.org/statistics

National Council on Aging. (n.d.a). *Elder abuse facts: How many older Americans are abused?* Retrieved from www.ncoa.org/public-policy-action/elder-justice/elder-abuse-facts/

National Council on Aging. (n.d.b). *What are the effects of elder abuse?* Retrieved from www.ncoa.org/public-policy-action/elder-justice/elder-abuse-facts/

National Health Care Anti-Fraud Association. (2018). *What is health care fraud?* Retrieved from www.nhcaa.org/resources/health-care-anti-fraud-resources/consumer-info-action.aspx

National Institute for Occupational Safety and Health. (2002). *Violence occupational hazards in hospitals.* Retrieved from www.cdc.gov/niosh/docs/2002-101/default.html

National Institute on Aging. (n.d.). *Spotting the signs of elder abuse.* Retrieved from www.nia.nih.gov/health/infographics/spotting-signs-elder-abuse

National Institute on Aging. (2016). *Elder abuse.* Retrieved from www.nia.nih.gov/health/elder-abuse

National Institutes of Health. (2017). *Elder abuse.* Retrieved from https://medlineplus.gov/elderabuse.html

National Safety Council. (2019). *Is your workplace prone to violence?* Retrieved from www.nsc.org/work-safety/safety-topics/workplace-violence

Neuman, J., and Baron, R. (1998). Workplace violence and workplace aggression: Evidence concerning specific forms, potential causes, and preferred targets. *Rensselaer Polytechnic Institute Journal of Management, 24*(3), 391–419.

Niolon, P. H., Kearns, M., Dills, J., Rambo, K., Irving, S., Armstead, T. L., and Gilbert, L. (2017). *Preventing intimate partner violence across the lifespan: A technical package of programs, policies, and practices.* Atlanta, GA: National Center for Injury Prevention and Control, Centers for Disease Control and Prevention.

Nugent, P. (2013, April 13). Social isolation. *Psychology dictionary.* Retrieved from https://psychologydictionary.org/social-isolation/

Occupational Safety and Health Administration. (2014). *Guidelines for preventing workplace violence for healthcare and social service workers.* OSHA 3148-06R. Retrieved from www.osha.gov/Publications/osha3148.pdf

Occupational Safety and Health Administration. (2015). *Enforcement summary.* Retrieved from www.osha.gov/dep/2015_enforcement_summary.html

Peek-Asa, C., Casteel, C., Allareddy, V., Nocera, M., Goldmacher, S., O'Hagan, E., . . . Harrison, R. (2009). Workplace violence prevention programs in psychiatric units and facilities. *Archives of Psychiatric Nursing, 23*(2), 166–176.

Ploeg, J., and Markle-Reid, M. (2018, April 5). Stressed and exhausted caregivers need better support. *Conversation.* Retrieved from https://theconversation.com/stressed-and-exhausted-caregivers-need-better-support-92340

Rai, S. (2002). Preventing workplace aggression and violence—a role for occupational therapy. *Work, 18,* 15–22.

Ramsey-Klawsnik, H., Dayton, C., Gregorie, T., and Koontz, B. L. (2018a). *Understanding and working with Adult Protective Services (APS): Part I: Overview of APS programs.* Retrieved from www.napsa-now.org/get-help/

Ramsey-Klawsnik, H., Dayton, C., Gregorie, T., and Koontz, B. L. (2018b). *Understanding and working with Adult Protective Services (APS): Part III: Intervention collaboration.* Retrieved from www.napsa-now.org/get-help/

Reitz, S. M., Scaffa, M. E., Campbell, R. M., and Rhynders, P. A. (2010). Health behavior frameworks for health promotion practice. In M. E. Scaffa, S. M. Reitz, and M. A. Pizzi (Eds.), *Occupational therapy in community-based practice settings* (pp. 46–69). Philadelphia, PA: F. A. Davis.

Scaffa, M. E., Chromiak, S. B., Reitz, S. M., Blair-Newton, A., Murphy, L., and Wallis, C. B. (2010). Unintentional injury and violence. In M. E. Scaffa, S. M. Reitz, and M. A. Pizzi (Eds.), *Occupational therapy in community-based practice settings* (pp. 350–375). Philadelphia, PA: F. A. Davis.

Schafer, M., Korn, S., Smith, P., Hunter, S., Mora-Merchan, J., Singer, M., and Van Der Meulen, K. (2004). Lonely in the crowd: Recollections of bullying. *British Journal of Developmental Psychology, 22,* 379–394.

Springer, K. W., Sheridan, J., Kuo, D., and Carnes, M. (2003). The long-term health outcomes of child abuse: An overview and call to action. *Journal of General Internal Medicine, 18*(10), 864–870. Retrieved from www.ncbi.nlm.nih.gov/pmc/articles/PMC1494926/

Spivak, R. (2017). Undue sacrifice: How female sexual assault victims fight the military while fighting in the military. *Duke Journal of Gender Law and Policy, 25*(77), 77–127.

Stoddard, S. A., Whiteside, L., Zimmerman, M. A., Cunningham, R. M., Chermack, S. T., and Walton, M. A. (2013). The relationship between cumulative risk and promotive factors and violence behavior among urban adolescents. *American Journal of Community Psychology, 51,* 57–65. doi:10.1007/s10464-012-9541-7

Teresi, J. A., Ramirez, M., Fulmer, T., Ellis, J., Silver, S., Kong, J., . . . Pillemer, K. (2018). Resident-to-resident mistreatment: Evaluation of a staff training program in the reduction of falls and injuries. *Journal of Gerontological Nursing, 44*(6), 15–23.

Thomas, K. A., Goodman, L., and Putnins, S. (2015). "I have lost everythin": Trade-offs of seeking safety from intimate partner violence. *Journal of Orthopsychiatry, 85*(2), 170–180.

Thomson, P., and Jaque, S. V. (2018). Shame and anxiety: The mediating role of childhood adversity in dancers. *Journal of Dance Medicine and Science, 22*(2), 100–108.

Thornberg, R. (2011). "She's weird!"—the social construction of bullying in school: A review of qualitative research. *Children and Society, 25*(4), 258–267.

Twinley, R., and Addidle, G. (2012). Considering the violence: The dark side of occupation. *British Journal of Occupational Therapy, 75*(4), 202–204.

United Nations Department of Economic and Social Affairs. (2017, June 21). *World population prospects: The 2017 revision: Lower fertility leads to ageing populations.* Retrieved from www.un.org/development/desa/publications/world-population-prospects-the-2017-revision.html

United Nations Development Programme. (2016). *Human development reports.* Retrieved from hdr.undep.org/en/data

U.S. Department of Housing and Urban Development. (2016). *Neighborhoods and violent crime.* Retrieved from www.huduser.gov/portal/periodicals/em/summer16/highlight2.html

U.S. Bureau of Labor Statistics. (2014). *Injuries, illness, and fatalities: Workplace homicides.* Retrieved from www.bls.gov/iif/oshwc/cfoi/workplace-homicides.htm.2014

U.S. Department of Veterans Affairs Office of Mental Health and Suicide Prevention. (2018). *VA national suicide data report.* Retrieved from www.mentalhealth.va.gov/docs/data sheets/OMHSP_National_Suicide_Data_Report_2005-2016_508.pdf

van Geel, M., Vedder, P., and Tanilon, J. (2014). Bullying and weapon carrying: A meta-analysis. *Journal of the American Medical Association Pediatrics, 168,* 714–720. doi:10.1001/jamapediatrics.2014.213

Van Noorden, T. H., Haselager, G. J., Cillessen, A. H., and Bukowski, W. M. (2015). Empathy and involvement in bullying in children and adolescents: A systematic review. *Journal of Youth and Adolescence, 44*(3), 637–657. doi:10.1007/s10964-014-0135-6

Verlinden, M., Veenstra, R., Ringoot, A. P., Jansen, P. W., Raat, H., Hofman, A., and Tiemeier, H. (2014). Detecting bullying in early elementary school with a computerized peer-nomination instrument. *Psychological Assessment, 26*(2), 628. doi:10.1037/a0035571

Volk, A. A., Veenstra, R., and Espelage, D. L. (2017). So you want to study bullying? Recommendations to enhance the validity, transparency, and compatibility of bullying research. *Aggression and Violent Behavior, 36,* 34–43. doi:10.1016/j.avb.2017.07.003

Waldman-Levi, A., and Weintraub, N. (2015). Efficacy of a crisis intervention in improving mother-child interaction and children's play functioning. *American Journal of Occupational Therapy, 69,* 6901220020, 1–11.

World Health Organization. (n.d.). *Violence against women: Prevalence* [Fact sheet]. Retrieved from www.who.int/reproductivehealth/publications/violence/VAW_Prevelance.jpeg?ua=1

World Health Organization. (2002). *World report on violence and health: Summary.* Retrieved from https://apps.who.int/iris/bitstream/handle/10665/42512/9241545623_eng.pdf;jsessionid=F52EA8FA9EDE2FADD7F6E81A254DC7DB?sequence=1

World Health Organization. (2014a). *Global health observatory data repository: Child maltreatment global estimates.* Retrieved from http://apps.who.int/gho/data/node.main.VIOLENCECHILDMALTREATMENT?lang=en

World Health Organization. (2014b). *Global status report on violence prevention 2014.* Retrieved from www.who.int/violence_injury_prevention/violence/status_report/2014/en/

World Health Organization. (2016). *INSPIRE: Seven strategies for ending violence against children.* Retrieved from https://apps.who.int/iris/bitstream/handle/10665/207717/9789241565356-eng.pdf;jsessionid=3BC87273085941756F7E649717C6754C?sequence=1

World Health Organization. (2017). *Violence against women* [Fact sheet]. Retrieved from www.who.int/en/news-room/fact-sheets/detail/violence-against-women

World Health Organization. (2018). *Suicide* [Fact sheet]. Retrieved from www.who.int/en/news-room/fact-sheets/detail/suicide

World Health Organization. (2019a). *Mental health: Suicide data.* Retrieved from www.who.int/mental_health/prevention/suicide/suicideprevent/en/

World Health Organization. (2019b). *Violence and injury prevention.* Retrieved from www.who.int/violence_injury_prevention/violence/en/

Zablotsky, B., Bradshaw, C. P., Anderson, C. M., and Law, P. (2014). Risk factors for bullying among children with autism spectrum disorders. *Autism, 18*(4), 419–427. doi:10.1177/1362361313477920

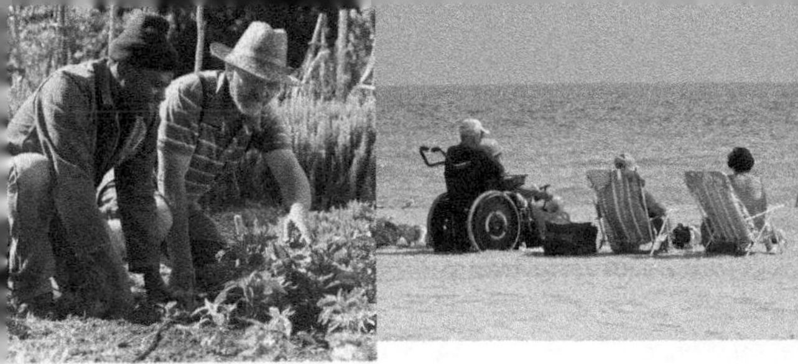

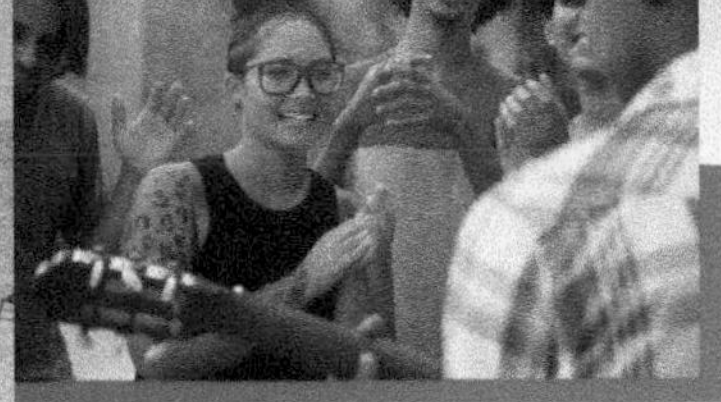

SECTION IX

Looking Ahead

Chapter 28

Future Directions in Community and Population Health Practice

Marjorie E. Scaffa, PhD, OTR/L, FAOTA, S. Maggie Reitz, PhD, OTR/L, FAOTA, and Patricia A. Crist, PhD, OTR/L, FAOTA

Occupational therapy maximizes health, well-being, and quality of life for all people, populations, and communities through effective solutions that facilitate participation in everyday living.

—American Occupational Therapy Association (2018b).

Learning Outcomes

This chapter is designed to enable the reader to:

28-1 Discuss the principles of futurist thinking.

28-2 Describe the characteristics of an ecological worldview, applying it to community and population health practice.

28-3 Explain the concept of sustainability and how it applies to occupational therapy.

28-4 Provide examples of potential occupational therapy contributions to livable communities.

28-5 Analyze the influence of artificial intelligence and other technological advances on the practice of occupational therapy.

28-6 Discuss the impact of globalization on the profession of occupational therapy.

28-7 Describe potential curricular and fieldwork options for teaching community and population health concepts.

28-8 Describe the role of community and population health participatory action research in occupational therapy practice and scholarship.

Key Terms

Ambient intelligence
Artificial intelligence
Collaborative practice
Collective violence
Community-based participatory action research
Community service learning
Community violence
Diffusion of innovation
Ecological worldview
Food security
Food waste
Globalization
Innovation
Integration
Interprofessional education
Invisible workloads
Living wage
Low food security
Mass violence
Microaggressions
Mixed methods research
Occupational justice
Robotics
Self-assertion
Sustainability
Three-dimensional printing
Very low food security
Virtual reality
White fragility
White privilege

Introduction

In ancient Greece and Rome, an oracle was a place where, or a medium by which, deities were consulted for advice or prophecy about the future. The modern futurist movement, which began in the 1960s, was fueled by the desire to understand and shape the future and is guided by three basic principles (Cornish, 1980). The first principle, or conviction, is the unity or interrelatedness of reality. It is the perception that the whole is greater than the sum of its parts, an insistence on the interconnectedness of everything in the universe (Cornish, 1980).

The second principle that directs futurist thinking is the crucial importance of time. The world of the future is shaped by the decisions made today and the determinations made in the past (Cornish, 1980). Futurists believe that almost anything can be accomplished in a period of 20 years.

The third principle on which futurists rely is the importance and power of ideas, particularly ideas about the future. The future is created out of ideas, the tools of thought. Without them, change is not possible. Futurists believe that human achievement is constrained more by conceptual restrictions or limitations in ideas than by access to material resources (Cornish, 1980).

Some advocate that the profession should recreate or reinvent itself. However, this is not the only available choice of action. An alternative is to embrace a vision that incorporates the fundamental principles of the profession, with its focus on occupation, and one that expands the scope of practice to include populations not typically served and settings not commonly utilized. The profession would not be where it is today if it had not survived the challenges of the past century. Thus, it is not desirable to discard what has been part of the profession's successful heritage.

Some predictions can be made about the future of occupational therapy based on current trends. The following statements reflect the authors' beliefs regarding the future of occupational therapy and are offered as "food for thought." It is anticipated that there will be:

- An increased role for occupational therapy in community and population health practice
- A significant shift in services from medical institutions to decentralized, coordinated, community-based settings
- Increased cultural diversity of the U.S. population, requiring a need for increased cultural competence among occupational therapy practitioners and recruitment of a more diverse workforce
- Increased numbers of elderly with a full range of health statuses, illnesses, and disabilities
- Increased emphasis on mental health and quality of life

- Increased need for occupational therapy in preventing and addressing social problems such as sustainability, intolerance of marginalized groups, violence, crime, and alcohol and drug abuse

What occupational therapy needs most to move forward in the 21st century are creative ideas and thoughtful, ethical decisions put into action. Only in this way can the profession fulfill its destiny as a "health agent" (Finn, 1972), enhance community health, and facilitate "community occupational development" (Bockhoven, 1968).

Engage Your Brain 28-1

Review the AOTA *Occupational Therapy Code of Ethics (2015)*. Which principles and related standards support future-forward thinking?

An Ecological Worldview

To become health agents, occupational therapy practitioners must make a paradigm shift from a holistic perspective to an **ecological worldview.** "An ecological worldview is holistic, but it's more than that. It looks not only at something as a whole, but also how this whole is embedded into larger wholes" (Capra and Steindl-Rast, 1991, p. 69). Ecological awareness recognizes the interrelatedness and interdependence of all phenomena.

The root of the word "ecological" comes from the Greek "oikos," which means "house." In a broader context, it refers to "the inhabited world, the house of humanity" (Capra and Steindl-Rast, 1991, p. 70). The house of humanity includes the biological, psychological, and spiritual aspects of life embedded in a physical, social, and cultural reality. The shift to an ecological paradigm reflects not only a change in thinking but also a change in values. Overall, the shift in values is characterized by a shift from self-assertion to integration (Capra and Steindl-Rast, 1991). **Self-assertion** is a living system's tendency toward domination in an effort to preserve and protect itself, while **integration** is the tendency to partner with other systems in order to fulfill the greater good and create sustainability. Table 28-1 provides a synopsis of the changes in values required by the ecological paradigm.

Table 28-1 Change in Paradigm, Change in Values

From a Holistic Perspective With an Emphasis on	To an Ecological Paradigm With an Emphasis on
Self-assertion	Integration
Rational thought	Intuitiveness
Analysis	Synthesis
Competition	Cooperation
Expansion	Conservation
Quantity	Quality
Domination	Partnership
Individuality	Community

Self-assertion is not completely lost in the ecological paradigm because it is essential for survival. However, left unchecked, self-assertion can become destructive, evidenced by the variety of community and population health problems experienced today such as violence, poverty, racism, homelessness, substance abuse, and destruction of the environment. Self-assertion must be tempered with integration to be useful and healthy. Koestler (1978) spoke of this dichotomy as the *Janus* nature. A living system is an integrated whole that asserts itself to protect its individuality. However, as part of a larger whole, the living system is required to integrate itself into the larger system. According to Capra and Steindl-Rast (1991), "it is important to realize that those are opposite and contradictory tendencies. We need a dynamic balance between them, and that's essential for physical and mental health" (p. 74).

Creating Opportunities in Community and Population Health Practice

Occupational therapy practitioners are by nature and training innovative thinkers who translate creative ideas into action. These ideas and actions expand the scope of practice. Some involve the expansion of professional roles, some include populations not typically served, and others describe practice in settings not typically utilized. For example, Sepulveda (2019), a pediatric occupational therapist, recognized the burden parents endure caring for their babies with medically complex diagnoses. Mothers who brought their infants in for therapy often expressed feelings of worry, fear, helplessness, guilt, and sadness. When she referred these mothers for postpartum depression screening, many results returned positive. Sepulveda realized that the more time she spent supporting mothers in meeting their own mental health and self-care needs, the more progress the children made and the more mother-child bonding occurred. As a result, Sepulveda (2019) began advocating for a "two-generation" approach to care in which occupational therapy practitioners and other providers address not only the child's health needs but also the parents'. This goes beyond teaching caregivers the skills needed to manage their children at home; it requires attention to and intervention for the physical and mental health needs of parents.

Occupational therapy in community and population health practice "aims to improve community-level occupational performance, participation, health and wellbeing" and addresses the "social and political factors that influence occupational participation at the community level" (World Federation of Occupational Therapists [WFOT], 2019b, p. 2–3). The WFOT (2019b) identified the following principles of a community-centered approach to population health:

- Community engagement is underpinned by trust, respect, and reciprocity.
- Asset and strengths-based approaches inform community-level service provision.
- Practice is occupation-centered and aims to increase community participation in occupations that are health promoting and socially and culturally meaningful.
- Services are provided with communities or as directed by them to support and enable the achievement of shared occupational goals.
- Interventions and enabling strategies are selected with or by communities that address barriers to occupational participation, health, and well-being.
- Outcomes of community-centered practice are demonstrated through improvements in community-level health, well-being, and inclusion (p. 1).

To be successful in community and population health practice, practitioners must see themselves providing a wide range of interventions. Direct service to individuals is only a small part of what occupational therapy has to offer. In community and population health practice, the client is often not an individual but rather a group, organization, agency, community, or population. Potential interventions may include case management, training, consulting, program coordination, policy development, and advocacy. These levels of intervention and others with corresponding strategies and goals are described in Table 28-2.

Many of the emerging areas of community and population health practice are predicated on the construct of **occupational justice,** which is based on the belief that humans are occupational beings and that participation in occupation is essential for health, well-being, and quality of life. Therefore, all persons should have the right to engage in meaningful occupation; this is their occupational right. Occupational injustice exists when this right is violated or goes unfulfilled (Stadnyk, Townsend, and Wilcock, 2010). When occupational injustice persists, occupational dysfunction is often the result.

Risk factors that cause occupational dysfunction due to occupational injustice include occupational imbalance, deprivation, and alienation (Wilcock, 1998). Occupational imbalance is a lack of balance among self-sustaining, productive, and leisure occupations that fails to meet an individual's physical or psychosocial needs, thereby resulting in decreased health and well-being. Occupational deprivation is the result of external circumstances or limitations that prevent a person from participating in necessary and meaningful occupations. Conditions that lead to occupational deprivation may include poor health, disability, poverty, isolation, and homelessness. Occupational alienation is a lack of satisfaction in one's occupations that leads to experiencing life as purposeless and meaningless. Tasks that are perceived as stressful, meaningless, or boring may result in an experience of occupational alienation. Occupational therapy practitioners are ethically

Table 28-2 Strategies, Goals, and Levels of Occupational Therapy Intervention

Intervention Type	Strategy or Process	Goals/Outcomes	Target/Level
Direct service	Providing occupational therapy intervention	Improved occupational performance	Individual
Counseling	Helping people learn how to achieve personal goals, resolve problems, make decisions, or change behaviors	Goal attainment, healthy behaviors, empowerment	Individual, interpersonal
Case management	Coordinating care plans	Improved client outcomes, comprehensive, coordinated care	Individual, interpersonal, organizational
Education	Providing information and employing the methods, strategies, and tools that facilitate learning	Positive change in knowledge, attitude, or behavior	Individual, interpersonal, organizational, societal/community, governmental/policy
Training	Providing information to enhance a skill or process	Competence in targeted skills, processes, techniques	Individual, interpersonal, organizational
Consulting	Using the knowledge and experience of an "expert" to help a person or organizational leaders make better decisions or deal more effectively with situations	Problem-solving in area of concern	Individual, interpersonal, organizational, societal/community, governmental/policy
Program development	Assessing the need for, planning, and evaluating programs and services	Improved services/care for target population	Organizational, societal/community
Program coordination	Managing the resources (e.g., staff, materials, space, finances, etc.) to accomplish the objectives of a program	Effective and efficient use of resources	Organizational, societal/community, governmental/policy
Policy development	Formulating rules, laws, policies, procedures	Laws, rules, policies, and procedures that are favorable to area of concern	Organizational, governmental/policy
Advocacy	Using the power of persuasion to alter public opinion and mobilize resources in favor of a policy or issue	Favorable change in policies, regulations, resource allocation	Organizational, societal/community, governmental/policy
Research	Building knowledge through systematic study	Improved practice, evidence-based practice	Organizational, governmental/policy

bound to address occupational injustice and inequity wherever it exists in health-care institutions, communities, and populations and in social and political policies and practices.

The Future of Population Health

Improving population health requires attention to the social determinants of health and the corresponding underlying structural factors. According to research, the most effective and efficient policies and practices are those that

> *address making access to health care and social services equitable; raising the quality of education, diet, and housing, and encouraging individual physical activity; increasing the availability of jobs that offer a living wage and security; reducing and remediating drug and domestic abuse; and eliminating toxins from the environment. (Fox and Grogan, 2017, p. 32)*

Multilevel, transdisciplinary population health approaches have demonstrated efficacy for improving health behavior, health-care delivery, and health policies (Croyle and Srinivasan, 2016).

Edington, Schultz, Pitts, and Camilleri (2015) predict increasing emphasis on the influence of environment, physical and social, on health, and the development of interventions designed to create healthier homes, workplaces, schools, and communities. Creating healthier milieus for all can have a significant impact on population health. The characteristics of healthy milieus include sustainability, livability, equity, and full inclusion.

Sustainable Communities

Sustainability is based on a simple principle:

> *Everything that we need for our survival and well-being depends, either directly or indirectly, on our natural environment. Sustainability creates and maintains the conditions under which humans and nature can exist in productive harmony, that permit fulfilling the social, economic and other requirements of present and future generations. (Environmental Protection Agency, 2016, para. 1)*

Sustainability is the capacity to endure. Human sustainability is the long-term maintenance of responsibility, which has environmental (ecological), economic (livable), and social (equitable) dimensions. Typically, the sustainability ecosystem emphasizes environmental (e.g., physical resources such as air, land, and water) and economic (e.g., goods, services, disaster response, and health care) issues, utilization, and preventative resource planning.

In order to create the optimal environment to facilitate the long-term sustainability of an initiative, one must consider the "three pillars" (Opp and Saunders, 2013; see Fig. 28-1). The economic, environmental, and social equity pillars all need to be addressed when determining sustainability initiatives. First, the economic pillar implies that each initiative needs to be economically viable for the community affected by it. The fiscal restrictions of community members, planners, and the budgetary demands of the local government are important considerations when addressing this pillar. Community occupational engagement increases the likelihood of limiting economic costs while ensuring maximum use and increasing cost benefits.

Second, the environmental pillar suggests that in an ideal situation minimal harm for the natural environment would result. Focusing on creating green spaces and community gardens, using recyclable materials, and minimizing land use are just a few

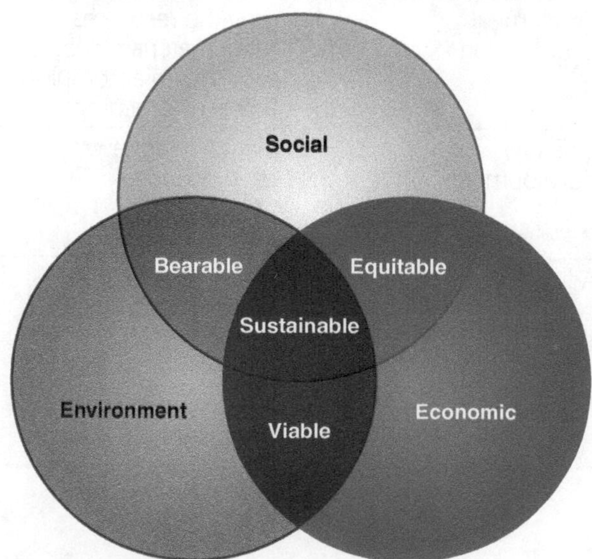

Figure 28-1 Sustainability model.

examples of the considerations associated with this pillar. In fact, man-environment considerations offer the most potent opportunity for sustained lifestyle integration.

The social equity pillar recommends creating initiatives that can benefit and be enjoyed by the greatest possible number of community members. This pillar incorporates one of the foundational beliefs of occupational therapists, accessibility for everyone to promote inclusion and empower community engagement regardless of needs or limitations. Since all three pillars must be addressed for long-term sustainability, ignoring one of the pillars in the design stage will likely create irreversible harm in the future. The traditional definitions of sustainability that were focused on avoiding exploitation, depletion, and irreversible alteration have evolved into a new definition that focuses on promoting enrichment (empowerment), growth (regeneration), and flexible change (resilience).

Human sustainability is based on the social capacity to tolerate environmental changes in lifestyle through managing goods and services as well as supporting sustainability as a form of person-environment stewardship. Human beings are the essential resource to ensuring that sustainability thrives. Improvements in consumer education, health, nutrition, and environmental accessibility allow individuals to better use their resources, daily and in emergencies. One explanation for the lack of attention to social and human health is that until recently the major disciplines driving the sustainability movement (i.e., engineering, architecture, climatology, and business) dismissed the social pillar as recipients and not equally important in sustainability planning. The importance of the social pillar is no longer being ignored with the recognition that people and populations must "buy-in" and implement sustainability routines in lifestyle and community development. For instance, the Rockefeller Foundation's 100 Resilient Cities project requires every fundable city plan to have a robust social (social intelligence) component as part of the required holistic resilience strategy (100 Resilient Cities, 2019).

Occupational Therapy Role

Occupational therapy's value to promote person-environment well-being through occupational engagement encourages the profession's participation in building sustainable, healthy communities and populations. Applying the profession's values and mission, occupational therapy practitioners are uniquely prepared health-care professionals able to contribute to sustainability planning in order to determine ecologically valid local and global community needs (Crist, 2018). Dorsey and Miller (2013) propose the concept of green ergonomics as one mechanism through which occupational therapy practitioners might contribute to sustainability. Green ergonomics refers to the integration of "ergonomics into sustainable development to enhance human performance, productivity, health and well-being, thereby promoting sustainability at both the individual and systems level" (p. 10). Opportunities exist for occupational therapy participation in the design and development of green buildings, green industry jobs, and green schools (Dorsey and Miller, 2013).

The WFOT (2012) published an official document titled *Environmental Sustainability: Sustainable Practice Within Occupational Therapy* that shifted discussions centered only on the medical model to also incorporate the social model. The position paper also broadened the focus on individual health to encompass population health, and evolved practice from institution-based to community settings, which positions the profession of occupational therapy to be a contributor to sustainability efforts. The intent was to realign occupational therapy with global issues to promote sustainable individual and environmental well-being and to address economic, social, and environmental agendas that meet population needs. In occupational therapy, "sustainability refers to the ability of human beings to live and thrive without threatening the ability of future generations to similarly live and thrive" (WFOT, 2018, p. 19).

In 2018, the WFOT developed guiding principles on sustainability for the profession. These include:

1. "Occupational therapy practitioners shall be encouraged to educate themselves about issues of ecosystem sustainability as it impacts ability to pursue chosen meaningful occupations and subsequently human health and well-being" (p. 19).

2. "Occupational therapy practitioners shall work with interested service users and communities to help them explore ways of participating in healthy, meaningful occupations in such a way that they contribute towards mitigation of environmental damage due to unsustainable lifestyles" (p. 21).
3. "Occupational therapy practitioners shall be encouraged to work collaboratively with service users to help them adapt to deleterious and health-impacting effects of environmental degradation due to unsustainable lifestyles so that they can continue to participate in meaningful occupations in a sustainable manner" (p. 23).
4. "Occupational therapy practitioners shall be encouraged to develop competences for empowering communities to find ways of facilitating meaningful occupations in a sustainable manner among community members, taking into account the need to maintain equitability and occupational justice" (pp. 25–26).
5. "Occupational therapy practitioners shall be encouraged to develop and maintain competence in administering occupation-based interventions to help interested service users and communities address ecosystem sustainability issues" (p. 27).

The WFOT embraces the implementation of sustainability practice to include capacity building, community-based rehabilitation, social entrepreneurship, human rights, and disaster preparedness and response.

Occupational therapy organizations around the world have adopted position papers or statements regarding sustainability, including Australia, Canada, England, and Sweden. These vary from engagement in the traditional model of sustainability (e.g., climate change) to sustaining programs (such as global access to durable medical equipment and health-care technology) to more recent sustainability issues centered around social justice, inclusion, and community resilience. At this time, the American Occupational Therapy Association (AOTA) has not adopted a position statement related to sustainability.

The increasing global awareness regarding the importance of promoting sustainable action plans provides a platform for occupational therapy to modify future practice. The future of the earth and its populations is unsustainable without significant change to promote human survival and best practices in environmental resource utilization. The WFOT's scholarly discourse on this topic encourages occupational therapy practitioners to explore possible approaches to addressing sustainability. Toward this end, the WFOT (2018) published sustainability recommendations (see Box 28-1).

Human sustainability is the result of a cohesive, responsive group of stakeholders—individuals, professionals, scholars, communities, and countries—working toward a shared vision. Beneficial human sustainability is a long-term responsibility forged through human and community partnerships reflecting a diverse group of community development planners, many with backgrounds not previously acknowledged (such as health-care providers). However, input is needed now from all fields to successfully implement sustainability goals.

Livable Communities

Many ways exist to make a community more livable, including adaptations to its physical and social fabrics. The AOTA developed a *Societal Statement on Livable Communities* in 2009 and updated it in 2016. In this statement, occupational therapy's role in promoting livable communities is detailed and includes:

- Identifying and eradicating barriers to equal health and quality of life
- Addressing architectural barriers in homes and communities to maximize occupational engagement
- Promoting the availability of participation in a variety of "physical, social, vocational, and cultural activities" (AOTA, 2016, p. 1)

Three examples of the many areas for future growth in occupational therapy's contributions to livable communities will be shared in greater detail. These include supporting people who serve as foster parents for children and youth, reducing food waste, promoting living wage policies, and creating safe and secure environments for occupational participation.

Box 28-1 World Federation of Occupational Therapy's 2018 Sustainability Recommendations

Occupational therapy practitioners, educators, scholars, and national organizations are encouraged to explore the possibilities of:

- Widening their scope of practice to incorporate sustainability in activity analysis and consider the health co-benefits of a low carbon lifestyle, and to include interventions that promote health while contributing toward sustainability among their clients
- Aligning their work with the United Nations Sustainable Development Goals
- Working with service users individually and in groups in the community to help them adapt to the adverse effects of climate change (an outcome of unsustainability) using occupation-based interventions
- Including content in curricula to help occupational therapy students acquire knowledge and develop competence in working with individuals and communities to help interested service users adopt sustainable occupational lifestyles and adapt to the adverse consequences of climate change
- Conducting research to clarify the relationships among meaningful occupational performance, sustainability, health, and well-being
- Conducting research to inform development of evidence-based and occupation-based models to guide occupational therapy interventions for interested service users and groups to help them develop sustainable occupational lifestyles and adapt to the negative consequences of climate change
- Including competence in promoting sustainability and helping people adapt to the adverse consequences of climate change in occupational therapy educational standards
- Including sustainability within national associations' ethical principles
- Encouraging occupational therapy practitioners to widen their scope of practice to include a "well" population to promote sustainable occupational lifestyles and adaptation to the adverse effects of climate change

Source: Sustainability Matters: Guiding Principles for Sustainability in Occupational Therapy Practice, Education and Scholarship (p. 41), by World Federation of Occupational Therapists, 2018. Retrieved from https://wfot.org/resources/wfot-sustainability-guiding-principles

Foster Care

A livable community accepts responsibility for those children and youth who do not have parents or family able to care for them. Occupational therapy can assist families and communities in meeting this responsibility, which includes facilitating the development and mitigating the impact of being fostered. The most frequent precipitating factors of being placed in foster care include neglect (61%), parental drug abuse (34%), caretaker inability to cope (14%), physical abuse (12%), child behavior problems (11%), and housing (10%). A child or youth may be placed in foster care because of one or more of these factors (Administration on Children, Youth and Families [ACYF], 2017), all of which can have a significant impact on mental health. Fostered children and youth have one of the highest rates of posttraumatic stress disorder (PTSD; AOTA, 2017) in the United States. The impact of homelessness is discussed in Chapter 20 and domestic violence is described in more detail in Chapter 17 of this text.

According to the ACYF, the number of children and youth in foster care in September 2016 totaled 437,465. In September 2012, 396,966 children and youth were in foster care. The number of children and youth in foster care has increased each year since 2012. As of 2016, 52% were male and 48% were female. The mean age was 8.5, with 7% being less than one year old. The most frequent placements in September 2016 included foster family, nonrelative (45%); foster family, relative (32%); institution (7%); and group home (5%). The case plan goal for children and youth in foster care in 2016 was for 55% of these children and youth to be reunified with their parent(s) or principal caretaker (ACYF, 2017).

Paul-Ward (2009) described the experience of foster children and youth as a type of occupational apartheid, as these children and youth are often segregated from the broader community and face

Box 28-2 Examples of Intensive-Level Services in Foster Care

- Advocacy at Individualized Education Plan (IEP) meetings
- Parenting skills and education for birth parents
- Social and play groups
- Developmental task and skill intervention for children and youth within foster care
- Developmental task and skill intervention for youth transitioning from foster care to adult independent living

From *Occupational Therapy's Role in Mental Health Promotion, Prevention, and Intervention With Children and Youth: Foster Care* (pp. 2–3), by the American Occupational Therapy Association, 2017.

additional stigmas beyond that of their foster status. In Paul-Ward's study of adolescent transitioning from foster care to independent living, she found that the average number of foster placements of study participants was 15. This disruption to daily life had a significant impact on these youths' ability to complete their education and meet other developmental tasks of adolescence in preparation for adult independent living (Paul-Ward, 2009).

The role of occupational therapy in foster care is summarized below using material from an AOTA (2017) information sheet. Services are described at three different levels—intensive, targeted, and universal. The intensive level is directed toward individual children and youth, foster parents, and biological parents (see Box 28-2). The targeted level involves developing services for children and youth within the foster care system who are in at-risk family living situations and those preparing for reunification (AOTA, 2017). Resources for reunification are available for parents and health professionals (Child Welfare Information Gateway, n.d., 2017). Developing partnerships with child welfare agencies and related institutions, screening resources, and creating programs are examples of universal intervention (AOTA, 2017).

Food Security and Food Waste

The challenges of gaining access to food and occupations surrounding the acquisition of food, food storage, and maximizing food use will continue to grow globally. This creates an opportunity for occupational therapy and occupational science to address this critical occupational justice challenge. The high volume of food waste in current times has a negative environmental impact on communities, as well as a detrimental economic impact on families (Stancu, Haugaard, and Lähteenmäki, 2016). In addition, critical food shortages are projected for the future, as crop production is unlikely to keep pace with global population growth (Ray, Mueller, West, and Foley, 2013) and will have an impact on food security. **Food security** is realized when "all people, at all times, have physical, social, and economic access to sufficient, safe, and nutritious food that meets their food preference and dietary needs for an active and healthy life" (International Food Policy Research Institute, n.d., para. 1). Thus, the reduction of food waste is a moral imperative and a matter of occupational justice.

Food waste includes both edible and what was once edible food that has been purposefully discarded once it reaches the consumer (Zepeda and Balaine, 2017). It can also refer to unintended food loss during the distribution phases (Porpino, Parente, and Wansink, 2015). Global estimates of food waste are staggering: "Roughly one third of the food produced in the world for human consumption every year—approximately 1.3 billion tonnes—gets lost or wasted" (Food and Agriculture Organization of the United Nations [FAO], 2019, para. 1). The rate of food waste is higher in North America and Europe (95 kg to 115 kg per year) than in sub-Saharan Africa and South and Southeast Asia (6 kg to 11 kg per year). In less industrialized countries, the majority of the waste occurs in the production and storage phases, early in the food production chain, while in industrialized countries the waste occurs later in this chain (FAO, 2019).

Engage Your Brain 28-2

How much is a tonne? How much food do you think you discard in a week?

Food waste rates in the United States mirror that of global estimates, with one-third of food going "uneaten through loss or waste. This waste adversely impacts food security and the environment. When food is tossed aside, so too are opportunities for healthier communities, economic growth, and environmental prosperity" (U.S. Department of Agriculture [USDA], n.d., para. 1). A pilot study of U.S. college students found the students to be knowledgeable about food waste and the environmental impact of that waste. The participants were concerned about food safety but were unaware of food insecurity (Zepeda and Balaine, 2017), which is interesting, as universities have started programs to combat food insecurity among college students (Bradshaw, 2017). Approximately one-third of college students experience food insecurity, with over half of these students working and 75% of them receiving financial aid (College and University Food Bank Alliance, 2018). In the United States, two terms are used to categorize degrees of food insecurity—low food security and very low food security. **Low food security** is defined as "reports of reduced quality, variety, or desirability of diet" with "little or no indication of reduced food intake" (USDA, 2018b, para. 2). **Very low food security** is defined as "reports of multiple indications of disrupted eating patterns and reduced food intake" (USDA, 2018b, para. 2). The impact of low food security and very low food security on people's daily meal preparation activities is displayed in Figure 28-2.

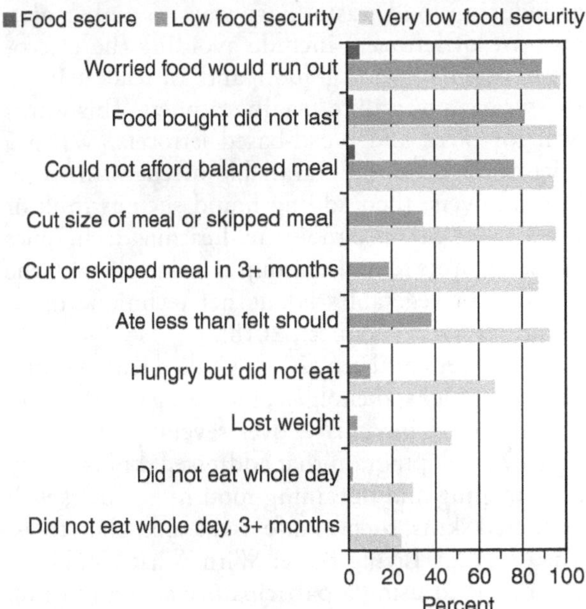

Figure 28-2 U.S. food security status.
(From Characteristics of Households With Very Low Food Security, *by U.S. Department of Agriculture, 2018.)*

A combination of interprofessional and professional strategies is needed to comprehensively address eradicating food waste and food insecurity. Occupational scientists can study the differing perceptions and actions related to food waste by age, identity (e.g., the "mother identity"—see Ioniță, 2017), geography, and nationality, thereby helping to inform community and population health strategies, including the policy advocacy and implementation undertaken by occupational therapy practitioners within interprofessional teams. Other interdisciplinary team members could include nutritionists, food economists, human geographers, and supply chain experts, among other professionals. Examples of potential interventions could be providing cooking classes and nutritional education at food banks and pantries (Porpino et al., 2015) to maximize the use of food and plant-based meals and advocating for policy changes such as in France, where retailers are mandated to donate food merchandise with close-to-expiring use-by dates to food banks (Zepeda and Balaine, 2017). Other potential actions include participating in media campaigns, such as the Love Food, Hate Waste initiative from the United Kingdom (Zepeda and Balaine, 2017) and supporting local farmers markets and farm-to-table businesses in a visible manner (e.g., using vendors for professional meetings and conferences).

Meal preparation and cleanup is an instrumental activity of daily living (IADL), which includes "planning, preparing, and serving well-balanced, nutritious meals and cleaning up food and utensils after meals" (AOTA, 2014a, S20). Occupational therapy practitioners can work with individual clients and communities to address the development of skills, routines, and habits in meal preparation that discourage food waste and address low levels and very low levels of food security. For example, one of the widely identified sources of food waste is the failure to use leftovers (Porpino et al., 2015; Stancu et al., 2016). People do not know how to leverage yesterday's leftovers to be today's and tomorrow's dinners—saving time and money as well as reducing food waste. Easy ways to make palatable use of leftovers include avoiding the microwave when reheating food and instead using a toaster oven or grill to regain crispness. This works well for pizza and bread-based leftovers. When a microwave is the only available mechanism to reheat leftovers, then adding liquid such as milk or water helps enhance moisture. Learning techniques to use leftovers to make a soup or casserole with the addition of vegetables is another technique to leverage leftovers (Bennett, 2018).

Scmelzeer and Leto (2018) worked with a group of community stakeholders, including people experiencing food insecurity, over several years to design a 7-week program that addressed skill building in managing and obtaining food resources as well as related skills, such as safe usage of kitchen tools. The program, Living Better With What You Have, was designed using a participatory action research process and the model of human occupation as a theoretical framework. Initial results indicate that the program was successful in improving food resource management. Scmelzeer and Leto (2018) concluded "programming that considers context and volition, habituation, and skill development in occupations helps address the underlying causes of food insecurity and highlights the distinct value of occupational therapy" (p. 7).

Living Wage

A **living wage** is defined as "a subsistence wage" or "a wage sufficient to provide the necessities and comforts essential to an acceptable standard of living" (Merriam-Webster Dictionary, 2019, para. 1). For a community to be considered livable, its inhabitants need access to a living wage in order to procure housing, food, and other necessities, as well as to support access to leisure and recreation occupations. One method to assess the livability of a community in terms of salary is the Living Wage Calculator designed by Glasmeier in 2004. This "is a market-based approach that draws upon geographically specific expenditure data related to a family's likely minimum food, childcare, health insurance, housing, transportation, and other basic necessities" (Glasmeier, 2019, para. 2).

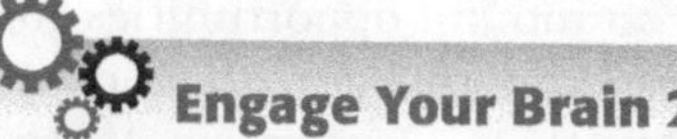

Engage Your Brain 28-3

What do you think is the livable hourly wage in your state, county, or city? Compare it to the results from the Living Wage Calculator by Glasmeier (2019). See the References for more information.

Although there is debate about the impact of living wage legislation on businesses and employees, research suggests positive outcomes. Fairris (2005) studied the result of legislation requiring city contractors in Los Angeles to provide a living wage to employees. Businesses affected by the ordinance were compared to businesses not covered by the legislation. Absenteeism, employee turnover, overtime, and job training hours all were reduced in the city-related businesses affected by the ordinance. All of these reductions would have positive financial gain for these businesses and the employees.

Living wage legislation has been implemented by more than 120 local governments within the United States (Fairris, Runsten, Briones, and Goodheart, 2015). Fairris et al. (2015) conducted a broader study of the impact of Los Angeles instituting living wage legislation, which debunked some of the fears regarding negative impacts on businesses. As in Fairris's earlier study, decreased business expenditures were realized due to increases in worker attendance and retention. In addition, the majority of businesses adapted to the law without the elimination of positions, using other methods instead to offset additional expenditures, such as increasing the cost of services, cutting profits, and reducing overtime.

Supporting polices and advocacy for a living wage is in alignment with the profession's core values and code of ethics. While respecting individual privacy, acting on documented wage gaps by job and advocating for living wages is supported by Principle 6, Fidelity (AOTA, 2015c). A separate study of the impact of increasing living wages of home-care workers in San Francisco (Howes, 2005) found positive results in terms of employee retention. In addition to supporting Principle 6, promoting the retention of experienced home-care workers can enhance patient and family care broadly and, more specifically, follow through with occupational therapy practitioners' recommendations. According to the AOTA (2015a), 19% of occupational therapy practitioners work in the school system, where there is a documented teacher wage gap (Allegretto and Mishel, 2016). The Principles of Beneficence, Nonmaleficence, and Fidelity (AOTA, 2015c) support occupational therapy practitioners' acknowledgment of wage gaps and advocacy for living wages for teachers and other colleagues.

Safe Environments for Occupational Participation

A large proportion of the global population lacks a safe environment for occupational participation due to community violence, pollution, or a lack of basic necessities such as access to water. A lack of safe places to walk, play, and socialize inhibits occupational participation and has a negative impact on the health of individuals and communities.

Community violence, a global public health problem and a social determinant of health, refers to "exposure to intentional acts of interpersonal violence committed in public areas by individuals who are not intimately related to the victim(s)" (National Child Traumatic Stress Network, n.d., para. 1). Community violence often happens suddenly and without warning. The most common types of community violence are shootings in schools, workplaces, houses of worship and other venues; terrorist attacks, riots, gang fights, and civil wars in foreign countries; or warlike conditions in U.S. cities. Another term frequently used in this context is "mass violence." Congress defines **mass violence** as "a multiple homicide incident in which four or more victims are murdered with firearms, within one event and in one or more locations in close proximity" (National Mass Violence and Victimization Resource Center [NMVVRC], 2018, para. 2).

People living in conditions of community violence typically experience their surroundings as unsafe, and this negatively affects occupational participation and community engagement, resulting in occupational deprivation. Exposure to community violence is a significant source of toxic stress, can shape people's perspectives on the future, and can reduce their sense of control. Children exposed to toxic stress in the absence of protective relationships have a higher risk for depression, anxiety, PTSD, substance use, and aggressive behavior. In addition, living in constant fear can have a profound negative impact on learning and development, leading to academic failure. Community violence is also associated with high rates of smoking, sleep disturbance, unhealthy eating habits, and low levels of physical activity resulting in obesity, asthma, heart disease, and diabetes (Violence Policy Center, 2017).

Factors that increase the likelihood of community violence include domestic violence, child maltreatment, gun availability, poor family functioning, substance abuse, inadequate emotion regulation, poverty, toxic levels of stress, and a lack of school/community cohesion. Reducing any combination of these risk factors is likely to decrease community and mass violence. Enhancing protective factors—for example, community collective efficacy, school connectedness and engagement, socioemotional competency, and positive role models in the media—can have the same effect. Reducing risk factors while simultaneously increasing protective factors will produce synergistic results.

The most efficacious approaches to community violence prevention will likely be multilevel, multisectorial, and multidisciplinary. Collaborative involvement of the educational, health, justice/law enforcement, and community sectors will be necessary. The United States has higher levels of community violence compared to other countries. This may "suggest that there are beliefs, values, and policies underlying our national culture that, if better understood and thoughtfully discussed, could reduce violence" (Moore et al., 2015, p. i). Occupational therapy practitioners can contribute the profession's unique perspective and expertise regarding the interplay between occupational participation and context to the solution of this community and population health concern.

On a larger scale, **collective violence** refers to "the instrumental use of violence by people who identify themselves as members of a group—whether this group is transitory or has a more permanent identity—against another group or set of individuals, in order to achieve political, economic, or social objectives" (Krug, Dahlberg, Mercy, Zwi, and Lozano, 2002). Collective violence typically involves "violent conflicts between nations and groups, state and group terrorism, rape as a weapon of war . . . and gang warfare" (World Health Organization

[WHO], 2019, para. 1). Collective violence usually results in complex emergencies or humanitarian crises where there is a breakdown in governmental authority and service provision. The outcomes of collective violence—for example, population dislocation, human rights abuses, and destruction of social networks and ecosystems—have profound consequences for community and population health.

Risk factors for collective violence include, but are not limited to, unequal access to power, inequitable distribution of resources, rapid demographic change, excessively high population densities, insufficient supply of food and/or safe water, and the intensification of ethnic, racial, national, or religious group fanaticism. These problems are extremely complex and will require a coordinated, global response.

Thriving Professional Communities

Thriving professional communities require an inclusive and equitable environment where all practitioners can work without fear of discrimination, bias, or other harm. The profession, especially given the demographics of the profession's members, must take time to reflect on the power and privilege differential between occupational therapy practitioners and the clients served. Themes of occupational and social justice have been woven through many of the chapters in this book. Most of these discussions have been outwardly focused, examining injustices and the role of occupational therapy and occupational science in combating those injustices. It is important to also look inward and examine whether the profession consciously or unconsciously participates in or ignores justice within its ranks.

A review of the demographics of occupational therapy practitioners shows an overwhelmingly female and white workforce. According to the last AOTA (2015a) *Salary and Workforce Survey,* 91.1% of occupational therapists and 90.5% of occupational therapy assistants were females, and 85.3% of occupational therapy practitioners were white. While many white women in the profession have faced discrimination or harassment based on their gender in the larger world, they have also been protected by being privileged. Although men are a minority within the profession of occupational therapy, they have identified privileges associated with their gender in their employment, specifically, "from a practical and a financial standpoint" (Maxim and Rice, 2018, p. 3). On the other hand, it has been observed by at least one of the chapter's authors that men in the profession can be subjected to comments and requests that if made by them to a woman colleague would be met with scorn and cries of harassment or misogyny. To be true to the *AOTA Occupational Therapy Code of Ethics (2015),* Principle 6, Fidelity (AOTA, 2015c) all occupational therapy practitioners need to be conscious of how colleagues are treated and speak up if bias is observed.

Drawbacks of the AOTA (2015a) *Salary and Workforce Survey* include the absence of relevant data either on gender beyond a binary construct or on occupational therapy practitioners with differing ability levels. Occupational therapy practitioners have reported feelings of isolation and bias based on differences (Heffron, The, and Harrison, 2018). This is inconsistent with the profession's commitment to inclusion and diversity articulated in the AOTA (2014b) *Occupational Therapy's Commitment to Nondiscrimination and Inclusion* and should be addressed in the future as the profession further evolves to meet its commitment.

Four important constructs to consider in the daily work lives of occupational therapy practitioners and of great significance to establishing and evolving a thriving professional community include white privilege, white fragility, microaggression, and invisible workload. These constructs are complex, and people's reaction to them can be intense. Readers are encouraged to read the sources cited in this section and to also look for other resources in their workplace or educational institution to assist in reflecting on and unpacking how professional actions are influenced by privilege.

White privilege has been debated over the last three decades and has been defined by a nonwhite family physician as "a long-standing concept defining a set of privileges available to white people because of their race and unavailable to others" (Hobbs, 2018, p. 197). The use of the term "white privilege" does not suggest "that white people have never struggled" and that all whites have access to health care and other resources. "White privilege should be viewed as a built-in advantage, separate from one's level of income or effort" (Collins and Wolski, 2018, p. 39). Examples of white privilege in daily life were developed by a white professor (McIntosh, 1989) within the specific context of her life in that time and space; they are autobiographical. The purpose of her writing was not to have people feel guilt or shame but for people to consider what advantages they realize due to their race. McIntosh's examples of privilege are helpful for individuals' reflection regarding their potential advantages within their own place, space, and time. Examples of McIntosh's (1989, p. 2) self-perceived privilege that may resonate with white occupational therapy practitioners include:

- "I can go shopping alone most of the time, pretty well assured that I will not be followed around or harassed."
- "I can easily buy posters, postcards, picture books, greeting cards, dolls, toys, and children's magazines featuring people of my race."
- "I can choose public accommodations without fearing that people of my race cannot get in or will be mistreated in the places I have chosen."

Ajayi (2016) asks white people to acknowledge that while white privileges are not under their control, that part of their identity places them at an advantage. "Knowing our privilege does not make us villains, but it should make us more conscious about the parts we play in systems that are greater than us. It should make us be more thoughtful; it should humble us" (Ajayi, 2016, p. 86).

White fragility is the construct that describes the manner in which some white individuals respond to discussions regarding race or white privilege. It is helpful to be aware of this potential reaction prior to providing professional development regarding race, either in an all-white space or a space with multiple races, including white individuals. White fragility

> *is a state in which even a minimum amount of racial stress becomes intolerable, triggering a range of defensive moves. These moves include the outward display of emotions such as anger, fear, and guilt, and behaviors such as argumentation, silence, and leaving the stress-inducing situation. These behaviors, in turn, function to reinstate white racial equilibrium. (DiAngelo, 2011, p. 54)*

An understanding of white fragility is also important in forming a response to observed microaggressions.

Microaggressions are intentional and unintentional slights or attacks directed toward individuals from a less powerful or privileged group. A common example and experience is for a black person to be applauded for their verbal skills—how "well spoken" or articulate they are (Ajayi, 2016). Other examples include asking a nonwhite person "No, where are you really from?" or asking a biracial person "What are you?" These examples and others were documented by a photographer at Fordham University (Nigatu, 2013). The accompanying photographs are compelling representations of how the flow of daily life is interrupted when deciding whether to ignore or respond to such comments.

Engage Your Brain 28-4

Review the University of Fordham photographs (Nigatu, 2013). Have you ever asked or been asked any of the questions displayed? What would be more appropriate questions to ask to start to get to know someone?

An awareness of and removal of **invisible workloads** is another important step in fostering a thriving professional community. One example of an invisible workload is the extra burden faculty from underrepresented groups shoulder as unofficial advisers and mentors of students from similar groups. This time burden can be especially difficult for tenure-track faculty, who must meet other service responsibilities and scholarship production in addition to this uncounted service to students and the institution. The Faculty Workload and Rewards Project (University of Maryland, n.d.) is an initiative to "improve organizational policies and practices that shape equity in workload for all faculty, including women and underrepresented minority faculty" (para. 2). Moule (2005) described the burden of the invisible workload through a 5-year study of her work as a faculty member. Although there is no formal literature documenting the extension of this phenomenon to health care, it would behoove occupational therapy practitioners to be vigilant of any additional drain that practitioners from underrepresented groups experience with mentoring and supporting students or new staff from underrepresented groups. If such work is being performed, it should be identified, valued, and compensated.

Diffusion of Innovations

An **innovation** is an idea, method, practice, or object that is perceived to be new or novel. Some innovations are not really new from an objective historical perspective but are new to the perceiver by virtue of a lapse of time since their initial discovery or introduction (Rogers, 1995).

Innovations often require a significant period of time for diffusion before being adopted by practitioners, academics, and researchers in a discipline. **Diffusion of innovation** refers to "the process by which an innovation is communicated through certain channels over time among the members of a social system" (Rogers, 1995, p. 5). Diffusion of innovation produces changes, both planned and unplanned, in the structure and function of a social system. See Chapter 3 for additional information on the diffusion of innovations theoretical framework.

Time is a factor in the diffusion process. Some individuals are early adopters of innovation, while others tend to lag behind. Some innovations are adopted very quickly. Others may take significantly longer periods of time. In a profession, diffusion of innovation requires a "critical mass" of adopters before the innovation becomes the standard. It is interesting to note that four of the topics that appeared in this chapter as future trends in the previous edition of this text have either a partial or full chapter dedicated to the topic in the current edition—transition services, aging in place, driving and community mobility for the older adult, and telehealth.

The occupational therapy profession is at an important crossroads in its history. Should the profession readopt the innovation of community and population health practice and all it entails and move ahead quickly and deliberately or accept the status quo and work within the narrower, existing parameters of practice? Emerging practice areas in community and population health are very much in harmony with the founders' visions of the profession. At the turn of the century, Fidler (2000) clearly supported change and suggested moving "beyond the therapy model." She advocated that practitioners become "occupationalists" who have the capability to practice and conduct research in a variety of areas, including but not limited to:

- Services and programs of wellness, of prevention, of learning enhancement, and lifestyle counseling
- Community planning and design
- Organizational, agency, and institutional design and operations
- Treatment, restorative interventions, and rehabilitation (Fidler, 2000, p. 101)

The next section describes future trends or innovations that already, or will soon, have an impact on occupational therapy practice.

Future Trends

It is always challenging to predict the future, but it seems extremely clear that at least two major trends will likely have an impact on occupational therapy practice in the coming decades: technology and globalization. Technologies, particularly artificial intelligence, virtual reality, robotics, and three-dimensional printing, have already changed the delivery of health-care services and will continue to do so at a rapid rate. These technologies as they might apply to occupational therapy practice will be briefly discussed here. Globalization has wide-ranging, complex effects on many aspects of life, and health care is no exception. The potential impact of globalization on the occupational therapy profession will be highlighted.

Artificial Intelligence, Virtual Reality, and Robotics

Artificial intelligence (AI) can be defined as a machine's "ability to correctly interpret external data, to learn from such data, and to use those learnings to achieve specific goals and tasks through flexible adaptation" (Kaplan and Haenlein, 2019, p. 15). Applications of AI are being designed for use in health care with a variety of populations. For example, "intelligent" assistive devices are being developed to support persons with decreased cognitive abilities due to dementia. Intelligent assistive devices

(IAD) are contextually aware and can provide assistance when appropriate (Bharucha et al., 2009). Prototypes using artificial intelligence have been developed to assist with hand washing, blood glucose monitoring, and kitchen activities. These devices use cameras and audio and video prompts to provide feedback to the user (Czarnuch and Mihailidis, 2011). AI can also be used for chronic disease prevention and management. For example, a diabetes prevention program can be delivered through AI using cognitive behavioral strategies. The AI coach is available 24 hours a day, 7 days a week and targets both nutrition and physical activity behavior change. AI is capable of monitoring and customizing care to accommodate an individual's unique needs (Stein, 2017). The applications of AI technology in occupational therapy practice seem endless.

Ambient intelligence (AmI) is a specific form of AI that refers to digital environments that are sensitive and responsive to the presence of people. This is technology that is typically used in "smart homes" that enables devices networked and integrated into the environment to anticipate and adapt to a person's specific needs. Ambient assisted living technology can allow persons with disabilities to live more independently and older adults to age in place longer while reducing the burden on caregivers (Cook, Augusto, and Jakkula, 2009; Rashidi and Mihailidis, 2013). Occupational therapy practitioners are acutely aware of the impact of environment on occupational performance and participation. As a result, the profession can make significant contributions to the development of home, work, and school AmI technology.

Virtual reality (VR) is "a computer-based technology that allows users to interact with a multisensory simulated environment and receive real-time feedback on performance" (Saposnik and Levin, 2011, p. 1380). VR interventions have been used in rehabilitation for traumatic brain injury (Man, Poon, and Lam, 2013), stroke (Laver, George, Thomas, Deutsch, and Crotty, 2011), and upper-extremity motor impairment (Sucar et al., 2013). In addition, VR has been found effective in improving the social cognition and social functioning of young adults with high-functioning autism (Kandalaft, Didehbani, Krawczyk, Allen, and Chapman, 2013). When occupational therapy interventions cannot be provided in vivo, where people live, work, and play, VR simulated environments are a good alternative. Occupational therapy practitioners can be involved in the development of VR simulations for therapeutic use.

Robotics is the science of engineering, building, and programming machines (robots) to perform jobs and tasks autonomously without human intervention (LEO Centre for Service Robotics, n.d.). Robots can assist older adults and persons with disabilities in their daily activities. For example, robots have been designed and built to retrieve dropped items from the floor; detect, grasp, and retrieve household items; and lift and transfer a person from a bed or wheelchair (Rashidi and Mihailidis, 2013). Combining AI with robotics makes autonomous, or self-driving, automobiles and "smart" wheelchairs and scooters possible, which can enhance mobility for persons with disabilities (Scudellari, 2017).

Socially assistive robots (SARS), machines that interact primarily though social cues, have been used therapeutically with individuals with autism spectrum disorder to generate motivation and social engagement and as therapy assistants in stroke rehabilitation (Obiedat, Ardehali, and Smith, 2018). Humanoid robots can provide automated coaching, encouragement, and task-specific feedback. These robots can engage in simple games (tossing a ball); demonstrate range-of-motion exercises; and monitor, measure, and report client performance to the therapist (see Fig. 28-3). An interdisciplinary effort between rehabilitation professionals and engineers can produce future applications of this technology for clinical and home use (Obiedat et al., 2018).

SARS are also used for companionship. These robots may take the form of a human, an animal, or a machine. Companion robots may fill the role of a pet to reduce stress and depression without the burden of caregiving. Some robots are capable of making eye contact, recognizing and responding to human emotions, conversing on a variety of topics, and even telling jokes (Medical Futurist, 2019).

Three-Dimensional Printing

Three-Dimensional Printing (3-DP) is a new technology that has great potential for use by occupational therapy practitioners and their clients. Based on computer-aided designs (blueprints), 3-DP manufactures solid objects using a variety of

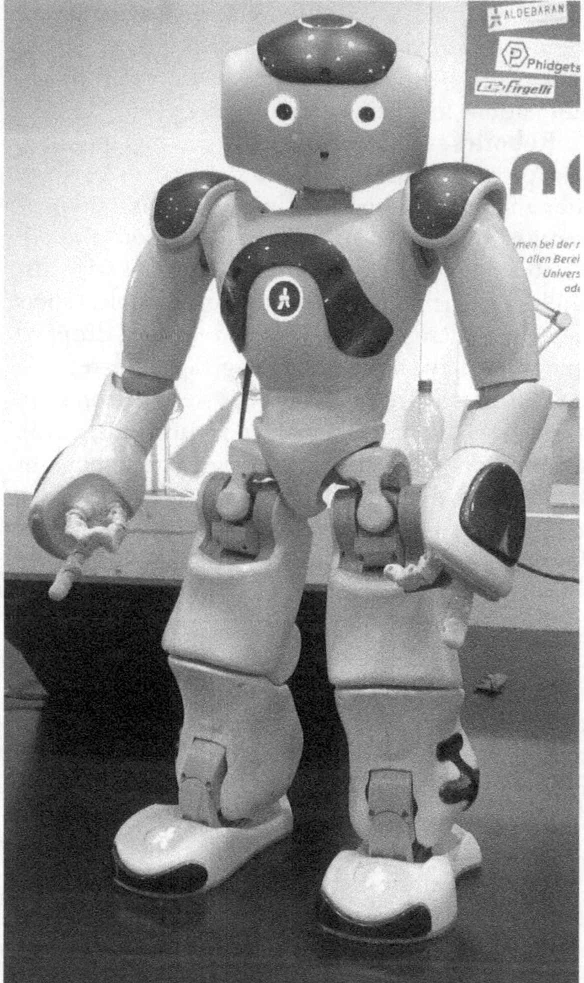

Figure 28-3 Therapy assistant robot. *(Photo courtesy of Ubahnverleih via https://en.wikipedia.org/wiki/Nao_(robot).)*

materials, including thermoplastics, metal, rubber, paper, and nylon in filament form. Health-care providers are increasingly using 3-DP technology for a variety of purposes. However, the research evidence on efficacy is scant at present, and reimbursement mechanisms are lacking. In physical medicine and rehabilitation, 3-DP is being used to fabricate orthoses and prostheses (Lunsford, Grindle, Salatin, and Dicianno, 2016). In occupational therapy, 3-DP makes the codesign (therapist and client) and production of customized assistive devices feasible. Commercially available devices are often expensive and may not meet a client's unique needs. Client participation in the design and personalization of the product enhances long-term use and satisfaction with the device (Schwartz, 2018).

Occupational therapy students at Spalding University were instructed on the basics of computer-assisted design technology and 3-DP and then paired with a community-dwelling older adult through the Elder Mentor Project. Students met with older adults over a period of 6 weeks to gather information regarding their needs, habits, roles, and routines. Using 3-DP, students and older adults cocreated designs and produced customized assistive devices. Examples of devices created include a paddle light switch, card holder, television remote holder, pill case, cell phone holder, and thumb ring page holder (Story, 2018).

Ganesan, Al-Jumaily, and Luximon (2016) describe the advantages of using 3-DP for the construction of splints over traditional methods—for example, for comfort, fit, durability, and proper ventilation. 3-DP splints are also lightweight and more aesthetic than handmade thermoplastic splints and in many cases can be constructed at a lower cost. Once designed, the data can be stored and the splint reproduced at any time. All of these features are likely to improve adherence to wearing schedules.

Thingiverse.com is a website that provides 3-DP resources, including how to customize a 3-D printable design, teach using a 3-D printer, and create 3-D models. There is an occupational therapy group on the website where practitioners can interact and post information and photos of objects and devices produced via 3-DP (MakerBot Industries, 2019).

Globalization

Globalization refers to the "growing interdependence of the world's economies, cultures, and populations brought about by cross-border trade in goods and services, technology, and flow of investment, people and information" (Peterson Institute for International Economics, 2019, para. 2). It is important to distinguish globalization from globalism. Globalism is an ideology that prioritizes a global order over the interests of individual nations. There is evidence worldwide of a backlash of nationalism and protectionism against globalism. However, many believe we are entering into a new wave or era of globalization. Due to the unprecedented pace of technological change, systems of health care, transportation, energy, communications, production, and distribution will all be transformed on a global level (Schwab, 2018).

Three aspects of globalization as it relates to the profession of occupational therapy are discussed here. The first is the incorporation of globalization in the profession's paradigm. The concepts of environment and context are very familiar to occupational therapy practitioners and are embedded in evaluation and intervention strategies. Expanding these ideas beyond the local to a global perspective is a natural extension of occupational therapy practice. This may include consideration of adopting a more sustainable lifestyle by practitioners and clients—for example, by walking and cycling more and driving less, which can not only improve individual health by reducing cardiovascular disease, depression, and diabetes but also simultaneously improve air quality and reduce the emissions that cause global warming (Hocking and Kroksmark, 2013). Through adapting and grading, occupational therapy can enable clients "to engage in alternatives to unsustainable occupations" (Whittaker, 2012, p. 436). Integrating the perspective of sustainable, global well-being into the occupational therapy paradigm can provide exciting new opportunities and venues for occupational therapy practice.

The second aspect is the globalization of professional interaction. The AOTA and the WFOT are committed to fostering a globally connected profession that is responsive to the occupational needs of diverse societies (AOTA, 2007; WFOT, 2019a). The WFOT (2019a) is a global network established in 1952 that currently includes 101 member associations representing over 550,000 occupational therapists. The WFOT is a recognized nongovernment organization by the WHO and the United Nations. Every 4 years through an international congress, the WFOT brings together occupational therapists from around the world for an exchange of ideas and research.

The third aspect is the relationship between globalization and occupational justice. According to the WFOT (2006) position statement on human rights, occupational therapists have an obligation to facilitate the achievement of a global, occupationally just society. The position statement is concerned with all people, not just patients or clients of occupational therapy services. "Global conditions that threaten the right to occupation include poverty, disease, social discrimination, displacement, natural and man-made disasters and armed conflict" (WFOT, 2006, p. 1). Occupational therapy practitioners can work with groups, communities, and populations to eliminate barriers to occupational performance, enhance occupational participation, and reduce occupational injustice throughout the world. The position paper provides a vision of an ideal world where people are free to engage in occupations that simultaneously provide personal meaning and serve the common good (Bryant, 2010). In order to participate effectively in the globalization of occupational therapy, practitioners need knowledge and skills in global and population health.

Implications for Professional Preparation and Education

Vision 2025 explicitly states "occupational therapy maximizes health, well-being, and quality of life for all people, ***populations, and communities*** [emphasis added]" (AOTA, 2018b, para. 1). In order for occupational therapy practitioners and other healthcare professionals to effectively participate in community and population health promotion and prevention efforts, educational programs need to facilitate the development of competencies for this area of practice. A primary challenge will be to balance the need to prepare students for traditional biomedical practice with the new demands of community and population health roles and the awareness of global health needs. McColl (1998) identified the knowledge needed by occupational therapy students and practitioners in order to participate effectively in the community (see Box 28-3).

In 2018, the Accreditation Council for Occupational Therapy Education (ACOTE), the organization responsible for accrediting entry-level occupational therapy educational programs, adopted new standards for occupational therapy assistant (associate and bachelor's level) and occupational therapist (master's and doctoral level) preparation programs to be implemented by July 31, 2020 (AOTA, 2018a). The 2018 accreditation standards for occupational therapy programs brings increased attention to community and population health

Box 28-3 What Students and Practitioners Need to Know to Participate Effectively in Community Programs

- What a community is
- How organizations and communities form
- How organizations and communities are governed
- How to identify community resources
- How to identify community needs
- How to facilitate change
- How persons with disabilities live in the community
- How persons develop and pursue occupations in the community
- What supports and barriers to participation in occupation exist in the community

From "What Do We Need to Know to Practice Occupational Therapy in the Community?," by M. A. McColl, 1998, *American Journal of Occupational Therapy, 52*(1), pp. 11–18.

practice competencies as compared to previous versions of the standards. For example, the word "community" appears 36 times and "population" appears 90 times in the 2018 *ACOTE Standards and Interpretative Guide.*

One section of the accreditation standards (the minimum essential requirements for accreditation of educational programs) is devoted to the context of service delivery. This section describes, in some detail, the competencies required for practicing in a variety of environments, with a major emphasis on community and social systems. Community-related competencies also can be found as minor components in other sections of the standards, including:

- Foundational content requirements
- Occupational therapy theoretical perspectives
- Basic tenets of occupational therapy
- Referral, screening, evaluation, and intervention plan
- Intervention plan formulation and implementation
- Leadership and management of occupational therapy services
- Professional ethics, values, and responsibilities
- Fieldwork education
- Doctoral capstone

Box 28-4 provides examples of standards that emphasize community and population health from the *Standards for an Accredited Educational Program for the Occupational Therapist* (AOTA, 2018a).

A number of educational approaches can be developed, implemented, and evaluated for their effectiveness in meeting the demands of emerging practice arenas. The accreditation standards allow the flexibility to create a variety of curricular models that qualify for accreditation. As every community and population is different, so, too, may educational programs differ in how they meet the need to produce a new type of occupational therapy practitioner.

Some educational programs are meeting the challenge by infusing community and population health practice content throughout the curriculum, while others are creating new courses that focus entirely on community and population health concerns. Some programs are using community-based sites in creative ways for level I fieldwork. Other programs place students in community programs for both level I and level II fieldwork. In addition, community service learning has become an attractive educational methodology within occupational therapy programs to address the competencies needed for effective community and population health practice. Integrating community service-learning opportunities in occupational therapy curricula can facilitate students' understanding and appreciation of social, economic, and environmental factors and their impact on occupational participation, health, and quality of life (Horowitz, 2012). The next section describes the role of community service learning, interprofessional education, and the clinical prevention and population health curriculum (CPPHC) framework in preparing students for community and population health practice.

Community Service Learning

Community service learning (CSL) is defined as "a teaching and learning strategy that integrates meaningful community service with instruction and reflection to enrich the learning experience, teach civic responsibility, and strengthen communities" (National Service Learning Clearinghouse, 2012, para. 1). Through CSL, occupational therapy students have the opportunity not only to practically

Box 28-4 ACOTE Standards Related to Community and Population Health Practice*

Section B: Content Requirements

1.0 Foundational Content Requirements

1.2 Apply and analyze the role of sociocultural, socioeconomic, and diversity factors as well as lifestyle choices in contemporary society to meet the needs of persons, groups, and populations.

1.3 Demonstrate knowledge of the social determinants of health for persons, groups, and populations with or at risk for disabilities and chronic health conditions. This must include an analysis of the epidemiological factors that impact the public health and welfare of populations.

2.0 Occupational Therapy Theoretical Perspectives

2.1 Apply, analyze, and evaluate scientific evidence, theories, models of practice, and frames of reference that underlie the practice of occupational therapy to guide and inform interventions for persons, groups, and populations in a variety of practice contexts and environments.

3.0 Basic Tenets of Occupational Therapy

3.4 Apply and analyze scientific evidence to explain the importance of balancing areas of occupation; the role of occupation in the promotion of health; and the prevention of disease, illness, and dysfunction for persons, groups, and populations.

4.0 Referral, screening, evaluation, and intervention plan and intervention plan: formulation and implementation

4.10 Recommend and provide direct interventions and procedures to persons, groups, and populations to enhance safety, health and wellness, and performance in occupations.

4.14 Evaluate the needs of persons, groups, and populations to design programs that enhance community mobility, and implement transportation transitions, including driver rehabilitation and community access.

4.18 Assess, grade, and modify the way persons, groups, and populations perform occupations and activities by adapting processes, modifying environments, and applying ergonomic principles to reflect the changing needs of the client, sociocultural context, and technological advances.

4.19 Demonstrate, evaluate, and plan the consultative process with persons, groups, programs, organizations, or communities in collaboration with inter- and intra-professional colleagues.

4.20 Demonstrate, evaluate, and plan care coordination, case management, and transition services in traditional and emerging practice environments.

4.21 Demonstrate, evaluate, and utilize the principles of the teaching-learning process using educational methods and health literacy education approaches:

- To design activities and clinical training for persons, groups, and populations
- To instruct and train the client, caregiver, family, significant others, and communities at the level of the audience.

4.23 Identify occupational needs through effective communication with patients, families, communities, and members of the interprofessional team in a responsive and responsible manner that supports a team approach to the promotion of health and wellness.

4.25 Demonstrate knowledge of the principles of interprofessional team dynamics to perform effectively in different team roles to plan, deliver, and evaluate patient- and population-centered care as well as population health programs and policies that are safe, timely, efficient, effective, and equitable.

4.26 Evaluate and discuss mechanisms for referring clients to specialists both internal and external to the profession, including community agencies.

4.27 Evaluate access to community resources, and design community or primary care programs to support occupational performance for persons, groups, and populations.

Continued

Box 28-4 ACOTE Standards Related to Community and Population Health Practice*–cont'd

4.28 Develop a plan for discharge from occupational therapy services in collaboration with the client and members of the interprofessional team by reviewing the needs of the client, caregiver, family, and significant others; available resources; and discharge environment.

5.0 Context of Service Delivery, Leadership, and Management of Occupational Therapy Services

5.1 Identify, analyze, and evaluate the contextual factors; current policy issues; and socioeconomic, political, geographic, and demographic factors on the delivery of occupational therapy services for persons, groups, and populations to promote policy development and social systems as they relate to the practice of occupational therapy.

5.2 Identify, analyze, and advocate for existing and future service delivery models and policies, and their potential effect on the practice of occupational therapy and opportunities to meet societal needs.

5.4 Identify and evaluate the systems and structures that create federal and state legislation and regulations and their implications and effects on persons, groups, and populations, as well as practice.

Section C: Fieldwork Education

1.1 Ensure that the fieldwork program reflects the sequence and scope of content in the curriculum design, in collaboration with the faculty, so that fieldwork experiences in traditional, non-traditional, and emerging settings strengthen the ties between didactic and fieldwork education.

* These abbreviated examples are drawn from the Master's Degree-Level Accreditation Standards.
From *Accreditation Council for Occupational Therapy Education (ACOTE) Standards and Interpretative Guide (effective July 31, 2020)*, by American Occupational Therapy Association, 2018a.

apply what they have learned in the classroom to a real-world problem but also to increase the awareness of occupational therapy in the community and provide much-needed services to underserved populations.

CSL has several characteristics that distinguish it from volunteerism. Volunteerism, although a highly valued occupation, is not an educational pedagogy. The purpose of volunteerism is to serve one's neighbors and communities in order to enhance the quality of life for all. Volunteers donate their time, effort, and talents to a need or cause they value out of a sense of social responsibility. In high-quality community service-learning programs, students are involved in identifying community needs, planning and implementing a service project, and engaging in structured reflection on what was learned through the service experience. CSL is designed to meet a community need while facilitating the development of skills in the learner.

Much research has been conducted on the effects of community service learning. The effects on the learner, many of which are congruent with occupational therapy's history and philosophical base, appear to be broad based and enduring. Regardless of the discipline, service-based learning appears to have a positive effect on:

- Self-efficacy and personal identity
- Interpersonal development, leadership, and communication skills
- Cultural understanding
- Social responsibility and citizenship skills
- Ability to apply learning to real-world situations
- Problem-solving and critical thinking skills (Brondani, 2012; Buff et al., 2015; Clark, McKague, McKay, and Ramsden, 2015; Gardner and Emory, 2018; Peters, McHugh, and Sendall, 2006; Steffes, 2004)

In addition, several potential benefits specific to the discipline of occupational therapy are evident. CSL can increase students' understanding of the role of occupational therapy in community and population health practice. CSL also provides opportunities to integrate theory with practice and network with professionals in a variety of disciplines. CSL allows community-based organizations, which currently may not include occupational therapy services, to experience the benefits of occupational therapy firsthand, thereby increasing the potential development of new job opportunities for occupational therapy practitioners in community and population health programs.

CSL also increases the probability that students might choose a community-based setting for future practice. What students learn in school is most likely how they will practice. It has been demonstrated that practitioners who are trained in institutions want to work in institutions (Weissert, Knott, and Steiber, 1993). Providing students early in their academic careers with opportunities to experience the potential for community and population health practice is one strategy to develop future practitioners for new roles.

The overall goal of a CSL program is to develop students' skills and competencies in the provision of community-based occupational therapy services to agencies and organizations in the local community, which have typically been underserved. An effective program is designed to:

- Respond to actual community needs
- Provide community-based organizations with the opportunity to experience occupational therapy services firsthand
- Increase the potential for the development of new job opportunities in community-based programs
- Increase the probability that students will choose a community-based setting for future practice

According to Horowitz (2012), "service learning provides occupational therapy education with a flexible, relatively low-cost pedagogy that advances the Centennial Vision *(now Vision 2025)* and provides opportunities for community practice through reflective, active learning experiences" (p. 3).

Interprofessional Education

Interprofessional education (IPE) is defined as "when students from two or more professions learn about, from and with each other to enable effective collaboration and improve health outcomes" (WHO, 2010, p. 7). Effective IPE prepares students to become health-care workers who are capable of working on an interprofessional team and providing collaborative care. **Collaborative practice** occurs "when multiple health workers from different professional backgrounds provide comprehensive services by working together with patients, their families, careers, and communities to deliver the highest quality of care across settings" (WHO, 2010, p. 13). Interprofessional collaborative practice requires mutual trust and respect, open communication, shared decision-making, mutual accountability, and a synergistic interaction of knowledge and skills. Sufficient evidence now exists to conclude that IPE enables effective collaborative practice, which in turn has been shown to optimize health services and improve health outcomes (WHO, 2010).

IPE can take a variety of forms. However, research has shown that IPE is most effective when principles of adult learning are employed, learning reflects real-world practice experiences, and interaction among students is facilitated. IPE can be delivered face-to-face, online, and/or in virtual contexts. IPE learning activities may include simulation exercises, problem/case-based discussion sessions, presentations, and community service-learning experiences (Bridges, Davidson, Odegard, Maki, and Tomkowiak, 2011). Some IPE programs are using social media tools and developing learning communities online as a means of overcoming limitations in space and time for face-to-face meetings. The social media applications and tools most often used include virtual simulation platforms, blogs, discussion boards, Wikis, Ning, and Second Life (Rankin, Truskey, and Chisolm, 2018).

The Interprofessional Education Collaborative (2011) convened a panel of experts to develop a set of competencies for interprofessional collaborative practice that could be used by all health-care disciplines to redesign their curricula to better prepare practitioners to engage in team-based care. The four categories of competencies are values and ethics, roles and responsibilities, communication, and teams and teamwork. Research on outcomes of IPE has demonstrated positive changes in perceptions and attitudes toward increased knowledge and skills in communicating with and changes in behavior regarding other health professions (Reeves et al., 2016).

IPE language and objectives are now included in the accreditation standards for occupational therapy education programs and supported by the AOTA. In an official document, the AOTA Commission of Education asserts that "entry-level occupational therapy curricula should include interprofessional education in which students have opportunities to learn and apply the knowledge and skills necessary for interprofessional collaborative practice" (AOTA, 2015b, p. 1). As a result, there are numerous examples in the literature of the use of IPE in occupational therapy programs, three of which will be briefly described here. The approaches used vary from fairly simple single IPE experiences to complex several-semester course sequences.

One approach to IPE at Idaho State University involved occupational therapy students and students from eight other health disciplines (both undergraduate and graduate level programs). Students attended discipline-specific lectures, assisted with interdisciplinary evaluations of pediatric clients, reflected on what they observed, and participated in interprofessional team meetings. The students received course credit, and the family received a comprehensive evaluation of their child's current level of functioning (Gee et al., 2016). At the University of Florida, students from 10 professions participated in team-based learning using cases that addressed patient safety, health-care ethics, and health systems. For each case, team members collaboratively made choices regarding patient care. An evaluation of the IPE experience indicated an increase in students' knowledge and application of teamwork skills (Black, Blue, and Foss, 2015).

At Saginaw State University, first-year students from six health-related professions participated in roundtable case study discussions to share their respective roles in the care of persons with medical and psychosocial conditions. Second-year students participated in four case-based simulations that provided opportunities to identify professional roles and practice collaboration and teamwork. Scenarios included in-home care, acute hospital care, a poverty simulation, and a disaster response simulation. All students attended a research showcase that displayed scholarly projects from each of the programs to expose them to evidence-based practices in other health-care disciplines. In addition, the occupational therapy students participated in a seminar-type discussion focusing on leadership skills, ethics, and teamwork within the context of an interprofessional team (Prast, Frederick, Herlache-Pretzr, and Lachter, 2015). Concerns regarding the IPE currently provided in occupational therapy programs include: (1) the limited number and types of professionals included on the team and (2) the lack of interprofessional opportunities in community and population health practice settings. Expanding the diversity of interprofessional teams to include non-health-care members and providing IPE experiences outside of the health-care environment will help prepare students for work in community and population health arenas.

Clinical Prevention and Population Health Curriculum Framework

Although the terms "community" and "population health" are frequently used in the accreditation document, ACOTE does not provide specific curricular content requirements. Braveman (2016) asserts that practice models to guide occupational therapy intervention at the population level are not well developed and that population health is not well understood by members of the profession. Braveman recommends that the profession of occupational therapy identify the specific competencies needed to work in population health and incorporate these into the educational accreditation standards more explicitly. Fortunately, an interdisciplinary curriculum framework has already been developed that can provide structure for occupational therapy education in this area.

The CPPHC framework was developed by the Healthy People Curriculum Task Force (Task Force) instituted by the Association for Prevention Teaching and Research (APTR). The APTR (2015) is a membership organization of educational institutions and faculty devoted to advancing prevention and population health education and research. The CPPHC framework for health professions education serves as the foundation for two *Healthy People 2020* objectives. These educational objectives include:

- Increase the inclusion of core clinical prevention and population health content in health professions education
- Increase the proportion of academic institutions with health professions education programs whose prevention curricula include interprofessional educational experiences (APTR, n.d., para. 2)

Task Force members assert that if *Healthy People* goals and objectives are to be achieved, all health-care professionals should be educated and interprofessionally trained in population health principles and practices. The CPPHC framework provides a common core of knowledge relevant for all health professions regarding prevention and health promotion for individuals and populations. The content guidelines in the CPPHC framework are compatible with a range of learning outcomes and competencies. This easily allows its application to a variety of health professions and to community-service learning and interprofessional educational experiences.

The CPPHC framework consists of four components: foundations of population health, clinical preventive services and health promotion, clinical practice and population health, and health systems and health policy (APTR, 2015). A brief description of each component follows:

- *Foundations of Population Health* includes "the quantitative and analytic skills used to assess, compare, describe, and monitor the health of populations."
- *Clinical Preventive Services and Health Promotion* highlights "evidence-based, health promotion and disease prevention interventions in the clinical setting."
- *Clinical Practice and Population Health* describes "opportunities and disciplines that require individual- and population-based health perspectives."
- *Health Systems and Health Policy* includes "the systems and policies that help to govern the health and healthcare system including collaborations between the clinical care and public health communities" (APTR, 2015, pp. 2–3).

The adoption of this framework by occupational therapy educational programs could enhance the knowledge and skills of students needed for future health-promotion practice.

The APTR (2015) Task Force recommends that all health professions education programs:

- Incorporate clinical prevention and population health educational content in their curricula.
- Evaluate students' knowledge and skills with regard to clinical prevention and population health.
- Use diverse teaching and learning methods to incorporate clinical prevention and population health content into degree and continuing education programs, including service-learning, problem/case-based learning, and simulation methods.
- Integrate innovative, interprofessional educational experiences and approaches focused on clinical prevention and population health (p. 4).

Implications for Research in Community and Population Health Practice

Baum and Law (1998) outlined a number of research areas that are relevant for community and population health practice. Occupational therapy researchers need to:

- Identify the factors that contribute to successful employment, self-sufficiency, and social integration
- Determine the conditions that enable persons with chronic disabilities to participate fully in their families, schools, work settings, and communities
- Investigate how the interaction of biopsychosocial and environmental factors contribute to the development of functional limitations, disabilities, and impairments
- Identify the personal, developmental, and environmental attributes that contribute to successful community living

Traditional approaches to quantitative research may not be the most effective ways of investigating the impact of occupational therapy in community settings or the impact of occupational therapy on community health. Typically, quantitative studies do not capture the unique experiences of community members or the complex interactions that affect health (Christiansen and Matuska, 2010). As a result, researchers in public and community health have advocated for the use of community-based participatory action approaches and mixed methods research. Kielhofner (2005) eloquently argues that participatory action research may be one strategy for bridging the divide between scholarship and practice in occupational therapy.

Community-based participatory action research (CBPAR) takes place in real-world contexts and is client centered, collaborative, action oriented, and designed to solve a community health problem.

In CBPAR, participants are involved in a collaborative relationship with the researcher to identify the problem to be addressed, determine the research questions, design the research methods, conduct data collection and analysis, and interpret and apply the results. Letts (2003) argues that participatory research is an approach that is consistent with the values of the profession and can make significant contributions to the knowledge base in occupational therapy.

Many applications of CBPAR use mixed methods research. **Mixed methods research** combines elements from both the quantitative and qualitative research traditions in an attempt to expand understanding of a phenomenon and confirm findings from a variety of data sources. Using mixed methods helps to neutralize the inherent biases and draw on the respective strengths of each, thereby increasing the validity and usefulness of the information obtained. Researchers intentionally combine the quantitative and qualitative data in order to gain a larger perspective on the phenomenon of interest. Mixed methods studies incorporate both deductive and inductive reasoning. Depending on the research questions, mixing quantitative and qualitative methods may be done sequentially, with one method following the other, or concurrently, where both methods are used simultaneously. Mixed methods research provides multiple perspectives on a problem, contextualizes the information obtained, and allows for an examination of the relationships between processes and outcomes (Office of Behavioral and Social Sciences Research, National Institutes of Health, 2011).

Although there are few examples of CBPAR in the occupational therapy literature, its use is growing. Taylor, Braveman, and Hammel (2004) describe two case examples of how community-based services for persons with AIDS and individuals with chronic fatigue syndrome were developed and evaluated using participatory action research. One CBPAR project, involving occupational therapy faculty and students, was based on the principles of occupational justice and addressed the importance of clean water in the ability of persons in Appalachian Kentucky to carry out the necessary and desired occupations of family and community life (Blakeney and Marshall, 2009).

Photovoice has been used as a CBPAR method for data collection. Photovoice combines "photography and group work to give people an opportunity to record and reflect on their daily lives" (Lal, Jarus, and Suto, 2012, p. 181). It was first used to identify community health issues and provide evidence to policy-makers. The process is participatory in that stakeholders identify issues of concern in their community or population group and determine the research questions. Participants are recruited and trained in the methodology, provided with cameras, and directed to take photos related to the research questions. They come together again to discuss the ideas and meanings represented in the photographs. Photovoice has been used by a variety of disciplines, including public health, education, nursing, and social work. Lal et al. (2012) identified four studies by occupational therapists using Photovoice; these included Andonian (2010), Andonian and MacRae (2011), Berinstein and Magalhaes (2009), and Zecevic, Magalhaes, Madady, Haylligan, and Reeves (2010). Photovoice is a unique research methodology that "provides a framework for occupational therapy researchers to apply a participant-centered approach and to identify participant solutions to barriers in occupational participation" (Lal et al., 2012, p. 1889).

More recently, Turcotte, Carrier, and Levasseur (2019) used CBPAR to create interventions that would foster older adults' social participation. The researchers created a CBPAR steering committee made up of stakeholders, including therapists, community members, service users, and health-care managers. The research objectives and methodology were formulated collaboratively, promoting an equitable relationship between the researchers and community partners. Nonacademic members of the steering committee participated in data collection and analysis, interpretation of the findings, and dissemination of the results through conferences and publications. Data were collected from four focus groups: (1) occupational therapists, (2) older adults, (3) community workers, and (4) caregivers. The participants identified the need for a continuum of services including personalized, group-based, and community-based interventions.

Envisioning the Future

Many of the complex socioenvironmental problems humans face have an impact on individual, community, and population health—for example, climate change, obesity, and collective violence. According to Wicks and Jamieson (2014), addressing these "wicked" problems that have defied the usual attempts to solve will require a transdisciplinary approach, cultural shifts, and transformative, higher-order change. Transformative change "results from re-patterning the way people do things rather than merely extending current patterns" (Wicks and Jamieson, 2014, p. 84).

To paraphrase Barker (1992) in *Future Edge: Discovering the New Paradigms of Success,* the three keys to the successful achievement of *Vision 2025* (AOTA, 2018b) are excellence, innovation, and anticipation. Excellence refers to the ability to do whatever it is one does with the utmost quality, in a cost-effective manner, while seeking continuous improvement. Innovation is the ability to initiate or introduce something new and different and in unison with excellence makes for a powerful combination. Anticipation is the ability to be in the right place at the right time with an excellent, innovative product or service. Anticipation allows one to predict or foresee future needs, trends, and priorities. If, in some small way, one can anticipate the future, then there is no need to fear it. The future can be embraced as an opportunity for growth and revitalization.

The ideas presented in this chapter serve as a catalyst to stimulate further dialogue and the dissemination of community and population health practice in these and other emerging practice areas. Successful entry into community and population health practice will require occupational therapy practitioners to expand their:

- Conceptualization of the usefulness of occupation
- Perspective on the role of occupational therapy
- View of the profession, nationally and globally
- Identification of potential opportunities
- Capabilities as program planners, policy developers, consultants, advocates, and grant writers

The only real barriers are the limits of one's creativity. Occupation is fundamental to human life. It improves physical and mental health, contributes to a sense of well-being, enhances life satisfaction, and provides meaning to everyday existence. Opportunities for professionals with expertise in occupational performance are evident in all spheres of human endeavor. One need only look with fresh eyes and an open mind.

Summary

- Futuristic thinking is based on three principles: (1) the unity or interrelatedness of reality, (2) the future is shaped by the decisions made today and in the past, and (3) the power of ideas to create the future.
- An ecological worldview is characterized by a shift in values from self-assertion to integration. Integration refers to the tendency to partner with other systems in order to fulfill the greater good and create sustainability. This change in values has implications for occupational therapy in community and population health practice.
- Sustainability refers to the ability to live and thrive today without threatening the ability of future generations to do the same. The WFOT encourages occupational therapy practitioners to incorporate sustainability principles into their practice.
- Technologies, particularly AI, VR, robotics, and 3-DP, have already changed the delivery of health-care services and will significantly affect the provision of occupational therapy services in community and population health practice.
- Globalization can provide exciting new opportunities and venues for occupational therapy practice by: (1) integrating the perspective of sustainable, global well-being into the occupational therapy paradigm, (2) fostering a globally connected profession that is responsive to the occupational needs of diverse societies, and (3) obligating occupational therapists to facilitate the achievement of a global occupationally just society. In order to participate effectively in the globalization of occupational therapy, practitioners need knowledge and skills in global and population health.
- A number of educational approaches can be developed, implemented, and evaluated for their effectiveness in meeting the demands of emerging practice arenas, including

community and population health practice. These include, but are not limited to, community service-learning opportunities, interprofessional educational experiences, and the incorporation of elements of the CPPHC framework into occupational therapy curricula.

- Traditional approaches to quantitative research may not be the most effective ways of investigating the impact of occupational therapy in community settings or the impact of occupational therapy on population health. CBPAR is a viable alternative that takes place in real-world contexts and is client centered, collaborative, action-oriented, and designed to solve a community health problem and can make significant contributions to the knowledge base in occupational therapy.

Learning Activities

1. Reflect and identify your levels of privilege as they relate to being a member of a health profession and a sustainable community.
2. The ability to process "big data" and data analytics offers cities and communities in the United States tools to assist in community efforts to promote healthy environments for occupational participation. One such example is the 500 Cities project (Centers for Disease Control and Prevention, 2017). Explore this website: www.cdc.gov/500cities/index.htm.

   How could you use this data to design forward-thinking population-based initiatives?
3. Develop a brief research proposal incorporating the principles of community and population health participatory action research and mixed method designs.
4. Compare your occupational therapy educational program to the CPPHC framework (APTR, 2015) to determine content areas that need to be enhanced for effective participation in community and population health services.

REFERENCES

Administration on Children, Youth and Families. (2017). *The AFCARS report.* Retrieved from www.acf.hhs.gov/sites/default/files/cb/afcarsreport24.pdf

Ajayi, L. (2016). The privilege principle. In *I'm judging you: The do-better manual* (pp. 82–91). New York, NY: Holt.

Allegretto, S. A., and Mishel, M. (2016). *The teacher pay gap is wider than ever: Teachers' pay continues to fall further behind pay of comparable workers.* Washington, DC: Economic Policy Institute.

American Occupational Therapy Association. (2007). AOTA centennial vision and executive summary. *American Journal of Occupational Therapy, 61,* 613–614.

American Occupational Therapy Association. (2014a). Occupational therapy practice framework: Domain and process (3rd ed.). *American Journal of Occupational Therapy, 68*(Suppl. 1), S1–S48. http://dx.doi.org/10.5014/ajot.2014.682.006

American Occupational Therapy Association. (2014b). Occupational therapy's commitment to nondiscrimination and inclusion. *American Journal of Occupational Therapy, 68*(Suppl. 3), S23–S24. doi:10.5014/ajot.2014.686S05

American Occupational Therapy Association. (2015a). *2015 AOTA salary and workforce survey.* Bethesda, MD: AOTA Press.

American Occupational Therapy Association. (2015b). Importance of interprofessional education in occupational therapy curricula. *American Journal of Occupational Therapy, 69*(Suppl. 3), 691341020. http://dx.doi.org/10.5014/ajot.2015.696S02

American Occupational Therapy Association. (2015c). Occupational therapy code of ethics (2015). *American Journal of Occupational Therapy, 69*(Suppl. 3), 6913410020p14. http://dx.doi.org/10.5014/ajot.2015.696S032

American Occupational Therapy Association. (2016). Societal statement on livable communities. *American Journal of Occupational Therapy, 70*(Suppl. 2), 1–2.

American Occupational Therapy Association. (2017). *Occupational therapy's role in mental health promotion, prevention, and intervention with children and youth: Foster care* [Information sheet.] Retrieved from www.aota.org/~/media/Corporate/Files/Practice/Children/SchoolMHToolkit/Foster-Care-Info-Sheet-20170320.pdf

American Occupational Therapy Association. (2018a). *Accreditation Council for Occupational Therapy Education (ACOTE) standards and interpretative guide (effective July 31, 2020).* Retrieved from www.aota.org/~/media/Corporate/Files/EducationCareers/Accredit/StandardsReview/2018-ACOTE-Standards-Interpretive-Guide.pdf

American Occupational Therapy Association. (2018b). Vision 2025. *OT Practice, 23*(1), 18–19.

Andonian, L. (2010). Community participation of people with mental health issues within an urban environment. *Occupational Therapy in Mental Health, 26,* 401–417.

Andonian, L., and MacRae, A. (2011). Well older adults within an urban context: Strategies to create and maintain social participation. *British Journal of Occupational Therapy, 74,* 2–11.

Association for Prevention Teaching and Research. (n.d.). *APTR Healthy People Curriculum Task Force.* Retrieved from www.aptrweb.org/?page=HPC_

Association for Prevention Teaching and Research. (2015). *Clinical prevention and population health curriculum framework.* Retrieved from www.teachpopulationhealth.org/

Barker, J. A. (1992). *Future edge: Discovering the new paradigms of success.* New York, NY: Morrow.

Baum, C., and Law, M. (1998). Community health: A responsibility, an opportunity and a fit for occupational therapy. *American Journal of Occupational Therapy, 52*(1), 7–10.

Bennett, P. (2018, September 4). *9 ways to make leftover food taste brand new.* Retrieved from www.thisisinsider.com/reheating-leftovers-taste-better-2018-8

Berinstein, S., and Magalhaes, L. (2009). A study of the essence of play experience to children living in Zanzibar, Tanzania. *Occupational Therapy International, 16,* 89–106.

Bharucha, A. J., Anand, V. B. S., Forlizzi, J. D., Dew, M. A., Reynolds, C. F., Stevens, S., and Wactlar, H. (2009). Intelligent assistive technology applications to dementia care: Current capabilities, limitations, and future challenges. *American Journal of Geriatric Psychiatry, 17*(2), 88–104.

Black, E. W., Blue, A. V., and Foss, J. J. (2015). Using team-based learning in interprofessional education to promote content knowledge and team skills applications. *American Journal of Occupational Therapy, 69,* 6911510222p1. doi:10.5014/ajot.2015.6951-PO7094

Blakeney, A. B., and Marshall, A. (2009). Water quality, health and human occupations. *American Journal of Occupational Therapy, 63,* 46–57.

Bockhoven, J. S. (1968). Challenge of the new clinical approaches. *American Journal of Occupational Therapy, 22,* 23–25.

Bradshaw, M. (2017). *Helping students with food insecurity earns TU a prestigious honor.* Retrieved from www.towson.edu/news/2017/2017caseaward.html

Braveman, B. (2016). Health policy perspectives—population health and occupational therapy. *American Journal of Occupational Therapy, 70*(1), 7001090010.

Bridges, D. R., Davidson, R. A., Odegard, P. S., Maki, I. V., and Tomkowiak, J. (2011). Interprofessional collaboration: Three best practice models of interprofessional education. *Medical Education Online, 16*(1). Retrieved from https://doi.org/10.3402/meo.v16i0.6035

Brondani, M. A. (2012). Teaching social responsibility through community service-learning in predoctoral dental education. *Journal of Dental Education, 76*(5), 609–619.

Bryant, W. (2010). Global voices, local lives: Human rights and occupational therapy. *World Federation of Occupational Therapists Bulletin, 62*(1), 5–6.

Buff, S. M., Jenkins, K., Kern, D., Worrall, C., Howell, D., Martin, K., . . . Blue, A. (2015). Interprofessional service-learning in a community setting: Findings from a pilot study. *Journal of Interprofessional Care, 29*(2), 159–162.

Capra, F., and Steindl-Rast, D. (1991). *Belonging to the universe: Explorations on the frontiers of science and spirituality.* San Francisco, CA: HarperCollins.

Centers for Disease Control and Prevention. (2017). *500 cities: Local data for better health.* Retrieved from www.cdc.gov/500cities/index.htm

Child Welfare Information Gateway. (n.d.). *Reunifying families.* Retrieved from www.childwelfare.gov/topics/permanency/reunification/

Child Welfare Information Gateway. (2017). *Supporting successful reunifications.* Washington, DC: U.S. Department of Health and Human Services, Children's Bureau. Retrieved from www.childwelfare.gov/pubPDFs/supporting_reunification.pdf#page=2&view=National statistics

Christiansen, C. H., and Matuska, K. M. (2010). Health promotion research in occupational therapy. In M. Scaffa, S. M. Reitz, and M. Pizzi (Eds.), *Occupational therapy in the promotion of health and wellness* (pp. 528–540). Philadelphia: F. A. Davis.

Clark, M., McKague, M., McKay, S., and Ramsden, V. R. (2015). Deeper learning through service: Evaluation of an interprofessional community service-learning program for pharmacy and medicine students. *Journal of Research in Interprofessional Practice and Education, 5*(1), 1–25.

College and University Food Bank Alliance. (2018). *Truth in numbers.* Retrieved from http://cufba.org/resources/

Collins, C., and Wolski, M. (2018). What is white privilege, really? Recognizing white privilege begins with truly recognizing the term itself. *Teaching Tolerance, 60,* 39–41.

Cook, D. J., Augusto, J. C., and Jakkula, V. R. (2009). Ambient intelligence: Technologies, applications, and opportunities. *Pervasive and Mobile Computing, 5*(4), 277–298.

Cornish, E. (1980). Toward a philosophy of futurism. *Health Education, 11,* 10–12.

Crist, P. A. (2018). *Moving the concept of sustainability into a deeper environmental dimension that engages occupational therapy.* Paper presented at the Connected in Diversity: Positioned for Impact, World Federation of Occupational Therapists Congress, Capetown, South Africa.

Croyle, R. T., and Srinivasan, S. (2016). Informing future population health interventions. *Cancer Epidemiology, Biomarkers and Prevention, 25,* 583.

Czarnuch, S., and Mihailidis, A. (2011). The design of intelligent in-home assistive technologies: Assessing the needs of older adults with dementia and their caregivers. *Gerontechnology, 10*(3), 169–182.

DiAngelo, R. (2011). White fragility. *International Journal of Critical Pedagogy, 3*(3), 54–70.

Dorsey, J., and Miller, L. (2013). Green ergonomics: Occupational therapy's role in the sustainability movement, *OT Practice, 18*(15), 9–13.

Edington, D. W., Schultz, A. B., Pitts, J. S., and Camilleri, A. (2015). The future of health promotion in the 21st century: A focus on the working population. *American Journal of Lifestyle Medicine, 10*(4), 242–252.

Environmental Protection Agency. (2016). *Learn about sustainability.* Retrieved from www.epa.gov/sustainability/learn-about-sustainability

Fairris, D. (2005). The impact of living wages on employers: A control group analysis of the Los Angeles Ordinance. *Industrial Relations, 44*(1), 84–105.

Fairris, D., Runsten, D., Briones, C., and Goodheart, J. (2015). *Examining the evidence: The impact of the Los Angeles Wage Ordinance on businesses and workers.* Los Angeles: University of California Institute for Research on Labor and Employment.

Fidler, G. S. (2000). Beyond the therapy model: Building our future. *American Journal of Occupational Therapy, 54*(1), 99–101.

Finn, G. L. (1972). The occupational therapist in prevention programs. *American Journal of Occupational Therapy, 26,* 59–66.

Food and Agriculture Organization of the United Nations. (2019). *Key facts on food loss and waste you should know!* Retrieved from www.fao.org/save-food/resources/keyfindings/en/

Fox, D. M., and Grogan, C. M. (2017). Population health during the Obama administration: An ambitious strategy with an uncertain future. *American Journal of Public Health, 107*(1), 32–34.

Freudenberg, N., Eng, E., Flay, B., Parcel, G., Rogers, T., and Wallerstein, N. (1995). Strengthening individual and community capacity to prevent disease and promote health: In search of relevant theories and principles. *Health Education Quarterly, 22*(3), 290–306.

Ganesan, B., Al-Jumaily, A., and Luximon, A. (2016). 3D printing technology applications in occupational therapy. *Physical Medicine and Rehabilitation International, 3*(3), 1085–1088.

Gardner, J., and Emory, J. (2018). Changing students' perceptions of the homeless: A community service learning experience. *Nurse Education in Practice, 29,* 133–136.

Gee, B. M., Holst, J., Baron, K., Kendall, E., Knudson, S., McKnight, L., and Streagle, K. (2016). Interprofessional education in occupational therapy: The Idaho State University model. *Open Journal of Occupational Therapy, 4*(2), article 11.

Glasmeier, A. K. (2019). *Living wage calculator.* Retrieved from http://livingwage.mit.edu/

Heffron, J., The, K., and Harrison, E. (2018, April). *Room for change? Experiences of occupational therapy practitioners with disabilities.* Poster session presented at the 2018 AOTA Annual Conference and Expo, Salt Lake City, UT.

Hobbs, J. (2018). White privilege in health care: Following recognition with action. *Annals of Family Medicine, 16,* 197–198.

Hocking, C., and Kroksmark, U. (2013). Sustainable occupational responses to climate change through lifestyle choices. *Scandinavian Journal of Occupational Therapy, 20,* 111–117.

Horowitz, B. P. (2012). Service learning and occupational therapy education: Preparing students for community practice. *Special Interest Section Quarterly: Education, 22*(2), 1–4.

Howes, C. (2005). Living wages and retention of homecare workers in San Francisco. *Industrial Relations, 44*(1), 139–163.

International Food Policy Research Institute. (n.d.). *Topic: Food security.* Retrieved from www.ifpri.org/topic/food-security

Interprofessional Education Collaborative. (2011). *Core competencies for interprofessional collaborative practice: Report of an expert panel.* Washington, DC: Interprofessional Education Collaborative.

Ioniţă, I. (2017). No crumbs left behind: Perceptions of food waste across generations. *Journal of Comparative Anthropology and Sociology, 8*(2). Retrieved from http://compaso.eu

Kandalaft, M. R., Didehbani, N., Krawczyk, D. C., Allen, T. T., and Chapman, S. B. (2013). Virtual reality social cognition training for young adults with high-functioning autism. *Journal of Autism and Developmental Disorders, 43*(1), 34–44.

Kaplan, A., and Haenlein, M. (2019). Siri, Siri, in my hand: Who's the fairest in the land? On the interpretations, illustrations, and implications of artificial intelligence. *Business Horizons, 62*(1), 15–25.

Kielhofner, G. (2005). Scholarship and practice: Bridging the divide. *American Journal of Occupational Therapy, 59,* 231–239.

Koestler, A. (1978). *Janus.* London, United Kingdom: Hutchinson.

Krug, E. G., Dahlberg, L. L., Mercy, J. A., Zwi, A. B., and Lozano, R. (2002). *World report on violence and health.* Geneva, Switzerland: World Health Organization.

Lal, S., Jarus, T., and Suto, M. J. (2012). A scoping review of the Photovoice method: Implications for occupational therapy research. *Canadian Journal of Occupational Therapy, 79,* 181–190.

Laver, K., George, S., Thomas, S., Deutsch, J. E., and Crotty, M. (2011). Virtual reality for stroke rehabilitation. *Stroke, 43*(2), e20–e21.

LEO Center for Service Robotics. (n.d.). *Defining robots and robotics.* Retrieved from www.leorobotics.nl/definition-robots-and-robotics

Letts, L. (2003). Occupational therapy and participatory research: A partnership worth pursuing. *American Journal of Occupational Therapy, 57,* 77–87.

Lunsford, C., Grindle, G., Salatin, B., and Dicianno, B. E. (2016). Innovations with 3-dimensional printing in physical medicine and rehabilitation: A review of the literature. *PM&R, 8*(21), 1201–1212.

MakerBot Industries. (2019). *Thingiverse.* Retrieved from www.thingiverse.com

Man, D. W. K., Poon, W. S., and Lam, C. (2013). The effectiveness of artificial intelligent 3-D virtual reality vocational problem-solving training in enhancing employment opportunities for people with traumatic brain injury. *Brain Injury, 27*(9), 1016–1025.

Maxim, A. J. M., and Rice, M. S. (2018). Men in occupational therapy: Issues, factors, and perceptions. *American Journal of Occupational Therapy, 72,* 7201205050p1-7201205050p7. doi:10.5014/ajot.2018.025593

McColl, M. A. (1998). What do we need to know to practice occupational therapy in the community? *American Journal of Occupational Therapy, 52*(1), 11–18.

McIntosh, P. (1989). *White privilege: Unpacking the invisible knapsack.* National SEED Project on Inclusive Curriculum, Wesley Centers for Women, Wellesley College. Retrieved from www.nationalseedproject.org/Key-SEED-Texts/white-privilege-unpacking-the-invisible-knapsack

Medical Futurist. (2019). *The top 12 social companion robots.* Retrieved from https://medicalfuturist.com/the-top-12-social-companion-robots

Merriam-Webster Dictionary. (2019). *Living wage.* Retrieved from www.merriam-webster.com/dictionary/living%20wage

Moore, K., Stratford, B., Caal, S., Hanson, C., Hickman, S., Temkin, D., Schmitz, H., Thompson, J., Horton, J., and Shaw, A. (2015). *Preventing violence: A review of research, evaluation, gaps, and opportunities.* Retrieved from www.childtrends.org/wp-content/uploads/2015/03/2015-15FuturesWithoutViolence1.pdf

Moule, J. (2005). Implementing a social justice perspective in teacher education: Invisible burden of faculty of color. *Teacher Education Quarterly, 32*(4), 23–42.

National Child Traumatic Stress Network. (n.d.). *Community violence.* Retrieved from www.nctsn.org/what-is-child-trauma/trauma-types/community-violence

National Mass Violence and Victimization Resource Center. (2018). *Definitions of mass violence crimes.* Retrieved from www.nmvvrc.org/About/MassViolence

National Service Learning Clearinghouse. (2012). *What is service learning?* Retrieved from http://servicelearning.org/what-service-learning

Nigatu, H. (2013, December 9). 21 racial microaggressions you hear on a daily basis. *BuzzFeed.* Retrieved from www.buzzfeed.com/hnigatu/racial-microagressions-you-hear-on-a-daily-basis

Obiedat, Q. M., Ardehali, M. S., and Smith, R. O. (2018). *Next generation of assistive social robotics: Therapeutic applications.* Retrieved from www.resna.org/sites/defaut/fikles/conference/2018/other/Obiedat.html

Office of Behavioral and Social Sciences Research, National Institutes of Health. (2011). *Best practices for mixed methods research in the health sciences.* Retrieved from http://obssr.od.nih.gov/mixed_methods_research

100 Resilient Cities. (2019). *About us.* Retrieved from www.100resilientcities.org/about-us/

Opp, S. M., and Saunders, K. L. (2013). Pillar talk: Local sustainability initiatives and policies in the United States—finding evidence of the "Three E's": Economic development, environmental protection, and social equity. *Urban Affairs Review, 49*(5), 678–717.

Paul-Ward, A. (2009). Social and occupational justice barriers in the transition from foster care to independent adulthood. *American Journal of Occupational Therapy, 63*(1), 81–88.

Peters, T., McHugh, M. A., and Sendall, P. (2006). The benefits of service learning in a down-turned economy. *International Journal of Teaching and Learning in Higher Education, 18*(2), 131–141.

Peterson Institute for International Economics. (2019). *What is globalization?* Retrieved from https://piie.com/microsites/globalization/what-is-globalization.html

Porpino, G., Parente, J., and Wansink, B. (2015). Food waster paradox: Antecedents of food disposal in low income households. *International Journal of Consumer Studies, 39,* 619–629.

Prast, J., Frederick, A., Herlache-Pretzer, E., and Lachter, L. G. (2015). Learning to work together: Strategies for integrating interprofessional collaborative practice into MSOT curriculum. *American Journal of Occupational Therapy, 69,* 6911510041p1. doi:10.5014/ajot.2015.6951-PO2084

Rankin, A., Truskey, M., and Chisolm, M. S. (2018). The use of social media in interprofessional education: Systematic review. *JMIR Medical Education, 5*(1). Retrieved from https://mededu.jmir.org/2019/1/e11328/pdf

Rashidi, P., and Mihailidis, A. (2013). A survey on ambient-assisted living tools for older adults. *IEEE Journal of Biomedical and Health Informatics, 17*(3), 579–590.

Ray, D. K., Mueller, N. D., West, P. C., and Foley, J. A. (2013). Yield trends are insufficient to double global crop production by 2050. *PLoS ONE, 8*(6), e66428. doi:10.1371/journal.pone.0066428

Reeves, S., Fletcher, S., Barr, H., Birch, I., Boet, S., Davies, N., . . . and Kitto, S. (2016). A BEME systematic review of the effects of interprofessional education: BEME Guide No. 39. *Medical Teacher, 38*(7), 656–668.

Rogers, E. M. (1995). *Diffusion of innovations* (4th ed.). New York, NY: Free Press.

Saposnik, G., and Levin, M. (2011). Virtual reality in stroke rehabilitation: A meta-analysis and implications for clinicians. *Stroke, 42,* 1380–1386.

Schwab, K. (2018). *Globalization 4.0—what does it mean?* Retrieved from www.weforum.org/agenda/2018/11/globalization-4-what-does-it-mean-how-it-will-benefit-everyone

Schwartz, J. (2018). A 3D printed assistive technology intervention: A phase I trial. *American Journal of Occupational Therapy, 72,* 7211515279p1. doi:10.5014/ajot.2018.7251-RP302B

Scmelzeer, L., and Leto, T. (2018). Promoting health though engagement in occupations that maximize food resources. *American Journal of Occupational Therapy, 72,* 7204205020p1-7204205020p9. doi:10.5014/ajot.2018.025866

Scudellari, M. (2017). *Self-driving wheelchairs debut in hospitals and airports.* Retrieved from https://spectrum.ieee.org/the-human-os/biomedical/devices/selfdriving-wheelchairs-debut-in-hospitals-and-airports

Sepulveda, A. (2019). *Why it makes more sense to care for kids and parents at the same time.* Retrieved from www.centerforhealthjournalism.org/2019/01/16/why-it-makes-more-sense-care-kids-and-parents-same-time

Stadnyk, R. L., Townsend, E. A., and Wilcock, A. A. (2010). Occupational justice. In C. Christiansen and E. Townsend (Eds.), *Introduction to occupation: The art and science of living* (2nd ed., pp. 329–358). Upper Saddle River, NJ: Pearson.

Stancu, V., Haugaard, P., and Lähteenmäki, L. (2016). Determinants of food waste behaviour: Two routes to food waste. *Appetite, 96,* 7–17.

Steffes, J. (2004). Creating powerful learning environments beyond the classroom. *Change, 36*(3), 46–50.

Stein, N. (2017). The future of population health management: Artificial intelligence as a cost-effective behavior change and chronic disease prevention and management solution. *MOJ Public Health, 6*(5). doi:10.15406/mojph.2017.06.00188

Story, S. (2018). Elder Mentor project: Using CAD and 3D printing to improve quality of life. *OT Practice, 23*(5), 24–25.

Sucar, L. E., Orihuela-Espina, F., Velazquez, R. L., Reinkensmeyer, D. J., Leder, R., and Hernandez-Franco, J. (2013). Gesture therapy: An upper limb virtual reality-based motor rehabilitation platform. *IEEE Transactions on Neural Systems and Rehabilitation Engineering, 22*(3), 634–643.

Taylor, R. R., Braveman, B., and Hammel, J. (2004). Developing and evaluating community-based services through participatory action research: Two case examples. *American Journal of Occupational Therapy, 58,* 73–82.

Turcotte, P-L., Carrier, A., and Levasseur, M. (2019). Community-based participatory research remodeling occupational therapy to foster older adults' social participation. *Canadian Journal of Occupational Therapy,* 1–15. https://doi.org/10.1177/0008417419832338

University of Maryland. (n.d.). *The Faculty Workload and Rewards Project.* Retrieved from https://facultyworkloadandrewardsproject.umd.edu/about.html

U.S. Department of Agriculture. (n.d.). *Food loss and waste.* Retrieved from www.usda.gov/foodlossandwaste

U.S. Department of Agriculture. (2018a). *Characteristics of households with very low food security.* Retrieved from www.ers.usda.gov/topics/food-nutrition-assistance/food-security-in-the-us/definitions-of-food-security.aspx

U.S. Department of Agriculture. (2018b). *USDA's labels describe ranges of food insecurity.* Retrieved from www.ers.usda.gov/topics/food-nutrition-assistance/food-security-in-the-us/definitions-of-food-security.aspx

Violence Policy Center. (2017). *The relationship between community violence and trauma.* Retrieved from www.vpc.org/studies/trauma17.pdf

Weissert, C., Knott, J., and Steiber, B. (1993). *Health professions education reform: Understanding and explaining states' policy options.* East Lansing: Michigan State University Department of Political Science and the Institute for Public Policy and Social Research.

Whittaker, B. (2012). Sustainable global wellbeing: A proposed expansion of the occupational therapy paradigm. *British Journal of Occupational Therapy, 75*(9), 436–439.

Wicks, A., and Jamieson, M. (2014). New ways for occupational scientists to tackle "wicked problems" impacting population health. *Journal of Occupational Science, 21*(1), 81–85.

Wilcock, A. (1998). *An occupational perspective on health.* Thorofare, NJ: SLACK.

World Federation of Occupational Therapists. (2006). *Position statement: Human rights.* Retrieved from www.wfot.org/resources/human-rights

World Federation of Occupational Therapists. (2012). *Position statement: Environmental sustainability, sustainable practice within occupational therapy.* Retrieved from https://wfot.org/resources/environmental-sustainability-sustainable-practice-within-occupational-therapy

World Federation of Occupational Therapists. (2018). *Sustainability matters: Guiding principles for sustainability in occupational therapy practice, education and scholarship.* Retrieved from https://wfot.org/resources/wfot-sustainability-guiding-principles

World Federation of Occupational Therapists. (2019a). *About.* Retrieved from www.wfot.org/about

World Federation of Occupational Therapists. (2019b). *Position statement: Occupational therapy and community-centred practice.* Retrieved from www.wfot.org/resources/occupational-therapy-and-community-centred-practice

World Health Organization. (2010). *Framework for action on interprofessional education and collaborative practice.* Retrieved from www.who.org.int/hrh/resources/framework_action/en/

World Health Organization. (2019). *Violence and injury prevention: Collective violence.* Retrieved from www.who.int/violence_injury_prevention/violence/collective/en/

Zecevic, A., Magalhaes, L., Madady, M., Haylligan, M., and Reeves, A. (2010). Happy and healthy only if occupied? Perceptions of health sciences students on occupation in later life. *Australian Occupational Therapy Journal, 57,* 17–23.

Zepeda, L., and Balaine, L. (2017). Consumers' perceptions of food waste: A pilot study of U.S. students. *International Journal of Consumer Studies, 41,* 627–637.

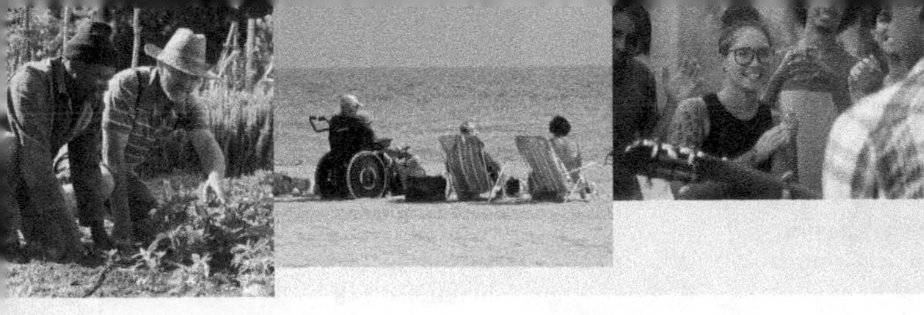

Index

Page numbers followed by "f" denote figures, "t" denote tables, and "b" denote boxes.

B

C

D

E

F

N

P

Q

R

S

T

U

V

W